HEALTH ASSESSMENT & PROMOTION STRATEGIES
Through the Life Span

sixth edition

HEALTH ASSESSMENT & PROMOTION STRATEGIES
Through the Life Span

sixth edition

Ruth Beckmann Murray, RN, MSN, EdD, N-NAP

Professor
Coordinator, Psychiatric/Mental Health Nursing Graduate Specialty
School of Nursing
Saint Louis University
St. Louis, Missouri

Judith Proctor Zentner, RN, MA, CFNP

Director of Health Services
Hickory Hill Furniture Corporation
Valdese, North Carolina

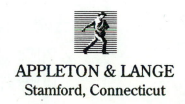

APPLETON & LANGE
Stamford, Connecticut

Copyright © 1997 by Appleton & Lange
A Simon & Schuster Company
Copyright © 1993, 1989 by Appleton & Lange
Copyright © 1985, 1979, 1975 by Prentice-Hall, Inc.

97 98 99 00 01 / 10 9 8 7 6 5 4 3 2 1

Prentice Hall International (UK) Limited, *London*
Prentice Hall of Australia Pty. Limited, *Sydney*
Prentice Hall Canada, Inc., *Toronto*
Prentice Hall Hispanoamericana, S.A., *Mexico*
Prentice Hall of India Private Limited, *New Delhi*
Prentice Hall of Japan, Inc., *Tokyo*
Simon & Schuster Asia Pte. Ltd., *Singapore*
Editora Prentice Hall do Brasil Ltda., *Rio de Janeiro*
Prentice Hall, *Upper Saddle River, New Jersey*

Editor-in-Chief: Sally J. Barhydt
Production Editor: Jeanmarie M. Roche
Designer: Libby Schmitz

ISBN 0-8385-6987-0

PRINTED IN THE UNITED STATES OF AMERICA

This book is dedicated to
  Our students—for their inspiration
  Our families—for their patience

Contents

Contributors

Mildred Heyes Boland, RN, MSN
Assistant Professor, Retired
College of Nursing
University of Arizona
Tucson, Arizona

Joyce Patricia Dees Brockhaus, RN, PhD
Child/Family/Marital Therapist (private practice)
Consultant to family businesses
Associate Clinical Professor
Department of Psychiatry
Saint Louis University School of Medicine
St. Louis, Missouri

Robert Herold Brockhaus, PhD
Professor
School of Business and Administration
Bob Coleman Professor of Entrepreneurship
Saint Louis University
St. Louis, Missouri

Elaine Cox, RN, MSN(R)
Acting Director, BSN Completion Program
Department of Science
Missouri Baptist College
St. Louis, Missouri

Dorothy Fox, RN, PhD
Assistant Vice President
Henry Ford Health System
Detroit, Michigan
Assistant Dean
Oakland University School of Nursing
Rochester, Michigan

Mary Ellen Grohar-Murray, RN, PhD
Associate Professor of Medical–Surgical Nursing
School of Nursing
Saint Louis University
St. Louis, Missouri

Joan Haugk, RN, BSN, MSW
In private counseling practice
Director of Stephen Ministries
St. Louis, Missouri

Ruth Beckmann Murray, RN, MSN, EdD, N–NAP
Professor
Coordinator, Psychiatric/Mental Health Nursing
    Graduate Specialty
School of Nursing
Saint Louis University
St. Louis, Missouri

Norma Nolan Pinnell, RN, MSN
Lecturer, Medical–Surgical Nursing
School of Nursing
Southern Illinois University
Edwardsville, Illinois
Adjunct Instructor
Department of Nursing
McKendree College
Lebanon, Illinois
Faculty
Deaconess College of Nursing
St. Louis, Missouri

Carolyn Samiezadé-Yazd, RN, PNP, MSN
Researcher in Transcultural Nursing
Evergreen, Colorado

Eleanor Sullivan, RN, PhD, FAAN
Professor
School of Nursing
College of Health Sciences
Professor
Department of Psychiatry
School of Medicine
University of Kansas
Kansas City, Kansas

Nina Kelsey Westhus, RN, MSN(R)
Doctoral Student and Instructor
School of Nursing
Saint Louis University
St. Louis, Missouri

Judith Proctor Zentner, RN, MA, CFNP
Director of Health Services
Hickory Hill Furniture Corporation
Valdese, North Carolina

Reviewers

Mary Ann Draye, ARNP, MPH
Assistant Professor
University of Washington
Seattle, Washington

Teresa Hanrahan La Monica, CPNP, MSN
School of Nursing
Georgetown University
Washington, DC

Arlene Miller, RN, PhD, CS
Assistant Professor
Department of Public Health, Mental Health,
   and Administrative Studies in Nursing
College of Nursing
University of Illinois at Chicago
Chicago, Illinois

Alice Obrig, MSN, MPH, EdD
Assistant Professor
School of Nursing
Fairfield University
Fairfield, Connecticut

Margaret G. Schultz, RN, MS
Associate Professor and Vice Chairperson
of the Division of Nursing Studies
Marian College of Fond du Lac
Fond du Lac, Wisconsin

Preface

To provide holistic care, we believe the nurse and other health care providers must consider all dimensions of development and the total health of the person and family. The physical, mental, emotional, sociocultural, and spiritual needs and characteristics are interrelated. Your emphasis must be on comprehensive assessment of the whole person and on health promotion and appropriate interventions and strategies rather than on patchwork remedies or fragmented understanding. This has been an emphasis in each of our previous editions. We are gratified to see the emphasis of nursing and health care dramatically follow our projection. Now in the sixth edition we have retained and updated the most important of these concepts.

This text introduces you to the person and the family during the entire life span—from birth to death. Birth is considered the first developmental stage, death the last. In Part I, Chapters 1, 2, and 3, you will explore the influences on the developing person—sociocultural, environmental, and spiritual and religious. In Part II, Chapters 4, 5, and 6, you will study the family as the basic unit for the developing person, theories of human development, and basic principles of growth and development. Both Parts I and II have been updated and expanded in this edition.

Parts III and IV have been expanded and reorganized in this sixth edition to incorporate both health assessment and health promotion strategies for each developmental stage. (See table on next page.) Each chapter is presented in a consistent format:

- Family development and relationships
- Physiologic concepts including physical characteristics, special considerations in physical assessment, nutrition, exercise, rest and sleep, and play or leisure
- Psychosocial concepts including cognitive, emotional and moral/spiritual development and health promotion, and individual developmental tasks
- Health care and nursing applications, including common health problems and special concerns

Research abstracts and case situations further highlight significant findings for the individual and family throughout the life span. Appendices give additional information about nutritional requirements, sources and functions of nutrients, stress management strategies and evaluation of their use, and American Academy of Family Practice guidelines. We believe that the integrated, holistic approach of this text provides the most comprehensive review possible of each developmental stage and, in a sense, a critical pathway paradigm for health.

As you use this book, keep in mind that although each person is unique, the uniqueness occurs in the predictable patterns discussed in this text. You can allay fears, give sound information, and make objective predictions with this knowledge. For example, a mother may be unduly distressed by the stubborn behavior of her toddler whom you are assessing. Your explanation that this behavior is characteristic of that age, with suggestions on how to deal positively with the behavior and what behavioral changes to expect in the future, can change a crisis into a workable situation. Also, your knowledge of normal mental and physical health at this and other developmental stages can help you detect deviations from the norm.

Your understanding of normal growth and development is used as a reference point not only for assessment but also for intervention measures appropriate to the person's or family's development. In this text, intervention focuses on measures that foster and maintain health as well as major points of care for common health problems.

We do not cover diseases, their treatment, or specific manual assessment techniques in detail. These are covered in many books that can be used in conjunction with this text. Instead we present knowledge of the highly complex normal and well person along with common health problems. Before you can understand the ill person and the family, you must understand the well person in the usual family and community setting. Only then can your assessment be thorough and your intervention individualized. Only then will you be prepared to give the community-focused care that is now emphasized.

Although nurses have always had to cope with death, usually it has been written about on a superficial

EXAMPLES OF HEALTH PROMOTION STRATEGIES TO DIMENSIONS OF THE WHOLE PERSON

Physical/Physiologic	Emotional	Cognitive	Social	Spiritual/Moral
Proper nutrition/fluid balance	Consistent warm, tender, nurturing of offspring	Promotion of curiosity and learning	Socialization processes	Values clarification
Balance of exercise—rest	Effective communication	Coping methods	Family, friend, peer relations	Acknowledgment of meaning and purpose of life
Immunizations	Effective guidance/discipline	Visualization	Group associations and processes	Establishment of belief system
Safety measures	Promotion of self-esteem, self-confidence, security	Imagery	Maintenance of cultural ties	Establishment of moral and ethical behaviors
Temperature control	Anxiety reduction measures	Health education		
Prevention of environmental hazards and pollution	Play, use of toys, leisure activities			
Cessation of habits destructive to health (smoking, alcohol or drug abuse, overeating)	Crisis resolution			
Health screening				

basis. An in-depth study of the phases of dying, how to assist the person and family in making decisions related to death, and specific care measures will enhance your ability to foster a naturalness about this last event in life.

Before reading any chapters, you should orient yourself by (1) reading the table of contents, (2) looking at the list of objectives that precedes each chapter, (3) glancing at chapter headings, and (4) noting the key terms that appear at the beginning of each chapter.

This text has been used successfully both at the beginning of clinical experience and at the graduate level in nurse practitioner programs in which a holistic life-span approach is featured. Wherever you encounter this text, we invite you to be an active participant as you read. Our ideas are presented with conviction and directness. But we want you to integrate and modify our ideas into your specific circumstances. Each of you will have to adapt this information to your setting—be it independent practice, health maintenance organization, hospital, clinic, or home.

ACKNOWLEDGMENTS

As we have moved from young adults to middle-aged adults and as our children have moved from the preschool era to young adulthood, we have experienced a good deal of the life-span development as well as the inclusion of comprehensive health promotion in nursing practice. That experience is incorporated throughout this text. However, a book is the result of collaborative thinking and efforts on the part of many people; authors do not work in isolation. We appreciate feedback from students, colleagues, and reviewers; we have incorporated their ideas and maintained the basic direction of the book, based on their comments. We are grateful, also, to a number of people who have helped in manuscript preparation.

To our typists, JoAnn Jenkins, Nancy Wied, Rebecca McMichael, and Michael Cahill, who each came to our rescue, we are grateful. Their conscientious work with handwritten material is commendable and appreciated. Without the conscientious assistance of Ruth's friends, Michael Cahill, Elaine Cox, Rachel and Michael Henrichs, Katharine Lehmann, and Sharon Stecher, the manuscript would not have been completed. They lovingly gave up time to assist with paste-up of the updated reference lists, reference numbering, and a variety of other such tasks. Another friend, Jearlean Ross, assisted with proofreading the *Instructor's Manual.*

Equally important was the support and assistance given by our families. Postal deliveries by Judy's husband, Reid, and the words of encouragement by various family members enabled us in our work.

Our thanks, too, to the members of the editorial and production staff of Appleton & Lange who gave valuable guidance and who most ably shepherded our book through the production process.

Ruth Beckmann Murray, RN, MSN, EdD, N-NAP
Judith Proctor Zentner, RN, MA, CFNP

I

Influences on the Developing Person and Family Unit

chapter one

Sociocultural Influences on the Person and Family

The culture and subcultures into which we are born encompass us and direct us for life. We learn an identity, values, beliefs, norms and habits of life, language(s), relationships, time, space, work, play, right, wrong, and physical and mental health practices.

Ruth Beckmann Murray

Key Terms

Culture	Family culture	Overclass	Pluralistic society
Manifest culture	Ritual	Poverty	Racism
Ideal culture	Status	Acute	Stereotyping
Subculture	Roles	Chronic	Prejudice
Ethnic	Dialect	Migrant family	Mongolian spots
Ethnicity	Evil eye	Refugees	Lactose intolerance
Hispanic	Acculturation	Immigrants	Caring
Latino	Hot-and-cold theory of disease	Underclass	Health
Regional culture	Mal ojo	Culture-bound illness or	Wellness
Rural	Susto	syndromes	Biopsychosocial or holistic health
Urban	Empacho	Maldicion	Health promotion
Socioeconomic level	Caida de la mollera	Transcultural nursing	Health protective behavior
Value system	Mollera caida	Cultural relativity	Primary prevention
Emic approach	Resfriado	Ethnocentrism	Secondary prevention
Religious culture	Catarro constipado	Culture shock	Tertiary prevention

Cultural care preservation	Nontraditional methods	Curandera	Coinage
Cultural care accommodation	Alternative methods	Cao gio	Health education
Cultural care repatterning	Quack	Cupping	Nurse entrepreneur

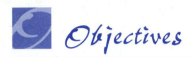 *Objectives*

Study of this chapter will enable you to:

1. Identify population groups in the United States.

2. Define *culture* and *subculture* and describe various types of subcultures.

3. Discuss the general components of any culture and how they affect the persons under your care.

4. Identify the dominant cultural and socioeconomic level values in the United States and discuss how they influence you as a health care worker as well as the client and family.

5. Contrast dominant traditional and emerging values with values of other racial or ethnic groups in the United States.

6. Compare the cultural values of the traditional Greek, the Spanish-speaking American living in the southwestern United States, and the Japanese in relation to the family unit, male and female relationships, childrearing patterns, the group versus privacy, time orientation, work and use of leisure, education, and change.

7. Contrast attitudes toward health and illness of persons living in the main cultures of the United States, Greece, Spanish-speaking American neighborhoods in the southwestern United States, Japan, and the Middle East.

8. Interview a person from another culture and contrast his or her values with those described in this chapter.

9. Discuss the influences of culture and socioeconomic level on the health status of the person and group.

10. Describe how knowledge of cultural and socioeconomic level values and attitudes toward daily living practices, health, and illness can contribute to the effectiveness of your health care.

11. Discuss ways to meet the needs of a person with cultural values and a socioeconomic level different from your own.

12. Apply knowledge about the teaching–learning process to a health education program for a person or family from another culture or socioeconomic level.

13. Assess and care for a person or family from another culture and socioeconomic level and identify your own ethnocentric tendencies.

When people talk or act differently from you, consider that to them you may also seem to talk or act differently. Many such differences are cultural and should be understood rather than laughed at or ignored.

The great divide between humans and animals is culture. Culture includes using language, art forms, and games to communicate with others; cooperating in problem solving; deliberately training children; developing unique interpretations; forming organizations; and making, saving, using, and changing tools. Humans are heir to the accumulation of wisdom and folly of preceding generations, and, in turn, they teach others their beliefs, feelings, and practices. The client, family, and you are deeply affected by the culture learned during the early years, often more so than by that learned later. An understanding of cultural and socioeconomic class systems and their influence on development of behavior is essential to understanding yourself and the person under your care.

CULTURAL POPULATIONS IN THE UNITED STATES

According to the 1990 census, one of every four persons in the United States is a person of color; 12.1% are black (11.8% are African-American or non-Hispanic black); 9.0% are Hispanic; 2.9% are Asian and Pacific Islander; and 0.4% are Native American, Eskimo, and Aleut. Each of these groups has increased since the 1980 census;

Asians and Pacific Islanders are often considered the "model minority," without need for social or governmental services (32, 39, 84, 226, 250).

The Asian, Asian-American, and Pacific Islander population is the fastest growing in the United States (10.8% from 1980 to 1990) and is diverse, composed of more than 30 cultures in the United States. Asians include Japanese, Chinese, Filipino, Korean, Vietnamese, Asian Indian, Thais, Hmong, Indonesians, Pakistani, Cambodians, and Laotians. Pacific Islanders include Polynesians (Hawaiians, Samoans), Micronesians (such as Chamorros, the indigenous people of Guam), and Melanesians (such as Fijians) (32, 84).

The Hispanic population, the second fastest growing population, rose 53% from 1980 to 1990. Many are young; the median age is 26 years; 30% are children under 15 years. More than 26% have incomes below the poverty level; 39.9% of Hispanic children live in poverty; however, there is a growing middle class. Thirty percent of Hispanic families are single-parent (39, 226).

The other two populations did not increase as much from 1980 to 1990 (13.2% for African American and 38% for American Indian, Eskimo, and Aleuts). Yet, despite the growth patterns, nonwhites continue to be separate from the white population and mainstream culture. Even if they are not separated physically, they may not really understand each other.

Almost 20 million (8%) of Americans were born in other countries. More than 32 million speak a language other than English at home. By the year 2000 it is estimated that one-third of the population will be nonwhite. There are also many nationalities represented among whites. The United States has been proclaimed as the First Universal Nation—a truly multicultural society (250).

DEFINITIONS

Culture *is the sum total of the learned ways of doing, feeling, and thinking, past and present, of a social group within a given period. These ways are transmitted from one generation to the next or to immigrants who become members of the society.* **Culture** *is a group's design for living, a shared set of socially transmitted assumptions about the nature of the physical and social world, goals in life, attitudes, roles, and values.* **Culture** *is a complex integrated system that includes knowledge, beliefs, skills, art, morals, law, customs, and any other acquired habits and capabilities of the human being. All provide a pattern for living together.*

Cultural behavior has two forms: manifest and ideal. **Manifest culture** *refers to patterns of actions, beliefs, and feelings that are readily identified by outsiders.*

It reveals what people are actually saying and doing daily. **Ideal culture** *refers to beliefs, practices, and feelings which people believe in or hold as desirable but do not always live by in actual practice* (149).

A **subculture** *is a group of persons within a larger culture of the same age, socioeconomic level, ethnic origin, education, or occupation, or with the same goals, who have an identity of their own but are related to the total culture in certain ways.* Mexican-Americans, Latinos or Spanish-speaking Americans, American Indians, African-Americans, and Asians or Asian-Americans such as Chinese, Filipino, and Japanese people represent subcultures within the overall culture of the United States. Ethnic, regional, socioeconomic, religious, and family subcultures also exist. A description of each follows.

The term **ethnic** *pertains to a group of people, distinguished from other people by race or nationality, who possess common physical and mental traits as a result of heredity, cultural traditions, language or speech, customs, and common history.* **Ethnicity** *refers to a national group.* In the United States, there are many European ethnic subcultures, for example, German, Italian, Polish, Slavic (representing a number of Slovakian countries), Scandinavian (Danish, Norwegian, Icelandic, Finnish, or Swedish), Swiss, French, Dutch, and Russian. There are also ethnic subcultures from the United Kingdom: English, Irish, Welsh, and Scotch. According to Spector, there are at least 106 different ethnic groups in the United States plus several hundred American Indian tribes (234).

The markers of racial or ethnic identity are every conceivable hue of color and sometimes as much a matter of socialization, ideology, and attitude as pigmentation. As the February 13, 1995, issue of *Newsweek* headlined, "What Color Is Black?" the faces on the cover were indeed every conceivable hue; eye color and facial appearance varied. Just as there are differences among Hispanics and Asian-Americans, so there is uniqueness in background, appearance, and lifeways among African-Americans. Morganthau reported that in one poll, one-third of African-Americans stated that blacks should not be considered a single race. In fact, the dark-skinned East Indians, Pakistanis, and Bangladeshis, despite their color, are Caucasians (189).

Further, an increasing number of African-Americans can claim to be biracial (189). Courtney describes the challenges and hurts that he has encountered because he is biracial. He states that being biracial has frequently meant denying half of his identity; which half depended on whether he was with Caucasians or African-Americans (52).

The Association of MultiEthnic Americans is a group lobbying in Washington to add a multiracial category to the questionnaire for the next census. Such a category would help depict the country's fluid demographics but may undermine laws or policies enacted to help racial minority groups with federal aid, voting districts, or in other ways.

Hispanic, referring to Spain, Hispania, or Spanish, is often a term reserved for **Latinos** or Spanish or Latin Americans who have mixed ancestry, without identifying country of origin. Most of those who are called Latino or Hispanic speak Spanish or Portuguese. *Among the Latino or Hispanic population, however, there are wide differences in genetic background, culture, tradition, lifestyle, and health behavior, depending on culture of origin, ancestry, and current socioeconomic status. The person who is designated Latino or Hispanic may be olive or dark complexioned and have come from Spain, Mexico, Puerto Rico, Cuba, Dominican Islands, or any Central American or South American country.* Those of Mexican-American origin constitute the largest group of Latinos or Hispanics. The term **Latino** is preferred by some Hispanics. For statistical purposes, specific birthplace should be recorded: Mexico, Puerto Rico, Cuba, Central or South America, or the United States (226). *For a general discussion of culture in this text the term Latino or Spanish-speaking will be used* (272).

Regional culture *refers to the local or regional manifestations of the larger culture.* Thus, the child learns the sectional variant of the national culture, for example, rural or urban, Yankee, Southern, Midwestern. Regional culture is influenced by geography, climate, natural resources, trade, and economics; variations may be shown in values, beliefs, housing, food, occupational skills, and language. One type of regional culture is *rural,* a term that is difficult to define, partially because it prompts different images for different people. Cattle ranchers, migrant workers, coal miners, loggers, American Indian reservations, and grain farmers each bring to mind life in rural America. Population density, population size, and distance from health care facilities are criteria frequently used in defining rural areas. The numerical values defining rural areas vary from one governmental agency to another (19, 135).

Rural *refers to an area or town with less than 2500 people, or a county that has less than 100,000 population.* **Urban** *is defined as a city of 50,000 or more people or an area of at least 50,000 persons that is part of a county with at least 100,000 population* (250).

Socioeconomic level *is a cultural grouping of persons who, through group consensus and similarity of financial position or wealth, occupation, and education, have come to have a similar status, lifestyle, interests, feelings, attitudes, language usage, and overt forms of behavior.* The people belonging to this group meet each other on equal terms and have a consciousness of cohesion. Socioeconomic level is not only economic in origin.

Other factors also contribute to superior status, such as age, gender, personal endowment, influence of the person or family in the community of residence in various organizations or politics, and reliance on tradition versus adoption of norms of dominant American culture (213).

The more the economic level of a group becomes fixed, the more predictable are its patterns of attitudes and behavior. Children learn the patterns of their own group and the group's attitude toward another level. The attitude patterns make up a culture's **value system,** *its concept of how people should behave in various situations as well as which goals they should pursue and how.* The value systems of the general culture and of the subculture or socioeconomic level may conflict at times. Further, in the United States or other westernized countries, all except the affluent members of several generations may at times change their economic or prosperity levels, but the values of the original level are likely to be maintained.

All cultures, subcultures, and ethnic groups possess certain values, customs, and practices common to every culture; share certain values, customs, and practices with some other cultures; and have certain values, customs, and practices unique only to that group of people. Cultures can best be studied from an **emic approach,** *by examining each culture based on the adaptiveness of behavior within its own perspective or frame of reference* (152).

Religious culture also influences the person, for a *religion constitutes a way of living, behaving, and thinking and therefore is a kind of culture.* Religious influences on values, attitudes, and behavior are discussed in Chapter 3.

Family culture *refers to family life, which is part of the cultural system.* The family is the medium through which the large cultural heritage is transmitted to the child. *Family culture consists of ways of living and thinking that constitute the family and sexual aspects of group life.* These include courtship and marriage patterns, sexual mores, husband–wife relationships, status and relationships of men and women, parent–child relationships, childrearing, responsibilities to parents, and attitudes toward unmarried women, children, divorce, homosexuality, or various health problems (68).

The family gives the child status. The family name gives the child a social position as well as an identity; the child is assigned the status of the family and the reputation that goes with it. Family status has a great deal to do with health and behavior throughout life because of its effect on self-concept (68).

Family rituals are the collective way of working out household routines and using time within the family culture, and are indicators of family values. **Ritual** *is a* *system of definitely prescribed behaviors and procedures. It provides exactness in daily tasks of living and has a sense of rightness about it.* The more often the behavior is repeated, the more it comes to be approved and therefore habitual. Thus, rituals inevitably develop in family life as a result of the intimacy of relationships and the repetition of continuity of certain interactions. Rituals change from one life cycle to another, for example, at marriage, after childbirth, when children go to school, and when children leave home. *Rituals are important in child development for several reasons:*

- They are group habits that communicate ways of doing things and attitudes related to events, including family etiquette, affectionate responses between family members, organization of leisure time, and education for group adjustment.
- They promote solidarity and continuity by promoting habitual behavior, unconsciously performed, that brings harmony to family life. Many rituals continue to the next generation, increasing the person's sense of worth, security, and family continuity or identity.
- They aid in maintaining self-control through disciplinary measures.
- They promote feelings of euphoria, sentimentality, or well-being, for example, through holiday celebrations.
- They dictate reactions to threat, such as at times of loss, illness, or death (68).

Family influences are dealt with more extensively in Chapter 4.

CHARACTERISTICS OF CULTURE

Culture as Learned

Culture has three basic characteristics. First, *culture is learned.* People function physiologically in much the same way throughout the world, but their behavior is learned and therefore relatively diverse. Because of culture, a child is ascribed or acquires a certain **status** *or position of prestige.* The child also learns or assumes certain **roles,** *patterns or related behaviors expected by others, and later by oneself, that define behavior and adjustment to a given group.* The behavior, values, attitudes, and beliefs learned within the culture become a matter of tradition, even though the culture allows choices within limits. What the person learns during development is of great significance. Culture determines the kinds of experiences the person encounters and the extent to which responses to life situations will be

either unhealthy, maladaptive, and self-defeating or healthy, adaptive, constructive, and creative (178, 213). What the person has learned from the culture determines how and what you will be able to teach him or her, as well as your approach during care.

Culture as Stable but Changing

The second characteristic of culture is that *it is subject to and capable of change to remain viable and adaptive, although it is basically a stable entity.* The culture of a society, like a human body, is dynamic but maintained at a steady state by self-regulating devices. In the United States and westernized countries throughout the world, there is often much overt change occurring. Yet underneath the manifested lifestyle changes, certain basic values of most people within the group are unlikely to be changed because behavior is defined by the culture. *Stabilizing features are traditions, group pressure, and the ready-made solutions to life's problems* that are provided for the group, enabling individuals to anticipate the behavior of others, predict future events, and regulate their life within the culture. *Everyone within the same culture does not behave in exactly the same way.* Norms and customs that persist may have a negative influence on the group (213). Food taboos during illness and pregnancy, pica, a high-animal-fat diet, and crowding of people into a common dwelling that provides an apt incubator for spread of contagious disease are examples.

A culture makes change, stability, or adaptation possible through its ideas, inventions, and customs. Together with physiologic adaptive processes, culture is a powerful force. Humans, for example, are able to live in a wide variety of climates because the body has adjusted gradually to permit survival. We have constructed a variety of lifestyles and patterns of social relationships to guarantee our survival and free ourselves from the limits of physical environments. Prescribed cultural norms are the most effective adaptive mechanisms that humans use. They affect physical, social, and mental well-being; aid adaptation to diverse situations, environments, and recurring problems; and teach about other environments to which we may have to adapt. In addition, some adaptive modifications are achieved through genetic, physiologic, and constitutional capacities that have been transmitted for generations through natural selection or cultural conditioning. This combination of change and stability can be seen in the United States (78). Elliott describes the stability of American institutions even with technologic change and the diversity of cultural people, or multiethnicity (74).

Another stabilizing aspect of culture is the use of language, even though the meanings of words also change over time. Although language forms vary from culture to culture, the terms for *mother* and *father* sound very much alike across cultural lines, perhaps because certain vocalizations are easy for a child to articulate and learn (78).

Learning cultural and family language is primarily by ear. In addition, use of language is determined considerably by age and sex, for example, baby talk, child talk, adult talk, girl talk, and boy talk. The language that is learned is a major part of one's identity. Subcultural groups, particularly the family, people from various geographic areas, and people from different ethnic or racial backgrounds differ in conversational conventions, that is, permitted topics of conversation; proper situations for discussing certain topics, such as during mealtime or before bedtime; level of vocabulary used; reaction to new words used; number of interruptions permitted; who can be interrupted; and who talks most (68).

The meeting ground between cultures is in language and **dialect,** *a variety of a language spoken by a distinct group of people in a definite place.* All immigrants to the United States brought their own ethnic/racial and cultural heritage and language. No doubt all had problems being acculturated to mainstream America, but generally their different lifestyles and accents were considered interesting and eventually accepted (93).

A number of dialects, in addition to native languages, are spoken in the United States. This is not uncommon in many countries of the world. Dialects are related to racial and ethnic background, geographic region, as well as neighborhood. If the words are not understood in relation to the culture, communication and relationship breakdown will occur. Choice of words, syntax, intonation, and level of emotion in speech all convey meanings (22, 68, 93).

Black English is a highly stylized, rhythmic, spontaneous language which relies on memory, avoids a rigid pattern, and often involves a participatory audience. African-Americans have more dependence on the ear (listening) for the spoken word than the eye (reading) for the written word (22). African-American culture can be viewed in the language and its usage—the pace, emotions, activity level, awareness, and very being that are expressed through words. To speak is to be active and participating. The vocabulary, grammar, and syntax of African-American dialect or language is natural, free flowing, and consistent with body gesture and movement. Black dialect provides an organization for the African-American to communicate unique cultural ideas. Black dialect will vary from region to region and with the age, sex, and economic level of the user. Some African-Americans avoid using Black dialect, especially those more highly educated and in higher socioeconomic levels (22, 93, 189, 240).

You will find a variety of regional dialects in the United States, for example, "Brooklynese," Southern mountain, "Tex-Mex" or "Spanglish" along the Texas–Mexico border, Texas cotton country, Missouri Ozarkian, and Pennsylvania Dutch. Variations can include aspects of pronunciation (*park, pahk, pawk*), usage (quarter *of, 'til, to* nine*),* or vocabulary (*sack* or *bag; submarine sandwich* or *po' boy*).

Language differences may give a false impression about the intelligence of a person, for some people have difficulty switching from native language or dialect to standard American English. Listen carefully to the language spoken, be accepting of the dialect, and validate meanings of words when necessary. In the United States, an estimated 3 million schoolchildren speak little or no English; Spanish is the most common native tongue (70%), followed by Asian languages (15%). School systems struggle with bilingual versus English-only classes (101).

Language emphasizes the values of a culture. For example, neither the language of the Nootka Indians on Vancouver Island nor that of the Hopi has a separate subject and predicate or parts of speech, as does English. These languages describe an event as a whole with a single term. Americans are complex, abstract, and fragmentary in their descriptions of the world around them. The Indo-European languages, of which English is one, emphasize time. Cultures using these languages keep records, use mathematics, do accounting, use clocks and calendars, and study archeology to learn of their historical past. In contrast, past, present, and future tenses do not exist in the Hopi language; the validity of a statement is not based on time or history but on "fact," memory, expectations, or customs. The Navaho language has little mention of clock time and instead emphasizes type of activity, duration, or aspects of movement. Moreover, Indo-European languages, like English, describe nonspatial relationships with spatial metaphors, for example, *long* and *short* for duration; *heavy* and *light* or *long* and *short* for intensity; *rise* and *fall* for tendency. In the Hopi language psychological metaphors are used to name mental processes; for example, *heart* can be used for *think* or *remember.* The Hopi language has limited tenses, makes no reference to time as an entity distinct from space, and is rich in verbs (in contrast to English, which is rich in nouns). It is a language that projects a world of movement and changing relationships (161, 253).

The natives in Alaska have numerous concepts about the varieties of space, whereas Americans have more words for the concept of time. The Eskimo language is seasonal—terms for many varieties of snow emerge in winter and for whaling in spring. Whole areas of the language are disappearing in the younger generations because the words refer to activities no longer much practiced, such as traveling with dogs and the intercession of a shaman (true for people in many lands). Certainly in the Arctic (and among farmers in the United States), the order of the language, the ecology of its sound and thoughts, derives from the mind's intercourse with the landscape. To learn a language is to know how its speaker perceives the land (161).

Conceptualizations and language influence the values, behavior, stability, strength, connectedness, and progress of a culture. Assessment of the person's intellectual ability must consider culture as well as age. People from non-Western cultures may learn differently and at a different rate because of different language and perceptual skills and value orientations (93). Most cultures are less technical and verbal than ours.

Analyses of the habits and practices of various peoples show that traditional language and behavior patterns practiced between parent and child within a culture are related to the interactions within that culture between employer and employee, among peers, and between nurse and patient, making for predictability and stability. Stability of culture promotes adaptability and economy of energy (100, 178).

Cultures also change, sometimes imperceptibly, so that norms, the usual rules for living, are modified to meet the group's needs as new life challenges arise. *Cultures change for various reasons:*

- Technologic change or innovation
- Competition among groups for geographic regions to meet members' sustenance and safety needs
- Use of another culture's inventions, art forms, or lifeways
- Education of the group
- Use of deferred gains for members to induce them to work for the good of the culture, as in Communist countries
- Change in political leadership, as in China, Russia, Iran, and Central America
- Increased scientific and industrial complexity
- Increased or decreased population growth
- Change in economic practices and standards, such as the change from feudalism to industrialism seen in some African and Asian countries
- Use of behavior modification techniques by groups in power
- Promotion of values, lifestyles, and products through mass media programming and advertisements (100)

Culture is continually shaped by forces and people outside our awareness. The United States is moving into a *Postindustrial* or *Post–Modern* society, where there are no universal criteria, such as moral standards, truth, and beauty, to guide or stabilize a culture. Yet there is also an emphasis on conformity or normalization. The following are some of the *problem areas of such a society:*

- Need for more professional knowledge
- Greater expectations by the public
- More goods considered to be public goods
- Lack of measurements to show what is actually needed and thus where money and resources should be directed
- A changing demography with more urban concentration
- Increased life expectancy
- Changing values, with little understanding of historical roots of the culture
- Power struggles between groups (194, 245)

Adaptational breakdown is likely to occur unless people come to grips with rapid social change: frequent shifting of families from one place to another, alterations in bureaucratic structures that may speedily engulf the worker in change, and diversity of options and continuing novelty in many life situations. A disposable, transient culture makes it difficult for people to establish roots or pass on culture as a guideline to future generations. Not all people have adjusted to the continual rapid change (78, 135, 213).

Risk of illness can be predicted from the amount of change. If a person is in the equivalent of the Alarm Stage of the stress syndrome continually, body defenses weaken (see Chapter 5). Extreme examples of persons caught in rapidly changing environments are the combat soldier, the disaster victim, the culturally dislocated traveler, the homeless person, the migrant worker. Other examples include the aged who are uprooted and the person who moves from a rural to an urban environment.

Resulting problems in health care include rising costs with efforts to contain costs, maldistribution and cross-training or nontraditional use of health personnel, greater demand by the consumer for the latest technology in care and professional competence, more regulation of health care services, movement to standardized care across different types of agencies and regions, and accountability and more procedures for ensuring it (245).

When significant numbers of people begin to respond differently to one or more facets of a culture, this factor may cause others in the society to realize that a particular custom or norm is no longer useful. Such customs might pertain to marriage, burial, childrearing, or moral codes. If a group of people (or isolated persons) can consistently adapt and at the same time follow the norm imperfectly, they may establish a new norm, which may be gradually adopted by others until it becomes the generally established pattern. Thus the culture and the people in it can be changed in spite of initial resistance. Such changes can have a positive or negative influence on health (178).

Each culture is a whole, but not every culture is integrated in the same way to the same extent. Some cultures are so tightly integrated that any change threatens the whole. Other cultures are characterized by traditional patterns that are easy to manipulate and change.

Cultural Components and Patterns

The third characteristic of culture is that *certain components or patterns are present in every culture,* regardless of how "primitive" or "advanced" it may be (100). Understanding them can help you understand yourself, your client, and the health care system in which you work. Table 1–1 describes components of all cultures and gives examples of the components (64, 78, 100, 165, 194, 213, 245).

All the foregoing components and patterns influence and are influenced by adaptation to climate, use of natural resources, geography, sanitation facilities, diet, group biological and genetic factors, and disease conditions and health practices.

COMPARISON OF CULTURES

Cultural Values in the United States

Perhaps the best indicator of what we really are and value is to observe what we watch on television, who we consider to be our heroes, how we spend our money, and how we use our time. Values also are influenced by the historical time in which a person was reared (the decade of childhood) and, thus, the person's age, as well as religion or philosophy, socioeconomic level, and ethnic/racial background.

The United States has been characterized as a *melting pot,* in that many cultural groups make up the population and have contributed to the value system. Over the years, many ethnic minorities have resettled in the United States and obtained citizenship. Many immigrants worked in bondage for 3 to 7 years in the United States to pay for their passage. In the late 1700s, the 1800s, and through the 1940s, numerous Germans, as well as other Europeans, emigrated to North America in search of religious or political freedom, for economic reasons, as refugees, and as a result of wars. Germans, for example, arrived having been sold as mercenaries to fight with the British or the colonists in the Revolutionary War (218). Approximately 50 million Americans are directly descended from German immigrants. Census records indicate that there have been more immigrants of German ancestry than of any other European nation; the next largest European groups are the Irish, English, and Italians (133, 250). Thus, German values and lifeways have seeped into all of American life, contributing to the mainstream value system (218).

Since the turn of the century, the United States has witnessed major immigrations of people from many lands seeking freedom and a better life. Causes include war and other military engagements, postwar reparations, economic disaster, the Communist takeover of countries, and political changes that cause hardship.

Several orientations and value systems may be simultaneously present in a given society or culture, but usually only one orientation dominates over a given period. Both *traditional* (middle-class or mainstream) and *emerging* (changing) *values,* however, are increasingly seen in the United States. Table 1–2 lists both traditional and emerging values. Some values show conflict between ideal and manifested values and behavior, based on values held by different generations, and the erosion of some basic values over the years (2, 54, 78, 88, 89, 165, 213).

One way to understand members in *mainstream culture* in the mid-1990s is to divide Americans into *three generations:* (1) the Silent Generation, aged 50 and older, (2) Baby Boomers, aged 30 to 49, and (3) Generation 13, aged 11 to 29, so called because this age group is the 13th generation to live in America. Core values of the Silent Generation are discipline, hard work, sacrifice, obligation, family relationships, faith, thrift, future time and goals, and financial and social conservatism. For them, life has been a mix of hard times and good times. Values of Baby Boomers include entitlement, no limits (anything goes), assumptions of success, work as a means to self-fulfillment, spontaneity, instant gratification, and focus on the present. The core values of Generation 13 tend to be a combination of the values of the Silent Generation and the Baby Boomers. Survival as a goal, need to achieve, hard work as a pragmatic necessity, self-protection, do-it-yourself skills, sense of community as a safety net, caution, planning, guarantees for results of efforts, and demand for pleasure and leisure are all important (78, 132).

African-American cultural values differ from the dominant cultural values in several ways, as shown in Table 1–3. No one person is embodied by all the characteristics listed in Table 1–3 (9, 20, 22, 86, 147, 154, 165,

TABLE 1–1. COMPONENTS OF ALL CULTURES

Component of the Culture	Purpose or Meaning	Examples
Provision of Physical Welfare; Feeding, Clothing, and Shelter Patterns	Survival and maintenance of population. Health promotion.	Production and processing of food, shelter, clothing. Personal and health care patterns. Production and use of tools. Manufacturing, industrialization. Change of land terrain for home building, farming, industry. Health care services.
Communication Systems	Basis for interaction and cohesion. Vehicle for transmission and preservation of the culture. Distinguishes groups from each other.	Language and dialects. Vocabulary and word taboos. Nonverbal behavior. Voice tone, rhythm, speed, pronunciation. Facial expressions, gestures, symbols. Mass media. Computers. Music. Art. Satellites.
Exchange of Goods and Services	Production and distribution of goods and services. Work roles. Payment. Obtain at least necessities or luxury, depending on culture.	Barter. Trade. Commerce. Financial institutions. Economic policies. Regulatory mechanisms. Health care institutions and services.
Travel and Transportation	Provision for obtaining goods and services. Mobility within and across cultures, societies, nations.	Walk. Use of animals, such as dog llama, horse, oxen. System of car, truck, railway, air travel/transport.
Social Controls; Institutions of Government	Maintenance of order. Organization of people, society, government. Regulation of time and activity. Power systems.	**Mores,** *morally binding attitudes.* **Customs,** *long-established practices having force of unwritten laws.* Value systems. Laws. Policies. Regulations. Public or group opinion. Political offices; kingships; dictators.
Forms of Property	Necessities to maintain survival. May contribute to person's worth, status, social position.	Personal belongings. Personal property. Real estate. Financial . institutions and systems.
Human Response Patterns	Family relationships structure other relationships and "taken-for-granted" activities to maintain the group. Values, beliefs, attitudes taught for socialization of person into culture. Ready-made solutions to life problems and goal achievements. Relationships structured by age, sex, status, wealth, power, number of kin, wisdom.	Rules for all social interaction, handling competition, conflict, cooperation, and games. Intimate habits of daily living personally and in groups. Manner in which one's body, home, property perceived. Daily "taken-for-granted" activities and interactions. Use of time and space. Health care roles and practices.
Family and Sexual Patterns	Maintain structure for care and support of others. Regulate relationships for survival, harmony, generational longevity.	Wedding ceremonies. Birth, childbearing practices. Family division of labor. Roles assigned to men, women, children. Inheritance rights. Care of elderly. Guardianship. Forms of kinship. Divorce proceedings, or removal of undesired member, such as infanticide, burial of woman with husband, or elderly leaving tribe to die. Use of time and space.
Knowledge	Survival and expansion of group and desired practices. Contributes to improved living standards through inventions, products, practices, services. Technologic innovation, mobility to higher social status.	Reasoning process. Education system — informal and local; formal and national. Skills. Values. **Science,** *systematized knowledge based on observation, study, experimentation.* Traditions. Folklore. Folk and scientific medical, nursing, and health care practices.
Belief System	Guides behavior of individuals and group during daily life, at special events, occasions, celebrations. Provide meaning to life and death. Indicates priorities. Guides health and illness behavior.	Religion. Ethical codes. Magical ideas and practices. Taboos. Rituals. Methodology. Philosophy. Organized institution of the church. Values and norms.
Artistic and Aesthetic Expression	Expression of meaning in life and death, feelings ranging from joy to sorrow, depending on situation. Spiritual expression. Expression of individual talents. Health promotion. Therapy and rehabilitation in illness.	Painting. Music. Dance. Architecture. Sculpture. Literature. Aesthetic expressions also in body adornment. Use and decoration of space and surrounding environment, such as floral gardens.
Recreation and Leisure Activities	Socialization. Use of leisure time. Travel to other cultures.	Play activities and tools. Games. Organized sports. Leisure activities depend on climate, terrain, available time, resources.

TABLE 1–2. VALUES OF DOMINANT CULTURE IN THE UNITED STATES

Traditional Values	Emerging Values
1. Marriage and children. Romantic love basis for marriage. Family stability*; try to resolve or live with issues.	1. Variety of alternate lifestyles. Marriage not considered permanent or only way of life. Divorce expected, a way out of issues or if lack of self-satisfaction.
2. Sexual activity in relationships if there is affection and commitment. Heterogeneous relationships acceptable.	2. Sexual relationships for self-satisfaction. Same-sex and bisexual relationships acceptable.
3. Willingness to sacrifice for good of family members, children. Role of parents/family to discipline and guide children, help children find answers.*	3. Less investment in having children; less sacrifice for children. Children given less discipline and guidance, expected to care for self, solve problems.
4. Work ethic*. Commitment to cause. Goal of work is provisions for life, status, success. Loyalty to employer. Follow routine. Quality workmanship.*	4. Decreasing work ethic, increasing emphasis on leisure and recreation. Freedom to indulge self. Routine work seen as dull, to be avoided. Work should be fun. Loyalty to self and technology.
5. Rules of conduct, etiquette. Socially acceptable behavior.* Formal responses.* Sensitive to effect of behavior on others.	5. Decreased emphasis on etiquette. Informal approach; disregard rules of behavior. Lack of respect for others. Don't care about effect of behavior on others. Less gentleness.
6. Puritanical. Preferred way to behave. Concern about effect on others. Cleanliness.*	6. Sensual. Societal obsession with sex, alternate lifestyles, experimentation, violence. Less concern with cleanliness in environment or life.
7. Materialistic. Thrift.* Economic security for present and future.	7. Materialistic consumerism for present excitement, enjoyment, prestige. Money taken for granted.
8. Equality of people* an ideal. Recognize differences. Inequality accepted based on personal abilities or background.	8. Equal opportunity for people. Differences accepted and diversity expected. More freedom for personal choices. Respect for ability to perform. Desire to reduce inequality.
9. Rugged individualism but also cooperate with group on larger projects. Superordinate–subordinate relationships.	9. Do your own thing. Group conformity during school and teen years, while seeking individuality. Peer relationships.
10. Competition; emphasis on individual. Achievement*. Success.* Status consciousness.	10. Competition, with emphasis on team. Aggressive behavior. Manipulate others to be successful. Disrespect for social status of others.
11. Authoritarian outlook*. Accept institutional and political leadership. Patriotism. Democracy. Freedom.	11. Democratic outlook. Question all leadership and institutions. Apathy to or disrespect for leaders and country. Freedom means self-gratification.
12. Self-reliance*. Responsible behavior.	12. Increasing dependency. Lack of planning. Use others in system. Irresponsible behavior.
13. Youth; beauty; health*; strength.*	13. Youth; beauty. Health is a right.
14. Future orientation.* Interest in long-term goals. Willing to defer immediate satisfaction.	14. Present outcome emphasized. Immediate answers and satisfaction expected.
15. Education* for social, geographic, economic, occupational mobility. Basic subjects. Science.* Advanced degrees.	15. Education for immediate goals. Experiment with methods. Mass media as an education tool, used to manipulate ideas and values, create desire for products, change practices.
16. Problem-oriented; systematic; specific. Thoughtfulness valued; time for thinking.	16. Process oriented; concerned about process even if no solutions. Focus on external and immediate experience. Inner experience or contemplation not valued. Power oriented.
17. Use of practical or functional goods or products. Keep objects considered valuable or sentimental. Maintain basic knowledge and skills.	17. New products. Technology. Automation. Use of disposable goods; recycle items for environment or for book fairs. Constant updating of knowledge and skills.
18. Speed. Change. Progress. Efficiency.* Time* important, scheduled.	18. Increasing demand for immediate output. Change even more rapid. Sense of hurry and no control over time or schedules.
19. Exert will over environment. Use of environmental resources for societal and own needs.	19. Environment represents a course; effort to save environment and resources in conflict with demand for products, waste.
20. Sense of humanitarianism, concern for others in trouble or disaster. Continued caretaking.	20. Depersonalization. Robot or machinelike performance by people is expected. Concern about effects on self from helping others (legal or codependency).
21. Books, media used to develop social conscience.	21. Mass media, information systems, electronic games used for personal enhancement and to influence masses. Education potential.

*Values that have been influenced historically by German values and lifeways (218, 219).

171, 197, 265). Intragroup variations of African-Americans arise because of geographic location, degree of acculturation and assimilation, socioeconomic status, and educational level.

Leininger's research indicated the following *values to be held by rural southern African-Americans and Caucasians* (147):

- Religion (following the Bible) (spiritual health is related to other aspects of health and involves a total way of living and acting.)
- Doing right, following a code of conduct
- Work ethic, sense of responsibility in work
- Care and concern for others, sharing food and other goods, being able to receive help in return
- Involvement, participating in activities to assist others, being aware of and feeling responsible for needs in the community
- Presence of self or remaining with another in times of trouble or need
- Health preservation; concern about others' health first, then personal health; use of traditional medicine if ill

Although research indicates that value differences exist for different racial/ethnic groups and economic levels, Lewis and Looney in their research found similarities as well as differences between most working class African-American families and affluent Caucasian families in the same geographic area (154). Billingsley provides information about interrelationships between Caucasian and African-American families (20).

In the 1990s, we see increasing nostalgia for the apparent, though not necessarily real, serenity of past eras and for pastoral images. There is a return by some people in the United States to family life. Others are returning to the clothing styles, music, dance steps, and entertainment themes of an earlier era. It is a way for the adult generation to expose their children to a way of life that young adults, adolescents, and children have not experienced.

In the past (and to some degree still for elderly and middle-aged adults), the Puritan or Protestant ethic described by sociologist Max Weber was the prime influence on American culture, even for those Americans who were not Protestants.

The *Puritan or Protestant ethic* upholds the five following assumptions (257):

1. The person is basically imperfect and must struggle against imperfection.
2. The person was placed on earth to struggle and so struggle must be valued. Any sign of surrender or softness denotes weakness in the person and is bad.
3. Self-sacrifice and aspiring to good conduct are essential to overcome evil and gain personal salvation.
4. Emotions cannot be overtly expressed.
5. The world is seen as useful and should provide for material satisfaction. Mastery of the environment is emphasized. Conservation of natural resources is secondary, for the resources of the world (which are supposedly inexhaustible) were put there to be used.

Earlier in this century Puritanical values and rigid Christian morality upheld the tenet of God's judgment. A strong conscience was developed in fear of punishment and social disfavor. Society was stable because traditions were adhered to and proverbs were taken seriously. Your understanding that many elderly and middle-aged persons still live by these values can help you better accept them and plan their care.

You need only look around at what Toffler calls our superindustrial society to realize that the Puritan or Protestant ethic has lost its hold (245). Yet parts of this ethic are being revived by some of the growing fundamentalist religious groups. *Major cultural shifts* in the United States, according to Naisbitt and Aburdene (194), include moving from:

- Industrialization to an information society
- Forced technology to a combination of high technology and high touch or interaction
- Short-term to long-term considerations in business, the economy, health practices, and social services
- Centralization to decentralization of management and services
- Institutional to self-help practices
- Representative democracy to participatory democracy
- Use of hierarchies to the practice of networking (interacting with others), to solve problems and achieve goals
- Either/or to multiple options in solving problems or seeking services

Naisbitt and Aburdene also note the rise of more women as leaders, a renaissance of the arts, sweeping worldwide religious movements, and decline of the welfare state (194).

Several of these trends are important to health care: the emphasis on an information society, high technology/high touch in care, the long-term perspective, decentralization of services, use of self-help practices, use of networking, seeking of multiple options, the rise of more women in leadership positions, and decline of the welfare state.

TABLE 1–3 COMPARISON OF SELECTED AFRICAN-AMERICAN VALUES AND DOMINANT CULTURAL VALUES

Value	African-American Culture	Dominant Caucasian Culture
Psychological connectedness	Individual secondary to group; individuality cannot be separated from group. Progress of group more important than that of individual. All members of group share disappointments or concerns of group. Both positive and negative feelings shared by group.	Primacy of the individual. Each person master of own destiny. Each citizen to carry own weight and be rewarded according to abilities and effort expended. Person esteemed for achievements. Group benefits from combined efforts of individual members; person only peripherally accountable for group's faults.
Rhythm: openness to feelings and emotionality	Rhythm: a natural flow of emotional release that can be looked into by others close to self; a source of all actions, song, dance, poetry, drama, sculpture. Engage in emotionality, such behavior is "real."	Emotional outbursts regarded as unsightly. Behavior cognitively examined for motives in order to understand another or self. Left-brain dominance fostered. Behavior governed by cognitive emphasis.
Social values	Home and family are centers of values rather than workplace.	Workplace, achievement, and material innovation valued as highly as home and family.
Time perspective	Time divided into natural units—day and night, seasons. Meetings and get-togethers scheduled around natural cycles. Emphasis on time is not a behavior of choice, but clock time is used to receive appropriate rewards (pay) or avoid punishment (low grades). Exactness about time not expected or required.	Time dissected into seconds, minutes, hours. Activities and meetings scheduled. Exactness about time expected and often required.
Direct experience	Person experiences reality through direct involvement; learning constantly occurs in interaction with environment. Learning not confined to classroom but gained through living. Book knowledge not as important as being able to put knowledge "to the test" of behaving.	Knowledge from experience and books valued. Abstract learning and problem solving emphasized.
Oral tradition	Themes in the language are: (1) emotional vitality, (2) realness, (3) resilience, (4) interrelatedness, (5) value of direct experience, and (6) distrust and deception. Black English provides organization to communicate unique cultural ideas. Body posture validates language used.	Standard English follows different grammatical rules and syntax.
Spirituality	Reality of the spirit acknowledged and accepted as a basic part of self; religion highly valued. Each person expected to know God personally. Many have a strong attachment to religion. Prayer and supernatural forces outside realm of cognitive/conscious awareness often attributed causal properties.	Religion as value varies with group. Spirituality often overlooked by mainstream psychological thought. Often less open expression about spirituality even if person has deep faith.
Creative improvisation	All creation is believed to return to former being. A group may perform as an act while each member creates his or her own reality. Everyone united by thematic material of eternity and thus behavior should be able to be understood and new relationships formed. No mental state is static or entrenched. Everything is part of a larger process, functionally connected.	Concept not present in Western thought.
Family	Strong, close bond and loyalty to family, including elders. Intricate family bonds include more than blood relatives; members may speak for each other and simultaneously.	Focus on nuclear family, but may include extended family. Stepparent family may create complex network with ambiguous bonds of support.
Education	Education emphasized as way to improve social status.	Education valued as way to improve self and achieve success.

Another phenomenon in the United States is the increasing number of a *new class of migrant workers*—mostly well-educated professionals and highly paid blue-collar workers who move around the country, following job relocations and business and economic trends. Frequent migrations prevent the family from establishing roots. Changing addresses may help the family and children be more flexible, if there is a strong family cohesion and identity, or it may create a sense of anomie, isolation, and identity diffusion. The family must realize that its problems will move with them, and often a change in lifestyle and higher cost of living awaits them in the new job/residential area. In the transition, there may be loss of friends, familiarity, and finances, and sometimes treasured items as well (9, 226, 255).

Other cultural lifestyles are often perceived as problematic by mainstream America. Various cultural groups may have values and behaviors or a lifestyle that are in conflict with the dominant values of society. For example, *American Indian* and *Alaskan Native people* value nature. Mainstream America believes that environmental resources are to be used. A persistent sense of family responsibility is traditional to American Indians, for example. Although family members leave the reservation to find work, they are expected to return to visit relatives or for emergencies and life cycle, or tribal, events. When cultural values of sharing, cooperation, and mutual dependence conflict with the demands of a job, American Indians face a difficult choice. If the call to attend a funeral or help a sick relative comes when a worker cannot take time off, the decision may be to give up the job. Employers are not always understanding of the values underlying the behavior (9, 86, 112, 113, 114, 270).

In contrast to the movies, myths, and legends about the *American Indian,* early settlers survived because of the good will and assistance of various Indian people. That most American Indians, like most Caucasians, are peaceful and helpful to others must be taught to the public. *Values* such as assistance to others, family harmony, gentleness to and love of the natural environment, inclusion in community roles and respect for and care of the elderly, and cooperation instead of competition are values that would be useful for all of our society to learn and practice. American Indian tribes were quite ahead of our Women's Liberation Movement in many ways. For example, marriage customs do not treat women and children as property, and homosexuality has been better accepted. In some tribes, such as the Iroquois, women have had a central role in community and governmental affairs (9, 86, 93, 270).

For many *second- and third-generation Latin or Spanish-speaking Americans,* educational and socioeco-nomic advances have paralleled a reduction in the size of their households and the development of individual and family rather than community orientation. But for the majority, loyalty to the family and a preference for large kin groups that act as support networks are very strong. Thus the competitiveness against others that is part of the educational system is avoided, and children may not make the high grades in school that are likely to ensure continued educational and employment success.

Many *non-Jewish, Caucasian U.S. ethnic cultures* inherited work and family *values from European Catholic peasant societies*—values that seem to set family interests against individual achievement. Generations of underemployment, fear of losing what little wealth the family had managed to accumulate, and the constant struggle to feed ever-growing families encouraged European immigrants to favor economic security over risk taking.

The *Southern Appalachian* person may have a value system that is almost on the opposite end of the continuum from the upper-middle-class professional as shown by Table 1–4 (127, 128).

Issues of violence are to this generation in the United States what the issue of sex was to the Victorian world. Today's young adults have grown up with the ever-present possibility of instantaneous death or permanent maiming by thermonuclear, chemical, or biological warfare agents. The threat and fear of violence are therefore constant facts of life. Fear of violence has led to a fascination with violence that further surrounds people with its symptoms. U.S. society is preoccupied with, almost mesmerized by, the violence of individual assault, homicide, teen gangs, organized crime, urban rioting, and political assassinations. Violence on television and in the movies shows the potential for brutality and aggression in all (100, 213).

People react differently to constant exposure to violence: they may tolerate it, develop disease symptoms, project their own aggression onto others, develop a neurotic preoccupation with it, or act violently themselves to discharge rage. We see examples of each reaction in our society in the form of physical, emotional, and social illness.

Persad (209) discusses how *concepts of aggression and dependency vary from culture to culture.* In U.S. culture, aggression is regarded as an innate force that has survival value and that requires appropriate channels for its expression; it is considered an integral part of social success. If aggression is not dealt with appropriately, however, the person becomes psychopathic. In some cultures, aggression is considered the result rather than the cause of psychopathy. Americans teach their children to be independent and emphasize the im-

TABLE 1–4. BASIC VALUES OF CULTURES WITH SELECTED CULTURAL EXAMPLES

Value	Range of Beliefs	Example of Cultural or Subcultural Group Adhering to Value
Human Nature (What is innate nature of man?)	The person is basically *evil but capable of achieving goodness* with self-control and effort.	Puritan ancestors. Protestants of Pentecostal or Fundamentalist background. Appalachian subculture.
	The person is a *combination of good and evil,* with self-control necessary but lapses in behavior understood.	Most people in the United States.
	The person is basically *good.*	Some religious groups, such as Society of Friends. Some philosophical groups, such as humanistic psychologists and members of Ethical Society.
Person–nature (What is relation of person to nature or supernatural?)	The person is *subjugated* to *nature* and cannot change whatever is destined to happen.	Spanish-speaking cultures. Appalachian subculture. Japanese and other Asian cultures.
	The person is to gain *mastery* over *nature;* all natural forces can be overcome.	Middle- and upper-class and highly educated people in the United States.
Time (What is temporal focus of human life?)	*Past time* is given preference; most important events to guide life have happened in the past.	Historic China.
	Present time is the main focus; people pay little attention to the past and regard the future as vague.	Spanish-speaking cultures. Appalachian subculture.
	Future is the main emphasis, seen as bigger and better; people are not content with the present.	Educated, professional, and middle-class people in the United States.
Activity (What is the main purpose in life?)	*Being orientation.* The person is important just because he or she is and may spontaneously express impulses and desires.	Appalachian subculture. Although no culture allows complete expression of impulses and all cultures must have some work done, the Mexican fiesta and Mardi Gras in New Orleans are manifestations of this value.
	Becoming-in-being orientation. The person is important for what he or she is, but must continue to develop.	Most religious cultures. American Indian subcultures. Greek culture.
	Doing orientation. The person is important when active or accomplishing something.	Most people in the United States.
Relational (What is one's relation to other people?)	*Individualistic relations.* These emphasize autonomy; the person does not have to fully submit to authority. Individual goals have primacy over group goal.	Most Gemeinschaft societies, such as folk or rural cultures. Yankee and Appalachian subcultures. Middle-class America, with emphasis on nuclear family.
	Collateral relations. These emphasize that the person is part of a social and family order and does not live just for oneself. Group or family goals have primacy.	Most European-American ethnic groups, especially Italian-American, Spanish-speaking cultures. American Indian tribal subcultures. Most cultures adhere somewhat through sibling relations in family.
	Lineal relations. These emphasize the extended family and biological and cultural relationships through time. Group goals have primacy.	Cultures that emphasize hereditary lines. Upper-class America. Oriental cultures. Middle East cultures. British culture.
	Relations are impersonal, focused on role behavior.	Business interactions, upper middle class, and those moving up the social ladder.

Data from references 127 and 128.

portance of the adolescent or young adult leaving home. Psychiatric therapy in the United States is often directed toward these goals. In Asian and many Asian-American cultures, however, indirect communication, modesty, cooperation with the team, and conformity to the group are valued rather than assertiveness of the individual. Touch or physical contact between business colleagues is avoided. Young adults may be castigated for abruptly leaving home or striving for independence.

Consideration for family elders is more important than one's desires to pursue personal goals. In our culture, a well-developed ego is considered necessary for maturity. In Asian cultures, personal preoccupation with the ego is considered absurd. In the Saudi Arabian culture, behavior that is normal for a U.S. businessperson is considered offensive, such as abrupt or interrupting speech, asking about a man's wife, and emphasizing a time schedule (209).

Use of time varies with the culture and historical era. For example:

- Ancient Greeks saw time as an eternal cycle.
- The Eskimo once stood motionless for hours in subzero temperature, waiting for a seal to surface to obtain food.
- Christianity changed the view of time because it was based on historical events and its history had a purpose. Church bells tolled the hours.
- Clocks appeared in Europe in the 14th century and were sold in city markets in the mid-16th century.
- The Gregorian, rather than the Julian, calendar was initiated in England in 1752. Time became a commodity.
- The Washington Meridian Conference in 1884 divided the world longitudinally into 24 equal time zones.
- Before the Industrial Revolution, the smallest unit of time was a day.
- After the Industrial Revolution, time became a commodity—money and minutes became important.
- In the Western world, time is seen as a progression of events, of new beginnings. Timetables are important. Appointments are to be kept by patients; mass transportation and mass media have timetables.
- Currently in America, people are hasty and impatient; they want things quickly, now, and easily acquired. Americans have lost the ability to sit still.
- Measurement of time is now in milliseconds; the societal clock tyrannizes and may be counter to the person's internal clock (236).

Health may be compromised by how the person uses time, or lets time use him or her. Nurses and health care providers must be attuned to the effects of use of time on themselves and the people they attend.

Comparison of Cultures: Greek, Latino or Spanish-Speaking, Japanese, and Middle Eastern

Tables 1–5 through 1–11 contrast Greek culture, Spanish-speaking American culture in the southwestern United States, and Japanese culture. Although many nationality groups fit under Spanish-speaking, and each nationality group has its unique values and customs, the values, norms, customs, and behaviors described in the tables are applicable to people who have a Spanish or Latino background, whether they are from Spain, Mexico, Puerto Rico, the Caribbean Islands, or Central or South America. There are variations in these values as the person or family is integrated into mainstream American culture. Furthermore, values may be lived differently, outwardly, if the person resides in Greece, Mexico, or Japan rather than the United States. Middle Eastern culture is described in the following section. References for these cultures are listed on page 30 along with other cultural groups.

Yet much of the behavior of a third- or fourth-generation family or person from a country reflects the original cultural and/or ethnic values. That fact explains differences among groups of people and should not be considered abnormal. Discussion centers on the family unit, male and female relationships, childrearing, the group versus privacy, time orientation, work and use of leisure time, education, and attitudes regarding change. The following discussion then compares the attitudes of U.S. residents toward health and illness with the corresponding attitudes in each of these cultures.

Table 1–4 summarizes Kluckhorn's presentation of five basic value questions, the range of beliefs derived from these questions, and examples of some (sub)cultural groups adhering to these beliefs (128). You may wish to assess your clients and their families according to these values as well as the characteristics presented in Tables 1–5 through 1–11. *Although neither a comprehensive study nor a stereotype of everyone in these cultures,* these comparisons indicate that subtle as well as obvious differences, along with some similarities, exist among different groups' values and behavior. *Understand that these cultural patterns will be followed by different persons in each culture to varying degrees,* denied by some, and not identified yet taken for granted by others. Chapter 4 discusses some of these values in relation to the family culture of the United States.

Focus: Middle Eastern Culture*

More people from the Middle East† are migrating to the United States because of political unrest in the region and somewhat easier travel possibilities. Many first-generation immigrants come here to study and then become permanent residents in America. These people strongly maintain their culture and religious values and practices; this makes them a unique set of clients to be cared for. Even though many of these clients identify with their country of origin, many also identify with a

---

*This section is written by Caroline Samiezadé-Yazd, RN, PNP, MSN.
†We are referring here to Lebanon, Syria, Jordan, Arabia, Egypt, Central Asia, Turkey, Afghanistan, Iran, and Palestine.

TABLE 1–5. A COMPARISON OF CULTURES: THE FAMILY UNIT

Component	Greek	Spanish-speaking	Japanese
Basis for marriage	Social and family welfare. All of society patterned on family.	Family welfare central.	Value family and household lineage. Family gives sense of purpose.
Type of family system	Paternalistic. Extended family. Monogamy. Marriage bond strong.	Paternalistic. Extended. Monogamy. Marriage bond strong. Family cares for ill, needy. Closely knit.	Traditional value on authority of father and elderly. Family strongly identified with father. Subordinate position of women and arranged marriage still accepted by older generation.
Family size	Want many children.	Children validate marriage. Large so parents not alone in old age.	Home, family, children are focus of women. Family planning, including use of abortion to control size in modern family.
Pattern of interaction	Authoritarian; man dominant in conversation and decision making. Man head of house and disciplinarian. Sex roles traditional male and female. Mother powerful in own way; credited with sustaining child with moral strength. Children subordinate. Oldest son responsible for family if husband not present. Child not focus of family activity. No special activities for child; even birthday a time to wish family long happiness with child rather than focus on child. Family together most of time with child learning to enjoy adult behavior and anticipate adulthood. Peer contacts through family.	Authoritarian. Man head of house. Woman subordinate socially, carries out family decisions. Sex roles traditional male and female. Child not sole focus of attention. Avoid admiration of child for fear of "evil eye." Child proud of home responsibilities. Familism reinforces attachment. Needs of family more important than needs of individual. Age and authority figures highly respected. Family loyalty strong. Obedience emphasized. Emphasize affiliation over confrontation; cooperation over competition. Interdependence over independence. Family ties may extend beyond biological relatives, including godparents (compadres), the boss. Modesty about body care and functions and sexuality.	Family revered as an institution. Close family relationship although may not express spontaneous companionship and warmth. Major decisions made by family. Subordination of individual to family interest. Traditional autocratic family system stronger in rural areas, with eldest son inheriting family property and hesitant to rebel against father. Young generation choosing own marriage partner, establishing own household, and daughter-in-law gaining freedom from mother-in-law's dominance. Increasing premarital and extramarital sexual affairs.

family, such as the Seyeds of Iran, or a city or a village they lived in, or a religion.

Roles. In Middle Eastern countries, Islam is a dominant religion, and roles in families are dictated by the religion of Islam, as well as by the culture of the country. Men tend to have earning positions in the household, and thus they either cannot or refuse to help with most or all household duties. Women, on the other hand, tend to be in control of household affairs. These roles are divided but complementary. There are some women in Islamic culture who maintain professional roles through the performance of a professional job outside the home. But in a traditional society and environment, roles tend to hold a status quo; the woman is at home and the man is the wage earner.

Muslim society tends to be paternalistic. Children carry throughout their entire life the last name of their father as their legal name. Even on marriage, women continue to maintain the last name of their father's family. Men have a great need to feel in control of situations relating to self and the family, and this may be viewed in Western culture as excessive control of women or family members. The controlling male brings great compliance into the family system through his role of leader.

Therefore, in the health care setting it is best to ask the man's permission or opinion when it relates to

TABLE 1–6. A COMPARISON OF CULTURES: CHILDREARING PATTERNS

Component	Greek	Spanish-speaking	Japanese
Process of childbirth	Considered normal process, not to be feared.	Considered normal process. Husband little involved. Prefer woman's presence. Special practices surrounding process.	Considered normal process.
Philosophy of childrearing	Effectiveness sought as parent, not as pal. Child raised to be strong, hard, firm, straight, for that is ideal personality. Wishes of elders put before child's wishes.	Effectiveness sought as parent, not as a pal. Child taught to do as parents do, to listen to parents' advice, learn from their experience, and not advance further than their parents.	Traditionally child to be dutiful, disciplined, responsible, respectful to elders. Young urban generations not bound as firmly by traditions.
Practices of childrearing	Mother firm, not overprotective. Baby kept in straight position when carried or in bed. Follow rigid schedule, consistent.	Consistent, traditional, faith in own judgment. Tradition of breastfeeding needs reinforcement if in Anglo health care setting.	Mother enveloping child in warmth during early years, but when child older, relationship more distant. Oldest son reared differently from other brothers, and brothers from sisters, so every child aware of his or her place.
Responsibility for child care	Primarily mother, but older children involved in daily activities, including care of younger siblings. Attitude of love and responsibility among siblings; new baby not seen as competition.	Husband ultimately responsible as head of household. Any family member, including siblings and cousins, responsible at times.	Mother primarily, but all of family involved.
Discipline	Consistent. Obedience very important and taught to child at early age. Child praised when good and told when bad; taught that it is important to be good and not shame family. Use group pressure to set limits on behavior.	Consistently correct child when behavior is bothersome and warned not to act in a way to provoke father. Instill fear of consequences. Instill pride in self-control and fear of being shamed. Seldom told he or she is "good" or "bad."	Firm, consistent, lack strong emotional expression. Emphasis on responsibility, duty, loyalty, patience, and orderliness. Promote feeling of insecurity when doing wrong.
Training of child	Taught to value interdependence, cooperation. Sibling rivalry when new baby arrives but does not last long. Mother delighted with new baby but shares self equally with older child, including offer of free breast during feeding. Older child invited to share excitement about baby. Parents never clown for child's amusement or give many material things.	Taught to value interdependence, companionship. Little sibling jealousy. Freely show affection and attention. May use child as translator for family if they are not bilingual.	Taught to value interdependence but responsible for own behavior. Taught to carry out obligation regardless of personal cost and to control behavior to avoid personal shame and disgrace of group. Develop strong sense of responsibility, loyalty to family or work group. Poor communication between generations because of differences in experiences, education, language comprehension, and values, fostering problems in modern society. Women's etiquette differs from that for men. Women taught to be passive, modest.

TABLE 1–7. A COMPARISON OF CULTURES: INTERACTION WITH OTHERS VERSUS PRIVACY

Component	Greek	Spanish-speaking	Japanese
Basic values of person and behavior	Strong sense of self-esteem. Inner core of personality not to be exposed or shamed. Value equality, individuality. Aloneness not sought, but borne with fortitude. Pride in glorious past of Greece.	Anxiety about being alone and concern for people who are alone. Not considered proper to compete, push self forward in group through achievements. Better to submit than provoke anger in another. Self-restraint emphasized. Violence atypical.	Strong sense of self-respect and important to be treated respectfully by others. Privacy defined differently than in United States; seen as loneliness. Group relationships sought and valued.
Personal possessions	Value in shared living and sharing possessions, especially with family and friends.	Sharing of possessions. One's own house nebulous; frequent unannounced visiting among family and friends.	Possessions not highly valued. Shared living space and possessions in family.
Status of person	Valued for what he or she is rather than position or achievement. Family unit valued, not individual.	Valued for what he or she is, depends on family. Child has mother and father's surname, respectively; hyphenated name common.	Belonging to right clique or faction important to status and future success. Try to join influential group at early age.
Interaction among persons	Resentment when treated impersonally, mechanically, or like a number on a chart. No word for "group," but born into group of family and friends. Extended family working together for benefit of each other. Units of cooperation retained from past, not created. Work to achieve common goal with those to whom individual feels loyalty. Speech important because it establishes interactions; expressive of feelings.	Much neighborhood socializing, especially among women to borrow, help, consult, discuss, or exchange gifts. Interchange of gifts and services frequent. Accepting as gracious as giving, and person not satisfied until he or she has returned a gift to show appreciation; return gift not necessarily same kind or form. Strangers not completely accepted unless related to established family by marriage. Interdependence between family and close friends does not extend to broader community.	Suppression of emotion in many situations. Most docile with strong urge to conform. Pleasant, polite, correct but aloof behavior to others in all classes. Use of polite, honorific, correct language to avoid being rude, to show respect and modesty. Concern about language use. Avoids handshake or body contact. Restrained, formal, hierarchal relationships in family, company, and political party rather than horizontal, comradely behavior. Ceremonious, at ease, and apologetic to acquaintances and friends but less so with strangers. Man unappreciative of domineering woman. Wish to avoid confrontation; strive to save face in conflictual situation.
Social activities	Family basic social group. Circle of friends important. Enjoy social affiliations, great loyalty to all groups to which one belongs. Food important with social activities.	Few formalized social groups. Suspicious of outsiders. Dependency on others accepted. Family basic social group. Women thought of as one social group, men another. Remain close to own social group for job or marriage partner. Use of diplomacy, tact, concern, respect for other's feelings. May appear to agree when does not. Child may avoid eye contact or not verbalize feelings, out of deference to elder.	Fondness for crowds and physical proximity of people. Participation and spectator roles in social activities and sports enjoyed.

TABLE 1–8. A COMPARISON OF CULTURES: TIME ORIENTATION

Component	Greek	Spanish-speaking	Japanese
Concept of time	Present important but prepare for something in future that is sure part of the life. No automatic faith in future. Distasteful to organize activities according to clock. Life regulated by body needs and rhythms, daily pattern of light and dark, and seasons.	Present important but validated by past. Expect future to be like present. Perform with distinction in present rather than emphasize efficiency, quantity. Life not regulated by clock but by body needs and rhythms, light and dark, seasons, religious holidays.	Time neither an absolute nor objective category but a process—the changing of nature with the person as part of it. Planning for future valued. Present considered important, and past priceless. Time is eternal, subjective.
Use of time	Time used spontaneously; not time conscious. Elastic attitude toward time; governed by cycles of nature. "Tomorrow" thought of as tomorrow, next week, or never. Activities and appointments usually not starting on time, person not hurried.	Time used spontaneously; not time conscious. Little emphasis on long-range planning. "Right now" means now or later. May arrive after scheduled appointment time.	Appreciation and effective use of time. Calmness and time for daily ceremony highly valued. Ceremony carried out in spite of rush of work. Emphasize long-range planning.

TABLE 1–9. A COMPARISON OF CULTURES: WORK AND USE OF LEISURE TIME

Component	Greek	Spanish-speaking	Japanese
Concept of work	Work thought of as life, a joy and dignity, not drudgery. Work interrupted primarily for religious reasons, not as claim to idleness or leisure. Women work as hard as men. Tenacious and resourceful at making the best of what they have and coping with difficulty. Person not to be hurried but works efficiently at own pace.	Work considered inevitable part of daily life. Not done just to keep busy or earn more money if present needs met. No moral corruption in being idle. Work at own pace and no specially defined working hours if possible. Everyone expected to cooperate and do his or her part. Work shared to decrease loneliness. Work roles of sexes and age groups distinct but each aware of tasks performed by others. Able to take over work roles of other family members. Child a part of work, of home and family, and feels important. No special rewards.	Enjoyment of work more important than money earned. Industriousness and hard work emphasized. Strong ties between person, the job, and the company. Work hard for success. Job mobility frowned on; loyalty to company. Independence in work traditionally valued but younger workers adjusting to Western concept of employment. Seek perfection on job. High sense of responsibility for job; quiet achievement. Consensus management emphasized.
Concepts of leisure	Leisure an attitude, a dimension of all life and work. Not confined to certain time but a continual expression of internal freedom, at work or rest.	Leisure synonymous with free time. No emphasis on leisure for own sake. Intersperse work with rest, socialize during work. Free time spent visiting.	Some leisure time used in solitude. Much leisure time spent in traveling with peers and family. Freer expression of emotion in recreational pursuits. Leisure should be useful or educational activity. Little leisure time for children; school studies and work emphasized.

TABLE 1–10. A COMPARISON OF CULTURES: EDUCATION

Component	Greek	Spanish-speaking	Japanese
Value on education	Highly prized, especially professional education. Curiosity and creativity valued. Educated person accorded much respect. Use of creative intellect and being a cultured citizen valued, but can be achieved through life's experiences and work as well as by education.	Learns that which interests him or her. Absent from school if learning little or if something more interesting going on elsewhere. Not seen as only way to achieve.	Respect for school and teacher. Education highly valued, with emphasis on scientific information. Parents involved in education. Eager to learn. Memorization emphasized. Believe in value of practical experience as well. Choice of college influences status in life. Much competition in education.
Educational methods	Emphasize quickness, curiosity, cleverness, realism, reason. Education applied to matters of life.	No emphasis on excelling or competing against other family members for high grades or honors. Use of native language may interfere with success in school. Competition in learning is avoided if possible.	Educational reform by U.S. occupation after World War II counter to traditional methods. Rote memorization, moral training, unquestioning acceptance of authority, strict discipline, competition for grades, and work rather than leisure activities emphasized.

family members. If this aspect is neglected, the man may feel insulted, and mistrust may develop in the relationship. In Western culture, this practice is viewed as a type of ownership by the man over his family. It is not viewed in this way by Muslims. The man rather perceives this as protecting the family for which he is responsible. This protection can be seen especially with a new mother and baby. In the absence of the husband, the health care provider can communicate through the woman's father or father-in-law, a designated brother or uncle of the husband, or the husband's mother.

In the Middle East, a large portion of a traditional village's female population is illiterate. Therefore, the role of mother and ability to bear and raise children are a major source of sense of self-esteem and identity. This affords one of the greatest opportunities for a woman to

TABLE 1–11. A COMPARISON OF CULTURES: ATTITUDES REGARDING CHANGE

Component	Greek	Spanish-speaking	Japanese
Value of change	Not valued for itself. Progress hoped for but not taken for granted. Change does not necessarily bring progress or improvement.	Change condemned if simply because it is change. Patience and postponing personal desires emphasized. Appreciate gentle approach. Little faith in progress or control over own destiny.	Physical world considered transient. Person appreciative of but does not cling to things; thus change accepted. Traditional activities, religion, family, and ancestors valued.
Pace of change	Deliberate.	Deliberate. Slow. Fearful or suspicious of change.	Able to adjust lifestyle to rapid economic, industrial, and urban changes.
Effect of change	No value on unlimited progress. Wants what is better than present but what is known and can be achieved. A plan to an American is synonymous with a dream to a Greek. Use material goods. Do not discard useful articles. Repair objects to maintain usefulness. Traditional Greek culture changing, becoming Westernized, affecting behavior of young.	Value system seen as constant. Feel many individuals not amenable to change by human endeavor. Adjust to environment. Use material goods to capacity. Generally remain near traditional home, maintain stable relationships with people. Change in main culture affecting behavior of young, causing insecurity in elders.	Urgency of Western-like activity a new phenomenon. Breaking traditional patterns and solidarity; increased individualism, competition, and individual insecurity. Youth seeking new values to replace old dogmas. Parent's generation generally reveres ancestors and authority of family and state—now rejected by younger generation to some extent.

realize her potential as a person. Because women are very respected for their role as mother, children, even into adulthood, place their mother's needs as paramount. Often this is done before considering even the wife's or family's needs, which can place an internal strain within the family structure.

Parenthood. Women do not practice contraception in the Middle East as often as in the West because the traditional role of the female is to bear children. Many misconceptions center around conception, for instance, that conception will not occur during breastfeeding. Such misconceptions are held even by the most educated people. When contraception is used, it must be, by Islamic law, a form that will not destroy an already united egg and sperm, such as birth control pills or a condom, because Muslims hold to the belief that life begins at conception. Arabs and Iranians may use abortion as a form of birth control, although it is not openly recommended or talked about and is clearly prohibited by Islamic law. Selective abortions are used in the case of an illegitimate child, as an attempt by the individual to maintain the society's integrity, as illegitimate children and unsanctioned sexual practices carry grave consequences (180).

Sexuality and childrearing practices differ from those of the West. Middle Eastern clients possess a feeling of fatalism; they do not plan excessively for future events but rather leave them to the will of God. Many women do not seek prenatal care in the Middle East; only when the baby is ready to be born do they go to the hospital or call a midwife to come to the home for the birth. Often women do not plan the layette or select a name until after the infant is born. Traditional as well as modern Middle Eastern women tend to breastfeed for extended periods; it is written as a requirement in the Koran to breastfeed for 2 years (130).

Children in the Middle East are viewed not only as a commodity but also as a blessing to the family. They are something to be cherished; therefore, families invest a great deal emotionally into their children and tend to practice lenient discipline measures. Children are usually not physically hit or verbally abused. Rather they are distracted away from whatever they are doing that is bad and encouraged to do good things.

Many Middle Eastern clients tend to base the success of their parenthood not on the cognitive skills of children, but rather on the weight gain, health, and normality of their children. They do not accept deviation of health status in others compared with the normal population. This author knew a woman from Kuwait who had a younger sister with Down's Syndrome. On introduction of her family, she said "This is my mother and this is my abnormal sister." She does not feel her sister is worthy enough to be called by her name.

Need for Affiliation. An important aspect of caring for Middle Eastern clients is to recognize their need for affiliation and belonging, which is central and critical to survival. The strength and importance of the individual are directly related to family members and friends; they are an integral part of life. Although men and women may be segregated, socialization is extensive. Middle Eastern people are known for their hospitality, and they emphasize family relations. Visiting among members of the extended family and their friends is a social obligation on all occasions, and children of all ages are included as part of the visits.

Cleanliness. Although Middle Easterners may live in crowded family situations within their homes, they use basic measures to ensure cleanliness. The client's body and clothes must be clean of bodily secretions, and most of these clients' homes are very clean and are always being cleaned. The expression, "You can eat off the floor," is literally true, because the family does eat from the floor, as well as sit, lie down, and sleep on the floor. These homes generally have no furniture or are sparsely or very selectively furnished. When you walk into such a home, you are required to remove your shoes to keep the carpet clean so events of the home may take place on a clean area. This produces for the Middle Easterner a definite feeling of separation between the external world and the internal world of their home.

Health Care. Muslims and Middle Eastern people often have home cures for common health problems. If it does not harm the client, let the person carry out the home or cultural remedies. It will serve to build trust in the relationship and show respect for the client. They believe that cures can be obtained through the use of home remedies, such as herbs, concentrated sugar preparations, and hot/cold foods. Although they believe in the superiority of Western medicine, they do not always trust it; therefore, they practice home-remedy medicine side by side with modern Western medical practices. When prescribing medical treatment or dispensing medicine, these clients believe that intrusive measures are of more value than nonintrusive measures. For example, intravenous medication is better than that given intramuscularly, injections are better than pills, and colored pills are better than white ones. Another example of a cultural practice is that at the time of delivery, parents want to say a prayer in the newly born child's ears. Muslims believe that the first sounds a child hears should be from the Koran in praise and supplication to God. This practice does not hurt the baby, but allowing its practice will go a long way to build trust into the relationship with the parents and family.

In the health care setting, the extensive visiting by family and friends can become very difficult for the institution to accommodate because visiting is usually restricted by policy. But for the Middle Eastern client, this visiting becomes extremely important in how the person perceives the disease and adapts to it. Lack of visitors can imply to the client that he or she is gravely ill and close to death when this may not be the case at all, but instead is the result of the hospital policy about visitors. Visiting should be allowed on a liberal basis. Visits from family members are also important because Middle Eastern clients do not expect personal care from health care providers; the role of the family members is to physically care for the person who is in the hospital.

Communication. Islam dictates that family affairs remain in the family; they are not affairs for the rest of the world. This can be seen in many situations, with modesty as one example. Women dress differently outside the home than they do inside the home. The body tends to be covered and only the face, hands, and feet show. For Muslim women residing in the West, this manner of dress is usually modified but still retains the quality of conservative fashion.

Respecting the client's modesty during health care or implementation of procedures is essential. Because of modesty, there is a difference in the information that a person gives to various people. Very personal information is shared only with intimate contacts; nonintimate or general information can be shared with almost anyone. Thus assessment must be done gradually and respectfully. Certain information may never be obtained from the client or family.

Communication in the Middle East is an elaborate system. It can be either very intimate in terms of content and word usage, or it can be very stilted, using only proper nouns and formal forms of verbs. The choice depends on whom you are talking to and the subject. A person may knowingly say the opposite of what he or she is thinking to avoid being rude. There are communication methods to avoid, especially in nonintimate conversations, because they are perceived as offensive and rude. First, outwardly showing anger or insulting someone is considered bad manners. Emotion can be shown with intimate persons but not with nonintimate contacts. Second, do not be abrupt or interrupt, especially with elders or when another is speaking. Third, in preliminary casual conversation that is part of business or professional association, if you are a man, do not ask the man about the female members of his family, including his wife, sisters, or daughters after they reach the age of puberty. For a woman to ask about female members is acceptable. It is important to use the person's title (Mr., Mrs., Dr.) until permission is given by the client to do otherwise.

As in all populations, communication and teaching become critical issues related to health outcome. Individuality should never be viewed as noncompliance. There are generally reasons for a Muslim's behavior or choice of action. Not carrying out a health care professional's teachings does not mean the Muslim is being uncooperative. You should reassess the situation in terms of its cultural totality.

Language Barriers. Interpreters or family members can be used to assist with teaching when the client's language is not known by the health care worker; however, family members may withhold information that they feel is too threatening for the client to hear or inappropriate to disclose about the client. If interpreters are used, they should be of the same language, religion, and country of origin. A mistake was made in one agency by having a female Muslim from Iraq interpret in Arabic to a new Muslim mother from Arabia, without first having obtained the husband's consent. When the father of the baby discovered this arrangement for his wife to learn newborn care through the Iraqi woman, he became angry and would not allow it. Involve family members when doing client teaching and always attempt to involve both the husband and wife together in discussions. If in the event the health care provider needs to talk to a woman about her husband, extreme tact should be used at all times in the discussion.

Language barriers can cause a great amount of misunderstanding. Listen to the themes of the content being discussed rather than to the exact words being used. It can take many years for a foreign person to learn a language, and usually building a vocabulary is the most difficult part of any language mastery. As an example, this author's husband has been in the United States for 15 years and is a doctorally prepared scientist, as well as a college instructor; he still is learning vocabulary that I take for granted. Ironically, with many foreigners, even though their vocabulary is not strong, their grammar and word usage are perfect.

When you do teaching with an individual or a family, remember that foreign people, to avoid embarrassment and save face, may appear to be understanding your communication, when in reality they are not understanding what you are saying. Some Middle Eastern persons are very good at convincing others that they know what to do when in reality they do not understand enough to take responsibility for their own or their family's health needs or care. It is best in these situations, if an interpreter cannot be procured, to use short simple sentences containing easy-to-understand vocabulary and to speak slowly and clearly. It is also best to communicate with the client using the same sentence each time. Saying, "How are you today?" one day, and then, "How are you feeling?" the next time may not be confusing to some one who speaks fluent English. But for someone who is struggling with the language it can be very confusing. It is also best to avoid slang and unconventional English because most Middle Easterners, when learning English, learn and cling to the security of proper English.

You may also rely on nonverbal means of teaching. Although there may be cultural differences in body language, some nonverbal communication may express similar emotions in any culture, such as fear, pain, and sadness. Teaching can also occur by physically moving the body of the person or showing what you want the person to learn by demonstrating in yourself. Pictures can be drawn to illustrate points of learning, or bilingual flash cards can be made to aid teaching. The cards should be bilingual so that the teacher and the learner each know what the card says and therefore have some basis for communication. These cards can be used at other times when interpreters and family are not available to communicate basic needs of the client, such as on night shift when the client wants to use the bathroom. Although this appears to be a simplistic means of communication, it can be very efficient and serve to decrease frustration and anxiety in both the client and the health care professional.

Differences in Values. Middle Eastern clients do not emphasize a time schedule; this Western value and practice is imposed on Middle Eastern people. Time factors for these people tend to be in terms of what is important at that moment rather than projecting rigidly into the future as to what is important.

This can cause conflicts in a health care setting where tests or health care appointments are scheduled at particular times and the client does not feel it is a priority. The client may view taking a bath and being clean as more of a priority and that the test can wait or be rescheduled for later.

Middle Eastern clients expect health care practitioners to find effective cures without asking many questions or using numerous diagnostic tests, which are often needed for a correct diagnosis. They believe if a doctor or nurse asks too many questions or orders too

many tests that the practitioner is naive, lacks experience, should not be trusted, or is narrow in perspective and understanding. These clients prefer older male doctors, preferably heads of departments in their specialty area, rather than younger or female doctors. The exception is that a female obstetrician or gynecologist is usually required for a female client who is pregnant or has a gynecologic disorder. Generally, Middle Eastern clients do not trust doctors completely because they feel doctors are too expensive, ask too many questions, and often lack experience.

Because of strict Islamic law, Muslims are not allowed to engage in deviant sexual practices, premarital sex, or adultery or to use illegal drugs or alcohol. Thus, the associated diseases (i.e., AIDS, sexually transmitted diseases, alcoholism, fetal alcohol syndrome) are virtually nonexistent.

These clients prefer the same caretaker each day; the same caretaker increases trust and acceptance in the relationship and decreases suspicion of the health care provider by the client and the family. Having the same caretaker also helps decrease mistrust of the world of medicine that these clients really do not understand thoroughly. A nurse can capitalize on this situation by being the same caregiver and consistently offering help.

The Middle Eastern client believes that if somebody compliments a person about something that is good or of value, such as jewelry or a new baby, or even looks at it with admiration, this behavior will bring out the evil eye. The **evil eye** *is a form of superstitious jealousy and mistrust of the admirer by the owner of the object being complimented.*

In the health care setting, avoid suspicion of the evil eye in Middle Eastern clients by directing compliments to the owner or to God (Allah), rather than to the object itself. Such action converts the possibility of the evil eye and misfortune into a blessing instead.

Legal Documents. The last area of client concerns is legal documents. It is recommended that birth certificates and legal documents be signed by both the father and mother of the baby. In the United States, statistical agencies of state governments feel that only the mother is the verifiable parent of a child. This can be very insulting to a patrilineal father. By having both parents sign the birth certificate or legal documents, the problem of the father being insulted is remedied and both the state and family have their interests met.

Consent forms are generally not used in the Middle East. First, the client does not feel he or she has the knowledge to assume responsibility for health decisions and therefore leaves this responsibility to the health care professional who has been trained to make these decisions. Second, in Islam, especially in front of witnesses, a man's word and agreement are considered binding and written documentation is therefore not necessary. When a consent form needs to be signed after an agreement has been made, it can be interpreted with mistrust and suspicion toward the health care provider. To avoid this, one physician found that, if the consent form was just presented in an institutionally oriented, matter-of-fact way, mistrust was minimized, and clients carried through with the required procedures.

Religious Beliefs. Middle Eastern clients may be Muslims, or they may adhere to other religions. Lifestyle and health care practices will be influenced by their religious beliefs. Chapter 3 discusses additional practices to be considered in the person's care, based on religious beliefs.

Without your understanding of Middle Eastern culture, these patients can be very frustrating to work with, but when you understand the culture and reasons for the cultural values, and realize that these values have meaning for the individual, Middle Eastern clients become enjoyable and rewarding clients to work with. When you have established trust with the person and family, you will see other aspects of their lives open up to you. This new view can be rewarding.

Attitudes Toward Health and Illness

How health is identified, physically and emotionally, varies from culture to culture, as do ideas about the factors related to health and disease. American definitions are emphasized later in the box on Key Definitions Related to Health and Health Promotion.

Dominant U.S. Culture. Attitudes in the United States toward health are influenced considerably by society's emphasis on mastery of the environment as opposed to adjustment to it. Illness is seen as a challenge to be met by mobilizing resources: research, science, funds, institutions, and people. Because independence is highly valued, the weak are expected to help themselves as much as possible. Self-care is emphasized. A person is evaluated on productivity or "doing good." Because the ability to be productive depends in part on health, individual health is highly valued. Health in the broadest sense is considered necessary for successful interaction with others, educational accomplishment, ability to work, leadership, childrearing, and capacity to use opportunities. Medical, nursing, and other health sciences and technology are considered important. The physical cause of illness is generally accepted. Only recently

have the psychological and sociocultural causes of disease also been emphasized.

The United States boasts of its medical research, technologically advanced medical care, and well-educated health care professionals. It devotes a higher share of national income to medical care than do other countries. Yet, by some measures, Americans live shorter and less healthy lives than citizens of most other industrialized nations. The United States ranked 18th in life expectancy in 1992. Infant mortality in 1993 was 8.4 per 1000 births, putting the United States behind 18 other nations. Heart disease deaths occur at a greater rate than in 17 other nations. The immunization rate is less than for many other industrialized countries. It is more economical, more effective, and easier to keep people healthy than it is to cure disease. Doctors, researchers, and medical care facilities have little effect on general health if the population lacks basic disease prevention and health promotion measures (190).

Common trends affecting health and health care in the United States and England include the following (83):

- Increasing numbers of elderly, both well and ill
- High mortality from cancer, stroke, and heart disease
- Use of advanced technology in medicine and nursing
- Increasing medical specialization in education and a new emphasis on family practice
- Greater acuity of illness in hospitalized patients
- Reduced length of stay in hospitals
- Greater need for aftercare in the community
- Expansion of hospital-based practice into the community
- Continuing inequities in health care

In the United States, and to some extent England and other countries, there is a health care crisis, with 1) escalating costs, 2) shifting of burden of payment from the federal to state and local governments, 3) less regulation of health care planning, 4) increasing supply of physicians, 5) expanding corporate enterprise in health care services, 6) greater competition between health care facilities and higher enrollment in prepaid group medical practices or health maintenance organizations, and 7) rising level of consumer activism in individual and community health matters. People are increasingly concerned about and involved in caring for themselves and others as health care faces decreasing economic resources (83).

There is increasing emphasis on prevention, primary health care, care delivered in the community rather than in the hospital, and changing the health care delivery system. Often problems are addressed quickly and massively, as if the problem can be solved immediately; this is based on the dominant value system. Yet, health values and care trends are not always evident or maintained. For example, in 1983, there were 1500 known cases of measles in the United States. In 1990, there were an average of 500 cases and one death a week from measles in the United States because many preschool children were not vaccinated at the recommended ages. Thus, 1991 was declared the Year of the National Immunization Campaign. Nine cities in the United States were chosen to participate in this national campaign, which targeted immunizing children under 2 years of age and those in the 2- to 6-year age group who missed previous immunizations. Community agencies and health care professionals had to collaborate in delivering education and immunization services in the community. The campaign was successful in reaching children who needed to be immunized and in alerting the nation to the need for continuing this public health measure (13, 104).

The *PEW Health Professions Commission Report,* based on study by an interdisciplinary group, emphasized the following points for health care in the United States (65, 104):

- For health care practitioners to be responsible for changes in the health care system and health care based on societal changes
- To increase the focus on wellness
- To increase the focus on care of populations
- To increase awareness of risk factors; reduce risk factors
- To make intensive use of information
- To increase the focus on consumer or client
- To increase the focus on outcomes of intervention rather than on process
- To do the same or better with fewer resources, for example, with Medicare, Medicaid, and Welfare reform
- To increase the focus on coordination and integration of services
- To reconsider human values and increase emphasis on interdependence

The PEW Health Professions Commission Report (65, 104) also stated that *competencies needed by ALL practitioners* by the year 2005 will be:

- Ability to care for community populations
- Focus on accountability
- Ability to provide preventive services
- Focus on healthy lifestyles
- Ability to manage information

Trends that are affecting health care providers in the United States in the 1990s, based on the economy and managed care emphasis, include the following (13, 65, 104):

- Health plans must be more flexible.
- Health care workers must have multiple skills.
- Nurses, doctors, and other health care providers must integrate services and focus on interdisciplinary rather than own identity, being in a team rather than individual practice.
- Nurses must increase focus on leadership training, as nurses traditionally have been the leaders in team coordination.
- Nurses must tell other practitioners about our value on primary and preventive care.

Greek Culture. In Greece, health is important and desired, but it is not a preoccupation. One should not pamper the self. Straight living gives a healthy body; thus fortitude, hardness, and a simple standard of living are pursued. Excesses in living—in eating, drinking, or smoking—are avoided, and, in general, the level of public health is high. Because children are prized, their health needs take precedence over adults' needs.

Going to bed is a sign of weakness except for recognized disease. People do not go to a physician unless there is something seriously wrong; but then they expect the physician, who is a father figure, to have the answers to their problems. Home remedies and the services of an herbalist are tried first as treatment. Prayers are said and vows are made. Illness is thought to arise from evil or magical sources that can be counteracted through magical practices. Entering the hospital is a last resort. The whole family is involved when a member is sick; each person has a specific role and a role gap exists during illness.

The organs of highest significance are the eyes, for they reflect the real person. Next in importance are the lips because of the words that come out of them. A girl's hair and a man's mustache are important symbols of sexual identity and attractiveness. The genital organs are not freely talked about but are respected for their reproductive functions. The body is meant to be covered and exposed only when necessary. Dress and ornamentation are essential to complete one's body image.

Childlessness is unfortunate and in the past the woman was held responsible. Women dislike any examination or treatment of the reproductive organs and accept gynecologic problems rather than seek medical care for fear fertility will be affected. An illness that may occur is hysteria, when the woman has bizarre complaints and behavior because it is believed that the uterus leaves the pelvis for another part of the body. Special care is given to women during pregnancy, when special regulations about hygiene, rest, activity, and a happy environment are followed.

The handicapped are not easily accepted because of the emphasis on a whole, strong, firm body. To be crippled, blind, or lame means that one is not a whole person, is dependent, and is unable to do anything for oneself.

Greek-Americans adhere to some or many of the aforementioned values and practices, depending on closeness to cultural ties. References pertinent to this section are found on page 30.

Latino Culture. Attitudes among Latinos in the American Southwest (or other Spanish-speaking people) are very unlike attitudes in mainstream America. Spanish-American people consider the self to be a whole person; thus, "better health" has no meaning. Good health is associated with the ability to work and fulfill normal roles, for one gains and maintains respect by meeting one's responsibilities. Criteria of health are a sturdy body, ability to maintain normal physical activity, and absence of pain. A person does not have to have perfect health; as long as the family is around, he or she is all right. Thus, preventive measures are not highly valued. A person does seek to care for oneself, however, through moderation in eating, drinking, work, recreation, and sleep, and by leading a good life (202).

Acculturation, *the process of change occurring as a result of contact between cultural groups,* is demonstrated by a minority group's adoption of the larger group's cultural mores. Lack of assimilation on the part of Latinos has been described as a strong barrier to their optimal use of health services. It is assumed that Latinos who retain Spanish as their first language, who are proud of their ethnic heritage, and who do not follow American norms and values are much less likely than their more assimilated counterparts to use health services or engage in preventive health behaviors. Marks et al., as a result of their study of elderly Latino women in Los Angeles, believe that cultural factors may have little impact on the health care-seeking behavior of Hispanics. Access to and availability of services, feelings toward screening processes, values about privacy, and sociodemographic factors are stronger determinants of Latino health practices (167).

Latino people believe that hardship and suffering are part of destiny, and that reward for being submissive to God's will and for doing good will come in the next life. Ill health is accepted as part of life and is thought to be caused by an unknown external event or object, such as natural forces of cold, heat, storms, and water, or as the result of sinning—acting against God's will. Latinos, for example, think that one cause of illness is bad air, especially night air, which enters through a cavity or opening in the body. Thus a raisin may be placed on the cord stump of the newborn and surgery is avoided if possible; both practices help prevent air from entering the body. Avoiding drafts, keeping windows closed at night, keeping the head covered, and following certain postpartum practices have the same basis. Other causes of disease (according to Hispanic beliefs) include overwork, poor food, excess worry or emotional strain, undue exposure to weather, uneven wetting of the body, taking a drink when overheated, and giving blood for transfusion. Underlying this thinking is the concept held by Asians of *yin* or "cold" and *yang* or "hot" or the hot-and-cold theory of disease that stems from the Hippocratic humoral theory and was carried to the Western Hemisphere by the Spanish and Portuguese in the 16th and 17th centuries (9).

The **hot-and-cold theory of disease** *does not always refer to physical temperature or foodstuff, but also to the effects that certain substances have or are thought to have on the body.* Basically all diseases are classified as hot and cold. Arthritis, pregnancy, postpartum period, cancer, pneumonia, colds, head- and ear aches, and teething are cold diseases. Hot diseases are fever, infections, diarrhea, rashes, ulcers, and constipation. It is considered dangerous to be outdoors at night if one's body is warm. Beliefs about which foods are warm and cold vary from one geographic region and culture to another. For example, prenatal vitamins may be a hot food and will not be taken during pregnancy, a hot condition, unless swallowed with fruit juice, a cold food. All foods, herbs, and medicines are classified as hot or cold. Avocado, fresh vegetables, dairy products, fish, and chicken are cold foods. Aspirin, cornmeal, eggs, beef, waterfowl, cereal grains, and chili peppers are considered hot. A goal is to balance the body: a hot disease is cured with a cold food and a cold disease is cured with a hot food, herb, or medication. Thus, aspirin could be taken for arthritis, which also fits into the Western medical system (9, 10, 86, 202).

Mal ojo, evil eye, *is a cause of disease that results when a person looks admiringly at the child of another. Symptoms include headaches, fever, crying, diarrhea, weight loss, insomnia, and sunken eyes.* Usually children are not openly admired, but precautions against illness include patting the child on the head or a light slap. A common illness in this culture, **susto,** with *symptoms of agitation and depression, results from traumatic, frightening experiences and may result in death.* Psychosocial forces causing disease are also seen in **empacho,** *a gastrointestinal disease that results from eating food that is disliked, or from overeating, or from eating hot bread.* **Caida de la mollera** or **mollera caida** *(fallen fontanels) is caused by a child falling or someone pulling the nipple out of the mouth too quickly, and results in cry-*

ing, vomiting, diarrhea, fever, restlessness, sunken eyes, and inability to grasp the nipple. Hydration is essential in treatment. **Resfriado** *(chilled) results from getting wet and not changing to dry clothes.* In turn, **catarro consti-pado** *(head cold or sinusitis)* may result. Disease may also result from organs or parts of the body moving from the normal position. Little attention is paid to colds, minor aches, or common gastrointestinal disorders (9, 10, 28, 86, 202, 264).

The role of the family is important in time of illness. The head of the house, the man, determines whether illness exists and what treatment is to be given. The person goes to bed when too ill to work or move. Treatment from a lay healer is sought if family care does not help. A physician is called only when the person is gravely ill; this is combined with visiting so the sick person does not get the rest and isolation advised by health care professionals in the majority culture. The sick person does not withdraw from the group; doing so would only make him or her feel worse. Acceptance of fate amounts to saying "If the Lord intends for me to die, I'll die." The discomfort of the present is considered, but not in terms of future complications. Being ill brings no secondary advantage of care or coddling. Communicable diseases are hard to control, for resistance to isolation is based on the idea that family members, relatives, and familiar objects cannot contaminate or cause illness. Taking home remedies, wearing special articles, and performing special ceremonies are accepted ways of getting and staying well. The person feels he or she will keep well by observing the ritual calendar, being brotherly, and being a good Catholic and member of the community. If the health care provider uses any procedure, such as an x-ray, it is considered to be the treatment and hence the person should be cured (9, 10, 86, 202).

Accidents are feared because they disrupt the wholeness of the person. In addition, Latinos fear surgery, the impersonality of the hospital and nurses, and any infringement on modesty.

The hospital represents death and isolation from family or friends. The "professional" (Anglo) approach of the majority culture is regarded as showing indifference to needs and as causing anxiety and discomfort.

Several authors describe specific health care practices of Spanish-speaking people and families and nursing implications, including for childbirth, childrearing, and prevention of communicable diseases. They also discuss customs related to use of folk medicine, use of surnames, and customs of interaction (9, 10, 86, 202).

Japanese Culture. Attitudes in Japan toward health strongly reflect the belief in a body–mind–spirit interre-

lationship. Spiritual and temporal affairs in life are closely integrated; thus, health practices and religion are closely intertwined, influenced considerably by the magicoreligious practices of Shinto, Japan's ancient religion. Bathing customs stem from Shinto purification rites, for example, and baths are taken in the evening before eating not only for cleanliness but for ceremony and relaxation as well.

There is strong emphasis on healthy diet (low fat, low sugar), physical fitness, an intact body, physical strength, determination, family and group relationships, and long life. Self-discipline in daily habits is highly valued, as are the mental, spiritual, and esthetic aspects of the person. All of these values and traits promote health and remain equally important to the sick person to promote recovery.

As a child, the individual is taught to minimize reactions to injury and illness. Hence to the Westerner a sick person may appear stoic. Part of the reserve in expressing emotion and pain is also influenced by childrearing and interaction practices, which emphasize correct behavior and suppression of emotion. Yet the sick person, as much as one who is well, expects to be treated with respect and resents being addressed abruptly or informally by first name. The person also resents people entering the hospital room without knocking. The Japanese male resents being dominated by women and he may feel uncomfortable with an American female health care professional because he interprets her behavior as overbearing. The person is eager to cooperate with the medical care program and wishes to be included in planning and decisions regarding care. The so-called professional approach of the average U.S. health care provider is likely to insult the average Japanese, although he or she may be too polite to say so. References pertinent to this section are found on page 30.

By studying life patterns of people in various cultures (especially those of patients for whom you care) and by taking into account the factors discussed in the following chapters on religion and family, you can better understand and handle varying levels of health, health problems, and care of different groups.

You may obtain additional information about people from various (sub)cultures and their specific nursing needs from references on page 30. Also, Vargus and Koss-Chioino, in their edited book, present strategies with children and adolescents of a number of ethnic and racial cultures, including foster-care children and middle-class adolescents who are African-American, American-Indian youth, Asian-American youth and first-generation members, Hispanic children and Latino gang members, and Southeast Asian families (251).

FOR FURTHER INFORMATION ON CULTURES

The references cited provide information about (sub)cultures and their specific health care and nursing needs:

African-American (9, 22, 29, 33, 37, 38, 46, 51, 52, 70, 73, 86, 87, 116, 126, 140, 147, 154, 168, 171, 189, 191, 195, 197, 203, 214, 231, 235, 240, 242, 243, 265)
Alaska Native (21, 33, 48, 67, 86, 161, 168, 172, 173, 184, 188, 230)
American Indian (9, 16, 33, 48, 75, 86, 107, 112, 113, 114, 136, 140, 168, 172, 173, 204, 205, 210, 217, 229, 234, 240, 270, 275)
Amish (9, 111, 263, 269)
Appalachian (9, 33, 86, 146, 177, 216, 256, 268)
Arabian (14, 117, 162, 168, 179, 180, 182, 185, 196)
Asian-American (9, 84, 86, 98, 120, 125, 155, 159, 168, 172, 173, 232, 240, 243, 258, 273, 276)
Asian-Pacific Islander (32, 84, 98, 173, 232)
British (83, 168, 173)
Canadian (86, 139, 173)
Caribbean (33, 86, 116, 153, 173)
Chinese (9, 31, 33, 63, 85, 86, 137, 156, 168, 173, 240)
Euro-American (9, 33, 80, 102, 173)
Filipino (9, 11, 15, 33, 86, 175, 237, 240)
German (33, 76, 102, 133, 140, 173, 215, 218, 219)
Greek-American (9, 86, 105, 168, 173, 223, 266)
Gypsy (8, 33)
Haitian (1, 33, 59, 86, 123, 173)
Iranian (121, 173, 183, 192)
Irish-American (33, 86, 95, 102, 173, 200, 277)
Italian-American (33, 102, 140, 169, 277)
Japanese (9, 33, 63, 86, 96, 129, 155, 168, 186, 198, 244)
Jewish (9, 86, 173, 193, 202, 222, 272)
Korean (9, 33, 42, 86, 240)
Mexican-American (10, 33, 71, 86, 92, 131, 140, 166, 168, 173, 174, 226, 239, 259)
Middle Eastern (14, 33, 134, 157, 158, 163, 168, 181, 183, 261)
Migrant Farmer (9, 43, 115, 226, 255)
Polish-American (122, 129, 140, 160, 168, 173, 199, 225)
Puerto Rican (9, 33, 63, 86, 153, 172)
Rural (19, 77, 132, 135, 147)
Southeast Asian (9, 28, 33, 45, 57, 79, 82, 92, 168, 212, 224)
Spanish-speaking or Latino (7, 9, 10, 33, 36, 39, 48, 61, 86, 90, 91, 110, 119, 167, 168, 172, 173, 208, 214, 240, 278)
Vietnamese (9, 33, 41, 66, 86, 141, 173, 243, 254)

SOCIOECONOMIC CLASS SUBCULTURE

Research about social stratification indicates that a person's class position is influenced by economic and social status and political power of the family and affects formation of values, attitudes, and lifestyle. Each class in any country tends to have a more or less specified set of values and role expectations regarding practically every area of human activity: sex, marriage, male–female and parent–child responsibilities and behavior, birth, death, education, dress, housing, home furnishings, leisure, reading habits, occupational status, politics, religion, and status symbols (129). In turn, health status in the United States is closely linked to income level. Poor people are more likely to have poor health and chronic illness (9, 86). Social class includes a group consciousness. Most persons can be objectively placed within a certain class (100), but they are sometimes accorded a status by others around them that might be different. Furthermore, they may see themselves at yet a different status level, based on race, sex, religion, ancestry, ethnic origin, or wealth in material goods. What seems natural and logical in determining status to some people may be rejected by others.

As you gain general knowledge about values and lifestyles of people in various economic levels, realize also that no one person encompasses all that the literature describes. Knowledge about lifestyles is generally useful to your practice, but *avoid stereotyping people* because of this knowledge.

Profile of Socioeconomic Levels

The Upper-Upper, Affluent, or Corporate Level

This level consists of a relatively small number (3–4%) of people who own a disproportionate share of personal wealth and whose income is largely derived from ownership. About 6 million or 6% of all households in the United States have an annual gross income above $100,000. Three percent of all children and less than 1% of all people over 65 years of age are among the wealthy. The surest way to get rich in America has been to own a business. New legislation makes the way even smoother (17, 18, 250).

Their work, profession, or business provides prestige, status, honor, wealth, and power. This group has both money and power and it can control how its assets are used as well as various other economic and political aspects of society. The decisions made by this group affect everyone else. These are the people who have had lineage, inherited wealth, and power for several generations. They are acknowledged by the general public and themselves as influential and as conservative leaders locally, nationally, and internationally. They feel obliged to tend their own financial and material resources well, to obtain the best possible education, to demonstrate impeccable tastes, and to take care of their health so that they can meet their obligation of giving of themselves personally and philanthropically to society (47, 49, 55, 106, 211, 246). The affluent family is almost clanlike; the individual and family has many connections. All members, including the women and youth, belong to elite clubs or organizations and also participate in and contribute considerably to the community and society as a whole through financial contributions and volunteer activities to various social, welfare, health, and political organizations. Frequently the affluent woman is actively committed to a cause, or several causes, and she makes time for and directs her volunteer efforts toward charitable organizations or chairing major civic and fund-raising events. Yet the very rich remain anonymous to most Americans (55).

This person or family lives in an exclusive residential area in a house whose atmosphere is spatial, elegant, and formal, and that affords privacy from the masses. This person or family may own several estates in different areas of the country (or world) that are located in the best areas, are furnished with family heirlooms and works of art, and are used in different seasons or for different purposes. The family may have a number of people to help it maintain its lifestyle, such as a maid, butler, gardener, and other staff members (47, 49, 55, 60, 78, 106, 211).

The children are educated in schools with fine reputations and reared by a governess or maid as well as by the parents. The mother usually is selective in her teaching, guiding, and care. Certain aspects of rearing are done only by the mother, others only by the maid or nanny. The children may feel closer to the parent surrogates than to the parents. They, like the parents, live with choices, for they have more animate and inanimate objects and possessions than others and many opportunities to follow the arts; to learn certain sports, such as horseback riding, tennis, swimming, or skiing; and to travel worldwide. But even the children know the importance and value of the objects and opportunities that surround them. They recognize the importance of self-control, behaviorally and in their various activities and sports, and of following family wishes and upholding the family name. They seek privacy and disciplined activity even though in the public view. They are busy and able to move smoothly from one activity to another. Yet they expect, and are expected, to be competent and successful at their chosen academic, recreational, and social pursuits (47, 49, 60, 78, 106, 211, 246).

Although the upper economic level is adult oriented, children know at an early age that they are special and parents try to instill a feeling that the children must do well because they have special responsibilities to society on reaching adulthood. The child, like the parent, associates with others from the same level, observing the average person from the sidelines, never really understanding what life is like for the average citizen or why people from lower economic levels live as they do. Although both adults and children take a lot for granted and feel entitled to the fine things in life, they feel a sense of responsibility, are discrete in behavior, and try to live up to their ideals. Destiny is abundance and limitless possibility. They are confident that life will be rewarding. Even crisis, such as illness or surgery, can be made into something basically pleasant, for the best of specialized health care professionals and comprehensive facilities can be obtained, and convalescence frequently involves a trip to and rest at a secluded place (47, 49, 106, 211, 213).

Table 1–12 lists *values* that are commonly held by people who are in the upper economic level in the USA (78, 165, 213).

The Lower-Upper Level

This group consists of people whose *wealth is more recently acquired and who have become well-known* (actors, famous doctors or lawyers, athletes), or they may be less famous but have large incomes, homes, and

TABLE 1–12. COMPARISON OF VALUES OF PERSONS IN UPPER AND UPPER-MIDDLE ECONOMIC LEVELS

Upper Level Values	Upper-Middle Level Values
Family name, lineage, traditions, position, home.	Family stability and prestige.
Privacy, seclusion (person is prey to publicity, slander)	Friendliness, sociability, pleasantness, patience in relationships, honesty.
Education, knowledge in breadth and depth respected, knowledge for knowledge sake.	Education, problem solving, concepts, and abstractions used and enjoyed.
Philanthropy with the arts, civic causes, societal projects for improvement.	Service to one or several causes.
Professional/career achievements, success.	Professional/career success, achievement.
Service to others, the wider community, civic events, nationally and even internationally; altruism.	Community involvement and leadership; local or regional focus.
High expectations and goals for family; initiative.	High goals; being responsible; initiative.
Influence; power; prestige; patriotism.	Democracy; patriotism.
Economic achievements.	Upward economic and social mobility; economic security.
Being strong; willpower; control or discipline over emotions, appearance, actions. Being self-directed but flexible; responsible.	Ability to withstand stress; spontaneous in emotions and actions. Appearance influenced by societal trends.
Excellence of performance; competence, success in activities.	Hard work; competence; success.
Traditional patterns.	Change, societal progress.
Possession of cultural artifacts and art pieces; consumption of material goods.	Material comfort; consumption of material goods; value objects gained by hard work.
Travel widely to seek intellectually stimulating experiences; wide association with others.	Leisure activity; travel for enjoyment and educational opportunity.

lifestyles that show off their money. They have social position and prestige because of what they *do*. The upper-upper-level person has position and prestige because of *who* he or she is; the person does not lose them even if encountering financial setbacks. The lower-upper-level person may slide down into middle-level anonymity if wealth is lost. The lower-upper-level (or newly rich) person or family also has an abundance of possessions and opportunity, but may be less humble about or more self-conscious of it than the upper-upper-level person. Although this person or family may attend the same activities, travel to the same areas, or send children to the same schools as the upper-upper-level family, this person or family is seen by the long-established wealthy as being different. Often a fine line separates these two levels in a community; such intangibles as social charm or likeability, family background, religion, area and value of residence, and schooling often make the difference. Money is only loosely related to social standing in many communities. Both women and men of this level are working—entering a profession, starting a business, or doing consultant work—for fun, for a sense of identity, to be worthwhile, to provide structure to the day or to life, to avoid the image of being intellectual (they are usually college educated), or to avoid being important only through the spouse (47, 49, 60, 78, 165, 213).

The Overclass

In America, we are witnessing the birth of a new social class: the **overclass,** *professionals and managers, who are upwardly mobile,* in some ways like the yuppies of the early 1980s. Although people in this group have interests and a culture in common, they are a new American elite, a part of businesses or fields of work that bright and ambitious people want to enter (not political leadership). They claim an increasing share of the national income (household income averages about $114,000), and they spend a proportionate amount of their income on themselves. They do not like to give money to causes. People in this group tend to be transnational, although they tend to live on either the East or West coast. They judge people on merit, which is demonstrated to them by a continual accumulation of academic and professional credentials.

This group rejects middle class values. The overclass leads a distinctive lifestyle that reflects yuppie tastes updated, that reveals a greater affluence and sophistication, and that is founded on privileges. Individuals in this group are likely to believe they are doing important things that no one else can do and that they merit privileges. More than money, this group values

competitive achievement on the job and in leisure, the number of books published or products launched, the art collection, the vehicles driven, the exotic food eaten. Members of this group are likely to be urban singles and couples without children. If the couple has children, they are likely to employ a nanny instead of using day-care. As one young mother said, "Oh yes, my child has called the nanny 'Mother', but that's OK. She's with her more than I am." Children will be sent to the Ivy League schools from which the parents have graduated. They prefer their children not to associate with children from other social classes, just as they prefer to live in gated, walled communities. They feel contemptuous toward ordinary workers, the middle class, or the poor, if they think of them at all. They may be totally unaware that those people may believe that members of the overclass have sold their souls. They may also speak of their quiet desperation (3, 12, 18).

The Upper-Middle Level

This group, the top third of the middle class, is described as *those who are well off and is considered to be the backbone of the community.* Income is high but varies, depending on occupation and geographic area, and investments are important. Each spouse is college educated and at least one is a professional—doctor, dentist, engineer, business manager, or lawyer. The main work of these people is intellectual instead of manual, requires professional training, and offers upward mobility. The workplace is as important to the spouse as to the employed member. They may begin family life in an apartment, but when financially able, they move to a large house in a better part of town or a suburb. Property and investments are gradually accumulated. They may have a maid and gardener, own more than one car, travel nationally and abroad, belong to a semielite country club, and frequently send their children to private schools and colleges (49, 78, 100, 165, 213). Both family stability and community leadership are valued. They often play a role in local civic and political affairs. The children have a number of opportunities educationally and culturally; in return, they are expected to be successful academically and socially. The children are often involved in a number of prestigious out-of-home activities and organizations, as are parents, and the children may actually have fewer home responsibilities than the upper-class child. Childrearing is permissive; children are given explanations instead of punishment. The parents will exert more direct influence on the child's schooling than will parents of the middle or working class (49, 78, 213). The work ethic is different for this group from the work ethic of the rich. Thus, children may do tasks to earn an allowance and may work at various jobs, such as babysitting, lawnmowing, or fast-food service, in the teen years to earn extra money. (By contrast, parents at higher economic levels do not expect their children to work while attending school.) This group has a relatively carefree lifestyle because money is not a major issue. Movement, gaiety, creativity, leisure activities, fun in indoor or outdoor sports, dancing, theatre, museums, travel or educational experiences, acquiring a deeper self-knowledge and self-control, and remaining youthful are major foci. One image is that of the serious-minded sportsman (55, 78, 165, 213).

Table 1–12 lists commonly held *values* of the upper middle economic level.

The Middle Level

According to pollsters, 90% of adults in America identify themselves as middle class (2). The middle economic level sometimes is divided in two categories: those who reached the American dream and those who have a comfortable existence. Members of the *American dream* group have education above the high school level in a professional or specialized school and include business people with small or medium-sized enterprises, self-employed business people, artists, skilled workers, office and sales workers, and public or private school teachers. Nurses and other health care professionals typically are in this level. These people have a special status because of education and occupation (many *work with* people), and have some status in the community, although they do not have much wealth. Typically they work in occupations that involve thinking rather than hard physical labor. They live in a pleasant residential section or suburb, in a nicely furnished house that they own, have two cars, sometimes including a van or four-wheel-drive vehicle. The family eats out weekly and vacations annually. This family is usually a nuclear family. It has linkages through kin for social and family goals as well as close friendships with neighbors. The family is active in community activities and organizations, and members may have some positions of power. They pursue some sports or other leisure activities as a family unit, but the family members frequently go to separate activities several evenings a week. They have a sense of success and security. Members of the *comfortable existence* group tend to have less education and fewer material goods than the first group, but they live comfortably. They have more than the necessities and are somewhat active in the community (17, 23, 53, 64, 78, 86, 154, 165, 213, 246, 247).

Parents in this group are child-oriented; family life often revolves around children and their interests. At work, the person typically deals with manipulation of symbols, ideas, or interpersonal relationships, has to be self-directed, and must use initiative to get ahead. Thus, families (single- or two-parent) have high aspirations for children and take pride in their accomplishments. Parents emphasize education, self-actualization, creativity, interpersonal sensitivity, and they value and encourage verbal and problem-solving skills. The middle (and upper) economic level(s) uses an elaborate code of speech, which is characterized by precision, differentiation of ideas, and extensive use of modifiers and clauses. Its verbosity may bury the meaning, and the abstractness of such speech causes lack of understanding among the working and lower economic levels. Parents teach the importance of hard work, self-reliance, thrift, patience, planning ahead, postponing immediate rewards for later rewards, and compassion for those who are less fortunate (68, 213).

These parents are typically more responsive to the advice of experts and research results. They accept the advice of experts, because it is based on their values and therefore offers what they want. Thus, for example, the parents change childrearing practices, perhaps several times on one child and, because of education, are more likely to feel insecure in childrearing and view it as problematic. They discuss childrearing practices with neighbors and friends, consult the physician, nurse, or child's teacher about what they are doing wrong (seldom do they see themselves doing anything right), and join various community organizations, such as the PTA, where they learn even more about childrearing. Parents are consistently more concerned about the child's feelings and try to understand the dynamics of the child's behavior and mix discipline with permissiveness. Discipline is often in the form of withdrawal of privileges or of disapproval, threats, or appeals to reason. Punishment is based on the parent's interpretation of the child's intent behind his or her action. If the child loses control, punishment results. If the outburst represents a release of feeling, the child is less likely to be punished. Additionally, the parent is more likely than a working-class parent to feel and be supportive, accepting, and egalitarian to the child. Children are expected to be expressive verbally and emotionally, be happy and cooperative, confide in parents, want to learn, have self-control, share readily, be self-directed, and stay well and healthy (23, 33, 52, 58, 68, 80, 86, 100, 165, 183, 213).

The parents do many activities together, and roles are not as sharply differentiated. Both parents are supportive of the children, especially of same-sex children, and the father's role as disciplinarian is secondary to that of supportive figure. This is in accordance with his wife's wishes. Father tends to agree with mother and plays a role close to that desired by her. The parent has greater stability of income and takes for granted much of what a poor parent works hard to achieve. As a result, this parent is freer to give attention to the child (23, 64, 68, 78, 86, 100, 165, 213).

Overall, the people in this group use the internist, family-practice physician, and pediatrician for routine health care, but the services of specialists are used when indicated. They respect health professionals and want thorough and scientific diagnosis and treatment. They see themselves as knowledgeable about health, and appreciate and will try to use additional information. They tolerate, although they do not like, high medical costs (68).

The group's *values* correspond closely to those of the dominant society previously described (see Table 1–2.)

The Lower-Middle or Working Level

This group is often perceived as those who are *just getting by*. Generally both spouses have graduated from high school and may attend community college. They both have jobs as industrial or blue-collar workers, clerical or service workers, agricultural wage earners, technicians, skilled or semiskilled workers, telephone operators, or waitresses (68, 213). Many of this group work with machines, tools, or objects. Chances for advancement are minimal unless the person pursues further education. Job security is threatened by the effects of automation in the workplace. Opportunity for job advancement is minimal without additional education or an apprenticeship. Many workers who are a part of this economic level are proud of their work, do it very well, and know that *they make an important contribution to society*. Society must have carpenters, plumbers, secretaries, farmers, garbage collectors, and all of the other workers who are in this group (201).

The family rents either a small home with two or three bedrooms or an apartment and takes good care of its home and belongings, including an older car. It has some conveniences but may not own many luxuries. The family depends on the extended family instead of social agencies for economic and emotional support and may be active in church but not in the PTA or other community organizations. The husband is typically head of the house and the woman is considered responsible for the home and child care. The family enjoys recreational activities as a family unit, such as bowling, attending the movies, and eating at fast-service or local "home-style" restaurants (23, 68, 78, 213).

The members of this group have watched and feel concern about the steady degradation and erosion of values and customs they consider essential to their perception of a real America (201). They value traditional values listed in Table 1–2. They believe people with money are not happy, and they are grateful for their parents' sacrifices. They accept their position and are basically proud of their hard work, homes, and accomplishments, even with less education. They believe that on-the-job, collective action is important. They believe that the poor deserve their poverty and should not be given welfare. (A natural economic depression and forced unemployment are the only two causes for poverty without moral blame.) Being higher in the social scale than the poor and some minorities gives them a social identity and a measure of social worth. They feel that equality of all people, including the poor, minorities, and women, is threatening and would pose problems of social adjustment. Another danger of equality is that friends or neighbors might surpass them. The present inequality allows the affluent or supervisors to be an elite group, to take care of people, to be friendly, helpful leaders. Equality of income would deprive people of their incentive to work. These people are stable breadwinners, churchgoers, voters, and family men and women. They may have two jobs and little leisure. Leisure is usually focused on activities that help the person temporarily forget the life situation and work. Many do not like their jobs but fear not finding another; therefore they keep the job because of family responsibilities and the hold on respectability that the job brings. What they want most is a decent standard of living (23, 64, 68, 78, 165, 201, 213).

The adult in this level typically has less education, reads less, and is therefore less responsive to research results and the advice of experts. Further, expert advice usually is not relevant to this value system. Childrearing is taken for granted and is not perceived as something that you do with a preset plan, nor as something that is problematic or to be discussed with others. These parents rely heavily on the extended family, retaining traditional methods of parenting and keeping the same goals that they perceived in their homes and parents. Desirable characteristics in the child, according to the parent, include the following: the child should be neat, clean, honest, obedient, respectful to parents, pleasant to adults, and trustworthy; conform to externally imposed standards; and respect the rights of others (64, 68, 100, 201, 213).

That the parent has the traditional values and views on childrearing can be related to how he or she was raised and educated and the present occupational role. The person typically deals with the manipulation of things and is subjected to standardization and direct supervision and authority; and getting ahead depends on collective action rather than individual initiative. Congruence exists between the adult's occupational requirements and values about the behavior of children. The occupational experience affects the parent's concept of what is desirable behavior—on or off the job, for adults or children. The parents value conformity of behavior; they have learned to conform to get ahead. Thus they punish nonconforming behavior, including what experts would call the natural curiosity of the child, as well as behavior that is extreme or disturbing. The preferred discipline technique is physical punishment rather than emphasis on reasoning. The child should not break rules that are externally imposed, but should remain orderly and obedient. And so the child of the working-class parent is prepared for a position in society as an adult, and in the future as a parent will impose constraints on his or her children in much the same manner (68, 213).

In this level, work and social roles and the roles of mother and father are more sharply differentiated, and the man and woman lead separate social lives. The mother is the more supportive parent, wanting the father to help with discipline. Frequently, the father views himself as the economic provider but sees no reason to help shoulder the responsibility of childrearing. He thinks it is important that the child be taught not to transgress, and because the mother has the primary responsibility for child care, discipline should also be her job. Because he is less involved in childrearing, the father also has less real authority and status in family affairs. In the process, the male and female children learn what it is to be a father and mother, and as adults, their expectations and behavior are influenced, at least to some degree, by what they unconsciously learned as children. If they have the opportunity of enough education and advantage to move into the middle level, they may slowly change their values and childrearing practices as they outwardly imitate other middle-class parents around them. Yet very often, values do not change and even overt behavior is nearer to that of their parents than that of their newly found middle-class friends (64, 68, 100, 213).

Health care is sought when a person is too sick to work—the group's definition of illness. Prevention is emphasized less than in the foregoing economic levels. People may try home or folk remedies first and then go to a general practitioner. The neighborhood health center will be used if one exists. Dental care is more likely to be neglected than other medical care. People in this level respond well to an approach that is respectful, personable, prompt, and thorough. They do not understand why health care should be so costly, and they may omit very expensive treatments or drugs whenever possible (68, 201).

The Upper-Lower Level

This group is perceived as those who are *having a real hard time.* The family is often only one step away from poverty and welfare. An individual has fewer chances of acquiring education. Thus people work at menial tasks, usually in nonunion jobs, but are proud to be working. Wages and job benefits are a concern (213). These people may work as domestics, gardeners, hospital or school maintenance or cafeteria workers, junk collectors, garbage collectors, or street cleaners. Often neither husband nor wife has completed high school and sometimes one may not have completed junior high. The family lives in a substandard flat in an older building, usually with an absentee landlord. The family is patriarchal; the woman works but also has all house and child responsibilities. Children are an asset; they leave school early and help support the family (213). The family enjoys picnics in the park and other free diversions. The family's only long trips are for funerals of relatives (213). Often the family had its beginning in lack of motivation for education, resulting in high school dropout for pregnancy or lack of academic success, early parenthood, a poor first job, a rapid succession of children, or an early separation or divorce. As life progresses, the chance to advance becomes even less likely (170, 213, 247).

Values of people in this level are similar to the traditional values of the lower-middle level, with greater emphasis on thrift and conformity to external authority (see Table 1–2).

The Poor

Poor people, the *underclass,* include those who are in acute poverty and those in chronic poverty. First, poverty has two definitions. **Poverty** is *having inadequate pre-tax money or source of income to purchase a minimum amount of goods and services.* Poverty is also a power issue. *It is the relative lack of an individual's access to and control over environmental resources.* Poverty reflects class and racial stratification and hopelessness and is seen in increasing homelessness and health problems that result from the conditions of poverty (213). The person or family in **acute poverty** *has reduced economic means for a limited time because of given circumstances* but anticipates being able to return to work and a better lifestyle. The person or family in **chronic poverty** *has a long family history of being unemployed and without adequate economic means and is unlikely to see much opportunity for improvement* (187).

The lines are not always so clearly drawn, however. Because of the unemployment problems of the 1980s and 1990s, more people who were in the middle economic level now are economically classified as poor. A single parent raising several children, although middle class by birth, may become acutely poor when a job is not available or a prolonged illness or other crisis occurs (72). The current government *poverty level* is $8076 per year for a couple, $9985 for a three-member family, $12,675 for a four-member family, $14,990 for a family of five, and $29,529 for a family of nine. Minimum income to be above poverty levels is $7363 for a single person. The median net worth of a poor family is $3900 (77). More than one in seven Americans live in poverty (39.6 million of 253 million) in the United States. Twelve percent of all households, 23% of elderly, and 22% of all children live in poverty (247).

Rural poverty is on the rise, especially in the South and Midwest of the United States. For example, in Illinois, 20% of the residents in eight nonmetropolitan counties live in poverty conditions. Poverty is more prevalent among rural females than males; 45.8% of the female-headed households in Illinois are at or below poverty level. Almost 50% of the children in rural areas in Illinois live in households with incomes less than half the poverty level. Because of the economic losses of farmers during the past decade, an increasing number now also work off the farm at least part-time (77). Having lost money because of weather conditions and consequent poor crops, falling prices for grain and livestock, and increasing costs for machinery, land, seed, and fertilizer, the farm family, once able to provide for basic needs, may rather suddenly lose the farm land and home and everything in it. Homelessness and destitution may follow. In a rural area, economic losses to farmers in turn affect the businessmen in small towns. The circle of poverty grows larger.

One of every five American *children* is poor; the rate is higher than for any other group in our society (250). This is a tragedy for millions of children and our country. Many poor children live in one-parent families, dependent on welfare and whatever social services can be secured. In one meeting for children living in a housing project for poor people, 9 of the 12 children who attended did not live with either parent or any adult. They survived on their own! Too many children born and reared in poverty never grow up to be economically productive members of society. Thus, all of us become poorer (126).

Elderly people continue to be at risk for poverty because of legislative and economic trends in the United States. *Elderly people in rural areas* are more likely to be poor than are urban elderly, and the poverty increases with age. People over 85 years are especially vulnerable. Poverty rates are higher for all rural demographic subgroups, including ethnic minorities, than for all urban demographic subgroups because of past employ-

ment experiences, education, and living arrangements. Often the rural elderly have had less pension or insurance coverage and less lifetime earnings, and thereby, they have less accumulated economic resources and lower Social Security benefits. Older women are particularly dependent on the marital union for economic well-being. To prevent poverty in the future elderly, employment prospects and strategies for retirement planning for today's young adults and middle-agers are key. Policies related to death and divorce benefits are also critical (176).

Homeless people are also among the poor, sometimes the acutely or newly poor. The duration of homelessness varies from a short time to many years, depending on the cause and the type of social services and assistance available to the person. People of all ages and all walks of life are among the homeless. It is not unusual that someone who was middle class lose a job and remain unemployed and then lose a home. Becoming a single parent or working at low-paying jobs adds to the risk of living on the street, especially if living with family members is not an alternative. The homeless population is younger and better educated; there are an increasing number of women with children and even entire family units. The homeless are represented by all racial groups and geographic areas. About one-third are chronically mentally ill, and about one-third are chemically dependent; however, being homeless for some period also brings stressors that contribute to a decline in both physical and mental health.

Migrant workers and their families also suffer poverty and its effects. The **migrant family** *is one with children under age of compulsory school attendance that moves from one geographic region to another for the purpose of working in agricultural production and harvest of tree and field crops and that receives 50% of its income from this activity.* There are three migrant streams:

1. East Coast states, traveled mostly by African-Americans who make their home in Florida
2. Mid-Western and Western states, traveled mostly by Mexican-Americans
3. West Coast states, traveled by Mexican-Americans

There are an estimated 4.2 million migrant workers; 60% are under 25 years; 25% are less than 6 years old. Because more Hispanic migrants are traveling as units in cars, vans, and pickup trucks, an increased number of children are exposed to the stresses of migrant life. Work crews without family are more common in the Eastern states and are composed of primarily African-American workers (226).

Refugees from other lands may suffer poverty although they are sponsored by a group, family, or resettlement agency. Because they *were fleeing war or persecution,* they often arrive with little. Many face an economic struggle, bringing few readily transferrable work skills. **Immigrants** from other lands *choose to come to a specific location,* drawn by jobs or family reunification. They may have economic struggles but are less likely to be in poverty (9).

The **underclass** is defined as *an urban census tract where 40% or more of the residents live below the poverty line, as part of a ghetto. The neighborhood typically has a high rate of female-headed families, welfare dependency, and labor force and high school dropouts.* The *white underclass* is composed of less than 2% of all non-Hispanic whites; between 5 and 17% of African-Americans live in underclass neighborhoods. America has always housed the poor, including poor white immigrants; however, the white underclass neighborhoods or white slums are found in the Midwest and Northwest, in areas of manufacturing decline or in areas where residents from the South have migrated but found no work. The white and black ghettos have many characteristics in common, including men who abandoned the work force and residents who dropped out of school. White underclass neighborhoods contain fewer high-rise tenements than black underclass neighborhoods, but all underclass neighborhoods feel isolated from the remainder of the city (267).

Images of crime, drugs, gangs, out-of-wedlock births, AIDS, and unemployed men are as much a part of the white underclass as they are a part of any group that is poor and in the inner city, including the black underclass. In 1991, 22% of children born to white women were born to single mothers. Many of those mothers have below-average IQs; outcomes for the child(ren) are not likely to be successful. Health care providers for poor whites are aware that some females are content to have babies out of wedlock. They have easy access to contraception; they do not believe in abortion or adoption. Pregnant elementary and high school students insist having a baby will give them someone to love and someone who loves them. The father of the baby disappears after the child's arrival—many times before the arrival. Often the girl is fleeing an abusive family, to find abuse in the new relationships with men. The cycle can be repeated in the next generation (267).

Characteristics of the poor, in general, include the following:

- *They are less educated* than most Americans. Only 56% of poor household heads have high school education, in contrast to 81% of all household heads. Only 16% have attended college.
- *Most of the poor do not work.* A total of 51% of working-age poor are unemployed; 40% work part-time, compared with 69% of all adults. Only 9% of poor working-age adults work full-time year-round, in contrast to 42% of all working-age adults. Lack of education contributes to the kind of jobs available or inability to get work.
- *Most of the poor live in single-parent households headed by women.* More than half (52%) of poor families, compared with 18% of all U.S. families, are headed by single females.
- *Few welfare recipients who work their way off welfare will also work their way out of poverty.* Often states do not allocate their share of the expense of operating job training programs. For example, the Family Support Act of 1988 called for more than half of the nation's Aid to Families with Dependent Children (AFDC) recipients to participate in Job Opportunities and Basic Skills Training (JOBS) programs. In 1992, only 16% of those eligible were participating in JOBS because states did not allocate money for the program. Sixty percent of the women who leave the AFDC roles do so because they get back together with their husbands or marry, not because they find jobs.
- *Most of the elderly are not poor.* The rate of poverty among the elderly has declined from 28.5% in 1966 to 12.9% in 1992 (246, 247, 250).

Table 1–13 summarizes *common myths about poor people* and presents contrasting facts (246, 247). Certainly, being poor and living in a homeless shelter, housing project, low-income area, ghetto, or slum means the person often is a school dropout and is isolated from the world of industry and work. Further, the person who applies for a job may be perceived as unreliable or unwilling to work by the employer. Some industries are trying to develop programs that create networks and teach poor people who have been out of work the habits that fit into today's work world (126).

Patterns of childrearing and family relationships of the very poor affect the next generation of parents. These characteristics may include the following:

- Misbehavior is regarded in terms of overt outcome; reasons for behavior are infrequently considered.
- Lack of goal commitment, impulsive gratification, fatalism, and lack of belief in long-range success result from effects of chronic poverty on a person's motivations and lifestyle. Immediate needs must be met first.
- Communication between family members is more physical than verbal; explanations may not be given to the child, affecting curiosity and learning.

TABLE 1–13. MYTHS AND FACTS ABOUT POOR PEOPLE IN THE UNITED STATES

1. **Myth:** The Great Society's war on poverty made the problem worse.

   Fact: The poverty rate in 1964, when President Lyndon Johnson formally promised to end poverty, was 19%. It is now 14.5%, a rise from 11.1% in 1973.

2. **Myth:** Welfare dependence passes from one generation to the next.

   Fact: In 1994, a prospective, longitudinal study of 700 families from 1968 to 1988 found that nearly two of every three children whose parents collected welfare benefits did not receive them as adults.

3. **Myth:** Welfare costs are a major burden on the middle class.

   Fact: A family earning $50,000 annually typically contributes $615 annually ($1.69 daily) to federal programs that support poor, elderly, and disabled people. Approximately 12% of the federal budget is spent on entitlement programs for the poor. Medicaid tops all other welfare programs in number of recipients and cost annually.

4. **Myth:** Work is a guaranteed way out of poverty.

   Fact: No. People on welfare who find jobs typically earn too little to support a family. Often the poor person has less education, which results in employment in low-paying jobs with no job security. To pull above the poverty level, a woman with children would have to earn $17,449, or $8.38 an hour.

5. **Myth:** The poor have too many children.

   Fact: The average poor family receiving ADC consists of 2.9 people; the average American family consists of 3.2 people.

6. **Myth:** Most of the poor live in inner-city ghettos.

   Fact: One in eight poor Americans lives in a census tract with poverty rates of 40% or above. Poor people live in better areas of a city, the rural areas, and all geographic regions of the United States.

7. **Myth:** Most of the poor are African-American.

   Fact: African-Americans are overrepresented among the poor; they represent 13% of the population and make up 29% of the poor. Caucasians make up 67% of America's poor and 83% of the total population.

8. **Myth:** Poverty is a lifelong situation.

   Fact: One in every five people in poverty leaves the poverty status each year. One-third of the nation's poor are impoverished temporarily because of job loss, illness, or divorce.

- Families are frequently large; each member acts to get whatever gratification he or she can. Previously unmet needs in the parent cause the parent to be poorly equipped to meet the dependency needs of many children. The child, as adult, continues the cycle of previously unmet needs and inability to nurture.
- Mother is the chief child-care agent; father is often a punitive figure. The milieu of the home is authoritarian, even though father may be frequently out of the home.
- Discipline is harsh, inconsistent, and physical, often makes use of ridicule, and is based on whether or not the child's behavior annoys the parent.
- Aggressive behavior is alternately encouraged and restrained, depending primarily on the consequences to the parent of the child's behavior. Such inconsistency causes the child to learn how to get away with certain behavior and does not teach impulse control.
- Sex is viewed as an exploitative relationship. Questions about sex and sexual experimentation are met with a punitive attitude (9, 40, 68, 169, 170, 187, 213).

Poor parents often have low self-esteem. Studies indicate that parents with low self-esteem provoke feelings of shame, guilt, defensiveness, and decreased self-worth in children by overestimating their ability to conform, by inappropriately or forcefully punishing or restraining them, denying necessities, and withdrawing love. Such childhood experiences cause low self-esteem in children and these feelings continue into adulthood, so that as parents these individuals inflict the same feelings they suffered as a child (40, 68).

Authoritarian or harsh childrearing practices, which may be called discipline, have as their explicit objective the development of toughness and self-sufficiency for survival; however, parents are warm and expressive. A loving attachment exists between parent and child. In their own home children are also likely to be expressive, although they may seem restrained with strangers. Children are often given adult responsibilities early; they are not the focus of the family in the way that middle-class children are. They must fend more for themselves (9, 33, 58, 68).

Most minority and ethnic cultures value kinship ties and the emotional, social, and economic support that the extended family provides, in contrast to dominant middle-class America, which values individualism and independence. Much visiting goes on between relatives in the lower and working levels; assistance is sought and appreciated. All get along better by sharing meager resources or by working together to gain resources. The grandmother (and grandfather if living) is valued as caretaker for the child if the mother works. But the grandmother is also valued because she is the carrier of the culture; she is wise and can teach the young a great deal. The grandparent also benefits from being valued as a person (33, 170).

Ability to delay gratification appears related to the situation. Frequently poor people learn early that they are at the mercy of the system, whether the system is legal–political, economic, educational, or health (33). Then, too, if hungry, cold, or without necessities, small wonder that a person takes whatever possible to appease hunger or feel more comfortable. Children learn to delay gratification if they can trust that what is needed will be there when needed. Poor children may seldom have this opportunity because of economic problems in the family. If meager resources are used to meet today's needs, it is difficult or impossible to plan ahead, save, or anticipate that planning and saving have merit. The poor person is present-oriented, in contrast to the future perspective of people in the middle and upper levels, because of necessity, cultural values, or inability to trust what is not tangible (9, 33, 40, 170).

Often the poor person appears to need an authoritarian, directive approach. The poor person (or the parents) may work in a situation in which he or she takes orders; the poor person's expectancy is to be *told* rather than *invited to talk with* someone about his or her ideas, problems, tentative solutions, or insights. Or the person may not understand the health care provider's professional jargon but is too polite or fearful to ask for an explanation. Also, if previous attempts to share ideas were met with rejection or ridicule by a parent, teacher, or health care professional, the person learned that it was safer not to respond. Finally, the poor person values action—getting something accomplished—more than words or promises (33, 169, 187).

Impaired verbal communication and problem-solving ability may be present, not because the poor person is cognitively deficient but for other reasons. Many ethnic or minority groups speak a dialect in the home; the child then has difficulty understanding standard English or being understood. Essentially the child must become bilingual to be successful in school (51, 52). The poor person uses a restricted code that is characterized by short sentences, lack of specificity, and lack of subordinate clauses for elaboration of meaning. The poor person speaks directly to the point. Such language is said to be concrete and to indicate lack of abstract thinking. In contrast to middle-class elaborate and sometimes vague speech, the speech of the poor person is logical and expressive. Thought is not buried in verbosity and vagueness. The blunt speech may be uncomfortable to listen to, both in words and in ideas (51, 187, 213). The same words in professional and folk terminology may have a different meaning. For example, some African-Americans use the term "high blood" to mean that they believe there is too much blood in the body. Ingestion of large amounts of salty foods is believed to be helpful for an astringent effect. You must clarify that high blood pressure is different so that the person does not increase the hypertensive state further by excessive eating of salty foods (9).

Linguists have found that dialects do have grammatical structure. Use of a dialect does not necessarily inhibit abstract thinking. Children must be taught problem solving and abstract thinking, however. If parents are seldom at home because of work, if the subculture values action more than words, if parents talk little with their children or brush aside questions, and if children associate more with peers than with adults, they are not likely to be stimulated to try new speech forms or new thought patterns. Schoolteachers try, but unfortunately they often have classes too large to give the needed individual instruction, to form a motivating relationship, or to assess fully what a child does not know. Parents often wish to help children learn more; in fact, most poor parents repeatedly emphasize that their children must get an education so that they can achieve more than their parents did. Unfortunately, good intentions and admonitions are not enough. Poor parents often lack the education, energy, time, or resources to help their children advance educationally or even keep up minimally. The farther behind a child gets, the less the likelihood of ever catching up with cognitive skills. The cycle is repeated each generation. Yet most poor parents are receptive to suggestions on how to make the best possible use of their limited resources or what specific measures to follow to enhance child development (51, 93, 170).

There is a clear relationship between poverty and ill health. Long-term ill health may contribute to poverty. Poverty predisposes to certain illnesses or causes a person to suffer adverse consequences of illness. As income level drops, health status declines. The ill child who is poor is less likely to attend school. The poor have higher infant and maternal mortality rates and a higher number of deaths from accidents. Preventive measures are less likely to be carried out in the family; children are less likely to be immunized (40, 108).

A poor person defines illness as being unable to work for days or weeks, and first uses folk or home remedies when ill or may go to a cultural healer. Reluctantly, and only when absolutely necessary, does he or she enter the scientific health care system. A person in chronic poverty may not go for professional, scientific care at all because of lack of knowledge, money, transportation, or an inadequate sense of self-worth. A poor person is suspicious of health care professionals or feels that there is a distance between the practitioner and self. These feelings can be overcome only by a gentle, respectful, courteous, prompt approach and straightforward speech. Although many people feel that much financial assistance is available for the poor and sick, such assistance is limited. Moreover, poor people are unfamiliar with or unlikely to use community agencies without your assistance. Because they often do not have the resources to practice preventive physical or dental care, they may be very ill—even irreversibly—on entry to the health care system (33, 147, 169, 187). Living in poverty takes its toll physically, emotionally, and mentally. Consequent behavior and health patterns should not be viewed as the fault of the victims.

INFLUENCES OF CULTURE ON HEALTH

Because every culture is complex, it can be difficult to determine whether health and illness are the result of cultural or other elements, such as physiologic or psychological factors. Yet there are numerous accounts of the presence or absence of certain diseases in certain cultural groups and reactions to illness that are culturally determined.

Culture-bound illness or syndrome *refers to the features of an illness that vary from culture to culture.* (See Table 1–14 for examples (35, 138, 264). Cultural influences may include food availability, dietary taboos, methods of hygiene, and effects of climate—all factors related to culture. Several examples of the influences of culture on health and illness follow. The examples are necessarily limited. The influence of other cultural folkways on health has been studied. Race, social class, ethnic group, and religion influence distribution of disease and death.

Differences exist among cultural populations and people from different races and socioeconomic levels with respect to risk for disease and distribution of disease and death. These broad factors influence education, occupation, lifestyle, and decisions about health care. These differences are important in planning health promotion programs for a community and a nation (233, 241). For example, a comparison of behavioral risk factors for 652 Latinos and 584 non-Latinos in San Francisco revealed that Latino men were less likely to have consumed alcoholic beverages and more likely to be sedentary in the prior month than their non-Latino counterparts. Latino women were less likely than non-Latino women to smoke cigarettes or to have ever had a Pap smear or clinical breast examination. Promotion of regular physical activity and use of screening tests would be part of a health promotion program for Latinos (208).

African-Americans have higher coronary disease mortality than do Caucasians between the ages of 25

TABLE 1–14. CULTURE-BOUND ILLNESS OR BEHAVIORS

1. **Latah:** In Southeast Asian females. Minimal stimuli elicit an exaggerated startle response, often with swearing. This is also reported among the Ainu of Japan, the Bantu of Africa, and French-Canadians.

2. **Grisi siknis:** Miskito Indians of Nicaragua. Headache, anxiety, irrational anger toward people nearby, aimless running, and falling down.

3. **Amok:** Southeast Asian males. Sudden mass assault by groups and, sometimes, death.

4. **Bulimia:** North American European-Americans, mostly females. Food binging is followed by self-induced vomiting. Sometimes associated with other conditions, such as depression, anorexia, and substance abuse.

5. **"Falling out":** African-Americans and Blacks in the Caribbean. Sudden collapse and paralysis and inability to see or speak; hearing and understanding intact.

6. **Lusto** (soul loss): Spanish-speaking societies. An expression of emotional stress, helplessness, and role conflict; caused by a frightening experience; consists of anorexia, listlessness, apathy, depression, and withdrawal.

7. **Voodoo** (being fixed or hexed): African-Americans. Gastrointestinal or behavioral symptoms and a sense of great helplessness; may cause death because of stimulation of both sympathetic and parasympathetic nervous system response.

8. **Bouffées delirantes:** French. Type of acute psychosis; transient psychosis with elements of trance or dream state.

9. **Shinkeisbitsu:** Japanese. A syndrome marked by obsessions, perfectionism, ambivalence, social withdrawal, neurasthenia, and hypochondriasis.

10. **Involutional paraphrenia:** Spanish and Germans. A midlife condition with paranoid features; "paraphrenia" distinct from schizophrenia and depression while containing elements of both.

and 64 years. African-Americans have been shown to have longer delay times than the majority population in seeking care for acute cardiac disease. Interviews with African-Americans admitted to a public hospital ($n = 254$) and to a private hospital ($n = 194$) for suspected acute myocardial infarction showed that several factors affected the decision to seek care. People in the lower socioeconomic level, in contrast to the middle socioeconomic level, take longer to seek care and have less access to care, both in mode of transportation and in responsive services. Those with limited education further delay the decision to seek care. African-American women delay longer in seeking hospitalization following symptoms than do men and they are at greater risk for poor coronary heart disease outcomes. Care-seeking behavior is also influenced by self-medication with symptom progression, degree of incapacitation and involvement of family or laypersons, all of which may further delay going to medical services (73).

These findings are consistent with studies of poor and middle class white populations. Public education about the importance of cardiac symptoms may help re-

Research Abstract

Ahijevych, K., and L. Bernhard, *Health Promoting Behaviors of African-American Women*, Nursing Research, 43, no. 2 (1994), 86–89.

The purposes of this study were to describe health-promoting lifestyle behaviors reported by 187 African-American women and to compare the findings with other reported findings from studies that utilized the Health Promoting Lifestyle Profile (HPLP) questionnaire. There is limited information about health care practices and beliefs within cultural populations. The health of women and people in cultural populations has only recently been addressed with as much concern as the health of Caucasian males. To implement and evaluate culturally competent care, it is critical to assess lifestyle behaviors of the populations being served.

The sample included 187 African-American women recruited from neighborhood health centers, a community center, a job training program, and health care and office work sites in a major Midwestern city. The women ranged in age from 18 to 69 years; almost two-thirds were single or divorced; more than half were employed full-time. Seventy-two percent had at least a high school education; 9% were college graduates. One-fourth reported a current medical diagnosis; hypertension and heart disease were most frequently reported.

The HPLP, a questionnaire based on a wellness framework, was used to determine the likelihood of the women engaging in health-promoting behaviors. The 48-item instrument employs a 4-point Likert scale (routinely to never); subscales include self-actualization, health responsibility, exercise, nutrition, interpersonal support, and stress management.

Results showed the highest mean scores for the subscales self-actualization and interpersonal support and the lowest mean score for exercise. Health-promoting behaviors for women in this study tended to be slightly higher than those reported for Hispanic women and lower than those reported for Caucasian women of all ages. African-American women reported higher performance on health responsibility (paying attention to and being educated about one's health, seeking assistance when necessary) than most other groups. Women in this study with a medical diagnosis had higher HPLP scores; health problems may be an incentive to increase efforts toward a sense of well-being and fulfillment.

Health care implications include the need to assess and enhance health-promoting behaviors and to reinforce assumption of responsibility for health. Development of questionnaires to measure health promotion in situations where individuals have limited resources may be warranted. Creative strategies to strengthen nutrition, exercise, interpersonal support, stress management, and self-actualization among African-American women are indicated by this study.

duce delay in seeking care. Education related to the perception of symptoms and cause of the symptoms is important (13). Assurance of access to a source of medical care, such as membership in a health maintenance organization, may also reduce delay.

The most dramatic change in the health of the American population in the last decade has been the sharp decline in the health of African-Americans. The most disadvantaged person in the nation in terms of health is the African-American male, whose life expectancy dropped from 65.2 years in 1987 to 64.9 years in 1988 and is steadily decreasing (46). The exact causes of the worsening health of African-Americans have not been conclusively identified, but strong evidence suggests that they are at greater risk because of smoking, high blood pressure, high cholesterol levels, alcohol and other drug intake, excess weight, and diabetes—health problems often associated with lower income and stressful life circumstances (46).

Other ethnic and racial differences occur in the risk for disease. For example, the risk for ischemic heart disease is lowest for Chinese-Americans and highest for person of South-Asian origin, according to one study (125). The American Indian is at risk for certain diseases, including diabetes, tuberculosis, alcoholism, and complications from these illnesses (16, 114). Fair-skinned individuals have a higher risk of cutaneous and ocular melanomas, probably because of protective effect of melanin against sun exposure, whereas both fair-skinned and dark-skinned people have similar rates of visceral melanoma (195).

Education and income level affect seeking of health care. Wells and Horn found that both poor, less educated African-American and Caucasian women sought diagnostic and treatment services for breast cancer later than did their counterparts who had higher median income and education levels. Thus, cancer screening programs are needed for these populations; however, women of the lower socioeconomic level also have less access to preventive and medical care, and asymptomatic women may not make use of preventive health services unless they are created specific to their outlook (262). Nurses are in a good position to institute screening procedures, teach about warning signs, and explain mammography and other cancer screening tests.

There is a growing awareness that variations in dietary practices among ethnic groups may explain some interethnic differences in morbidity and mortality. For example, research suggests that dietary practices and nutrient intake of Mexican-American women may protect them against lung and breast cancer. Dietary practices may also explain their low rates of low birth weight despite low income and education. Dietary behaviors are sensitive to cultural changes that occur with migration. With acculturation, food choices begin to resemble those of white non-Hispanics. For example, whole-fat milk and corn tortillas are replaced by low-fat milk and bread. Alcohol and tobacco consumption increases. These dietary changes may be responsible for the greater number of low-birth-weight babies being born to acculturated Hispanics. In one study, first-generation Mexican-American women were of lower socioeconomic status than were the second-generation counterparts or white non-Hispanic women. Yet, they had a higher average intake of protein, vitamins A, C, and folic acid, and calcium than women in the other two groups. For white, non-Hispanic women, risk for a poor diet is increased by poverty, youthful age, low education, small stature, large body mass, and smoking (97).

Occupations held by certain cultural groups predispose the people to illness. For example, in the United States, migrant farm workers of all races are at risk for malnutrition, skin diseases, reactions to chemicals used on the land, domestic violence, depression, tuberculosis, and other respiratory diseases, and high-risk pregnancies are not uncommon (43, 226).

Culturally induced belief in magic can cause illness and death. The profound physiologic consequences of intense fear, including inability to eat or drink, may be responsible. Yet there may be no physiologic changes except in the terminal moments. If the behavior of friends and relatives—what they say or do—strongly reinforces the person's conviction of imminent death, the victim becomes resigned to fate and soon meets it (164).

Gomes and Carazos (90) describe the sudden death of a 21-year-old Mexican-American male following a **maldición** (hex) uttered by his mother. Toxicology and drug screening were negative in autopsy; only

chronic bronchitis was evidenced. There was no indication of suicide. The mother admitted to having delivered a curse on the son the evening before his death and that he trembled and sobbed all night. When she called an ambulance to take the son to a local hospital, he died enroute. The woman's husband died of a heart attack while crossing the street 10 days later. It was then that relatives and neighbors designated her as a *bruja* or witch. She blamed the local hospital for both deaths.

Ethnic differences exist in the use of diagnostic and health care services. For example, Suarez found use of Pap smear and mammogram screening for cancer increased in Mexican-American women as they became more proficient in English and more acculturated to the United States (239). In the United States, Parker found American-Indian, African-American, and Hispanic mothers were most likely, and Caucasian and Asian-American mothers least likely, to obtain midwifery care. Local availability of midwives, however, also determines a woman's choice for provider (205). Lack of health care access was suggested as the reason for a significant increase in deaths from asthma among African-Americans, in contrast to the number of deaths from asthma among Caucasians, in Chicago from 1968 through 1991 (242).

Immigration is a complex crisis that exacts a great toll from the migrant in terms of mental and physical health, occupational and socioeconomic status, and total lifeways. Of all migrants, the lot of the refugee is the most difficult. Memories of torture, losses, and culture shock are major components. The *crisis of immigration* appears to be manifested as follows:

- During the first year, the refugees experience relief, euphoria, and relatively high levels of happiness and life satisfaction.
- During the second year, exile shock occurs, with high levels of depression and unhappiness.
- During the third year, emotional improvement and increased adaptability are manifested (224).

Southeast Asian students who came to the United States may experience feelings that have been described in a *five-stage model* by Fernandez (79):

1. **Conformity stage:** *Characterized by a preference for American culture over own culture, feelings of racial self-hatred, negative beliefs about own culture,* ashamed of family, positive feelings toward American culture, desire to be American citizen.
2. **Dissonance stage:** *Characterized by struggle over loyalty to family versus desire to be independent.* Person sees advantage of and wants to in-

corporate both cultures within personal life. Person experiences considerable cultural confusion and conflict.

3. **Resistance and immersion stage:** *Characterized by rejection of American culture and retreat into own culture, avoidance of contact with American people and cultural artifacts* to the extent possible. Person experiences difficulty in student or worker role because of others' expectations.

4. **Introspection stage:** *Characterized by careful observation and thoughtful consideration as the person learns to balance the demands of both cultures,* gains language fluency, and adapts behavior for the situation, either home or outside the home.

5. **Synergistic articulation and awareness stage:** *Characterized by feeling a clear cultural identity, feelings of self-acceptance and esteem as a member of the cultural group, and resolution of the cultural conflict* by either maintaining and being content with the familial bond or becoming socialized to be more independent and individual, resulting in less closeness to family (79).

Smith describes conditions of Inuit Indians in the Canadian Arctic, people in refugee camps, Ethiopians in the Sudan, and Cambodians on the Thailand–Cambodian border. Health agencies give service but do not seek justice on behalf of the people they are serving. Yet the health of people is influenced far more by politics and power, and by distribution of land and wealth, than by treatment or preventive health measures. If a population loses control and feels powerless or despairs, the essence of the people, as well as their health, will begin to disintegrate (230).

► HEALTH CARE AND NURSING APPLICATIONS

Importance of Cultural Concepts

Mainstream Americans have not been adept at understanding people from other countries and cultures, although the United States has been an open society to immigrants. Those of minority cultures in the United States and people from other lands typically, and of necessity, have carefully observed and become familiar with the mainstream Caucasian culture in the United States.

Because of the rise of scientific medical practices and specialization, many consumers of health care in the United States are voicing a preference for caring behaviors and cultural practices. Especially the poor, middle-to-lower socioeconomic groups, and rural populations find the cosmopolitan approach to medical care too com-plex, too questionable, too difficult to understand and attain, and too expensive. Further, human dignity and normal developmental processes may be sacrificed in the process (143), and there is concern about lack of privacy for self, family, and health records (274).

A poor person or a person from an ethnic minority usually does not seek medical help until the problem is a serious one, for various reasons: finances, child-care problems, fear of hospitals and medical personnel, fear of becoming a "guinea pig," and fear of death. Often the person relies first on various family and cultural remedies and folk healers. Or the person may rely on religious beliefs for healing. The response to what is perceived as poor or indifferent health care or inhumane treatment is to stay away (169).

Transcultural nursing, developed by Madeleine Leininger in the mid-1960s, is increasingly a focus in nursing education and practice. **Transcultural nursing** *is the study and comparative analysis of different cultures/subcultures throughout the world in relation to caring, health, illness, beliefs, values, lifeways, and practices, so that this knowledge can be used in practice to provide culture-specific and cultural-universal nursing care to people.* The goal is to develop a body of knowledge so that transcultural nursing concepts, theories, and practices are an integral part of nursing education, service, and research (140–152). Leininger has developed *general principles* to guide transcultural practice, education, and research. She has emphasized the importance of knowing and respecting the cultural background, values, and practices of people to provide appropriate, meaningful, and satisfying care to people. These principles emphasize human rights and ethical considerations related to cultural care. They have been published in the *Journal of Transcultural Nursing,* Vol. 3, no. 1, Summer 1991, pp. 21–22 (151). Leininger describes the importance of the nurse being prepared for worldwide nursing and that transcultural nursing education should be worldwide (152). Other authors have also written about educational and practice models that build on cultural concepts (9, 22, 28, 34, 62, 87, 202).

Essential to practice is awareness of cultural values, sensitivity to different beliefs and practices, and the concept of **cultural relativity** *(behavior that is appropriate or right in one culture may not be so defined in another culture)* versus **ethnocentrism** *(behavior based on the belief that one's own group is superior)* (143).

Attitudes Related to Culture

If you live or work in a culture different from your own, you may suffer **culture shock,** *feelings of bewilderment, confusion, disorganization, frustration, and stupidity, and* *the inability to adapt to differences in language and word meanings, activities, time, and customs that are part of the new culture* (261).

Brink and Saunders describe four phases of culture shock (29):

1. *Honeymoon phase:* This stage is characterized by excitement, exploration, and pleasure. This phase may be experienced by a short-term visitor.
2. *Disenchanted phase:* The person feels stuck, depressed, irritated, and that the environment is unpredictable and no longer exotic. The normal cues for social intercourse are absent and the person is cut adrift. The person may become physically ill.
3. *Beginning resolution phase:* New cultural behavior patterns are adopted. Friends are found. Life becomes easier and more predictable.
4. *Effective function phase:* The person has become almost bicultural and may experience reverse culture shock on return home.

An antidote for culture shock is to look for similarities between your native and new cultures. To adapt to a new culture, be interested in the culture and be prepared to ask questions tactfully and to give up some of your own habits. Learn the language, customs, beliefs, and values to the greatest extent possible. Seek a support system—someone with whom you can be yourself and validate and who can help you to adapt (29, 261). Leininger (142) and Weiss (261) give a number of specific suggestions for adapting to another culture. Brislen, Cushner, and Young also discuss techniques that assist individuals in making the transition from one culture to another (30).

In the United States, you are working in a **pluralistic society** *in which members of diverse ethnic, racial, religious, and social groups maintain independent lifestyles and adhere to certain values within the confines of a common civilization.* Knowledge of other cultures helps you examine your own cultural foundations, values, and beliefs, which, in turn, promotes increased self-understanding. Avoid ethnocentricity; **racism,** *assumptions that a certain group is inferior;* and **stereotyping,** *fixed beliefs that do not permit an individual view of a person or group.* For example, emphasizing daily bathing to a group that has a severely limited water supply is useless, for the water will be needed for survival. Recognize that your patterns of life and language are peculiar to your culture; your judgment of another group may be inaccurate.

Caucasian health professionals may label Asian parents as noncompliant because they are not as forceful as Caucasian parents in having the chronically ill child carry out prescribed exercises when the exercises caused pain. In turn, Asian parents may be less responsive to the health professionals. Health professionals are often unaware of the complex factors that influence client responses to treatment and care. Clients may not follow the treatment because they have different priorities (9). In fact, many cultural groups do not respond like the average middle-class American. American Indians value cooperation and patience, and respond quietly, even passively. Do not misinterpret this behavior as apathy about health or health care. They believe each living thing follows a cycle; illness is defined in relation to a personal inner cycle and seasonal cycles, in contrast to the emphasis on germ theory by the health care system. Thus, the medicine man is seen as more helpful than the physician (9, 107, 240, 275).

All people have some **prejudice,** *unfavorable, intolerant, injurious preconceived ideas formed before facts are known.* It emerges in such expressions as "Those upper-crust people always . . . " or "Those welfare people never. . . . " Examine your thinking for unconscious prejudice, understand your own class background, and distinguish your values from those held by people under your care. Try to withhold value judgments that interfere with your relationship with the patient and with objective care. *There are too many unknown factors in people's lives to set up stereotyped categories.* A family may be in the middle class or upper class in terms of income, education, and goals, for example, and yet live in an upper-lower-class neighborhood because they refuse to emphasize material wealth. A farmer, according to our criteria, may be categorized in the upper-lower economic level and yet regard himself or herself as very much a part of the middle class. A person who lives in an economically depressed section of the United States and is poor may have an adequate public education, a middle-class value system, and upper-class graciousness.

If you feel you are stooping by helping poor people, you may be labeled a "do gooder" and be ineffective. Recognize the behavior of poor people not as pathologic but as adaptive for their needs. Realize, too, that not only the poor need your help. A rich person also may need a great deal of help with care, health teaching, or counseling. Having money does not necessarily mean one is knowledgeable about preventive health measures, nutrition, and disease processes. Persons of all classes deserve competent care, clear explanations, and a helpful attitude.

The misinterpretation of behavior typical of a social class does not always go in one direction, from upper to lower. Suppose that you are a nurse with a working-class background whose patient is a 50-year-old corporation president, a member of the newly rich class, admitted for coronary disease. This person seems obsessed with finding out when he or she can resume professional duties, exactly how many hours can be worked daily, and chances for a recurrence. An understanding of socioeconomic position, along with possible motives, values, and status (which this individual feels must be maintained), will enable you to work with the seeming obsession rather than simply label the client an "impossible patient."

Try to accept people as they are regardless of culture or social class. Picture the world through the eyes of others—those you care for. In this way, you can maintain your own personal standards without being shocked by theirs.

Self-Assessment of Cultural Attitudes is a questionnaire that can help you assess your own cultural attitudes and perceptions.

Assessment

Realize when you assess a client that your questions may seem intrusive. For example, among some American-Indian tribes, the question carries with it assumptions and

---

▶ **SELF-ASSESSMENT OF CULTURAL ATTITUDES**

- To become more aware of your attitudes toward and feelings about people of other racial/ethnic backgrounds, ask yourself the following questions:

1. What is your cultural or subcultural background?

2. What is your earliest remembrance of racial or ethnic differences?

3. What are the messages you have received in your life about African-American, Asian-American, American-Indian, and Latino people?

4. What messages have you received in your life about Caucasians of different nationality backgrounds?

5. How much experience did you have with any person from a racial/ethnic minority group different from your own while you were growing up?

6. In what way have these experiences affected your behavior toward people from the group(s)?

7. Describe people from other racial/ethnic minority groups with whom you have felt comfortable or uncomfortable.

8. What features or characteristics are dominant in people from other racial/ethnic minority groups with whom you have had contact?

9. What have you observed about the racial/ethnic composition of your community?

10. What have you observed about the interaction of people from diverse cultural backgrounds at your school, church, or workplace or in organizations you attend?

11. Do you consider yourself to be nonracist or racist? (A member of any race can be a racist against a different racial group.)

12. What do you plan to do to increase your understanding of a person different from you?

---

obligations. If the person is asked a question, it implies that he or she has the answer and that the answer is needed by you. Otherwise, there is no reason to ask the question. If the person does not know the answer, the person starts to talk about something else to maintain cultural practice and to save face and dignity. You may be able to obtain information by more indirect means, without putting the person on the spot (136). You may also need to use an interpreter (see Table 1–15).

Learning about another's cultural background can promote feelings of respect and humility as well as enhance understanding of the person and the family—needs, like and dislikes, behavior, attitudes, care and treatment approaches, and sociocultural causes of disease.

Leininger described *nine major domains to consider while doing a cultural assessment:* (1) patterns of lifestyle, (2) specific cultural norms and values, (3) cultural taboos and myths, (4) world view and ethnocentric tendencies, (5) general features that the client perceives as different or similar to other cultures, (6) health and life care rituals and rites of passage to maintain health, (7) folk and professional health–illness systems that are used, (8) degree of cultural change and acculturation needed, and (9) methods of caring for self and others in regaining health (141, 142).

According to Tripp-Reimer, Brink, and Saunders, a *thorough cultural assessment guide would include* the following components (248):

- *Values:* Health, human nature, person–nature, time, activity, relational, and other
- *Beliefs:* Health (health maintenance, causes and treatment of illness), religious, other
- *Customs:* Communication (verbal and nonverbal), decision making, food/diet, grief/dying, religious, family roles, and sick role/patient
- *Social structure:* Family lines of authority, education, ethnic affiliation, physical environment, religion, use of economic resources, health care facilities, use of art and history, and cultural change
- *Preferences about their health care situation*

Orque's Ethnic/Cultural System Framework shows how basic human needs are influenced by various aspects of a culture: (1) value orientation, (2) family life processes, (3) diet, (4) religion, (5) language and communication processes, (6) healing beliefs and practices, (7) the social group's interactive patterns, and (8) art and history of the social group (202).

Assessment must *consider the complexity and coherence* between (1) the individual life span; (2) development and aging; (3) biological and physiologic factors; (4) contextual and interaction models of intellectual

TABLE 1–15. GUIDELINES FOR USING A LANGUAGE INTERPRETER

1. Hospital translators, in contrast to family members, may not be as familiar with a particular dialect, but may be more neutral and better at interpreting technical aspects of health care.

2. Patients and family members may be embarrassed to answer some questions or reveal some information in the presence of each other but would be willing to talk with an interpreter. Clients may request a specific translator or bring their own.

3. Family members, in contrast to an interpreter, have knowledge of the patient and may be able to insert additional information in context, but may be guarded with personal information.

4. Family members, in contrast to an interpreter, may have issues about what is meant, how much is translated, and how much is condensed or omitted (248).

5. Plan what you want to say ahead of time. Avoid confusing the interpreter by backing up, inserting a proviso, rephrasing, or hesitating. Be patient.

6. Address the person/family directly. Avoid directing all comments to and through the interpreter.

7. Assure the person/family and interpreter of confidentiality.

8. Use short questions and comments. Technical terminology and professional jargon (e.g., like "psychotropic medication") should be reduced to plain English.

9. When lengthy explanations are necessary, break them up and have them interpreted piece by piece in straightforward, concrete terms in the foreign language by the interpreter.

10. Use language and explanations the interpreter can handle.

11. Make allowances for terms that do not exist in the target language.

12. Try to avoid ambiguous statements and questions.

13. Avoid abstractions, idiomatic expressions, similes, and metaphors. It is useful to learn about the use of these grammatical elements in the target language.

14. Avoid indefinite phrases using "would," "could," "if," and "maybe." These can be mistaken for actual agreements or firm approval of a course of action.

15. Ask the interpreter to comment on the client's word content and emotions.

16. Invite correction and induce the discussion of alternatives: "Correct me if I'm wrong, I understand it this way . . . Do you see it some other way?"

17. Pursue seemingly unconnected issues raised by the client. These issues may lead to crucial information or may uncover difficulties with the interpretation.

18. Return to an issue if you suspect a problem and get a negative response. Be certain the interpreter knows what you want. Use related questions, change the wording, and come at the issue indirectly.

19. Provide instructions in list format. Ask clients to outline their understanding of the plans. If alternatives exist, spell each one out. Check the quality of translated health-related materials by having them backtranslated.

20. Clarify your nursing limitations. The willingness to talk about an issue may be viewed as evidence of "understanding" it or the ability to "fix" it.

Adapted from Murray, R., and M. Huelskoetter, Psychiatric/Mental Health Nursing: Giving Emotional Care (3rd ed.). Stamford, CT: Appleton & Lange, 1991, p. 109.

functioning; (5) personality development, and expression; (6) social interaction; and (7) family and social support systems in relation to racial, ethnic, and cultural status and spiritual/religious/philosophical beliefs and values. Racial/ethnic minorities may experience a very different process of development and aging and manifest illness differently from Caucasians. Variability within racial/ethnic groups and for female/male are also apparent. There is lack of research data on normative development and mental health characteristics over the life course and on manifestation of psychiatric symptoms among various racial and ethnic groups (141, 142).

Cultural differences should be anticipated not only for refugees, immigrants, and first-generation immigrants but also for persons even further removed in time from their country of origin and for persons from other regions within your country. A person's behavior during illness is influenced by *cultural definitions* of how he or she should act and the meaning of illness. Understanding this situation and seeking reasons for behavior help avoid stereotyping and labeling a person as uncooperative and resistant just because the behavior is different. As you *consider alternate reasons for behavior,* care can be individualized. People from different cultural backgrounds classify health problems differently and have certain expectations about how they should be helped. If cultural differences are ignored, your ability to assess and help the clients and their ability to progress toward a personally and culturally defined health status may be hampered. You should be able to translate your knowledge of the health care system into terms that match the concepts of your clients.

Knowledge about socioeconomic levels and cultural groups may help explain late or broken agency appointments that result from fear or inferiority feelings, lack of transportation, or someone to care for the children at home rather than from lack of interest in health. A reservation American Indian, poor African-American, or recent immigrant, for instance, may not be accustomed to keeping a strict time schedule or appointments if unemployed, for a strict clock-time orientation is not valued as highly as in the industrialized work force. Take time to talk with the person and you will learn of fears, problems, aspirations, and concerns for health and family and human warmth.

Assessment involves observing, listening, and talking with the client and, frequently, the family. *Some people communicate best in their first (or native) language when they are ill.* Further, the elderly person from a nationality group may always speak the national language at home, having never learned English. There is currently an emphasis on a group maintaining its national language, because language provides the strength and connectedness of a community. For example, Slate writes that the Navajo culture and Nation, its values, beliefs, and customs, can be kept alive only if the language is preserved for the Navajo people, especially children (229). Linguist Leap concurs for other American Indian communities, but acknowledges that tribal people must also know the English language (136). Because of the diversity of cultures found in the United States, and the number of people for whom English is not the first language, you may need to use an *interpreter* to assist you with assessment, care planning, and intervention. Become acquainted with people in the community who speak another language fluently and can be an interpreter for health care professionals. Table 1–15 gives guidelines for an interpreter. Learn key words of his or her language. Use language dictionaries or a card file of key words. Breach the language barrier so that your assessment is more accurate and care measures will be understood by the person. As you assess clients and do a physical assessment, remember that *people differ not only culturally but also biologically* (Table 1–16). Studies on biological baselines for growth and development or normal characteristics have usually been done on Caucasian populations. These norms may not be applicable to nonwhites. Biological features, such as skin color, body size and shape, and presence of enzymes, are the result of biological adjustments made by ancestors to the environment in which they lived (9, 86, 220).

Pain assessment must consider cultural factors: different population groups have *about the same physical thresholds of pain,* although there is individual variation in each group; however, *how different populations express pain varies* according to whether or not the individuals were taught to speak about or give evidence of their pain (physical and emotional). It is necessary to look for subtle cues of pain among Northern European, Asian, and American-Indian people and not to overmedicate people who tend to be more expressive, such as Italian or Jewish people. Family members may also react differently when they see the patient in pain. Families of Eastern European groups tend to be proactive and assertive on behalf of the patient. Patients also respond differently when family members are present. In some cultures, the patient is not expected to talk about the pain to the family (9, 63, 276).

Various physical differences are known to exist. **Mongolian spots,** *the hyperpigmented, bluish discoloration* occasionally seen in Caucasian neonates, are normal for many Asians, American Indians, and African-Americans. Type of ear wax varies and may determine the presence of ear disease in preschoolers. Dry ear wax is recessive and is found primarily in American Indians and Asians. Wet ear wax is found in most African-Americans and Caucasians. Also, people with dry ear wax have fewer apocrine glands and perspire less; they usually do not have as much body odor. Thus, presence

TABLE 1–16. ASSESSMENT OF SKIN COLOR

Characteristic	White or Light-skinned Person	Dark-skinned Person
Pallor Vasoconstriction present	Skin takes on white hue, which is color of collagen fibers in subcutaneous connective tissue.	Skin loses underlying red tones. Brown-skinned person appears yellow-brown. Black-skinned person appears ashen gray. Mucous membranes, lips, and nailbeds are pale or gray.
Erythema, Inflammation Cutaneous vasodilation	Skin is red.	Palpate for increased warmth of skin, edema, tightness, or induration of skin. Streaking and redness are difficult to assess.
Cyanosis Hypoxia of tissues	Skin, especially in earlobes, as well as in lips, oral mucosa, and nailbeds, has bluish tinge.	Lips, tongue, conjunctiva, palms, soles of feet are pale or ashen gray. Apply light pressure to create pallor; in cyanosis tissue color returns slowly by spreading from periphery to the center.
Ecchymosis Deoxygenated blood seeps from broken blood vessel into subcutaneous tissue	Skin changes from purple-blue to yellow-green to yellow.	Oral mucous membrane or conjunctiva will show color changes from purple-blue to yellow-green to yellow. Obtain history of trauma and discomfort. Note swelling and induration.
Petechiae Intradermal or submucosal bleeding	Round, pinpoint purplish red spots are present on skin.	Oral mucosa or conjunctiva show purplish-red spots if person has black skin.
Jaundice Accumulated bilirubin in tissues	Skin, mucous membranes, and sclera of eyes are yellow. Light-colored stools and dark urine often occur.	Sclera of eyes, oral mucous membranes, palms of hand, and soles of feet have yellow discoloration.

of body odor may be indicative of disease. Pelvic shape of the woman, shape of teeth and tongue, fingerprint pattern, blood type, keloid formation, and presence of the enzyme lactase vary among groups. Persons with certain blood types are more prone to certain illnesses (9, 22, 86, 202).

Adults who have **lactose intolerance** are *missing lactase, the enzyme for digestion and metabolism of lactose in milk and milk products;* they become ill on ingestion of these foods. Symptoms include flatulence, distention, abdominal cramping, diarrhea, and colitis. Milk intolerance because of enzyme deficiency occurs in more than 80% of Chinese, Japanese, and Eskimo adults and in 60 to 80% of American-Indian, African-American, Jewish, and Mexican-American adults. Only people of Northern European Caucasian extraction and members of two African tribes tolerate lactose indefinitely, even some aged Caucasians will have lactose deficiency.

Other biological variations exist. Susceptibility to disease varies with blood type. Rh-negative blood type is common in Caucasians, rarer in other groups, and absent in Eskimos. Myopia is more common in Chinese; color blindness is more common in Europeans and East Indians. Nose size and shape correlate with ancestral homeland. Small noses (seen in Asians or Eskimos) were produced in cold regions, high-bridged noses (common to Iranians and American Indians) were common in dry areas; and the flat, broad noses characteristic of some Blacks were adaptive in moist, warm climates (9, 22, 86, 202).

To aid assessment, learn about the significant religious practices and the everyday patterns of hygiene, eating, types of foods eaten, sleeping, elimination, use of space, and various rituals that are a part of the person's culture. Because the client and the practitioner may have different perspectives of health and illness, the following *questions can enhance understanding about the client's viewpoint:*

- What do you think caused your problem?
- Why do you think it started when it did?
- What do you think this illness does to you? What problems has it caused for you?
- What do you fear most about your illness?
- How severe is your illness?
- What kind of treatment have you already tried? What else would help?
- What would you like for health care providers to do for you? What results do you wish for from treatment?

For persons from another country, a thorough physical examination should include the components listed in Physical Examination of Foreign-born Immigrants (81).

► **PHYSICAL EXAMINATION OF FOREIGN-BORN IMMIGRANTS**

Screening Tests

- PPD for tuberculosis, even if there is a history of Bacillus Calmette-Guerin (BCG) vaccine
- Chest x-ray if the tuberculosis skin test is positive or if there are symptoms of pulmonary disease
- Hepatitis B serology, surface antigen, and core antibody tests, to determine if the person is infectious
- Hemoglobin and hematocrit (Anemia may be caused by parasites, malaria, and malnutrition.)
- Stool tests for ova and parasites (Giardiasis, ascariasis, amebiasis, pinworms, hookworms, tapeworms, whipworms, and fluke are not rare.)

Complete History and Physical Examination

- Include gross nutritional status, vision and hearing, dental examination, and identification of high-risk pregnancy. Question bowel habits and abdominal pain to detect salmonella, shigella and parasites.

Immunization Update

- Persons 18 years and older are often overlooked for history of vaccination for measles, mumps, rubella, tetanus, diphtheria, hepatitis B, and polio.

Nursing Diagnoses

The nursing diagnoses in Selected Nursing Diagnosis Related to Transcultural Nursing may be applicable to work with people in various cultures. Leininger discusses the importance of including non-Anglicized cultural concepts in the North American Nursing Diagnosis Association (NANDA) taxonomy, rather than focusing on Anglo-American Western cultural values. Further, the diagnostic categories should include positive health descriptors and assets of cultures in dealing with human conditions (148).

Concepts of Culturally Based Intervention

Caring *is assistive, supportive, or facilitative actions toward another person or group with evident or anticipated needs in order to ameliorate or improve a human condition or lifeway* (143, 146). Nurses in different cultures tend to know and emphasize different care constructs such as support, comfort, and touch. Caucasian nurses

► SELECTED NURSING DIAGNOSES RELATED TO TRANSCULTURAL NURSING*

Pattern 5: Choosing

Ineffective Individual Coping

Decisional Conflict

Health-Seeking Behaviors

Pattern 6: Moving

Altered Health Maintenance

Pattern 7: Perceiving

Powerlessness

Pattern 8: Knowing

Knowledge Deficit

---

*Many of the NANDA nursing diagnoses are applicable to an individual in any culture who is ill. From North American Nursing Diagnosis Association, NANDA Nursing Diagnoses Definitions & Classification 1995–1996. Philadelphia: North American Nursing Diagnosis Association, 1994.

---

in the United States generally believe that care involves use of technologic aids, medicines, and psychophysiologic comfort measures. Generally, Caucasian and some non-Caucasian clients agree. In several non-Western cultures, nurses and clients perceive care as protective with a sociocultural emphasis. For example, nurses in Turkey and Israel emphasize restorative caring functions because of war activities. Samoan caregivers are expected to protect the person from breaking cultural or social rules to prevent illness or harm. Chinese nurses perceive surveillance and protection as dominant caring modes. Depending on the culture, Leininger states, the concept *care* can mean many different things (143–145):

Comfort	Restoration
Support	Direct assistance
Attention	Helping the dependent
Compassion	Tenderness
Touch	Trust
Love	Instruction
Stimulation	Succorance
Presence	Empathy
Protection	Medical/technical
Surveillance	Assistance

Personalized help   Maintaining well-being
Nurturance
Stress alleviation

Care and caring are basic to health, health promotion, and illness prevention. For more information see Key Definitions Related to Health and Health Promotion. Health is a desire universally, and in most societies health is linked with goals of human development, satisfaction of basic needs, work, quality of life, and social well-being. Yet in the war-torn or very poor countries of the world, health may scarcely be a memory, let alone a perceived state in the current reality.

At the 1978 Alma-Ata Conference, sponsored by the World Health Organization and UNICEF, the World Assembly declared the goal "Health for All by the Year 2000." This goal called for radical health improvements; primary health care was the strategy to achieve health.

► KEY DEFINITIONS RELATED TO HEALTH AND HEALTH PROMOTION

- **Health:** State of well-being in which the person is able to use purposeful, adaptive responses and processes, physically, mentally, emotionally, spiritually, and socially, in response to internal and external stimuli (stressors) to maintain relative stability and comfort and to strive for personal objectives and cultural goals.

- **Wellness:** Ability to adapt, to relate effectively, and to function at near-maximum capacity and includes self-responsibility, nutritional awareness, physical fitness, stress management, environmental sensitivity, productivity, expression of emotions, self-expression in a variety of ways, creativity, personal care, and home and automobile safety (44, 69).

- **Biopsychosocial or holistic health:** High level and total view of health; unity of body, mind (feelings, beliefs, attitudes), and spirit; and person's interrelatedness with others and the environment (5).

- **Health promotion:** Activities that increase the levels of health and well-being and actualize or maximize the health potential of individuals, families, groups, communities, and society (207).

- **Health protective behavior:** Any behavior performed by a person, regardless of the perceived or actual health status, to protect, promote, or maintain health, whether or not that behavior is actually effective (103).

- **Primary prevention:** Activities that decrease the probability of occurrence of specific illness or dysfunction in an individual, family, group, or community and reduce incidence of new cases of disorder in the population by combating harmful forces that operate in the community and by strengthening the capacity of people to withstand these forces (44, 207).

- **Secondary prevention:** Early diagnosis and treatment of the pathologic process, thereby shortening disease duration and severity and enabling the person to return to normal function as quickly as possible (44, 207).

- **Tertiary prevention:** Restoring the person to optimum function through rehabilitation and within the constraints of the problem when a defect or disability is fixed, stable, or irreversible (44, 207).

The Declaration of Alma-Ata asserted that health is a fundamental human right and that people, individually and collectively, have the right and duty to participate in their care (4).

Economic, political, and environmental factors that contribute to poor health must be addressed in health planning and policy formation. Community participation increases access to health care; provides for greater efficiency, effectiveness, and coordination of services; and leads to equity in and self-reliance of a population. It requires time, energy, cultural knowledge, trust and respect, common goals, and constant dialogues. Nurses are in a key position to foster this model of health and the consequent empowerment (99, 104, 238).

Healthy People, 2000, the latest U.S. guide, presents three goals: (1) to increase the healthy life span, (2) to reduce health disparities, and (3) to achieve universal access to preventive services. In the United States a national health program is needed to achieve equity in access to health care for the individual and family (99, 104, 238). For these goals to be reached with *all* people in the United States, health care providers must become competent in giving culturally based care.

Leininger, in her Theory of Cultural Care Diversity and Universality, proposes that client therapy goals should be congruent with cultural values, beliefs, and lifeways. Cultural care congruence will explain and predict outcomes. Three *principles for client therapy goals* are: (1) cultural care preservation or maintenance, (2) cultural care negotiation or accommodation, and (3) cultural care repatterning or restructuring. These *principles are defined* as follows:

1. **Cultural care preservation** *refers to assistive, facilitative, or enabling acts that preserve cultural values and lifeways viewed as beneficial to the client.*
2. **Cultural care accommodation** *refers to assistive, facilitative, or enabling acts that reflect ways to adapt or adjust health care services to fit client's needs, values, beliefs, practices.*
3. **Cultural care repatterning** *refers to altered designs to help clients change health or life patterns that are meaningful; the cognitive way that one recognizes different attributes and features of a culture for new patterns of care to become evident and for retention or preservation of selected values, beliefs, or practices of the culture* (145–147, 152).

Assumptions underlying *traditional* medical care in the United States are not consistent with culturally based care (see Table 1–17). Thus, people seek other methods of care (44, 69, 207).

TABLE 1–17. COSMOPOLITAN, WESTERN CONVENTIONAL, OR TRADITIONAL SCIENTIFIC MEDICAL CARE ASSUMPTIONS

1. An illness has an organic or biological beginning, which is the result of a distinct etiology outside the person.
2. The illness is involuntary and brought on by an invasion of the victim by an excess amount of the causal elements. The powerful influence of the psyche in the body is ignored.
3. Treatment must be accomplished by a scientific rationale and a medium that counterattacks or neutralizes the cause.
4. The cure must be prescribed or administered by a competent specialist.
5. The patient must defer to the services of the specialist because the special skills and understanding of the specialist are unavailable to the patient.
6. The patient is usually divided into parts: the specialist possesses increasing knowledge about smaller fragments or units of the person.
7. The physician or specialist absolves the sick from moral responsibility for the illness.
8. Procedures and technology are designed to treat serious illness and diseases but not to maintain health.
9. Some health treatment procedures and programs may become harmful and cause disease.

Nontraditional and Alternative Methods to Health Care

About a third of all Americans rely to some extent on nontraditional methods to prevent or treat illness, even if they see a physician regularly. Often these methods are used without the doctor's knowledge. Ten percent of Americans rely on nontraditional methods exclusively (6).

Nontraditional methods *are a variety of practices not used by the traditional medical system, many of which have their basis in nontechnologic or cultural methods of prevention or healing,* and may include non-Western methods. For example, nontraditional methods of treatment for chronic low back pain, which is surgically treated, include acupuncture and chiropractic treatment. These methods have been used successfully in the past, and there has been at least some descriptive research reported on the use of these methods. Dr. Dean Ornish, founder and director of the Preventive Medicine Research Institute in Sausalito, California, is conducting a 2-year study on 200 volunteers on use of a nontraditional, noninvasive regimen to reverse heart disease. Instead of angioplasty or bypass surgery, he prescribes a lifestyle-based regimen of exercise, meditation, group support, and strict vegetarian diet. To date, 95% have maintained the regimen, and only one person has required surgery (53). In a study by a Harvard University team, the folk remedy cranberry juice for urinary tract infections has been found to prevent recurring infection (6).

Alternative methods *include a variety of unrelated practices that are promoted as having health benefits but have not been subjected to scientific review and may have had little objective observation or study.* For example, a physician may suggest excision for precancerous cells on the cervix. The woman who uses alternative methods may visit a naturopath biweekly to have her cervix swabbed with an enzyme to break down abnormal cells, use a specially prepared vaginal suppository, and drink herbal teas daily (6, 53).

Homeopathy is an increasingly popular alternative treatment method; however, there is no scientific evidence that it is anything more than a placebo. The placebo effect can play a major role in the success of all medical treatments (109).

Some insurance bills are now paying for nontraditional and alternative methods because they are less costly. These methods avoid hospitalization and focus on nontechnologic methods. The danger is that some people will not get the needed medication or surgery, at least not soon enough.

Congress established the Office of Alternative Medicine at the National Institutes of Health in 1992. It has organized workshops to teach alternative practitioners how to conduct experiments, write reports, compose grant proposals, and satisfy Food and Drug Administration requirements (6).

Teach clients to be cautious when undergoing unproven treatments; see Reasons to Avoid Use of Unproven Treatments (6). Unproven treatment and quackery are not the same, but the methods used to promote the treatment may be similar. Other characteristics of a *quack, one who makes pretentious claims about the ability to treat others with little or no foundation,* include the following (249):

- Promises an easy or quick cure
- Offers only testimonials as proof of healing power
- States that he or she is ridiculed or persecuted by traditional health professionals
- Promotes products through faith healers, door-to-door health advisors, or sensational ads
- Refuses to accept proven methods of research
- Claims the treatment is better than any prescribed by a physician

Be willing to compare approaches with the client. Do not ridicule the person who has gone the nontraditional route. Above all, this person needs your listening ear and understanding guidance. Remember that people think in terms of having symptoms and eradicating them. If the latter takes place to their satisfaction, they will place their trust in the health care provider who was responsible for their improvement, regardless of his or her credentials. What you call a *hoax* others may call *hope.* Refer people who have been a victim of a quack to their local Better Business Bureau, local medical society and nursing organization, and The National Council Against Health Fraud, P.O. Box 1276, Loma Linda, CA 92354, (714) 824–4690.

Specific Culturally Based Interventions

Your *approach to* and way of *speaking to* the client will set the tone for how the client reacts to you and everyone else on the team. *Call the person by title and last name* until the person tells you to call him or her by first name. Calling someone by his or her first name can suggest that he or she is in a subservient role to you. Be sensitive also to how you *speak about* the person.

Dark-skinned people in the United States are divided about what to be called. "Black" is the term used by the Census Bureau. Only 30% of Blacks, usually younger persons, prefer the term "African American"; the older generation prefers the terms "Afro-American" and "Black." In some rural areas of Southern states, older black people refer to themselves as "Colored" or "Negro." Blacks from the Caribbean may prefer being called "Jamaican" or "Haitian-American" (70).

Learn what the client has as a priority in care. Include the person's ideas in planning and giving care. Often you may have to negotiate with the individual or family to carry out the essential medical treatments and nursing care, as well as include the cultural practices, the medicine man or spiritualist, or spiritual healing rituals they hold most dear.

▶ **REASONS TO AVOID USE OF UNPROVEN TREATMENTS**

- Claims of a secret or miracle cure with no side effects or pain
- Claims from practitioners that the medical community is trying to keep their cure from the public
- Demands that the client use only alternative treatment
- Claims that the treatment is better than approved treatment because it is natural
- Confirmation that the drugs or devices do not have Food and Drug Administration approval
- Proposal of a single, simple solution for diagnosing or treating all illnesses

Respecting the person's need for privacy or need to have others continually around is essential. Understand that some clients or families will not be expressive emotionally or verbally. Respect this pattern, recognizing that *nonverbal behavior is also significant.* The meaning of a gesture differs from country to country. A friendly wave of the hand may be an insult, depending on hand position. Be aware, too, that word meanings may vary considerably from culture to culture so that the person may have difficulty understanding you and vice versa. Be sure the gesture or touch you use conveys the message you intend. If you are unsure, avoid nonverbal behavior to the extent that you can.

Interference with normal living patterns or practices adds to the stress of being ill. You will encounter and need to *adapt care to the following customs:* drinking tea instead of coffee with meals, eating the main meal at midday instead of in the evening, refusing to undress before a strange person, doing special hair care as described by Grier (94), avoiding use of the bedpan because someone else must handle its contents, maintaining special religious or ethnic customs, refusing to bathe daily, refusing a pelvic exam by a male doctor, moaning loudly when in pain, and showing unreserved demonstrations of grief when a loved one dies.

A client with a strict *time orientation* must take medicines and receive treatments on time or feel neglected. You are expected to give prompt and efficient, but compassionate, service to the patient and family. Time orientation also affects making appointments for the clinic and plans for medication routine or return to work after discharge, and influences a person's ideas about how quickly he or she should get well. Clients with little future-time orientation have difficulty planning a future clinic appointment or a long-range medication schedule. They cannot predict now how they will feel at a later date and may think that clinic visits or medicines are unnecessary if they feel all right at the moment.

For some clients, the *hurrying behavior of the nurse or other health care providers* is distressing; it conveys a lack of concern and lack of time to give adequate care. In turn, the person expresses guilt feelings when it is necessary to ask for help. Although you may look very efficient when scurrying, you are likely to miss many observations, cues, and hidden meanings in what the person or family says.

Examine your own attitude about busyness and leisure in order to help others consider leisure as part of life. The disabled person, whose inability to work carries a stigma, must develop a positive attitude about leisure and may seek your help.

Your knowledge of cultures will enable you to practice *holistic care,* including cultural values and norms as part of the nursing process. Holistic healing practices combine the best of two worlds: the wisdom and sensitivity of the East and the technology and precision of the West. Although holistic practitioners use conventional therapies in many cases, the emphasis remains on the whole person: physical, emotional, intellectual, spiritual, and sociocultural background. The focus is on prevention and overall fitness, and on the individual taking responsibility for his or her own health and well-being. Multiple techniques are used to restore and maintain balance of body energy. These techniques include exercise, acupuncture, massage, herbal medicine, nutritional changes, manipulation of joints and spine, medications, stress management, and counseling. The nurse–client relationship is the key to holistic nursing care, for the person has come to expect a caring interaction from the healer. The **curandera** *(herb healer)* of the Spanish-speaking Southwest makes a tea from herbs, for example, and the patient slowly sips the tea. The pain is gone. The client's faith is a major factor in herbal cures— faith in God, the plants, and the curandera. The curandera also has faith in recovery as she shows caring, looks at and listens to the patient, and heals.

When you care for *Hispanic families,* including *Mexican-American migrant families,* the information about Spanish-speaking populations in Tables 1–5 through 1–11 will be useful. Further, note the degree of acculturation, as decision-making patterns in some Cuban-American and migrant farm worker families are evolving to be more equal between husbands and wives. Men have power and authority outside the family; women are responsible for the daily affairs of the family life. Bearing and rearing children are highly valued; girls learn that helping to care for younger siblings and to help with housework is part of their role. Respectful or deferential behavior is expected toward others on the basis of age, sex, social position, economic status, and position of authority. Health care providers are respected, but you are also expected to be respectful. Personal relationships are more important than institutional relationships; talk with the person about daily life events. Assess language preference of the person, who may be unwilling to speak about a problem if he or she cannot describe it in the native language, even though the person speaks English as well. If a translator is necessary, an adult of the same sex as the client is preferred. Avoid using a child in the family as an interpreter because that places the child in a superior position, which is unacceptable. Parents are unlikely to expose family problems to the child or expect the child to assume responsibility for family difficulties (226).

Herbs used by various cultural groups are increasingly found to have medicinal value; they are chemically similar to drugs used by scientific practitioners. Also, a culture's favored drink may have implications for health. Health practitioners in a remote Mexican village found that the only available beverage was an alcoholic drink made from the juice of a local plant. A safe water supply was brought in, but the people did not fare well on it. The local drink was a rich source of essential vitamins and minerals not otherwise present in the local diet. Although it may have appeared desirable to change a cultural pattern for certain health reasons, the unanticipated consequences proved detrimental to health in another way.

Do not automatically teach everyone to drink milk because *lactose intolerance* may exist. Calcium can be obtained in other ways: seafoods (cook fish to yield edible bones), leafy vegetables, yogurt, buttermilk, aged cheese (lactose has been changed to lactic acid during aging), or homemade soup (add vinegar to the water when cooking a soupbone to decalcify the bone). Most ethnic groups have adapted ways of cooking to ensure calcium intake from nondairy sources; listen carefully to their dietary descriptions. If the lactase-deficient person wishes to ingest considerable milk foods, an enzyme product to add to milk, called Lact-Aid, may be purchased from drug or health food stores. An acidophilus milk, which contains a controlled culture of *Lactobacillus acidophilus* bacteria, is also easily digested (9, 86).

A woman in labor may want to rely on lay medical help; she may be suspicious of the impersonal hospital and professional-looking nurses and ask for cultural practices such as to have a knife placed under the bed to help "cut labor pains." While implementing scientific health care, you can be more prepared to act on this belief that psychologically helps the patient.

Folk medicine practices help people gain a sense of control over their fate. Often the practice does no real harm but can be misinterpreted (9, 86). In one example, a Vietnamese mother used the ancient Chinese practice of **cao gio** *("scratching the wind")* to care for her child's cold. In this practice, the child's chest or back is covered with mentholated oil and then rubbed with a coin or hard object. The striations left on the child's skin, although causing no harm or injury, were interpreted by a health care provider as signs of child abuse. The health care provider reported the family, as required by law, based on her perceptions. The parents were charged, and the father, in fear of a jail term and in humiliation, hung himself. Be aware of possible folk medicine practices and their terminology, and explore these practices prior to making conclusions about the client.

Some recent immigrants may adhere closely to traditional practices. Others may not. Your care cannot be based on assumption or stereotype. Immigrants may combine traditional cultural and Western practices. Many *Chinese-Americans* practice Western-oriented activities of exercise, religious practices, lifestyle, and illness behavior activities. In the health behavior activities of dietary practices and the sick behavior measures, use of a mixture of Chinese and Western practices have been reported by more than 50% of Chinese-Americans. Chinese-Americans described more Western practices the longer they lived in the United States. Four influencing variables—(1) the familiarity of the participant with Western health care systems, (2) language, (3) occupation, and (4) religion—are significant to their described health beliefs, dietary practices, and sick behavior measures (86, 258, 273). Yep shares information on how nurses can better care for clients from an *Asian culture* (273):

- Talk to the person in a way that shows respect. Call the person by title and last name. Do not talk down to the person or family.
- Older people may not be fluent in English, even if they have lived in the United States for many years. Speak slowly to the client; invite the family to help interpret to the client and communicate feelings or questions to the health professional. The client is unlikely to admit that he or she is not understanding.
- Asian clients probably will not want to bother the practitioners with their complaints and problems. Most Asians believe suffering is part of life and must be accepted; however, the client is likely to complain to family members. Include family in your assessment, and question the client repeatedly and in several different ways to assess pain.
- Illness may be viewed as the result of an imbalance between yin and yang, an evil spirit, improper food, or by something bad in the family.
- Having the family bring familiar foods will make the hospital stay more comfortable for the Asian client. Some are accustomed to having rice at every meal.
- Most Asians highly respect and even fear authority; doctors and nurses represent authority. Thus, the client expects a formal relationship and may become confused by an informal approach.
- Explanations should be given slowly and repeatedly in simple language; the client is likely to be too intimidated by the authority figure to ask questions. The family should also be given the explanations so they can clarify for the client, if necessary.

- Older Asian people may associate hospitals with death; it's the last place to go. On the other hand, hospitals also represent power and dominion. Hospital routines may not be understood. For example, an Asian person views his or her blood as finite in supply, vital energy, and a life source; thus, repeated blood samples may cause much fear.

- Asian adults do not touch much and are not usually demonstrative about affection. A smile conveys caring much better than a touch, as does performing little extras for the client without being asked, such as filling the water pitcher.

- Use the family as an important resource. Request they visit frequently and for long hours, if they desire. They can assist in care; in fact, the client may expect them to. Cooperation with treatment and care routines will be fostered through communication with and involvement of the family (273).

These points are pertinent to people in other cultures as well. Among the nearly one million *Southeast Asian Vietnamese, Hmong, Cambodian, and Laotian refugees* in the United States, adjustment difficulties are manifested in anxiety, family abuse, posttraumatic stress disorder, intergenerational conflict, psychotic episodes, suicidal threats, substance abuse, and other antisocial behaviors that may be masked by physical symptoms. High levels of dysfunction occur for the first and second years, often into the third year of resettlement. If culturally focused health care is given, with appropriate psychotherapeutic intervention and *low* doses of antidepressant medication, emotional health shows improvement in the third or fourth year (224).

A part of transcultural care is providing health care services for *immigrant populations.* In 1992, the United States was the new home for 1,105,545 people; political refugees, adopted children from other countries, and others. Several medical conditions legally exclude immigrants, including untreated sexually transmitted diseases, positive HIV serology, active tuberculosis, infectious Hansen's disease (leprosy), and some mental disorders. The local public health department should do the screening tests on foreign-born immigrants at the initial checkup (see the box on Physical Examination of Foreign-born Immigrants) (9, 81).

Be aware that newcomers to this country may be suspicious about the screening process; extra time must be spent in explaining why each component is necessary. You may need to use an interpreter (see Table 1–15). Many immigrants find jobs as food workers. When they first come to America, it is essential that they be in good health and not carriers of disease. Foreign exchange students, visitors with visas, and tourists are not required to undergo medical clearance; however, the exposure to disease that these individuals have had may in turn affect others around them (81).

Nursing intervention is key for the *refugees,* in that the nurse focuses on the needs of the whole person as well as medical and psychiatric symptoms, in contrast to the emphasis of physicians. Often, 24-hour caretaking is required by the ill person; thus, other family members may also become debilitated and are unable to go to work and school. The refugees may be desperate for help and seek medical care, diagnostic tests, and medication prescriptions from multiple physicians and care centers, each quite unaware of the others. This results not only in duplication of services and increased costs, but often in conflicting instructions, sacks full of medication in the home, confusion and fragmentation for the person, and no alleviation of the problems (224).

Culturally, these clients acknowledge a belief in a supernatural or magical etiology of their illness and consult regularly with indigenous healers. Nearly all display evidence of healing methods such as **cupping** (*applying a heated jar to the skin to form a vacuum to suction out illness*) and **coinage** (*rubbing a coin or spoon over the skin to rub out illness*) for physical symptoms. Polypharmacy is the norm. They use substances from many sources: herbal medications, over-the-counter and prescription drugs from the United States as well as other countries, and remedies sent by relatives in Southeast Asia and France. Use of prescription drugs ranges from total noncompliance to self-regulated drug use (224).

Mental illness carries shame and stigma in the *Southeast Asian community;* social support systems tend to disappear as the patient become less manageable. Hospitalization is often for threatened or attempted suicide. Barriers to health care, in addition to cultural and family attitudes, include lack of transportation to or inaccessibility of services, job schedules, family demands, and financial limitations. A culturally appropriate mental status examination form is a priority to determine effects of folk beliefs and healing modalities (212, 224).

Some cultures, such as the *traditional Filipino,* believe that illness is the result of evil forces and that treatment involves protection from or removal of these evil forces. For example, the body is viewed as a container that collects debris, so flushing involves stimulating perspiration, vomiting, flatus, or menstrual bleeding to remove evil forces from the body. Use of heat and control of cold through herbs, teas, water, and fire help maintain a balanced internal temperature. Protection involves a gatekeeping system against the invasion of natural and supernatural forces. Mental illness may be thought to be the result of a witch casting a spell; carrying an oval stone or wearing a cross, if the person is a Christian, will act as an antidote or protection. Using direct eye contact with the sick person is also believed to remove a witch's spell (175). Snyder describes folk healing among *older Asian-Americans and Hawaiians in Honolulu* and the implications for health education and nursing care (232). Die and Seelback describe the importance of the family and church or temple for elderly Vietnamese immigrants in securing health and other services (66).

You can *incorporate indigenous folk medicine* and *practitioners* into professional and scientific health care practices. The two are not automatically exclusive. For example, in one *Navaho* nursing care service, the medicine man is an active participant, and Navaho mothers are encouraged to use their infant cradle boards and to be home for the blessing ceremonies (143). Having an Indian corn ceremony, where corn is ritualistically deposited around the patient's bed in the hospital, meets a cultural need and is not difficult for housekeeping to clean up (248, 252).

Bell (16) and Huttlinger and Wiebe (114) describe beliefs, values, and practices related to health and illness among the *Navajo*. Bell also gives a sensitive account of her reactions to living among, as well as caring for, the Navajo and she gives a broader understanding of the culture from an Anglo perspective (16). Huttlinger and Wiebe describe specific research about Navajo men and women who had diabetes (114).

As you care for clients from different cultures, be aware of *barriers* to accessibility or receptivity *to health care services*. For example, barriers to health care in a *rural* community may include the following (19):

- Heavy work schedule
- Economic difficulties
- Lack of health insurance coverage, high deductibles
- Lack of accessible health care services, long distances to services
- Negative attitudes toward health care services
- Lack of information about prevention or health maintenance, ignorance of warning signs of disease
- Inadequate prenatal care
- Less attention to or care for chronic illnesses
- Value of self-reliance and risk-taking behaviors

As you intervene, teach, or counsel, adjust your communication approach with and behavior toward clients from another cultural background, as people from most ethnic/racial groups feel uncomfortable initially when interacting with someone who is different. Although you may be communicating in a way that is natural to you, someone from another culture may perceive that behavior as too forward or aggressive, too passive, or unempathic. While you cannot assume a different mask for each person you interact with, be aware that the client may misinterpret your well-intentioned behavior. Use general knowledge about a culture while you simultaneously see the individual and unique differences of people. Unfortunately, many nurses are not bilingual. The client who uses English as a second language may not speak or understand English adequately for you to effectively assess, teach, or intervene in other ways.

In *male-dominated households (Spanish-speaking, Asian, Middle Eastern)*, the male head of house must be included in all decisions and health teaching if you expect to solicit cooperation. In most such families, and African-American and Jewish families, there is also an older female relative such as an aunt, mother-in-law, or grandmother who is the designated health care provider for that family. She must also be included in decision making and health teaching. Speaking to the important family elder with respect will gain you a staunch ally; the desired behavior change will almost certainly be assured (9, 86).

Relations between the client and the family may at times seem offensive or disharmonious to you. Differentiate carefully between patterns of behavior that are culturally induced and expected and those that are unhealthy for the persons involved.

The changing society may cause families to have a variety of problems. Be a supportive listener, validate realistic ideas, prepare the family to adapt to a new or changing environment, and be aware of community agencies or resources that can provide additional help. See Table 1–18 for *guidelines on making referrals*. When a client has no family nearby and seems alone and friendless, you may provide significant support. Develop a personal philosophy that promotes a feeling of stability in your life so that you, in turn, can assist the client and family to explore feelings and formulate a philosophy for coping with change.

One way to have a lasting effect on the health practices of a different cultural group is through *health teaching* that includes a philosophy of prevention. **Health education** *specifically transmits information, motivates the inner resource of the person, and helps people adopt and maintain healthful practices and lifestyles.* Outsiders cannot make decisions for others, but people should be given sufficient knowledge concerning alternate behavior so that they can make intelligent choices themselves. See Table 1–19 for teaching principles and methods.

Various pressures interfere with attempts at health teaching. Behind poor health habits lie more than ignorance, economic pressure, or selfish desires. Motivation

TABLE 1–18. GUIDELINES FOR MAKING A REFERRAL

1. Know the available community resources and the services offered.

2. Recognize when you are unable to further assist or work with the client; be honest about your own limits and your perceived need for a referral. Avoid implying rejection of the client.

3. Explore client readiness for referral. The client may also have ideas about referrals and sources of help or may be unwilling to use community agencies.

4. Determine what other professionals had contact with the client and confer with them about the possibility of referral. Various ethnic and racial groups prefer using the extended family or church.

5. Discuss the possibility of referral with a specific person at the selected agency prior to referral.

6. Inform parents of your recommendations and obtain their consent and cooperation if the client is a minor.

7. Be honest in explaining services of the referral agency. Do not make false promises about another agency's services or roles.

8. Describe specifics about location, how to get to the referral place/person, where to park and enter, and what to expect on arrival.

9. Have the client (or parent) make the initial appointment for the new service if he or she is willing to do so; some people may prefer you to make the initial contact. Tell the person that you have called the agency and that he or she is expected.

10. Do not release information to the referral agency or person without written permission from the client (or parent).

11. Ask the client to give you feedback about the referral agency/person to help you evaluate your decision and to help you make a satisfactory referral selection if needed for future needy individuals or families.

plays a great part in continuing certain practices even though a person has been taught differently by you. Motivation, moreover, is influenced by a person's culture, status, and role in that culture and by social pressures for conformity. Starting programs of prevention can be difficult when people place a low value on health, cannot recognize cause-and-effect relationships in disease, lack future-time orientation, or are confused about the existence of preventive measures in their culture. Thus preventive programs or innovations in health care must be shaped to fit the cultural and health profiles of the population. Long-range prevention goals stand a better chance of implementation if combined with measures to meet immediate needs. A mother is more likely to heed your advice about how to prevent further illness in her sick child if you give the child immediate attention.

IMPROVING HEALTH CARE PRACTICE AND ADVOCACY

You may talk with members of the National Association of Hispanic Nurses, the American Indian/Alaskan Indian Nurses Association, and the Black Nurses Association to gain information about how to give care that includes cultural values and customs. Refer to the reference list also.

With knowledge about cultures and ways to care for people from different cultures, you can be an advocate for a client from a different culture to ensure accessibility and appropriateness of services. In turn, you can help the health care system to be more culturally sensitive to care of clients, or several agencies can work together for that goal.

You can use modern technology to continue learning about cultural care as well as contribute to improved care. The AJN Network, an international computer network, has made the following situations feasible: You can get answers from nurses around the world for a difficult treatment problem. You can release an announcement to nurses all over the country. You can talk to the author of the nursing journal article that you just read.

The AJN network provides continuing education credit offerings in text and computer-assisted instruction formats, patient information on various topics, national and international news related to health care, resource databases for conference and nursing organizations, a nurse consultant feature where users can ask questions and get responses, and forums where current topics and clinical issues are posted for discussion among all the network users (24–26).

Additionally, computer software is being developed specifically for nurse practitioners so that not only all the medical procedures that physicians also use and document are visible, but the things that are uniquely nursing can be documented in the database. This will educate other nurses, physicians, other health providers, and administrators about what is uniquely nursing, thereby showing its value (25). Such software related to other health care disciplines is also becoming available so that all members of the team can work together for optimum client care and advocacy.

Sites for Health Promotion and Wellness Programs

Traditionally the main health concerns for employees in the workplace were safety and accident prevention. A yearly physical examination was also included in many industries.

Today industries and some hospitals and other work settings are adding programs for their *employees* that generally include emphasis in four areas: stress reduction, exercise, smoking cessation, and nutritional and weight guidance, particularly for obesity and sodium and cholesterol reduction. Some industries have also established employee assistance programs to help the chemically dependent employee reduce alco-

TABLE 1–19.   PRINCIPLES AND METHODS OF TEACHING

General Approach
1. Convey respect; be genuine.
2. Reduce social distance between self and others as much as possible.
3. Promote sense of trust and an open interaction; a trusting relationship fosters self-understanding and motivation to follow a teaching plan.
4. Elicit description of feelings from the client about the subject matter or situation to relieve tension and meet the learner's needs.
5. Be organized in presentation.
6. Use a comfortable setting and audiovisual aids as indicated.
7. Encourage questions, disagreement, and comments to ensure that your presentation stays focused on client needs and meets teaching goals.
8. Encourage, support, and reinforce as you present content.

Teaching Specific Content
1. Begin at knowledge level of client; consider readiness to learn.
2. Determine what client wants to know and already knows.
3. Answer the client's questions first; the client will then be more receptive to the information presented.
4. Build on what the client knows. Gently refute myths or misunderstandings.
5. Relate information to behavior patterns, lifestyle, and sociocultural background to increase likelihood of their being followed by the client.
6. Assist client in reworking your ideas to fit cultural, religious, or family values and customs to ensure that the material to be learned will be practiced.
7. Be logical in sequence of content.
8. Present more basic or simpler content prior to more advanced or complex information.
9. Present one idea, or a group of related ideas, at a time, rather than many diverse ideas together.
10. Demonstrate as you describe directions, suggestions, or ideas, if possible.
11. Break content into units and a series of sessions, if necessary. Do not present too many ideas at one time.
12. Teach the family as thoroughly as the client to ensure that suggestions on interpersonal relationships and other concerns will be followed.
13. Present the same information to friends, employer, occupational health nurse, schoolteacher, clergyman, or significant community leader, if possible and relevant.
14. Provide written instructions in addition to oral presentations.
15. Provide feedback and reinforcement to the client as you provide opportunity for practice and review.

Individual Teaching

Programmed Learning
Material is presented in carefully planned sequential steps through program instruction books or a teaching machine, a simple manually operated machine or a complex computer. One frame of information is presented at a time. The learner then tests his or her grasp of the information in the frame by writing, or in the case of a computer, keying, a response to a question, usually a multiple-choice type. The book or machine then gives the correct response. If the learner's response was incorrect, the program presents (or, in the case of a book, directs him or her to turn to) a repetition of the information or a more detailed explanation.

Literature
Pamphlets and *brochures* describe preventive measures, signs and symptoms of disease, and major steps of intervention. These are published by many health care organizations and agencies, often for specific diseases or groups.
Autobiographies of persons with certain disease processes and "how-to" books by persons who have experienced certain health problems directly or indirectly pass along suggestions to others.

Audiovisual Material
A recorder and cassettes explaining preventive measures, disease processes, or specific instructions can be loaned to the client. He or she can stop the cassette at any point and replay necessary portions until satisfied with the learning. "Talking Books" is a program that records information for the visually impaired. Closed-circuit television or videotape setups allow the person to hear and view material.
Note that these methods of individual instruction are only individual to a certain point. Only when the client can check learning with a *resource person,* ask further questions as necessary, and have help in making personal applications will learning become more significant. That process involves you. The person does not learn from a machine alone.

Computer
Instructions for prevention and health care for any condition, information related to growth and development and care of the child, adolescent, and adult of any age is available through computer-assisted instruction formats. Computer programs for client teaching are available for home and health care agencies. For example, a graph along with instructions can teach a patient about bypass surgery. A parent can be shown exactly how tubes will be placed in a child's ear.

(*continued*)

TABLE 1–19. PRINCIPLES AND METHODS OF TEACHING (continued)

Group Teaching

Client groups provide a channel through which feelings and needs can be expressed and met, especially if the people have similar problems, such as colostomy and diabetes. Thus you can use the group process to enhance health teaching or for therapy to aid coping with problems (Fig. 1–1). You may work with a group that has formed to accomplish some specific goal such as losing weight, promoting research to find a cure for cancer, or providing guidance to parents with mentally retarded children. In some cases information is not enough. Social support is also necessary, especially when engaging in a lesser-valued activity—such as not eating excessive sweet foods.

Evaluation of Teaching

1. Check frequently to determine if content is of interest or being understood.
2. Have client repeat content or give examples of application of content.
3. Have client review previously covered content, and its application, at each teaching session.
4. Determine the amount of learning that has occurred.

hol or drug intake and remain a safe, dependable worker. Some settings offer day-care for workers with young children—to reduce the worker's stress related to child care. Others have stress management programs for their employees and their clients. Facilities may boast nearly 24-hour availability of a fully equipped exercise room, gymnasium, handball court, and whirlpool baths or, for example, a rough running track that has been measured out around a furniture factory in rural North Carolina. In some cities the employer uses existing exercise facilities in various clubs or organizations such as the local chapter of the American Heart Association for screening or teaching programs.

In 1982, one of the authors (J.Z.) started a *health clinic in an industry* which included not only safety and accident prevention and health promotion activities, but also primary care for all workers and insured family members. A physician consults once weekly to review

any medical questions/problems. In addition to being very user friendly, this program has conservatively estimated a savings of $250,000 to $500,000 each year of its existence (worker numbers have ranged from 300 to 600). This calculation is based on what the services would have cost in the traditional health care system versus what they actually cost in this program. The program has been written up in two national journals, a state journal, and the local media (277).

Health promotion sites could also be established in stores, housing projects, neighborhood community centers, schools, churches, laundry facilities, or senior nutrition sites. Such sites would be more acceptable for health screening, well-child checkups, immunizations, or counseling to many cultural populations than is the hospital or traditional outpatient setting. Innovative city and county public health agencies have for years used nontraditional settings for health promotion and illness

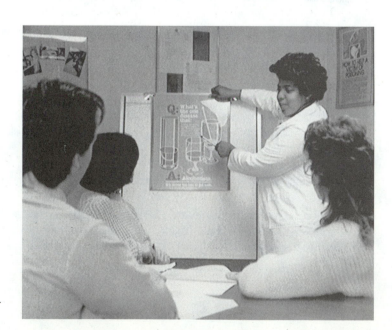

Figure 1–1. Group teaching provides an opportunity to provide health teaching to individuals with similar health concerns and problems. *(From Berger, K.J., and M.B. Williams,* Fundamentals of Nursing: Collaborating for Optimal Health. *Stamford, CT: Appleton & Lange, 1992, p. 181.)*

prevention. The nurse practitioner frequently works in a nontraditional site or, like other graduate-prepared nurses in any specialty, engages in entrepreneurial opportunities or faculty practice, combining practice, research, and academic roles.

Health care services must be given in nontraditional sites to reach the *homeless, refugees,* or *migrant workers.* Consistency in services and personnel will help such individuals develop a trusting relationship and seek and accept health care. The health clinic, adjacent to the day treatment program or walk-in meal site, must be open at flexible hours and employ staff who are accepting and provide a variety of services besides health screening, primary care, or referral to other care agencies. Of greater importance than health services are available food, clothing, showers and personal care supplies, a safe place to rest, shelter from the weather and especially at night, and laundry facilities. In addition, the site should provide telephone and either employment counseling or referral to employment services. Available information on housing and paralegal services to assist with obtaining entitlements such as Social Security, disability benefits, or pensions are also helpful. Giving the person a personal identification card that also includes name, address, and phone number of a treatment facility is beneficial. One author (R. M.) has worked for more than 10 years with a community service agency in a metropolitan area that provides the above services for the poor and homeless, including the severely and persistently mentally ill and chemically dependent.

The **nurse entrepreneur** is changing the future of health care. Entrepreneurial opportunities are available for those with foresight and a desire to apply nursing skills in a different fashion (27).

Among the factors causing a need for nurse entrepreneurs is the change in the public attitudes and values and growing emphasis on prevention. The present trend of reducing hospital use and curtailing Medicare and Medicaid costs is presenting a need for more cost-effective health care providers. Nurses are the perfect professional group to participate in the expansion of primary health care and prevention services.

Nurse entrepreneurs are doing well in several areas. One nurse practitioner in North Carolina has a business providing health care for industries. She employs another nurse practitioner, several part-time registered nurses, a part-time physician, and a part-time health educator. The firm provides whatever is needed in health care, from screenings to primary health care and care of chronic problems, with a great emphasis on wellness and preventive programs. Another nurse practitioner has opened a family practice office in a small North Carolina town. A community health advanced practice nurse in a metropolitan area in Missouri has a consultant business for child-care centers. A psychiatric advanced practice nurse in the same city consults for extended-care facilities for elderly. A nurse in Southern California provides acute hemodialysis service. A Florida nurse provides a day-care center for children with medical problems. Another nurse practitioner in Florida opened a private practice called Women's Health Watch.

These are only a few examples. Each state differs in the legal authority, reimbursement practices, and the prescription authority given to nurses in advanced practice. These factors greatly influence how much of an entrepreneur a nurse can be. A 1994 survey found that only three states have no statutory prescribing authority for nurse practitioners. In all but two states nurse practitioners can be reimbursed directly for Medicaid clients. And 35 states allow third-party reimbursement within the statute or have an any-willing-provider type of statute applicable to nurse practitioners (206). As of mid-July 1995, nurse practitioners could open their own practices, without physician backup, in Maine, Oregon, Washington, Alaska, New Hampshire, and Washington, DC (26).

Because of change and uncertainty, a whole new set of career opportunities are available. The future belongs to those who are able to respond to new demands and who have the courage to follow their convictions. In turn, people with diverse background will have a choice in selecting the type of health care service that best meets their needs. Then, culturally based care can be a reality.

SUMMARY

1. You will encounter diverse value systems and customs in your care of clients.
2. To understand your own and others' cultural backgrounds is interesting and enhances your care of the client, family, group, and community.
3. People from the same culture are uniquely different from each other while they also share similarities.
4. People from different cultural backgrounds share similarities as well as differences in various life patterns and values.
5. Cultural background has a major influence on development and health.
6. You will practice principles of cultural care, based on concepts in this chapter, in every health care setting.

7. Engage in lifelong learning about your own and others' cultures to, as effectively as possible, communicate with, relate to, assess, intervene with, and comprehensively care for the client.

► REFERENCES

1. Adhikara, N., and R. Menzies, Community-Based Tuberculin Screening in Montreal: A Cost Outcome Description, *American Journal of Public Health,* 85, no. 6 (1995), 786–790.
2. Adler, J., What Is An American? Sweet Land of Liberties, *Newsweek,* July 10 (1995), 16–23.
3. Adler, J., The Rise of the Over-class, *Newsweek,* July 31 (1990), 32–46.
4. *Alma-Ata: Primary Health Care.* Geneva: World Health Organization, 1978.
5. Alster, K., *The Holistic Health Movement.* Tuscaloosa: University of Alabama Press, 1989.
6. Alternative Medicine, *Harvard Women's Health Watch,* 1, no. 10 (1994), 2–3.
7. Alvarez, J., *The Other Side.* New York: Button, 1995.
8. Anderson, G., and B. Tighs, Gypsy Culture and Health Care, *American Journal of Nursing,* 73, no. 2 (1973), 282–285.
9. Andrews, M., and J. Boyle, *Transcultural Concepts in Nursing Care.* Philadelphia: J.B. Lippincott, 1995.
10. Anthony-Tkach, C., Care of the Mexican-American Patient, *Nursing and Health Care,* 2, no. 8 (1981), 424–432.
11. Aranata, F., and J. Carroll, *Philippine Institutions.* Manila: Solidaridad, 1988.
12. Baldwin, D., The Doctor (Robert Coles) Is in, *Common Cause Magazine,* May/June (1988), 25–30.
13. Barnes, D., et al, Primary Health Care and Primary Care: A Confusion of Philosophies, *Nursing Outlook,* 43, no. 1 (1995), 7–16.
14. Beare, P., Nursing Education Comes into Its Own in Saudi Arabia, *Nursing and Health Care,* 8, no. 5 (1987), 272–274.
15. Behind Those Smiles Lies Deep Frustration, *Philippine News,* March 13–19 (1991), 14.
16. Bell, R., Prominence of Women in Navajo Healing Beliefs and Values, *Nursing & Health Care,* 15, no. 5 (1994), 232–240.
17. Belsky, G., Americans Are Doing Better but Feeling Less Secure, *Money,* May (1995), 24–26.
18. ———, Why Most of the Rich Will Get Richer, *Money,* May (1995), 134–138.
19. Bigbee, J.L., The Uniqueness of Rural Nursing, *Nursing Clinics of North America,* 28, no. 1 (1993), 131–144.
20. Billingsley, A., *Black Families and the Struggle for Survival: Teaching Our Children to Walk Tall.* New York: Friendship Press, 1974.
21. Birkert-Smith, K., *Eskimos.* New York: Crown, 1971.
22. Bloch, B., Nursing Care of Black Patients, in Orgue, M., Bloch, B., and Monrrey, L., eds. *Ethnic Nursing Care: A Multicultural Approach.* St. Louis: C.V. Mosby, 1983, pp. 81–113.
23. Blumin, S.M., *The Emergence of the Middle Class.* Cambridge, England: Cambridge University Press, 1991.
24. Bovender, N., Computers: The Newest Tool Available to Nurses, *Nursing Matters,* 5, no. 7 (1995), 16.
25. ———Computer Software Developed for Nurse Practitioners, *N.P. News,* 3, no. 4 (1995), 5, 11.
26. ———Nurse Practitioners Could Fill Medical Gap in Areas Where Doctors Are Scarce, *Rocky Mountain News,* July 23 (1995), 34a.
27. ———The Nurse Practitioner as Entrepreneur, *N.P. News,* 3, no. 3 (1995), 1, 5.
28. Brink, P., Value Orientations as an Assessment Tool in Cultural Diversity, *Nursing Research,* 33, no. 4 (1984), 198–203.
29. ———, and J. Saunders, Culture Shock: Theoretical and Applied, in Brink, P., ed. *Transcultural Nursing: A Book of Readings,* Englewood Cliffs, NJ: Prentice-Hall, 1978, pp. 128–138.
30. Brislen, R., K. Cushner, and M. Young, *Intercultural Interactions: A Practice Guide.* Beverly Hills, CA: Sage, 1986.
31. Brower, H.T., Culture and Nursing in China, *Nursing and Health Care,* 5, no. 1 (1984), 26–31.
32. Browne, C., and A. Broderick, Asian and Pacific Island Elders: Issues for Social Work Practice and Education, *Social Work,* 39, no. 1 (1994), 252–259.
33. Bullough, V.L., and B. Bullough, *Health Care for the Other Americans.* New York: Appleton-Century-Crofts, 1982.
34. Bunkers, S., The Healing Web, *Nursing and Health Care,* 13, no. 2, (1992), pp. 68–73.
35. Campinha-Bacote, J., Culturological Assessment: An Important Factor in Psychiatric Consultation Liaison Nursing, *Archives of Psychiatric Nursing,* 2, no. 4 (1988), 244–250.
36. ———, Voodoo Illness, *Perspectives in Psychiatric Care,* 28, no. 1 (1992), 11–17.
37. Capers, C., Nursing and the Afro-American Client, *Topics in Clinical Nursing,* 7, no. 3 (1985), 1–17.
38. ———, Mental Health Issues and African-Americans, *Nursing Clinics of North America,* 29, no. 1 (1994), 57–64.
39. Castex, G., Providing Services to Hispanic/Latino Populations: Profiles in Diversity, *Social Work,* 39, no. 3 (1994), 288–296.
40. Catalano, R., The Health Effects of Economic Insecurity, *American Journal of Public Health,* 81, no. 9 (1991), 1148–1152.
41. Ching, C., Vietnamese in America: A Case Study in Cross-Cultural Health Education, *Health Values: Achieving High-Level Wellness,* 8, no. 3 (1984), 16–20.
42. Choi, H., Cultural and Noncultural Factors as Determinants of Caregiver Burden for the Impaired Elderly in South Korea, *The Gerontologist,* 313, no. 1 (1993), 8–15.
43. Ciesielski, S., D. Esposito, J. Protiva, and M. Piehl, The Incidence of Tuberculosis Among North Carolina Migrant Farmworkers, 1991, *American Journal of Public Health,* 84, no. 11 (1994), 1836–1838.
44. Clark, C. *Wellness Nursing: Concepts, Theory, Research, and Practice.* New York: Springer, 1986.
45. Coakley, T.A., P. Ehrlich, and E. Hurd, Southeast Asian Refugees: Health Screening in a Family Clinic, *American Journal of Nursing,* 80, no. 11 (1980), 2032–2036.
46. Cockerham, W., *Medical Sociology* (5th ed). Englewood Cliffs, NJ: Prentice Hall, 1992.
47. Coles, R., The Children of Affluence, *The Atlantic Monthly,* September 1977, 53–66.
48. ———, *Eskimos, Chicanos, Indians.* Boston: Little, Brown, 1978.
49. ———, *Children of Crisis: Vol 5. Privileged Ones, The Well Off, and Rich in America.* Boston: Little, Brown, 1978.
50. Collado, C., Primary Health Care: A Continuing Challenge, *Nursing & Health Care,* 13, no. 8 (1992), 408–413.
51. Comer, J., and A. Poussaint, *Black Child Care.* New York: Simon & Schuster, 1975.
52. Courtney, B., Freedom From Choice, *Newsweek,* February 13 (1995), 16.
53. Cowley, G., P. King, M. Hager, and D. Rosenberg, Going Mainstream, *Newsweek,* June 26 (1995), 56–57.

54. Coyle, J., How to Beat the Squeeze on the Middle Class, *Money,* May (1995), 106–112.

55. Crane, M., Queen of the Charity Ball, *St. Louis Magazine,* May (1991), 39–41.

56. Cravener, P., Establishing Therapeutic Alliance Across Cultural Barriers, *Journal of Psychosocial Nursing,* 30, no. 12 (1992), 10–14.

57. D'Avanzo, C., B. Frye, and R. Froman, Stress in Cambodian Refugee Families, *IMAGE: Journal of Nursing Scholarship,* 26, no. 2 (1994), 101–105.

58. Dacey, J., and J. Travers, *Human Development Across the Lifespan* (3rd ed.). Dubuque, IA: Brown & Benchmark, 1996.

59. Danticut, E., *Breath, Eyes, Memory.* New York: Vantage, 1995.

60. Danner, P., *An Ethic for the Affluent.* Lanham, MD: University Press of America, 1980.

61. Darabi, K., and V. Ortuz, Childbearing Among Young Latino Women in The United States, *American Journal of Public Health,* 77, no. 1 (1987), 25–28.

62. Davis, L., et al., AAN Expert Panel Report: Culturally Competent Health Care, *Nursing Outlook,* 40, no. 6 (1992), 277–283.

63. Davitz, L., Y. Sameshima, and J. Davitz, Suffering as Viewed in Six Different Cultures, *American Journal of Nursing,* 76, no. 8 (1976), 1296–1297.

64. DeMott, B., *The Imperial Middle.* New York: William Morrow, 1990.

65. DeTornyay, R., Reconsidering Nursing Education: The Report of the PEW Health Professions Commission, *Journal of Nursing Education,* 31, no. 7 (1992), 296–301.

66. Die, A., and W. Seelback, Problems, Sources of Assistance, and Knowledge of Services Among Elderly Vietnamese Immigrants, *The Gerontologist,* 28, no. 4 (1988), 448–452.

67. Dumond, D.E., *The Eskimos and the Aleuts.* London: Thames & Hudson, 1977.

68. Duvall, E., and B. Miller, *Marriage and Family Development* (6th ed.). New Yorker: Harper & Row, 1986.

69. Edelman, C., and C. Mandel, *Health Promotion Throughout the Life Span* (2nd ed.). St. Louis: C.V. Mosby, 1990.

70. Edminston, B., What Do You Call a Dark-Skinned Person, *American Demographics,* 71, no. 11 (October 1993), 9.

71. Ehling, M.B., The Mexican American (el chicano), in Clark, A.L., ed., *Culture and Childrearing.* Philadelphia: F.A. Davis, 1981.

72. Ehrenreich, B., and K. Stallard, The Nouveau Poor, *The New Day,* 14, no. 4 (1982), 1.

73. Ell, K., J. Haywood, E. Sobel, M. deGuzman, D. Blumfield, & J.P. Ning, Acute Chest Pain in African Americans: Factors in the Delay in Seeking Emergency Care, *American Journal of Public Health,* 84, no. 6 (1994), 965–970.

74. Elliott, M., Here to Stay: An Adopted Son Embraces the Land of 'More,' *Newsweek,* July 10 (1995), 36–37.

75. Emeigh, T., Native American Heroines: The Biography in the Curriculum, *The Educational Forum,* 52, no. 5, (Spring 1988), 255–268.

76. Evans, R.J., *German Family Life.* London: Croom Helm, 1982.

77. Face of Rural Poverty, *Farmweek,* December 5 (1994), 7.

78. Farley, J.E., *Sociology* (3rd ed.). Englewood Cliffs, NJ: Prentice-Hall, 1994.

79. Fernandez, M.S. Issues in Counseling Southeast-Asian Students, *Journal of Multicultural Counseling and Development,* (1988), 157–164.

80. Finn, J., Culture Care of Euro-American Women During Childbirth: Using Leininger's Theory, *Journal of Transcultural Nursing,* 5, no. 2 (1994), 25–37.

81. Fisher, L., Health Care Recommendations for Treating Immigrant Populations, *Health Line Ink,* Fall (1994), 1, 7.

82. Floriani, C., Southeast Asian Refugees: Life in a Camp, *American Journal of Nursing,* 80, no. 11 (1980), 2028–2030.

83. Flynn, B., The Caring Community: Primary Health Care and Nursing in England and the United States, in Leininger, M., ed., *Care: Discovery and Uses in Clinical and Community Nursing.* Detroit: Wayne State University Press, 1988, pp. 29–38.

84. Fong, R., and N. Mokuau, Not Simply "Asian Americans": Periodical Literature Review on Asians and Pacific Islanders, *Social Work,* 39, no. 3 (1994), 298–305.

85. Fraser, J., *The Portrait of a Chinese People.* New York: Summit Books, 1980.

86. Giger, J., and R. Davidhizar, *Transcultural Nursing: Assessment and Intervention* (2nd ed.). St. Louis: C.V. Mosby, 1995.

87. ——, & G. Turner, Black American Folk Medicine Health Care Beliefs: Implications for Nursing Plans of Care. *The Association of Black Nursing Faculty Journal,* 3, no. 2 (1992), 42–46.

88. Gilbert, D.A., *Compendium of American Public Opinion.* New York: Facts on File, 1989.

89. Gingrich, N., *To Renew America.* New York: Harper/Collins, 1995.

90. Gomez, E., and N. Carazos, Was Hexing the Cause of Death? *American Journal of Social Psychiatry,* 1, no. 1 (April 1981), 50–52.

91. Gonzalez, J., The Religious World of Hispanic Americans, in Neusner, J., ed., *World Religions in American: An Introduction.* Louisville, KY: Westminster/John Knox Press, 1994.

92. Gordon, V., I. Matonsek, and T. Lang, Southeast Asian Refugees: Life in America, *American Journal of Nursing,* 80, no. 11 (1980), 2031–2036.

93. Graham, J., *Another Mother Tongue.* New York: Beacon Press, 1990.

94. Grier, M., Hair Care for the Black Patient, *American Journal of Nursing,* 76, no. 11 (1976), 1781.

95. Griffin, W.D., *A Portrait of the Irish in America.* New York: Macmillan, 1983.

96. Grossberg, K.A., ed., *Japan Today.* Philadelphia: Ishi Institute for Study of Human Issues, 1981.

97. Guendelman, S., and B. Abrams, Dietary Intake Among Mexican-American Women: Generational Differences and Comparison with White Non-Hispanic Women, *Journal of Public Health,* 85, no. 1 (1995), 20–25.

98. Guild, K., Asian and Pacific Islander: Myth and Reality, *Social Work,* 33, no. 2 (1988), 142–147.

99. Haddon, R., An Economic Agenda for Health Care, *Nursing and Health Care,* 11, no. 1 (1990), 21–30.

100. Haferkamp, H., ed., *Social Structure and Culture.* Berlin: Walter de Gruyter & Co., 1989.

101. Hancock, L., and P. Katel, The Bilingual Bog, *Newsweek,* October 23 (1994), 89.

102. Hand, D., *Magical Medicine: The Folklores and Ritual of the People of Europe and America.* Berkeley: University of California Press, 1980.

103. Harris, D., and S. Guten, Health Protective Behavior: An Exploratory Study, *Journal of Health and Social Behavior,* 20 (1979), 17–29.

104. Healthy America: Practitioners for 2005—Executive Summary, *Journal of Allied Health,* (1992), 3–22.

105. Hecker, M., and F. Heike, eds., *The Greeks in America, 1528–1977.* Dobbs Ferry, NY: Oceana, 1978.

106. Henry, B., and E. Di Giacomo-Geffers, The Hospitalized Rich and Famous, *American Journal of Nursing,* 80, no. 8 (1980), 1426–1429.

107. Hobus, R., Living in Two Worlds: A Lakota Transcultural Nursing Experience, *Journal of Transcultural Nursing,* 2, no. 1 (1990), 33–36.

108. Hogue, C.J., and M. A. Hargraves. Class, Race and Infant Mortality in the United States. *American Journal of Public Health, 83,* (1993), 9–12.

109. Homeopathy: Is Less Really More? *Harvard Health Letter,* 20, no. 7 (1995), 1–3.

110. Horn, B., Cultural Concepts and Postpartal Care, *Nursing and Health Care,* 2, no. 11 (1981), 516–517, 526–527.

111. Hostetler, J.A., *Amish Society* (3rd ed.). Baltimore: John Hopkins University Press, 1980.

112. Hutchinson, S., The American Indian Senior Citizens View of Women, *Bulletin of American Association of Social Psychiatry,* 1, no. 3 (1980), 13–15.

113. Huttlinger, K., and D. Tanner, The Peyote Way: Implications for Culture Care Theory, *Journal of Transcultural Nursing,* 5, no. 2 (1994), 5–11.

114. Huttlinger, K., and P. Wiebe, Transcultural Nursing Care: Achieving Understanding in a Practice Setting, *Journal of Transcultural Nursing,* 1, no. 1 (1989), 27–32.

115. Jacobson, M., M. Mercer, L. Miller, et al., Tuberculosis Risk Among Migrant Farm Workers on the Delmarva Peninsula, *American Journal of Public Health,* 77, no. 1 (1987), 29–31.

116. James, S., When Your Patient Is Black West Indian, *American Journal of Nursing,* 78, no. 11 (1978), 1908–1909.

117. Johnson, H., Psychiatric Mental Health Consultation and Nursing in the United Arab Emirates, *Journal of Psychosocial Nursing,* 30, no. 5 (1992), 25–28.

118. Jones, J., and C. Block, Black Cultural Perspectives, *The Clinical Psychologist,* 37, no. 2 (1984), 58–62.

119. Juark, T., Access to Health Care for Hispanic Women: A Primary Health Care Perspective, *Nursing Outlook,* 43, no. 1 (1995), 23–28.

120. Keefe, S., *Appalachian Mental Health.* Lexington, KY: University Press of Kentucky, 1988.

121. Kendall, K., Maternal and Child Care in an Iranian Village, *Journal of Transcultural Nursing,* 4, no. 1 (992), 29–36.

122. Kimball, S., The Polish Presence in Illinois, *Alumnus— Southern Illinois University at Edwardsville,* Fall (1986), 5–7.

123. Kirkpatrick, S., & A. Cobb, Health Beliefs Related to Diarrhea in Haitian Children: Building Transcultural Nursing Knowledge, *Journal of Transcultural Nursing,* 1, no. 2 (1990), 2–12.

124. Kitnano, H., *Race Relations* (4th ed.), Englewood Cliffs, NJ: Prentice-Hall, 1991.

125. Klatsky, A., I. Tekawa, M. Armstrong, and S. Sidney, The Risk of Hospitalization for Ischemic Heart Disease Among Asian Americans in Northern California, *American Journal of Public Health,* 84, no. 10 (1994), 1672–1675.

126. Klein, J., A Tale of Two Cities, *Newsweek,* August 15 (1994), 57.

127. Kluckhorn, F., Family Diagnosis: Variations in Basic Values of Family Systems, *Social Casework,* 32 (February–March 1958), 63–72.

128. ——, and E. Strodtbeck, *Variations in Value Orientations.* New York: Row, Petersen, 1961.

129. Kohn, M., A. Naoi, C. Schoenback, C. Schooler, et al., Position in the Class Structure and Psychological Function in the United States, Japan, and Poland, *American Journal of Sociology,* 95, no. 4 (1990), 964–1008.

130. *Koran* 2:223. Translation and commentary by A. Yusef Ali.

131. Kosko, D., and J. Flaskerad, Mexican American Nurse Practitioner, and Lay Control Group Beliefs About Cause and Treatment of Chest Pain, *Nursing Research,* 36, no. 4 (1987), 226–231.

132. Kruse, L., Changing Faces in Our Land, *Successful Farming,* 91, no. 11 (1993), 1.

133. Largest Ethnic Group is German-Americans, *Clinton County Historical Society,* 16, no. 1 (1993), 32–33.

134. Larson-Presswalla, J., Insights into Eastern Health Care: Some Transcultural Nursing Perspectives, *Journal of Transcultural Nursing,* 5, no. 1 (1994), 21–24.

135. Latimer, G., A Threat to American Values: The Disparity Between Urban and Rural Cities, Towns, *Nation's City Weekly,* 11 (August 8, 1988), 4.

136. Leap, W., *American Indian English.* Salt Lake City: University of Utah Press, 1993.

137. Lee, L.Y., *The Winged Seed.* New York: Simon & Schuster, 1995.

138. Leff, J., The Cross-Cultural Study of Emotions, *Culture and Medical Psychiatry,* 1 (1977), 317–330.

139. Lei, A., Nursing in Today's Multicultural Society: A Transcultural Perspective, *Journal of Advanced Nursing,* 20 (1994), 307–313.

140. Leininger, M., *Nursing and Anthropology: Two Worlds to Blend.* New York: John Wiley & Sons, 1970.

141. ——, *Transcultural Nursing: Concepts, Theories, and Practices.* New York: John Wiley & Sons, 1978.

142. ——, *Transcultural Nursing.* New York: Masson, 1979.

143. ——, Caring: A Central Focus of Nursing and Health Care Services, *Nursing and Health Care,* 1, no. 10 (1980), 135–143.

144. ——, *Transcultural Care Diversity and Universality: A Theory of Nursing.* Thorofare, NJ: Charles B. Slack, Inc., 1985.

145. ——, ed., *Care: Discovery and Uses in Clinical and Community Nursing.* Detroit: Wayne State University Press, 1988.

146. ——, ed., *Care: The Essence of Nursing and Health.* Detroit: Wayne State University, 1988.

147. ——, Southern Rural Black and White American Lifeways With Focus on Care and Health Phenomena, in Leininger, M., ed., *Care: The Essence of Nursing and Health.* Detroit: Wayne State University Press, 1988, pp. 133–159.

148. ——, Issues, Questions, and Concerns Related to the Nursing Diagnosis Cultural Movement from a Transcultural Nursing Perspective, *Journal of Transcultural Nursing, 2,* no. 1 (1990), 23–32.

149. ——, The Significance of Cultural Concepts in Nursing, *Journal of Transcultural Nursing, 2,* no. 1 (1990), 52–59.

150. ——, (ed.), *Ethical and Moral Dimensions of Care.* Detroit: Wayne State University Press, 1990.

151. ——, Transcultural Care Principles, Human Rights, and Ethical Considerations, *Journal of Transcultural Nursing,* 3, no. 1, (1991), 21–22.

152. ——, *Culture Care Diversity and Universality: A Theory of Nursing.* New York: National League for Nursing, 1991.

153. Leonard, M.A., and C.A. Joyce, Two Worlds United, *American Journal of Nursing,* 71, no. 6 (1971), 1152–1155.

154. Lewis, J., and J. Looney, *The Long Struggle: Well-Functioning Working Class Black Families.* New York: Brunner/Mazel, 1983.

155. Lin, E., W. Carter, and A. Kleinman, An Exploration of Somatization Among Asian Refugees and Immigrants in Primary Care, *American Journal of Public Health,* 75, no. 9 (1985), 1081–1084.

156. Lin, Y.C., China: Health Care in Transition, *Nursing Outlook,* 31, no. 2 (1983), 94–99.

157. Lipson, J.G., and A. Meleis, Issues in Health Care of Middle Eastern Patients, *The Western Journal of Medicine,* 139, no. 6 (1983), 854–861.

158. ———, Culturally Appropriate Care: The Case of Immigrants, *TCN,* 7, no. 3 (1985), 48–56.

159. Lomund, B., *Asian Americans: Social and Psychological Perspectives,* vols. I and II. Los Angeles: Science and Behavior Books, 1980.

160. Lopata, H., *Polish Americans: Status Competition in an Ethnic Community.* Englewood Cliffs, NJ: Prentice-Hall, 1976.

161. Lopez, B., *Arctic Dreams.* Toronto: Bantam Books, 1986.

162. Luna, L., Transcultural Nursing Care of Arab Muslims, *Journal of Transcultural Nursing,* 1, no. 1 (1989), 22–26.

163. Luna, L., Care and Cultural Context of Lebanese Muslim Immigrants: Using Leininger's Theory, *Journal of Transcultural Nursing,* 5, no. 2 (1994), 12–20.

164. MacDonald, A., Folk Health Practices Among North Coastal Peruvians: Implications for Nursing, *IMAGE: Journal of Nursing Scholarship,* 13, no. 6 (1981), 51–56.

165. Macionis, J., *Sociology* (3rd ed.). Englewood Cliffs, NJ: Prentice-Hall, 1991.

166. Markidis, K., J. Boldt, and L. Roy, Sources of Helping and Intergenerational Solidarity: A Three Generations Study of Mexican-Americans, *Journal of Gerontology,* 41, no. 4 (1986), 506–511.

167. Marks, G., et al., Health Behavior of Elderly Hispanic Women: Does Cultural Assimilation Make a Difference? *American Journal of Public Health,* 77, no. 10 (1987), 1315–1319.

168. Marsella, A., and P. Pedersen, *Cross Cultural Counseling and Psychotherapy.* New York: Pergamon Press, 1981.

169. Mason, D., Perspectives on Poverty, *IMAGE: Journal of Nursing Scholarship,* 13, no. 3 (1981), 82–88.

170. Mayer, S., and C. Jencks, Growing Up in Poor Neighborhoods: How Much Does It Matter? *Science,* 243 (March 17, 1989), 1441–1445.

171. Mbiti, J., *African Religions and Philosophies.* Garden City, NY: Anchor Books/Doubleday, 1970.

172. McAdoo, H., *Family Ethnicity: Strength in Diversity,* Newbury, CA: Sage, 1993.

173. McGoldrick, M., J. Pearce, and J. Giodano, eds. *Ethnicity and Family Therapy.* New York: Guilford Press, 1985.

174. McKenna, M., Twice in Need of Care: A Transcultural Nursing Analysis of Elderly Mexican Americans, *Journal of Transcultural Nursing,* 1, no. 1 (1989), 46–52.

175. McKenzie, J., and N. Chrisman, Healing Herbs, Gods, and Magic: Folk Health Beliefs Among Filipino-Americans, *Nursing Outlook,* 26, no. 5 (1977), 326–329.

176. McLaughlin, D., and L. Jensen, Poverty Among Older Americans: The Plight of Nonmetropolitan Elders, *Journal of Gerontology,* 48, no. 2 (1993), S44–S54.

177. McNeil, W.K., *Ozark Mountain Humor.* Little Rock, AR: August House, 1989.

178. Mead, M., ed. *Cultural Patterns and Technological Change.* New York: Greenwood Press, 1985.

179. Meleis, A., The Arab American in the Health Care System, *American Journal of Nursing,* 81, no. 6 (1981), 1880–1883.

180. ———, Arab American Women and Their Birth Experience, *MCN,* 6, no. 3 (1981), 171–176.

181. ———, and A.R. Jansen, Ethical Crisis and Cultural Differences, *The Western Journal of Medicine,* 138, no. 6 (1983), 889–893.

182. ———, and C. LaFever, The Arab American and Psychiatric Care, *Perspectives in Psychiatric Care,* 22, no. 2 (1984), 72–86.

183. ———, J. Lipon, and S. Paul, Ethnicity and Health Among Five Eastern Immigrant Groups, *Nursing Research,* 41, no. 2 (1992), 98–103.

184. Middaugh, J., Cardiovascular Deaths Among Alaskan Natives, *American Journal of Public Health,* 80, no. 3 (1990), 282–283.

185. Mills, A., Saudia Arabia: An Overview of Nursing and Health Care, *Focus on Critical Care,* 13, no. 1 (1986), 50–56.

186. Mitsubishi Motors Corporation, *Introduction To Japan.* Tokyo: Sanseido, 1988.

187. Moccia, P., and D. Mason, Poverty Trends: Implications for Nursing, *Nursing Outlook,* 34, no. 1 (1986), 20–24.

188. Morgan, L., *And the Land Provides: Alaskan Natives in a Year of Transition.* Garden City, NY: Anchor Press/Doubleday, 1974.

189. Morganthau, T., What Color Is Black? *Newsweek,* February 13 (1995), 63–65.

190. Moving on the Challenge of Health, *Parameters for Health,* 19, nos. 3 & 4 (1994).

191. Mui, A., Caregiver Strain Among Black and White Daughter Caregivers: A Role Theory Perspective, *The Gerontologist,* 32, no. 2 (1992), 203–212.

192. Mura, P., and A. Mura, Cyclical Evolution of Nursing Education and Profession in Iran: Religious, Cultural, and Political Influences, *Journal of Professional Nursing,* 11, no. 1 (1995), 58–64.

193. Naimann, H., Nursing in Jewish Law, *American Journal of Nursing,* 70, no. 11 (1970), 2378–2379.

194. Naisbitt, J., and P. Aburdene, *Megatrends 2000: Ten New Directions for the 1990s.* New York: William Morrow, 1990.

195. Neugut, A., S. Kizelnik-Freilich, and C. Ackerman, Black–White Differences in Risk for Cutaneous, Ocular, and Visceral Melanomas, *American Journal of Public Health,* 84, no. 11 (1994), 1828–1829.

196. Nichols, P., Transplanted to Saudi Arabia, *American Journal of Nursing,* 89, no. 8 (1989), 1048–1050.

197. Nobles, W., African Psychology: Foundations for Black Psychology, in Jones, R.L., ed., *Black Psychology.* New York: Harper & Row, 1980.

198. Norbury, P., ed., *Introducing Japan.* New York: St. Martin's Press, 1977.

199. Obedinski, E., and H. Stankiewiczand, *Polish Folkways in America.* Lanham MD: University Press of America, 1987.

200. O'Grady, J., *How the Irish Became American.* Boston: Twayne Publishers, 1981.

201. Olson, S., Year of the Blue Collar Guy, *Newsweek,* November 8 (1989), 16.

202. Orque, M., B. Bloch, and L. Monrroy, *Ethnic Nursing Care: A Multi-cultural Approach.* St. Louis: C.V. Mosby, 1983.

203. Paris, P., The Religious World of African Americans, in Neusner, J., ed., *World Religions in America: An Introduction.* Louisville, KY: Westminster/John Knox Press, 1994.

204. Parker, J., The Lived Experiences of Native Americans with Diabetes Within a Transcultural Nursing Perspective, *Journal of Transcultural Nursing,* 6, no. 1 (1994), 5–11.

205. Parker, J., Ethnic Differences in Midwife-Attended US Births, *American Journal of Public Health,* 84, no. 7 (1994), 1139–1141.

206. Pearson, L., Annual Update on How Each State Stands on Legislative Issues Affecting Advanced Nursing Practice, *The Nurse Practitioner,* 20, no. 1, (1995), 13–51.

207. Pender, N., *Health Promotion in Nursing Practice* (2nd ed.). Stamford, CT: Appleton & Lange, 1987.

208. Perez-Stable, E., G. Marin, and B. Van Oss Marin, Behavioral Risk Factors: A Comparison of Latinos and non-Latino Whites in San Francisco, *American Journal of Public Health,* 84, no. 6 (1994), 971–976.

209. Persad, E., Some Cultural Factors in Psychiatric Training, *Canadian Mental Health,* 19, nos. 3 & 4 (1971), 11–15.

210. Phillips, S., and S. Lobar, Literature Summary of Some Navajo Child Health Beliefs and Rearing Practices within a Transcultural Nursing Framework, *Journal of Transcultural Nursing,* 1, no. 2 (1990), 13–20.

211. Phipps, L. Confusion of a Young WASP, *New York,* 21, no. 34 (1991), 24–31.

212. Pickwell, S., The Incorporation of Family Primary Care for Southeast Asian Refugees in a Community-Based Mental Health Facility, *Archives of Psychiatric Nursing,* 3, no. 3 (1989), 173–177.

213. Popenoe, D., *Sociology* (10th ed.). Englewood Cliffs, NJ: Prentice-Hall, 1995.

214. Porter, C., and A. Villarruel, Nursing Research with African-American and Hispanic People: Guidelines for Action. *Nursing Outlook,* 41, no. 2 (1993), 59–67.

215. Prittie, T., *Germany.* New York: Time, Inc., 1981.

216. Rafferty, M., *The Ozarks: Land and Life.* Tulsa: University of Oklahoma Press, 1980.

217. Reidhead, V., Odyssey to Navajo-Hopi Land, *Discovery,* Fall (1986), 8–11.

218. Ripples, L.J., *Of German Ways.* New York: Barnes & Noble, 1970.

219. ———, *The German-Americans.* Boston: Twayne Publishers, Division of G.K. Hall, 1976.

220. Roach, L., Assessment: Color Changes in Dark Skin, *Nursing '77,* 7, no. 1 (1977), 48–51.

221. Rojas, D., Leadership in a Multicultural Society: A Case in Role Development, *Nursing & Health Care,* 15, no. 5 (1994), 258–261.

222. Rosenbaum, J., Mental Health Care Needs of Soviet-Jewish Immigrants, in Leininger, M., ed., *Care: Discovery and Uses in Clinical and Community Nursing.* Detroit: Wayne State University Press, 1988, pp. 107–121.

223. Rosenbaum, J., Cultural Care of Older Greek Canadian Widows Within Leininger's Theory of Culture Care, *Journal of Transcultural Nursing,* 2, no. 1 (1990), 37–47.

224. Rumbaut, R., How Well Are Southeast Asian Refugees Adapting? *Business Forum,* 10, no. 4 (1985), 26–31.

225. Sanders, I., and E. Morawska, *Polish American Community Life: A Survey of Research.* Boston: Boston University Press, 1975.

226. Sciantz, M., The Mexican-American Migrant Farm Worker Family, *Nursing Clinics of North America,* 29, no. 1 (1994), 65–73.

227. Seidell, J., K. Bakx, P. Deurenberg, et al., The Relation Between Overweight and Subjective Health According to Age, Social Class, Slimming Behavior, and Smoking Habits in Dutch Adults, *American Journal of Public Health,* 76, no. 2 (1986), 1410–1415.

228. Seley, J., 10 Strategies for Successful Patient Teaching, *American Journal of Nursing,* 94, no. 11 (1994), 63–65.

229. Slate, C., Finding a Place for Navajo, *Tribal College,* Spring (1993), 10–14.

230. Smith, S., Speaking Out: People Without Land, *American Journal of Nursing,* 89, no. 2 (1989), 208–209.

231. Snow, L., Traditional Health Beliefs and Practices Among Lower Class Black-Americans, *The Western Journal of Medicine,* 139 (1983), 830–838.

232. Snyder, P., Health Service Implications of Folk Healing Among Older Asian Americans and Hawaiians in Honolulu, *The Gerontologist,* 24, no. 5 (1984), 471–476.

233. Sorlie, P., E. Backland, and J. Keller, US Mortality by Economic, Demographic, and Social Characteristics: The National Longitudinal Mortality Study, *American Journal of Public Health,* 85, no. 7 (1995), 949–956.

234. Spector, R.E., *Cultural Diversity in Health and Illness* (4th ed.). Stamford, CT: Appleton & Lange, 1996.

235. Spitze, G., and S. Miner, Gender Differences in Adult-Child Contact Among Black Elderly Parents, *The Gerontologist,* 32, no. 2 (1992), 213–218.

236. Steinhart, P., Time Passes. *Audubon,* January (1984), 8–11.

237. Stern, P., Solving Problems of Cross-cultural Health Teaching: The Filipino Childbearing Family, *IMAGE: Journal of Nursing Scholarship,* 13, no. 6 (1981), 47–50.

238. Stoto, M., and J. Durch, National Health Objectives for the Year 2000: The Demographic Impact of Health Promotion and Disease Prevention, *American Journal of Public Health,* 81, no. 11 (1991), 1456–1465.

239. Suarez, L., Pap Smear and Mammogram Screening in Mexican-American Women: The Effects of Acculturation, *American Journal of Public Health,* 84, no. 5 (1994), 742–746.

240. Sue, D., *Counseling the Culturally Different: Theory and Practice* (2nd ed). New York: John Wiley & Sons, 1990.

241. Susser, M., Editorial: Social Determinants of Health-Socioeconomic Status, Social Class, and Ethnicity, *American Journal of Public Health,* 85, no. 7 (1995), 903–904.

242. Targonski, P., V. Persky, P. Orris and W. Addington, Trends in Asthma Mortality Among African Americans and Whites in Chicago, 1968 Through 1991, *American Journal of Public Health,* 84, no. 11 (1994), 1830–1833.

243. Tien-Hyatt, J., Keying in on the Unique Care Needs of Asian Clients, *Nursing and Health Care,* 8, no. 5 (1987), 269–271.

244. Tierney, M., and L. Tierney, Nursing in Japan, *Nursing Outlook,* 42, no. 5 (1994), 210–213.

245. Toffler, A., *The Third Wave.* New York: Bantam Books, 1980.

246. Topolnicki, D., Five Trends to Bank on, *Money,* May (1995), 102–103.

247. ———, No More Pity for the Poor, *Money,* May (1995), 122–127.

248. Tripp-Reimer, T., P. Brink, and J. Saunders, Cultural Assessment: Content and Process, *Nursing Outlook,* 32, no. 2 (1984), 78–82.

249. Uretsky, S., and C. Birdsall, Quackery: A Thoroughly Modern Problem, *American Journal of Nursing,* 86, no. 9 (1986), 1030–1032.

250. *Statistical Abstract of the United States: 1990 National General Population Characteristics.* Hyattsville, MD: U.S. Bureau of Census, 1990.

251. Vargus, L., and J. Koss-Chioino (eds.). *Working With Culture: Psychotherapeutic Interventions With Ethnic Minority Children and Adolescents.* San Francisco: Jossey-Bass, 1992.

252. Villaire, M., Interview—Toni Tripp-Reimer: Crossing Over the Boundaries, *Critical Care Nurse,* June (1994), 134–141.

253. Von Bertalanffy, L., *General System Theory.* New York: George Braziller, 1968.

254. Vuong, G.T., *Getting to Know the Vietnamese.* New York: Frederick Unger, 1976.

255. Walker, G.M., Utilization of Health Care: The Laredo Migrant Experience, *American Journal of Public Health,* 69 (1979), 667–672.

256. Wang, J., Caretaker–Child Interaction Observed in Two Appalachian Clinics, in Leininger, M., ed. *Care: The Essence of*

Nursing and Health. Detroit: Wayne State University Press, 1988, pp. 195–216.

257. Weber, M., *The Protestant Ethic and the Spirit of Capitalism,* trans. Talcott Parsons. New York: Charles Scribner's Sons, 1930; students' edition, 1958.

258. Webster, R., Asian Patients in the CCU, *Nursing 4,* no. 31 (March 28–April 10, 1991), 16–19.

259. Weiss, J., The U.S./Mexico Border, *Nursing and Health Care,* 13, no. 8 (1992), 418–424.

260. Weiss, M., *The Clustering of America.* New York: Harper & Row, 1988.

261. Weiss, O., Cultural Shock, *Nursing Outlook,* 19, no. 1 (1971), 40–43.

262. Wells, B., and J. Horn, Stage at Diagnosis in Breast Cancer: Race and Socioeconomic Factors, *American Journal of Public Health,* 82, no. 10 (1992), 1383–1385.

263. Wenger, A., and M. Wenger, Community and Family Patterns of the Old Order Amish, in Leininger, M., ed., *Care: Discovery and Uses in Clinical and Community Nursing.* Detroit: Wayne State University, 1988, pp. 39–54.

264. Westermeyer, J., Psychiatric Diagnosis Across Cultural Boundaries, *American Journal of Psychiatry,* 142, no. 7 (July, 1985), 278–805.

265. White, J., and P. Thana, *The Psychology of Blacks.* New York: Prentice-Hall, 1990.

266. White, P., To Be Indomitable, To Be Joyous: Greece, *National Geographic,* 157, no. 3 (1980), 360–393.

267. Whitman, D., D. Friedman, A. Linn, C. Doremus, and K. Hetter, The White Underclass, *U.S. News and World Report,* October 12 (1994), 4ff.

268. Wigginton, E., *The Foxfire Books,* Vols. 1–5. Garden City, NY: Anchor Press/Doubleday, 1979.

269. *Wisdom of Amish Folk Medicine.* North Canton, OH: The Leader Co., p. 19.

270. Wisdom of the Elders: Mississippi Choctaws, *AARP News Bulletin, 27,* no. 11 (December 1986), 5.

271. *Global Strategy for Health by All by the Year 2000.* Geneva: World Health Organization, 1981.

272. Yankauer, A., Hispanic/Latino—What's in a Name? *American Journal of Public Health,* 77, no. 1 (1987), 15–17.

273. Yep, J., An Asian Patient. How Does Culture Affect Care? A Family Member Responds, *Journal of Christian Nursing,* 6, no. 5 (1991), 5–8.

274. Your Health Records: Is Your Privacy at Risk? *Living Right,* Fall (1995), 12–17.

275. Yuki, T., Caring for the Urban American Indian Patient, *Journal of Emergency Nursing, 7,* no. 3 (1981), 110–113.

276. Zborowski, M., Cultural Components in Response to Pain, in Apple, D., ed., *Sociological Studies of Health and Sickness.* New York: McGraw-Hill, 1960, pp. 118–133.

277. Zentner, J., C. Dellinger, W. Adkins, and J. Greene, Nurse Practitioner Provided Primary Care: Managing Health Care Costs in the Workplace, *AAOHN Journal,* 43, no. 1 (1995), 52–53.

278. Zimmerman, R., W. Vega, A. Gil, G. Warheit, E. Apospori, and F. Biafora, Who Is Hispanic? Definitions and Their Consequences. *American Journal of Public Health,* 84, no. 12 (1994), 1985–1987.

chapter two

Environmental Influences on the Person and Family

Earth does not belong to us; we belong to the earth.

—*Chief Seattle*

Key Terms

Perfect or complete combustion	Photochemical smog	Synthetic chemicals	Pica
Imperfect or incomplete combustion	Pollutant Standards Index	Sediment	Caution
Carbon monoxide	Greenhouse effect	Heat	Corrosive
Hypoxic state	Refrigerator effect	Biologic oxygen demand	Danger
Sulfur oxides	Acid rain	Pesticides	Ignitable
Sulfur dioxide	Radioactive substances	Dioxin	Nontoxic
Sulfuric acid	Sick building syndrome	Food additives	Reactive
Nitrogen oxides	Formaldehyde	Zoonoses	Toxic
Nitrogen dioxide	Radon	Sound overload	Warning
Suspended particles	Common sewage	Decibels	Teratogenic
Hydrocarbons	Pathogenic organisms	Recycled	Mutagenic
Ozone	Plant nutrients	Hazardous waste	Therapeutic milieu

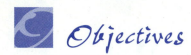

Objectives

Study of this chapter will enable you to:

1. Explore the scope of environmental pollution, both outdoors and indoors, and the interrelationship of different kinds of pollution with one another and with people.

2. Observe sources of air pollution in your community and identify resulting hazards to human health.

3. List types of water pollution and describe resultant health problems.

4. Describe substances that cause soil pollution and the effect of those substances on the food web and on other facets of health.

5. Discuss types of food pollution and ways to prevent food contamination.

6. Listen to noise pollution in various settings and discuss its long-term effects on health.

7. Contrast different types of surface pollution and resultant health problems.

8. Discuss health hazards encountered in the home and on the job and the major effects of these contaminants.

9. Discuss and practice ways that, as a citizen, you can reduce environmental pollution.

10. Discuss your professional responsibility in assessing for illness caused by environmental pollutants and in taking general intervention measures.

11. Demonstrate an ability to help establish a therapeutic milieu for a client.

Although ecology is a well-publicized subject, often the physical environment in which we live is taken for granted and overlooked as a direct influence on people and their health. You may wonder why a book discussing major influences on the developing person, family unit, and their health contains a chapter about humans and their environment. Yet where we live and the condition of that area—its air, water, and soil—determine to a great extent how we live, what we eat, the disease agents to which we are exposed, our state of health, and our ability to adapt. This chapter focuses primarily on noxious agents to which many people in the United States are exposed in the external environment. Because of the interdependence of people, only those living in isolated rural areas escape the unpleasant effects of our urban, technologically advanced society. Yet even the isolated few may encounter some kind of environmental pollution, whether through groundwater contaminated from afar, food shipped into the area, smog blown from a nearby city, or contaminated rain or snow. Further, the pollutants that are discussed are observed worldwide.

Nursing in the past was concerned primarily with the client's immediate environment in the hospital or home. Today nursing and health care are extended to include assessment of the family and community as well as the individual. Interventions are directed toward promoting a healthy environment for individuals and families, well or ill, and maintaining public health standards and federal regulations. Understanding some specific environmental health problems and their sources and effects will enable you to function both as a citizen and as a professional to help prevent or correct those problems. Teach about prevention of and effects from the pollutants described in this chapter as you care for people in the agency, home, or community. There are links between various pollutants and between pollutants and disease.

HISTORICAL PERSPECTIVE

The natural components of the environment were once considered dangerous. In most instances people dealt successfully with any environmental problems encountered. In their quest to conquer nature, early people discovered fire and the wheel. Fire was essential to survival; but with its advent, natural or man-made sparks and pollutants were sent into the atmosphere—the beginning of environmental pollution.

The fire and the wheel played major roles in early civilization and industrialization of the world. With the industrial revolution came many technologic advances that gave people increased power and comforts. These advances also introduced artificial, chemical, and physical hazards into the environment. Soon after the start of the Industrial Revolution, the population of cities grew; disease spread with the crowding of people, and food distribution became more complex. It became apparent that the natural components of the environment were not as dangerous as the man-made components.

The entire environment has been and is a vital part of our existence. Human skill in manipulating the environment has produced tremendous benefits; but none has been without a price, the high price of pollution. Pollution of our environment not only is a health threat but also offends esthetic, spiritual, social, and philosophic values. Environmental pollution is a complex, significant problem requiring multiple solutions (Fig. 2–1).

Antipollution legislation in the United States can be traced back to the early 1900s. In 1906 the first federal Food and Drug Act was passed, and in 1914 drinking water standards were enacted to serve as guides for water supplied on interstate carriers. Congress passed the federal Water Pollution Control Act in 1948. Most of these legislative moves were poorly funded and supported, however, and so had little effect on growing pollution problems. Finally in the early 1960s Congress began taking a firm and leading role in combating environmental pollution. The Clean Air and Solid Waste Disposal Act of 1965 and the Clean Water Restoration Act of 1966 are examples of this attempt to fight pollution (28, 51, 54). The U.S. Environmental Protection Agency (EPA) was created in 1970 to consolidate, strengthen, and coordinate federal efforts. Several important laws were passed after the formation of the EPA (e.g., Clean Water Act [1972], Pesticides Control Act [1972], Safe Drinking Water Act [1974], Resource Conservation and Recovery Act [1976], and Toxic Substances Control Act [1976]). The Toxic Substances Control Act was the first attempt to provide comprehensive regulation of potentially dangerous chemical substances. The Resource Conservation and Recovery Act gave the EPA the power to track hazardous wastes from generation site to final disposal (51, 54, 181).

During the 1980s the EPA reversed some earlier decisions and postponed implementation of some of their requirements. Nevertheless, enactment of important laws did occur, including Asbestos School Hazard Detection and Control Act (1980), Consumer-Patient Radiation and Health Safety Act (1981), Nuclear Waste Policy Act (1982), International Environmental Protection Act (1983), and Asbestos Hazard Emergency Response Act (1986) (28, 51). In the 1990s attempts are being made to develop environmental impact statements based on health-risk assessment (69), and legislation such as the Clean Air Act of 1990 has tightened previous regulations (65).

The following is divided into discussions of air, water, soil, food, noise, and surface pollution; however, these categories overlap. To illustrate, when a person inhales harmful particles from the soil that have become airborne, soil pollution becomes air pollution; and soil or surface pollution becomes water or food pollution if the harmful particles are swept into the water, consumed first by fish and then by people.

AIR POLLUTION

This most excellent canopy, the air, look you, this brave o'erhanging firmament, this majestical roof fretted with golden fire—why, it appears no other thing to me than a foul and pestilent congregation of vapors.

Hamlet (II, ii, 314–315)

Problems of Air Pollution

Air pollution is not a new problem; people have known for centuries that air can carry poisons. Miners would take canaries with them into the mines—a dead bird meant the presence of lethal gas. Natural processes such as forest and prairie fires, volcanic eruptions, and wind erosion have long contaminated the air. A dramatic example of natural air pollution in the United States was caused by the 1980 eruption of Mount St. Helens in the state of Washington. Gases and dust from the volcano were spewed into the atmosphere, and local communities were covered with volcanic ash. Human activities such as burning of fossil fuels, surface mining of coal, incineration of solid wastes, and manufacturing

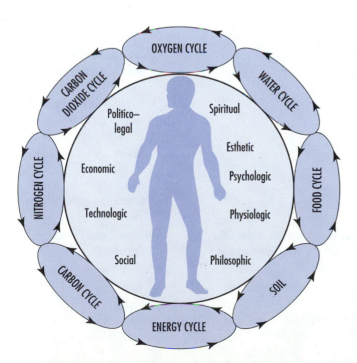

Figure 2–1. Human interrelationship with the environment.

processes are recognized as sources of pollution. The current problem of toxic air pollution came sharply into focus in late 1984 when more than 2500 people died and as many as 100,000 were left with permanent disabilities as a result of a gas leak from a Union Carbide Corporation fertilizer plant in Bhopal, India (183).

Air pollution and water pollution act interchangeably; together they present a world problem. All people on the earth share the oceans and the air. Significant local pollution of either can greatly affect distant areas, especially if the oceans cannot, by the processes of precipitation, oxidation, and absorption, cleanse the atmosphere before harmful effects occur. Given enough time, the oceans can cleanse the atmosphere; but if the amount of pollution exceeds the ocean's capacity to neutralize the waste, harmful materials are dispersed into the atmosphere, and we realize the effects by breathing contaminated air (32).

Sources of Air Pollution

The five most common pollutants found in the air are carbon monoxide, sulfur oxides, nitrogen oxides, suspended particles, and hydrocarbons. The sources of these air pollutants vary, and the effects on humans differ according to length and degree of exposure to the pollutant. Air pollution is most harmful to the very young, the very old, and persons with respiratory and cardiac disease (see Table 2–1) (2, 4, 22, 25, 33, 35, 48, 60, 63, 75, 81, 82, 97, 123, 133, 149, 151, 152).

A major cause of air contamination is imperfect or incomplete combustion. **Perfect or complete combustion** exists only in chemistry books and is the *result of hydrogen and carbon uniting completely with oxygen, thereby relinquishing heat, water vapor, light, and carbon dioxide to the air.* **Imperfect or incomplete combus-**

TABLE 2–1. COMMON AIR POLLUTANTS

Pollutant	Characteristics	Source	Where Found	Effects
Carbon monoxide (CO)	Colorless Odorless Tasteless Poisonous Contributes to photochemical smog	Motor vehicle—car exhaust Cigarette smoking Forest fires Faulty or unvented furnaces or kerosene or wood space heaters	Garages Tunnels Heavy traffic areas Basements and homes that are poorly ventilated CO detector monitors excess levels, prevents poisoning	*Hypoxia, decreased oxygen level in blood* Dizziness Hypotension Tachycardia Headaches Cherry red lips and skin Fatigue Drowsiness Impaired perception and thinking; odd behavior; brain damage Dangerous to people with heart or respiratory disease or anemia; pregnant women; children Fetal growth retardation and brain damage Death: Exposure to 0.05% CO air concentration can be fatal in 30 minutes from respiratory or heart failure
Sulfur oxides		Factories that burn coal or oil that contains sulfur	Coal that contains sulfur Industrial and urban areas	Irritation of mucous membranes: eyes, nose, throat, lungs
Sulfur dioxide (SO_2)	Heavy poisonous gas			Causes or aggravates respiratory disease
Sulfuric acid (H_2SO_4)	Heavy, corrosive colorless liquid	Sulfur trioxide (SO_3) reacts with water vapor to form mist		Death Damage to plants Corrosion of metals

(continued)

TABLE 2–1. COMMON AIR POLLUTANTS

Pollutant	Characteristics	Source	Where Found	Effects
Nitrogen oxides Nitrogen dioxide	Gaseous end products Visible, red-brown gas Toxic Foul-smelling	Burning fossil fuel Motor vehicles Other transportation modes Burning natural gas, oil and coal in power plants	Coal Oil Natural gas Urban areas Rural areas if power or industrial plants present Nitrous oxide reacts in sunlight to produce smog and ozone	Irritation of mucous membranes of throat Altered night vision Respiratory disease Heart disease Cancer
Suspended particles	Minute particles Dust Dirt Soot Aerosols Fly ash	Industrial processes Power and heating plants Wood or coal burner in homes Wind erosion Forest or building fires Incineration of solid wastes Surface mining	Urban industrial areas Rural mining areas Observable on surfaces in homes	Irritation to mucous membranes: eyes, nose, throat Respiratory disease Damage to surfaces
Asbestos particles	Asbestos material deteriorates, releases fibers in air	Factories Homes Public buildings Roadways Brake linings Clutch facings Now regulated or prohibited	Building insulation Shingles Sidings Floor and ceiling tiles Patching compounds Textured paints Appliances	Respiratory disease Rate of lung cancer 5 times greater in person with asbestosis than if no asbestos scarring; person with asbestosis who smokes 1 pack of cigarettes daily is 50 times more likely to develop lung cancer.
Tobacco smoke	Direct or passive smoke in environment	Tobacco cigarettes	Anywhere someone smokes tobacco products	Cardiac disease Respiratory disease Cancer Low birth weight in infants Paternal smoking affects birth weight of baby
Hydrocarbons	Volatile organic compounds of hydrogen and carbon	Natural sources—85% Decomposition of organic matter Evaporation of gasoline from motor vehicles Vapors from chemical solvents Incomplete combustion	Atmosphere Forests Coal, gas, and petroleum fields Industrial and chemical manufacturing plants	React in presence of sunlight to produce smog or ozone
Ozone	Pungent Colorless Toxic gas	Lower atmosphere—formed in air by chemical reactions between nitrogen oxide and hydrocarbons	Upper atmosphere—a protective barrier against excess sunlight Lower atmosphere	Irritates eyes and mucous membranes of nose and throat Respiratory distress Cardiac distress Nausea Headaches Decreased tolerance to exercise Affects venous system Severely affects children, elderly, chronically ill Causes plants to turn yellow, reducing photosynthesis
Photochemical smog	Chemical reaction between nitrogen oxides and hydrocarbons stimulated by sunlight			Eye irritation Cardiac distress Lung damage Decreased tolerance to physical activity

tion refers to the *additional liberation of carbon monoxide, sulfur oxides, nitrogen oxides, and hydrocarbons into the air.*

The EPA has developed the **Pollutant Standards Index (PSI)** as a *means of reporting daily air pollution concentrations.* The PSI converts the pollutant concentrations measured in a community's air to a number on a scale of 0 to 500. Intervals of the PSI scale are related to the potential health effects of the daily measured concentrations of the five major pollutants previously described. The intervals and terms used to describe the air quality levels are as follows: 0 to 50—good; above 50—moderate; above 100—unhealthful; 201 to 300—first stage alert, very unhealthful; 301 to 400—second stage alert, hazardous; 401 to 500—third stage alert, significant harm. When the pollution index is greater than 100, individuals with existing heart or respiratory ailments should reduce physical exertion and outdoor activity (174).

Four additional air pollution problems should be mentioned: (1) depletion of the upper atmosphere ozone layer; (2) increasing levels of atmospheric carbon dioxide; (3) acid rain; and (4) radioactive substances. As noted, a thin layer of ozone surrounds the earth and blocks much of the sun's ultraviolet radiation from reaching the earth's surface. The ozone layer is in danger of being depleted by the continued use of fluorocarbons (Freon) and chlorofluoromethanes that release chlorine into the stratosphere to combine with ozone. The continued use of fluorocarbon-propelled aerosol products and supersonic transport planes adds to that danger (55, 60, 91, 122).

In Caucasians short-wavelength ultraviolet sunlight is thought to cause melanoma and nonmelanoma skin cancer that would increase in incidence if there were a reduction of the ozone layer. In addition, studies have shown that an increase in ultraviolet radiation damages the immune system of humans (55, 60, 133).

Increasing Carbon Dioxide

The atmospheric content of carbon dioxide has increased significantly in the past century. Carbon dioxide is added to the atmosphere by burning fossil fuels. The increased level of atmospheric carbon dioxide alters the heat balance of the earth. Sunlight passes through the carbon dioxide, but the *radiation of heat away from the earth is slowed, producing what is known as the* **greenhouse effect.** Such changes might eventually result in melting of the polar ice caps, flooding of large coastal plain areas, and disruption of food production (55, 77, 91). Some scientists fear the *opposite may*

occur—the **refrigerator effect.** The carbon dioxide concentration would eventually prevent enough of the sun's rays from reaching earth that cooler temperatures would occur, again affecting food production and health factors (55, 77). Scientists find signs of a shift in distribution of invertebrate species that suggest a rapid warming of the Northern Hemisphere, which affects the food chain overall.

Acid Rain

Acid rain is the *end product of chemical reactions that begin when sulfur dioxide and nitrogen oxides enter the atmosphere from coal-, oil-, and gas-burning power plants, iron and copper smelters, and automobile exhaust.* These gases undergo changes and eventually react with moisture to form sulfuric acid and nitric acid. One-half to two-thirds of the pollution falls as acid rain or snow; some of the remainder is deposited as sulfate or nitrate particles that combine with dew and mist to form dilute acids (190). Most of northeastern United States; portions of the upper Midwest, Rocky Mountains, and West Coast; and parts of Ontario, Quebec, Nova Scotia, and Newfoundland in Canada now receive strongly acidic precipitation (122, 140). The United Kingdom, continental Europe, Poland, and central Russia have reported environmental damage from acid rain or snow. Although the full effect on the environment is not understood as yet, increased acidity in soil, streams, or ponds can be documented. Certain freshwater ecosystems are particularly sensitive to acid; fish, frogs, and some aquatic plants die. Acid rain leaches compounds out of soil, damaging the root systems of plants. Forests die. Crops are damaged. With continued episodes of acid rain, limestone and marble statues and buildings are dissolved, and homes and other structures weather more quickly (61, 140, 144, 153, 190). It will be years before the full effect of acid precipitation is known. At present, the only solution is to decrease the emissions of sulfur and nitrogen oxide into the atmosphere.

Radioactive Substances

Radioactive substances are *produced by mining and processing radioactive ore and by nuclear fission and radiation procedures* used in industry, medicine, and research. Pollution from radioactive materials poses a serious threat to our ability to reproduce and to our gene structure. It is also related to an increase in leukemia and other cancers, as demonstrated in persons working with radioactive materials over long periods without adequate safeguards and in survivors of the bombings in

Hiroshima and Nagasaki, Japan. A small fraction, 1 to 3%, of all cancers in the general population is attributable to natural radiation. Occupational irradiation produces an increase over the natural incidence (18, 34, 164).

Indoor Air Pollution

Some significant indoor pollutants are carbon monoxide, asbestos particles, nitrogen oxides, formaldehyde, and radon. Office workers and others in North America and Europe who work in poorly ventilated buildings regularly report a *variety of nonspecific but illness-producing symptoms*. The buildings have been referred to as "sick buildings," giving rise to the "**sick building syndrome**". Symptoms include the following:

- Irritation of the skin, eyes, nose, and throat
- Mental fatigue
- Headache
- Dizziness
- Frequent respiratory infections
- Hypersensitivity reactions

Exposure to other indoor pollutants, such as cigarette smoke and inhalants, increases the symptoms (15, 17, 70, 78, 103, 108, 117, 158).

Formaldehyde, a *colorless gas characterized by a strong, pungent odor,* escapes into the air from foam insulation, particle board, plywood, and fiberboards. Formaldehyde gas in newly insulated homes has reached concentrations high enough to cause dizziness, drowsiness, nausea, vomiting, rashes, nosebleeds, and diarrhea. It is extremely hazardous and probably is a carcinogen. Nitrogen oxides are released from unvented gas stoves and space heaters. As they accumulate in the home, these pollutants can affect sensory perception and produce eye irritation (153).

Radon, a *natural radioactive gas produced by the decay of uranium-238,* is the most serious health threat of the common indoor pollutants, causing serious respiratory problems. It seeps into basements through cracked floors and diffuses out of brick and concrete building materials. The EPA estimates that radon is responsible for 5,000 to 20,000 deaths from lung cancer each year (15, 17, 34, 48, 78, 103, 117, 124, 138, 141, 158).

Particles such as dust, soot, ash, and cigarette smoke may be inhaled into the lungs. Many household products such as cleansers, drain openers, and paint removers have toxic ingredients and cause respiratory irritation and eye or skin irritation on contact. Some are carcinogenic when fumes or particles are inhaled over

time. Fungi and bacteria from humidifiers and air conditioning systems can cause allergies or Legionnaires' disease and aggravate asthma (130).

Indoor air pollution can be controlled by several measures: proper venting of gas stoves, heaters, and wood stoves; painting over materials that emit radon and formaldehyde; and daily airing of the house. House plants, especially spider plants, can be used to absorb air pollutants in the home.

All forms of air pollution are physically irritating and present a potential hazard to long-range health either by direct harm to the mucous membranes of the respiratory tract or by the indirect effects of continuously breathing contaminated air. Only in becoming aware of these factors as personal health threats will we seriously consider alternatives to using two or three cars, seek to know the serious hazards in our jobs, become concerned about houses downwind from an industrial site or the amount of ultraviolet light we receive, and use natural products instead of chemicals for many household tasks.

WATER POLLUTION

Pollution of the water from the natural processes of aquatic animal and plant life, combined with man-made waste, constitutes another hazard to the delicate state of human health. Man-made water pollution has two major origins, *point sources* and *nonpoint sources*. Point sources are those that discharge pollutants from a well-defined place (e.g., outlet pipes of sewage treatment plants and factories). Nonpoint sources consist of runoff from city streets, construction sites, farms, and mines.

Types of Water Pollution

The most common water pollutants are common sewage, pathogenic organisms, plant nutrients, synthetic chemicals, inorganic chemicals, sediment, radioactive substances, oil, and heat (see Table 2–2) (20, 29, 37, 47, 59, 61, 81, 85, 86, 94, 150, 166). Because humans are dependent on water and the lower forms of life in water for food, any of these water pollutants can affect well-being and health (see Fig. 2–2). In addition, as for air pollution, water pollution has economic implications. Further, water pollution is a global problem, as is air pollution. Faced with an expanding world population, we must increasingly be aware of the significance of every organism in the food web (see Fig. 2–2) and its relationship to us (81).

TABLE 2–2. COMMON WATER POLLUTANTS

Pollutant	Characteristics	Source	Where Found	Effects
Common sewage	Traditional waste from domestic or industrial sources	Sewage disposal system: septic tanks, cesspools, outdoor toilets	Sewage drains into water source, and water unable to deal with waste	Waste uses oxygen needed by aquatic plant and animal life Water rendered useless Aquatic death Human gastrointestinal diseases Infectious diseases
Pathogenic organisms	Various disease-producing microorganisms	Sewage contamination	Rivers, lakes, streams Drinking water Farm areas Rural or urban areas where population is dense and public utilities are limited	Infectious gastroenteritis Hepatitis Typhoid fever Giardiasis, cholera
Plant nutrients	Nutrients, especially phosphates and nitrates, that nourish plant life	Sewage Livestock and human excrement Soil erosion Industrial wastes Chemical fertilizer	Rural ground water and drinking supplies Nutrients not easily removed by water treatment centers may inadvertently change substances into usable mineral form, causing more plant growth	Unpleasant odor and taste in water Disturbs normal food web in body of water Infant illness and death from nitrate-induced methemaglobinemia
Synthetic chemicals	Synthetic chemical substances such as detergents, cleaning agents, pesticides	Homes Industries	Widespread	Poisonous to aquatic life Unpleasant taste and color in water Possible disease
Inorganic chemicals	Mineral substances Toxic materials	Mining Manufacturing processes	Water supplies Toxic waste materials may be dumped into water or land areas	Corrodes water treatment equipment Kills plant and animal life Disease in humans
Sediment	Particles of dirt or sand	Soil erosion		Reduced photosynthesis for aquatic plants in water where soil suspended; causes reduced food chain for animals Disrupts reproductive cycles of aquatic animals: clogs streams Prevents natural reservoirs from filling with rain Increased cost of water treatment
Radioactive material	Synthetic or natural	Waste from nuclear power plant Industrial or research facilities using radioactive materials Uranium mines	Widespread	Contamination of water and food Cancer
Oil spills		Natural seepage Dumping of waste oil Flushing ship bilges Oil refinery discharge Accidental spills account for small percentage of spill	Widespread	Death to bird and other aquatic life Presence in food web of humans—unknown effects
Heat	High temperature Reduces ability of water to absorb oxygen	Industrial processes	Widespread	Death of aquatic life Ecologic balance of lakes and rivers permanently upset Interference with food chain for humans and animals

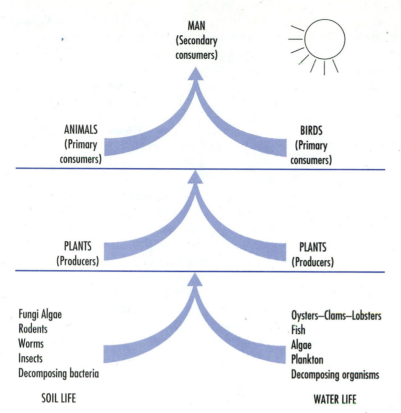

MAN
(Secondary
consumers)

ANIMALS
(Primary
consumers)

BIRDS
(Primary
consumers)

PLANTS
(Producers)

PLANTS
(Producers)

Fungi Algae
Rodents
Worms
Insects
Decomposing bacteria

Oysters–Clams–Lobsters
Fish
Algae
Plankton
Decomposing organisms

SOIL LIFE

WATER LIFE

Figure 2–2. Food web.

One of the most frightening results of water pollution is the threat to the oceans. The collective practice of the world's nations of ocean dumping of sewage may permanently pollute the oceans. The Ocean Dumping Act was amended in 1977 so that ocean dumping would not be allowed after December 31, 1981. Yet ocean dumping of garbage, sewage, toxic chemicals, radioactive wastes, and medical wastes not only continues but is increasing. When the Act was amended in the 1970s, most people were concerned about the environment. In the 1980s the major concern was the cost of enforcing environmental standards. Now the results from failure to enforce the Ocean Dumping Act are apparent. Paper, boxes, cans, glass bottles, egg cartons, fishing nets, plastic products, syringes, vials of blood, and other debris clutter the shore line. Some beaches have closed because of the health hazard. In addition to the danger to humans, the pollution is endangering wildlife; dolphins, gulls, turtles, shellfish, fish, and sea lions mistake the waste for food or become entangled in the debris (34, 61, 81, 99, 110).

Problems in Water Purification

The common denominator of all major water pollution is called **biologic oxygen demand (BOD),** *the amount of free oxygen that extraneous substances absorb from*

water (61). The natural water purification process involves the action of bacteria, which use oxygen to decompose organic matter. If too much waste is dumped into a given body of water, this natural cleansing process cannot take place or at least does not take place fast enough. Further, once the water in the underground aquifer is contaminated, it is nearly impossible to guarantee a safe water supply.

The ultimate problem of water pollution stems from our using natural resources in greater and greater amounts because of additional industrialization, population growth, a greater dependence on appliances, and a subsequent increase in the need for sewage disposal. The problem of dissolving waste has put a strain on waste-disposal systems. Even excessive amounts of treated waste now obstruct the waterways. Current engineering research is attempting to solve some of the problems of water pollution by developing different types of waste-disposal systems.

When water contains pollutants in ever-increasing amounts, it becomes a threat to human health. At present, the quality of water service for countless people must be improved; many inhabitants of rural areas and small towns obtain their drinking water from polluted sources (21, 44, 61, 85, 129). In several areas of the United States wastewater is being used for irrigation. This water contains low levels of organic chemicals. Although it is considered safe for human use, the water is not meant for drinking purposes; however, indirect human consumption does occur when surface waters are used for water supply (61, 81, 85, 179). Keeping drinking water separate from water for other uses would help conserve water supplies and ensure greater purity, as water used for other purposes could be refiltered at less expense (81, 150).

Pollution of marshes and shorelines has severely impaired breeding habitats for many types of shellfish and deep-water species, thereby subsequently affecting the food supply. Polluted water cannot be used for recreational purposes; backpackers, campers, swimmers, windsurfers, and waterskiers have all felt the impact of water pollution. In addition to the health risk, the odor of decay and the unsightliness of polluted water destroy the beauty of any natural setting.

Misuse of our water has far-reaching consequences, threatening people all over the world from every age group and culture. We must take personal responsibility for stopping needless pollution of the water by exercising careful personal use of agents that can ultimately destroy it and by using legal procedures to prevent undue dumping of wastes into lakes, rivers, and streams. Some health problems associated with contaminated water could be eliminated by proper legislation, and needless sickness and death could be avoided. Such legislation as the Clean Water Act of 1987 and the revised Safe Drinking Water Act of 1986, which promote water quality standards and impose a system of control on all sources of pollution, are effective and worthy of support. More importantly, the health of future generations and their chance to enjoy the beauty, taste, and power of the water depend on those of us who are so carelessly polluting it. Water, like oxygen, is essential to life, development, and health.

SOIL POLLUTION

As early as 1950 the federal Food and Drug Administration announced that the potential health hazards of compounds containing chlorinated hydrocarbons such as dichlorodiphenyltrichloroethane (DDT) had been underestimated. The Federal Environmental Pesticide Control Act, passed in 1972 and amended in 1975 and 1978, requires that all pesticide products sold or distributed in this country must be registered with the EPA (49, 185).

The EPA's pesticide control program has three major components: registration of pesticides, training of pesticide applicators, and monitoring and research. All pesticides must be registered with the agency before being marketed. The agency approves labeling and sets maximum safe levels for pesticide residues in human and animal food. The EPA has developed an applicator training program, certifying individuals permitted to apply restricted-use pesticides. In addition, the agency sponsors research on pesticides and monitors pesticide levels in the environment. Both acute and long-term pesticide effects are considered in the epidemiologic studies (49, 185). See Table 2–3 for a summary of sources, locations, and effects of pesticides (6, 12, 14, 52, 62, 68, 106, 115, 131, 134, 143, 185).

Despite the EPA's efforts, evidence indicates that the EPA receives insufficient funding, and standards are not being followed; long-term effects are yet unknown. According to a report from the National Research Council of the National Academy of Sciences, industrial wastes are being dumped on or pumped into the earth's crust, and few studies are being done to determine whether the sites are safe. It may be possible to contain wastes safely and to lessen toxicity in wastes in the natural systems of the earth if the chemical nature of the waste and the geologic nature of the disposal area are understood. Geologic mapping is needed as a guide to safe disposal sites and for research on reactions between chemicals and rock or soil, fracture patterns in rocks, fluid flow, and hydrodynamics of deep basins (81, 178).

The widespread contamination by **dioxin** in Missouri in 1983 following massive flooding illustrates the complexity and extent of the problem. Chemicals were used without awareness of harmful effect. Unregulated use of chemicals and dumping of various chemicals by industries had occurred for some time and had only become apparent later. Furthermore, chemicals did not remain where originally used or dumped. Flood waters, underground water, and wind transported chemicals or their residues from one soil site to another. People are now learning that their past and present symptoms and diseases are related to or caused by hazardous pollutants in the environment to which they did not know they were being exposed (155).

Dioxin is considered a toxic synthetic complex organic chemical compound. It is insoluble in water but dissolves in organic solvents mixed with water. It is strongly attracted to lipids: fatty tissues in the body, oils, related lipid substances, and soil particles. The chemical remains in lipids or soil for many years and during a flood or soil erosion can move through water with solvents, soil particles, or colloids to which it is attached. Dioxin is also part of many other chemical compounds (e.g., chlorophenols, herbicides, and the antiseptic hexachlorophene). It can be generated by incineration of industrial, commercial, and municipal wastes that contain chlorinated aromatics, chlorophenols, or polychlorinated biphenyls (PCBs) (41, 42, 53, 155, 178).

TABLE 2–3. EFFECTS OF PESTICIDE SOIL POLLUTANTS

Pollutant	Characteristics	Source	Where Found	Effects
Pesticides Insecticides Herbicides Fungicides	Substances used to kill weeds, rats, mice, worms, fungi, and insects	Pesticide manufacturing plants Exposure by inhalation of dust or spray, direct skin contact, ingestion of contaminated food and water, contact with contaminated equipment	Farms Industry Homes Gardens Federal, state, and local agencies Storage bags Spray equipment Surface water contamination by dust or spray Rain washes into streams and lakes, affecting food supply	May be undiagnosed Toxic effects vary, but most remain in soil long periods, causing water, soil, and food pollution, and disease Cholinesterase inhibition Central nervous system depression or stimulation: Forgetfulness Attention impairment Short attention span Anxiety Depression Nervousness Hyperirritability Insomnia Skin rashes and diseases Eye disease Respiratory disease Digestive disorders Reproductive problems Birth defects Cancer Leukemia Destruction of insects, bees, and birds reduces cross-pollination essential in food chain Water pollution from spray, dust, or rain affects food chain Destruction of earthworms and rodents interferes with food cycle for animals and people Farmers, workers in pesticide-manufacturing plants, agricultural workers, commercial pest-control operators are at high risk

Dioxin produces a wide range of harmful effects in animals and humans; some are chronic and long-term (41, 42, 53, 155, 178):

- Liver damage
- Birth defects
- Spontaneous abortions and sterility
- Some types of cancer
- Nerve and brain damage; decreased sensory perception
- Disturbed enzyme production
- Reduced immunity to infections
- Chloracne, a disfiguring and painful affliction of the skin that may last many years
- Damage to the gastrointestinal tract, with weight loss
- Damage to the immune system

Dioxin is not only a problem for residents along rivers outside of St. Louis, Missouri, the scene of much publicity in 1983. Dioxin is a contaminant in Agent Orange, the herbicide sprayed in Vietnam. Many U.S. service personnel and their families were exposed and are suffering a variety of health problems. Where additional sites of dioxin contamination may be found is not yet known, but dioxin is being found in many areas of the United States (41, 178, 180, 188).

FOOD POLLUTION

Some of the same chemicals found in pesticide preparation are used as **food additives**. These purposely used additives are not designed to be toxic but rather to *preserve, improve, and protect nutritional value.*

Although the average person in the United States consumes a significant amount of additives every year, it is difficult to determine the potential health risk over a life span. Certain food additives interfere with intestinal mucosa absorptive ability and therefore affect availability of nutrients and drugs. Also, some nontoxic substances or chemicals used as food additives are metabolized into toxic substances in the body. Adverse reactions to synthetic flavors and colors include gastrointestinal, respiratory, neurologic, skeletal, and skin disorders. Removal of artificial flavors and colors from the diet has been found to reduce hyperkinesis and certain learning disabilities in children with these disabilities (13, 18, 56, 154, 168, 182).

Unexpected side effects have resulted from *antibiotic and hormone residues from drugs given to animals for growth promotion and disease prevention.* In people these residues have resulted in (1) allergy and increased drug toxicity or resistance to pathogens when the *same* family of antibiotics is later administered therapeutically and (2) change of normal bacterial flora in a body area so that invasion by pathogens is more likely, causing infection or disease (170). Synthetic estrogen, diethylstilbestrol (DES), was used in cattle feed to promote rapid weight gain. Studies have linked DES to increases in a rare reproductive tract tumor in young women whose mothers were given DES while pregnant. As a result of these studies, use of DES has been restricted. An attempt to ban its use and the use of other sex hormones as feed supplements is underway (38, 170).

A considerable amount of pesticides is ingested by most families in the United States from eating fruits and vegetables grown in Mexico and the United States where large amounts of chemicals are used repeatedly to control insects, weeds, rodents, and other agricultural pests. The U.S. consumer wants to purchase fruits and vegetables that are without blemish and appear as perfect as a picture. Blight, rust, fungus, or other causes of discoloration can most quickly be controlled by chemical application; however, the farmers are caught in a pesticide treadmill. Each year it takes more and different poisons to accomplish the same task, and the insects continue to produce hybrid strains that are resistant to the chemicals. Even those banned by the EPA in the United States are likely to be used in other countries where they usually are shipped by U.S. chemical manufacturers. Examples of disease-producing chemicals that contaminate foodstuffs include chlordane; toxaphine; 2,4-D; DBCP; paraquat (a small amount on the skin causes asphyxiation); EDBC (a fungicide that breaks down into a potent carcinogen, ETU); aldicarb (methyl isocyanate, which converts to hydrogen cyanide gas, and killed and injured people at Bhopal,

India); and parathion (an organophosphate pesticide so lethal that a tablespoon on the skin is fatal) (114). The pesticide market is so large that production is estimated to equal 1 pound of chemicals annually for every person—men, women, and children—on earth. Although DDT, chlordane, Dieldren, and 2,4,5-T are banned in the United States and Europe, they are sold to many developing countries that are increasingly a source of some of our food products. People in Third World countries do not know how to use chemicals to avoid widespread contamination, and the number of deaths and injuries attributed to agrichemicals in those countries is increasing. For example, in rural Brazil, DDT levels 10 times that considered safe have been found in mother's milk. Ten percent of that population suffers symptoms of mild chronic poisoning. Levels of DDT 90 times higher than that in U.S. milk have been found in milk sold in Guatemala. Stomach and colon cancers have increased five times in African countries where large amounts of agrichemicals have been used. Drinking paraquat has become a popular form of suicide in Sri Lanka and Central and South America, although careless handling causes the most deaths of agricultural workers. In addition to causing human misery, the pesticides and herbicides are ravaging the ecosystems by killing birds, plants, and marine life (106, 115, 131).

Pesticide use could be reduced greatly by using better agricultural techniques (114, 115):

- Crop rotation
- Intercropping—alternating small plots of different plants
- Avoidance of monocropping—planting huge fields of only one crop season after season
- Polyculture—diversifying species within the same crop type
- Providing habitat for beneficial insects
- Selecting plants for their resistance to pests
- Timing planting of crops to avoid pest attacks or to plant them in their optimal climate
- Development of biological controls (some insects and pests are natural predators on other insects and pests)
- Developing improved hardware for safer application when pesticides and herbicides are applied.

Farmers in the United States are decreasing pesticide use (167); however, a toxin often remains in the food chain even after a toxic chemical has been banned because the toxins bioaccumulate in the environment. Chlordane, used widely in the Midwest in the 1970s as a soil insecticide for corn, was banned for that use because studies showed it produced cancer; however, it was allowed until recently to remain in the market as a termiticide. Through groundwater contamination, it has accumulated in the sediments of rivers and lakes. In the spring of 1987, residents of Missouri and other nearby states that receive river flow from Missouri were warned not to eat fish from a number of the Missouri rivers and lakes because the fish were contaminated with chlordane (120).

In St. Louis and the surrounding area, the soil, water, and air remain contaminated from the processing of uranium oxide for the world's first nuclear reaction 45 years ago. Several radioactive waste sites are in the St. Louis metropolitan area. Nearby people live and children play without knowledge of the radioactive levels, the impending danger, or the long-term effects in health development. Only recently have the sites and their potential dangers become known (86).

This situation is not too different from that of residents of the Great Lakes regions: millions of people who live near the Great Lakes have as much as 20% higher levels of toxic chemicals in their bodies than other U.S. residents. Over the years they have ingested many toxins (benzine, hexachloride, PCBs, DDT, toxaphene, mercury) from contaminated water and fish (81, 155).

The effects on present and future generations of the 900 identified leaking hazardous waste sites in the United States remain unknown. Other sites, as yet unidentified, may be contaminating soil and, in turn, water, food, and air (81, 153).

In addition to the additives, synthetic pesticides, and other man-made chemicals that may appear in trace amounts in processed foods, natural toxic compounds are in huge concentrations in the food supply; for example, apples, cabbage, celery, lettuce, peaches, pineapple, and turnips are all considered natural carcinogens. Regulatory agencies pay little attention to the dangers of these natural toxic chemicals (153, 188).

Other food pollution hazards are *radioactive materials* such as strontium 90, which has been traced in milk; mercury found in swordfish; worms; and mold, which may be present without noticeable change in the food's appearance, taste, or smell. Food handlers may introduce their infectious diseases into food by touching it or the equipment with soiled hands or by coughing onto it. Prolonged storage of highly acidic foods in aluminum cookware or aluminum foil may cause more aluminum than usual to enter the body. Using unlined copper utensils for cooking or storing food may also be harmful (72, 170). Food sources may become contaminated by the chemicals and metals used in fertilizers and pesticides. In the future, diseases from food additives may assume as much significance in humans as do the **zoonoses**, *diseases transmitted between animals and humans,* such as trichinosis, brucellosis, tuberculosis, psittacosis, salmonellosis, typhus, roundworms, and rabies (153).

Because of the endless contamination possibilities from bacteria, toxins, viruses, parasites, and protozoa, the Food and Drug Administration and the Department of Agriculture enforce laws passed by Congress, impose various regulations of their own, and, in general, monitor the food industry nationwide. Various state and local authorities also attempt to regulate standards within their respective jurisdictions (51). Yet these agencies cannot possibly determine every breach of regulation.

Astute observations must be made about standards in the food store. Demanding to know the growing, cleansing, processing, and handling procedures is not out of line. Reporting suspected breaches is your responsibility for health.

NOISE POLLUTION

Sensory stimulation plays a major role in psychological and physiologic development and is therefore directly related to physical and mental health. Sound is but one form of sensory stimulation. **Sound overload**, *unwanted sound that produces unwanted effects,* and sound deprivation can be hazards to health (5, 18, 34, 66, 187).

Sound overload can produce temporary or permanent hearing loss by affecting the tympanic membrane, sensory cells in the cochlea, and auditory nerve, and by slowly deteriorating the microscopic cells that send sound waves from the ear to the brain. The effects produced on each person's hearing vary, depending on the sound intensity and pitch, the location of the source in relation to the person, the length of exposure, and the person's age and history of previous ear problems. Hearing can be permanently damaged after only a few intense exposures to noise. Millions of Americans either have measurable hearing deficits or are exposed to occupational noise levels capable of producing permanent hearing loss (5, 18, 66).

One means of determining the potential hazard of any sound is to measure its loudness. The *measurement of sound loudness is stated in* **decibels.** The faintest audible sound is designated 1 decibel; ordinary conversation, measured at 40 to 60 decibels, is considered adequately quiet. The EPA identifies 55 decibels as the level above which harmful effects occur. Studies have shown that moderately loud sounds of 75 to 80 decibels such as those produced by a clothes washer, tabulating machine, or home garbage-disposal unit can be discomforting to human ears and can, over a period, produce temporary or permanent hearing loss. Table 2–4 lists examples of common sound pollutants and their decibel readings. Sound louder than 130 decibels (e.g., that produced by a nearby jet plane, gunshot blast, or a rocket at the launching pad) may cause actual pain (18, 34,

TABLE 2–4 COMMON SOUND POLLUTANTS AND THEIR DECIBEL READINGS

Sound	Decibels
Rustle of leaves	10
Library whisper	30
Normal conversation	60
Electric shaver	60–86
Car	60–90
Office (busy)	70–85
Vacuum cleaner	72–75
Dishwasher	76–96
Minibike	76
Shop tools	80–95
Loud street noise	80–100
Alarm clock	80
Video arcade	80–105
Subway	80–114
Snowmobile	85–120
Heavy city traffic	90–95
Food blender in home	93
Pneumatic hammer	95
Air compressor	95
Power lawnmower	80–95
Dirt bike	95
Farm tractor	98
Chain saw	100–110
Outboard motor	102
Jet flying at 1000 ft	103
Ambulance siren	105
Stereo headset	110
Riveting gun	110
Jackhammer	113
Motorcycle	115
Live rock music	120
Firearm	130–140
Jet plane at takeoff	150
Rocket engine	180

174). Persons who work regularly with any of the machines listed should realize the potential long-range effects of such noise levels.

The Noise Control Act was passed in 1972 and amended in 1978 as the Quiet Communities Act. Under this Act the EPA set noise emission standards for the transportation vehicles and products that are major sources of noise. The Act also provides for research into the psychological and physiologic effects of noise on people. State and local governments have been given primary responsibility for enforcing these standards (119). The Occupational Safety and Health Administration (OSHA) requires hearing protectors be provided to workers who are exposed for 8 hours to a noise level of 85 decibels or higher. There are no regulations for recreational noise, which may be hazardous (5).

Effects of Noise Pollution

Sound overload affects everyone at some time by intruding on privacy and shattering serenity. In addition to hearing loss, it can produce impaired communication and social relationships, irritability, chronic headache, tinnitus, insomnia, depression, fatigue, and tension. Noise has also been associated with elevated blood cholesterol levels, atherosclerosis, and accident proneness. Research indicates that less obvious physiologic changes in the digestive, cardiovascular, endocrine, and nervous systems also can occur. These changes can produce blood vessel constriction, pallor, dilated pupils and visual disturbance, increased and irregular heart rate, hypertension, headache, gastrointestinal spasm with nausea and diarrhea and eventual peptic ulcer, hyperactive reflexes, and muscle tenseness. These responses do not subside immediately but continue up to five times longer than the actual noise (16, 174). Humans do not adapt to excessive sound, as was once thought, but learn to tolerate it. Even when a person is asleep, noise cannot be shut out completely. He or she awakens exhausted by the efforts to sleep in the midst of excessive external stimuli. Awareness of environmental stress factors can aid an individual to reduce or cope with them.

Although not every harmful form of sound can be avoided, certain measures can decrease the risk of hearing loss:

- Wear protective ear coverings.
- Shorten exposure time.
- Have regular hearing examinations.
- Seek immediate medical attention for any ear injury or infection.
- Wear ear plugs when exposed to loud noise for a long time or intense sound even for a short time.
- Use sound-absorbing materials to reduce noise at home and at work.
- Do not use several noisy machines at one time.
- Do not drown out unwanted noise with other noise.

You can educate the public about the hazards of excess noise and ways to reduce noise in the home environment:

- Hang heavy drapes over windows closest to outside noise sources.
- Use foam pads under mixers and blenders.
- Use carpeting in areas of heavy foot traffic.
- Use upholstered instead of hard-surfaced furniture.
- Install sound-absorbing ceiling tile in the kitchen.

The hospital, considered a place to recuperate and rest, may actually contribute to symptoms because of the noise levels in certain areas. Noise levels in infant incubators, the recovery room, and acute care units are high enough to act as a stressor and stimulate the hypophyseal-adrenocortical axis. Peripheral vasoconstriction affecting blood pressure and pulse, threats to hearing loss in patients receiving aminoglycosidic antibiotics, and sleep deprivation may occur. Noise pollution in the operating room, causing vasoconstriction, pupil dilation, fatigue, and impaired speech communication, has also been found.

SURFACE POLLUTION

Until the mid-1960s U.S. residents were not concerned with problems of waste disposal or recycling. Raw materials were plentiful, and the open-dump method of disposal was convenient and economical. In the early 1970s, however, people became more concerned with the decreasing supply of natural resources and the health problems created by open dumps.

The Solid Waste Disposal Act was passed by Congress in 1965. The primary focus of this act was on the disposal of waste, not collection or street cleaning. In 1970 Congress passed the Resource Recovery Act, which shifted the emphasis of federal involvement from disposal to recycling, resource recovery, and the conversion of waste into energy. Subsequent laws such as the Resource Conservation and Recovery Act of 1976 have been passed to facilitate further the safe disposal of waste (51).

The total quantity of solid waste is large and increasing. Every day the average American generates approximately $3\frac{1}{2}$ pounds of trash. More than 160 million tons of solid wastes per year, not including sludge, construction debris, factory wastes, and dumped cars, are produced in the United States (65). Most present disposal methods for this waste pollute land, air, or water. This pollution appears many places: in open air, foul-smelling dumps, smoking incineration centers, junkyards, and poorly covered landfills.

Solid-Waste Disposal Methods

Solid waste is discarded in four basic ways: (1) in open dumps, (2) in landfills, (3) by incineration, and (4) as salvage.

Open Dumps

The open dump (now illegal in most states) is the oldest, most convenient, and most economical method. It creates many health problems, however, and is esthetically undesirable. Dumps serve as breeding grounds for rodents, flies, and other insects such as cockroaches; they also attract seagulls, notorious as thieves and litterers. Houseflies carry poliomyelitis, tuberculosis, diarrhea, dysentery, hepatitis, and cholera. Rats carry plague, tapeworm, Rocky Mountain spotted fever, and rat-bite fever. Water running off from these dumps pollutes local streams and lakes. Rain and surface water can seep through the wastes and pollute underground water. Any attempt to burn the surface waste in the dumps emits large quantities of foul-smelling fumes that increase air pollution and thus respiratory problems among local inhabitants. Dumps invite accidents and fires in addition to lowering the value of surrounding property (81, 99).

Landfills

Landfills are the final destination for 80 to 86% of the trash generated in the United States. Of the total amount of trash in a landfill, 35.6% is paper, 20.1% is yard wastes, 8.9% is food wastes, 8.7% is metal, 7.3% is plastics, and 8.4% is glass. Many of these materials are biodegradable; they are reduced to their basic components through natural actions of the environment (6, 11, 65, 81, 99).

Landfills are not the answer to the problem of surface pollution. In fact, landfills are closing at the rate of almost one a day. Some older landfills are closing because they are full. Others are being closed because they leak toxic fluids. Even though landfills, especially sanitary landfills, are more acceptable than open dumps, they can produce dangerous health hazards. Local groundwater can be contaminated by chemical mixtures that leak out of the landfill area. In addition, as the trash ferments, methane gas is produced. When this gas accumulates, explosions and spontaneous combustion can occur. The methane gas can also migrate underground and kill nearby vegetation (81, 91, 99).

When handled properly, landfills can be economical, sanitary, and aesthetically acceptable. Landfills should be placed far from water sources, and the waste should be quickly covered to avoid foul smells, spontaneous combustion, breeding of rats and flies, and scavenging by rodents.

Incineration

A significant amount of household solid wastes is combustible and therefore suitable for incineration. Decentralized incineration is usually poorly controlled and frequently produces gaseous emissions and particulates that pollute the air and damage our health. Central incineration conducted by federal, state, or local governmental bodies is expensive, although necessary for large urban areas. The controlled-combustion process used in these centers prevents the emission of harmful gases and uses the by-product, heat, for an energy source. Through incineration, the volume of waste can be reduced by 90% of its original bulk. The remaining material can be removed to landfills or compressed for use in soil conditioners or construction material (34, 91, 99).

Salvage

The composition of solid waste has changed in past years; today it includes larger amounts of paper, plastics, aluminum cans, and other packaging and wrapping materials. Many such materials will not decompose or rust; therefore they present new problems in disposal. If these products are *salvaged*, they can be **recycled**, *treated by mechanical, thermal, or biologic means so that they can be used again*, thus promoting resource recovery and reuse (81, 99, 125).

Hazardous-Waste Disposal

The EPA has defined **hazardous waste** as *discarded material that may pose a threat or hazard to human health or the environment*. These wastes can be solids, liquids, sludges, or gases. They are toxic, ignitable, corrosive, infectious, reactive (react with air, water, or other substances, resulting in explosions and toxic fumes), or radioactive. It is estimated that 10 to 15% of all garbage produced in the United States is considered hazardous (30, 47, 91, 99, 104, 176, 178). According to the EPA, the United States generates approximately 300 million tons of hazardous waste annually (99).

Although most hazardous wastes are generated by the manufacturing industries, the Armed Forces, with their obsolete explosives, herbicides, and nerve gases, contribute significantly to the total volume. Hospitals, medical research laboratories, mining operations, ser-

vice stations, retailers, and householders also contribute to the problem of hazardous-waste production. Only a small percent of the hazardous waste currently generated is disposed of in an environmentally sound manner. The rest threatens our water and air quality and our water and land ecosystems. The EPA has identified approximately 1200 sites where improper disposal of hazardous wastes has occurred. These sites are on a priority list for cleanup action (34, 187).

Hazardous wastes can become a threat to human health in various ways: direct exposure of persons at or near the disposal site; direct exposure to persons as a result of accidents during transportation of the wastes; exposure to polluted air during improperly controlled incineration; and contamination of groundwater and food (34, 187).

In an attempt to prevent such happenings and to protect U.S. citizens from the dangers of hazardous waste, The Comprehensive Environmental Response, Compensation and Liability Act was passed in 1980. One objective of this Act was to establish a fund—Superfund—for the purpose of responding to emergency situations involving hazardous substances and of performing remedial cleanups. In 1986 a new Superfund was established and the program strengthened. After 13 years, however, less than 15% of the waste sites are fully cleaned, although more than $30 billion has been spent (52, 126).

Nuclear Waste

One type of hazardous-waste product that has attracted considerable attention is radioactive waste. Some fission products that must be stored are cesium-137, strontium-90, iodine-131, and plutonium-239. Some decay rapidly in hours or days, whereas others require thousands and millions of years to lose their radioactive potency. No satisfactory method of permanent disposal has been developed; the cost and fear of leakage from the storage area have been stumbling blocks (116).

The use of nuclear energy or power produced by fission reactors has caused much concern and debate among the people of the United States. The concerns center around two major issues: the long-term disposal of radioactive wastes and the safety of the actual reactors.

When a utility shuts down a reactor at the end of its period of usefulness, the utility is faced with the problem of what to do with intensely radioactive materials. At present, only three means of disposal exist: dismantlement of the reactor with the debris shipped to a burial site; entombment of the reactor in a concrete structure; and protective storage that would prevent public access for 30 to 100 years. Even though nuclear power is a quarter-century old, the problem of safe disposal of radioactive waste has not been solved.

The seriousness of problems associated with the safety of nuclear reactors for generating electricity is well illustrated by the following highly publicized events. In Pennsylvania in March, 1979, an accident occurred at the nuclear reactor site known as Three Mile Island. In retrospect, the accident was preventable and was less severe than originally reported. It is estimated that residents near the site were exposed to 0.10 rad, the equivalent of four x-ray studies (95). The major health effect of the accident was on the mental health of the people in the region. Another accident occurred in April, 1986, at a nuclear power plant at Chernobyl in the former Soviet Union. A fire in the plant's nuclear reactor sent a cloud of deadly radiation into the air. Some people in the plant died immediately, and hundreds of people in the vicinity developed radiation sickness. Contamination was so severe that the escaped radiation was detected around the world by monitoring devices (91, 145).

The fear, anger, and confusion felt by the Three Mile Island and Chernobyl communities are shared nationally and internationally. The majority of citizens now have serious second thoughts about the safety and reliability of nuclear power (95, 187). Diminishing resources lead to the need for alternative energy sources such as coal and the sun. The problems in this area must be explored.

Hospital Waste

The amount of solid waste produced by hospitals should be a primary concern to health workers. The average citizen accumulates and disposes of many pounds of solid waste daily. The average hospital patient also accumulates many pounds of solid waste daily. Hospitals add tons of pathologic materials yearly to the waste load. This increase in hospital wastes can be attributed to the increase in disposable products: syringes, needles, surgical supplies, styrene dishes and utensils, various plastic products, linens, uniforms, and medication containers. Many hospitals use disposable products because they are considered cheaper, easier to store, and less likely to produce cross-infection. Yet hospitals often fail to consider the cost or inconvenience of transporting or discarding large quantities of these contaminated objects. In the past, much of a hospital's solid waste, often contaminated by infectious organisms, was removed to open dumps or sanitary landfills without proper initial sterilization, thus spreading pathogens to land, water, and air (54, 153). Most hospital workers did

not consider the implications of casually using disposable items (153, 171); however, the laws have been tightened on the disposal of infectious and related waste. The mandates and consequent fines for not following the mandates have made a significant difference in this issue (see Fig. 2–3).

One study conducted in an urban area with 16 participating hospitals revealed that the nurse influences decisions about the purchase of patient care items more than any other hospital worker. If these decisions are largely your responsibility, know how much trash your hospital creates, where the waste goes, the decontamination procedures used before disposal, the cost of disposal, why your agency uses disposable products, and how much your agency contributes to environmental pollution. Form an interdepartmental committee, perhaps of administrators, nurses, doctors, and patients. Report your findings to them, and together consider all the advantages and drawbacks of various products. Consider cost, convenience, infection control, and quality. Give each new product a careful clinical trial and adopt it for use only after careful consideration about contributions to patient care. Avoid using disposable items if nondisposables will do the job as well. Pass this information on to the patients and families. Encourage health workers in homes to demonstrate and teach proper disposal of such items as syringes and dressings, especially at this time of increasing incidence of infectious diseases, including AIDS. Work to reduce the huge volume of solid waste that is taking space and depleting natural resources (54, 80) and for disposal of infectious wastes in non-air-polluting incinerators, which many cities and hospitals do not have.

The effectiveness of nonpolluting incinerator conversion of trash into hot gases, which then transforms water into steam, has been demonstrated for years by St. Louis University Hospital, St. Louis, Missouri. The Hospital's incinerator conversion project, which heats and cools the entire St. Louis University Medical Center and also sterilizes all hospital equipment, received national attention at the U.S. Department of Energy's Technology Transfer 80's Program. The hospital received a national award for the project from the Department of Energy in November 1984.

Lead Poisoning

Lead is another surface pollutant. The two principal routes of exposure to lead are ingestion and inhalation. Sources contributing to the ingestion of lead are lead-based paint chips or flakes, lead solder in plumbing, lead solder in seams of food cans, lead from dietary sources that were contaminated while being grown or

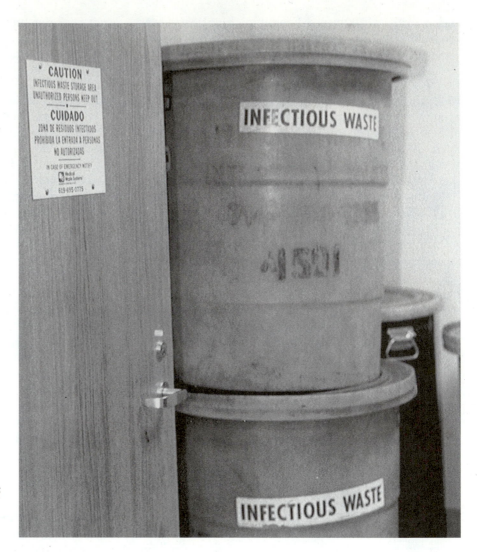

Figure 2–3. Hospitals accumulate large amounts of infectious wastes, which pose a health hazard if not stored and disposed of properly. *(Photograph by Patrick Watson.)*

cooked, lead from improperly glazed earthenware or ceramic ware, and lead-contaminated "moonshine." Sources contributing to the inhalation of lead are leaded gasoline, contaminated dust or soil particles, cigarette smoke, and industrial sites such as battery plants. Since the airborne levels of lead significantly decreased (87% between 1975 and 1986) with the phaseout of leaded gasoline, other sources of lead are being closely studied (18, 28, 91, 93, 127, 142, 174).

Although lead poisoning is seen most frequently in children from inner cities, no economic or racial subgroup of children is exempt from lead toxicity. Children in some ethnic groups are exposed to lead through folk remedies used by their families; other children living in the "lead belt" (i.e., cities of the Northeast and Midwest) are especially at risk.

Another urgent problem arises when young children, mainly in urban slums, form the *habit of eating nonfood substances, including peeling paint, plaster, or putty containing lead, a behavior called* **pica.** The precise cause of pica is not completely understood, but it may be related to nutritional, cultural, and emotional factors. Acute or chronic lead poisoning, an insidious disease, results from this eating pattern and is a major source of brain damage, mental deficiency, and behavior problems. The pathologic changes that occur affect the nervous, renal, and hematopoietic systems. Kidney damage is usually reversible, but chronic lead poisoning in childhood may lead to gout or kidney disease later in life. Damage to the hematopoietic system is evident by the reduction in the number and quality of red blood cells produced, thus leading to severe anemia. The most serious effects are on the nervous system (7, 24, 28, 93, 142).

Although the trend apparently is toward reduced lead screening, child health programs should consider routine screening of all children from 1 to 5 years of age, as high blood levels of lead have been found in children in all areas (141). Reduction of leaded gasoline and establishment of autoemissions standards set by the EPA have been steps in the right direction.

OCCUPATIONAL HAZARDS

Increasingly we learn of the health hazards that many workers face daily at their jobs. Monotony, paced work, and performance pressures are major sources of stress in many jobs and can contribute to disease pathology. The muscle strains, backaches, fractures, burns, eye injuries, and other accidental emergencies are taken for granted by the public. But workers may not suffer the consequences of the hidden environmental hazards—the chemicals or radiation they work with directly or indirectly—until years later. Often in the past the cause of the physical illness remained unsolved. Not only do

miners and factory workers become ill because of their work environment, hospital workers also may suffer. Those who work regularly with certain anesthetics, for example, may develop cancer, leukemia, or lymphoma. Those who work with high levels of radiation risk sterility or defective offspring if adequate protection is not maintained. Nurses may suffer infections, back and muscle injuries, varicose veins, and any of the other physical or emotional effects of stress.

The Occupational Safety and Health Act of 1970, the Coal Mine Health and Safety Act of 1969, and the Toxic Substances Control Act of 1976 are some of the laws passed by Congress that have been responsible for making occupational safety and health a public health concern rather than a private matter. Through these laws the federal government works to prevent work-related accidents and disease, to correct hazardous working conditions, to promote good health for working men

Research Abstract

Kelter, J., Latex Allergies on the Rise Among Health Care Workers, The American Nurse, January–February (1995), 8.

The Occupational Safety and Health Administration has collected information about and held hearings on the hazards of latex from workers in various health professions and geographic areas. Latex is found in surgical gloves, catheters, intubation tubes, enema tips, and anesthesia masks.

Up to 17% of health care workers may exhibit some allergic reaction to extended latex exposure; persons with acute reactions are no longer able to work. Constant exposure to latex is reported to cause various symptoms: contact dermatitis, itching, runny nose, conjunctivitis, sneezing, wheezing, asthma, and fatal anaphylaxis. The cornstarch powder in latex gloves causes dispersion of latex proteins into the air and provides a respiratory route of exposure in addition to skin exposure to offending proteins. Once sensitization to latex has occurred, individuals often react to latex products commonly found in the home, such as latex rubber in clothing and shoes, balloons, rubber bands, and automobile parts. Department stores and grocery stores contain many latex products as well.

All workers who have regular contact with latex products must protect themselves from sensitization through the following strategies:

1. Use vinyl gloves or low-protein gloves that are powder-free or lightly powdered.
2. Wash hands after wearing gloves.
3. Report symptoms of contact dermatitis immediately and pursue determination of the causative agent.
4. Do not use oil-based emollients with glove use, as this significantly increases the absorption of latex proteins and can increase sensitization.
5. The worker who is latex sensitive has a right to have an alternative product made available for use.

Societal implications of the data gathered so far are for hospitals and other health care settings to test and use nonlatex alternative products. The Food and Drug Administration should fulfill its promises to require all manufacturers to label all products containing latex and to develop guidelines about safe protein levels and manufacturing processes.

Health care implications include asking patients/clients during the assessment, or history, about latex sensitivity, to wear nonlatex gloves over latex gloves to protect patients, and to be aware of one's own possible sensitivity.

and women, and to improve compensation. The Occupational Safety and Health Act established the Occupational Safety and Health Administration, which conducts inspections of industries to force compliance and research to establish the hazardous levels of various chemicals. Relatively few of the many chemicals in industry have been researched, but the standards and prevention and treatment measures are published periodically in the *Federal Register,* which can be obtained from the Department of Labor.

The Occupational Safety and Health Act has forced industries to become more active in seeking health services for employees and has assisted the occupational health nurse to offer additional services related to disease prevention and education of employees (28). Health screening is also being emphasized, for contamination from some substances can be detected early enough to prevent disease.

To promote early screening and prevent long-term effects of noise pollution on hearing, the *Federal Register* publishes updated guidelines on occupational hearing conservation. Basically, each hearing program must consist of five parts:

1. Employee education (each employee must be told the significance of the program)
2. An analysis of the noise in the workplace, now required every 2 years or as noise levels change
3. Engineering and administrative controls (environmental noise must be altered if possible)
4. Audiometric testing (all employees exposed to 85 decibels or more [over a period of 8 hours] must be tested yearly and before employment)
5. Personal protective equipment (a variety of hearing protectors must be available)

Along with these guidelines are specific requirements for those who administer and interpret tests, circumstances in which tests are administered, and instruments for measuring noise levels and hearing.

Another group of health hazards are related to the large cosmetics industry in the United States. Aerosol preparations, hair dyes, and feminine sprays increasingly are related to skin and other diseases, including cancer. As with other occupational chemicals, effects of the use of these products are usually not known until years after their regular usage (28,191).

Often occupational hazards are taken for granted. They are seen as part of the job. Employees in laundry and dry cleaning establishments, for example, suffer hazards of excess heat, humidity, and noise; falls and accidents from slipping on wet floors; back injury and muscle strains from lifting; and circulatory problems from standing. Janitorial workers may have contact with

dangerous chemicals in cleaning agents. Asthma is an occupational hazard for animal workers, veterinarians, farmers, bakers, carpenters, welders, and many other workers.

Industrial nurses and safety engineers emphasize wearing protective clothing and using protective equipment. Yet there are problems. The employee may not want to be bothered with cumbersome protective clothing; or the protective clothing and equipment given to a female worker may be too large and heavy and thus be ill-fitting and not protective, for they are designed for the male employee. (A few companies do specialize in protective clothing designed for females.) Hard hats, safety shoes and gloves, and ear muffs that fit improperly may actually contribute toward an accidental injury.

To compound the problem of prevention, length of exposure to an industrial substance often determines if it will cause disease. The amount of exposure to the worker often depends on the production phase involved. Additionally, each substance appears likely to produce a disease such as cancer in a specific body part; such information becomes available after workers become ill. Sex is also a factor, for some substances affect the reproductive organs of the female (or fetus) but do not affect the male. Some substances do not affect the male reproductive organs, but the father's genes may contribute to fetal damage.* Each year an estimated 10,000 American workers die of work-related injuries.

In a review of death certificates of 348 Texas women whose deaths resulted from injury at work, the median age of the women at death was 37 years (range, 17–92 years), resulting in a premature loss (death before age 65) of 9078 potential years of life. Homicide was the leading cause of death (53%), followed by injuries from motor vehicles, falls, fires and flames, machinery or tools, explosions, and other causes. Injuries from firearms caused 70% of the homicides. The remaining homicides were caused by injuries from cutting or piercing instruments, strangulation, drowning, and other means. The retail trade industry had the highest workplace homicide rate. Three retail trade subindustries had especially high workplace homicide rates: gasoline service stations; food-bakery-and-dairy stores, and eating-and-drinking places. Of the occupations, female drivers of heavy trucks had the highest fatal occupational injury rate, with motor vehicle incidents accounting for 89% of their fatal injuires. Three oc-

---

*Information about health hazards for female employees and preventive or corrective measures is available from the Woman's Occupational Health Resource Center, American Health Foundation, 320 East 43rd Street, New York, NY 10017.

cupations had markedly elevated workplace homicide rates: stock handlers and baggers, food counter and fountain workers, and supervisors and proprietors in sales occupations. Of the 85 confirmed workplace homicides, 47% occurred during robberies, 7% during arguments between victims and customers, 21% in other known circumstances, and 25% in unknown circumstances. The offenders were either of unknown relationships or strangers to the victims in 71% of the homicides; spouses or other intimate acquaintances in 16% of the homicides; customers in 8% of the homicides; and co-workers in 5% of the homicides. Injuries from firearms caused 81% of the confirmed workplace homicides. Similar results have been found in studies in Wisconsin and Maryland; however, these studies probably underestimate fatal occupational injuries of women (39, 40).

Studies of causes of occupationally related death in California and Texas showed a higher percentage of homicides, particularly for police, security guards, taxi drivers, supervisors or clerks in gas stations, and waiters in food and dairy stores and eating and drinking places. In California homicide rates for females were highest among service occupations (eating and drinking places). Firearms accounted for 77% of all work-related homicides. Workers 65 years or older were at higher risk for homicide than younger workers. Homicides are more likely to occur between 3 PM and 3 AM (39, 40, 90).

Controlling exposures of high-risk individuals and developing strict standards for reducing such exposures (e.g., handgun control laws) might greatly reduce assaults and prevent senseless loss of life in the workplace. Employees in food-bakery-and-dairy stores are a high-risk group. The number of homicide-related robberies in convenience stores can be reduced by making the cash register area more visible from the street; by making it known that as little money as possible is kept in the cash register; by using a drop safe into which, at night, all bills of value greater than $1 are placed; and by keeping the store clean of potential hiding places. Bulletproof barriers between the driver and passenger compartments in taxicabs, enclosed cashier booths in gasoline service stations, and protective vests for law-enforcement officers and private-security personnel are other possible techniques to prevent workplace homicides. The extent to which these techniques are already practiced and their efficacy at preventing these homicides, however, are unknown (39, 90).

Hazards of the factory or mine can extend beyond the workplace and endanger the workers' families and other residents of the community. Workers carry out dust particles on skin and clothing; wind currents also deposit particles. Even if workers shower before leaving work, the total removal of all dust particles of some chemicals or elements is difficult. As a result, some communities become known for a high incidence of certain types of cancer or skin or respiratory disease.

Knowing that the worker may come in contact with a variety of harmful substances and that presenting symptoms may often seem unrelated to the occupation should help you be more thorough and careful in assessment. Also, as a citizen you can work for enforcement of preventive measures for known hazards and for continued research.

Table 2–5 summarizes common industrial agents (various substances, elements, or chemicals) and their major known effects. Refer to the references at the end of the chapter for more information (3, 23, 26, 38, 46, 54, 70, 71, 76, 86, 91, 107, 111–113, 120, 132, 137, 161–163, 171, 172, 186).

Excessive heat, cold, humidity, sunlight, noise, and/or vibration are health hazards in many occupations. Examples are listed below. These hazards are further aggravated by smoking or alcohol or drug abuse in these occupations (132):

Agriculture	Highway/street construction
Airlines	
Auto mechanics	Laundry
Commercial fishing	Lumbering/sawmill operations
Construction	Meat butchering/wrapping
Cosmetology	
Dry cleaning	Mining
Extermination	Painting
Factory assembly line production	Police/security
	Postal
Firefighting	Shipping industry
Forestry	Shipyard
Foundry/smelter	Transportation
Garden/nursery	Welding
Gasoline station	Woodworking

Other occupational hazards exist for women and men. Clerical and other workers who regularly use video display terminals and computers have higher stress-related illnesses, more eyestrain, neck and back strain, headaches, and greater emotional burnout (161).

► HEALTH CARE AND NURSING APPLICATIONS

Global Responsibility

In maturing countries, people are again focusing on the fundamentals: redefining goals and values, supporting the family, working cooperatively to achieve a healthier

TABLE 2–5. EFFECTS OF SOME COMMON INDUSTRIAL AGENTS ON THE WORKER

Agent	Type of Industry or Occupation	Body Area Affected
Acetaldelhyde	Chemical; paint	All body cells, especially brain and respiratory tract
Acetic anhydride	Textile	Exposed tissue damage, especially eye and respiratory tract (ulceration, irritation)
Acetylene	Welding; plastic; dry cleaning	Respiratory tract asphyxiant; explosive, especially when combined with certain substances
Acrolein	Chemical	Skin. Eye. Respiratory tract
Allyl chloride	Plastic	Skin. Respiratory tract. Kidney
Ammonia	Chemical; leather; wool; farmers; refrigeration workers	Eyes. Skin. Respiratory tract (ulceration, irritation)
Anesthetic gases (leakage from equipment, exhalation of patients)	Surgical nurses; medical, hospital, dental, veterinary workers	Reproductive organs (spontaneous abortions, infertility, congenital abnormalities and cancer whether male or female exposure) Neurologic system (drowsy, irritable, headache) Respiratory tract (infections, cancer)
Aniline	Paint; rubber; dye manufacture	Skin. Hematopoietic system. Respiratory system
Arsenic	Mines; smelters; leather; chemical; oil refinery; ship builders; insecticide and pesticide makers and sprayers; pottery workers; agriculture; brass and bronze makers	Skin (ulcerations, cancer) Lung. Liver (cancer) Neurologic damage. Gastrointestinal symptoms Reproductive system (birth defects, chromosome alterations); if acute exposure, death in 1–7 days
Asbestos	Brake mechanics; mines; textiles; insulation; paint; sheet metal workers; shipyard workers; construction; plastics; pipe fitters; maintenance workers; millers; present on city streets	Respiratory tract (cancer, asbestosis, bronchitis, emphysema). Laryngeal cancer. Gastrointestinal tract (cancer) More harmful to people who smoke
Benzene	Rubber; chemicals; explosives; paints and paint strippers; shoemakers; dye users; office workers; chemists; hospital workers; solvent cleaner users; coke oven workers; furniture finishers; artists; degreasers	Skin. Liver. Brain (carcinogenic). Respiratory system Hematopoietic system (anemia, leukemia). Reproductive system (chromosome mutations in males, menstrual irregularities, stillbirths)
Beryllium	Foundry; metallurgic; aerospace; nuclear; household appliance; production, metal cans; shipbuilding	Skin and eye (inflammation, ulcers). Respiratory tract (acute inflammation and berylliosis—chronic lung infection). Systemic effects on heart, liver, spleen, kidneys
Butyl alcohol	Lacquer; paint	Eye. Skin. Respiratory tract
Cadmium	Smelters; storage battery workers; silver industry; plastics; dental; pigment makers; artists; electrical workers; households (silver cleaner, ice cube trays); plating; alloys	Gastrointestinal tract (irritation, cancer). Reproductive system (decreased sperm, impotence). Kidney Respiratory Tract. Hematopoietic system
Carbon disulfide	Rubber; viscose rayon workers; plastics; soil treaters; wax, glue, or resin makers; medical; laboratory workers; agriculture	Gastrointestinal tract. Cardiovascular. Liver. Kidney. Brain Reproductive system (decreased sperm, decreased libido, impotence, infertility, menstrual changes, stillbirth, spontaneous abortion)
Carbon tetrachloride	Solvent; dry cleaning; paint; chemical laboratory; household (fire extinguishers)	Skin. Gastrointestinal tract. Liver. Kidney. Bladder Brain. Respiratory tract (irritation and carcinogen)
Chemotherapy (antineoplastic) medications	Medical; nurses	Skin and cornea (irritation, ulcers). Reproductive system (fetal damage, cancer). Liver and other organs (may be carcinogenic) (some need special handling; effects vary with specific agent)
Chlorine	Industrial bleaching; laundry; chemical industries; swimming pool maintenance	Eyes. Respiratory tract. Skin (irritation, ulcerations, infections, cancer) Skin discoloration (orange)
Chloroform (chlorinated hydrocarbons)	Chemical; plastics; dry cleaners; drug workers; electronic equipment workers; insect control	Heart degeneration. Liver. Kidney. Reproductive system (infertility male and female). Brain. Skin

(continued)

TABLE 2–5. EFFECTS OF SOME COMMON INDUSTRIAL AGENTS ON THE WORKER (continued)

Agent	Type of Industry or Occupation	Body Area Affected
Chromium	Chrome plating; chemical; industrial bleaching; glass and pottery; linoleum makers; battery makers; metal cans and coatings	Irritating to all body cells, skin, eye, respiratory tract (cancer, ulcerations), liver, kidney
Cleaning agents, solvents	Maintenance workers; painters; households	Respiratory tract (irritation, allergy, asthma, cancer) Eyes (irritation, ulcers) Skin (ulcers, dermatosis, cancer)
Coal cumbustion products (soot, tar, coal tar products)	Gashouse workers; asphalt, coal tar, or pitch workers; coke oven workers; mines; plastics; roofers; waterproofers; metal coating workers; ship building	Skin. Respiratory tract. Larynx. Gastrointestinal tract Scrotum. Urinary tract. Bladder (carcinogenic to all areas) Hyperpigmentation of skin
Cotton, flax, hemp, lint	Textile	Respiratory tract (byssinosis—chest tightness, dyspnea, cough, wheezing; chronic bronchitis) Cigarette smokers especially affected
Creosol	Chemical; oil refining	Denatures and precipitates all cellular protein Skin. Eye. Respiratory Tract. Liver. Kidney Brain
Dichloroethyl ether	Insecticide; oil refining	Respiratory tract
Dimethyl sulfate	Chemical; pharmaceutical	Eye. Respiratory tract. Liver. Kidney. Brain
Dyes	Dyeworkers	Urinary bladder (cancer)
Ethylene oxide	Hospital workers (sterilization); workers using epoxyresins	Skin. Eyes (infection, ulcers, burns) Neurologic system (drowsy, weak). Leukemia; lymphoma Respiratory tract (dyspnea, cyanosis, pulmonary edema, cancer) Gastrointestinal tract (vomiting, cancer) Reproductive organs (chromosome damage, spontaneous abortion, fetal damage, infertility—male and female)
Exhaust fumes	Mechanics; gas station and garage workers	Respiratory tract. Urinary bladder (cancer)
Formaldehyde	Laboratory workers; medical (cold sterilization); mechanics; textile; home insulators; mobile home owners; households (wet-strength paper towels, permanent press clothing, foam insulation)	Liver. Lung. Skin (infection, ulcers, cancer) Eye, nose, throat (irritation) Neurologic system (headache, fatigue, memory loss, nausea) Reproductive tract (gene mutation)
Freon	Refrigeration; aerosol propellants	Respiratory tract. Cardiovascular system
Fungus, parasites, microorganisms	Food; animal; outdoor workers; clinical laboratory workers	Skin. Respiratory tract (infection, including hepatitis B)
Germicidal agents	Health care providers; maintenance/cleaning workers	Skin (contact allergy, dermatosis)
Hydrogen chloride	Meat wrappers	Respiratory tract (irritation and asthma)
Hydrogen sulfide	Mines; oil wells; refineries; sewers	Respiratory tract (respiratory paralysis in high concentrations). Eye
Iron oxide	Mine, iron foundry; metal polishers and finishers	Respiratory tract (cancer). Larynx
Lead	Auto; smelters; plumbing; paint; metallurgic; battery workers; paint; plumbers; plastics; pottery; ceramics; gasoline station attendants; electronics; manufacture; shipbuilding; shoemakers; households; exposure in 120 industries	Hematopoietic. Cardiovascular (hypertension) Liver. Kidney. Central nervous system and brain (behavioral change). Muscles; bone. Gastrointestinal tract. Reproductive system (decreased sperm count, chromosome mutation, causes fetal damage or spontaneous abortion during first trimester of pregnancy, infertility—male and female, stillbirth, impotency, menstrual irregularities)
Leather	Leather; shoe	Nasal cavity and sinuses. Urinary bladder (carcinogenic). Larynx
Lye	Households (drain openers, oven and other cleaners)	Eyes (corneal ulceration) Skin (ulcerations) Respiratory tract (irritation)
Manganese	Mine; metallurgic; welders; shipbuilding	Respiratory tract. Liver. Brain

(continued)

TABLE 2–5. EFFECTS OF SOME COMMON INDUSTRIAL AGENTS ON THE WORKER (continued)

Agent	Type of Industry or Occupation	Body Area Affected
Mercury	Electrical and laboratory workers; dye makers; explosives; drug workers; plastics; paint; pesticide workers; households; exposure in 80 different types of industries	Toxic to all cells. Skin (ulcers, dermatosis, hyperpigmentation). Respiratory tract. Liver Brain damage. Reproductive system (infertility — male and female, spontaneous abortions, birth defects). Reduced vision. Psychic changes Exposure of pregnant women causes congenital defects and retardation in child
Methylene chloride	Paint removers	Respiratory tract (irritant, carcinogen). Skin. Eye. Liver. Brain. Cardiac. Gastrointestinal tract
Mica	Rubber; insulation	Respiratory tract
Naphthalene	Textile cleaners	Larynx (cancer). Eyes. Lungs.
Nickel	Metallurgic; smelter; electrolysis workers	Skin. Respiratory tract (infection and cancer). Reproductive tract
Nitric acid	Chemical industries; electroplaters; jewelers; lithographers	Skin (ulcerations, orange discoloration) Eye (ulcerations)
Nitrobenzene	Synthetic dyes	Skin. Hematopoietic system. Brain
Nitrogen dioxide	Chemical; metal; arc welding; explosives; silos	Eye. Respiratory tract. Hematopoietic system
Organophosphates (pesticides; insecticides)	Agriculture; pesticide manufacturers and sprayers; exterminators	Reproductive system (congenital anomalies) Brain dysfunction and neurologic damage (memory loss, disorientation, ataxia, liver and convulsions). Kidney (cancer) Respiratory tract (infections, cancer). Cardiovascular
Pentachlorophenol	Wood preservative industry	Liver. Kidney. Nervous system. Reproductive system. Carcinogenic to all systems
Petroleum products	Rubber; textile; aerospace; workers in contact with fuel oil, coke, paraffin, lubricants Dry cleaning; diesel jet testers	Skin. Respiratory tract. Larynx. Scrotum. Carcinogenic to all systems. Dermatosis. Hyperpigmentation of skin
Phenol	Plastics	Corrosive to all tissue, liver, kidney, brain Skin (ulceration)
Polyurethane	Plastics and most other industries	Respiratory tract (asthma, cancer) Dermatosis
Printing ink	Printers	Respiratory tract (irritation). Larynx (cancer). Urinary bladder (cancer)
Radiation	Health care providers: doctors, nurses, dentists, radiologists, and x-ray technicians (diagnostic, fluoroscopy, treatment, isotopes), physical therapists (diathermy), microbiologists and laboratory technicians (electron microscope); office workers (some types of computers and office machines); radar systems (police, weather, airport workers); nuclear generating stations; AM, FM, TV broadcasting stations; atomic workers; food workers; fiber workers; households (microwave ovens, some computers)	Reproductive system (chromosome irritation, sterility in men and women, birth defects, impotence, cancer) Hematopoietic system (leukemia) Thyroid (cancer) Other body systems, bone and skin (cancer)
Rubber dust	Rubber	Respiratory tract (chronic disease, cancer). Dermatosis.
Silica	Mine; foundry; ceramic or glass production	Respiratory tract (silicosis, pneumoconiosis, emphysema)
Sulfur dioxide	Oil refining; ore smelting; brewery workers; flour bleachers; paper; sulfuric acid workers	Respiratory tract (acute exposure causes laryngospasm, circulatory arrest, death)
Talc dust	Mine	Respiratory tract (cancer). Calcification of pericardium
Tetraethyl lead	Chemical	Hematopoietic system. Brain
Thallium	Pesticide; fireworks or explosives	Skin. Eye. Respiratory and gastrointestinal tracts. Kidney. Brain

(continued)

TABLE 2–5.   EFFECTS OF SOME COMMON INDUSTRIAL AGENTS ON THE WORKER (continued)

Agent	Type of Industry or Occupation	Body Area Affected
Toluene	Metal coatings; rubber; paint; clerical workers; printers; cosmetologists; plastics	Skin. Respiratory tract. Liver. Hematopoietic system. Brain (may cause drunken state and accidents). Reproductive system (infertility, birth defects, chromosome damage in male). Kidneys
Trichloroethylene	Chemical-metal degreasing; contact cement; paint; plastics; upholstery cleaners	Skin. Liver. Kidney. Brain (carcinogen). Cardiac system
Vinyl chloride	Plastic; rubber; insulation; organic-chemical synthesizers; polyvinyl-resin makers	Skin. Respiratory tract (asthma). Cancer in the liver, kidney, spleen and brain. Reproductive system (chromosome mutation, stillbirth, spontaneous abortion); exposure of pregnant woman to polyvinyl chloride causes defective fetus
Wood products	Furniture	Respiratory tract (asthma). Larynx (cancer).
Zinc	Plating; in brass, bronze, other alloys	Respiratory tract. Neurologic system. Hematopoietic system

course and higher quality of life, and recognizing that the environment and people are interdependent.

In 1992, the United Nations held the Earth Summit in Rio de Janeiro for representatives from 170 countries. Delegates drafted treaties to protect mothers and children, small farmers, neighborhoods, families, communities, and indigenous people and to preserve cultural diversity and biodiversity. Sessions focused on causes of poverty and joblessness, environmental ethics, and acknowledgment of humans as one species within the web of all life on the planet. The Healthy Cities Movement emphasizes a healthy, well-educated, responsible citizen, high literacy rates, effective prenatal care, low infant mortality, low criminal rate, a stable, demographically balanced population, and personal security (153).

What we do to the environment and how we live affects everyone, eventually worldwide, as we see with destruction of rainforests to obtain their products. What is destroyed cannot be regained, and synthetic development may not be adequate (19, 153, 184).

The size, concentration, and mobility of populations have greatly increased. The spread of diseases, such as HIV/AIDS, Ebola hemorrhagic disease, pulmonary syndrome virus, hepatitis C, Lyme disease, bubonic plague, and yellow fever, has also increased, according to WHO. At least 29 new diseases have emerged in the past 20 years and are a threat to all countries. There are several reasons for new and reemerging diseases (184):

- Changes in lifestyle, including overcrowded cities where population growth has outpaced supplies of clean water and adequate housing
- Dramatic increases in national and international travel, whereby a traveler may spread the disease from one country to another before falling ill

- Deterioration of traditional public health activities needed to quickly recognize emerging problems, such as surveillance and diagnostic laboratories
- Complacency, despite numerous warnings in recent years
- Antibiotic resistance, so that effective treatment of the simplest infection is difficult
- Existence of unrecognized microorganisms in nature that are as deadly as the Ebola virus and will be distributed as people go into remote areas

The following are the main reemerging diseases (184):

- Tuberculosis, up 27.8% in 1990–1993 versus 1984–1986
- Diphtheria, up 141% in 1994 from 1990
- Cholera, up 154% in 1994 from 1990
- Dengue fever, now reported in many Latin American and Caribbean countries for the first time in 50 years
- Yellow fever, now reported for the first time in decades in Latin America
- Bubonic plague, with more than 2000 cases reported in 1993–1994, the highest total since in 1954
- Gonorrhea, staphylococcal infections, dysentery, malaria, and other diseases that show growing resistance to antibiotics

Personal Responsibility

Consider the environment, the various social institutions, and the population as a complex of interacting, interdependent systems. Environmental problems are a concern to everyone and are of equal consequence to every part of the world. Each of us shares the earth, so we are all responsible for its well-being. Environmental pollution is our collective fault and requires our collective solutions. In the United States alone discarded materials amount to billions of tons yearly, and the quantity is growing annually.

A fourfold environmental protection system is useful for continuously identifying, analyzing, and controlling environmental hazards (28, 153):

1. Surveillance—maintaining an awareness of what people and industries are doing to the air, water, and land and of the effect of these actions on health; monitoring exposure
2. Development of criteria for the detection of pollution; detection
3. Research, including data from various records
4. Compliance—getting local government and industry to accept and implement new standards

Citizen Role

An informed public can help establish such a system, but the financial support and legislative and administrative guidance of federal, state, and local governments provide the most feasible solutions. Encourage your local, state, or federal government officials to pass legislation that would protect the environment (e.g., installation of scrubbers in factories to decrease the release of sulfur dioxide, use of low-sulfur or "washed" coal, and control of or safe disposal of nuclear or other hazardous wastes). Support production of biodegradable products

from potato scraps, corn, molasses, beets, and castor oil. These nonpetroleum ingredients can be transformed into a strong, flexible plastic that will degrade completely.

The Resource Conservation and Recovery Act of 1976 (PC 94-580) provides for recycling of our natural resources, safe disposal of discarded materials, and management of hazardous wastes, those that contribute to increased mortality or pose a substantial present or potential threat to human health or environment. But these goals are not possible without individual effort. Refer to Table 2–6 for disposal of hazardous products. See Conservation Solutions for a summary of conservative strategies (14, 31, 54, 74, 81, 105, 130, 142, 153, 155, 164, 180).

As a citizen, you should conserve natural resources to the best of your ability and learn about the environmental pollution in your own area. Remember that metallurgic and chemical companies are the greatest sources of hazardous waste. Campaign for minimized waste and for safe disposal of unavoidable waste. Encourage the development of additional burial sites for long-term safety and the monitoring of present sites for escape of wastes (9, 54, 74, 125, 133, 150, 180, 188).

Lifestyle Changes

Conservation Solutions summarizes activities to conserve, reduce pollution, and change lifestyle that can be accomplished by the citizens to conserve natural resources. For some people, following the suggestions will mean major changes—in shopping, in not care-

TABLE 2–6. COMMON TOXIC AGENTS AND HOW TO DISPOSE OF THEM

Product	Danger	Disposal
Pest-control chemicals (insecticides, mothballs, flea and roach powder, weed killer)	Poisonous, carcinogenic	Offer leftovers to a nursery or garden shop or local business. Pesticides may be accepted by a chemical waste company or county agricultural agency.
Oil-based paints	Flammable	Call your local health department; ask if it has a policy for disposal of paint (some agencies have free cleanup days). Paint you cannot use can go to a neighbor, friend, or local organization or theatre group.
Solvents (paint thinner, turpentine, rust remover, nail polish remover, furniture stripper)	Flammable and poisonous; respiratory, eye, and skin irritant	Use all of them or give them away. Paint thinner can be reused by letting the liquid set (in a closed jar) until paint particles settle out. Strain off and reuse the clear liquid. Wrap the residue in plastic and put in trash.
Waste motor oil	Poisonous if ingested	Recycle at a gas station or auto service center.
Car batteries	Corrosive to skin and eyes	Check area gas stations. Some will take old batteries. A few offer cash for them.

► CONSERVATION SOLUTIONS

Energy Solutions

- Use public transportation; carpool; bike, walk rather than drive a car if feasible.
- Invest in ample insulation, weatherstripping, and caulking for home and workplace.
- Use electricity and hot water efficiently. Buy energy-saving household appliances.
- Reduce demand for energy by turning off lights, radio, and television when no one is using them; run dishwasher and washer and dryer only when they have full loads.
- Make the most of oven heat—bake foods in batches; turn oven off shortly before baking is finished and use remaining heat to complete the job.
- Dry clothes outdoors on a line.
- Use clothes dryer efficiently; separate loads into heavy- and lightweight items as lighter ones take less time.
- In winter turn down thermostat a few degrees, especially at night and when house is empty. In summer if using air conditioning, turn thermostat up a few degrees. Regularly service the furnace and air conditioner.
- Close off and do not heat or cool unused rooms; use insulating shades and curtains on cold winter nights and hot summer days.

Food Solutions

- Eat foods lower on the food chain—vegetables, fruits, and grains; decrease consumption of meat and animal products.
- Read the labels on food; buy foods that have not been heavily processed. Learn which additives are harmful.
- Support laws that ban harmful pesticides, drugs, and other chemicals used in food production. Support markets that offer contaminant-free food.
- Avoid food from endangered environments, such as rain forests.

Water Solutions

- Install sink faucet aerators and water-efficient showerheads, which use two to five times less water with no noticeable decrease in performance.
- Take showers, not baths, to reduce water consumption.
- Do not let water run when it is not actually being used while showering, shaving, brushing teeth, or hand washing clothes.
- Use ultra low-flush or air-assisted toilets, saving 60 to 90% water. Composting toilets use no water and recycle organic waste.
- Buy phosphate-free, biodegradable soaps and detergents; ask your supermarket to carry them if it does not.
- Do not run the tap until the water is cold to get a drink. Instead, keep water in a refrigerator bottle.
- Economize water when washing the car, sprinkling the lawn, and removing debris from surfaces; repair leaks.

Toxins and Pollutants Solutions

- Read labels; buy the least toxic products available; find out the best disposal methods for toxic products. Use nonharmful substitutes.

- Avoid purchasing clothes that require dry cleaning, which uses toxic chlorinated solvents. Dry clean only when necessary.
- Avoid contact with pesticides by thoroughly scrubbing or peeling foodstuffs; if possible, maintain your own garden without use of pesticides.
- Test your home for radon, especially if you live on the East Coast or in Wisconsin, Minnesota, North Dakota, Colorado, or Wyoming.
- Ask your service station to use CFC recovery equipment when repairing auto air conditioners.
- Use more energy-efficient cars.
- Keep your automobile in top working condition with a regular tuneup; make sure antipollution controls are working properly.
- Operate your vehicle properly; do not idle or rev engine; drive at steady pace; obey speed limits.
- Support legislative initiatives that encourage industry to modify manufacturing processes to eliminate the production of hazardous wastes and to reuse and recycle wastes when possible.

Waste Reduction and Recycling Solutions

- Buy products in bulk or with the least amount of packaging. (A major contributor to acid rain is sulfur dioxide, one of the chemicals used to process virgin paper. In the very low oxygen environment of the trash dump, paper or plastic may take 40 or more years to degrade.)
- Buy products that are recyclable, repairable, reusable, and biodegradable; avoid disposables. (Every 3 months enough aluminum cans are thrown away to rebuild an entire commercial fleet.)
- Separate your recyclable garbage such as newspaper, glass, paper, aluminum, and organic waste if you have a garden. Send to the landfill what cannot be used. (Only 10% of garbage is recycled in the United States.)
- Recycle newspapers through paper drives. Each Sunday thousands of trees are made into newspapers that are not recycled.
- Use recycled products. Landfills are rapidly being exhausted, and the cost of recycling must be recovered.
- Buy recycled paper for all uses. (It takes 16,320 kilowatt-hours of electricity to produce 1 ton of paper from virgin wood pulp. It takes 64% fewer kilowatt-hours (5919) to produce 1 ton of recycled paper from waste paper.)
- Use curbside pickup for recyclables if available.
- If you do not have a recycle center, ask your city council to establish one. Find local groups that can use your recyclables.

Housekeeping Solutions

- Use simple substances for cleaning. An all-purpose cleaner, safe for all surfaces, is 1 gallon hot water, $\frac{1}{4}$ cup sudsy ammonia, $\frac{1}{4}$ cup vinegar, and 1 tablespoon baking soda. After use, wipe surface with water to rinse.
- Keep drains open by using the following mix once weekly: 1 cup baking soda, 1 cup salt, $\frac{1}{4}$ cup cream of tartar. Pour $\frac{1}{4}$ cup of the mixture weekly into the drain; follow with a pot of boiling water. If drain is clogged, pour in $\frac{1}{4}$ cup baking soda followed by $\frac{1}{2}$ cup vinegar. Close drain until fizzing stops. Then flush with boiling water.
- Use low-phosphate or phosphate-free detergents to wash clothes and dishes.
- Use natural furniture and floor polish products; such products use lemon oil or beeswax in a mineral oil base.
- Use nontoxic products to control pests. Control ants by sprinkling barriers of talcum powder, chalk, bone meal, or boric acid across their trails. Control cockroaches by dusting lightly with borax. Control ticks and fleas on pets by applying an herbal rinse. Boil $\frac{1}{2}$ cup of fresh or dried rosemary in a quart of water: Steep herb 20 minutes, strain, and cool. Then sponge on pet. Air-dry.

(continued)

► CONSERVATION SOLUTIONS (continued)

Housekeeping Solutions (cont.)

- Maintain air circulation and clean ventilation systems and ducts to remove fungi, mold, pollen, toxic residues, sprays, and other contaminants. Avoid hair spray and cleaning sprays.

- Manage household hazardous waste: buy only what is needed; do not store with household products; give unused product to someone else who may be able to use it rather than disposing of it. Do not pour oil, grease, or hazardous chemicals down the drain.

Tree-saver Solutions

- Plant trees; as trees grow, they remove carbon dioxide from the atmosphere through photosynthesis, slowing buildup of carbon dioxide. (Carbon dioxide causes over 50% of the greenhouse effect.)

- Join efforts to save forests from being cleared or burned. When forests are burned, carbon is released, adding to carbon dioxide buildup and global warming.

Preservation of Life and Environment Solutions

- Do not burn leaves or garbage; instead, compost organic materials.

- Do not buy endangered plants, animals, or products made from overexploited species (furs, ivory, reptile skin, or tortoise shell).

- Avoid buying wood from the tropical rain forests unless it was propagated by sustainable tree farming methods.

- Buy products from companies that do not pollute or damage the environment.

- Join, support, volunteer your time to organizations working on environmental causes.

- Contact your elected representatives through letters, telegrams, calls, or visits to communicate your concerns about conservation and environmental issues.

---

lessly disposing of articles, or in transportation—or it could mean planting a patio or rooftop garden or limiting the number of pets.

Quiet surroundings are a natural resource, too. Make your own quieter through personal habits. Help plan for local recreation sites that offer natural surroundings. Campaign for adequate acoustical standards in homes, apartments, hospitals, and industrial buildings and for noiseless kitchen equipment. Participate in local government planning to decrease town and city noise in relation to transportation routes, zoning, and industrial sites.

Support for Conservation

Ecological principles can be applied to urban renewal. Chattanooga, Tennessee, is an example of how city leaders, city planners, environmentalists, businessmen, and the local Audubon Society collaborated to reduce air pollution, create green areas, make the city more attractive and convenient, and develop a sustainable city to reduce flight to the suburbs (57).

Join citizens' crusades for a clean environment or a conservation organization and attend workshops given by the Cancer Society, Sierra Club, Conservation Foundation, and League of Women Voters to learn more about problems, preventive measures, and means of strengthening legislation. Support antipollution and noise-control laws. Support your city and health agencies in their attempts at pollution control and recycling (9, 122, 133, 175, 180). Be an involved citizen!

Environmental regulations are needed to protect lives, health, and economic livelihood. Some corporations, and in turn Congress, press to weaken environmental protection. Yet studies show that regulations have changed economic incentives; responsible companies are rewarded, which means that businesses can prosper and that tourism will return to an area that has reduced pollution and is ecologically and aesthetically maintained. For example, tourists do not visit a seashore area where there is sewage discharge, runoff, burning, and garbage and sludge dumping. Sharper environmental regulation will protect all life, including wilderness and beautiful areas and endangered species. We can prevent humans from becoming an endangered species. The *National Wildlife Journal*, February/March/1996 issue, presents more information, as does the Winter 1995–1996 issue of *Missouri Resources*.

The various national wildlife organizations are studying the environment and alerting citizens about hazardous wastes and toxins in the environment. These organizations, such as National Wildlife Federation, Audubon Society, Sierra Club, Nature Conservancy, and Coalition for the Environment in St. Louis, have worked closely with Congress and state legislators to pass protective legislation, have held public hearings to initiate protective measures, and have conducted citizen education. Often neither the legislators nor the citizens are as attentive as they should be. Support given to this type of organization and to legislative efforts is important as a citizen. In the process you are contributing to the health of your family, your community, and your nation.*

---

*For more information on specific measures for wasting less and practicing ecologically sound living, see Saltonstall, R. *Your Environment and What You Can Do About It: A Citizen's Guide.* New York: Walker & Co., 1970, and the booklets published by the U.S. Department of Labor and the EPA that are listed in the references.

Professional Responsibility

Although health care and nursing responsibilities have been interwoven throughout this chapter, consider that your primary responsibilities are detection through thorough assessment, making suggestions for intervention, and health teaching.

Assessment and Nursing Diagnosis

Screening for occupational diseases resulting from exposure to contaminants is most accurately done by occupational health nurses and physicians rather than by employees in corporate medical groups. Increasingly there are improved radiologic and blood chemistry diagnostic tests to detect diseases that are related to the occupation, including a blood test to detect pesticide contamination. Keep abreast of medical advances (54, 147, 153, 172).

You can play a significant role in the early detection of lead poisoning, for example. Assessment of a child's health should include observation for physical signs such as tremors, abdominal discomfort, decreased appetite, and vomiting and questions related to a pica behavior. Ask the mother about her child's interest in play, ability to get along with playmates, coordination, and level of developmental skill attainment. Phrase your questions and comments carefully, in a nonjudgmental manner, so that the mother will not feel that her fitness as a parent is being judged. If the persons for whom you are caring live in unsatisfactory, low-income housing, work for improvement through local legislation. Emphasis must be placed on repair and deleading of dwelling places, not just on moving the present dweller to a new house or apartment. You can encourage the formation of screening and case-finding programs, already started in many cities, and you can assist with their activities. Be as thorough in assessment as possible. An example of questions usually not asked on standard health history forms that you could use in assessment of the employed client is presented in Fig. 2–4. See Selected Nursing Diagnoses Related to Environmental Considerations. Exposure to lead is also seen in other areas such as indoor firing ranges. Such recreation raises blood lead levels (177).

Intervention

Health teaching and advocacy can increase client and community awareness and contribute to prevention of illness from pollutants or hazards. Encourage people to read labels and current literature (see Educate the Consumer: Signal Words on U.S. Labels).

► SELECTED NURSING DIAGNOSES RELATED TO ENVIRONMENTAL CONSIDERATIONS*

Pattern 1: Exchanging
Risk for Injury

Pattern 3: Relating
Social Isolation

Pattern 5: Choosing
Health-Seeking Behaviors

Pattern 6: Moving
Altered Health Maintenance

Pattern 7: Perceiving
Powerlessness

Pattern 8: Knowing
Knowledge Deficit

---

* Many of the NANDA nursing diagnoses are applicable to the person who is ill as a result of environmental pollution or hazards, or occupational causes.
From North American Nursing Diagnosis Association, NANDA Nursing Diagnoses Definitions & Classification 1995–1996. Philadelphia: North American Nursing Diagnosis Association, 1994.

Natural or man-made chemical pollution in soil, water, and food products can produce various adverse effects, ranging from slight health impairments to death. Although local public health officials are responsible for maintaining safe nitrate levels in the water supply, your responsibilities are to aid in the education of the public concerning the health hazards of such pollutants and to use the epidemiologic method in your work. Be aware of such symptoms as fatigue, listlessness, and sleepiness that may indicate an untoward reaction to this particular form of pollution.

You may have an opportunity to teach people who earn a living as **pesticide applicators** and handlers. They should follow the following *precautions*:

- Wear rubber or neoprene gloves while handling pesticides to avoid skin contact.

1. Occupational history (start with last job first).

	COMPANY	DATE EMPLOYED	JOB
(a)	_____	_____	_____
(b)	_____	_____	_____
(c)	_____	_____	_____
(d)	_____	_____	_____

2. In these jobs, have you ever been exposed to:
Excessive radiation or radioactive material?
Excessive noise? _____   Excessive heat or light? _____

3. Have you worked in dusty trades? _____
With any specific chemicals? _____
In any vapors or fumes? _____
If your answer is yes to any questions in (2) and (3), please elaborate. _____
_____
_____

4. Has a job ever made you "sick"? _____   If so, which job? _____
Explain how you were sick. _____

5. Have you ever worn any protective equipment or a specific support? _____
If so, what? _____

6. Have you ever had a serious work injury? _____   If so, please describe. _____
_____

7. Have you ever had several minor work injuries? _____   If so, please describe. _____
_____

8. Have you ever applied for, or received, workers' compensation? _____

9. Have you ever had a pension for disability? _____
_____

Figure 2–4. Occupational history form.

- Keep pesticide-soiled clothing separate from other family laundry.
- Empty all cuffs and pockets before doing laundry so trapped pesticide granules do not dissolve in wash water.
- Daily wash all clothing worn while applying pesticides. The longer the garments are stored before laundering, the more difficult it is to remove the pesticide.
- Prerinsing is an effective way to dislodge pesticide residue.
- Wash only a few items at a time, and wash for a 12- to 14-minute cycle. Use the recommended amount of heavy-duty detergent. Liquid detergents are more effective than powders in removing oil-based pesticides.
- The hotter the water (preferably 140° F), the more effectively pesticide is removed.

- It may be necessary to discard heavily contaminated clothing.
- To remove possible pesticide residues from the washing machine tub, run the washer through a complete cycle using detergent and a full level of hot water (157).

Another dangerous problem associated with chemical pollution is its possible carcinogenic effect (as seen in Table 2–5). Incidence of specific forms of cancer can be higher or lower, depending on exposure to specific compounds, a common example being the high incidence of lung cancer in the United States and England because of heavy tobacco use. Be aware and knowledgeable about the incidence of chemically produced cancer in your particular locale. Health teaching can then be directed at trying to eliminate or control the responsible carcinogenic chemical. Radiation is also carcinogenic.

► EDUCATE THE CONSUMER: SIGNAL WORDS ON U.S. LABELS

- **Caution:** fatal dose is more than 1 oz (32 mL); low-level toxicity
- **Corrosive:** may chemically "eat" through standard containers
- **Danger:** a few drops can be fatal; highly toxic; requires specific protective measures
- **Ignitable:** may pose a fire hazard
- **Nontoxic:** only an advertising word; can mean anything from safe when swallowed to less than 50% of tested animals died within 2 weeks of testing
- **Reactive:** may be explosive or produce poisonous substances
- **Toxic:** a poison to humans or environment
- **Warning:** fatal dose is somewhere between 1 tablespoon (16 mL) and 1 oz (32 mL); moderately toxic

Encourage the use of protective clothing and sunscreen lotions to prevent overexposure to the sun. Prevent overexposure to ionizing radiation by making certain that unnecessary x-ray studies are not taken, by keeping a record of the frequency of such studies, and by using a lead shield when x-ray examinations are given.

The biochemical response to chemical pollution or radiation can influence the cells in various ways. **Teratogenic** (*producing fetal malformations*) and **mutagenic** (*producing hereditary changes*) are two such changes in cells. Be aware that these changes can occur in both the client and the health care provider who are exposed to radiation. Genetic counseling might be indicated for couples who have been exposed to radiation. Citizens should know of the possibility for dealing effectively and therapeutically with biochemical changes, whether prenatally or in any stage of growth and development (18, 34, 91, 187).

In 1977 the National Institute for Occupational Safety and Health (NIOSH) issued a document, "The Right to Know: Practical Problems and Policy Issues Arising From Exposure to Hazardous Chemicals and Physical Agents in the Workplace." It proceeded from the premise that workers have a right to know about risks to which they have been exposed. For political and economic reasons and because of constraints from the Department of Health and Human Services, NIOSH officials were reluctant to create a regulation based on the document; however, pressure from workers, consumer and conservation groups, and unions persisted (10).

Under the Hazardous Communication Rule passed in 1983, workers must be informed about any hazardous chemicals to which employees are exposed in the workplace. The rule is limited, however; it covers only manufacturing companies, and employers may claim a chemical is a trade secret and release the name only to a health professional who has a right to know. Health care professionals, the unions, and conservation and consumer groups must continue to advocate for all workers so that the rule will be applied in a broader perspective (10, 148). You are also a worker and are exposed to a variety of health hazards, including musculoskeletal injuries, infectious diseases, antineoplastic agents administered to cancer clients, laser injuries, smoke inhalation, and stress (79, 186).

As a professional and as a citizen, you can encourage officials and consumers in your community to develop innovative technologies to cope with the hazardous effects of aspects of our current lifestyle. For example, the city of Muskegan, Michigan, constructed an innovative facility that recycles wastewater so that it can be used safely and economically to irrigate farmland. Sewage residues given conventional treatment become more toxic with each step. Wastewater and sewage residues that are gradually percolated through natural soil filters use fewer chemicals to treat sewage and generate less sludge. The resulting water residues are high in plant nutrients and can be recycled as fertilizer. Land-treatment facilities use energy only for pumping, allow communities to reuse water, and can make money for the community (101).

Join the Nurses Environmental Health Watch, a nonprofit organization, with chapters in most states. The organization seeks to educate nurses and the public about current issues influencing health and the environment, including environmental toxins and pollutants, nuclear energy and energy alternatives, resource recovery and recycling, chemical and biologic warfare, and occupational hazards for nurses. A quarterly newsletter, *Health Watch,* includes items about national and local activities and resources on environmental issues. Educational forums are sponsored by local chapters.

In the past 100 years disease and death have been reduced because of preventive public health measures in the form of environmental control, such as water and waste management, rodent and insect control, development of housing codes. Now we are again faced with problems and diseases that have an environmental impact. Prevention can begin with informed consumer groups who have educational and work projects as their goals. It can begin with your responsibility for the client's environment.

Client's Immediate Environment

Besides a feeling of responsibility for the community and physical environment in which the client lives, you also have a responsibility for that individual's immediate environment while receiving health care. The client's *surroundings should constitute a* **therapeutic milieu** *free of hazards and conducive to recovery, physically and emotionally.*

The client's surroundings should be clean and adequately lighted, ventilated, heated, and safe. Precautions should always be taken to prevent injury, such as burns from a hot water bottle. Falls should be prevented by removing obstacles and electric cords from walking areas and having the person wear well-fitted shoes and use adequate support while walking. Lock the bed or wheelchair while the client is moving to and from them. In the home be sure that electric cords and scatter rugs are not placed so that the person could fall. Wipe up spilled liquids immediately. Use sterile technique and proper handwashing methods to ensure that you bring no pathogenic organisms to the client. Avoid excessive noise from personnel and equipment to the degree possible. Various equipment used in client care must also be monitored for safe function.

The aesthetic environment is also important for rest. Arrange articles on the bedside table in a pleasing manner if the client is unable to do so. Keep unattractive equipment and supplies out of sight as much as possible. Electric equipment should be in proper repair and function. Minimize offensive odors and noise. Place the person's bed or chair by a window or door so that the person can watch normal activity rather than stare at the ceiling or walls. As a nurse, involve yourself in making the entire ward and the clients' rooms look pleasing. Consider color combinations and the use of drapes, furniture, clocks, calendars, pictures, and various artifacts to create a more homelike atmosphere. The committee in charge of decorating and building should include at least one nurse. You may need to volunteer to ensure that nursing and, indirectly, clients are represented in such programs.

The client's surroundings should not only be safe and attractive, but the emotional climate of the unit and entire institution affects clients and staff as well. The client and family are quick to respond and react to the attitudes and manner of the staff. Here are some questions you might ask yourself. How do I treat delivery workers who bring gifts and flowers to clients? Do I participate in the joy such remembrances bring to the client? Do I help arrange the flowers into a pleasant pattern or just stick them quickly into whatever can be found? Do I treat visitors as welcome guests or as foreign intruders? The emotional climate should radiate security and acceptance. A warmth should prevail that promotes a sense of feeling of trust, confidence, and motivation within the client as he or she and the staff work together to cope with problems. The emotional relationship between the client and the health care staff should help the client reach the goal of maximum health.

In a truly therapeutic milieu the staff members also feel a sense of harmony among themselves. There are mutual trust and acceptance between staff and supervisors, and supervisors recognize work well done by the staff. As a result, staff members feel motivated to continue to learn and to improve the quality of client care. Staff members are not likely to give individualized, comprehensive, compassionate care in an agency where they are not treated like individuals or where their basic needs are not met.

Be aware of environmental pollution in the health care environment. "No smoking" should be the rule, not only when oxygen is in use but also in most health care settings. Conference or dining rooms or lounges for health care providers may have either a "no smoking" rule or a limited "smoking" area. Sometimes there are designated smoking areas outside the building so that employees or visitors who smoke must go outdoors. In the past it was difficult to teach a client the adverse effects of smoking and nicotine when an odor of cigarette smoke hung on the uniform. Moreover, health care providers benefit from practicing what they teach others. Health care providers and clients may also come in contact with agents listed in Table 2–5. Constant vigilance is necessary to detect harmful agents and prevent or reduce their usage. Early assessment of harmful effects to reduce the symptoms and proper interventions for dermatoses, allergens, or other symptoms is essential.

Be aware that a "sick building syndrome" exists; however, it is the people in the building that suffer. The source of the problem is an inadequate ventilation system that creates poor mechanical air flow. Equipment such as the ozone from the photocopier and furnishings such as fiberboard and carpet that contain formaldehyde add to the problem when there are no windows or windows do not open. Volatile organic compounds (benzene, chloroform, and formaldehyde) may be given off by paints, vinyls, printed documents, telephone cable, solvents, and some furniture or carpets. Biological agents, including mold, dust, mites, algae, fungus, and pollen, may be in the humidifier or vent system. Tobacco smoke, which contains volatile organic compounds and other gases and particles, is dirtier than the usual air the smoker inhales. Carbon dioxide levels may be well above that considered healthy. Common complaints are headaches, fatigue, coughing, sneezing, nausea, difficulty with concentration, bleary eyes, and irritation of the nose and throat. The symptoms clear when the person leaves the building. Vents must be cleaned and furniture arranged so that airflow can be maintained. Fresh air should be circulated indoors. Co-workers should unite to find and correct the problem. The

Occupational Health and Safety Administration has standards for various settings, and employees and clients have a right to a workplace free of recognized hazard (92, 106, 107, 117).

There are times when the treatment for the client's infection or the therapy modalities may also affect the health care provider, for example, radiotherapy and chemotherapy. Proper precautions should be taken to protect the provider from excess exposure and to protect the client. Follow the guidelines and universal precautions, developed by the Centers for Disease Control and Prevention to prevent infection spread. Follow guidelines for handling chemotherapeutic and radioactive materials. Several journals also present updated information regularly, such as *Hospital Employee Health, Nursing Quality Connection, Cancer Nursing,* and publications by the American Society of Hospital Pharmacists.

If you are caring for a person in the home, you are limited in the amount of change you can make. You can point out such hazards as electric cords in the walking area, however. You can suggest furniture rearrangement if you think that the person could function more easily with the change. You can put a clock in sight, pull the drapes, or place needed materials within the client's reach, if feasible.

Specific ways of meeting the client's environmental needs also differ for various developmental stages. The components of a therapeutic milieu are different for the baby than for the middle-aged man; however, a safe, secure environment, physically and psychologically, must be present for both. Accurately determining the factors that make up the environment and making appropriate changes may be the first step in promoting health.

It is past time for all of us to ask ourselves some basic questions. How much energy and natural resources do we need to sustain life, to maintain the high standard of living in the United States? How much are we willing to pay for benefits that will not poison us with side effects? How does population growth affect the use and abuse of natural resources? Will strictly controlled energy allocation be necessary because people refuse to abide by suggested limits? Must children continue to grow up with strontium-90 in their bones, DDT in their fat, and asbestos in their lungs? What more can each of us do personally and professionally to maintain a health-fostering environment?

SUMMARY

1. Health and development are adversely affected by air, water, soil, food, noise, and surface pollution.

2. Sources of air pollution are carbon monoxides; sulfur and nitrogen oxides; suspended particles, such as dust, ash, aerosols, and asbestos; tobacco smoke; hydrocarbons; ozone; photochemical smog; acid rain; radioactive substances; formaldehyde; and radon.

3. Sources of water pollution are sewage and pathogenic organisms; plant nutrients; synthetic and inorganic chemicals; sediment; radioactive material; oil spills; and heat from industrial processes.

4. Sources of food pollution include pesticides and food additives such as antibiotics and hormones administered to animals that are produced for food; contaminated water and soil used in food production; and contamination from pathogens during food processing or handling.

5. Noise pollution in the home and workplace produces numerous adverse health and safety effects.

6. Sources of surface pollution include open dumps; landfills; incineration of waste; salvage operations; unsafe disposal of hazardous, pathogenic, or radioactive wastes in the home or workplace; and lead found in soil, the home, and workplace.

7. Health workers must be aware of various health hazards in the workplace, both of the client and self.

8. Health care workers have global, local, personal, and professional responsibilities for controlling pollution effects and preventing further hazards to health and development populations.

9. Health care workers are responsible for promoting a therapeutic or healing milieu/environment for the client.

10. Health care workers must engage in legislative advocacy, public education, public policy changes, and creation of societal resources to foster a healthy environment.

► REFERENCES

1. A Primer on Pesticides, *Chemecology,* 22, no. 7 (1993), 3.
2. Ahlborg, G., and L. Bodin, Tobacco Smoke Exposure and Pregnancy Outcome Among Women: A Prospective Study at Prenatal Care Centers in Orebro County, Sweden, *American Journal of Epidemiology,* 133, no. 4 (1991), 338–347.
3. Arlien-Soborg, P., *Solvent Neurotoxicity.* Boca Raton, FL: CRC Press, 1991.

4. Ayres, J., R. Harrison, and V. Soyseth, Exposure to Air Irritants in Infancy and Prevalence of Bronchial Hyper-responsiveness in Schoolchildren, *Lancet,* 346 (1995), 128–129.

5. Bahadori, R., and B. Bohne, Adverse Effects of Noise on Hearing, *American Family Physician,* 47 (1993), 1219–1229.

6. Baker, J.L., Agricultural Chemical Management Practices to Reduce Losses due to Drainage, *American Journal of Industrial Medicine,* 18, no. 4 (1990), 477–483.

7. Barker, P., and D. Lewis, The Management of Lead Exposure in Pediatric Populations, *Nurse Practitioner: American Journal of Primary Health Care,* 15, no. 12 (1990), 8–10, 12–13, 16.

8. Barlett, D., and J. Steele, *Forevermore: Nuclear Waste in America.* New York: W.W. Norton, 1985.

9. Baxter, T., Spring Cleaning, *Sierra,* March–April (1993), 66–79.

10. Bayer, R., Notifying Workers at Risk: The Politics of the Right-to-Know, *American Journal of Public Health,* 76, no. 11 (1986), 1352–1356.

11. Biodegradable Plastics: Friend or Foe of Waste Management? *Chemecology,* 19, no. 8 (1990), 2–3.

12. Bode, L.E., Agricultural Chemical Application Practices to Reduce Environmental Contamination, *American Journal of Industrial Medicine,* 18, no. 4 (1990), 485–489.

13. Bradstock, M., et al., Evaluation of Reactions to Food Additives: The Aspartame Experience, *American Journal of Clinical Nutrition,* 43 (1986), 464.

14. Brand, C., Fifty Ways to Save Water, *St. Louis Society Audubon Newsletter,* April (1988), 3.

15. Briasco, M.E., Indoor Air Pollution: Are Employees Sick From Their Work? *AAOHN Journal,* 38, no. 8 (1990), 375–380.

16. Bruce, R.D., Noise Pollution, *Community Health Nursing.* Philadelphia: F.A. Davis, 1985.

17. Buckler, G., The Effect of Indoor Air Quality on Health, *Imprint,* 41, no. 3 (1994), 60–62, 65, 93.

18. Bullough, B., and V. Bullough, *Nursing in the Community.* St. Louis: C.V. Mosby; 1990.

19. Byrnes, P., Wild Medicine, *Wilderness,* Fall (1995), 28–33.

20. Calabrese, E., *Biological Effects of Low Level Exposures to Chemicals and Radiation.* Boca Raton, FL: Lewis, 1992.

21. Can You Still Drink the Water? *Environmental Health Perspective,* 102, no. 3 (1994), 286–288.

22. Caplan, R., *Our Earth, Ourselves.* New York: Bantam Books, 1990.

23. Castleman, M., Toxics and Male Infertility, *Sierra,* 70, no. 2 (1985), 49–52.

24. Centers for Disease Control, Childhood Lead Poisoning—U.S. Report to the Congress by the Agency for Toxic Substances and Disease Registry, *MMWR,* 37, no. 32 (1988), 481–485.

25. Children at Risk From Ozone Air Pollution—United States, 1991–1993, *Journal of the American Medical Association,* 273 (May 17, 1995), 1484–1485.

26. Choi-Lao, A., Trace Anesthetic Vapors in Hospital Operating Room Environments, *Nursing Research,* 30, no. 3 (1981), 156–160.

27. Clark, M., The Garbage Health Scare, *Newsweek,* July 20 (1987), 56.

28. Clemen-Stone, S., D. Gerber Eigsti, and S.L. McGuire, *Comprehensive Family and Community Health Nursing* (4th ed.). St. Louis: Mosby-Year Book, 1995.

29. Coffel, S., *But Not a Drop to Drink!* New York: Rawson, 1989.

30. Cohen, G., and J. O'Connor, *Fighting Toxics: A Manual for Protecting Your Family, Community, and Workplace.* Washington, DC: Island Press, 1989.

31. Collins, E., The Perils of Plastic, *Health* (June 1990), 36–37.

32. Commoner, B., *Making Peace with the Planet.* New York: Pantheon Books, 1990.

33. Cook, M., and R. Hoffman, Unintentional Carbon Monoxide Poisoning in Colorado, 1986 Through 1991, *American Journal of Public Health,* 85 (1995), 988–990.

34. Cookfair, J., *Nursing Process and Practice in the Community.* St. Louis: Mosby-Year Book, 1991.

35. Corcoran, E., Trends in Energy: Cleaning up Coal, *Scientific American,* 264, no. 5 (1991), 106–116.

36. Council on Scientific Affairs, American Medical Association, Environmental Tobacco Smoke: Health Effects and Prevention Policies, *Archives of Family Medicine,* 3, no. 10 (1994), 865–878.

37. *Cryptosporidium* in Drinking Water, *Missouri Epidemiologist,* XVII, no. 4 (1995), 1, 8.

38. Dacey, J., and J. Travers, *Human Development Across the Lifespan* (3rd ed.). Madison, WI: Brown & Benchmark, 1996.

39. Davis, H., Workplace Homicides of Texas Males, *American Journal of Public Health,* 77, no. 10 (1987), 1290–1293.

40. ———, P. Honchar, and L. Suarez, Fatal Occupational Injuries of Women, Texas 1975–84, *American Journal of Public Health,* 77, no. 12 (1987), 1524–1527.

41. Dioxins: A Polychlorinated Perplexity, *Health and Environment Digest.* Navarre, NM: Freshwater Foundation, 1990, p. 1.

42. Dioxin's Threat to Human Health, *MOPIRG Reports,* 10, no. 1 (1995), 2.

43. Do Pico, G., Farm-Related Lung Diseases: Toxic Gases and Chemicals, *The Journal of Respiratory Diseases,* 15, no. 7 (1994), 603–618.

44. Drinking Water Guidelines, *Environmental Health Perspective,* 102, no. 3 (1994), 271.

45. Edwards, R., Leaky Drums Spill Plutonium on Ocean Floor, *New Scientist,* 147 (July 22, 1995), 5.

46. Egginton, J., Menace of Whispering Hills, *Audobon,* January (1989), 28–35.

47. Eisenbud, M., *Environmental Radioactivity: From Natural, Industrial, and Military Sources.* Orlando: Academic Press, 1987.

48. Environmental Protection Agency, *Asbestos Fact Book,* Washington, DC: Office of Public Affairs, May 1986.

49. ———, Pesticides and the Consumer, *EPA Journal,* 13, no. 4 (1987), 2–47.

50. ———, *Environmental Progress and Challenges: EPA's Update.* Washington, DC: Environmental Protection Agency, 1988.

51. ———, *An Introductory Guide to the Statutory Authorities of the United States Environmental Protection Agency.* Chicago: U.S. Environmental Protection Agency, 1988.

52. ———, *Our Air, Our Land, Our Water.* Chicago: U.S. Environmental Protection Agency, 1988.

53. EPA Study Confirms Dioxin Health Threat, *MOPIRG Reports,* 10, no. 1 (1995), 1.

54. Federal and State Regulation of Medical Waste, *Journal of Legal Medicine,* 15, no. 1 (1994), 1–89.

55. Fisher, D., *Fire and Ice: The Greenhouse Effect, Ozone Depletion and Nuclear Winter.* New York: Harper & Row, 1990.

56. Food for Thought and Health, *Chemecology,* 24, no. 6 (1995), 2–3.

57. Frenay, R., Chattanooga Turnaround, *Audubon,* 98, no. 1 (1996), 82–85, 88.

58. Fuel for Thought: Examining Alternatives. *Chemecology,* 22, no. 6 (1993), 2–5.

59. Gallagher, M.M., et al., Cryptosporidiosis and Surface Water, *American Journal of Public Health,* 79, no. 1 (1989), 39–42.

60. Gay, K., *Ozone.* New York: Franklin Watts, 1989.

61. ———, *Water Pollution.* New York: Franklin Watts, 1990.

62. Geiss, J., and D. Savitz, Home Pesticide Use and Childhood Cancer: A Case–Control Study, *American Journal of Public Health,* 85 (1995), 249–252.

63. Glantz, S.A., and W.W. Parmley, Passive Smoking and Heart Disease: Epidemiology, Physiology, and Biochemistry, *Circulation,* 83, no. 1 (1991), 1–12.

64. Gorham, E., An Ecologist's Guide to the Problems of the 21st Century, *The American Biology Teacher,* 52, no. 8 (1990), 480–483.

65. Green Watch, *Good Housekeeping,* April (1991), 71, 73–74, 78–80, 84, 88, 90–92, 94.

66. Grossman, J., The Quest for Quiet, *Health,* February (1990), 57.

67. Gustafson, D.I., Field Calibration of Surface: A Model of Agricultural Chemicals in Surface Waters, *Journal of Environmental Science and Health. Part B. Pesticides, Food Contaminates, Agricultural Wastes and Environmental Letters,* 25, no. 5 (1990), 665–687.

68. Hallenbeck, W.H., *Pesticides and Human Health.* New York: Springer-Verlag, 1985.

69. Harvey, P.D., Educated Guesses: Health Risk Assessment in Environmental Impact Statements, *American Journal of Law and Medicine,* 16, no. 3 (1990), 399–427.

70. Hedge, A., P. Burge, A. Robertson, S. Wilson, and J. Harris-Bass, Work-Related Illness in Offices: A Proposed Model of "Sick Building Syndrome," *Environment International,* 15 (1989), 143–158.

71. Henderson, D., Cookware as a Source of Additives, *FDA Consumer,* 16, no. 2 (1982), 11-B.

72. *Home Personal Action Guide.* Washington, DC: Humane Society, 1990.

73. Household Waste Need Not Trash the Environment, *Chemecology,* 20, no. 5 (1991), 2–3.

74. How Agricultural Nurses Are Improving Safety and Health, *Successful Farming,* April (1995), 64.

75. Huston, C., Carbon Monoxide Poisoning, *American Journal of Nursing,* 96, no. 1 (1996), 48.

76. Inh, R.W., and N. Asal, Mortality Among Laundry and Dry Cleaning Workers in Oklahoma, *American Journal of Public Health,* 74, no. 11 (1984), 1278–1280.

77. Is the Earth Heating Up? *National Wildlife,* 33, no. 5 (1995), 5.

78. Jaakkola, J., P. Tuomaala, and O. Seppanen, Air Recirculation and Sick Building Syndrome: A Blended Crossover Trial, *American Journal of Public Health,* 84 (1994), 422–428.

79. Jacobson, E., New Hospital Hazards: How to Protect Yourself, *American Journal of Nursing,* 90, no. 2 (1990), 36–41.

80. Jennings, B., and S. Gudermuth, Hospital Solid Waste: A Challenge for Nurses, *Missouri Nurse,* 47 no. 2 (1973), 5–7.

81. Johansson, A., *Clean Technology.* Boca Raton, FL: Lewis, 1992.

82. John, E.M., D.A. Savitz, and D.P. Sandler, Prenatal Exposure to Parents' Smoking and Childhood Cancer, *American Journal of Epidemiology,* 133, no. 2 (1991), 123–132.

83. Johnson, C.J., and B.C. Kross, Continuing Importance of Nitrate Contamination of Groundwater and Wells in Rural Areas, *American Journal of Industrial Medicine,* 18, no. 4 (1990), 449–456.

84. Jones, C.J., et al., Elevated Nicotine Levels in Cervical Lavages from Passive Smokers, *American Journal of Public Health,* 81, no. 3 (1991), 378–379.

85. Jorgensen, E., ed., *The Poisoned Well: New Strategies for Groundwater Protection.* Washington, DC: Island Press, 1989.

86. Kaufman, S., Radioactive Wastes in St. Louis: The Waste Pile Grows to 45 Years High, *Alert,* 18, no. 1 (1987), 4, 8.

87. Kent, G.J., et al., Epidemic Giardiasis Caused by a Contaminated Public Water Supply, *American Journal of Public Health,* 78, (1988), 139–143.

88. Ketter, J., Latex Allergies on the Rise Among Health Care Workers, *The American Nurse,* January–February (1995), 9.

89. Klonoff-Cohen, H.S. Edelstein, E. Lefkowitz, et al., The Effect of Passive Smoking and Tobacco Exposure Through Breast Milk on Sudden Infant Death Syndrome, *Journal of the American Medical Association,* 273, no. 10 (1995), 795–798.

90. Kraus, J., Homicide While at Work: Persons, Industries, and Occupations at High Risk, *American Journal of Public Health,* 77, no. 10 (1987), 1285–1289.

91. Kronenwetter, M., *Managing Toxic Wastes,* New York: Julian Messner, 1989.

92. Laliberte, R., The Truth About Sick-Building Syndrome: Breathing Uneasy, *Health,* September (1990), 63–65, 82.

93. Landrigan, P.J., and A.C. Todd, Lead Poisoning, *Western Journal of Medicine,* 161, no. 2 (1994), 153–159.

94. Lanyon, L.E., Dairy Manure and Plant Nutrient Management Issues Affecting Water Quality and the Dairy Industry, *Journal of Dairy Science,* 77, no. 7 (1994), 1999–2007.

95. Last, J.M., *Public Health and Human Ecology,* Stamford, CT: Appleton & Lange, 1987.

96. Lead in the Modern Workplace, *American Journal of Public Health,* 80, no. 9 (1990), 907.

97. Leahy, J.G., and R.R. Colwell, Microbial Degradation of Hydrocarbons in the Environment, *Microbiology Review,* 54, no. 3 (1990), 305–315.

98. Lee, S.D., Risk Assessment and Risk Management of Noncriteria Pollutants, *Toxicology and Industrial Health,* 6, no. 5 (1990), 245–255.

99. Lee, S., *The Throwaway Society.* New York: Franklin Watts, 1990.

100. Lehmann, P., What Are Those Additives in Food? *Consumer's Research Magazine,* 65, no. 3 (1982), 13–17.

101. Licht, J., and J. Johnson, Sludge is an Awful Thing to Waste, *Sierra,* March–April (1986), 29–32.

102. Lipscomb, J., B. Burgel, L. Wotowic McGill, and P. Blanc, Preventing Occupational Illness and Injury: Nurse Practitioners as Primary Care Providers, *American Journal of Public Health,* 84, (1994), 643–645.

103. Little, S.P., F. Lewis, C. Yang, and F.A. Zampiella, Worksite Indoor Air Quality Management, *AAOHN Journal,* 42, no. 6 (1994), 277–283, 296–299.

104. Losi, M.E., C. Amrhein, and W.T. Frankenberger, Environmental Biochemistry of Chromium, *Review of Environmental Contamination Toxicology,* 136 (1994), 91–121.

105. MacEachern, D., *Save Our Planet.* New York: Dell Trade Paperback, 1990.

106. Maizlish, N., L. Rudolph, and K. Dervin, The Surveillance of Work-Related Pesticide Illness: An Application of the Sentinel Event Notification System for Occupation Risks (SENSOR), *American Journal of Public Health,* 85 (1995), 806–811.

107. Mancino, D.J., Radiation in the Nurse's Workplace, *Imprint,* 30 (1983), 35–39.

108. Marino, P., et al., A Case Report of Lead Paint Poisoning During Renovation of a Victorian Farmhouse, *American Journal of Public Health,* 80, no. 10 (1990), 1183–1185.

109. Marshall, G., Don't Be Shocked, *Nursing Times,* 77, no. 17 (1981), 721–722.

110. Marx, W., Cry of the American Coast, *Reader's Digest,* December (1988), 110–115.

111. Mattia, M.A., Hazards in the Hospital Environment: Anesthesia Gases and Methylmethacrylate, *American Journal of Nursing,* 83, no. 1 (1983), 73–76.

112. ———, Hazards in the Hospital Environment: The Sterilants, Ethylene Oxide and Formaldehyde, *American Journal of Nursing,* 83, no. 2 (1983), 241–243.

113. ———, and S. Blake, Hospital Hazards: Cancer Drugs, *American Journal of Nursing,* 83, no. 5 (1983), 758–762.

114. McConnell, R., A. Anton, and R. Magnotti, Crop Duster Aviation Mechanics: High Risk for Pesticide Poisoning, *American Journal of Public Health,* 80, no. 10 (1990), 1236–1239.

115. McCormick, J., Diet for a Poisoned Planet, *Greenpeace,* 12, no. 3 (1987), 17–20.

116. McCuen, G., *Nuclear Waste: The Biggest Clean-up in History.* Hudson, WI: GEM, 1990.

117. Mendel, A., and A. Smith, Consistent Pattern of Elevated Symptoms in Air Conditioned Office Buildings: A Reanalysis of Epidemiologic Studies, *American Journal of Public Health,* 80, no. 10 (1990), 1193–1199.

118. Meth, I., Electrical Safety in the Hospital, *American Journal of Nursing,* 80, no. 7 (1980), 1344–1348.

119. Miller, M., and C. Silverman, eds., *Occupational Hearing Conservation.* Englewood Cliffs, NJ: Prentice-Hall, 1984.

120. Miller, M., Chlordane in Missouri, *Alert,* 18, no. 1 (Spring 1987), 1, 6–7.

121. Moore, C., Does Your Cup of Coffee Cause Forest Fires? *International Wildlife,* 19, no. 2 (1989), 39–44.

122. Moore, C., Poisons in the Air, *International Wildlife,* 25, no. 5 (1995), 38–45.

123. Morris, R., and R. Munasinghe, Ambient Air Pollution and Hospitalization for Congestive Heart Failure Among Elderly People in Seven Large Cities, *American Journal of Public Health,* 85 (1995), 1361–1362.

124. Mossman, K.L., and M. Sollitto, Regulatory Control of Indoor Rn, *Health Physics,* 60, no. 2 (1991), 169–176.

125. Mowitz, D., Tires Turn to New Uses, *Successful Farming,* 1 (January 1995), Special Section.

126. Najem, G.R., T. Strunck, and M. Feuerman, Health Effects of a Superfund Hazardous Chemical Waste Disposal Site, *American Journal of Preventive Medicine,* 10, no. 3 (1994), 151–155.

127. *Toxicity of Lead in Children (TLC): Clinical Trial.* Research Triangle Park, NC: National Institute of Environmental Health Sciences, 1993.

128. Neufer, L., and D. Narkunas, Hazardous Releases at the Community Level: A Practical Approach to Analyzing Potential Health Threats, *AAOHN Journal,* 42, no. 7 (1994), 329–335.

129. Nyren, P., Testing the Waters: The Basics of Water Quality, *Flinn Scientific Inc.,* 95, no. 2 (1995), 1–4.

130. Obtaining an Exposure History, *American Family Physician,* 48, no. 3 (1993), 483–485.

131. Ordin, D., and L. Fine, Editorial: Surveillance for Pesticide-Related Illness: Lessons from California, *American Journal of Public Health,* 85 (1995), 762–763.

132. Ossler, C., Men's Work Environments and Health Risks, *Nursing Clinics of North America,* 21, no. 1 (1986), 25–36.

133. Ozone: It's in St. Louis and Facing Some Tough Air Quality Choices, *New Science,* 11, no. 3 (1995), 1–2.

134. Pesticides and the Human Condition, *Chemecology,* 17, no. 8 (1988), 2–4.

135. Pope, C., Respiratory Disease Associated With Community Air Pollution and a Steel Mill, Utah Valley, *American Journal of Public Health,* 79, no. 5 (1989), 623–628.

136. Potter, M.E., and J.L. Brudney, Risk Assessment for Infectious Foodborne Diseases: A Priority with Problems, *Journal of Agromedicine,* 1, no. 3 (1994), 11–22.

137. Precautionary Measures in the Preparation of Antineoplastics, *American Journal of Hospital Pharmacy,* September (1980), 1184–1186.

138. Precipitation Affects Indoor Radon Levels, *Chemecology,* 19, no. 8 (1990), 9.

139. Price, J.H., and S. Everett, Perceptions of Lung Cancer and Smoking in an Economically Disadvantaged Population, *Journal of Community Health,* 19, no. 5 (1994), 361–375.

140. Pringle, L., *Rain of Troubles: The Science and Politics of Acid Rain.* New York: MacMillan, 1988.

141. Probart, C.K., Issues Related to Radon in Schools, *Journal of School Health,* 59, no. 10 (1989), 441–443.

142. Public Health, Housing Agencies Work Together to Reduce Lead Hazard, *The Nation's Health,* January (1995), 11.

143. Putting Risk in Perspective: Pesticide Benefits Far Outweigh Risk, *Chemecology,* 19, no. 6 (1990), 2–3.

144. Ratoff, J., What's the Source of Acid Rain? *Science News,* March 3 (1990), 143.

145. ———, and D.E. Thomsen, Chernobyl May Be Worst Nuclear Accident, *Science News,* 129 (1986), 276.

146. Risks of Living Near Love Canal, *Science,* 217, no. 4562 (1982), 808–810.

147. RN's Facing New Dangers at Works, *American Journal of Nursing,* 95, no. 10 (1995), 78, 81.

148. Rule Finalized Last November: Suit Challenges OSHA Limits on Workers' Right to Know Hazards, *The Nation's Health,* July (1984), 1, 5.

149. Russell, A., J. Milford, and M.S. Bergin, Urban Ozone Control and Atmospheric Reactivity of Organic Gases, *Science,* 269 (July 28, 1995), 491–495.

150. Safe Drinking Water: Will Congress Weaken the Law That Protects Your Health? *National Wildlife,* 33, no. 3 (1995), 29–32.

151. Samet, J.M., New Effects of Active and Passive Smoking on Reproduction? *American Journal of Epidemiology,* 133, no. 4 (1991), 348–350.

152. Schwartz, J., Editorial: Is Carbon Monoxide a Risk Factor for Hospital Admission for Heart Failure? *American Journal of Public Health,* 85 (1995), 1343–1344.

153. Schuster, E., and Brown, C. (eds.). *Exploring Our Environmental Connections.* New York: National League for Nursing Press (Public No. 14-2634), 1994.

154. Sexton, K., and M.E. Radzikowski, The Environment and Our Health, *Healthcare Trends and Transition,* 5, no. 4 (1994), 22–23, 26.

155. Silver, J., The Past, Present, and Future of Times Beach, *Missouri Resources,* 12, no. 4 (1995–1996), 10–15.

156. Sockrider, M., and D. Coultas, Environmental Tobacco Smoke: A Real and Present Danger, *The Journal of Respiratory Diseases,* 15, no. 8 (1994), 715–733.

157. Sohn, M., Special Care Is Required with Pesticide Applicator's Clothing, *Union Banner,* May 23 (1990), 11.

158. Soine, L., Sick Building Syndrome and Gender Bias: Imperiling Women's Health, *Social Work in Health Care,* 20, no. 3 (1995), 51–65.

159. Specter, M., Sea-Dumping Ban: Good Politics, but Not Necessarily Good Policy, *Chemecology,* 22, no. 4 (1993), 9–12.

160. Steenland, K., and D. Brown, Silicosis Among Gold Miners: Exposure–Response Analysis and Risk Assessment, *American Journal of Public Health,* 85 (1995), 1372–1377.

161. Stellman, J., Occupational Health Hazards of Women: An Overview, *Preventive Medicine,* 7 (1978), 281–293.

162. ———, *Women's Work, Women's Health, Myths and Realities.* New York: Pantheon Press, 1978.

163. ———, The Effects of Toxic Agents on Reproduction, *Occupational Health and Safety,* April (1979), 36–43.

164. Sticklin, L.A., Strategies for Overcoming Nurses' Fear of Radiation Exposure, *Cancer Practice: A Multidisplinary Journal of Cancer Care,* 2, no. 4 (1994), 275–278.

165. Stigliani, W., et al., Chemical Time Bombs, *Environment,* 33, no. 4 (1991), 4–9, 26–30.

166. Stomach Cancer in Navahos and Uranium Link Suspected, *The Nation's Health,* July (1987), 9.

167. Survey: Farmers Using Fewer Pesticides, *Farm Week,* May 15 (1989), 9.

168. Takashi, S.T., et al., Mutagens in Food as Causes of Cancer, *Nutrition and Cancer: Etiology and Treatment.* New York: Raven Press, 1981.

169. Taming Toxics in Your Home, *National Wildlife,* 28, no. 3 (1990), 29.

170. Taylor, S.L., Food Allergies and Sensitivities, *Journal of American Diet Association,* 86 (1986), 599.

171. Technology Produced Occupational Hazards for Nurses, *The American Nurse,* April (1987), 7–8.

172. Test Can Detect Pesticide Poisoning in Farmers, *St. Louis Post-Dispatch,* February 1 (1987), Sect. C, p 12.

173. Topf, M., Theoretical Considerations for Research on Environmental Stress and Health, *IMAGE: Journal of Nursing Scholarship,* 26 (1994), 289–294.

174. Turk, J., and A. Turk, *Environmental Science.* Philadelphia: W.B. Saunders, 1988.

175. Udall, J., Turning Down the Heat, *Sierra,* July–August (1989), 26–39.

176. Uphold, C., and M. Graham, *Clinical Guidelines in Family Practice* (2nd ed.). Gainesville, FL: Barmarrae Books, 1994.

177. Valway, S., et al., Lead Absorption in Indoor Firing Range Users, *American Journal of Public Health,* 79, no. 8 (1989), 1029–1032.

178. Von Stackelberg, P., Whitewash: The Dioxin Cover-up, *Greenpeace,* March–April (1989), 7–11.

179. Waste Treatment That Pays Off in Water, Energy and Plants, *Chemecology,* 17, no. 8 (1988), 5–6.

180. Weaver, D., Our Global Community and You, *Missouri Resource Review,* Winter–Spring (1990), 18–27.

181. What Price Clean Up?, *Chemecology,* 22, no. 4 (1993), 2–7.

182. Whelan, E., Diseases and Misinformation. In Nutrition Myths and Misinformation: Special Report, *Nutrition and the MD,* 11 (1985), 1.

183. Whitaker, M., 'It Was Like Breathing Fire . . .', *Newsweek,* December 17 (1984), 26–32.

184. WHO Reports on New, Re-emerging Diseases Threatening World Health, *The Nation's Health,* 25, no. 10 (1995), 24.

185. Whyatt, R.M., Setting Human Health-Based Groundwater Protection Standards When Toxicological Data Are Inadequate, *American Journal of Industrial Medicine,* 18, no. 4 (1990), 505–510.

186. Williamson, K., et al., Occupational Health Hazards for Nurses, Part II, *IMAGE:Journal of Nursing Scholarship,* 20, no. 3 (1988), 162–168.

187. Wold, S., *Community Health Nursing: Issues and Topics.* Stamford, CT: Appleton & Lange, 1990.

188. Women Farmworkers Speak Out on Conditions, *The Nation's Health,* April (1993), 10.

189. Wright, A.L., et al., Relationship of Parental Smoking to Wheezing and Nonwheezing Lower Respiratory Tract Illnesses in Infancy, *Journal of Pediatrics,* 118, no. 2 (1991), 207–214.

190. Young, L., *Sowing the Wind: Reflections on the Earth's Atmosphere.* New York: Prentice-Hall, 1990.

191. Zahm, S., D. Weisenburger, P. Babbitt, R. Saal, J. Vaught, and A. Beaer, Use of Hair Coloring Products and the Risk of Lymphoma, Multiple Myeloma, and Chronic Lymphocytic Leukemia, *American Journal of Public Health,* 82 (1992), 990–997.

chapter three

Spiritual and Religious Influences on the Person and Family

Faith is the soul riding at anchor.

—*A. W. Shaw*

Key Terms

Religion

Spiritual dimension

Hinduism and Sikhism

Buddhism, Jainism, and Shintoism

Confucianism and Taoism

Islam

Judaism

Christianity

   Roman Catholicism

Greek/Eastern Orthodox faith

Protestantism

Seventh-Day Adventists

Church of Jesus Christ of Latter-Day Saints (Mormon)

Jehovah's Witnesses

Church of Christ, Scientist (Christian Scientists)

Society of Friends (Quakers)

Unity School of Christianity

Mennonites

Amish

Moravians

Waldenses

Unitarian Universalists

Neo-Pentecostalism

North American Indian religions

   Shamanism

     Spirit world

     Supreme Being

Culture hero

  New Age Movement

Agnostic

Atheistic

Cult

Devil or Satan worship

Voodo illness

Spiritual need

Spiritual distress

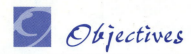

Objectives

Study of this chapter will enable you to:

1. Define the terms *religious* and *spiritual* and the connotations of each.

2. Contrast the major tenets of Hinduism, Sikhism, Buddhism, Jainism, Shintoism, Confucianism, Taoism, Islam, Judaism, Christianity, and North American Indian religions.

3. Compare the major tenets of the various branches of Christianity: Roman Catholicism, Eastern Orthodoxy, various Protestant denominations, other Christian sects.

4. Gain an overview of the variety of religions in the United States.

5. Discuss how religious beliefs influence lifestyle and health status in the various religious groups and subgroups.

6. Identify your religious beliefs, or lack of them, and explore how they will influence your practice.

7. Discuss your role in meeting the spiritual needs of client and family.

8. Describe specific nursing measures that can be used to meet the needs of persons with different religious backgrounds.

9. Work with a client who has religious beliefs different from your own or refer the client to an appropriate resource.

Until an illness occurs, the person may give no thought to the meaning of his or her life or spiritual beliefs. But when he or she feels vulnerable and fearful of the future, solace is sought. Religion can provide that solace.

A person sneezes. You say, "God bless you." Why? Perhaps unconsciously you are coordinating the medical–physical with the religious–spiritual. But you may feel afraid to work professionally with the combination. This fear comes in part from the long-lived schism between science and religion.

The attitude that medical science is superior to the spiritual dimension or to religion has affected us all. Yet the spiritual dimension and religion are there as they always have been. Each culture has had some organization or priesthood to sustain the important rituals and myths of its people. Primitive peoples combined the roles of physician, psychiatrist, and priest. The Indian medicine man and the African witch doctor combine magic with religion; with their herbs, psychosuggestion, and appeals to the gods, they realize that the person is a biopsychospiritual being (122).

I had the cancer patient visualize an army of white blood cells attacking and overcoming the cancer cells. Within 2 weeks the cancer had diminished and he was rapidly gaining weight. He is alive and well today.

Is this a priest or a faith healer talking? No, this is a prominent tumor specialist talking today. An internationally known neurosurgeon says, "In a very real sense, medicine is now—as it has always been—faith healing." Other health providers have seen life return after death. Thus, some health workers are trying to reunite the biopsychospiritual being.

History reveals that in the 5th century AD, Western society disintegrated and religion and scientific theory split. Through a long process, the two theories are now sharing dialogue. In her manuscript, "Suggestion for Thought," Florence Nightingale attempted to integrate science and mysticism. She felt the universe was an incarnation of a divine intelligence that regulated all things through law (65). She recognized that humans have spiritual needs; spiritual care enables the person to be conscious of the presence of God, the creator and sustainer of the universe (52).

The 1980s and 1990s have shown an increased awareness of the link between health and religion, and the subject is being discussed more openly. A study of 1077 students at Northern Illinois University suggested that students who attended church regularly and scored high in religiosity stayed healthier than students who did not attend church and scored low in religiosity. The students who attended church also used less alcohol, drugs, and cigarettes (23, 100). Several articles in medical and nursing journals and in the newspapers have discussed physicians and nurses who pray with their patients; the authors state that prayer has added to the effectiveness of therapy (3, 5, 23, 30, 122).

DEFINITIONS

Religion is defined on various levels: *a belief in a supernatural or divine force that has power over the universe and commands worship and obedience; a system of beliefs; a comprehensive code of ethics or philosophy; a set of practices that are followed; a church affiliation; the conscious pursuit of any object the person holds as supreme. In short, religion signifies that a group of people have established and organized practices that are related to spiritual concerns.*

This definition, however, does not portray the constancy and at times the fervency that can underlie religious belief. In every human there seems to be a **spiritual dimension,** *a quality that goes beyond religious affiliation, that strives for inspiration, reverence, awe, meaning, and purpose even in those who do not believe in any god. The spiritual dimension tries to be in harmony with the universe, strives for answers about the infinite, and especially comes into focus as a sustaining power when the person faces emotional stress, physical illness, or death. It goes outside a person's own power.*

Some authors subsume spirituality or spiritual needs under cultural traditions or philosophic beliefs, or describe spirituality as including all positive human qualities. Culture, philosophy, love, and reverence for another person are all *humanizing influences.* The feelings called forth by the consciousness of a presence of a higher nature than human, unconnected with material objects or qualities, are *spiritual influences* (56).

In the midst of our specialized health care you have an opportunity to go beyond the dogma to bring together the biopsychospiritual being through the study of the religions and religious symbols of your clients. Those are world religions, not your personal or country's basic religion. Mass media, rapid transportation, and cultural exchanges have nullified the provincial approach.

WORLD RELIGIONS

Studying world religions poses a semantic difficulty in that an expression in the Chinese-based religion of Confucianism may have no equivalent in the English language. Thus, language has dictated what people think, how they act, and how their religious beliefs are carried out (9).

Concepts, however, are often basically the same but are rephrased in each religion's own linguistic style. The saying "Love one another as I have loved you" will appear to the Hindu as "This is the sum of religion, do not unto other what causes pain to you"; to the Taoist as "Return goodness for hatred"; and to the Muslim as "No one is a believer unless he desires for his brother what he desires for himself."

Each religion also has other characteristics in common:

- A world view, a way of perceiving reality; a description of existence and life meaning; assumptions about the universe and life
- Basis of authority or source(s) of power
- A portion of scripture or sacred word
- An ethical code that defines right and wrong
- A psychology and identity so that its adherents fit into a group and the world is defined by the religion
- Aspirations or expectations
- Some ideas about what follows death

See Table 3–1 for key facts about eight major world religions. For additional information about philosophic and mystical aspects of Hinduism, Buddhism, Islam, Taoism, and Sikhism, see Rice (103), the descriptions in this chapter, and related references.

The major world religions can be divided into categories in an attempt to group characteristics even further (9). The *alpha* group includes Christianity, Judaism, and Islam. All adhere to a Biblical revelation of a supernatural, monotheistic God. People in these religions are "doers." They obey because God commands; they make covenants with God for protection; they have a historical fixed scripture that is canonized for public use, and they often proselytize. Into the *gamma* group go Taoism (pronounced "dowism"), Confucianism, and Shintoism. In these religions people believe either that everything is in the being of God or that there is no godhead (still a definite belief). These people try to be in harmony with the world around them. Their most immediate concern is in relationships with others. Scripture is a family affair. They can be characterized as simple in faith, spontaneous, and straightforward in feelings of affection for people, flowers, and birds. The final grouping is the *beta* group, which includes Buddhism and Hinduism. These religions have their roots in Indian soil, their world view is pantheism, and they teach that everything is in the being of God. Adherents are interested in "being" rather than "doing." They have a collective literature for private devotion. Control of mind and body is desired, as some of the yoga practices show. The beta and gamma groups do not define God

TABLE 3–1. KEY FACTS ABOUT THE EIGHT MAJOR WORLD RELIGIONS

Religion	Where Strongest	Supreme Being	Founder/ When Founded	Historical Leaders	Leadership	Sacred Writings	Holy Places	Typical Holy Days
Hinduism	India Ceylon	Brahman All Reality	No historical founder 3200 BC	Mahatma Gandhi Ramakrishna	Sannyasis (holymen) Guru (preacher)	Vedas Brahmanas Upanishads Great Epics	Benares (city) Ganges (river)	The Mela Holi Festival Dasera Divuli
Judaism	Israel Europe Western Hemisphere	Yahweh (Jehovah or God)	Abraham 1300 BC	Moses Amos Micah Other prophets	Rabbis	Torah Talmud	Jerusalem	Rosh Hashanah Yom Kippur Hanukkah Purim Passover
Taoism	China	Jade Emperor Many folk gods	Lao-Tzu (or Lao-Tse) 604 BC	Lao-Tse Chuang-Tse 350–275 BC	None	Tao-Te-Ching	Kiangsi and many holy mountains	Birthdays of Gods Festival of Souls Autumn Festival
Confucianism	China Japan Korea	Confucius Shang-Ti	Confucius 557 BC	Yang Chu Moh Tih	None	NuChing Sau Shu	None	None
Buddhism	China Japan India Burma	108 different names	Gautama 560–480 BC	Gautama Amitabha	Bhikkhus Monks Also nuns Lamas	Dharma (Sutta) Vinaya Abhidhamma	Sarnath Lumbini Buddh-Gaya Kusinara	Perahera Festival in Ceylon Wesak (Kason) in May
Christianity	Western Europe Western Hemisphere	God	Jesus AD 30	John the Baptist, 12 disciples, 4 gospel writers, writers of epistles	Varied Priests Ministers Layman	Bible Old Testament New Testament	Bethlehem Jerusalem Rome Nazareth	Christmas Good Friday Easter Pentecost
Shinto	Japan	Izanagi (Sky Father) Izanami (Earth Mother)	No founder AD 6th century	None	None	Nihongi Kojiki	Mt. Fujiyama	New Year Bon (Festival of Dead) Tenri-Kyo (January)
Islam	Arabia Middle East	Allah	Mohammed AD 570–632	Mohammed Husein (grandson) Abu Bakr Omar Othman Ali	None	Koran	Mecca Jerusalem	Ramadan (Sacred Month)

as clearly as the alpha group. The beta and gamma groups look inside themselves for answers: common sense rather than commands from God determines good. Salladay contrasts pantheistic with Christian beliefs (111).

The following discussion presents a more detailed insight into each major world religion through personality sketches. Each person has a fictitious name and represents not a single person but a composite of knowledge gained from the authors' interviewing, reading, and personal experience. Although these personalities are presented as acting and thinking in a certain way, remember that the person's culture, family background, and personality affect how that person lives out a religious experience. Thus, a particular Hindu and a given Roman Catholic may be more in agreement religiously than two Lutherans. You cannot make generalizations about a religion from knowing a single follower.

Hinduism and Sikhism

Rama tells us that nothing is typically **Hindu** and that anyone who puts religion in neat packages will have difficulty comprehending his outlook. Rama is named after Ramakrishna, the greatest saint of **Hinduism** of the 19th century. The history of Rama's religion goes back to approximately 1500 BC, when the **Vedas**—*divine revelations*—were written. His main religious texts are the **Upanishads,** or *scriptures,* and the **Bhagavad Gita,** a *summary of the former with additions. The most expressive and universal word of God is* **Om,** or **Aum,** providing the most important auditory and visual symbol in Rama's religion.*

Rama speaks of some of the worship popular in India today: of the family and local deities and of the trinity—**Brahma,** *the creator,* **Vishnu,** *the preserver and god of love,* and **Shiva,** *the destroyer.*

Rama tells of his own shrine in his home where, in the presence of various pictures of **incarnations** (*human forms of God*) and with incense burning, he meditates. He also thinks of Buddha, Muhammed, and Jesus as incarnations and sometimes reads from the scriptures inspired by their teachings, although they represent other major religions.

Despite this vast array of deities and the recognition that all religions are valid, Rama believes in one universal concept—**Brahman,** the *Divine Intelligence,* the *Supreme Reality.* Rama believes all paths lead to the understanding that this "reality" exists as part of all physical beings, especially humans. Rama's entire spiritual quest is directed toward uniting his *inner and real self,* the **atman,** with the concept of Brahman. So although Rama has gone through several stages of desire—for pleasure, power, wealth, fame, and humanitarianism—the last stage, his desire for freedom, for touching the infinite, is his main goal.

Rama is interested in health and illness only as a guide to this goal. He feels that the human love for the body is a cause for illness. He says, for example, that we overeat and get a stomachache. He views the pain as a warning—in this case, to stop overeating. He does not oppose medical treatment if absolutely necessary, but he believes that medicine can sometimes dull the pain and then the person overeats again, thus perpetuating the cause of the problem. Medical or psychiatric help,

Rama says, is at best transitory. The cause of the pain must be rooted out.

In order not to dwell on physical concerns, Rama strives for moderation in eating and in other body functions. He considers only the atman as real and eternal and the body as unreal and finite. The body is a temple, a vehicle, no more. He tries to take care of it so that it will not scream at him because of overindulgence or underindulgence. Rama is a vegetarian. He believes that meat and intoxicants would excite his senses too much. Yet the Hindu diet pattern is flexible; definite rules are not set. If Rama is sick, he tries to bear his illness with resignation, knowing its temporary nature. He believes that the prayer of supplication for body cure is the lowest form of prayer, whereas the highest form is devotion to God. To him, death and rebirth are nearly synonymous, for the atman never changes and always remains pure. He compares the atman to the ocean: as ocean water can be put into various containers without changing its nature, so can the atman be put into various physical and human containers without changing its nature.

Thus if death is imminent, Rama believes that the body, mind, and senses weaken and become lifeless but that the never-changing atman is ready to enter into a new form of life, depending on the person's knowledge, deeds, and past experiences. Full acceptance of death is encouraged. Death is a friend to be faced bravely, calmly, and confidently.

Rama says that as a devotee of God he is following a *training course* called **yoga.** As a preliminary, however, he must establish certain moral qualifications. He must strive for self-control, self-discipline, cleanliness, and contentment. He must avoid injury, deceitfulness, and stealing. His overwhelming desire to reach God can be implemented through one or a combination of the four yoga paths: (1) **inana yoga** through *reading and absorbing knowledge,* (2) **bhakti yoga** through the *devotion of emotion and love,* (3) **karma yoga** through *work dedicated to God,* and (4) **raja yoga** through *psychological experiments on oneself.* Rama combines the first three by reading and memorizing portions of the ancient scriptures, by meditating daily at his shrine, and by dedicating the results of his professional work to God.

Rama mentions that various forms of yoga have spread around the world to form hybrid groups with varied purposes. One branch that has appeared in medical centers is **hatha yoga,** meaning *sun and moon, symbolizing an inner balance that is achieved through muscle and breathing exercises.* Ultimately the body is prepared for meditation through these exercises.

From the bhakti emphasis comes **Sikhism,** founded by Nanak who was born in 1469. The Sikhs

---

*See the symbol at the beginning of this section. A transliteration of the script is *a, u, m.* It is written in English as *Om,* or *Aum. Om, God,* and *Brahman* are synonymous and mean a *consciousness* or *awareness* rather than a personified being.

had nine other gurus, or spiritual mentors, who sequentially taught that God was the one and only reality. The fifth guru compiled the scripture. Starting as a pacifist group, the Sikhs evolved to warriors.

Also from bhakti influence has come the **Hare Krishna** movement in the United States, starting in 1965 when A.C. Bhaktivedanta came to New York City. The first Krishna temple was established on the Lower East Side (31).

For Rama, religion is not something to be picked up and put down according to a schedule or one's mood. It is a constant and all-pervading part of his life, every value and action, and the life of his country. India's literature and art are witness to this fact. It also influences family life and structure. Basically marriage is for life, and people marry someone in the same social level. The husband is treated with respect, and the mother is thought of as ideal. The family is patrifocal; the father has final authority. He is like a god. All family members are close. Elders are respected, cared for when they are ill, and considered as experienced models; children and grandchildren seek their wisdom. Children have reverence for both father and mother, and back talk is unthinkable. Friends are to be treated as brothers and sisters, and visitors are always treated congenially.

Buddhism, Jainism, and Shintoism

Umeko Sato is a member of the sect of **Buddhism** called **Soka Gakkai.** This sect is a powerful religion in Japan, with a government party, a university, and a grand temple representing it. Now more than 70 years old, this organization that constitutes 10% of Japan's population, known previously as a militant proselytizer, has toned down this phase and is living more graciously with other sects and creeds. Based on the **Lotus Sutra,** *part of the Buddhist scriptures,* its doctrine advocates the three values of happiness: profit, goodness, and beauty. Sato is attracted by the practicality of the teaching, the mottoes that she can live by, the emphasis on small group study, and present world benefits, especially healing.

Although Sato's beliefs at some points seem in direct contrast to the original Buddhist teachings, she is happy to explain the rich multireligious tradition that her family has had for generations. She emphasizes that she is affected by the **Confucian** emphasis on the family unit, by Christianity's healing emphasis, by **Shintoism,** the state religion of Japan until 1945, and by Buddhism, which originated about 600 BC in India with a Hindu named Siddhartha Gautama.

Currently approximately 90% of Japan's 120 million people adhere both to Buddhism and to Shintoism, although the nation has never been known as devout. Less than 1% are Christian. Another small religion is **Jainism.** The "Jains" hark back to the 6th century BC, about the same time as Buddha. Their fundamental tenet is *ahimsa,* a refusal to injure any living thing. Jains believe every living thing has a soul.

There are two groups of Jains. A small group of approximately 100 are called *sky clad* because they wear no clothes. They renounce clothing and all earthly possessions. The other, larger group is called *white clad* because they wear white clothes. Together the groups contain monks, nuns, laymen, and laywomen who all take vows to guide them in all aspects of daily life.

Although the Jains are found in Japan and other countries, including the United States, they probably are known best for their bird hospital in Old Delhi, India, which treats 20,000 birds each year.

Gautama, shortly after a historic enlightenment experience during which he became the Buddha, preached a sermon to his followers and drew on the earth a wheel representing the continuous round of life and death and rebirth. Later eight spokes were added to illustrate the sermon and to provide the most explicit visual symbol of Buddhism* today. Sato repeats Buddha's four noble truths: (1) life is disjointed or out of balance, especially in birth, old age, illness, and death; (2) the cause of this imbalance is ignorance of one's own true nature; (3) removal of this ignorance is attained by reaching **Nirvana,** *the divine state of release, the ultimate reality, the perfect knowledge* via (4) the eightfold path.

The eight spokes of the wheel represent the eightfold path used to reach Nirvana. Sato says that followers subscribe to right knowledge, right intentions, right speech, right conduct, right means of livelihood, right effort, right mindfulness, and concentration. From these concepts has arisen a moral code that, among other things, prohibits intoxicants, lying, and killing of any kind (which explains why Buddhists are often vegetarians). She further explains that the Mahayana branch of Buddhism took hold in Japan as opposed to the Theravada branch. The **Theravada branch** emphasizes an intellectual approach through wisdom, people working by themselves through meditation and without ritual. The **Mahayana branch** emphasizes involvement with humankind, ritual, petitionary prayer, and concern for one's sibling. Sato believes that the Mahayana branch

---

*See the symbol at the beginning of this section.

provides the happier philosophy of the two, and she tells of the ritual of celebration of Gautama's birthday. But most Japanese believe in **Amitabha Buddha,** a god rather than a historical figure, who is replacing the austere image of Gautama as a glorious redeemer, one of infinite light. Also, the people worship **Kwannon,** a goddess of compassion.

Sato explains that she cannot omit mention of the one austere movement within the Mahayana branch, the **Zen sect.** Taking this example from Gautama's extended contemplation of a flower, Zen followers care little for discourse, books, or other symbolic interpretations and explanations of reality. Hours and years are devoted to meditation, contemplation of word puzzles, and consultation with a Zen master. In seeking absolute honesty and truthfulness through such simple acts as drinking tea or gardening, the Zen student hopes to experience enlightenment. In America, a version of Buddhism called *Buddhaharma* is emerging. Women and men are considered equal. This group provides meditations for the public on a CD-ROM disk.

Sato next turns to her former state religion, **Shintoism.** Whereas Buddhism produced a solemnizing effect on her country, Shintoism had an affirmative and joyous effect. Emperor, ancestor, ancient hero, and nature worship form its core. Those who follow Shintoism, she says, feel an intense loyalty and devotion to every lake, tree, and blossom in Japan and to the ancestral spirits abiding there. They also have a great concern for cleanliness, a carryover from early ideas surrounding dread of pollution in the dead.

Sato says that her parents have two god shelves in their home. One contains wooden tablets inscribed with the name of the household's patron–deity and a symbolic form of the goddess of rice and other texts and objects of family significance. Here her family performs simple rites such as offering a prayer or a food gift each day. In a family crisis, perhaps an illness, the family conducts more elaborate rites such as lighting tapers or offering rice brandy. The other god shelf, in another room, is the Buddha shelf; and if a family member dies, a Buddhist priest, the spiritual leader, performs specified rituals there.

Sato strongly emphasizes that if illness or impending death causes a family member to be hospitalized, another well family member will stay at the hospital to bathe, cook for, and give emotional support to the ill person. Sato believes that recovery depends largely on this family tie. If death occurs, Sato will be reminded of the Buddhist doctrine teaching that death is a total nonfunction of the physical body and mind and that the life force is displaced and transformed to continue to function in another form. Every birth is a rebirth, much as in the Hindu teaching, the rebirth happens immediately after death, according to some Buddhists. Others believe that rebirth occurs 49 days after death, during which time the person is in an intermediary state. The difference in quality of death, birth, and existence depends on whether the person lived a disciplined or undisciplined life.

Buddhism teaches the living how to die well. The elderly, or feeble, are to prepare themselves mentally for a state that would be conducive for a good rebirth. The person is to remain watchful and alert in the face of death, to resist distraction and confusion, to be lucid and calm. Distinct instructions are given in what to expect as life leaves the body, as the person enters an intermediary state, and as Nirvana is about to occur.

So although Sato has grasped a new religious path for herself, her respect for tradition remains.

In giving care to a person with Umeko Sato's background, be aware of the varied religious influences on life. The sect's emphasis on the here and now rather than on the long road to Nirvana may place a high value on physical health so that the person can benefit from the joys and beauty of his life. The person may readily voice impatience with the body's dysfunction. You can also respond to the great concern for cleanliness, the desire to have family nearby, and the need for family rites that are offered for the sick member. Should a family member be dying, you may see some ambivalence. The family member may want to prepare himself or herself in the traditional way, but someone with Sato's background, with emphasis on present world benefits and healing, may deny that there is a valid preparation for death.

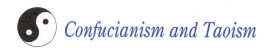

Confucianism and Taoism

Wong Huieng is a young teacher in Taiwan simultaneously influenced by **Taoism,** the *romantic and mystical,* and **Confucianism,** the *practical and pragmatic.* To provide insights into these Chinese modes of thinking, although it is more representative of Taoism, Wong Huieng uses the yin–yang symbol.* The symbol is a circle, representing **Tao** or the *absolute,* in which two tear shapes fit perfectly into one another, each containing a small dot from the other. Generally yang is light or red, and yin is dark. Ancient Chinese tradition says that everything exists in these two interacting forces. Each represents a group of qualities. Yang is positive or masculine—dry, hot, active, moving, and light. Yin is femi-

---

*See the symbol at the beginning of this section.

nine or negative—wet, bold, passive, restful, and empty. For example, fire is almost pure yang and water almost pure yin, but not quite. The combination of yin and yang constitutes all the dualisms a person can imagine: day–night, summer–winter, beauty–ugliness, illness–health, life–death. Both qualities are necessary for life in the universe; they are complementary and, if in harmony, good. Yang and yin energy forces are embodied in the body parts and affect food preferences and eating habits.

Huieng translates this symbol into a relaxed philosophy of life: "If I am sick, I will get better. Life is like going up and down a mountain; sometimes I feel good and sometimes I feel bad. That's the way it is." Though educated, she is not interested in climbing up the job ladder, accumulating wealth, or conquering nature. Her goal is to help provide money to build an orphanage in a natural wooded setting.

Huieng thinks of death as a natural part of life, as the peace that comes when the body is worn out. She admits, however, that when her father died, human grief took hold of her. Before his death, her mother went to the Taoist temple priest and got some incense that was to help cast the sickness from his body. After death, they kept his body in the house for the required time, 49 days. The priest executed a special ceremony every 7 days. Her mother could cry only 1 hour daily, 2:00 until 3:00 in the morning. Now her mother talks through the priest to her father's ghost. Although Huieng regards this practice as superstitious and thinks that painting a picture of a lake and mountain is a more fitting way to erase her grief, she looks at the little yellow bag, containing a blessing from the priest, hanging around her neck, and finds it comforting if not intellectually acceptable.

Now Huieng turns to her practical side and talks about **Confucius,** the *first saint of the nation.* Although **Lao-tzu,** the *founder of Taoism,* is a semilegendary figure said to have vanished after he wrote the *bible of Taoism,* **Tao-te-ching,** Confucius has a well-documented existence.

Confucius, born in 551 BC, wrote little. His disciples wrote the **Analects,** *short proverbs, embodying his teachings.* He is revered as a teacher, not as a god. Huieng does not ask him to bless her but tries to emulate him and his teachings, which she has heard since birth. The temple in his memory is a place for studying, not for praying. And on his birthday, a national holiday, people pay respect to their teachers in his memory.

Five important terms in Confucius' teaching are **Jen,** *a striving for goodness within;* **Chun-sui,** *establishing a gentlemanly or womanly approach with others;* **Li,** *knowing how relationships should be conducted and having respect for age;* **Te,** *leading by virtuous character rather than by force;* and **Wen,** *pursuing the arts as an adjunct to moral character.* Huieng stresses that in Li are the directives for family relationships. So strongly did Confucius feel about the family that he gave directives on proper attitudes between father and son, elder brother and junior brother, husband and wife. Also, Huieng believes she cannot harm her body because it was given to her by her parents. Her concept of immediate family includes grandparents, uncles, aunts, and cousins. Her language has more words for relationships between relatives than the English language does.

Huieng believes that in caring for her body, she cares for her family, the country, and the universe. Essentially, to her, all people are family.

Important in your understanding of a person with Wong Huieng's background is the dualism that exists in such thinking. Acceptance of the particular version of mysticism and practicality and of the yin and yang forces that are seen as operating within self will help in building a foundation of personalized care.

The person may have more respect for older than younger staff members and may respond well to teaching. There may be a strong desire to attain and maintain wellness. These factors are directly related to the religious teaching; you can use them to enhance care. Additionally, talk slowly to the person if language is an issue. Rely on family members to help you understand the person's feelings. Permit familiar foods. Remember that foods are also divided into appropriate groups for types of illness. Address the person by the proper name. Do not use excessive touch signals unless they are invited. Remember this person may be in awe of health care authority and may be intimidated.

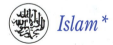 *Islam* *

Omar Ali is *Muslim,* a member of **Islam,** the youngest of the major world religions. "There is no God but Allah; Muhammad is His Prophet"[†] provides the key to Omar's beliefs. He must say this but once in his life as a requirement, but he will repeat it many times as an affirmation. Muslims believe in a final judgment day when everyone will be judged and sent either to Paradise or to the fire of hell, depending on how justly he or she

---

*A portion of this section was contributed by Caroline Samiezadé-Yazd, RN, MSN, PNP.
[†]These words are a translation of the sacred calligraphy in the symbol shown at the beginning of this section. The prophet's name is sometimes spelled *Muhammad.*

lived life according to God's laws. They believe everyone, except children before the age of puberty, are responsible for their own good and bad actions and deeds and that no one can intercede on behalf of another.

Omar has also been influenced by the 3000-year-old **Zoroastrianism,** *which is a religion of pre-Islamic Iran* that flourishes in Bombay today. Likewise, it was a monotheistic religion even though dualism was also espoused.

Omar is an Egyptian physician whose religious tradition was revealed through Muhammed, born approximately AD 571 in Mecca, then a trading point between India and Syria on the Arabian peninsula. Hating polytheism and paganism in any form, Muhammed recited God's revelation to him as is documented in the **Quran,*** *scriptures.* Omar believes in the biblical prophets, but he calls Muhammed the greatest—the seal of Prophets.

Through the Quran and the **Hadith,** *the traditions,* Omar has guidelines for his thinking, devotional life, and social obligations. He believes he is a unique individual with an eternal soul. He believes in a heaven and hell, and while on earth he wants to walk the straight path.

To keep on this path, Omar prays five times a day: generally on rising, at midday, in the afternoon, in the early evening, and before retiring. Articles needed are water and a prayer rug. Because the Quran emphasizes cleanliness of body, Omar performs a ritual washing with running water over the face, arms, top of head, and feet before each prayer. Omar explains that in the bedridden client this requirement can be accomplished by pouring water out of some sort of receptacle. If a Muslim's entire body is considered ritually unclean, he must wash the entire body. If water is unavailable or the person cannot bathe, clean soil may be used in place of the ritual washing. After this washing the Muslim needs either a ritually clean cloth or a prayer rug and a clean place to pray. He may not face a dirty area such as the bathroom when making his prayer, even if this area is in the line toward Mecca. The Muslim must physically readjust himself in this case to comply with Islamic regulations. Then, facing Mecca, he goes through a series of prescribed bodily motions and repeats various passages in praise and supplication.

Omar also observes **Ramadan,** *a fast month,*† during which time he eats or drinks nothing from sunrise to sunset; after sunset he takes nourishment only in moderation. He explains **fasting** (*abstinence from eating*) as a discipline aiding him to understand those with little food and more importantly, as a submission to Allah. At the end of Ramadan, he enters a festive period with feelings of goodwill and gift exchanges. The sick, the very old, pregnant and lactating mothers, children, and Muslims who require the ingestion or injection of substances throughout the day hours are exempt without penalty from practice of this belief.

Omar has made one pilgrimage to Mecca, another requirement for all healthy and financially able Muslims. He believes the experience created a great sense of brotherhood, for all the pilgrims wore similar modest clothing, exchanged news of followers in various lands, and reviewed their mutual faith. The 12th day of the Pilgrimage month is the **Feast of Sacrifice (Eida-Fita)** when all Muslim families kill a lamb in honor of Abraham's offering of his son to God.

In the line with the Quran's teaching, Omar does not eat pork (including such items as bologna, which might contain partial pork products), gamble, drink intoxicants, use illicit drugs, or engage in religiously unlawful sexual practices such as premarital sex, homosexuality, and infidelity. The emphasis on strict moral upbringing—dating, dancing, drinking, and sex outside marriage are forbidden—puts the Muslim on a common ground with conservative Christians. Abstinence from drug use also eliminates many potential health and social problems.

Omar worships no images or pictures of Muhammed, for the prophet is not deified. Nor does he hang or display pictures of any prophet or any god or worship statues or religious symbols. He gives a portion of his money to the poor, for Islam advocates a responsibility to society.

Omar points out that not all Arabs are Muslims and not all Muslims are Arabs. Arabs come from a number of nations stretching from Morocco to the Persian Gulf. Persons who are Arab Muslims speak Arabic and uphold the tenets of Islam. Omar emphasizes the importance of gaining specific knowledge about their complex social structure. The centrality of religion and the family are closely related and reflect many aspects of health care.

Omar mentions that parts of the basic Islam faith are used by a United States-based group commonly known as the **Black Muslims (Nation of Islam).** Known to have stringent, seclusionist rules, the Black Muslims are rapidly increasing in numbers and power. They seem to be moving away from orthodox Islam. Members may not get politically involved; membership is especially appealing to young African-American men who like the masculine focus, the structure, and the emphasis on self-help and self-esteem.

---

*Sometimes spelled *Koran.*

†Coming during the ninth month of the Muslim year, always at a different time each year by the Western calendar, and sometimes spelled *Ramazan.*

Omar outlines the ideas of his religion as it applies to his profession. He believes that he can make a significant contribution to health care but that essentially what happens is God's will. Submission to God is the very meaning of Islam. This belief produces a very fluid feeling of time and sense of fatalism. Planning ahead for a Muslim is not a value as it is in Western culture; to defy God's will brings on the evil eye.

Muslim clients who are ill are excused from many, but not all, religious rules, but many will still want to follow them as closely as possible. Even though in a body cast and unable to get out of bed, a client may want to go through prayers symbolically. The person might also recite the first chapters of the Quran, centered on praise to Allah, which are often used in times of crises. Family is a great comfort in illness, and praying with a group is strengthening, but the Muslim has no priest. The relationship is directly with God. Some clients may seem fatalistic, completely resigned to death, whereas others, hoping it is God's will that they live, cooperate vigorously with the medical program. Muslims do not discuss death openly because if they did, the client and family may lose all hope and the client could die as a result. Instead, Muslims tend to communicate grief in gradual stages rather than immediately and all at once. Further, they make it a point never to let the affected person lose hope. The family, even in the gravest of situations, will not attempt to prepare for the death even when it is imminent. After death, a body must be washed with running water by a Muslim and the hands folded in prayer. Muslims do not perform autopsies, embalm, or use caskets for burials. Instead, they wrap a white linen cloth around the dead person and place the body into the ground facing Mecca. Knowledge of these attitudes and traditions can greatly enhance your care.

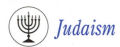

Judaism

Seth Lieberman, strongly influenced by the social concern emphasis in **Judaism,** is a psychiatrist. In the Jewish community each member is expected to contribute to others' needs according to his or her ability. Jews have traditionally considered their community as a whole responsible for feeding the hungry, helping the widowed and orphaned, rescuing the captured, and even burying the dead. Jewish retirement homes, senior citizens' centers, and medical centers are witnesses to this philosophy.

Seth cannot remember when his religious instruction began—it was always there. He went through the motions and felt the emotion of the Sabbath eve with its candles and cup of sanctification long before he could comprehend his father's explanations. Book learning followed, however, and he came to understand the fervency with which his people study and live the law as given in the **Torah,** *the first five books of the Bible,* and in the **Talmud,** *a commentary and enlargement of the Torah.* His spiritual leader is the *rabbi.* His *spiritual symbol* is the **menorah.***

His own *entrance into a responsible religious life and manhood* was through the **Bar Mitzvah,** a ceremony which took place in the synagogue when he was 13. (Girls are also educated to live responsible religious lives, and a few congregations now have a similar ceremony, the **Bas Mitzvah,** for girls.)

Although raised in an Orthodox home, Seth and his family are now Reform. He mentions another group, the Conservatives. The **Orthodox** *believe God gave the law;* it was written exactly as He gave it; *it should be followed precisely.* **Reform Jews** *believe the law was written by inspired men* at various times and therefore is *subject to reinterpretation.* Seth says he follows the traditions because they are traditions rather than because God demands it. **Conservatives** *are in the middle, taking some practices from both groups.* Overriding any differences in interpretation of ritual and tradition is the fundamental concept expressed in the prayer "Hear, O Israel, the Lord our God, the Lord is One." Not only is He one, He loves His creation, wants His people to live justly, and wants to bless their food, drink, and celebration. Judaism's double theme might be expressed as "Enjoy life now, and share it with God." Understandably then, Seth's religious emphasis is not on an afterlife, although some Jewish people believe in one. Although Jews have had a history of suffering, the inherent value of suffering or illness is not stressed. Through their observance of the law, the belief of their historical role as God's chosen people, and their hope for better days, Jews have survived seemingly insurmountable persecution.

Seth works with physically, emotionally, and spiritually depressed persons. He believes that often the spiritual depression is unnoticed, misunderstood, or ignored by professional workers. He cites instances in which mental attitudes have brightened as he shared a common bond of Judaism with a client.

He offers guidelines for working with a Jewish person in a hospital or nursing home. Although Jewish law

---

*See the symbol at beginning of this section. The seven-branched candelabrum stands for the creation of the universe in 7 days, the center light symbolizes the Sabbath, and the candlelight symbolizes the presence of God in the Temple.

can be suspended when a person is ill, the client will be most comfortable following as many practices as possible.

Every Jew observes the **Sabbath,** *a time for spiritual refreshment, from sundown on Friday to shortly after sundown on Saturday.* During this period Orthodox Jews may refuse freshly cooked food, medicine, treatment, surgery, and use of radio, television, and writing equipment lest the direction of their thinking be diverted on this special day. An Orthodox male may want to wear a **yarmulke** or *skullcap* continuously, use a *prayer book* called **Siddur,** and use **phylacteries,** *leather strips with boxes containing scriptures,* at weekday morning prayer. Also, the ultra-Orthodox male may refuse to use a razor because of the Levitical ban on shaving.

Some Orthodox Jewish women observe the rite of **Mikvah,** *an ancient ritual of family purity.* From marriage to menopause (except when pregnant) these women observe no physical-sexual relations with their husbands from 24 hours before menstruation until 12 days later when a ritual immersion in water renders them ready to meet their husbands again.

Jewish dietary laws have been considered by some scholars as health measures: to enjoy life is to eat properly and in moderation. The Orthodox, however, obey them because God so commanded. Food is called **treyfe** (or *treyfah*) if it is *unfit* and **kosher** if it is *ritually correct.*

Foods forbidden are pig, horse, shrimp, lobster, crab, oyster, and fowl that are birds of prey. Meats approved are from those animals that are ruminants and have divided hooves. Fish approved must have both fins and scales. Also, the kosher animals must be healthy and slaughtered in a prescribed manner. Because of the Biblical passage stating not to soak a young goat in its mother's milk, Jews do not eat meat products and milk products together. Neither are the utensils used to cook these products nor the dishes from which to eat these products ever intermixed.

Guidelines for a satisfactory diet for the Orthodox are as follows:

- Serve milk products first, meat second. Meat can be eaten a few minutes after milk, but milk cannot be taken for 6 hours after meat.
- If a person completely refuses meat because of incorrect slaughter, encourage a vegetarian diet with protein supplements such as fish and eggs, considered neutral unless prepared with milk or meat shortening.
- Buy frozen kosher products marked Ⓤ *K,* or *pareve.*
- Heat and serve food in the original container and use plastic utensils.

Two important holy days are Rosh Hashanah and Yom Kippur. **Rosh Hashanah,** *the Jewish New Year,* is a time to meet with the family, give thanks to God for good health, and renew traditions. **Yom Kippur,** the *day of atonement,* a time for asking forgiveness of family members for wrongs done, occurs 10 days later. On Yom Kippur, Jews fast for 24 hours, a symbolic act of self-denial, mourning, and petition. **Tisha Bab,** the *day of lamentation,* recalling the destruction of both Temples of Jerusalem, is another 24-hour fast period. **Pesach** or **Passover** (8 days for Orthodox and Conservative, 7 days for Reform) *celebrates the ancient Jews' deliverance from Egyptian bondage.* **Matzo,** *an unleavened bread,* replaces leavened bread during this period.

The Jewish person is preoccupied with health. Jews are future-oriented and want to know diagnosis, how a disease will affect business, family life, and social life. The Jewish people as a whole are highly educated, and although they respect the doctor, they may obtain several medical opinions before carrying out a treatment plan.

Although family, friends, and rabbi may visit the ill especially on or near holidays, they will also come at other times. Visiting the sick is a religious duty. And although death is final to many Jews except for living on in the memories of others, guidelines exist for this time. When a Jewish person has suffered irreversible brain damage and can no longer say a **bracha,** *a blessing to praise God,* or perform a **mitzvah,** *an act to help a fellow,* he or she is considered a "vegetable" with nothing to save. Prolonging the life by artificial means would not be recommended. But until then the dying client must be treated as the complete person he or she always was, capable of conducting his or her own affairs and entering into relationships.

Jewish tradition says never to leave the bedside of the dying person, which is of value to the dying and the mourners. The dying soul should leave in the presence of people, and the mourner is shielded from guilt of thinking that the client was alone at death or that more could be done. The bedside vigil also serves as a time to encourage a personal confession by the dying, which is a *rite de passage* to another phase of existence (even though unknown). This type of confessional is said throughout the Jewish life cycle whenever one stage has been completed. Confessional on the deathbed is a recognition that one cycle is ending and that another cycle is beginning. Recitation of the *Shema* in the last moments before death helps the dying to affirm faith in God and focus on the most familiar rituals of life.

Death, being witnessed at the bedside, helps to reinforce the reality of the situation. Immediate burial and specified mourning also move the remaining loved ones through the crisis period. (Note, however, that if a Jew dies on the Sabbath, he or she cannot be moved, except by a non-Jew, until sundown.) After the burial, the mourners are fed in a meal of replenishment called *se'udat havra'ah*. The step symbolizes the rallying of the community and the sustenance of life for the remaining. Also, Jews follow the custom of sitting *shiva* or visiting with remaining relatives for 1 week after the death (60).

Judaism identifies a year of mourning. The first 3 days are of deep grief; clothes may be torn to symbolize the tearing of a life from others. Seven days of lesser mourning follow, leading to 30 days of gradual readjustment. The remainder of the year calls for remembrance and healing. During that year a prayer called the mourner's *Kaddish* is recited in religious services. It helps convey the feeling of support for the mourner (60). At the annual anniversary of death, a candle is burned, and special prayers said.

So from circumcision of the male infant on the eighth day after birth to his deathbed and from the days of the original menorah in the sanctuary in the wilderness until the present day, the followers of Judaism reenact their traditions. Because many of these traditions remain an intrinsic part of the Jew while striving to maintain or regain wellness, the preceding guidelines offer a foundation for knowledgeable care.

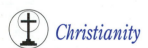 *Christianity*

Beth Meyer, a *Roman Catholic,* Demetrius Callas, an *Eastern Orthodox,* and Jean Taylor, a *Protestant,* are Christian American nurses representing the three major branches of Christianity. Although **Christianity** divided into Eastern Orthodox and Roman Catholicism in AD 1054, and the Protestant Reformation provided a third division in the 16th century, these nurses share some basic beliefs, most importantly that Jesus Christ as described in the Bible is God's son. Jesus, born in Palestine, changed "BC" to "AD." The details of His 33 years are few, but His deeds and words recorded in the Bible's New Testament show quiet authority, loving humility, and an ability to perform miracles and to visit easily with people in varied social positions.

The main symbol of Christianity is the cross,* but it signifies more than a wooden structure on which Jesus was crucified. It also symbolizes the finished redemption—Christ rising from the dead and ascending to the Father to rule with Him and continuously pervade the personal lives of His followers.

---

*See the symbol at the beginning of this section.

Christians observe **Christmas** *as Christ's birthday;* **Lent** as a *season of penitence and self-examination preceding* **Good Friday,** *Christ's crucifixion day;* and **Easter,** *His Resurrection day.*

Beth, Demetrius, and Jean rely on the New Testament as a guideline for their lives. They believe that Jesus was fully God and fully man at the same time, that their original sin (which they accept as a basic part of themselves) can be forgiven, and that they are acceptable to God because of Jesus Christ's life and death. They believe God is three persons—the Father, the Son, and the Holy Spirit (Holy Ghost), the last providing a spirit of love and truth.

Beth, Demetrius, and Jean differ in some worship practices and theology, but all highly regard their individuality as children of God and hope for life with God after death. They feel responsible for their own souls, the *spiritual dimension of themselves,* and for aiding the spiritual needs of their patients.

Roman Catholicism, according to Beth, is a religion based on the dignity of the person as a social, intellectual, and spiritual being made in the image of God. She traces the teaching authority of the church through the scriptures: God sent His Son to provide salvation and redemption from sin. He established the Church to continue His work after ascension into heaven. Jesus chose apostles to preach, teach, and guide. He appointed Saint Peter as the Church's head to preserve unity and to have authority over the apostles. The mission given by Jesus to Saint Peter and the apostles is the same that continues to the present through the Pope and his bishops. Beth notes that in the last several years, women in the Roman Catholic Church, both nuns and laywomen, are speaking out more on issues and are asking for more recognition and respect as God's spokespeople.

Beth believes that the seven *Sacraments* are grace-giving rites that give her a share in Christ's own life and help sustain her in her efforts to follow His example. The Sacraments that are received once in life are Baptism, Confirmation, Holy Orders, and usually Matrimony.

Through **Baptism** Catholics believe the *soul is incorporated into the life of Christ and shares His divinity.* Any infant in danger of death should be baptized, even an aborted fetus. If a priest is not available, you can perform the sacrament by pouring water on the forehead and saying, "I baptize thee in the name of the Father, of the Son, and of the Holy Spirit." The healthy baby is baptized some time during the first weeks of life. Adults are also baptized when they convert to Catholicism and join the church.

Confirmation *is the sacrament in which the Holy Spirit is imparted in a fuller measure to help strengthen* *the individual in his or her spiritual life.* **Matrimony** *acknowledges the love and lifelong commitment between a man and a woman.* **Holy Orders** *ordains deacons and priests.*

The Sacraments that may be received more than once are **Penance** (*Confession*), the **Eucharist** (*Holy Communion*), and the **Anointing of the Sick** (*Sacrament of the Sick*). Beth believes that **Penance,** *an acknowledgment and forgiveness of her sins in the presence of a priest,* should be received according to individual need even though it is required only once a year by church law. The **Mass,** often called the **Eucharist,** is the *liturgical celebration whose core is the sacrament of the Holy Eucharist.* Bread and wine are consecrated and become the body and blood of Christ. The body and blood are then received in Holy Communion.

The Eucharist is celebrated daily, and all Roman Catholics are encouraged to participate as often as possible; they are required by church law to attend on Sundays (or late Saturdays) and specified holy days throughout the year unless prevented by illness or some other serious reason.

Beth is glad that the Anointing of the Sick has been modified and broadened and explains the rite to client and family to allay anxiety. Formerly known as Extreme Unction or the last rites, this sacrament was reserved for those near death. Now **Anointing of the Sick,** *symbolic of Christ's healing love and the concern of the Christian community,* can provide spiritual strength to those less gravely ill. Following anointing with oil, the priest offers prayers for forgiveness of sin and restoration of health. Whenever possible, the family should be present to join in the prayers.

If the client is dying, extraordinary artificial measures to maintain life are unnecessary. At the hour of death the priest offers Communion to the dying person by means of a special formula. This final Communion is called *Viaticum.* In sudden deaths the priest should be called and the anointing and Viaticum should be administered if possible. If the person is dead when the priest arrives, there is no anointing, but the priest leads the family in prayer for the person who just died.

Beth divides the Roman Catholic funeral into three phases: the **wake,** *a period of waiting or vigil during which the body is viewed and the family is sustained through visiting;* the **funeral mass,** *a prayer service incorporated into the celebration of the Mass;* and the **burial,** *the final act of placing the person in the ground.* (This procedure may vary somewhat, for some Catholics are now choosing cremation.) The mourners retain the memory of the dead through a Month's Mind Mass, celebrated a month after death, and anniversary masses. Finally, the priest integrates the liturgy for the dead with the whole parish liturgical life.

Beth is convinced that her religious practice contributes to her health. She believes that the body, mind, and spirit work together and that a spirit rid of guilt and grievances and fortified with the strength of Christ's life has positive effects on the body. She believes that suffering and illness are allowed by God because of our disobedience (original sin) but that they are not necessarily willed by God or given as punishment for personal sin.

While in the hospital, a Roman Catholic may want to attend Mass, have the priest visit, or receive the Eucharist at bedside. (Fasting an hour before the sacrament is traditional, but in the case of physical illness, fasting is not necessary.) Other symbols that might be comforting are a Bible, prayer book, holy water, lighted candle, crucifix, rosary, and various relics and medals.

The **Greek Eastern Orthodox faith** is discussed by Demetrius. The Eastern Orthodox Church, the main denomination, is divided into groups by nationality. Each group has the **Divine Liturgy,** the *Eucharistic service,* in the native language and sometimes in English also. Although similar in many respects to the Roman Catholic faith, the Eastern Orthodox faith has no pope. The seven sacraments are followed with slight variations. Baptism is by triple immersion: the priest places the infant in a basin of water and pours water on the forehead three times. He then immediately confirms the infant by anointing with holy oil.

If death is imminent for a hospitalized infant and the parents or priest cannot be reached, you can baptize the infant by placing a small amount of water on the forehead three times. Even a symbolic baptism is acceptable, but only a living being should receive the sacrament. Adults who join the church are also baptized and confirmed.

The **unction of the sick** has never been practiced as a last rite by the Eastern Orthodox; it is a *blessing for the sick.* Confession at least once a year is a prerequisite to participation in the Eucharist, which is taken at least four times a year: at Christmas, at Easter, on the Feast Day of Saint Peter and Saint Paul (June 30), and on the day celebrating the Sleeping of the Virgin Mary (August 15).

Fasting from the last meal in the evening until after **Communion,** another term for the *Eucharist,* is the general rule. Other fast periods include each Wednesday, representing the seizure of Jesus; each Friday, representing His death; and two 40-day periods, the first before Christmas and the second before Easter.

Fasting to Demetrius means avoiding meat, dairy products, and olive oil. Its purpose is spiritual betterment, to avoid producing extra energy in the body and instead think of the spirit. Fasting is not necessary when ill. Religion should not harm one's health.

Demetrius retains the Eastern influence in his thinking. He envisions his soul as blending in with the spiritual cosmos and his actions as affecting the rest of creation. He is mystically inclined and believes insights can be gained directly from God. He tells of sharing such an experience with a patient, Mrs. A., also Greek Orthodox.

Mrs. A. had experienced nine surgeries to build up deteriorating bones caused by rheumatoid arthritis. She faced another surgery. On the positive side, the surgery promised hope for walking; on the negative, it was a new and risky procedure. Possibly she would not walk; possibly she would not live. Demetrius saw Mrs. A. when he started working at 3:30 PM. She was depressed, fearful, and crying. Later, at 6:30 PM, he saw a changed person—fearless and calm, ready for surgery. She explained that she had seen Jesus in a vision, and that He said, "Go ahead with the surgery. You'll have positive results. But call your priest and take Communion first." Demetrius called the priest, who gave her Communion. She went into surgery the next day with supreme confidence. She now walks.

In addition to Communion, other helpful symbols are prayer books, lighted candles, and holy water. Especially helpful to the Orthodox are *icons,* pictures of Jesus, Mary, or a revered saint. Saints can intercede between God and the person. One of the most loved is *Saint Nicholas,* a 3rd-century teacher and father figure who gave his wealth to the poor and became an archbishop. He is honored on Saint Nicholas Day, December 6, and prayed to continuously for guidance and protection.

Every Sunday morning Demetrius participates in an hour-long liturgy. Sitting in an ornate sanctuary with figures and symbols on the windows, walls, and ceiling, facing the tabernacle containing the holy gifts and scripture, Demetrius finds renewal. He recites, "I believe in one God, the Father Almighty, Maker of Heaven and Earth, and of all things visible and invisible. And in one Lord Jesus Christ, the only begotten Son of God."

Protestantism is divided into many denominations and sects. Jean Taylor is a member of the *Church of God* (Anderson, Indiana). She identifies the church by its headquarters because there are some 200 independent church groups in the United States using the phrase "Church of God" in their title. Her group evolved late in the 19th century because members of various churches felt that organization and ritual were taking precedence over direction from God. They banded together in a drive toward Christian unity, toward a recognition that any people who followed Christ's teachings were members of a universal Church of God and could worship freely together.

This example speaks of one of the chief characteristics of Protestantism: the insistence that God has not given any one person or group of persons sole authority to interpret His truth to others. Protestants use a freedom of spiritual searching and reinterpretation. Thus, new groups form as certain persons and their followers come to believe that they see God's teaching in a new and better light. Jean believes that reading the Bible for historical knowledge and guidance, having a minister to teach and counsel her, and relying on certain worship forms are all important aids. But discerning God's will for her life individually and following that will are her ultimate religious goals.

Jean explains that she "accepted Christ into her life" when she was 8 years old. This identified her as personally following the church's teaching rather than just adhering to family religious tradition. A later experience, in which the Holy Spirit gives the person more spiritual power and discernment, is called *sanctification.*

Jean defines her corporate worship as free liturgical, with an emphasis on congregational singing, verbal prayer, and Scripture reading. A sermon by the **minister,** *the spiritual leader,* may take half the worship period. As with many Protestant groups, two sacraments or ordinances are observed: (1) baptism (in this case, **believer's** or **mature baptism** by *total immersion into water* and (2) Communion. To Protestants, the bread and wine used in Communion are symbolic of Christ's body and blood rather than the actual elements. One additional ordinance practiced in Jean's church and among some other groups is **foot washing,** *symbolic of Jesus' washing His disciples' feet.* These ordinances are practiced with varied frequencies.

Because of the spectrum of beliefs and practices, defining Protestants, even within a single denomination or sect, is almost impossible. Some Protestant groups, retaining their initial emphasis on individual freedom, have allowed no written creed but expect members to follow an unwritten code of behavior. Jean does suggest some guidelines, however. She lists some of the *main Protestant bodies* in the United States, beginning with the most formal liturgically and sacramentally, the *Protestant Episcopal* and *Lutheran* churches. The inbetweens are the *Presbyterians, United Church of Christ, United Methodists,* and *Disciples of Christ (Christian Church).* The liturgically freest and the least sacramental are the *Baptists* and *Pentecostals.*

Among these groups, some of the opposing doctrines and practices are as follows: living in sin versus living above sin; predestination versus free will; infant versus believer's baptism; and loose organization versus tightly knit organization. Some uphold **fundamental precepts,** *holding to the Scriptures as infallible,* whereas others uphold **liberal precepts,** *using the*

Scriptures as a guide, with various interpretations for current living. Recently liberal and conservative Christians have become even more divided by subjects such as abortion, same-sex relationships, and what constitutes morality. The groups on the right, while proclaiming their absolute stands, have not exhibited the tolerance, forgiveness, or freedom of conscience that is part of Christianity, notes one Lutheran pastor (139).

With this infinite variety, Jean believes that learning the individual beliefs of her Protestant client is essential. When and if a client wants Communion, if an infant should be baptized, and what will be most helpful spiritually to the patient—these factors are learned by careful listening. Generally Jean believes that prayer, a scriptural motto such as "I can do all things through Christ who gives me strength" (Philippians 4:13) or a line from a hymn can give strength to a Protestant. Some patients will also want anointing with oil as a symbolic aid to healing.

Jean has discovered that there are wide differences in Protestantism, sometimes even within the same denomination, about the theology and rituals of death. Some Protestant theologies have come to grips with the realities and meaning of death; others block authentic expression of grief by denying death and focusing on "If you are a Christian, you won't be sad."

Some Protestants view death as penalty and punishment for sins; others see death as a transition when the soul leaves the body for eternal reward; and still others view death as an absolute end. All agree that death is a biological and spiritual event, a mystery not fully comprehended.

Rituals surrounding death vary widely. Some churches believe that the funeral service with a closed casket or memorial service with no casket present is more of a testimony to the joy and victory of Christian life than the open-casket service. Others believe that death is a reality to face instead of deny and that viewing the dead person promotes the grief process and confrontation with death in a Christian context.

Jean believes that for most Protestants the minister represents friendship, love, acceptance, forgiveness, and understanding. His or her presence seems to help the dying face death with more ease. She also believes that Protestants are becoming more active in ministering to the bereaved through regularly scheduled visits during the 12 to 18 months after the funeral, although there are no formal rituals.

OTHER GROUPS OF INTEREST

Practices or beliefs unique to certain groups should be part of every health provider's knowledge.

Seventh-Day Adventists rely on Old Testament law more than do other Christian churches. As in Jewish tradition, the Sabbath is from sundown Friday to sundown Saturday. Like the Orthodox Jew, the Seventh-Day Adventist may refuse medical treatment and use of secular items such as television during this period and prefer to read spiritual literature. Diet is also restricted. Pork, fish without both scales and fins, tea, and coffee are prohibited. Some Seventh-Day Adventists are **lacto-ovo-vegetarians:** *they eat milk and eggs but no meat.* Tobacco, alcoholic beverages, and narcotics are also avoided. Because Adventists view the body as the "temple of God," health reform is high on their list of priorities and they sponsor health institutes, cooking schools, and food-producing organizations. They are pioneers in making foods for vegetarians, including meatlike foods from vegetable sources. Worldwide they operate an extensive system of more than 4000 schools and 400 medical institutions and are active medical missionaries (9, 73). Much of their inspiration comes from Ellen G. White, a 19th-century prophetess who gave advice on diet and food and who stressed Christ's return to earth.

The **Church of Jesus Christ of Latter-Day Saints (Mormon)** takes much of its inspiration from the **Book of Mormon,** *translated from golden tablets found by the prophet Joseph Smith.* The Mormons believe that this book and two others supplement the Bible. Every Mormon is an official missionary. There is no official congregational leader, but a **seventy** and a **high priest** *represent successive steps upward in commitment and authority.*

The Articles of Faith of the Church of Jesus Christ of Latter-Day Saints, as given by Joseph Smith, include statements of belief:

- God and His Son, Jesus Christ, and the Holy Ghost
- The same organization that existed in the Primitive Church
- Worship of God according to personal conscience while obeying the law of the land
- People being punished for their own sins and not for Adam's transgression
- All people being saved, repentance, and obedience to the laws and ordinances of the Gospel
- Being honest, true, chaste, benevolent, virtuous, hopeful, persistent, and doing good to all people

Specific Mormon beliefs are that the dead can hear the Gospel and can be baptized by proxy. Marriage in the temple seals the relationship for time and eternity; families are forever and essential for one's eternal destiny. This celestial marriage permits husband and wife to become gods. This process, called *exaltation* or *eter-*

nal progression, allows the pair to populate other worlds by having newly created human souls as their offspring. After a special ceremony in the temple, worthy members receive a white garment. This garment, continuously worn under the clothes, has priesthood marks at the naval and at the right knee and is considered a safeguard against danger. The church believes in a whole-being approach and provides education, recreation, and financial aid for its members. A health and conduct code called *Word of Wisdom* prohibits tobacco, alcohol, and hot drinks (interpreted as tea and coffee) and recommends eating, though sparingly and with thankfulness, herbs, fruit, meat, fowl, and grain, especially wheat.

The Mormon believes that disease comes from failure to obey the laws of health and from failure to keep the other commandments of God; however, righteous persons sometimes become ill simply because they have been exposed to microorganisms that cause disease. They also believe that by faith the righteous sometimes escape plagues that are sweeping the land and often, having become sick, the obedient are restored to full physical well-being by the gift of faith.

Statistics indicate that the Mormon population succumbs to cancer and diseases of the major body systems at a much lower rate than the general population in this country. The death rate for patients suffering from cancer is less than 50% that of the general population; 50% less for those with diseases of the nervous, circulatory, and digestive systems; 33% less for kidney diseases; and 10% less for those with respiratory diseases. Mental illness occurs only half as often among Mormons as among the general population (73).

An explanation for these differences from the norm might be that the Mormons literally believe that the body is the "temple of God." They have programs of diet, exercise, family life, and work to help that "temple" function at optimum level.

Although the two groups just discussed—the Seventh-Day Adventists and the Mormons—generally accept and promote modern medical practices, the next two groups hold views that conflict with the medical field. The first group, **Jehovah's Witnesses,** refuses to accept blood transfusions. Their refusal is based on the Levitical commandment, given by God to Moses, declaring that no one in the House of David should eat blood or he or she would be cut off from his or her people, and on a New Testament reference (in Acts) prohibiting the tasting of blood. Jehovah's Witnesses in need of surgery may be fortunate enough to be near a surgeon who uses no blood transfusions because of reduced operating time. Other surgeons are becoming more willing to do surgery without using blood, using intravenous fluids similar to the body's fluid composi-

tion instead. The new plasma expanders can also be used.

Masulis (68) discusses the ethical dilemmas facing the nurse and other health care professionals when caring for the child of a family that is Jehovah's Witness. She believes the Jehovah's Witness argument against receiving blood transfusions (ingesting blood) (Genesis 9:3–6, 1 Samuel 14:31–35; Acts 15:19–21, 28–29) is based on false analogy. Transfused blood does not function as food and is not equivalent to ingested blood.

Every Jehovah's Witness is a minister. Members meet in halls rather than in traditional churches, and they produce massive amounts of literature explaining their faith.

The second group, **Church of Christ, Scientist (Christian Scientists),** turn wholly to spiritual means for healing. Occasionally they allow an orthopedist to set a bone if no medication is used. Parents do not allow their children to undergo a physical examination for school; to have eye, ear, or blood pressure screening; or to receive immunizations. In addition to the *Bible,* Christian Scientists use as their guide Mary Baker Eddy's *Science and Health With Key to the Scriptures,* originally published in 1875. The title of this work indicates an approach to wholeness, and those who follow its precepts think of God as Divine Mind, of spirit as real and eternal, of matter as unreal illusion. Sin, sickness, and death are unrealities or erring belief. Christian Scientists do not ignore their erring belief, however, for they have established nursing homes and sanitoriums, the latter recognized in the United States under the federal Medicare program and in insurance regulations. These facilities are operated by trained Christian Scientist nurses who give first-aid measures and spiritual assistance.

A Christian Scientist graduate nurse must complete a 3-year course of training at one of a number of accredited sanitoriums. The training includes, among other subjects, classes in basic nursing arts, care of the elderly, cooking, bandaging, nursing ethics, care of reportable diseases, and theory of obstetric nursing. The training is nonmedical, and in the work of a Christian Scientist nurse no medication is administered. The nurse supports the work of the **practitioner,** *who devotes full time to the public practice of Christian Science healing.* Healing is not thought of as miraculous but as the application of natural spiritual law.

The practitioner helps people apply natural spiritual law. Such a person is not a clergyman and does not necessarily hold special church office. Becoming a practitioner is attained largely through self-conducted study and a short course of intensive study from an authorized teacher of Christian Science, but daily study, prayer, application, and spiritual growth are the foundation of practice. The practitioner will treat anyone who comes for help and is supported, like other general practitioners, by clients' payments.

A Christian Scientist who is in a medical hospital has undoubtedly tried Christian Science healing first, may have been put there by a non-Scientist relative, or may be at variance with sacred beliefs. If brought in while unconscious, the person would want to be given the minimum emergency care and treatment consistent with hospital policy. The person may also appreciate having a Christian Science practitioner called for treatment through prayer.

Yet sometimes the Christian Scientist or family may feel so desperate about personal or a loved one's health status that they seek traditional medical care—sometimes too late. Case (18) describes how a Christian Scientist family, following their traditional beliefs and guidance of the sect elders, sought medical care too late to save the life of their son. The parents describe their anguish as they learned that earlier antibiotic treatment for bacterial meningitis could have saved their son's life and that Christian Science practitioners had no effective care measures. They also discuss the conflicts and guilt related to leaving Christian Science and seeking spiritual solace elsewhere. They discuss appreciation of the nonjudgmental and supportive approach of the nursing and medical team as they rendered treatment, explained, and tried to save the son's life.

Two more groups of special interest because of their positive personal and health emphasis are the Unity School of Christianity and the **Society of Friends (Quakers).** Whereas most Roman Catholics acknowledge the earthly spiritual authority of the Pope and most Protestants regard the Bible as their ultimate authority, the Society of Friends' authority resides in direct experience of God within the self. A Friend obeys the **light within,** the **inner light** or the **divine principle;** *this spiritual quality causes the Friend to esteem self and listen to inner direction.*

All Friends are spiritual equals. Without a minister and without any symbols or religious decor, unprogrammed corporate worship consists of silent meditation, with each person seeking divine guidance. Toward the end of the meeting, people are free to share their inspiration. The meeting closes with handshaking. Always interested in world peace, Friends have been instrumental in establishing organizations that work toward human brotherhood and economic and social improvements resulting in better health. Friends have staffed hospitals, driven ambulances, and served in medical corps, among numerous other volunteer services.

The **Unity School of Christianity** believes that health is natural and sickness is unnatural. Followers

think illness is real, but they believe it can be overcome by concentrating on spiritual goals. Late in the 19th century Charles and Myrtle Fillmore started this group after studying, among other religions, Christian Science, Quakerism, and Hinduism. Thus it blends several established concepts in a new direction. Today Unity Village in Missouri has a publication center that publishes several inspirational periodicals, is beautifully landscaped and open for guests to share in the beauty, and houses its real force, Silent Unity. **Silent Unity** *consists of staff who are available on a 24-hour basis to answer telephone calls, telegrams, and letters from people seeking spiritual help.* They offer prayer and counseling to all faiths with no charge.

Some religious groups have retained life style and geographic solidarity and theologic unity. These groups originated in other countries and immigrated to America.

The **Mennonites,** for example, some of whom settled in Pennsylvania, are part of a group called the Pennsylvania Dutch, who are of German, rather than Dutch, descent. The Mennonites generally emphasize plain ways of dressing, living, and worshipping. They do not believe in going to war, swearing oaths, or holding offices that require the use of force. Many of them farm the land or are inclined toward service professions. They are well known for their missionary efforts. Another group, the **Amish,** split from the Mennonite family.

A group with northern headquarters in Bethlehem, Pennsylvania, and southern headquarters in Winston-Salem, North Carolina, is the **Moravians.** These people have also been noted for their missionary work. A restored Moravian village is open for touring in Winston-Salem, and during Christmas and Easter special services are shared with non-Moravian friends.

The **Waldenses,** a Presbyterian group, have their headquarters in Rome but largely populate the town of Valdese, North Carolina. Each summer an outdoor drama portrays their pilgrimage to freedom.

Unitarian Universalists constitute yet another group of interest. The principal founder and leader in the early 19th century was William Ellery Channing. A Unitarian is considered a member of a universal church from which no person can be excommunicated except by the "death of goodness" in that person's heart. Freedom, democracy, positive faith, and saving the world from tyranny and oppression are major themes. Jesus is usually viewed by the members as a great prophet but not as part of the Trinity.

Another facet of Christianity in the United States is **Neo-Pentecostalism.** This is not a group but a trend or phenomenon that has gained support from small groups in all major denominations—some Roman

Catholics, Presbyterians, and Lutherans—and from those churches traditionally closer to the Pentecostal spirit.

The heart of the Pentecostal spirit is an enthusiastic personal relationship with Christ. Those who are a part of this trend tell about leaving a dead, organized religion or of leaving a religious tradition that no longer has meaning. They are anxious to share their insights. The hallmark of this experience is *"speaking in tongues"* or **glossolalia.** Christians trace this experience back to the 1st century A.D. In 1914, however, the phenomenon became institutionalized with the organization of the Pentecostal Assembly of God Church. This group placed its emphasis of a right relationship with God on glossolalia. Three other Pentecostal denominations have come into being: Church of God (Cleveland, Tennessee), Foursquare, and United Evangelical Brethren (73).

Neo-Pentecostalism is thought of as the renewed interest in glossolalia; it is sometimes called the **Charismatic Movement.**

Just what is *glossolalia?* Oral Roberts (82) describes it as the *prayer language of the spirit;* he believes that it is a release of thoughts so deep within the person that ordinary words do not suffice. Sounds made by the person are not in any known language, and the conscious mind, through prayer, should interpret the glossolalia after the experience so that the person can use the gained insight in everyday living (104).

Followers of the Neo-Pentecostal phenomenon have sometimes remained as part of the mainline churches in which their experience originated. Others have formed new organizational fellowships that are evolving into new mainline churches. For example, followers of a certain television evangelist will go to that person's religious training center or college. In turn, that religiously trained person will start a congregation following the tenets of that leadership. Eventually all those congregations will bind together in an overall identity membership.

North American Indian Religions

The **North American Indian religions** developed for centuries with very little influence from outside the continent. Power, Supreme Being, guardian spirits, totems, fasting, visions, **shamanism** (*belief in a priest who can influence good and evil spirits*), myth telling, and ritualism are all part of a varied belief system.

The location of the tribal group influenced its belief system. Indians of the Far North, Northeast Woodlands, Southeast Woodlands, Plains, Northwest Coast, California and the Intermountain Region, and Southwest make up the main tribal divisions.

Yet all belief systems have certain features in common: (1) **spirit world**—a *dimension that permeates life but is different;* (2) **Supreme Being**—*God who represents other lesser deities;* (3) **culture hero**—a *spirit who competes with the Great Spirit and who sometimes is a trickster;* (4) spirits and ghosts such as atmospheric spirits (wind) or underworld powers (snakes); (5) guardian spirits acquired by visions seen during fasting; (6) medicine men and medicine societies; (7) ritual acts such as the Sun Dance; (8) prayers and offerings.

A direct descendant from the Oglada Sioux outlines the belief of the Makaha (1, 39). The Great Spirit, or Wakan Tanka, which is in all and throughout all, manifests itself in the following 16 powers:

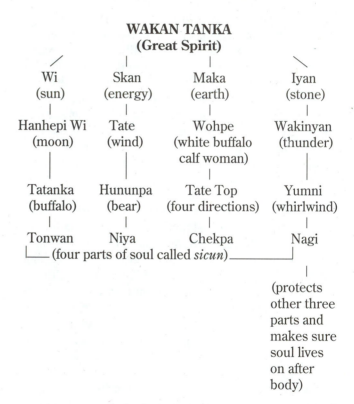

WAKAN TANKA
(Great Spirit)

Wi (sun)	Skan (energy)	Maka (earth)	Iyan (stone)
Hanhepi Wi (moon)	Tate (wind)	Wohpe (white buffalo calf woman)	Wakinyan (thunder)
Tatanka (buffalo)	Hununpa (bear)	Tate Top (four directions)	Yumni (whirlwind)
Tonwan	Niya	Chekpa	Nagi

└── (four parts of soul called *sicun*) ──┘

Nagi (protects other three parts and makes sure soul lives on after body)

Note that people (who have souls) rank at the bottom. This explains the reverence for aspects of nature and animals.

Harmony or spiritual balance is what North American Indians want to achieve in their relations with the supernatural powers.

When caring for an American Indian, it is wise to obtain access to the spiritual leader from that particular region and his or her tribe. Many healing rituals are kept secret, so the health care provider can be most effective by making the appropriate connection, rather than by trying to intervene in the belief system.

New Age Movement

Recently much media attention has been given to the **New Age Movement.** Despite the name, some of the philosophies and practices of this movement are generally old ideas and practices, such as the use of positive thinking. One author has said that aspects of the New Age are so old that it appears new (48). For example, the power of positive thinking and imaging was taught by Norman Vincent Peale for decades (87, 88, 89). A number of other religious leaders were also teaching similar concepts based on Biblical Scriptures during the same era.

In contrast, Salladay states that holistic health care, which many Christian nurses strive to implement in their practice, has its roots not in Christian Scripture, but in New Age thoughts and the writings of Edgar Cayce, called the father of holistic health by New Agers. There are nurses who would claim that nursing began caring for the whole person, physically, emotionally, mentally, and spiritually (holistic health practice) decades ago, but that often other practitioners claim as their own that which nursing has been quietly and appropriately doing and writing about. Historically, nurses who practiced by caring for the whole person did *not* talk about reincarnation or other concepts that are discussed in New Age literature, nor do most nurses who currently practice care of the whole person (111).

The New Age Movement also has claimed some of the terms that nursing has used. For example, our philosophy for the past 25 years in writing nursing textbooks has been holistic health. Unfortunately, some nurses who are leery of the New Age Movement are now renouncing these terms (27, 48). Yet, giving care to the whole person is a basic and essential concept of nursing.

Basically New Age thinking is pantheistic and does not dwell on sin or evil. In this view human beings are considered all divine, all good. All is God, so God is in everything. In Christian theism, humans are sinful and saved by God through Jesus. Carried to extreme, the pantheistic philosophy would have people healing themselves because they are God, and the Christian theism would have God doing all work without human cooperation or help. Both approaches, however, make use of optimism, holism, and synergism. New Age practices such as positive thinking, biofeedback, autosuggestion, and meditation can remain helpful adjuncts to healing as long as they do not become the "only way" for healing to take place (27, 48).

Agnosticism and Atheism

This chapter has concentrated so far on worship of God, the divine or other positive spirits, with an emphasis on traditional teaching. Some people live by ethical standards, considering themselves either **agnostic,** *incapable of knowing whether God exists,* or **atheistic,** *believing that God does not exist.*

Cults

In the 1970s various *cults* gained publicity. Some older cults are based on fundamental religions, but they are unique in their own way. The Snake People, for example, incorporate the holding of snakes into their services. Newer cults have arisen from communal groups whose goals are stated as religious. Some cults spring from the philosophy and schedule of a self-chosen leader who entices youth in search of identity from their parents and formalized church. The youth involved may evolve into robots. Parents have had to "kidnap" their children to get them home and "deprogram" them to recognize their original personalities. Attention has focused on cults that are attracting not only the young but also the elderly (7, 74, 85, 123). In the early 1990s, the number of cults was estimated at 5000. We have the recent memory of the inferno at Waco, Texas, that destroyed David Koresh and his fellow Branch Davidians. We also have learned that sexual abuse of women and children in cults is a common story, both as part of initiation into the cult and as part of their ongoing role. Not only in the United States are cults a phenomenon. In Japan a growing number of sects, such as the Supreme Truth, are gathering young people. The latter sect, led by Shaho Asahara, has stockpiled enough nerve gas to kill 4.2 to 10 million people (59).

Singer gives a comprehensive descriptive of cult life historically and currently (123). She defines **cult** as *any group that forms around a person who claims he or she has a special mission or knowledge, which will be shared by those who turn over their decision making to the self-appointed leader.* Not all cults are religious. Cults vary in philosophy, purpose, power, and structure. The personality, preferences, and desires of the leader are central in the evolution of the group, but the cult structure is basically authoritarian and the leader manipulative and powerful. Cults have the following effects (123):

- They take away personal freedom.
- They take away personal possessions.
- They are violent toward their members.
- They divide or tear apart families.
- They are harmful to children in multiple ways.

Singer describes how cults work: how they recruit people, their physically and psychologically persuasive techniques, the thought reform that occurs, their intrusion into the workplace and general society, the difficulty in leaving a cult, and their harassment of critics, citizens, and even state and national governments. As a psychologist who has counseled thousands of people who experienced cult life, she described at length how we can help survivors escape and recover. The effects of the abuse and forced neglect on the children and their parents and the guilt of adults about the behavior they participated in, without choice, can be devastating, but overcome. Exit counseling, deprogramming, support, love, and understanding—over time—are necessary; postcult adjustment involves every aspect of life. Comprehensive health care is essential to help the person regain identity (123).

Devil or **Satan Worship** is also practiced as a cult. The Satanic Bible was reportedly written by Anton Szandor LaVey who was part of the Church of Satan in San Francisco. The group is supposedly inactive but has splinter groups working, which are called *covens*. Reportedly there are various categories of worshippers: dabblers; self-styled, traditional satanists; and occult cult worshippers. The basic beliefs encompass power or energy in souls and bodies of animals and humans that can be absorbed through rituals. Rituals can be very powerful and macabre when they involve murder, dismembering body parts of animals and humans, and eating these organs. One young man spoke of how he became a precocious student of Satan. He read dozens of books on Satan as "Light-Bearer, the strongest and wisest angel in heaven, robbed of his rightful worship by a jealous God." He spoke of putting a hex on others, drinking ghoulish concoctions, and being obsessed with certain rites as he moved through the hierarchy to priesthood (123).

Signs associated with Satanism are "666"; an upside-down cross; the word *Satan;* a picture of a horned beast; skulls; hoods; goat heads; reversed words (*natas*); ashes; and obsession with black such as a black room, and black candles (25, 27, 123).

Adolescents are most likely to investigate Satanism. Usually they are unsure of their identity, need a group to accept them, and can find a sense of power in the rituals. Occasionally a teenager or college student will appear to have one life of being an outgoing honor student and another life of occult Satanism. Class lines, religion, and intelligence levels are crossed easily in cults (14, 123).

Counselors and psychiatrists and some ministers and priests have had to deal with devil possession in treating clients. Although we do not often speak in these terms in our scientific age, devil possession is a recurring theme in clients' self-diagnosis and one that you should listen for with the new wave of interest in psychic occultism and witchcraft and their various practices.

Summary of American Religions

The *Encyclopedia of American Religions* (1978, two volumes) by J. Gordan Melton (75) would be a good addition to the reference shelf in any health care facility in the United States. It is the first reference work to gather detailed information on all 1200 American religions from the well-known to the lesser cults. This work encompasses all religionists from mystical Hassidic Jews, metaphysicians, psychics, and witches to believers in the imminent end of the world, magic, unidentified flying objects (UFOs), traditional Catholics, Lutherans, and Methodists. The author places all 1200 groups into 18 families with common heritages and lifestyles and identifies these families as:

Liturgical	Liberal
Reformed Presbyterian	Holiness
Pietist Methodist	European Free Church
Pentecostal	Independent
Baptist	Fundamentalists
Adventist	Latter-Day Saints
Communal	Metaphysical
Psychic and New Age	Magick
Eastern	Middle Eastern
Lutheran	

Other references will also assist you in understanding the beliefs and spiritual needs of your clients (7, 57, 73, 74, 79, 80).

OTHER TRENDS IN THE SPIRITUAL DIMENSION

Only when Christianity combines its beliefs with the already existing beliefs of other religions does the blend have a chance of working in the nondominant culture in the United States. For example, Mormonism and Charismatics have had the most impact on American Indians' religion, and since the 1960s these groups have become more visible on Indian reservations. Likewise, the Peyote religion, in which the followers eat the peyote cactus, has added some Christian content such as God, Mary, Jesus, and heavenly angels—all with Indian symbolism.

In churches across the country, what formerly was known as "voodoo" is now called "spiritualism" and is testimony to blending of African and Catholic traditions.

Voodoo illness involves the belief that illness or death may occur as a result of a supernatural force. Various terms are used interchangeably with voodoo, including *rootwork, hex, black magic, witchcraft, spell,* and *conjuring.* Rootwork is part of the voodoo system associated with putting a hex on a person so she or he has good or bad experiences. There is a "misery hex" and a "lucky hex." Bags with dirt and roots may be hidden on a person's property. Mediating these experiences is a root doctor who can cast or remove spells (14, 50, 63). Campinha-Bacote describes the history of voodoo illness, the nonacceptance of Western medicine by voodoo believers, how the nurse may assess for this cultural phenomenon, and relevant nursing interventions for these clients, who are usually of African-Haitian, West African, or African-American descent (14).

In another trend, religion is being thought of by "mainline" Americans as a private affair. People may have strong personal beliefs but not want to rely on established institutions to control their religious life. Also, more religious programming is brought into the home, car, or work, via television, VCR, tapes, radio, and compact disks. People can listen in almost any setting via headphones without disturbing others.

A trend in mainline churches is to evaluate the role of women in the clergy and to consider gender-neutral and nonsexist language for the liturgy. For centuries Western religious thought has maintained the concept of the great chain of being—God, angels, men, women, animals, plants, inanimate objects—in which those above rule those below. This hierarchic concept was reflected in the traditional subordinate role for women in many churches. Along with a stronger role for women in our society has come an expanded role in many churches. For example, of 166 Christian denominations surveyed, 84 now ordain women.

As more women begin to lead the service and liturgy, the language issue will become more focused. Some people are unable to relate to the idea of God as male or God as the father. Proponents of nonsexist language for the liturgy are attempting to address these issues. One male author writes that he could never relate to God until he faced the issue that his feelings of relationship to God were exactly the same as to his biological father. He advocated that a positive spiritual life for him could come only after he separated the emotional background from the spiritual and cleared the emotional areas first (126). The same principle is applicable to women who may speak of God as parent (114, 115, 126).

Another trend in the 1990s is to use the 12-step program (originally developed by Alcoholics Anonymous) for overcoming several addictions and for building spiritual strength. This approach refers to "God" but may

view God as a higher power, deity, spiritual force, or even the collective power of the group (128).

Also families may be meeting their needs in nontraditional ways. One family of four—two parents and two children—decided at a family conference that their historical church was not providing an adequate spiritual diet for them. Rather than all look for another church together, they decided to pursue what was developmentally and spiritually appropriate for each. In time one child joined the Methodist Church, the other child an Interdenominational Church, one parent a Charismatic Church, and the other parent an Episcopal Church.

Another trend can be seen on university and college campuses. Despite talk of the cynical and materialistic 1990s, a fervency of religious spirit, along with well-planned and well-executed spiritual programs, has been funneled through such groups as Inter-Varsity and Campus Crusade for Christ as well as mainline Catholic, Muslim, Jewish, and Methodist groups.

Health care professionals, as well as religious leaders and lay people, are increasingly concerned about the erosion of values and the need to practice moral values and ethical principles. Smedes, a professor of ethics at Fuller Seminary, writes that the United States is experiencing a crisis of morals. The crisis is not that people engage in wrong acts—people have always done that; it lies, instead, in the loss of shared understanding of what is universally considered to be right behavior toward others and doubt about whether there is a moral right or wrong. Organized religion, families who follow moral precepts, and schools that teach moral values have a key role in formation of moral values. The FBI has studied the relationship of proportion of church members and nonchurch members to crime rates in various communities. Cities with higher proportions of church members have lower rates of crime than more secular cities. For example, the West Coast has a higher crime rate than other parts of the nation and has by far the lowest church attendance rates. We may be healthier in all dimensions and development may proceed more normally for our population if our nation continues to embody religious teachings (127). One study showed that church attenders, as compared with nonchurch attenders, reported better health, more happiness, and longer marriages than did their counterparts (49). One book, devoted largely to the "Boomers" in the 1990s, reported that many of the people of that age group were reaching out to religious organizations, but not with total acceptance. They reportedly would find some aspect of the church or organization to be valuable enough that they would join even though they could not embrace the total teachings. They seemed able to live with the ambivalence because of the perceived gain (105).

► HEALTH CARE AND NURSING APPLICATIONS

You can use the foregoing—basic beliefs, dietary laws, and ideas of illness, health, body, spirit, mysticism, pragmatism, pain, death, cleanliness, and family ties—as a *beginning*. Even more basic than understanding these concepts is respecting your client as a person with spiritual needs who has a right to have these needs met, whether he or she has formal religious beliefs. No one will respect your spiritual aid if you do not appear competent and thoughtful in your work. You are not expected to be a professional spiritual leader, for which lengthy training and experience would be required. You can, however, aid clients. You are the transition, the key person between the client and spiritual help.

If you feel inadequate, you may want to imitate several nurses who also felt the same. They decided that they could not meet the spiritual needs of others because they had not met—or even identified—their own. They had a series of discussions focusing on their own needs and used the book *Spiritual Care: The Nurses Role* (121), along with the accompanying workbook (118). When they had a clear vision of their own value system and made plans to meet their own needs, they could begin to focus on others. They also discussed appropriate and inappropriate spiritual intervention and learned to be comfortable making appropriate referrals when they believed that their lack of time or expertise did not allow them to intervene (11).

Also by one of the same authors are *The Spiritual Needs of Children* (119) and *Spiritual Dimensions of Mental Health* (120), both excellent guidebooks.

In considering another's spiritual needs, do not overwhelm or be antagonistic. The goal should be to allow the Divine Spirit to touch another person through the caregiver.

Assessment

Although you can learn a great deal by picking out points in case studies (see page 129), remember that they provide only a basis. You will have to accept each client's individual spiritual development. For example, the sacraments have a very different meaning to Susan than to a child. To a 10-year-old child the meaning of baptism might be carrying an ugly little baby on a pillow to the front of the church, pouring water on its head, and trying to believe that the baby emerges as a beautiful child of God.

Robert Coles (20) recounted anecdotes from Hopi, Christian, Muslim, Jewish, agnostic, and atheistic children. His conclusion was that they all have an immediacy of spiritual issues in their lives. An adolescent or young adult caught up in sorting out various facets of learned idealism and trying to fit them into more realistic daily patterns may temporarily discard religious teaching. He or she may reject the guidance of a spiritual leader because the latter is associated with the parents' beliefs; yet the adolescent is nevertheless searching and needs guidance. An elderly person suffering the grief of a recently lost mate may repeatedly question how a God of love could allow this loss. Some physiologically mature people are not religiously mature; they may expect magic from God. The spiritually maturing individual experiences the fruits of faith in God in behavioral terms of love, trust, and security. The external spiritual stimuli of God's word, sacraments, and relationships with other believers create an inner peace and love through which the person experiences God within and then reaches out to others in supporting relationships.

One author noted that the elderly, at a time when they were attending fewer organized religious functions, seemed to have improved inner spiritual strength (99). This is attributed to "transcendental operations" in which knowledge comes from personal ways of knowing rather than from a given external circumstance.

Furthermore, realize that people can use the same religious terms differently; *saved, sanctified, fell out, slain by the spirit,* and *deathbed conversion* all connote religious experiences. You should listen carefully, and you may have to ask questions to determine accurately the individual person's meaning.

Spiritual beliefs and beliefs about purpose in life and life after death are important dimensions of high-level wellness. Beliefs are related to feelings about self-worth, goals, interactions with others, philosophy of life, interpretations of birth, life events, and death. The value and meaning of life are not judged by its length but by the purpose for which the person lives, the principles by which they live, the reflection about a Being greater than self, and the love and joy obtained from relationships with others. All of these factors may directly affect health status.

Assessment for spiritual needs of any client, not just the terminally ill or dying, should be part of the nursing history. **Spiritual need** is defined as a *lack of any factor necessary to establish or maintain a dynamic, personal relationship with God, or a higher being, as defined by the individual.* Four areas of concern can be covered later in the interview as part of assessment after the client feels safe with the nurse. The following are the assessment areas:

- Person's concept of God or deity
- Person's source of strength and hope
- Significance of religious practices and rituals

• Perceived relationship between spiritual beliefs and current state of health

During this part of the assessment, be prepared for any answer. The agnostic or atheist may answer with as much depth and meaning from his or her perspective as someone with a specific religious background. The person who is part of a formal religion may not answer freely, reserving such conversation for the spiritual leader or hesitating until the nurse is better known to the client.

When determining medical background such as drug or food allergies, you could also ask about religious dietary laws, special rituals, or restrictions that might be an important part of the client's history. Recording and helping the client follow beliefs could speed recovery.

Perhaps you could share with the chaplain the responsibility for asking some of the following questions as you give client care. No specific set of questions will be right for every client, but the questions in Table 3–2 might draw helpful responses as you assess and diagnose in the spiritual realm (130).

TABLE 3–2. QUESTIONS FOR SPIRITUAL ASSESSMENT

1. Who is your God? What is He/She/It like? (Or, what is your religion? Tell me about it.)
2. Do you believe that God or someone is concerned for you?
3. Who is the most important person to you? Is that person available?
4. Has being sick (what has been happening to you) made any difference in your feelings about God? In the practice of your faith? If it has, could you explain how it has changed?
5. Do you believe that your faith is helpful to you? If it is, how? If it is not, why not?
6. Are there any religious beliefs, practices, or rituals that are important to you now? If there are, could you tell me about them? May I help you carry them out by showing you where the chapel is? By telling the dietary department about your vegetarian preference? By allowing you specific times for prayer or meditation?
7. Is there anything that would make your situation easier? (Such as a visit from the minister, priest, rabbi, or chaplain? Someone who would read to you? Time for reading your religious book or praying? Someone to pray with you?)
8. Is prayer important to you? (If so, has being sick made a difference in your practice of praying?) What happens when you pray?
9. Do you have available religious books or articles such as the Bible, prayer books, phylacteries, or crucifix that mean something to you?
10. What are your ideas about illness? About life after death?
11. Is there anything especially frightening or meaningful to you right now?
12. If these questions have not uncovered your source of spiritual support, can you tell me where you do find support?

Be sure to look for the person's strengths, not weaknesses. Remember that you must not preach or reconstruct. Allow the client to assume his or her own spiritual stance.

Because your relationship with the person may be of short duration, be sure to document well the results of this interview. Later, when you or others care for the client, you should watch for religious needs that may be expressed through nonreligious language. You must again let the client know what options are open for spiritual help. If you hide behind busyness and procedures, you may lose a valuable opportunity to aid in health restoration.

Your greater understanding of social class and cultural differences gleaned from Chapter 1 should help you comprehend some of the religious differences. For instance, a poor Protestant American who has grown up with the barest survival materials, who has no economic power, no money for recreation, no hope for significant gain, and no positive attitude about this life may center his or her whole being in the church. It provides as best it can for his or her emotional, recreational, and spiritual needs. When the person sings about heaven in terms of having beautiful clothes, a crown, and a mansion, he or she is singing with a much different meaning than the wealthy Protestant American who is really more concerned about mansions *here* than *over there*.

In a wider sense an Egyptian Christian and an American Christian, although voicing the same basic beliefs, will differ in their approaches to religion. The Egyptian, influenced by the Islamic attitudes of his or her country might say, "No matter what happens; it's God's will. I can do no more about it." The American Christian may be more influenced by the individual drive to guide his or her life, a philosophy prevalent in this culture. Another cultural difference centers on the influence of the family with an ill member. The Egyptian, accustomed to having family and friends around nearly constantly, will expect a continuation of such activity during illness. Their presence provides spiritual and emotional support. The American, more mobile and used to the American hospital system of limiting visitors in number and time, may be better able to detach self from the emotional and religious support given by the presence of family.

Religion influences behavior and attitudes toward:

• Work—whether you work to expiate sin, because it is there to do, or because of a conviction that it is a God-given right and responsibility
• Money—whether you save money to deny yourself something, buy on an installment plan, buy health insurance, consider money the root of all evil, or believe that it should be used for

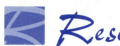

Research Abstract

Krause, N., Religiosity and Self-esteem Among Older Adults, Journal of Gerontology: Psychological Sciences, 50B, no. 5 (1995), 236–246.

Research indicates that self-esteem is an important correlate of psychological well-being in later life. Participation in religious practices and religious beliefs may foster self-esteem and well-being. Research indicates people become more religious as they age. Other sources of self-validation, such as employment, other activities, and contact with friends, may decline in later life. The purpose of this study was to examine the relationship between religiosity and self-esteem in later life.

The national U.S. sample consisted of 1005 participants between 65 and 100 years of age, retired, and living at home. Interviews were conducted with English-speaking individuals who had a social security number listed. Variables included religious organizational affiliation, practice of religion (reading Bible, listening to religious programs), religious beliefs or practices that promote coping, self-esteem measures, chronic health problems, contact with relatives, and contact with friends.

Findings suggest that religious belief and practices are related to one's feeling of self-worth in a complex way. Self-esteem is highest among older people with either greater or no religious involvement and lower among people with minimal commitment to their faith. Religious practices are a major coping mechanism among those who value their religion.

Health care implications include the importance of assessing religiosity, providing for ways for the client to practice religious beliefs, and involving clergy or religious peers in the care of the elderly person when warranted.

the betterment and development of persons and society

- Political behavior—ideas about the sanctity of the Constitution, effects of Communism, importance of world problems, spending abroad versus spending for national defense, school or residential desegregation, welfare aid, and union membership
- Family—kinds of interaction within the family, honoring of parents or spouse, children, or siblings
- Childrearing—interest in the child's present and future, attitudes toward punishment or rewards for behavior, values of strict obedience as contrasted with independent thinking, or how many children should be born
- Right and wrong—what is sin, how wrong is gambling, drinking, birth control, divorce, smoking, and abortion

Consider how essentially the same situation can be diversely interpreted by two teenagers of different faiths. One, a Fundamentalist Protestant, may spend an evening dancing and playing cards and suffer crushing guilt because she participated in supposed sinful acts. The other, a Jewish teenager, may participate in the same activities and consider it a religiously based function. Your knowledge of and sensitivity to such differences are important, for essentially similar kinds of decisions—right and wrong as religiously defined—will be made about autopsy, cremation, and organ transplants. Furthermore, although religious bodies may hand down statements on these issues, often the individual person alters the group's stand while incorporating individual circumstances into the decision.

Ideally, religion provides strength, an inner calm and faith with which to work through life's problems. But you must be prepared to see the negative aspect. To some, religion seems to add guilt, depression, and confusion. Some may blame God for making them ill, for letting them suffer, or for not healing them in a prescribed manner. One Protestant believed she had made a contract with God: if she lived the best Christian life she could, God would keep her relatively well and free from tragedy. When an incurable disease was diagnosed, she said, "What did I do to deserve this?" Another Protestant, during her illness, took the opposite view of her contract with God. She said, "I wasn't living as well as I should and God knocked me down to let me know I was backsliding."

Healing, too, has varied meanings. Some will demand that God provide a quick and miraculous recovery, whereas others will expect the process to occur through the work of the health team. Still others combine God's touch, the health providers' skill, and their own emotional and physical cooperation. Some even consider death as the final form of healing.

Sometimes you must deal with your own negative reactions. Your medical background and knowledge may cause you dismay at some religious practices. For instance, how will you react as you watch a postoperative Jehovah's Witness client die because she has refused blood? How will you react to a Christian Scientist client who, in your opinion, should have sought medical help a month ago to avoid present complications? Here is one response given by a Christian Scientist nurse: "People can be ruined psychologically by going against a long-held belief. They may live and get better physically but will suffer depression, guilt, and failure in not holding to their standard." Basically they prefer to die. Should you dictate otherwise? You may need to think through and discuss such situations with a spiritual leader.

Nursing Diagnosis

The spiritual needs of clients have become a part of the evolving nursing diagnosis system of classification under the value–belief category. **Spiritual distress,** *when the person experiences or could experience a disturbance in the belief system that is his or her source of strength,* is the main diagnostic category. This problem may be related to not being able to practice spiritual rituals or may be caused by a conflict between spiritual beliefs and the health regimen (94).

Other issues may be present also. For example, clients may question their belief system, may be discouraged or despairing, may feel spiritually empty, or may be ambivalent, first asking for spiritual assistance, then rejecting it.

The person's situation may be pathologic (losing a body part), treatment-related (abortion), or situational (death or significant person); however, all these areas are affected by spiritual beliefs. *As nurses become more attuned to these situations, perhaps meeting the client's spiritual needs will not be unattached from other care.* At

Case Situation: Spiritual Distress

Susan Santini is a 40-year-old, middle-class, Caucasian bank president. She lives in a small town with her husband and four children. She also deals in real estate, works with civic and Roman Catholic church groups, and is developing an advertising company. She seems constantly busy. She discusses business over lunch and competes with friends when playing golf or bridge.

One evening she started having severe chest pain. She was taken in an ambulance to a metropolitan hospital 75 miles away where a specialist successfully performed a triple-bypass surgery.

For the first time in her life, Susan was stopped. She was away from family and friends and was confined. Good and bad memories flooded her mind. She began to evaluate her activities, her emphasis on material gain and competition, how her children were growing so fast, how her religious activities were superficial, and how, without skilled surgery, she might have died.

At first she tried being jovial with the staff to strike out these new and troubling thoughts. But she could not sleep well. She was dreaming about

death in wild combinations with her past life. She began to mention these dreams, along with questions about how the surgery would affect her life span, diet, and activities. She mentioned a friend who seemed severely limited from a similar surgery. She also said she was worried about the problems her teenagers were beginning to face and about her own ability to guide them properly.

The staff members never forced Susan to express more than she wished but answered the questions and asked her if she would like to see the chaplain since her own priest was not available. Susan agreed. An appointed nurse then informed the chaplain of Susan's physical, emotional, and spiritual history to date. In the course of several sessions the chaplain helped Susan work through a revised philosophy of life that put more emphasis on spiritual values, family life, and healthy use of leisure.

the same time, the spiritual dimensions must be thought of as something in addition to the psychosocial dimension. Specific measures must be taken for spiritual care, which are not necessarily included in psychosocial care. One study showed that nursing educators were using only psychosocial intervention for spiritual care (95).

Intervention

Spirituality is an integral part of holistic health. In a study that indicated spiritual perspectives, hope, acceptance, and self-transcendence showed connectedness and a positive outcome when viewed together (46). There is a qualitative difference between giving spiritual care and supporting another person by sharing transcendent human qualities. Florence Nightingale described spiritual care as that which enables a person to be conscious of the presence of God, who is the creator and sustainer of the universe. Karns stated that nurses can only cooperate in spiritual care; they cannot give it. She explained that the highest form of spiritual care in the Christian tradition is to help the person be in a position to be conscious of God's touch and the presence of the Holy Spirit. To do that, the nurse must have had such an experience. *Thus, spiritual care will differ from person to person, for the Christian and non-Christian, for the believer and agnostic or atheist* (56).

Spiritual support can be given to the *ill and dying person* in various ways. Your warmth, empathy, and caring human relationship are essential. Respect for the person's beliefs, willingness to discuss spiritual matters, and providing for rituals and sacraments of religion are important. Be open to religious and philosophic beliefs other than your own. You may be uncomfortable discussing spiritual matters, yet it is for the client that you will try to overcome personal reluctance to discuss spiritual concerns. Often the intimacy of spiritual concerns is discussed by the client during the intimacy of physical care. Helping the person ask questions and seek solutions does not mean that you have to supply the answers.

With the dying client, the aspects of spiritual support considered most helpful are (1) calling the person directly by name, (2) talking directly to the person (realize everything may be heard by the dying person), and (3) supporting the family by staying with them as they say goodbye. Let family members know they can touch their dying loved one, offer your condolences, and offer to help them in any appropriate way.

Spiritual care of the *psychiatric patient* is often overlooked. Assessment must determine whether the person is describing a religious delusion, something most

people would consider false, such as "I am Jesus Christ" or "I am Mohammed." Or is the person stating conflicts between religious beliefs and rituals and the current situation or feelings? Such statements may sound like and be labeled as delusions, but the *nursing diagnosis of spiritual distress* would be more appropriate. The spiritual components that you can address through listening and counseling are the person's sense of not being loved by others, of having no meaning or purpose in life, and of feeling unforgiven or not being able to forgive another. These issues take time to resolve; referral to clergy may be indicated.

Interventions for the person who makes delusional statements include the following:

- Understand that what sounds delusional to you and contrary to your religious beliefs may have been religious fact taught to the person. For example, some religions teach that mental illness is demonic possession.
- Convey acceptance of the need for the delusion while you state that you do not agree with it.
- Do *not* argue with the person's belief; state doubt about the belief.
- Respond to the feelings or themes presented in the statements rather than to the exact words. For example, in response to "I am God," you may say, "I sense you are saying you want to be important."
- Avoid abstract discussion about religion or the delusional statements.
- Restate core beliefs that the person is conveying, such as, "You are special to God."

Be alert to subtle clues that indicate desire to talk about spiritual matters, need for expressions of love and hope, desire for your silent presence, and acceptance of behavior when the client labels self as bad.

Certain *norms for providing spiritual care* must be followed:

- Do not impose personal beliefs on clients or families. A sickbed or deathbed is not a proper time for proselytizing.
- Respond to the person out of his or her own background. Use knowledge about that background, but avoid acting on stereotypes. (For example, all Catholics believe _____ or all Hindus do _____.)
- If you cannot give the spiritual support being asked for by the person, enlist someone who can.

Often there is little communication between health care providers and pastoral care representatives. You can fill that gap. Such rapport can mean that the *whole* person is served rather than segmented parts. Chaplains are especially helpful to clients and to nurses when they assist with the expression of anger, death, and grief (33). You and the chaplain, however, need to know what to expect from each other; there is no substitute for talking about these expectations and agreeing on strategies.

Nine combinations of patient behavior that call for conferring with or referring to a spiritual leader unless contraindicated by the care plan are:

1. Withdrawn, sullen, silent, depressed
2. Restless, irritable, complaining
3. Restless, excitable, garrulous, wants to talk a lot
4. Shows by word or other signs undue curiosity, anxiety about self
5. Takes turn to worse, critical, terminal
6. Shows conversational interest, curiosity in religious questions, issues; reads Scripture
7. Specifically inquires about chaplain, chapel worship, Scripture
8. Has few or no visitors; has no cards, flowers
9. Has had, or faces, particularly traumatic or threatening surgical procedure

With all these aspects to consider, a *team approach* that includes the client, family, health care providers, and chaplain or other spiritual leader is imperative. Because Americans want weekends away from the job, the weekend hospital staff often has double responsibility. Furthermore, weekends are when most people attend corporate worship. Preparing the client for chapel service or seeing that the Sabbath ritual is carried out places a special responsibility on you, the nurse. Be especially sensitive to acceptance of the person's spiritual beliefs and try to provide the important factors, be they rituals, diet, quiet, group work, various articles, or family relationships.

Validate the appropriateness of proposed interventions with the client; for example, ask if the person wishes you to pray with him or her about the concerns that have been voiced. The person can then accept or reject your offer.

If a client is confined to a room, you can prepare a worship center or shrine by arranging flowers, prayer book, relics, or whatever other objects have spiritual meaning.

You should keep one or more calendars of various religious holidays. The Eastern Orthodox Easter usually does not coincide with the Roman Catholic and Protestant Easter. Jewish holidays usually do not fall on the same dates of the Western calendar in successive years. Remember, also, that holidays are family days and that ill people separated from the family at such times may be especially depressed.

Maintaining a list of available spiritual leaders, knowing when to call them, and knowing how to prepare for their arrival are other important responsibilities. If a client cannot make the request, consult with the family. One woman said, "If my sister sees a priest, she will be sure she is dying." Once a health care provider took the initiative to call an Eastern Orthodox priest who, unfortunately, represented the wrong nationality; the client's main source of comfort was to have come from discussion and prayers in the native language.

As you prepare the client and the setting for a spiritual leader, help create an atmosphere that reflects more than sterile procedure. Privacy has previously been emphasized by drawing curtains and shutting doors. Although acceptable to some, this approach may produce a negative response in others. Perhaps more emphasis should be given to cheerful surroundings: sunshine, flowers, lighted candles, openness, and participation by family and staff in at least an introductory way. Perhaps the client and spiritual leader could meet outdoors in an adjoining garden. The Shintoist and Taoist would especially benefit from the aesthetic exposure. If the client is a child on a prolonged hospitalization, a special area might be designated for religious instruction.

Brief the spiritual leader on any points that might provide special insight and be sure that the client is ready to receive him or her. Prepare any special arrangements such as having a clean, cloth-covered tray for Communion. Guard against interruption by health care providers from other departments who may be unaware of the visit. Finally, incorporate the results of the visit into the client's record.

Many will benefit from the sacraments, the prayers, Scripture reading, and counseling given by the spiritual leader, but others will want to rely on their own direct communication with God. The Zen Buddhist, Hindu, Muslim, and Friend might be in the latter category. All may wish reading material, however. Most will bring their sacred book with them, but if they express a desire for more literature, offer to get it. Some hospitals furnish daily and weekly meditations and a Bible.

Occasionally it may be helpful to give Scripture references for various stated spiritual needs. For example, reference to love and relatedness can be found in Psalm 23; reference to forgiveness in Matthew 6:9–15; reference to meaning and purpose in Acts 1:8.

A positive interfaith magazine is *Guideposts* (Guideposts Associates). A novel with religious insights is *Christy* (Avon Books, 1968) by Catherine Marshall. A spiritually based autobiography is *Joni* (World Wide

Publication, 1976) by Joni Eareckson. A delightful biography about a spiritually mature preschool-age child is *Mister God, This Is Anna* (Ballantine Books, 1974) by Fynn. *In Search of God: The Story of Religion* by Marietta Maskin is written for youth but is also recommended for adults who work with youth. Many other spiritually inspiring books, such as those written by Scott Peck, and journals, including *Journal of Christian Nursing,* are available for use by clients and health care providers. Do not overlook the opportunity to share the ministry of books.

If you feel comfortable doing so, you can at times say a prayer, read a Scripture, or provide a statement of faith helpful to the client. If you do not feel comfortable in providing this kind of spiritual care, you can still meet the client's spiritual needs through respectful conversation, listening to the client talk about beliefs, referral to another staff member, or calling one of the client's friends who can bolster his or her faith. If spiritual leaders are not available, you could organize a group of health workers willing to counsel with or make referrals for clients of their own faiths.

Shared prayer, if it is accepted by the client, counteracts the loneliness of illness or dying by offering the person intimacy with a Supreme Being and another person without the need for confession. It can be a means of bringing both human and divine love. It holds transcendent qualities and conveys both present and future hope. Prayer can focus on the conditions or emotions that the client is unable to talk about, allowing the person to handle the matter or vent in another way. Prayer should promote closeness, through closed eyes and hands that touch. Prayer should not strip the person of defenses. Nor should prayers be recited as a way to avoid the person or avoid questions raised by the person.

Use of life review can foster developmental, emotional, and spiritual maturity (not only in the elderly and dying person). Encourage the person to reminisce about past life experiences. Memories can be pleasurable or painful, but recalling them with a skilled listener can help resolve those ridden with shame, guilt, anger, or other feelings. Past sources of strength can also be identified, and sometimes they are useful in the present situation. Music can also be used to lift depression, convey calm, stimulate hope and joy, and promote physical and mental healing.

Several authors describe how counseling and mental and spiritual methods can be combined to help the client heal hurtful or traumatic memories, forgive self or others, work through unresolved grief, promote healing within self, and establish healthier relationships with others. Both non-Christian and Christian nurses may find these articles helpful (107, 116, 133).

Atheists should not be neglected because they do not profess a belief in God. They have the same need for respect as everyone else and may need you to listen to fears and doubts. The person does not need your judgment.

Moreover, just as health teaching is often omitted for health care providers who are clients, so is spiritual guidance often omitted for spiritual leaders who are clients. You must recognize that each person, regardless of religious stand or leadership capacity, may need spiritual help.

Various groups refuse medical or hospital treatment for illness, including members of Fundamentalist or Holiness groups, Jehovah's Witnesses, Amish, and Christian Scientists. Realize that if adults refuse treatment for themselves or their children, they are not deliberately choosing death. They are rejecting something objectionable, based on their beliefs. If at all possible, offer acceptable alternative treatments. Jehovah's Witnesses accept intravenous normal saline solution, Ringer's lactate solution, dextrose, Haemaccel, and hydroxyethyl starch solution. Members of rural Fundamentalist sects and the Amish are often willing to go to chiropractors and will allow physicians to set fractures and suture lacerations. Nurses may teach nutritional therapy or various stress management or relaxation techniques. Sometimes parents will accept the services of a home health nurse even though they refuse hospital and formal medical treatment.

Although a hospital setting has been used as a point of reference throughout this chapter, you can improvise in your setting—nursing home, hospice, school, industry, clinic, home, or other health center—to provide adequate spiritual assistance.

Table 3–3 summarizes interventions for many of the religions discussed in this chapter.

Research in Spiritual Care*

Exactly what constitutes spiritual care needs further research. In a recent research study, "Spiritual Care Interventions by Psychiatric Nurses" (using 300 professional, registered, hospital-based psychiatric nurses in Missouri), the most commonly recalled interventions were psychosocial rather than spiritual. Therapeutic communication/use of self ranked first; being cheerful and kind and use of touch were the most common interventions after that. The respondents were least comfortable doing specific spiritual care interventions such as

---

*Sections on Research in Spiritual Care and Evaluation were contributed by Elaine Cox, RN, MSN(R).

TABLE 3–3. SUMMARY OF MAJOR HEALTH CARE IMPLICATIONS OF SELECTED RELIGIOUS CULTURES/SUBCULTURES

Religion	Food Preference	Responsibility Related to Client Belief/Need
Hinduism	Vegetarian; no alcoholic beverages; other restrictions conform to sect doctrine; fasting important part of religious practice, with consequences for person on special diet or with diabetes or other diseases regulated by food	Medical care is last resort; client considers help will come from own inner resources. Nurse should treat client with respect and convey sense of dignity. Reinforce need for medical care and explain care measures. Client may reject help and be stoic. Assess carefully for pain. Provide privacy. Assist to maintain religious practices. Cleanliness and dietary preferences are important. Certain prescribed rites are followed after death. The priest may tie a thread around the neck or wrist to signify blessing; the thread should not be removed. Immediately after death, the priest will pour water into the mouth of the corpse; the family will wash the body. They are particular about who touches their dead. Bodies are cremated. Loss of limb is considered sign of wrongdoing in previous life.
Buddhism Zen, sect of Buddhism Shintoism, Japan's state religion	Vegetarian; no intoxicants; moderation in eating and drinking	Family help care for ill member and give emotional support. Religion discourages use of drugs; assess carefully for pain. Cleanliness important. Question about feelings regarding medical or surgical treatment on holy days. Prepare for death; help patient remain alert, resist confusion or distraction, and remain calm. Last rite chanting is often practiced at bedside soon after death. Contact the deceased's Buddhist priest or have the family make contact.
Islam	No pork and pork-containing products; no intoxicants	Members are excused from religious practices when ill but may still want to pray to Allah and face Mecca. There is no spiritual advisor to call. Family visits are important. Cleanliness is important. After 130 days, fetus is treated as fully developed human. Members maintain a fatalistic view about illness; they are resigned to death, but encourage prolonging life. Patient must confess sins and beg forgiveness before death, and family should be present. The family washes and prepares the body, folds hands, and turns the body to face Mecca. Only relatives or friends may touch the body. Unless required by law, no postmortem or no body part should be removed.
Black Muslim (Nation of Islam)		There is no baptism. Procedure for washing and shrouding dead and performing funeral rites is carefully prescribed. Cleanliness is important.
Judaism	Orthodox eat only kosher (ritually prepared) foods; milk consumed before meat, or meat eaten 6 hours before milk consumed; does not eat pig, horse, shrimp, lobster, crab, oyster, birds of prey if Orthodox. Others may restrict diet. Special utensils and dishes for Orthodox. Fasts on Yom Kippur and Tisha Bab; may fast other times but excluded if ill	There is no infant baptism. Baby is circumcised on eighth day if Orthodox. Preventative measures, avoiding illness, are important. Members are concerned about future consequences of illness and medication. They are preoccupied with health; will convey that pain is present and want relief. Nursing measures for pain are important. On Sabbath, Orthodox Jews may refuse freshly cooked foods, medicine, treatment, surgery, and use of radio or television. Orthodox male may not shave. Nurse should avoid loss of yamulka, prayer books, or phylacteries. Nurse must arrange for kosher or preferred food; food may be served on paper plates. Check consequences of fasting on person's condition. Visits from family members are important. If patient is without family, notify synagogue so other people may visit. Family or friends should be with dying person. Artificial means should not be used to prolong life if patient is vegetative. Confession by dying person is like a rite of passage. Human remains are ritually washed following death by members of the Ritual Burial Society. Burial should take place as soon as possible. Cremation is not permitted. All Orthodox Jews and some Conservative Jews are opposed to autopsy. Organs or other tissues should be made available to the family for burial. Parts of the body are not donated to medical science or removed, even during autopsy. Donation or transplantation of organs requires rabbinical consultation. A fetus is to be buried, not discarded.

(continued)

TABLE 3–3. SUMMARY OF MAJOR HEALTH CARE IMPLICATIONS OF SELECTED RELIGIOUS CULTURES/SUBCULTURES

Religion	Food Preference	Responsibility Related to Client Belief/Need
Christianity		All will wish to see spiritual advisor when ill and to read Bible or other religious literature and follow usual practices.
Roman Catholic	Nothing special, except fasting or abstaining from meat on Ash Wednesday and Good Friday; some Catholics may fast every Friday and other holy days	Client finds comfort in having rosary, Bible, prayer book, crucifix, medals. Infant baptism is mandatory, and especially urgent if prognosis is poor. Baptism is demanded if aborted fetus may not be clinically dead. For baptismal purposes, death is a certainty only if there is obvious evidence of tissue necrosis. Tell priest if you baptize baby; it is done only once. Inquire about dietary preferences and fasting. Members may want information on natural family planning. The Rite for Anointing of the Sick is mandatory. If the prognosis is poor, the patient or his family may request it. In sudden death, priest is called to anoint and administer Viaticum, if possible, or special prayers are said. Amputated limb may be buried in consecrated ground; there is no blanket mandate but it may be required within a given diocese. Donation or transplantation of organs is approved providing the recipient's potential benefit is proportionate to the donor's potential harm.
Orthodox		
Eastern Orthodox (Turkey, Egypt, Syria, Cyprus, Bulgaria, Rumania, Albania, Poland, Czechoslovakia)	Fasting each Wednesday, each Friday, and 40 days before Christmas and Easter; avoid meat, dairy products, and olive oil	Prayer book and icons are important. Infant is baptized if death is imminent. Check consequences of fast days on health; fasting is not necessary when ill. Blessing for the sick (unction) is not last rite but a form of healing by prayer. Last rites are obligatory if death is impending; cremation is discouraged.
Greek	Fasting periods on Wednesday, Friday, and during Lent; avoid meat and dairy products	Prayer book and icons are important. Infant is baptized if death is imminent. Patient prepares by fasting for Holy Communion and Sacrament of Holy Unction. Fasting is not mandatory during illness. Members oppose euthanasia. Every reasonable effort should be made to preserve life until terminated by God. Cremation or autopsies that may cause dismemberment are discouraged. Last rites are administered for the dying.
Russian Orthodox	Fasting on Wednesday, Friday, and during Lent; no meat or dairy products	Prayer book and icons are important. There is no baptism of infant. Check consequences of fasting on health. Cross necklace is important; it should be replaced immediately when patient returns from surgery. Do not shave male patients except in preparation for surgery. Patients do not believe in autopsies, embalming, or cremation. Traditionally, after death, arms are crossed, and fingers are set in a cross. Clothing at death must be of natural fiber so that the body will change to ashes sooner.
Protestantism (Many denominations and sects)		
Baptist	Some groups condemn coffee and tea; most condemn alcoholic beverages; some groups may fast on Sundays or other special days, especially in Black Baptist churches	There is no infant baptism. Client may be fatalistic; may believe illness is punishment from God; and may be passive about care. Inquire about effect of fasting if client is on special diet, is a diabetic, or has disease dependent on dietary regulation.
Brethren (Grace) (Plymouth)	Most abstain from alcohol, tobacco, and illicit drugs	There is no infant baptism. Anointing with oil is done for physical healing and spiritual uplift. There are no last rites.
Church of Christ, Scientist (Christian Scientist)	Avoid coffee and alcoholic beverages	There is no infant baptism. If hospitalized or receiving medical treatment, guilt feelings may be intense. Be supportive. Allow practitioner or reader to visit freely as desired. Use nursing measures to alleviate pain. Patient may refuse blood transfusions as well as intravenous fluids and medication. There are no last rites or autopsy, unless sudden death.
Church of Christ	Avoid alcoholic beverages	There is no infant baptism. Anointing with oil and laying on of hands are done for healing. There are no last rites.
Church of God	Most avoid alcoholic beverages	There is no infant baptism.

(continued)

TABLE 3–3. SUMMARY OF MAJOR HEALTH CARE IMPLICATIONS OF SELECTED RELIGIOUS CULTURES/SUBCULTURES

Religion	Food Preference	Responsibility Related to Client Belief/Need
Protestantism (cont.)		
Church of Jesus Christ of Latter Day Saints (Mormon)	Eat in moderation; limit meat; avoid coffee and tea; no alcoholic beverages; avoid use of tobacco	There is no infant baptism, but baptism of dead is essential; living person serves as proxy. Laying on of hands is done for healing. White undergarment with special marks at navel and right knee is to remain on; it is considered a safeguard against danger.
Episcopalian	May fast from meat on Friday	Infant baptism is mandatory, but not for aborted fetus or stillbirth. Patient fasts in preparation for Holy Communion, which may be daily; thus, check effects on disease. Rite for Anointing Sick (last rites) is not mandatory.
Friends (Quakers)	Moderation in eating; most avoid alcoholic beverages and drugs	There is no infant baptism. Health teaching is important. Give explanations about medical technology used in care. Share information about condition as indicated.
Jehovah's Witnesses	Avoid food to which blood is added, e.g., certain sausages and lunch meats	There is no infant baptism. Members are opposed to blood transfusion. (Hospital administrator or doctor may seek court order to be appointed guardian of child in times of emergency need for blood.) There are no last rites.
Mennonite	Most avoid alcoholic beverages	There is no infant baptism. Shock therapy, psychotherapy, and hypnotism conflict with individual will and personality.
Nazarene	Avoid alcoholic beverages	There is no need to baptize infant. Stillborn is buried. Laying on of hands is done for healing. There are no last rites.
Pentecostal	Avoid alcoholic beverages	There is no infant baptism. Prayer, anointing with oil, laying on of hands, speaking in tongues, shouting, and singing are important for healing of patient.
Unitarian/Universalist		Infant baptism is not necessary. Cremation is preferred to burial. Check before calling clergy to visit.
Seventh-Day Adventists	Vegetarian (no meat) or lacto-ovo-vegetarian (may eat milk and eggs but not meat); pork and fish without fins and scales prohibited; avoid coffee and tea; avoid alcoholic beverages	There is no infant baptism. Health measures, prevention, and health education are important. Some believe in divine healing and anointing with oil. Avoid administering narcotics and stimulants. Use nursing measures for pain; medication is last resort. Check on food preferences. Sabbath is Friday sundown until Saturday sundown for most groups. Client may refuse medical treatment and use of secular items, such as television, on Sabbath.

praying with the patient/family, discussing God, and reading Scripture to the patient. Although use of spiritual interventions was low, the nurses' attitudes toward doing them were positive. If obstacles, such as lack of time, unfavorable institutional policy, and lack of basic and inservice nursing education about spiritual care were removed, the nurses reported they would provide spiritual care. The majority of the nurses believed spiritual care was the responsibility of every nurse and the right of every patient, and that it provides holistic care. The core problem underlying these findings was that the majority of nurses in the study did not see the spiritual dimension as separate and distinct from the physical and psychosocial dimensions and this was reflected in their behaviors (24). The findings by Cox with psychiatric nurses were similar to the findings in a study with oncology nurses (4).

Evaluation

Exactly what aspects of spiritual care can be evaluated are difficult to determine. Evaluation of spiritual care interventions can best be analyzed by using both objective and subjective criteria, with spiritual well-being as the major criterion. The following questions with positive answers indicate a direction toward that criterion. Does this intervention: (1) bring peace or unity (129); (2) provide a source of help, comfort, relief, or strength (136); (3) promote transcendent values such as meaning, purpose, love, relatedness, and forgiveness of self/God/others (95, 96); (4) decrease or alleviate symptoms such as anxiety, withdrawal, helplessness, agitation, crying, hostility (21), guilt, shame, depression, and unforgiveness (129); (5) bring integration to the personality (93); (6) help the person to cope and problem-solve (71); and (7) promote hardiness, hope, and intrinsic spiritual values (76). The above would provide evidence of spiritual well-being. These questions can be measured on a continuum of 1 to 10 answered by both nurse and patient. Objective measures alone are inadequate, as the patient must realize the positive value of the outcome for continuing reinforcement and success.

Outcomes that we must strive for are those that (1) enhance trust, (2) allow people to carry on spiritual practices not detrimental to health, (3) decrease feelings of anxiety and guilt, and (4) cause satisfaction with their spiritual condition. To ensure these responses, spiritual care should be considered part of quality assurance. Sister Rosemary Donley suggests that this incorporation—with the addition of more mystery and more grace—will help foster support for the poor, the minorities, the very rich, that is, those who are sometimes blamed for their illnesses (29).

SUMMARY

1. You will encounter a variety of beliefs in your care of clients.
2. To understand your own and others' belief systems—spiritual, religious, philosophic—is interesting and enhances your care of the client, family, group, and community.
3. People who practice the same belief system or religion will differ from each other while they also share similar beliefs; extent of practice will vary from person to person.
4. People from different belief systems will have some beliefs and practices in common.
5. Spiritual/religious/philosophic background has a major influence on development and health.
6. Your own spirituality will be conveyed to the client as you care for him or her in any health care setting.
7. Engage in lifelong learning about your own and others' belief systems to, as effectively as possible, assess and comprehensively care for the client.

▶ REFERENCES

1. Adams, B., *Prayers of Smoke.* Berkeley, CA: Celestial Arts, 1990.
2. Adler, J., 800,000 Hands Clapping, *Newsweek,* June 13 (1994), 46–47.
3. Anderson, B., and A. Steen, Spiritual Care, Reflecting God's Love to Children, *Journal of Christian Nursing,* 12, no. 1 (1995), 12–17.
4. Are RNs Reluctant Spiritual Caregivers? *American Journal of Nursing,* 95, no. 8 (1995), 12–13.
5. Bair, J., Doctor's Mix Medicine/Prayer, *St. Louis Post Dispatch,* June 10 (1995), 50.
6. Bakken, K., *The Call to Wholeness: Health as a Spiritual Journey.* New York: Crossroad Publishing, 1990.
7. Beit-Hallahmi, B., *The Illustrated Encyclopedia of Active New Religious Sects and Cults.* New York: Rosen Publishing Group, 1993.
8. Berkowitz, P., and N. Berkowitz, The Jewish Patient in the Hospital, *American Journal of Nursing,* 67, no. 11 (1967), 2335–2337.
9. Braswell, G.J., *Understanding World Religion* (rev.). Nashville, TN: Broadman & Holman, 1994.
10. Butler, R., The Roman Catholic Way in Death and Mourning. In Grollman, E., ed., *Concerning Death: A Practical Guide for the Living.* Boston: Beacon Press, 1974, pp. 101–118.
11. Buys, A., Discussion Series Sensitizes Nurses to Patient's Spiritual Needs, *Hospital Progress,* 62 (October 1981), 44–45.
12. Caillat, C., Jainism. In Eliade, M., ed., *The Encyclopedia of Religion,* 15. New York: Macmillan, 1987, pp. 507–514.
13. Campbell, T., and B. Chang, Health Care of the Chinese in America, *Nursing Outlook,* 21, no. 4 (1973), 245–249.
14. Campinha-Bacote, J., Voodoo Illness, *Perspectives in Psychiatric Care,* 28, no. 1 (1982), 11–12.
15. Carpenito, L., *Handbook of Nursing Diagnosis* (4th ed.). Philadelphia: J.B. Lippincott, 1991, pp. 264–267.
16. Carson, V., Meeting the Spiritual Needs of Hospitalized Psychiatric Patients, *Perspectives in Psychiatric Care,* 18, no. 1 (1980), 17–20.
17. ———, et al., The Effect of Didactic Teaching on Spiritual Attitudes, *IMAGE: Journal of Nursing Scholarship,* 18, no. 4 (1986), 161–164.
18. Case, R., We Let Our Son Die, *Journal of Christian Nursing,* 4, no. 2 (1987), 4–8.
19. Clark, C.C., et al., Spirituality: Integral to Quality Care, *Holistic Nursing Practice,* 5, no. 3 (1991), 67–76.
20. Coles, R., *The Spiritual Life of Children.* Boston: Houghton Mifflin, 1991.
21. Collins, D., *Spiritual Distress: A Problem for Psychiatric Patients? A Survey of Psychiatric Nurses.* Unpublished master's thesis, 1992.
22. Conrad, N.L., Spiritual Support for the Dying, *Nursing Clinics of North America,* 20, no. 2 (1985), 415–426.
23. Cornell, G., Studies: Religious Faith, Health Linked, *The State Journal-Register,* November 28 (1992), 18.
24. Cox, E., *Spiritual Interventions by Psychiatric Nurses.* Unpublished master's thesis, St. Louis University, 1995.
25. Davis, R., Protect Your Family From Cults, *Home Life,* April (1991), 32–34.
26. Davis, T., The Truth about the Mormon Family, *Home Life,* May (1991), 48–49.
27. Dieter, M.E., The Gospel and New Age Thought, *Vital Christianity,* 111, no. 7 (1991), 27.
28. Dobmeier, T., Professionalizing Spiritual Care, *Journal of Christian Nursing,* 8, no. 2 (1990), 32.
29. Donley, Sr. R., Spiritual Dimensions of Health Care: Nursing's Mission, *Nursing and Health Care,* 12, no. 4 (1991), 178–183.
30. Duckro, P., Let Us Pray, *Here's News.* St. Louis: St. Louis University Health Science Center, August 8, 1994.

31. Eck, D., *Roots in Who Are They?* Los Angeles: Bhaktivedanta Book Trust, 1982.

32. Eich W., When Is Emergency Baptism Appropriate? *American Journal of Nursing,* 87, no. 12 (1987), 1680–1681.

33. Eickhoff, A., The Chaplain–Nurse Relationship. *Nursing Management,* 13, no. 3 (1982), 25–26.

34. Ellis, D., Whatever Happened to the Spiritual Dimension? *The Canadian Nurse,* September (1980), 42–43.

35. Ellwood, R., East Asian Religions in Today's America. In Neusner, J., ed., *World Religions in America: An Introduction.* Louisville, KY: Westminster/John Knox Press, 1994.

36. Esposito, J., Islam in the World and America. In Neusner, J., ed., *World Religions in America: An Introduction.* Louisville, KY: Westminster/John Knox Press, 1994.

37. Fleeger, R., and J. Van Heukelein, The Patient's Spiritual Needs: A Part of Nursing Diagnosis, *The Nurses Lamp,* 28, no. 4 (1977).

38. Gibney, F., Jr., Ritual Murder in Mexico, *Newsweek,* April 24 (1989), 55.

39. Gill, S., Native Americans and Their Religions. In Neusner, J., ed., *World Religions in America: An Introduction.* Louisville, KY: Westminster/John Knox Press, 1994.

40. Gill, S., and I. Sullivan, *Dictionary of Native American Mythology.* Santa Barbara, CA: ABC-CLIO, 1992.

41. Glustrom, S., *When Your Child Asks–A Handbook for Jewish Parents* (rev.). New York: Bloch, 1991.

42. Gordon, A., The Jewish View of Death: Guidelines for Mourning. In Kubler-Ross, E., ed., *Death, the Final Stage of Growth.* Englewood Cliffs, NJ: Prentice-Hall, 1975, pp. 44–51.

43. Greeley, A., The Catholics in the World and America. In Neusner, J., ed., *World Religions in America: An Introduction.* Louisville, KY: Westminster/John Knox Press, 1994.

44. Guoli, G., Zorastrianism. In Eliade, M., ed., *The Encyclopedia of Religion* (15th ed.). New York: Macmillan, 1987, pp. 579–591.

45. Gurka, A., How Did Anne Help? *Journal of Christian Nursing,* 8, no. 5 (1991), 23.

46. Haase, J., T. Britt, D. Coward, N. Leidy, and P. Penn, Simultaneous Concept Analysis of Spiritual Perspective, Hope Acceptance, and Self Transcendence, *IMAGE, Journal of Nursing Scholarship,* 24, no. 2. (1992), 141–145.

47. Hauerwas, S., *Nursing the Silences: God, Medicine, and the Problem of Suffering.* Grand Rapids, MI: Eerdman's, 1990.

48. Hensley, D.E., Old or New? Understanding the New Age Movement, *Vital Christianity,* 111, no. 7 (1991), 21–23.

49. Hering, M., Believe Well, Live Well, *Focus on The Family,* September (1994), 1–4.

50. Hillard, J.R., Diagnosis and Treatment of the Rootwork Victim, *Psychiatric Annals,* 12, no. 7 (1982), 709–714.

51. Hover, M., If a Patient Asks You to Pray With Him, *RN,* April (1986), 17–18.

52. Hultkrantz, A., North American Religions: An Overview. In Eliade, M., ed., *The Encyclopedia of Religion, 15,* New York: Macmillan, 1987, pp. 526–535.

53. Impoco, J., Japanese Religious Group Changing, *Hickory Daily Record,* December 16 (1987), Sect. D, p. 13.

54. Jordan, M., The Protestant Way in Death and Mourning. In Grollman, E., ed., *Concerning Death: A Practical Guide for Living.* Boston: Beacon Press, 1974, pp. 81–100.

55. Jorgensen, J.G., Modern Movements. In Eliade, M., ed., *The Encyclopedia of Religion, 15.* New York: Macmillan, 1987, pp. 541–544.

56. Karns, P.S., Building a Foundation for Spiritual Care, *Journal of Christian Nursing,* 6, no. 5 (1991), 11–13.

57. Kelsey, M., Faith: Its Function in the Wholistic Healing Process. In Otto, H., and Knight, J., eds., *Dimensions in Wholistic Healing: New Frontiers in the Treatment of the Whole Person.* Chicago: Nelson-Hall, 1979.

58. Kertzer, M., *What Is a Jew?* (rev. ed.). New York: Macmillan, 1969.

59. Kristof, N., From Manipulative Teen to Guru to Manipulative Cult Leader. *The Charlotte Observer,* March 26 (1995), 15a.

60. Kushner, H., *When Bad Things Happen to Good People,* New York: Schocken Books, 1989.

61. Lang, B., The Death that Ends Death in Hinduism and Buddhism. In Kubler-Ross, E., ed., *Death, The Final Stage of Growth.* Englewood Cliffs, NJ: Prentice-Hall, 1975, pp. 52–57.

62. Larson, G., Hinduism in India and America. In Neusner, J., ed., *World Religions in America: An Introduction.* Louisville, KY: Westminster/John Knox Press, 1994.

63. Lex, B., Voodoo Death: New Thoughts on an Old Explanation, *American Anthropologist,* 76 (1974), 819–823.

64. Luna, L.J., Transcultural Nursing Care of Arab Muslims, *Journal of Transcultural Nursing,* 1, no. 1 (1989), 22–26.

65. Macrae, J., Nightingale's Spiritual Philosophy and Its Significance for Modern Nursing, *IMAGE, Journal of Nursing Scholarship,* 27, no. 1 (1995), 8–14.

66. Martin, J., A Home Health Aide Responds: Seek Understanding, *Journal of Christian Nursing,* 4, no. 2 (1987), 10–16.

67. Marty, M.E., Native Americans, *Christian Churches in the United States* (1985), pp. 114–115.

68. Masulis, K., When Parents Refuse Treatment for Their Children, *Journal of Christian Nursing,* 4, no. 2 (1987), 10–16.

69. McConkie, B.R., *Mormon Doctrine.* Salt Lake City, UT: Bookcraft, 1966.

70. McGilloway, O., and F. Myco, eds., *Nursing and Spiritual Care.* London: Harper & Row, 1985.

71. McHolm, F., *A Nursing Diagnosis Validation Study: Defining Characteristics of Spiritual Distress.* Unpublished thesis, Kent State University, 1988.

72. McIntyre, S., Ritual as Spiritual Practice, *Woman of Power,* 19 (Winter 1991), 19–21.

73. Mead, F., and S. Hill, *Handbook of Denomination in the United States* (9th ed.). Nashville, TN: Abingdon Press, 1990.

74. Melton, J., *Encyclopedic Handbook of Cults in America.* New York: Garland, 1992.

75. Melton, J.G., *The Encyclopedia of American Religions,* I & II. Wilmington, NC: McGrath, 1978.

76. Mickley, J., K. Soeken, and A. Belcher, Spiritual Well-Being, Religiousness, and Hope Among Women with Breast Cancer. *IMAGE, Journal of Nursing Scholarship,* 24, no. 4 (1992), 267–272.

77. Miller, A., *The Major World Religions: Adult Education Class,* St. Louis, MO: September 25–November 7, 1994.

78. Munley, A., *The Hospice Alternative: A New Context for Death and Dying.* New York: Basic Books, 1983.

79. Neusner, J., ed., *World Religions in America: An Introduction.* Louisville, KY: Westminster/John Knox Press, 1994.

80. Neusner, J., Judaism in the World and America. In Neusner, J., ed., *World Religions in America: An Introduction.* Louisville, KY: Westminster/John Knox Press, 1994.

81. Occhiogrosso, P., *The Joy of Sects.* New York: Doubleday, 1994.

82. O'Driscoll, P., Muslims Fight Stereotypes of Their Faith, *USA Today,* April 7 (1989), 1–2.

83. Okamoto, A., Religious Barriers to World Peace, *Journal of Religion and Health,* 15, no. 1 (1976), 26–33.

84. Olson, M., The Out-of-Body Experience and Other States of Consciousness, *Archives of Psychiatric Nursing,* 1, no. 3 (1987), 201–207.

85. Opinions Vary on Status of Cults Today, *History Daily Record,* January 23 (1995), 4a.

86. Papovitz, L., Life/Death/Life, *American Journal of Nursing,* 86, no. 4 (1986) 416–418.

87. Peale, N.V., *The Power of Positive Thinking.* Pawling, NY: Foundation for Christian Living, 1952.

88. ———, *Positive Thinking for Times Like This.* Pawling, NY: Foundation for Christian Living, 1961.

89. ———, *Imaging: The Powerful Way to Change Your Life.* Carmel, NY: Guideposts, 1982.

90. Peck, M.L., The Therapeutic Effect of Faith, *Nursing Forum,* 20 (1981), 2153–2166.

91. Penrose, V., et al., Spiritual Need in Sickness: I Lack Myself, *Nursing Mirror,* 154 (March 10, 1982), 38–39.

92. Petersen, M., *A World of Wisdom.* Salt Lake City, UT: Church of Jesus Christ of Latter-Day Saints, n.d.

93. Peterson, E., and K. Nelson, How to Meet Your Client's Spiritual Needs, *Journal of Psychosocial Nursing,* 25, no. 5 (1987), 35–39.

94. Piles, C., Providing Spiritual Care, *Nurse Educator,* 15, no. 1 (1990), 36–41.

95. Piles, C., Putting Spiritual Care into the Curriculum, *Journal of Christian Nursing,* 6, no. 3 (1989), 18–21.

96. Piles, C., *Spiritual Care: Role of Nursing Education and Practice. A Needs Survey for Curriculum Development.* Unpublished doctoral dissertation, Saint Louis University, St. Louis, 1986.

97. Pill, R., The Christian Science Practitioner, *Journal of Pastoral Counseling,* 4, no. 1 (1969), 39–42.

98. Porath, T., Humanizing the Sacrament of the Sick, *Hospital Progress,* 53, no. 7 (1972), 45–47.

99. Reed, P.G., Spirituality and Mental Health in Older Adults: Extant Knowledge for Nursing, *Family and Community Health,* 14, no. 2 (1991), 14–25.

100. Religion: A Healthy Choice, *Intervarsity,* Fall (1992), 11.

101. Repass, D.D., Stolen Words, *Vital Christianity,* 11, no. 7 (1991), 29.

102. Richards, L., *A Marvelous Work and a Wonder.* Salt Lake City, UT: Deseret Book Company, 1975.

103. Rice, E., *Eastern Definitions.* Garden City, NY: Doubleday & Company, 1978.

104. Roberts, O., *A Daily Guide to Miracles.* Tulsa: Pinoak, 1975.

105. Root, W., *A Generation of Seekers.* San Francisco: Harper, 1994.

106. Rosten, L., ed., *Religions of America* (rev. ed.). New York: Simon & Schuster, 1975.

107. Rush, B., Healing A Hidden Grief, *Journal of Christian Nursing,* 3, no. 2 (Summer 1986), 10.

108. Russell, D.L., Personal letter on Christian Science beliefs and practices, December 1, 1975.

109. Ryan, J., The Neglected Crisis, *American Journal of Nursing,* 84, no. 10 (1984), 1257–1258.

110. Sachen, K.L., and V.J. Carson, Responding to the Spiritual Needs of the Chronically Ill, *Nursing Clinics of North America,* 22, no. 3 (1987), 603–611.

111. Salladay, S.A., World Views Apart: Nursing Practice and New Age Therapies, *Journal of Christian Nursing,* 6, no. 4 (1991), 15–18.

112. Satprakashananda, S., ed., *The Use of Symbols in Religion.* St. Louis: Vedanta Society, 1970.

113. Saunders, E.D., *Buddhism in Japan.* Philadelphia: University of Philadelphia Press, 1964, pp. 265–286.

114. Schroeder, J.A., Towards a Feminist Eucharistic Theology and Piety, *Dialog,* no. 30 (Summer 1991), 221–226.

115. Schutzius, M.J., Missing Voices of Women in Our Church, *Probe,* 25, no. 4 (1987), 1.

116. Seamonds, D., Healing of Memories: What Is It? Is It Biblical? *Journal of Christian Nursing,* 3, no. 2 (Summer 1986), 4–9.

117. Shannon, M., Spiritual Needs and Nursing Responsibility, *Imprint,* 27 (December 1980), 23.

118. Shelly, J.A., *Spiritual Care Workbook.* Downer's Grove, IL: Inter-Varsity Press, 1978.

119. ———, *The Spiritual Needs of Children: A Guide for Nurses, Parents and Teachers.* Downer's Grove, IL: Inter-Varsity Press, 1982.

120. ———, and S.D. John, *Spiritual Dimensions of Mental Health.* Downer's Grove, IL: Inter-Varsity Press, 1983.

121. ———, and S. Fish, *Spiritual Care: The Nurses Role* (3rd ed.). Downer's Grove, IL: Inter-Varsity Press, 1988.

122. Siner, H., "Doctor Claims It's Healthy to Pray," *Cappers,* May 10 (1995), 4.

123. Singer, M., *Cults in Our Midst.* San Francisco: Jossey-Bass, 1995.

124. Singh, K., Sikhism. In Eliade, M., ed., *The Encyclopedia of Religion, 15.* New York: Macmillan, 1987, pp. 315–320.

125. Slimmer, L., Helping Students to Resolve Conflicts Between Their Religious Beliefs and Psychiatric–Mental Health Treatment Approaches, *Journal of Psychiatric Nursing and Mental Health Services,* 18 (July 1980), 37–39.

126. Sloat, D.E., Why Can't I Relate to God? *Journal of Christian Nursing,* 5, no. 6 (1988), 11–15.

127. Smedes, L., *Caring and Commitment.* San Francisco: Harper & Row, 1988.

128. Stafford, T., The Hidden Gospel of the 12 Steps, *Christianity Today,* 35, no. 8 (1991), 14–19.

129. Stoll, R., Essence of Spirituality. In Carson, V., ed., *Spiritual Dimensions of Nursing Practice.* Philadelphia: W.B. Saunders, 1989.

130. ———, Guidelines for Spiritual Assessment, *American Journal of Nursing,* 79, no. 9 (1979), 1574–1577.

131. Suchetka, D., Ramaden, *The Charlotte Observer,* February 18 (1995), Sect. A, p. 12.

132. Suzuki, D.T., E. Fromm, and R. DeMartino, *Zen Buddhism and Psychoanalysis.* New York: Grove Press, 1960, p. 5.

133. Tawless, J., Visualizing the Healer, *Journal of Christian Nursing,* 3, no. 2 (Summer 1986), 12–14.

134. Those Who Preserve the Ritual Bath, *St. Louis Post-Dispatch,* January 9 (1977), Sect. H, p. 3.

135. Tinney, J.S., Black Muslims, *Christianity Today,* 20 (March 12, 1976), 51–52.

136. Toth, J., Faith in Recovery: Spiritual Support After an Acute MI. *Journal of Christian Nursing,* 9, no. 4 (1992), 29–30.

137. Tye, L., Pentecostal Churches Mushroom Around Globe, *The Charlotte Observer,* December 11 (1994).

138. *Unity School of Christianity.* Unity Village, MO: Unity School of Christianity, n.d.

139. Weber, G., A Radical Religious Crusade, *St. Louis Post-Dispatch,* February 22 (1995).

140. Wilson, J., *Religion in American Society.* Englewood Cliffs, NJ: Prentice-Hall, 1981.

141. Yep, J., An Asian Patient: How Does Culture Affect Care? *Journal of Christian Nursing,* 8, no. 5 (1991), 6–9.

II

Basic Concepts Related to the Developing Person and Family Unit

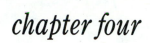
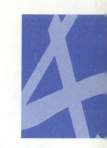

chapter four

The Family: Basic Unit for the Developing Person

The American family does not exist. Rather, we are creating many American families of diverse styles and shapes.

—J. Footlick

 Key Terms

Family	Patrifocal/patriarchal family	Personality	Family interaction
Compadrazgo	Matrifocal/matriarchal family	Adaptive responses in the family	Dyads
Padrinazgo	Same-sex/homosexual family	Courtship	Stepfamily
Compadre	Single state	Establishment stage	Stepgeneration parents
Nuclear family	Roles	Expectant stage	Family cultural pattern
Extended family	Physical functions	Couvade syndrome	Therapeutic or helping relationship/alliance
Single-parent family	Affectional functions	Parenthood or expansion stage	
Stepfamily	Social functions	Disengagement or contraction stage	Genogram

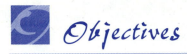 *Objectives*

1. Define *family* and discuss the family as a system and the implications for the developing person.

2. Summarize theoretic approaches for studying the family.

3. Describe the purposes, tasks, roles, and functions of the family and their relationship to the development and health of its members.

4. Describe family adaptive mechanisms and their purposes.

5. List stages of family life and developmental tasks for the establishment, expectancy, parenthood, and disengagement stages.

6. Discuss your role in helping the family achieve its developmental tasks.

7. Relate the impact of feelings about the self and childhood experiences on later family interaction patterns.

8. List and describe the variables affecting the relationship between parent and child and general family interaction, including single-parent, stepparent, and adoptive families.

9. Identify ways in which your family life has influenced your present attitudes about family.

10. Discuss the influence of 20th-century changes on family life and childrearing practices in the United States and other countries.

11. Predict how a changing culture may affect the development and health of the family system.

12. Describe therapeutic communication methods to be used when working with a family or other clients.

13. Describe characteristics and phases of a therapeutic relationship with a client such as the family.

14. Assess a family, constructing a genogram and using criteria listed in the chapter, to formulate a nursing diagnosis and plan of care.

15. Explore your role and various measures and resources to use in promoting physical and emotional health of a family in various situations.

It's an uncanny feeling—to suddenly know that I am answering my son's question with the same words—even the same tone—as my father used with me 30 years ago.

Even though I have a happy, successful marriage, two loving children, a nice home, and a profession in which I feel competent, I constantly fight a feeling of inferiority. A contributing factor must be that my parents never encouraged or complimented me. When I took a test, they emphasized the 2 wrong, not the 98 right.

I always admired my aunt. If my cousin, her son, had told her he wanted to build a bridge to the moon, she would have furnished the nails.

These three people are speaking of aspects of a social and biological phenomenon that is often taken for granted: the family. So strongly can this basic unit affect our development and health that we may live successfully or unsuccessfully because of its influence. Much that the person learns about loving, coping, and the various aspects of life is first learned in the family unit.

Some form of family exists in all human societies. Culture, not biology, determines family organization (96). Between society and the individual person, the family exists as a primary system and social group, for most people share many of life's experiences with the

family. Thus the family has a major role in shaping the person; it is a basic unit of growth, experience, adaptation, health, or illness.

The traditional family persists as a norm in the imagination, but today norms hardly exist with the fragility of marriage, the high incidence of divorce (and remarriage), the many styles of family life, the diversity of roles held by members, and the increasing number of homeless families. Thus today's children are being shaped differently—sometimes negatively—by the family unit. For many youngsters, the pain of family life, a changing family scene, having no permanent home, and being separated from other family members are compounded by poverty and neglect.

This chapter is not an exhaustive study of families or family life. Rather, it is an overview of the various forms, stages, and functions of contemporary American families and of how you can use this knowledge. Although various aspects of the family are discussed separately, keep in mind that family purposes, stages of development, developmental tasks, and patterns of interaction are all closely interrelated, all influenced by historical foundations, and all continually evolving into new forms. Thus the family should be viewed as a system, affected by the culture, the environment, religious–spiritual dimensions, and other variables, which in turn affects the person and society.

DEFINITIONS

Family

The **family** *is a small social system and primary reference group made up of two or more persons living together who are related by blood, marriage, or adoption or who are living together by agreement over a period of time.* The family unit is *characterized by face-to-face contact, bonds of affection, love, loyalty, emotional and financial commitment, harmony, simultaneous competition and mutual concern, a continuity of past, present, and future, shared goals and identity, and behaviors and rituals common only to the specific unit* (9, 75, 78).

The **family** may also be defined as *domestic partners, people who have chosen to share each other's life in an intimate and committed relationship of mutual caring.* This definition permits the extension of legal benefits usually accorded traditionally married heterosexuals, such as health and life insurance and pension benefits, property rights, hospital and prison visitation rights, and bereavement leave to homosexual or same-sex families or unmarried partners. Family may be defined differently by different cultures. For example, **compadrazgo** *is a form of social alliance embedded in the Latino culture.* It involves family-type links with roots back to the feudal European days. Compadrazgo can be identified as follows (35):

1. It is a family kin tie, but it is *not biologically or legally ascribed.* Once entered into, it assumes *dimensions of affection and responsibility similar to that of a family.*
2. It *has a ritualistic aspect;* the relationship is initiated via a religious blessing.
3. It is *coparenthood* in contrast to **padrinazgo** (*godparent*), *with a relationship like parent, grandparent, aunt, and sister.* Individuals call one another **compadre,** *a title imbued with great warm feeling and deep respect.* The relationship is only good, ideal, supportive, and caring.
4. *Caring in this relationship includes a reciprocity, expressed by gift giving, hospitality, economic aid, and assurance about assistance in the future.*

The family is a group whose members rely on each other for daily services. With the family, the person can usually let down his or her guard and be more himself or herself than with other people. The family comprises a household (or cluster of households) that persists over years or decades and that is characterized by value, role, and power structures; communication patterns; affective socialization, family coping, and health care functions; and developmental stages and tasks (44, 111). Internal and external structures exist in a family. *Internal structure* includes family composition, rank order, subsystems, and boundary. *External structure* includes culture, religion, social class status and mobility, environment, and extended family. *Instrumental function* refers to how routine activities of daily living are handled. *Expressive function* refers to nonverbal and verbal communication patterns, problem-solving roles, control aspects, beliefs, alliances, and coalitions (9).

Healthy families are characterized by (1) a sense of togetherness that promotes capacity for change; (2) a balance between mutual and independent action on the part of family members; (3) availability of nurturance and resources for growth and sustenance; (4) stability and integrity of structure; (5) adaptive functioning; and (6) mastery of developmental tasks leading to interdependence, progressive differentiation, and transformation to meet the requisites for survival of the system (103).

Sometimes families live together daily. Sometimes the adult partners are employed in different geographic areas, or one member is hospitalized or in prison. They maintain contact by telephone, correspondence, and visits. In the two-career family the partners share the same residence on weekends or on a consistent basis. These families carry out their functions and characteristics in their own unique way.

In this stressful time families may have difficulty in maintaining these characteristics. Your support, teaching, and counseling may assist them in maintaining health.

Family Composition

The family takes several forms. Table 4–1 defines traditional, as well as nontraditional family forms, such as the *same-sex,* or *homosexual family,* who may be childless, have custody of and care for biological children from a previous heterosexual marriage, or have adopted children. Alternately, one of the lesbian women may, through artificial insemination or one-time contact with a selected man, bear a child, and the other woman in the relationship also takes on the parenting role, clearly acknowledging that she is not the mother; or the gay couple may contract with a woman to carry a baby to term for them. Currently the homosexual who has had a biological child more frequently is exerting custody, visiting, and caretaking rights and responsibilities with the child after establishment of the same-sex relationship. Various references describe the same-sex family (21, 22, 30, 46, 48, 57, 69, 100). Or the family may com-

TABLE 4–1. TYPES OF FAMILY COMPOSITION

1. **Nuclear family:** Mother, father, child(ren).
2. **Extended family:** Nuclear plus other relatives of one or both spouses. Relatives of the nuclear family may or may not live with the nuclear family. May include great-grandparents and great-great-grandparents.
3. **Single-parent family:** Mother or father, living with either biological or adopted children, possibly tied emotionally but not legally to a partner.
4. **Stepfamily:** One divorced or widowed adult with all or some of his or her children and a new spouse with all or some of his or her children, and often, also, the children born to this union so that parents, stepparents, children, and stepchildren (or stepsiblings) live together.
5. **Patrifocal/patriarchal family:** Man has main authority and decision-making power.
6. **Matrifocal/matriarchal family:** Woman has main authority and decision-making power.
7. **Same-sex/homosexual family:** Gay or lesbian partners live together.
8. **Single state:** Never married, separated, divorced, widowed.

prise a childless couple; siblings, especially in middle or late life; friends in a commune; or a man and woman living together without being married, with or without children.

The family may be *symbolically duplicated in the work setting*: a woman may be perceived as a grandmother, mother, or sister, or a man may be perceived as a grandfather, father, or brother to an employee. The family member who is no longer present because of divorce or who is dead or missing may remain clearly in the other members' memory; they may refer to the person on special occasions. Or the deviant of the family—the alcoholic or runaway—may influence other family members to act in an opposite manner.

The family may also be a *series of separate but interrelated families*. The middle-aged parents are helping the adolescent and young adult offspring to be emancipated from the home while simultaneously caring for increasingly dependent parents and sometimes up to four pairs of grandparents plus older aunts and uncles. All related family members may not live under the same roof (in fact, they never did in America), but the extended family exists psychologically—in spirit. The middle-aged person's caregiving role is discussed in Chapter 13.

A real entity is psychic life of the family; the *extended* family affects thoughts and actions, provides sustenance, and contributes to identity. Present-day mobility of people, ease of communication over distance, freedom to evolve and think independently, freedom to develop in ways less restricted by strong or rigid ethnic or cultural mores, and ease of transportation allow families in the United States to be geographically distant yet emotionally close and often quite involved with each other, to the point of giving assistance.

The mass media presents a picture of family life dissolving in the United States. Although the divorce rate is approximately 50 to 70%, most divorced people remarry. Because of longer life expectancy and the young age at which people marry, the young couples of today enter and remain in marriage longer than did their grandparents. Family authorities estimate that the divorce rate, extremely high in the 1970s and early 1980s, may decline in the 1990s. People are beginning to realize that divorce does not necessarily improve life; the allure of creativity, growth, and expanding oneself emotionally through divorce is not necessarily realistic. Some families speak of trying harder, resolving to stay committed to each other in conflictual times.

OVERVIEW OF FAMILY THEORETIC APPROACHES

Theoretic approaches to the study of families include developmental, structural–functional, interactional, role, family systems, and crisis theories. These approaches are summarized in Table 4–2. Refer to several references at the end of the chapter for more extensive explanation (1, 44, 111, 124).

PURPOSES, TASKS, ROLES, AND FUNCTIONS OF THE FAMILY

Although the institution of the family is being scrutinized and predictions are made that it may pass into oblivion, the family has demonstrated throughout history that it is a virtually indestructible institution. Family structure, roles, and responsibilities have been influenced by technology and the resulting social changes. But technologic advances alone do not determine family structure and function. Family systems are endlessly adaptive and very resistant to outside pressure. In a society in which objects are often disposable and people feel uneasy and dispensable, individuals seek secure relationships. The family can be a source of security, although for some people it is not, with long-term detrimental consequences.

The U.S. family has passed through major transitions. The family was once a relatively self-contained, cohesive domestic work unit; it has become a group of persons dispersed among various educational and work settings. Various agencies have absorbed many purposes once handled solely by the family group. Schools educate; hospitals care for the sick; mortuaries prepare the dead for burial; churches give religious training; government and private organizations erect recre-

TABLE 4–2. SUMMARY OF MAJOR FAMILY THEORIES AND APPROACHES

Family Theory	Definition of Family	View of Person	Approach/Focus
Developmental theory: compilation of several frameworks	*Series of interacting personalities, intricately organized into paired positions* (father, husband, daughter, sister); *norms for reciprocal relations prescribe role behavior for each position; predictable natural history designated by stages*	Person is a member of group; each new member adds to complexity of interaction.	**Study family** in terms of role behaviors for each family life-cycle stage, along with the changing ages of each person; study quality and type of interaction as age and member composition of family changes. **Focus:** Analyze developmental needs and tasks of each family life-cycle stage; analyze family behaviors and changing developmental tasks and role expectations in terms of increasing complexity, analyze children, parents, and family unit as a whole. Cultural influences at each stage of family life cycle are considered.
Structural-functional theory: focus on family as a system	*Social system open to outside influences and transactions; maintains boundaries by responding to demands of system or acting under family constraints, passively adapting to external forces rather than acting as an agent of change in itself*	Person is seen as reactive in fulfilling roles and as having status in the social system.	**Study family** in relation to other social structures or social systems and in terms of roles. **Focus:** Determine how family patterns are related to other institutions and overall society; study family functions (reproduction, socialization of children, provision of physical needs, economics).
Interactional theory: reflection of role theory and psychodynamic theory	*Defined in terms of individual members, a unity of interacting personalities with assigned position and roles, expectations, and norms of behavior; seen as closed unit with little relationship to outside institutions, associations, or cultures*	Person is seen as fulfilling roles and as an interacting being. Messages sent by members to each other have multilevel meanings.	**Study family** in terms of overt interactions, fulfillment of interacting roles and ways of communicating. **Focus:** Analyze roles, interstatus relations, authority matters, action-taking communication processes, conflicts, problem solving and decision making. Teach most effective communication methods.
Role theory: life is structured according to roles that are ascribed or assumed by the person in interaction with others; roles are learned through socialization	*Defined in terms of members' role interaction;* roles contribute in the following way to the family unit: Circumscribe behavior; Define social position, responses, expectations; Influence group associations; Are purpose of interaction; Provide norms for the family or group	Person is seen in terms of roles, which are specialized or shared and depend on sex, age, social norms, status, complementarity. Roles change through development and negotiation, which depend on flexibility, stability, and congruence of expectations. Person experiences role reciprocity, complementarity, or strain. **Role reciprocity:** *mutual exchange; sharing affects decision making and cohesion; personal and family needs met; high mutual dependence in division of labor; potential for growth; commitment to family and reducing conflict* **Role complementarity:** *family members differentiate and define roles in relation to each other; opportunity*	**Study family** in terms of role interactions, differentiation, allocation, role change, and role strain. **Focus:** Analyze role reciprocity, complementarity, and strain.

(continued)

TABLE 4–2. SUMMARY OF MAJOR FAMILY THEORIES AND APPROACHES (continued)

Family theory	Definition of Family	View of Person	Approach/Focus
Role theory (cont.)		for growth; sometimes not a sense of mutual-gratification; can confirm identity of one at expense of other; if rigid roles, transitions are difficult **Role strain:** *occurs when individuals have difficulty meeting others' or own expectations and the obligations of the role and is manifested as:* 1. **Role conflict:** *unclear, incomplete, contradictory elements in role; performing one role makes it impossible to perform another; conflicting norms* 2. **Role overload:** *must consider impact of distribution of power; the greater the control over negotiation of roles, the more person can avoid role strain; person with less power assumes more unwanted burdens; person with more power has less dependency needs and can make role demands.*	
Family systems theory	*Intergral unit in society, made up of parts or members, with individual and family characteristics who are interacting and interdependent. Maintain equilibrium by developing repetitive techniques of interaction.*	Person is member of system and subsystem.	**Study family** as a whole unit; sum of whole is greater than its parts or subsystems. **Focus:** Analyze family's adaptive process, exchange between members and subsystems, and decision making, transactions, bargaining, cooperative, and coercive processes. Examine rules of family organization, patterns of interaction, traditions, whether boundaries are open and flexible or closed, and interaction with other systems.
Crisis theory	*Family made up of members who individually experience hazardous events*	Problems or illness of one member is expressed in conflict or problems of that family. All family members are affected by inability of one to cope.	Brief therapy **Study family** in terms of crisis impact on all, rather than just one. **Focus:** Analyze present situation. Identify role and conflicts, general coping skills. Avoid blame; focus on perception and reality. Specific tasks are to be mastered. Alternate plans for coping are attempted until effective ways to reduce tension and disorganization are found. Ways to handle future crisis are explored. Therapist uses a variety of cognitive, educational, behavioral, and communication approaches to help family cope with crisis and become more functional.

ational facilities; nursing homes care for the aged; and various manufacturing firms bake, can, or bottle food and make clothes.

Purposes and Tasks of the Family

When the family changed from a production unit to a consumption unit, it also lost some degree of authority to regulate its members' behavior. The emphasis now is on democratic sharing, togetherness, the child's potential as an individual, and the fun aspects of parenthood. Enjoyment and relaxation in every human relationship are considered important. Technology is seen as the reason for this view and the way to attain the happy state, but the person who believes too strongly in what technology can accomplish may have unrealistic expectations about living and thus undergo considerable stress in marriage and childrearing.

Yet the family is still considered responsible for the child's growth and development and behavioral outcomes; indeed, the family is a cornerstone for the child's competency development. Because the family is strongly influenced by its surrounding environment and by the child itself, the family should not bear full blame for what the child is or becomes. Few parents deliberately set out to rear a disturbed, handicapped, or delinquent offspring, although such failures occur.

The family is expected to perform the following tasks. *The tasks may be basically the same for most types of family composition, but how they are manifested often is related to the type of family structure:* nuclear, extended, single-parent, same-sex, patrifocal, or matrifocal. *Culture of the family group* (racial, ethnic, geographic, socioeconomic, religious) *also influences how the following tasks are achieved.* **Basic tasks** are as follows:

- Provide for physical safety and economic needs of its members and obtain enough goods, services, and resources to survive.
- Create a sense of family loyalty and a mentally healthy environment for the family's well-being.
- Help members to develop physically, emotionally, intellectually, and spiritually and to develop a personal and family identity.
- Foster a value system built on spiritual and philosophic beliefs and the cultural and social system that is part of the identity.
- Teach members social skills and to communicate effectively their needs, ideas, and feelings and to respect each other.

- Provide social togetherness simultaneously with division of labor and performance of family and sex roles with flexibility and cooperation.
- Reproduce and socialize the child(ren), teaching values and appropriate behavior, providing adult role models, and fostering a positive self-concept and self-esteem in the child(ren).
- Provide relationships and experience within and without the family that foster security, support, encouragement, motivation, morale, and creativity.
- Help the members to cope with crises and societal demands; create a place for recuperation from external stresses.
- Maintain authority and decision making, with the parents representing society to the family as a whole and the family unit to society.
- Promote integration into society and the ability to use social organizations for special needs when necessary.
- Release family members into the larger society—school, church, organizations, work, and politics.
- Maintain constructive and responsible ties with the neighborhood, school, and local and state government (1, 9, 18, 37, 83).

The family often has difficulty in meeting these tasks and needs assistance from external resources. The family's ability to meet its tasks depends on the maturity of the adult members and the support given by the social system—nursing and health care, educational, work, religious, social, welfare, governmental, and leisure institutions. The family that is most successful as a unit has a working philosophy and value system that is understood and lived, uses healthy adaptive patterns most of the time, can ask for help and use the community services available, and develops linkages with nonfamily units and organizations (37).

Roles of the Family

The family assigns **roles,** *prescribed behaviors in a situation,* in a way similar to society at large (78). In society there are specialists who enforce laws, teach, practice medicine, and fight fires. In the family there are also such performance roles: breadwinner, homemaker, handyman (or handywoman), the expert, political advisor, chauffeur, and gardener. There are also emotional roles: leader, nurturer, sustainer, protector, healer, arbitrator, scapegoat, jester, rebel, dependent, "sexpot," and "black sheep." Members may fill more than one role. The fewer people there are to fulfill these roles, as in the nuclear family, the greater the number of demands placed on one person. If a member leaves home, someone else takes up his or her role. Any member of the family can satisfactorily fulfill any role in either category unless he or she is uncomfortable in that role. The man who is sure of his masculinity will have no emotional problems diapering a baby or cooking a meal. The woman who is sure of her femininity will have no trouble gardening or taking the car for repair. Today many men and women no longer are restricted to carrying out only traditional sex roles. They enjoy sharing roles, working together to get the tasks done without worrying about what is man's or woman's work.

The emotional response of a person to the role he or she fulfills should be considered. Someone may perform the job competently and yet dread doing it. The man may be a carpenter because his father taught him the trade, although he wants to be a music teacher. Changes in performance roles also necessitate emotional changes (e.g., in the man who takes over household duties when his wife becomes incapacitated).

The child learns about emotional response to roles in the family while imitating adults. The child experiments with various roles in play and eventually finds one that is emotionally comfortable. The more pressure put on the child by the parents to respond in a particular way, the more likely that child is to learn only one role and be uncomfortable in others, as evidenced by the athletic champion who may be a social misfit. The child becomes less adaptive socially and even within the family as a result.

Exercising a capacity for a variety of roles, either in actuality or in fantasy, is healthy. The healthy family is the one in which there is opportunity to shift roles intermittently with ease (78). Through these roles family functions are fulfilled.

Functions of the Family as a Social System

The family is a system. It functions as a unit to fulfill its purposes, roles, and tasks. It provides shelter, stability, security, and a setting for nurturance and growth. It is a place to experiment with the dynamics and role behaviors required in a system. It has an energy that provides a support system for individual members. As the social system changes, the family system must also adapt if it is to meet individual needs and prepare its members to participate in the social system.

The organization of a family system is hierarchal, although it may not be directly observable. The usual family hierarchies are built on kinship, power, status, and privilege relationships that may be related to individual characteristics of age, sex, education, personality, health, strength, or vigor. We can infer a hierarchy by observing each person's behavior and communication. For instance, who talks first? Last? Longest? Who talks to whom? When? Where? About what? If one family member consistently approaches the staff about the client's health care, he or she probably holds an upper position in the family and has the task of being "expert." Your attempt to communicate with family members may meet with resistance if the communication inadvertently violates the family communication hierarchy (67).

Hierarchal relations in the family system determine the role behavior of family members. These hierarchal role relationships typically have great stability, and ordinarily family members can be counted on to behave congruently with their roles. When there are differences in behavior from situation to situation, they are almost inevitably in response to the family's expectations for that particular situation or circumstance (67). Families develop a system of balanced relationships. When one member leaves the family or experiences a change such as illness, other family members also must adapt. Roles and relationships are based on reciprocal interaction, with each member of the family contributing to the total unit in a unique and functional way. If a member should fail to meet the expectations of the roles established by his or her position in the hierarchy for the moment, the remaining members of the family generally react by using pressure (e.g., persuasion, punishment, argument, being ignored) on the "deviant" person (67). Ackerman (1) states that all family functions can be reduced to two basic ones: (1) ensuring the physical survival of the species and (2) transmitting the culture, thereby ensuring essential humanness. The union of mother and father, of parent and child, forms the bonds of identity that are the matrix for the development of this humanness.

Physical functions of the family are met by the parents' *providing food, clothing, and shelter, protection against danger, provision for bodily repairs after fatigue or illness, and reproduction.* In "primitive" societies these physical needs are the dominant concern. In Western societies many families take them for granted (1, 78).

Affectional functions are equally important. Although many traditional family functions such as education, job training, and medical care are being absorbed by other agencies, *meeting emotional needs and promoting adaptation and adjustment are still two of the family's major functions.* The family is the primary unit in which the child tests emotional reactions. Learning how to reach and maintain emotional equilibrium within the family enables him or her to repeat the pattern in later life situations. The child who feels loved is likely to contract fewer physical illnesses, learn more quickly, and generally have an easier time growing up and adapting to society (1, 78).

Satir believes a healthy family has five dominant attitudes (98):

1. No distinctions are made about worth of people; all members are perceived as equal.
2. All persons are seen as unique and developing.
3. When a disturbing situation arises, members understand that many factors were involved—people were not simply trying to be difficult.
4. Members accept that change is continuous.
5. Members freely share their thoughts and feelings with a minimum of blame and feel good about each other and themselves.

Other important attitudes are:

- The feeling of unity between man and woman and a separateness from their families of origins so that interfamily interference with the marriage is avoided
- An ability to invest in the marriage to a greater degree than in other relationships
- A feeling of balance or complementarity, for perfect equality is probably impossible
- A movement from a romantic "falling in love" to a warm, loving, companionable, accepting relationship
- An ability to maintain variety and frequent interactions with each other

Social functions of the modern family include *providing social togetherness, fostering self-esteem and a personal identity tied to family identity, providing opportunities for observing and learning social and sexual roles, accepting responsibility for behavior, and supporting individual creativity and initiative.* The family actually begins the indoctrination of the infant into society when it bestows a name and hence a social position or status in relation to the immediate and kinship-group families. Simultaneously, each family begins to transmit its own version of the cultural heritage and its own family culture to the child. Because the culture is too vast and comprehensive to transmit to the child in its entirety and all at once, the family selects what will be transmitted. In addition, the family interprets and evaluates what is transmitted. Through this process, the child learns to share family values (1, 5, 78).

Thus socialization is a primary task of the parents, for they teach the child about the body, peers, family, community, age-appropriate roles, language, perceptions, social values, and ethics. The family also teaches about the different standards of responsibility society demands from various social groups. For example, the professional person such as a physician, nurse, or lawyer, those in whom people confide and to whom they entrust their lives and fortunes, are held more accountable than the farmer or day laborer. There is also a difference in the type of contact that society has with a particular group: for example, the mail or milk deliverer does not enter the home, but the exterminator is free to enter a home and look into every corner.

The parent generation educates by literal instruction and by serving as models. Thus the child's **personality,** *a product of all the influences that have and are impinging on him or her,* is greatly influenced by the parents (75).

FAMILY ADAPTATION

Adaptive responses in the family represent the *means by which it maintains an internal equilibrium so that it can fulfill purposes and tasks, deal with internal and external stress and crises, and allow for growth of individual members.* Some capacity for functioning may be sacrificed to control conflict and aid work as a unit. But the best functioning family keeps anxiety and conflict within tolerable limits and maintains a balance between effects of the past and new experiences. Just as other social systems adapt, so must the family system (44).

Ideally, the family achieves equilibrium by talking over problems and finding solutions together. Humor, nonsense, shared work, and leisure all help relieve tension. The family members know that certain freedoms exist within their confines that are not available elsewhere.

Successful and happy families define their most important priority as the spouse and the family; the business or career of both or either of the partners comes second. Children may come second before the business or career; hobbies and volunteer activities are further removed priorities. Each spouse needs to serve as a comforter, listener, companion, and counselor to the other, to be supportive and fully committed, and to avoid being negative. That does not mean one person is a doormat, for each is supportive to the other. The spouses may wish to set aside one night a week, or a month, to be only with each other, sharing uninterrupted time and activity. Each parent may wish to have a day date with each child monthly, spending time together at lunch, shopping, or in some mutually favorite activity.

Yet even the most stable family will sometimes use various adaptive mechanisms to cope with stress, which, in turn, promotes more stress; however, these mechanisms are not overused in healthy families (70, 78).

Adaptive Mechanisms in Family Life

Various types of family coping strategies are discussed by Friedman. These internal strategies include relying on the family members and sharing together, using humor, working to control the stress by problem solving or to cognitively reframe it, and striving to be flexible in roles. Strategies that extend outside the family include (1) seeking information, (2) maintaining linkage with people or agencies in the community, (3) using self-help groups or informal or formal support networks, and (4) seeking spiritual support (44).

Dysfunctional or ineffective coping strategies used by families during stressful times include denial of problems, exploitation or manipulation of one or more family members, abuse of or violence toward children or adult members, use of authoritarianism or threats, changing to ineffective customs or traditions or family myths, use of alcohol or drugs, and abandonment of the family by one member through separation, divorce, or suicide (44). Family response to stressors and conflict between the spouses or the parents and children affect the personality development and behavior of children and adolescents, and may contribute to illness such as hyperactivity or behavioral acting out (39, 84).

Emotional conflicts in the family may be avoided, minimized, or resolved through scapegoating, coalitions, withdrawal of emotional ties, repetitive verbal or physical fighting, use of family myths, reaction formation, compromise, and designation of a family healer. Two or more of these mechanisms may be used within the same family. If these mechanisms are used exclusively, however, they become defensive and are unlikely to promote resolution of the conflict, so that the same issue will arise repeatedly (70, 78).

Scapegoating or Blaming. Scapegoating or blaming involves labeling one member as the cause of the family trouble and is expressed in the attitude, "If it weren't for you. . . . " Or one member may offer himself or herself as a scapegoat to end an argument by saying, "It's all my fault." Such labeling controls the conflict and reduces anxiety, but it prevents communication that can get at the root of the problem. Growth toward resolution of the problem is prohibited.

Coalitions or Alliances. Coalitions or alliances may form when some family members side together against other members. Antagonisms and anger result. Eventually the losing party tries to get control.

Withdrawal of Emotional Ties. Loosening the family unit and reducing communication may be used to handle conflict, but then the family becomes rigid and mechanized. Family members are also likely to seek affection outside the family so that the home becomes a hotel with everyone superficially nice. In some families there is no show of emotion, for such emotion signifies loss of control or giving in to unacceptable impulses.

Repetitive Fighting. Verbal abuse, physical battles, loud complaints, curses, or accusations may be used to relieve tension and allow some harmony until the next round. The fight may have the same theme each time stress hits the family. The healthy family allows some "blowing up" as a release from everyday frustrations, but it does not make a major case out of every minor incident or temporary disagreement.

Family Myths or Traditional Beliefs. These myths or beliefs can be used to overcome anxieties and maintain control over others, as illustrated in the following statements: "Children are seen, not heard." "We can't survive if you leave home." "Talking about feelings will cause loss of love." In contrast, the healthy family members encourage growth and creativity rather than rigid control.

Reaction Formation. Reaction formation is seen in a family in which there is superficial harmony or togetherness. Traumatic ideas are repressed and transformed into the opposite behavior. Everybody smiles, but nobody loves. No one admits to having any difficulties. Great tension is felt because true feelings are not expressed.

Resignation or Compromise. Temporary harmony may occur when someone gives up or suppresses the need for assertion, affection, or emotional expression to keep peace. The surface calm eventually explodes when unmet needs can no longer be successfully suppressed.

Designation of One Person as Family Healer or Umpire. This mechanism involves using a "wise one" (most often in the extended family) or a minister, storekeeper, bartender, or druggist to arrange a reconciliation between dissenting parties. Part of the dynamics sometimes underlying the helper role is that the referee gets great satisfaction from finding someone worse off than self. The healer feels a sense of heightened self-esteem or omnipotence. A variant of the healer role is that of family "protector," who takes on all the stresses to save other members stress or conflict. One person ends up fighting the battles for everyone else in the family.

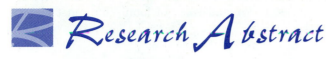

Research Abstract

D'Avanzo, C., B. Frye, and R. Froman, Stress in Cambodian Refugee Families, IMAGE: Journal of Nursing Scholarship, 26, no. 2 (1994), 101–105.

More than a million Southeast Asians from Cambodia, Laos, and Vietnam live in the United States, according to the U.S. Census Bureau in 1990. The experience of the Khmer people of Cambodia under the Khmer Rouge has been equated with the Jewish holocaust. Because of their prior stresses of starvation, rape, witness of murder punishment, and unremitting insecurity and exhaustion, Cambodian refugees continue to be at high risk for stress-related disorders. Somatization, clinical depression, posttraumatic stress syndrome, suicide, and unexpected death syndrome are commonly experienced. Yet, few Cambodian immigrants received mental health services, even when available, because of lack of knowledge about treatment.

The purpose of this comparative descriptive study was to improve understanding of the beliefs of Cambodian refugee women about stress in the family and how stress is handled.

Two samples of 60 Cambodian women were interviewed in their homes in two communities on the East and West coasts that contained large enclaves of Cambodian refugees. Translation was provided by a trusted, informal female community leader. Informants were identified by snowball or network sampling. Participants were told the research had nothing to do with the government and that they could refuse; they signed a consent form written in the Cambodian language.

Data were analyzed by determining the most frequently occurring responses and rank order of responses by frequency. Demographic variables on the total sample and two subgroups were summarized using descriptive statistics. Finally, the two subgroups were compared for similarities of ranked responses.

The two subgroups differed significantly on some demographic variables. The East Coast group had few years in the United States, less education before immigration, and a greater number of young children living at home. Almost 60% of the East Coast sample had lived in the United States for 6 years or less, in contrast to 55% of the West Coast sample who had lived here 8 years or longer. The East Coast group was more likely than the West Coast group to have a woman as head of household. Behaviors associated with stress or thinking too much included headaches, shouting, chest pain, palpitations, shortness of breath, and sleeping a lot. Less frequently cited stress responses were dizziness, inability to concentrate, loss of appetite, and neglecting spiritual beliefs. The most commonly perceived stressors were thinking about the war in Cambodia, financial concerns, loneliness, grief about family left behind, cultural losses, language problems, and health status. The women, especially single heads of households, felt responsible for reducing the stress felt by the family, but they also felt powerless or ineffectual in understanding stress.

The refugees' prior experiences and their feelings, accompanied by the process of acculturation, limited social supports, and low income may produce a cycle of stress. Because Cambodians are reluctant to seek mental health services, they will need culturally sensitive health care.

To remain adaptive, families maneuver to secure compliance of all members with the family rules through verbal and nonverbal communication to each other. Usually one member is designated as the one who must maintain a specific pattern of dependent behavior, sometimes negative or unhealthy, to keep all other family members comfortable. If the designated member tries to change behavior and become more independent, he or she receives no support. The feedback received is that he or she is disrupting the status quo and the other family members are uncomfortable. Thus sick behavior will be maintained at the expense of the development of the designated person and of the family.

Maladaptation

Signs of strained or destructive family relationships include the following (9, 19, 44, 75, 119):

- Lack of understanding and communication between members, resulting in unclear roles and conflict

- Each family member alternately acting as if the other did not exist or harassing through arguments
- Lack of family decision making and lines of authority
- Parents' possessiveness of the children or the mate
- Children's derogatory remarks to parents or vice versa
- Extreme closeness between husband and his mother or family or the wife and her mother or family
- Members not maintaining individuality, being too close or enmeshed or too distant
- Parent being domineering about performance of household tasks
- Few outside friends for parents or children
- Scapegoating or blaming each other for difficulties
- High level of anxiety or insecurity present in the home
- Lack of creativity and stability
- Pattern of immature or regressive behavior in parents or children
- Boundaries between generations not maintained; children carrying out parental roles because of parent's inability to function, illness, or abandonment

You may find yourself in the role of family healer. Help the family to develop harmonious ways of coping and avoid the protector or omnipotent role. The text by Kramer (70) gives in-depth information pertinent to assessment of and intervention with families.

STAGES OF FAMILY DEVELOPMENT

Like an individual, the family has a developmental history marked by predictable crises. The developmental crises are normal, but they are also disturbing or frightening because each life stage is a new experience. The natural history of the family is on a continuum: from courtship to marriage or cohabitation; choosing whether to have children; rearing biological or adoptive offspring, if any; and releasing children into society to establish homes of their own. In later life the aging parents or grandparents are a couple once again, barring divorce or death. The nurturing of spouse or children goes on simultaneously with a multitude of other activities: work at a job or profession, managing a household, participation in church and community groups, pursuit of leisure and hobbies, maintaining friendships and family ties. Or the person may decide to remain single but live with a person of the same or opposite sex; then the purposes, tasks, and roles of family life must also be worked out.

Initial or Establishment Stage

Courtship and engagement precede establishment of the family unit. Developmental tasks to accomplish during this courtship period include contending with partner-selection pressures from parents; giving over autonomy while retaining some independence; preparing for marriage, including a mutually satisfying sex life; and becoming free of parental domination. In the **establishment stage,** *the couple establishes a home of its own; main psychologic tie is no longer with family of orientation (parental family).* They commit themselves to living together, usually through marriage. (Readiness for marriage in U.S. society is discussed in relation to young adulthood in Chapter 12.) They must work out patterns of communication, daily living, sexual relations, a budget, and a philosophy of life. Relationships with family and friends are also different after marriage and must be worked out (37, 79, 119).

Today families may choose to have no children, one child and adopt others, or two or three children instead of a larger family. Some women believe that motherhood is not necessary for fulfillment. Certainly the man's chief fulfillment is not necessarily from fatherhood. Some people are wise enough to know that children do not automatically bring happiness to a marriage. Children bring happiness to parents who want them and who are selfless enough to become involved in the adventure of rearing them. Children bring trauma to a troubled marriage.

Limitation of family size and birth spacing yield substantial family health benefits. Certain associations in death, disease, and disability are apparent. Maternal deaths increase when maternal age is below 20 or above 40 years and after the third pregnancy for women of all age groups except those over 40. Increased maternal disease, obstetric complications, maternal deaths, and postnatal mortality occur with six or more pregnancies. Unwanted pregnancy increases maternal disease and death, especially if the pregnancy is terminated by abortion that results in infection or hemorrhage. Other effects of unwanted pregnancy include excessive nausea and vomiting, spontaneous abortion, toxemias, complications of labor and delivery, emotional illness prenatally or postnatally, marital friction, and divorce. Infant mortality rate increases for birth order above three in the lower social class and rises among women under 17 years of age. The safest years for a normal delivery are between ages 20 and 29. Infants of youngest mothers of highest parity are at greatest risk for disease and death regardless of social class. Mothers are less likely to have premature or low-birth-weight infants and therefore healthier infants when spacing is greater than 2 years but less than 6 years (102).

The establishment phase ends when the woman becomes pregnant or when the couple works out its living patterns and philosophy of life (which may include a decision not to have children).

Expectant Stage

During the **expectant stage,** or *pregnancy,* which is a developmental crisis, many domestic and social adjustments must be made. The couple (or the single mother and her significant other) is learning new roles and gaining new status in the community. Attitudes toward pregnancy and the physical and emotional status of the mother and father (and of significant others) will affect parenting abilities. Now the couple thinks in terms of family instead of a pair. They explore beliefs about childrearing and plan for the expanded family in terms of space, budget, and necessary supplies (37).

The woman may initially dislike being pregnant because it interferes with her personal plans, or she may feel proud and fulfilled. Sexual desire may either increase or decrease. She may be more or less interested in her surroundings. Usually she is more preoccupied with herself, her new feelings, and changing body image, and she experiences fantasies and fears about the baby and the childbirth experiences.

The man experiences a variety of feelings on learning of the pregnancy, feelings that change during the pregnancy. The reality of the pregnancy increases with time. Men may experience ambivalent feelings initially, but fatherly feelings develop. Men may feel guilty about the wife's pregnancy and her physical symptoms, anxious and depressed about their own adequacy, proud of their virility, and fearful of approaching the wife sexually. Concerns identified by fathers are caring for the infant, adequacy as a father, financial security, and the baby's effect on the marital dyad (62, 72, 73, 75, 102, 115).

Early and thorough prenatal care for the woman is essential. Both the woman and the man may experience similar physical and emotional symptoms such as nausea, indigestion, backache, distention, irritability, and depression. Symptoms may result from hormonal changes or feelings about the pregnancy in the woman. In the man they are part of the **couvade syndrome,** *which may be a reaction based on identification with or sympathy for the woman, ambivalence or hostility toward the pregnancy, or envy of the woman's childbearing abil-*

ity. The symptoms of couvade syndrome are symbolically a means for the father to participate in the client's development and birth, an early indication of interactions that will continue with the child, and a means of affording the pregnant woman and new infant protection (32, 49, 62). The physical symptoms, complex feelings, and changes in body image that accompany pregnancy are described by several authors (32, 49, 62, 88, 94, 95, 102, 115).

Major decisions for the couple are whether to attend childbirth preparation classes and whether the man should be present in the labor and delivery rooms. The woman may feel eager to have the man with her, or she may fear that he will think of her as sexually unattractive or be repulsed. The man may be curious about what is happening and want to attend his child's birth, or he may feel guilty about not wanting to when he feels others expect him to be there. He may be embarrassed about his wife's behavior and appearance during labor and delivery, or he may fear that he cannot cope with the childbirth event if present. Sexual fantasies triggered by labor and delivery may threaten the man who has tenuous emotional equilibrium. If the man has considerable unconscious conflicts or a weak self-image as a man, he may wish not to be involved in childbirth preparation, labor, or delivery. Some men and women cannot participate in childbirth preparation classes and should not be made to feel guilty about their decision. Participation may not enhance the couple's self-esteem and may create additional emotional crisis. Participation in Lamaze classes and childbirth does not change the woman's perception of her partner as ideal man, husband, or father, but it does improve her self-image as ideal woman, wife, and mother (62). In addition, the woman more likely will be in good physical condition for labor if she has had preparation.

Although the woman needs extra "mothering" from the partner (or others) during pregnancy, the man also needs extra attention and nurturing or he may be unable to continue to support the mother-to-be emotionally (62). You can listen to the woman's and man's concerns and help them understand that what they are experiencing is normal. Various teaching aids explaining pregnancy and what to expect during the birth experience are also useful. Your care should be family centered, directed toward both parents-to-be. You can help the woman to gain maternal feelings and the man to see the importance of his role as provider and nurturer.

The man must be prepared for fathering just as the woman is for mothering. Fathers also go through the five operations (mimicry, role play, fantasy, introjection–projection–rejection, and grief work) identified by Rubin (94) as necessary to attain the maternal role.

For additional information about prenatal influences on the mother and baby, see Chapters 6 and 7. Information about parenting and developmental tasks for the expectancy phase is also presented in Chapter 12. Several authors give further information on the fathers' reactions and responsibilities (53, 72, 73, 75, 102, 115).

The family that prepares for adoption of a child does not have the tasks associated with the physical aspects of pregnancy, but it does have to accomplish the other tasks of readiness.

Parenthood or Expansion Stage

In the **parenthood or expansion stage,** there is *birth or adoption of a child,* and the couple assumes a status that it will never lose as long as each has memory and life—that of parent. The *stages of parenthood* are (102, 115):

- *Anticipatory stage:* Pregnancy. The couple is learning the new roles and perceptions associated with pregnancy discussed earlier.
- *Honeymoon stage:* The time following birth when the parents feel excited about the new relationship but also uncertain about the meaning of parental love. A parent–child attachment is being formed. During this time difficult adjustments must be made. Because the parents lose sleep, husband–wife intimacy diminishes, and there is less freedom for the couple to follow their own interests.
- *Plateau or consolidation stage:* The years during the child's development when the parents are active in the role of mother and father. During this time the parents deal with problems in the family, community, church, school and immediate social sphere. They are concerned with family planning, socialization and education of the child, and participation in community organizations.
- *Disengagement or contraction stage:* The termination of the parent–child family unit that occurs when the last child marries or leaves home permanently and the parents let go of their major childrearing responsibilities to allow the offspring to be autonomous.

Americans value creativity and individuality; thus no set patterns of parenthood exist. Parents rely on their own uniqueness, wisdom, and skills, how their parents raised them, or on books. Youth are poorly prepared to make the transition to parenthood. Yet how parents treat a child is the single most important influence on the child's physical, emotional, and cognitive development and health.

The couple may accept the idea of parenthood but reject a particular child because of the child's sex, appearance, time of the birth in their life cycle, or the child's threatening helplessness; or the couple may reject the idea of parenthood but genuinely love the baby who was unplanned. Often parents have difficulty because pregnancy, childbirth, and parenting are romanticized in our society, and the romantic ideal differs considerably from the reality of 24-hour responsibility and submersion of their personal desires for many years to come.

How the parents care for and discipline the child is influenced considerably by the parents' own maturity; how they were cared for as children (as shown by studies on child abuse); their feelings about self; culture, social class, and religion (see Chapters 1 and 3); their relationship with each other; their perceptions of and experiences with children and other adults; their values and philosophy of life; and life stresses that arise. Moreover, the historical eras in which the parents were reared and in which they are now living and the prominent social values of each era subtly influence parental behavior.

Each critical period in the child's development reactivates a critical period in the parent. Demands made on the parent vary with the age of the child. The infant needs almost total and constant nurturance. Some parents thrive during this period and depend on each other for support. Other parents feel overwhelmed by the infant's dependency because their own dependent needs are stimulated but unmet. The baby's cry and behavior evoke feelings of helplessness, dependency, and anger associated with their unacceptable dependency needs and feelings and then guilt and fatigue. The toddler struggles with individuality and autonomy, exploring and vacillating between dependency and independency. At this stage the child is intense and often unreasonable in demands and refusal to obey commands. The parents may enjoy this explorative, independent behavior of the child, even though the toddler leaves the parent feeling tired and frustrated; or the primitive behavior of the child may stimulate primitive impulses in the parent, who may feel threatened by the will of the toddler. The parent who has difficulty controlling angry impulses may find the toddler's temper outbursts totally unacceptable. Parents who have difficulty caring for the dependent infant may do very well with the independent preschooler or adolescent, or the reverse may be true. The parent may be able to resolve personal conflicts and move to a more advanced level of integration as he or she works with the developing child, or the parent may be unable to cope with the aroused feelings (12).

Some parents believe that they must possess a child and will try to fit that child into a mold—their image. Other parents see their task of parenthood as stewards—to be a guide, a helping friend, a standard setter for the child. They invest themselves in the creative potentialities of their young, nurturing, educating, and protecting the child. They love but do not smother; guide but do not control; discipline but do not punish; offer freedom but do not abandon. They see the child as a lamp to light rather than a vessel to fill (14, 79).

Parents who possess their children believe they have the right to dictate the terms of their child's life. Then the child has only half a life; parental need to control is greater than real love for child. Too much pressure is placed on the growing child, disturbing his or her emotional development (14, 79).

Just as detrimental are the parents who abandon the child to rear itself—parents who spend too little time with and give too little affection to the child. Such children spend considerable time with television and peers; they learn that the adult world does not want them. In one study children who spend most of their time with peers were more influenced by the lack of the parents' presence, attention, and concern than by the attractiveness of the peer group. The peer-oriented child held negative views of self and peer group and expressed dim views of the future. The peer-oriented children rated parents lower in both expression of affection and support and in exercise of discipline control than did children who spent more time with adults. Peer-oriented children reported engaging in more antisocial behavior such as doing something illegal, playing hooky from school, or lying (14, 79).

Parents should rethink their priorities when they have children. Parents must invest time in such a way that it brings quality to their relationship with the child. Children need the encouragement of doing things and talking through things with adults (14, 79).

Developmental tasks for the couple, *which are reworked with the birth of each child, are to* (9, 37, 83, 102):

- Provide for the physical and emotional needs of the child, conveying love and security freely regardless of the child's appearance or temperament
- Reconcile conflicting roles—wife–mother, husband–father, worker–homemaker or family man, and parent–citizen
- Accept and adjust to the demands and stresses of parenthood, learning or relearning basics of child care, adjusting personal routines and needs to meet the child's needs, and trying to meet the spouse's needs as well

- Provide opportunities for the child to master competencies expected for each developmental stage, to allow the child to make mistakes and learn from them, to restrict the child reasonably and constantly for safety, and to attain the emotional developmental tasks described by Erikson (38)
- Share responsibilities of parenthood and together make necessary adjustments in space, finances, housing, lifestyle, and daily routines that are healthy for the family (meals, sleep)
- Maintain a satisfying relationship with spouse—emotionally, sexually, intellectually, spiritually, and recreationally—while maintaining a personal sense of autonomy and identity
- Feel satisfaction from being competent parents and the parenting experience but maintain contacts with relatives and the community
- Provide socialization experiences to help the child make the emotional shift from family to peers and society so that the child can become a functioning citizen
- Refine the communication system and relationships with spouse, children, and others and permit offspring to be autonomous after leaving home

Other authors also describe the reactions, roles, and responsibilities involved in parenting (1, 12, 14, 18, 23, 52, 67, 70, 72, 73, 75, 79, 98, 115).

As the children mature and leave home, the parents must rework their self-concepts as parents and people so they can assume new roles, responsibilities, and leisure activities to accomplish the last stage of parenthood, disengagement. You can assist the couple in meeting developmental tasks.

Disengagement or Contraction Stage

The last, or **disengagement or contraction stage** occurs *when children leave and the partners must rework their separateness.* The middle-aged woman may return to work after the children leave home if she was not employed while childrearing; new roles evolve for each of the spouses. This is often a time for maximum contact between the partners, especially when retirement occurs. Retirement planning and preparation for the spouse's death must occur. Eventual bereavement, loneliness, and further role changes and losses will occur.

Sometimes, however, this stage does not last too long. The young adult who is unemployed, a college dropout, or divorced may return home to live. Sometimes teenage or young adult offspring return with children of his or her own because of divorce, economic problems, or other crises so that grandparents may become involved in raising the grandchildren. The aged parents or other relatives may be unable to continue to live independently and are included in the household of middle-aged offspring. Consequently, the tasks, functions, roles, and hierarchical relationships of the family must be reworked. Space and other resources must be reallocated. Time schedules for daily activities may be reworked. Privacy in communication, use of possessions, and emotional space must be ensured. Old parent–child conflicts and ideas about who is boss and how rules are set and discipline accomplished may resurface and should be discussed and worked through. These families can benefit from counseling; your guidance may be crucial. The middle-aged family is more fully discussed in Chapter 13.

Table 4–3 lists suggestions to adult children and their parents to make living together more harmonious (68, 98, 106).

FAMILY INTERACTION

Family interaction is a *unique form of social interaction based on a set of intimate and continuing relationships. It is the sum total of all the family roles being played within a family at a given time* (37). Families function and carry out their tasks and lifestyles through this process.

Family therapists, psychiatrists, and nurses are giving increased attention to the emotional balance in family **dyads** or *paired role positions* such as husband and wife or mother and child. They have noted that a shift in the balance of one member of the pair (or of one pair) alters the balance of the other member (or pair). The birth of a child is the classic example (79). Dyads and emotional balance also shift in single-parent and stepparent families (23, 70, 97, 116, 117).

Interaction of the husband and wife or of the adult members living under one roof is basic to the mental, and sometimes physical, health of the adults and to the eventual health of the children. Two factors strongly influence this interaction: (1) the sense of self-esteem or self-love of each family member and (2) the different socialization processes for boys and girls (14).

Importance of Self-esteem

The most important life task for each person—to feel a sense of self-esteem, to love and have a positive self-image—evolves through interaction with the parents

TABLE 4–3. GUIDELINES FOR WHEN YOUNG ADULTS MOVE IN WITH PARENTS

1. Remember what it was like when a new baby came home. No matter how beloved the child, disruptions are bound to occur. Realize that another relative's homecoming will be the same.

2. Everyone involved should remember whose house it is.

3. Realize that no matter how many years sons or daughters have been away, family procedures do not change. Mom may still be critical. Dad may be the constant advice giver. Expect it.

4. Talk about resentments. Discuss problems if you think it will help.

5. Parents may say offspring are grown up. But that does not mean they believe it. Still, they cannot exert the same authority with a 30- or 40-year-old as with a youngster.

6. Offspring and elderly parents must be flexible. It is unfair to expect the middle-agers who are the "hosts" to change their household and life routines too much.

7. Even if parents refuse money, adult offspring should insist on paying something, no matter how minimal. Otherwise, the offspring are reinforcing the idea that parents are taking care of them. Elderly parents can also contribute financially most of the time.

8. When grandchildren are involved, set rules about who is in charge. To decrease dependency, babysitters should be hired when possible. Then family members do not feel obligated or constrained.

9. Determine length of the adult offspring's stay. It need not be a precise date, but future plans about leaving the home should be explicitly stated.

10. Both adult offspring and older relatives should share responsibilities if possible. But do not upstage mom or dad; for example, if mom loves cooking, do not make her feel useless by taking over in the kitchen.

11. Space permitting, privacy is important. The relative who has lived on his or her own is probably used to time and space alone.

12. Middle-agers should resist meddling in the affairs of either offspring or parents. They can advise. But grown offspring need to think for themselves, and older relatives expect to make their own decisions.

13. Realize that the living situation may be temporary. Living together may not be ideal for anyone. But some parents and offspring or middle-agers and their parents become closer during such periods.

from the time of birth onward and, in turn, affects how the person interacts in later life with others, including spouse and offspring.

The adult in the family who lacks self-acceptance and self-respect probably will not be a loving spouse or parent. Behavior will betray feelings about self and others because he or she will perceive no automatic acceptance and little love from others in the family. Because perception of an event is the person's reality, such a person in turn reacts in ways designed to defend self from the rejection that he or she *thinks* will be received: he or she may criticize, get angry, brag, demand perfection from others, or withdraw. In this way, he or she builds up self, the emotional reasoning being: "I may not be much, but others are worse." Such behavior is corrosive to any relationship but particularly one as intimate as the family's. Because of overt behavior, those intimate with him or her are not likely to appreciate or respond to the basic needs for love, acceptance, and respect. Indeed, the common responses to such behavior are counterattack or withdrawal, which, in turn, perpetuate the other's negative behavior. To remain open and giving in such situations is difficult for the mate but may be the only way to elevate the other's self-esteem. Perhaps only then can he or she reciprocate loving behavior. You can help family members realize the importance of respecting and loving one another and help them work through problems stemming from the low self-esteem of a family member (14, 75, 115).

Influence of Childhood Socialization

The second crucial influence on interaction between adults in the family is the difference in socialization processes for boys and girls. These differences are so embedded in the U.S. social matrix that until recently they had gone nearly unnoticed. There is a different social source for self-love in boys and girls. The girl is loved simply because she exists and can attract, as shown by the admiration pretty little girls receive. The girl is also taught to be subtle, for such behavior is part of her attraction. The boy is loved for what he can do and become; he must prove himself. Boys, especially from school age on, are given less recognition than girls for good looks and much recognition for what they can do. A boy learns to be direct, to brush aside distractions (sometimes including a woman's voice, for most disciplining will come from the mother and female schoolteachers and can be perceived as nagging after a while), and to get to the essence of things (14, 15, 65, 75, 115).

These concepts of what is appropriate boy and girl behavior are taught early and continue to affect heterosexual interactions throughout life. In traditional courtship, for example, the boy is expected to be in charge, to be dominant, to prove himself; the girl is expected to attract, to be passive. In marriage, however, these expectations cause problems, for the man is proving himself largely through his work, and this aspect of his earlier courtship behavior is now less visible to his wife. If the woman does not understand the dynamics of his behavior, she is likely to feel rejected and unloved, thinking she can no longer attract him. If the wife is also working, the husband may think of her as a competitor and work harder to keep his self-esteem. His physical self, including his involvement in lovemaking, is very much intertwined with his social, professional, and financial self, and failure in one is likely to cause feelings of failure in the total self, affecting his sense of masculinity, sexuality, and personhood (14, 65, 75, 115).

All these facts are compounded by the shift in balance between the man and woman found in modern marriage, especially with the advent of the women's liberation movement. The husband often labors under the illusion that he enjoys the rights and responsibilities inherent in a patriarchal family system. Yet he must recognize the qualifications and drive for independence, the basic humanness, of his wife. You can help the couple to recognize the effect of their early socialization on their behavior and expectations and to work through misunderstandings. Help parents to overcome sexual stereotypes so that they do not inflict them on their children. Carmichael's book *Nonsexist Childrearing* (29), may be helpful.

Variables Affecting Interaction Between the Child and Adult

Long before the child learns to speak, sensory, emotional, and intellectual exchanges are made between the child and other family members. Through such exchanges, and later with words, the child receives and tests instructions on how to consider the rights of others and how to respond to authority. The child also learns how to use language as a symbol, how to carry out certain routines necessary for health, how to compete, and what goals to seek. The games and toys purchased for and played with the child, the books selected and read, and the television programs allowed can provide key learning techniques.

The *child's spontaneity* can evoke in the adult fresh ways of looking at life long buried under habit and routine. The child says, "It's too loud, but my earlids won't stay down" or "I want one of those little red olives with the green around" or "Give me that eraser with the handle." The child can also recreate for the adult the difficulty of the learning process: "Is it today, tomorrow, or yesterday? You said when I woke up it would be tomorrow, but now you call it 'today.'"

Family interaction for the child and adult is also affected by the *ordinal position and sex of the children* and by the presence of an only child or of multiple births such as twins, of an adoptive child, or stepchild.

Parents tend to identify with their children and to treat them according to how they were treated as children. A parent can identify best with the child who matches his or her own sibling position. A man from a family of boys may not know how to interact with a daughter and may not empathize with her. In the process of identifying with the parent, the child picks up many of the parent's characteristics, especially if the child is the oldest or lone child. For example, the oldest boy may be dependent instead of independent if his father was the youngest sibling and retained his dependent behavior into adulthood. Using family constellation theory, Hoopes and Harper (60) and Toman (112) describe features of each child in a family, based on sex and ordinal position, how the child feels about and interacts with people, and which ordinal position spouse he or she will most happily marry.

Ordinal Position of the Child

Birth order is important to development. Table 4–4 lists characteristics of children in first, middle, and last ordinal positions, as well as of the only child. *Siblings, both same and opposite sex, have an important influence on each other* as buddies, bullies, or heroes, and the *early relationship often affects the adult relationship.* Whether the child has male or female siblings also affects personality development (60, 67, 75, 78, 112). For example, secondborn boys with an older sister are more feminine or empathic and nurturing than those with an older brother. If two siblings are more than 6 years apart, they tend to grow up like only children (60, 112).

Children are the logical targets for fulfilling many of the parents' frustrated ambitions and needs. In a large family these yearnings and aspirations can be parceled out among a number of children, but when there is only one child, this child can sense the parents' manipulation and expectations. Thus the only child usually is a peacemaker if he or she and the parents are the only household members. He or she is inadvertently brought into the parents' conflicts and is forced to help maintain harmony and preserve equilibrium in the household (78, 112). As you counsel parents who plan for or have only one child, emphasize the need for peer activity and the danger of too much early responsibility and pressure.

Family With a Large Number of Children

The family with more than three or four children is less frequently seen now than in the past. The lastborn child may be less wanted than the first or middleborn, although parents feel more skilled and self-confident in rearing the younger children. Large families have advantages. Of necessity, the children learn thrift and conservation of resources and material goods. Members know the hot water supply is not unlimited, that food is not to be wasted, and that toys and clothing can be recycled. Children learn to share time, space, and possessions. The children learn to do for themselves and each other; they learn responsibility. In a loving home, they

have not only their parents' love but also that of siblings, a listening ear, respect, support, compassion, and help. If the parent does not have time to read to the 3-year-old, the older sibling does. He or she gains more experience in reading, gains increased self-esteem from being helpful, and learns responsibility and caring. Each child learns cooperation, compromise, and tolerance and how to handle peer pressure. The effort, work, expense, and self-denial of having a large family can be offset by the rewards of watching children grow and develop and by a sense of contribution to the generations to come (75, 79, 103).

Your teaching and support can influence how well parents cope with responsibility of a large family.

Multiple Births

Twins or other multiple births have considerable impact on family interaction. If ovulation has been inhibited with contraceptive pills, multiple births are more likely once this method stops being used. Multiple fetuses in utero create many problems for the parents in relation to health of mother and babies, financial strain, ethical decisions if certain embryos may not live, and family relationships. The needs and tasks of these parents will differ from the parents who have a single birth.

Often these parents lack emotional and financial support and sufficient help with child care and household tasks. Your suggestions and support can influence how well the parents cope with their responsibility.

Because multiple births are often premature, the first 4 or 5 months are very demanding on the parents in terms of the amount of energy and time spent in child care; this means that the parents have less energy and time for each other or other children. The mother should have help for several months if possible—from the husband, a relative, friend, or neighbor. Financial worries and concern about space and material needs may also intrude on normal husband–wife relationships or on relationships with other children.

Although books discourage the mother of twins from breastfeeding or using alternate breast- and bottlefeeding, the mother may be able to breastfeed both twins successfully by alternating breast- with bottlefeedings. The babies will not necessarily be poor breastfeeders with this arrangement.

You can suggest shortcuts in, or realities about, care that will not be detrimental to twin babies and that will give the parents more time to enjoy them. A diaper service, for example, is well worth the investment, for 1000 diapers may be used in a month's time. The parents should not be made to feel guilty if they are not as conscientious with two babies as they would be with

TABLE 4–4.   INFLUENCE OF ORDINAL POSITION ON CHILD

Firstborn Children

1. Are most likely to be wanted
2. Enjoy advantages until second child comes along
3. Are subject to greater parental expectations for achievement in school, work at home, and adult success
4. Begin to speak earlier in life
5. Demonstrate higher intellectual achievement
6. Are more achievement-oriented and responsible
7. Are more goal directed, plan better, and experience fewer frustrations
8. Identify more with parents than with peers
9. Are more dominant with siblings and peers
10. Have stronger superego or conscience, more self-discipline, and inner direction
11. Are more socially insecure
12. Engage in less risk-taking
13. Tend to have responsible leadership or high-level positions and be successful in adulthood

Middle Children

1. Are more difficult to characterize because of variety of positions in family
2. Receive less of the parents' time
3. Are praised less often
4. Are less stimulated toward achievement
5. Learn to compromise, handle conflict, and be adaptable because they are caught between jealousy of older sibling and envy of younger sibling
6. Develop sense of humor as adaptive mechanism
7. Learn double or triple roles and are prepared for more relationships in adulthood because of sibling coalitions
8. May succeed in role of mediator or negotiator in adulthood

Youngest Children

1. Benefit from parents' experience with childrearing
2. Tend to identify more with peer group than with parents
3. Are less tense, more affectionate, more good-natured, possibly to gain parental attention and sibling acceptance
4. Are popular with peers
5. Are more flexible in thinking
6. Have fewer expectations for household tasks or school achievement from parents
7. More dependent in relationships

Only Children

1. Resemble first-born children
2. Experience greater parental pressure for mature behavior and achievement
3. Learn to fill many roles because fewer family members have more demands
4. May be forced to assume roles prematurely without adequate preparation
5. Are more mature, cultivated, serious, and goal-oriented than peers who have siblings
6. Are more assertive, responsible, and independent
7. May be adept at various roles but lack self-confidence
8. Are usually intellectually superior, curious, creative with rich fantasy life, and academically successful
9. May feel lonely but able to entertain self and find satisfaction in personal pursuits because of parental demands
10. Demonstrate superiority in use of language
11. Do not usually share feelings and experiences with someone close
12. Learn less about coping with jealousy, envy, and sibling rivalries and sharing adult attention than peers with siblings
13. Learn less about intimate interactions with opposite or same-sex peers
14. Develop into a well-adjusted, capable adult rather than the stereotype of spoiled, selfish child

one. Each can be given a total bath every other day instead of daily. Heating bottles before feeding is not necessary. The parents should try to avoid getting so wrapped up in meeting the babies' physical needs that resentment, anger, or excessive fatigue creeps in. Multiple offspring should be fun as well as work.

Encourage the parents of twins (or multiple offspring) to perceive the babies as individuals and to consider the long-term consequences of giving them similar-sounding names, dressing them alike, having doubles of everything, and expecting them to behave alike. Tell parents about the U.S. national organization, Mothers of Twins, whose local branch can be a place to share feelings and ideas and gain practical suggestions. In the United Kingdom there is a Twins Clubs Association, a self-help organization with local chapters that provide educational and advocacy services.

Multiple-birth children usually are closer than ordinary siblings. These children have lived with each other from before birth on, so experiences are different from that of having various aged siblings. Parents often force one to be older and one to be younger in behavior; it is difficult for the one to play role of "older" because neither has the advantage of extra years of experience over the other, who is developmentally on the same level. With paternal twins, authority preference of parents tends to determine what age ranks the girl and the boy will be ascribed. In contrast, identical twins meet the world as a pair; it is difficult to imagine life without each other. It takes longer to separate in adolescence and adulthood (they may not, emotionally or physically). Each tends to seek multiple-birth persons as friends or mates.

They soon learn about the extra attention resulting from their birth status and may take advantage of the situation. Interaction between them is often complementary; for example, one twin may be dominant and the other submissive. Each learns from reinforcement of his or her experiences about the advantages of the particular role chosen. They learn to resist control by others and to manipulate others by acting alike and "in collusion." They do not have to manage conflicts with parents or others alone.

Siblings of a multiple birth usually are more detached from other siblings, even from parents, than each other. Twins may each receive less parental affection and communication because parents have less time to devote to each child. Thus twins are often slower to talk and many have a slower intellectual growth unless parents work to prevent it (79, 115). Yet the bond and sharing that occurs between twins or multiple-birth individuals can have positive effects on development as well. The sense of security and identity and the ability to share may be stronger, and these people have a unique empathy and ability to switch roles that enhances interpersonal relationships (5).

Sex of the Child

Sex also influences development within the family (75). In most cultures a higher value is placed on male than on female children. Actually, in some cultures only a boy's birth is welcomed or celebrated, and the family's status is partially measured by the number of sons. A family with several girls and no boys may perceive another baby girl as a disappointment. The girl may discover this attitude in later years from overhearing adult conversations, and she may try to compensate for her sex and gain parental affection and esteem by engaging in tomboy behavior and later assuming masculine roles.

If a boy arrives in a family that hoped for a girl, he may receive pressure to be feminine. He may even be dressed and socialized in a feminine manner. If the boy arrives after a family has two or three girls, he may receive much attention but also the jealousy of his sisters. Often he will grow up with three or four "mothering" figures (some may be unkind) and in a family more attuned to feminine than to masculine behavior. Developing a masculine identity may be more difficult for him, especially if there is no male nearby with whom to relate. In spite of being pampered, he may be expected by his family to be manly. The boy may feel envious of his sisters' position and their freedom from such expectations.

The girl who arrives in a family with a number of boys may also receive considerable attention, but she may have to become tomboyish to compete with her brothers and receive their esteem. Feminine identity may be difficult for her.

You can help parents understand how their attitude toward their own sexuality and their evaluation of boys and girls influence their relationship with their children. Emphasize the importance of encouraging the child's unique identity to develop.

Adopted Child

The adopted child may suffer some problems of the only child. In addition, the adopted child may have to work through feelings about rejection and abandonment by the biological parents versus being wanted and loved by the adoptive parents. The child should be told that he or she is adopted as early as the idea can be comprehended. Usually by the preschool years he or she can incorporate the idea of being a wanted child.

Adopted children bring their own genes, birth experiences, biological family ties, and often an extensive life history to their adoptive family. The adoptive family is not the same as a biological family. Both adoptive parents and adopted children tend to feel they have less control over their situation than other families. Adoptive parents and adopted children are both likely to have experienced a sense of loss. It is not unusual for the adoptive child to seek his or her own biological parents in late adolescence or young adulthood, especially if the child was old enough to remember both parents when adopted, even when the adoptive parents are truly considered the parents. This search may be a threat to adoptive parents, or they may feel secure enough to even assist the offspring in the search.

The adoptive parents' personal qualifications, their marital harmony, their love of the child, their acceptance of the child as is, and the child's having friends are major determinants of the child's adjustment and development. Factors not predictive of adjustment are socioeconomic status, occupational status, presence or absence of biological siblings, age of parents, health of adopters, religion, or prior experience with children (67, 78, 91, 112, 115).

Definition of "suitable" adoptive parents has been liberalized. Adoption agency requirements of age, marital status, race, and mother's employment status are more flexible. The adoptive parent may be a man. Additionally, today's couples consider adoption even if they have their own children. Some believe they have a responsibility and enough love to provide a home for an existing child rather than add to the total population. Others are single persons who want to offer love and security to a child.

Social and legal changes have affected the kinds of children in need of adoption. Earlier adoption agencies served mainly unmarried Caucasian mothers who saw adoption as the only alternative for their babies. Today fewer infants are available because there is greater social acceptance of out-of-wedlock births; more unmarried mothers keep their babies. Contraceptives and abortions have also reduced the number of unwanted infants. A different category of adoptable children has grown in size, however. These children with "special needs" have at least one of the following characteristics: age over 5; black; biracial; or physically, emotionally, or cognitively handicapped. Increasingly, state legislatures terminate parental rights in cases of children in long-term foster care who have remained unvisited and ignored by their biological parents and when the likelihood of the child's returning to his or her own home is minimal. New legislation has allowed abused children to become eligible for adoption (24–26, 36, 50, 67, 122).

Because of fewer available children in the United States, families are more likely to consider adopting a foreign child. Foreign adoption raises cultural, social, interracial, and emotional issues for the adoptive parents, their families and friends, and the specific community. Warren (122) discusses issues and concerns, qualifications, and the process. Additional information is available from International Concerns Committee for Children, 911 Cypress Drive, Boulder, CO 80303.

Despite more liberal definitions of adoptability, the number of people applying to adopt a child, homes approved, placements made, and adoptions completed declined compared with the number of available children. Thus an increasing number of older or disabled children need permanent placement.

You may have an opportunity to educate adults about the opportunity for adopting an older child with special needs or to work with adoptive parents, who also have needs.

Adoption of a child with special needs involves four phases: (1) commitment of adults and child, (2) honeymoon or placement period, (3) storm period, and (4) adaptation and adjustment. The phases do not abruptly begin and end; each phase builds on the preceding phase and sometimes reversals occur. The phases, along with thoughts, emotions, and activities accompanying each phase, are summarized in Table 4–5. The adoptive process can terminate at any point. If termination is necessary, both sides—the family and child—need help to understand what happened and to understand that *no one person* is responsible. Future adoption procedures are enhanced if proper guidance is given with the first failure (24–26).

Stresses to adoptive families include the following (24, 26, 50, 67, 70, 71, 120):

- The parents may worry about the child's heredity.
- The parents choose to be parents; hence they are highly motivated to give parenting and thus will invest considerable expense and time.
- The parents see themselves as a chosen group because someone thought they should be good parents; the chosen group idea leads to problems such as difficulty in setting limits, increased stress in parenting role, and oversensitivity to problems in the child.
- Infertile couples may have feelings of hostility or inferiority that are projected on the child; the child is a constant reminder of their inability to conceive.
- The adopted child or adolescent may project normal feelings of anger onto "adoptive" parents; parents may think normal developmental problems are a fact of adoption.

TABLE 4–5. ADOPTIVE PROCESS*

Phases	Thoughts and Emotions	Activities
Commitment of adults and children	*Adults* make general decision to adopt (stage 1), leading to decision to adopt specific child(ren) (stage 2).	*Adults* prepare for adoption through dialogue with helpful people and agencies and sometimes attend sessions on adoption given by adoption agency.
"Courting stage"	*Child* expresses desire for adoption (stage 1), leading to decision on specific family (stage 2).	*Child* is counseled for potential adjustment by adoption agency staff. Visits are arranged and made between potential family and child. All members involved (including existing children in family) get to know each other.
Placement	*Parents* are on an "emotional high"; excitement.	Household routines are altered to accommodate child. Limit-setting is minimal. Parent(s) meet child's whims.
"Honeymoon period" (child[ren] come to live with parent[s])	*Child(ren)* are excited but somewhat scared. "Can I trust these people?" "Will they send me away when I don't act my best?"	*Child* is put on best behavior. Sometimes parents show of affection for child is not accepted because of child's past negative parenting.
"Storm period"	*Parents* are tired of permanent house guest, feel anger, disappointment and guilt, and displace these feelings on each other and the child. They may wish the child would leave.	*Parents* treat child or other family members with decreasing tolerance for behavior not in family norm.
	Child can no longer keep up good behavior but wants to be loved and accepted.	*Child* may have tantrums, run away, or try to reject parents before they reject him or her.
	Parents may feel sense of failure. They may have expected too much of themselves and child and now may strike out at each other and other family members. Spouses may be jealous of time and energy mate gives to child.	If the outcome is positive, the *parents* will use problem solving, limit setting with flexibility, sense of humor, ongoing empathy and caring, supportive others, and community resources.
	Child may think, "They don't want me. What's going to happen to me?" and may live with anticipatory grief, fears of rejection, and insecurity, based on past hurts. Parents and child test each other.	
Adaptation and adjustment phase (equilibrium occurs)	*All* believe they can live and work together; mutual trust is growing; family feels fused as a unit and able to handle frustrations and crisis.	Parents are consistent with child. *Parents* and *child* can attend to outside interests without threatening family status.

*"Adults" and "child" are used in this table; however, only one adult may be adopting (single parent), and more than one child may be adopted.

- If one child is adopted and one is biological, favoritism, insufficient rewards to adoptive child, or competition between children may result.
- Sanctions and regards for role performance differ from those for biological parents (e.g., the company may not have maternity leave for adoptive parents; there is little emotional support for adoptive parents in society).
- Role autonomy is lacking. Adoptive parents need someone to agree that they will be good parents but need someone else to bear a child. These requirements inject dependence into a role considered independent, which may undermine parental confidence.
- Community or school attitudes may be negative; one's "own" child is spoken of as a biological child. The child encounters these attitudes of distinguishing between "real" and "adoptive," which undermines the sense of belonging and can drive a wedge between parents and child.

What was once viewed as a process that ended when the adoption decree was granted is now recognized as a condition that affects those involved throughout their lives. It is a permanent change in legal status. Adoption is a unique way of building families. These families are different from other families because of the circumstances that bring people to adoption and because of the way adoption continues to affect their lives (91, 99).

Adoptive parents, adoptive children, and adoptive family dynamics are different from birth parents, birth children, and birth family dynamics. Sometimes these differences generate problems within a family, and sometimes the adoption becomes the focus of other

► INTERVENTION GUIDELINES FOR THERAPY WITH ADOPTIVE FAMILIES

- Conventional treatment may not work well with adoptive families.
- Adoptive parents need validation as parents and of their decision to adopt.
- Adoptive parents must be included in therapeutic interventions to empower them further and to reinforce the adoptive commitment.
- In treating child-rooted problems, often the job will be to help parents modify their expectations.
- A child cannot successfully mourn the past and integrate it into the present circumstances if preoccupied with emotional survival. Developing a sense of safety and security is of paramount importance.
- Child-rooted barriers can come from unfinished emotional business, attachment disorders, or poor preparation for adoption.
- Adult-rooted barriers may stem from unfinished business, marital problems, or individual pathologies.
- Environmental barriers include lack of support or active disapproval from the extended family or the broader community.
- Any assessment is useful only if the assessed family accepts it as valid.
- In deciding to terminate an adoption that is not working, one must be committed to preserving the family's integrity, yet open to the removal of the child as a viable option.
- When an adoption is terminated, avoid judgment about reasons for its failure. Plans for adoption of another child should not be made until grief over the loss is resolved.

conflicts or unresolved family issues. Any time there are problems in an adoptive family, the significance of the adoption must be considered. Changes in the nature of adoptions have meant that more adoptive families have been seeking professional assistance and that professionals are having to consider the kinds of services the families may need and how to deliver them. Intervention Guidelines for Therapy with Adoptive Families are summarized above (20, 24, 26, 36, 50, 67, 70, 71).

Stepchild

The monograph *The Future of Children: Children and Divorce* presents the history and current status of divorce in the United States, the role of and effects on each parent, the effects on children, and their adjustment through the life span, and legal considerations such as custody. The lack of information on how divorce affects nonwhite children and their parents is a serious omission in the research literature.

About 26% of all children under 18 years of age (17 million) live with a separated or divorced parent, or a stepparent. In 1991, 39% of divorced women with children lived in poverty; 55% of those with children under 6 years of age were poor. Employment of mother may not be a sufficient buffer against economic deprivation (45).

There is great need to educate parents, family members, attorneys, and judges about the impact of divorce and conflict on children. Public assistance programs and ensuring support from the father are critical to reduce effects of poverty on divorced women who are awarded child custody.

Interparental conflict after divorce, with verbal and physical aggression, overt hostility, and distrust, and the primary parent's emotional distress create problematic parent–child relationships and greater emotional and behavioral maladjustment in the child. Boys are more likely to be affected with disturbed emotions and behavior from high-conflict divorce. Court-ordered joint physical custody and frequent visitation arrangements in high-conflict divorce are associated with poorer child outcomes, especially for girls. Intervention programs are essential for the parents and child(ren) (31).

The stepchild grieves and mourns the loss of a biological parent from death or divorce and must also deal with problems associated with integration into a new family unit. The stepchild may have conflicting feelings of loyalty to the natural parent and to the stepparent, thinking that acceptance of the stepparent is rejection of the natural parent. The stepchild may also feel rejected by his or her remarried natural parent, seeing the stepparent as a rival for the parent's attention. Further, when there are stepsiblings, jealousy, conflict, and hate may be dominant feelings in the offspring. More on the stepparent family follows in the next section.

FAMILY LIFESTYLES AND CHILDREARING PRACTICES

There is no single type of contemporary U.S. family, but the lifestyles of many correspond to the factors discussed in this section, including family structure, family cultural pattern, and the impact of the 20th century. These factors, in addition to those already discussed, influence family interaction and so an understanding of them will assist you in family care.

Family Structure

Childrearing and family relationships are influenced primarily by family structure. The biological and reproductive unit considered typical in the United States is the mother–father–child group. Traditionally, the parents were married, had established a residence of their own, were viewed (along with their children) as an integral social unit, and lived in an intimate, monogamous relationship. Emphasis in U.S. marriage is on pursuit of love in a romanticized way and on individual happiness rather than on family bonds as in many other cultures. Yet kinship ties are usually recognized on both sides of the family.

In many situations, however, a child may grow up in a family that differs from the typical one. Some cultures believe it takes a village (or a whole community) to raise a child. In some cultures or families, an aunt, uncle, or grandparent may be a continuing member of the household unit; one or the other parent may be absent because of death, divorce, illegitimacy, military service, or occupation involving travel. The children may not suffer long-lasting effects, yet most studies show children fare better emotionally, and usually physically and economically, in homes with both biological parents, regardless of parents' education, race, or social status (45).

The *single-parent family* is increasingly common. Although death and illegitimacy may cause the family to have only one parent, divorce of the natural parents is the more common reason. In most cases these families have undergone a major change in lifestyle. A parent may have died either suddenly or after a long illness. If the parents are divorced, the family may have experienced considerable disruption before the breakup. Sometimes the single-parent family is a planned event. A woman, lacking a suitable partner but wanting to be a mother, will choose to have a child by artificial insemination; or a single man or woman may choose to adopt a child. Regardless of the reason for the situation, these families often encounter considerable stress, including financial strain, sometimes even poverty.

Hanson investigated *characteristics of healthy single-parent families* in a purposive nonrandomized sample of 42 families with at least one child between the ages of 12 and 18 years. Results indicated differences in health of parents and children according to sex. Boys living with the mother had the best overall health; girls living with the father had the worst overall health. Children in general had higher overall health living with the mother. Children living with father had a lower physical health score, even though the single fathers had a significantly higher level of socioeconomic status. Single mothers had poorer overall health than single fathers. Health of parents and children, problem solving, social support, and socioeconomic status varied according to custody arrangement, with joint custody most beneficial for the mother. The variables most predictive of mental and physical health of single parents were social support and communication, whereas social support, com-

munication, and religiousness were most predictive for children (56).

A study was conducted by Ford-Gilboe to determine which variables would predict *choice of health promotion options in single-parent and two-parent families.* The convenience sample in a midsize city in southern Ontario consisted of 138 families (68 single-parent families, 70 two-parent families) with at least one preadolescent child. Subjects included the mother and one child closest to age 12. The majority of subjects were Caucasian, identifying with the Canadian culture, but from a variety of ethnic backgrounds. A package of questionnaires, consisting of a number of self-report instruments, was completed by the mothers and children. Mother's education was the only demographic variable significantly related to choice of health options. Family pride, family cohesion, mother's nontraditional sex role orientation, general self-reliance, network support, and community support were significantly related to choice of health options. Family cohesion and mothers' sex role orientation were the best predictors of choice of health options. Single-parent families and two-parent family types were similar on all demographic variables, but two-parent families were found to have more community support, higher income, and more resources (43).

In many healthy persons, *emotional attachment to a dead or divorced spouse* (or to the lost parent), with recurrent episodes of painful grief, *may remain many years.* Mourning in later life may be qualitatively different from that in earlier life; may be more prolonged and more difficult to complete; and may be related to less flexibility in aging, more rigid ego, and enormity of loss (spouse, identity, peer and family relations, sex companionship, style of living, routines and habits, economic security). The attachment for the spouse, lost through either divorce or death, which lasts for many years, may be unknown to even the closest friends or family of the survivor. Yet most mourners resolve their loss and become involved in life in new ways and with new people. The loss also offers an opportunity for personal development (67).

In the *single-parent family the children may experience grief for the absent parent,* guilt for their real or imagined part in the loss, shame for the change in their family structure, and fear about what changes the future may bring. Roles are changed. Each person may need to assume additional responsibilities and tasks. Parents may change their lifestyles. Mother may go to work or school, for instance; father may move into an apartment; or both parents may begin dating. An adolescent may serve as a parent substitute to younger siblings, or other children may assume new household tasks. The initial task of this family is to accept its family structure as a workable option for family living.

Children living in this household often exhibit more adaptability, responsibility, and maturity than their peers; however, the child who lives with the parent of the opposite sex may have more difficulty with adjustment to the divorce or death of the other parent or to the remarriage of the parent than if the child lived with the same-sex parent. Inappropriate social behavior, difficulty with identity formation, depression, and poorer school performance may be manifested by the child. If there always was only one parent, the child may have evolved behavior and roles appropriate to the partner, regardless of the child's sex. This may also create later developmental problems (90).

Often an open discussion of the changed lifestyle, along with support from relatives, friends, and other single-parent families, enhances the problem-solving abilities of these persons. Family members may need professional help if they exhibit symptoms of more extreme dysfunction, grieving, or prolonged "acting-out" behaviors. The family may also need information about various community resources; a major concern for single-parent families is financial strain or poverty, especially for the woman, because of wage inequities, difficulty with divorce settlements and child support, or lack of preparation financially in case of parental death (90).

The stepfamily is also common. Statistics vary, but a television newscast in mid-1995 reported 50% of first marriages, 60% of second marriages, and 80% of third marriages with children end in divorce. *The remarriage of a divorced or widowed parent with children may form a composite family unit known as the* **stepfamily.** These families may be formed in a variety of ways: a mother with children may remarry; a father whose children visit may remarry; either of the new parents may have an ex-spouse or children from a previous marriage (children and stepsiblings), and, to complicate this family even more, the remarried couple may decide to have children of its own. Inlaws and several sets of grandparents complete the picture. This family is now a far cry from the typical nuclear family, and the interaction becomes increasingly complex. Because remarriages are fragile, the adults may divorce from the second marriage as well, creating more loss and devastation. If a third marriage or unmarried partnership occurs, there are more layers of relatives, many of whom hardly contact or know each other and who may not like each other at all. An unanswered question is whether the current generation of stepchildren will care for stepparents or other steprelatives in old age.

When a couple marries for the second or third time and either or both have children from a previous marriage, the new husband and/or wife become instant stepparents. This addition of children to a couple's life differs from the situation of first-marriage couples, whose children are added at a slower pace. Additionally, the myth that familial love occurs via the marriage ceremony is common but it is a myth.

Adjustment to a new, unique family unit is the major task of the stepfamily. *Stepfamilies go through stages of development* (117):

- *Fantasy stage:* The adults dream that past wrongs of the previous marriage will be fixed and everything will be fine; everyone will be made whole in the new marriage.
- *Reality stage:* Dreams of a unified family are destroyed, and the transition is seen as much more conflictual than anticipated. Everyone involved has lost something.

New members cannot be assimilated within an existing family; instead a new family unit is formed. New rules, customs, and activities must be developed. Conflictual values and family ghosts must be resolved. Table 4–6 summarizes stepfamily characteristics and tasks (116, 117).

All members of this new family bring a history of life experiences, relationships, and expectations to the stepfamily. Conflict often occurs when the values and rules of individuals or the former single-parent family differ from those of the second (117).

Conflicts about raising stepchildren can be the most explosive issue in remarriages. The partners must

TABLE 4–6. COMPARISON OF STEPFAMILY CHARACTERISTICS AND TASKS

Stepfamily Characteristics	Stepfamily Tasks
Begins after many losses and changes	Dealing with losses and changes
Incongruent individual, marital, family life cycles and needs	Negotiating different developmental needs; synchronizing life cycles
Children and adults come with values and expectations from previous families	Establishing new traditions and different expectations; clarifying roles and values
Parent–child relationships predate the new couple	Developing a solid couple bond and forming new relationships
Biological parent elsewhere in actuality or in memory	Creating a "parenting coalition": the couple works on its union first
Children often members of two households	Accepting continual shifts in household composition: changing people, personal space, residence, responsibilities, roles
Legal relationship between stepparent and children is ambiguous or nonexistent	Risking involvement despite little societal support

Data from References 116 and 117.

realize they cannot be "superparents" and they will not receive instant love from the stepchildren. In fact, the child may never be affectionate toward the stepparent; the divided loyalty between the birth parent and stepparent may be unresolvable. The adult may not really feel affection for the stepchild either, despite wanting to. Time must be spent between adult and child: it takes time and shared activity to build a trusting, caring relationship. Parents or children should not expect too much too fast. The stepparent should avoid criticism of or competition with the birth parent; a new niche must be fashioned. The stepparent should reach out to the child even if rejection is present, be fair and honest in interactions, and create time and space that is designated for only the stepchild. Discipline problems are best handled at first by the birth parent; later regulations and rules can be applied by either partner. As most children are part of a single-parent home before they merge into a stepparent home, they are not likely to relinquish roles easily. Lastly, partners should focus on their marriage relationship and present an undivided front to the children (116, 117).

In time family members develop agreement about what is "right." Such agreement may include the "correct" church to attend, the "right" time for dinner, and how to celebrate birthdays. Open communication between members is essential to make decisions that are livable for all members.

In addition to adjusting in the family, stepfamilies must adjust to expectations of the outside world. Often differences in the reconstituted family are ignored because the family appears intact. Feelings of frustration, inadequacy, and isolation in family members stem from expectations that they feel as close to one another as blood relatives are expected to. The absent parent may still be an active influence in the original family. For instance, a divorced father may still contribute to his children's support and spend time with them on a regular basis, but they may be living with a stepfather. Even a deceased parent is remembered, not always accurately, and sometimes the stepparent is compared to the memory.

The child's ability to work through these feelings is influenced by age, sex, level of development, adaptive capabilities, and the understanding and support received from significant adults. He or she may need professional help to work through the difficulties of integration into a new family structure.

The stepfamily, like the single-parent family, needs to accept itself and be accepted as a combination of persons living together in a unique family unit. It is a potentially stressful situation that requires flexibility and adaptability of its members. This family offers many opportunities for growth and friendship through the differ-

ing experiences of its members; yet studies show that children in stepfamilies generally do not fare better than children in single-parent families (45).

In response to the growing number of these families, support groups such as the National Stepfamily Association operate to help them face their unique situations. Despite the old adage that children are flexible and can "bounce back," the trauma of divorce is second only to death. Often the problems that arise in the second marriage are more devastating than earlier ones. The children know that the original parent will not return and they are faced with a new parent whom they often initially neither want nor accept emotionally. Counseling groups have started in schools, courts, and private practice to help these children (7, 47).

Another type of family structure has been termed *apartners*. Instead of getting married, a couple, who may have children by a previous marriage, choose to maintain separate residences, take care of their own children, professional life, and everyday affairs but share special times with each other on a regularly scheduled basis. Personal time and freedom, coupled with intimacy, are what the participants say they seek. Gay or lesbian couples may also have this arrangement, often because of social constraints rather than choice.

The single state (*never married, separated, divorced, widowed*) is another family structure. Today in the United States more individuals have chosen singlehood than in the past. Some would apply family developmental tasks to this person; however, it is no longer considered necessary to marry and bear children to be fulfilled and accomplished. The single state can promote development of creativity, object ties, and healthy narcissism through the following (9, 67, 115):

- *Privacy:* Being able to think and create in a peaceful atmosphere without interruption
- *Time:* Being able to travel, cultivate talents and interests, entertain and be entertained, and follow intellectual pursuits
- *Freedom:* Being able to choose and make decisions, form friendships, use time as desired, depend on self, have a healthy narcissism
- *Opportunity:* Being able to extend borders of friendship, develop skills and knowledge, enjoy geographic moves or job mobility and success (The single person is often preferred for certain jobs or positions.)

Yet singlehood is not always happy for the never-married, separated, widowed, or divorced individual. It can be lonely. There can be too much unoccupied time and resulting depression. There can be too much space and freedom and the inability to make decisions. The silence of the home when entering from a day's work may be overwhelming. Talking and sharing both the joys and stresses and the daily routine events may be needed, but there is no one who really wants to be contacted or who responds other than in his or her own narcissistic way. There may be financial concerns or unwise use of money because of prior lack of opportunity with financial affairs. Others may expect the single person always to be available to help because he or she "has no family or obligations," but the single person may have difficulty receiving help in return or even asking for it. It is as if society expects the single person to manage everything alone. The person is a nonentity until someone needs something, and the single person is seen as available. In like manner, the single person may be taken advantage of by home repairmen, by businesses, by acquaintances who pose as lovers, or by someone seeking an object interaction sexually. There may be places the single person cannot go because of cultural restrictions. We have a couple–oriented society. Special holidays and anniversary dates can be especially painful. The person may be alone and forgotten by friends who are busy with their families; or even in a crowd of merrymakers, and in spite of a smiling face, the person may feel isolated and alone (115).

Your acceptance, support, validation, and teaching are crucial in promoting health in the single person.

Stepgeneration parents constitute a different kind of family *when the mother will not, does not, cannot, or should not care for her offspring.* More than a million children live in households (sometimes five-generation) that are headed by one or both grandparents or great-grandparents. Circumstances that lead the grandparent generations to provide care for the grandchildren transcend race and economic level and reflect a number of factors that create instability in family life. The elder generation may provide a home to both grandchildren or great-grandchildren and their parent(s) if the parental generation (1) is unemployed; (2) if there has been separation, divorce, or death of one of the parents; (3) if one or both parents are physically or mentally ill; (4) if one or both parents are abusing or addicted to alcohol or drugs; (5) if physical, emotional, or sexual abuse of the child has occurred; or (6) if one or both parents are imprisoned. How well the situation works depends on the degree of respect and love shown and communication; how clearly rules are set and enforced in the home; who takes responsibility for child care and home maintenance tasks; and legal and financial problems for the family unit. In a stable home, all generations can benefit from each other and learn to appreciate each other. In a home with conflict, each person may carry scars. Some conflicts will be inevitable as the children and grandparent generations each grow older and have different needs. Yet, the grandparents can

▶ **NATIONAL ORGANIZATIONS FOR GRANDPARENT CAREGIVERS**

ROCKING: Raising Our Children's Kids: An Intergenerational Network of Grandparents

- Gives information on raising children.
- Links custodial grandparents with support groups.
- *Address:* Rocking, Inc., PO Box 96, Niles, MI 49120

Grandparents United for Children's Rights

- Addresses needs of custodial grandparents.
- *Address:* 137 Larkin St, Madison, WI 53705
- Telephone: (608) 238–8751

National Coalition of Grandparents

- Fosters legislation concerning custody and visitation.
- *Address:* 137 Larkin St, Madison, WI 53705

Grandparent Information Center

- Provides guidance in surrogate-parenting issues.
- Refers grandparents to local organizations that can help.
- *Address:* AARP Grandparent Information Center, 601 E St., NW, Washington, DC 20049

have real peace of mind as they realize their contribution to the young ones, which offsets the sense of burden that comes with the tasks of young child care. Several national organizations offer assistance to grandparent caregivers; they are listed in the National Organizations for Grandparent Caregivers (4, 28, 66, 107). The real concern is that the grandparent(s) may become ill or die before the child is reared. Most grandparents realize that the physical and emotional care and moral and spiritual guidance they give may prevent the grandchild from repeating the pattern the child was born into.

Family Size

Family size is related to distinctive patterns of family life and child development. Most children in the United States are members of a small family system, that is, one with three children or less. Some couples are choosing to have no children to pursue their own careers or professions or leisure interests, which become sublimation for children. Others make this choice because they believe the current world situation is not one into which to bring children.

The *small family system* has the following features: (1) emphasis is on planning (the number and the frequency of births, the objectives of childrearing, and educational possibilities); (2) parenthood is intensive rather than extensive (great concern is evidenced from pregnancy through every phase of childrearing for each child); (3) group actions are usually more democratic; and (4) greater freedom is allowed individual members. The child or children in the small family usually enjoy advantages beyond those available to children in large families of corresponding economic and social level, including more individual attention. On the other hand, these children may retain emotional dependence on their parents, grow up with extreme pressure for performance, and retain an exaggerated notion of self-importance.

The *large family,* generally thought of as one with six or more children, is not a planned family as a rule. Parenthood is commonly extensive rather than intensive, not because of less love or concern but simply because parents must divide their attention more ways. In the very large family emphasis is on the group rather than on the individual member. Conformity and cooperation are valued above self-expression. Discipline in the form of numerous and stringent rules frequently is stressed, and there is a high degree of organization in the activities of daily living (115). If parents lack initiative and use their resources unwisely, disorganization may exist. For additional information see the section on The Family with a Large Number of Children, p. 158.

Family Cultural Pattern

The ways of living and thinking that constitute the intimate aspects of family group life constitute the **family cultural pattern** (102). The family transmits the cultural pattern of its own ethnic background and class to the child, together with the parents' attitudes toward other classes.

Within the national cultural pattern of the United States, significant variations have been found in family cultural patterns and social systems (18). In Millstadt, Illinois, for instance, the German farm family provides a distinctive social system, with cultural features distinct from its Italian neighbors across the river in St. Louis. The Maine Yankee and the North Carolina rebel may speak the same language, but the meanings of the words used may be quite different because of regional variables. Thus, how families rear their children depends on ethnic group and class, region, nation, and historical period.

Influence of 20th-Century Changes

Shift From an Agrarian to a Complex Technologic Society. This shift has produced dramatic changes for the U.S. family. A greater percentage of children now survive childhood than in 1900, and a higher percentage of mothers survive childbirth. Some marriages occur at an earlier age. Some women marry during or after completing high school, and before completing college or becoming established in a career or profession, despite the trend for women to reject traditional roles. Some describe the negative reactions of young adult and middle-aged women, including the mother, toward the woman's decision to simultaneously pursue marriage and career plans during the last semester of college or before becoming employed. These young adults believe they can manage both; typically the husband-to-be encourages the young woman to be as committed to her profession as she is to him. Some women marry at a later age than in former generations. Fewer children are born to most parents, they are spaced closer together, and more first children are born to parents in their late thirties or early forties. There is an increasing number of women who are single mothers by choice, whether they are teenagers or in their late thirties or early forties. Middle-aged couples now typically have more years together after their children are grown and leave home. Because of an increased life expectancy, families now have more living relatives than formerly, especially elderly relatives, for whom the family may have responsibility.

Other Trends Related to Living in a Complex Industrial Society. Families live primarily in urban or metropolitan areas; more families than ever are homeless or at risk for homelessness. More women work outside the home. The U.S. woman who formerly stayed home and was the "homemaker" has also gone through several changes. Once homemaking took a good deal of time. Now modern conveniences make tasks easier. The woman who stays home today concentrates more on "mothering." Her outside activities may include volunteer work so she can control her hours and feel she has prime time at home yet is contributing outside the family unit. Or the father may be the house parent because he has an office in the home or is the unemployed member who thereby assumes child and home care responsibilities. Family members are becoming better educated. Family incomes may be unstable; acquisition of personal housing and equipment sought early in the marriage is not always possible. Greater individual freedom exists. Sexual mores are changing, with trial and serial marriages. Value changes and different patterns of living apparently are the norm.

The emphasis on the family-kinship group has been replaced by acceptance of the nuclear or other types of family. Because Americans are so mobile and are increasingly living in smaller homes or apartments, or in townhouses or condominiums, many ties with kin other than the immediate family are loosened or at least geographically extended. Sometimes close friends become "the family." Yet many Americans strengthen kinship ties through letters, telephone calls, and holiday and vacation visits. Religious influences affect family ties. For example, Jews or European Catholics, with their many family traditions, are generally more embedded in a network of relatives than are white Protestants. The four- and five-generation family and great-grandparent–great-grandchild (as well as grandparent–grandchild) relationships are gaining the attention of researchers.

Yet there are other trends to counter the technology, anonymity, the sense of being treated as an object and impersonally, and societal and family violence. There is a growing body of knowledge available to parents and to family members, for almost any type of situation. There are more parenting classes. There is more emphasis on need for tenderness and warmth in relationships and the importance of meeting psychosocial rather than materialistic needs. Promoting the maximum potential of each family member and preventing or breaking the cycle of family abuse and violence are of great concern. Health promotion rather than illness treatment is considered important socially as well as economically (106).

Rapid Change. Rapid change is a fact that families must acknowledge. Medical, pharmacologic, and scientific advances in birth technology and all areas of health, the increased number of single-parent families, the growing emphasis on the civil and economic rights of minority groups, and the women's liberation movement are only a part of the cultural expansion of this century. As people live longer, more older people will divorce, remarry, or cohabitate. Those who lack healthy emotional roots within their nuclear families, who have few or no kinship ties, who cannot adjust to rapid change, and who have little identity except as defined by job and income are more likely to become depressed, alcoholic, unfaith-

ful to mate, or divorced (9, 51, 67, 78, 115). Today's changing social environment makes it increasingly difficult for a parent to be certain of his or her identity. How, then, is he or she to provide emotional roots for the child?

U.S. Childrearing Practices. There is no one traditional national pattern, only the general concern that children develop "normally." Parents are encouraged through culture, education, and the mass media to use whatever the dominant childrearing theory is at the time. With each new wave of "knowledge," and through media influence, parents are bombarded by conflicting reports. Often the change in theory application occurs during the same parental generation so that parents do not trust their own judgment, and considerable inconsistency results. The inconsistency, rather than the theory, probably creates the main problems in childrearing. Sometimes parents strive to avoid rearing their children as they were reared but nevertheless do so unwittingly because of the permanency of enculturation. Children are often given approval and disapproval for their behavior and told they are "good" or "bad." This practice, along with inconsistency and other factors, contributes to competition and sibling rivalry. Research continues to show that children who experience consistent love, attention, and security will grow up to be adults who can better survive change and stressors, with self-reliance, optimism, and identity intact (106).

Father's Role. The father's role is being reconsidered, and he is more active in child care (73, 75, 115). Still, the mother is primarily responsible for the crying baby and young child care. The infant is often trained in privacy, individualism, and independence by childrearing practices. Fear of "spoiling" the infant if he or she is held too much or responded to spontaneously still exists. Thus the infant may develop behavioral extremes to get needs met.

When the children are old enough to be out of the home, parents often strive to do things for their children and center their activities around their children's activities. Work responsibilities are not necessarily demanded, but there is subtle pressure for the children to repay by pleasing the parents through use of talents, organizational achievements, or honors won. Because of the small size of the nuclear family, the school-age child or adolescent may spend more time with peers than with family members. Because of the youth idealization of our culture, seniority does not invoke special respect for the older person (parent). The childrearing parent must offer more than age if he or she wants to maintain control.

Day-care centers or babysitters who are usually not relatives continue to be important in child care. What happens if the mother and parent-surrogate differ greatly about childrearing practices? The child generally acknowledges the authority of parents or at least the mother, but parent-surrogates affect him or her nevertheless. Any adult who is with the child reinforces behavior in the child that conforms to the adult's own standard of behavior. The child conforms to the adult's desires to gain approval. If the parent-surrogate acts in a way contrary to the values of the parents, both parents and child probably will be distressed.

Renewed Focus on the Family

The United Nations proclaimed 1994 as the International Year of the Family. Certainly the health of a nation, and the world, depends on the health of the family.

The American family has changed. After World War II, 80% of children grew up in homes with two biological parents who were married to each other. In 1980, this figure had fallen to 50%, and the percentage has fallen even further. Today, 30% of all U.S. births are to single mothers, despite more than 1.6 million abortions annually. Families dissolve at a greater rate in the United States than in any other major industrialized country, and the United States leads the world in father absence from the home and in the abortion rate (45).

The poverty rate for children in single-parent homes is more than 10 times that for children in two-parent homes. Unilateral, no-fault divorce means the spouse who wants out holds all the rights; divorce plunges many women and their children into poverty or near poverty. Children are left with less time and less moral guidance from parents than ever before.

The American family is at a crossroads, undergoing enormous change and fracturing. With 72% of American adults recognizing that family life is decaying, there is renewed emphasis on making changes. There is more talk about family values. The key is for families to make sacrifices in their economic lifestyle to make time for each other and their children. Business can promote family values by providing opportunities for flex-time and using the home as the workplace, when it is feasible, and by providing paternity as well as maternity leave, the father who is at home 1 or 2 weeks with the new mother and baby provides necessary nurturing and help to mother with child-care and household tasks. There must be more media and cultural emphasis on the value that real freedom comes from fulfilling duties to the spouse and our children, rather than from pursuing personal pleasures (8).

Family Life Around the World

In *Canada,* a huge but sparsely populated country, one finds a cultural mosaic of different national and cultural groups. Thus, family life differs across the country. The far-eastern provinces are more conservative and have lower divorce and abortion rates than the western provinces; however, young people in Quebec, even though it is heavily Catholic, have the highest rate of premarital sex, cohabitation before marriage, and lowest birth rate in the nation because of abortion. Farm families in Alberta, Manitoba, and Saskatchewan have more children than do families in urban areas such as Calgary, Edmonton, and Toronto. Typically, both parents work (the tax rate is high in Canada to fund the health and social programs), but the emphasis is on activities with the children. Because of the influence of mass media and travel and decline in church attendance in Canada, Canadian and U.S. families appear to becoming more alike (54).

In the past 20 years, *Britain's* families have struggled with rising divorce, remarriage, lone parenting, mobility, and increasing cohabitation. Often both parents work. In some areas state education begins at age 4, but older family members or private institutional care is typically used for young children of working parents. Even afternoon tea, designed for family time, is gradually disappearing. Marriage seminars and literature and films supporting family life are popular as young families work to commit themselves to each other and their children (16).

In the multicultural society of *Australia,* marriages and children are valued, although families are experiencing an increasing divorce rate. The impact of divorce is seen in schoolchildren adjusting to visitation rights as well as in participation in church and social life. Teens are becoming more unsettled in behavior and more Western in appearance. The church has dropped some of the strong moral stands it took in the 1950s and 1960s; religious education in schools has had to fight for existence. Home schooling, typical in the Outback, is increasing in urban areas. Conflicts between generations over the old and new ways are common. Family life in urban areas differs considerably from family life in sparsely settled rural areas, on the huge ranches in the Outback, or for the Aborigines. Yet amidst the harshness of the sunburnt country is seen a gentleness in families (101).

In *Latin America,* from Mexico to the tip of Chile, a common family characteristic is that the mother is the core. Yet, family life is changing drastically in some countries. For example, in Mexico, there are daily about 4000 requests for divorce; 40% of children live with divorced parents; 25% are raised by single mothers. During the past 15 years there has been an increasing rate of murder, abortions, suicide, and addicted and runaway youths. There is renewed effort by the government, churches, and educational institutions to make family life an emphasis (13).

In *Costa Rica,* a small, democratic Central American country, the economy flourishes, and it offers some of the best health care and educational possibilities in Latin America. Religion is important. The typical Costa Rican family is composed of five to seven members, often including grandparents or other relatives. The father has traditionally been the sole breadwinner while mother stayed home to care for the children. Urbanization and industrialization, however, are changing the concept of family; there is less emphasis on family relations and more emphasis on employment, even for mothers. Many social problems seen in the United States, only 3 hours flying time away, are now seen in Costa Rica. There is a new concern about social and family issues and solutions (92).

In *Italy, Germany,* and *France,* family life is valued. A meal is cooked, not popped in the microwave. The family sits around the dinner table and converses. Young families with children stroll through the park on Sunday afternoon. Attitudes toward childrearing differ from those in the United States. Parents motivate children by fear and humiliation, in contrast to encouragement, which is commonly used in the United States. As a result, young people are more likely to feel insecure and hostile, which can spill over to how they relate in the family and with children. In Western Europe, there is greater emphasis on cohabitation before marriage, more open display of nudity, and declining church attendance. Thus, we see a combination of old customs and new morality, which will in turn influence family development (109).

In *Russia,* the family is considered the primary unit of society, just as in other countries. Under Communism, other maxims of official propaganda diminished the emphasis on family. Crime rates and unemployment soar; wages are below living minimum. The birth rate is falling as the abortion rate escalates. Often young families live in small apartments with the parents because of the housing shortage. Both parents work because of economic necessity; older members help with child care. Biblical principles have always been present, even under Communism. There are rapid and great social changes now. With the fall of Communism, parents are demonstrating renewed interest in the now available religious books and television programs to help them continue to teach moral principles (17).

Africa is made up of many countries, cultures, and lifestyles. Traditional culture is family oriented; the extended family has undergirded tribal society for centuries. In urban areas of South Africa, husbands commute to work, and the materialism and lack of family time seen in Western societies are evident. In the black townships of South Africa, the legacy of apartheid has split families for generations. Children live with grandparents while parents work the mines in far-off locales. Husbands live in single-sex hostels with minimal facilities. New relationships may be started; families are destroyed. Progress, materialism, high population growth, and the influence of Western culture have precipitated a massive influx of families from the country to the city; three generations are crowded into small living quarters. Because of employment and school conditions, parents and children may see little of each other. In some countries, drought, famine, migrations, and war have disrupted all life patterns and caused massive numbers of death, leaving no trace of a family and countless orphaned children or single survivors in a family. Whether families are black, white, or socially mixed, the turbulent political and social issues will continue to dominate and affect family life negatively (110).

In *Japan,* Westernization has taken its toll. An overly efficient, stressful work environment and focus on economic success have taken their toll. Fathers may work in a remote location with no opportunity for family life for months at a time. Both husbands and wives are tempted to be unfaithful. Fathers die suddenly in their forties from overwork (*Karoshi*). There is renewed emphasis on the family unit with construction of larger dwelling units so that extended families can live together with less crowding. Employers are beginning to refocus on the value of family and the importance of a male role model in the home for children (64).

► HEALTH CARE AND NURSING APPLICATIONS

The family as the basic unit for the developing person and health cannot be taken for granted. Although family forms have changed and will continue to change, each person, to develop healthfully, needs some intimate surroundings of human concern. "No man is an island."

You will frequently encounter the entire family as your client in the health care system, regardless of the setting. You may be asked to do family-centered care, to nurse the client and the family or to do "family therapy." Yet you will not be able to care for the family even minimally unless you understand the family system and the dynamics of family living presented in this chapter.

Rapid change, increasing demands on the person, technologic progress, and other trends mentioned seem to isolate people. Many families are not aware of the forces pulling them apart. More than ever, they need one place in their living where they can act without self-consciousness, where the pretenses and roles demanded in jobs, school, or social situations can be put aside. The living center should be a place where communication takes place with ease; where each knows what to expect from the other; where a cohesiveness exists that is based on nonverbal messages more than verbal; and where a person is accepted for what he or she is. The family may need your help in becoming aware of disruptive forces, of their maladaptive patterns, and of ways to promote an accepting home atmosphere.

Communication and Relationship Principles Basic to Client Care

Communication is the heart of the nursing process and health care, for it is one of the primary methods used to accomplish specific and general goals with many different kinds of people. It is used in assessing and understanding the client and family and in intervention. Communication helps people express thoughts and feelings, clarify problems, receive information, consider alternate ways of coping or adapting, and remain realistic through feedback from the environment. Essentially the client learns something about the self, how to identify health needs, and if and how he or she wishes to meet them.

Analysis of your communication pattern will help you improve your methods. Realize that you cannot become skilled in therapeutic communication without supervised and thoughtful practice. As you talk with another, however, do not get so busy thinking about a list of methods that you forget to focus on the person. Your keen interest in the other person and use of your personal style are essential if you are to be truly effective. To be effective while communicating with the person or family, use simple, clear words geared to the person's intelligence and experience. Develop a well-modulated tone of voice. Be attuned to your nonverbal behavior. *Methods basic for conducting purposeful, helpful communication* with a client/family along with their rationale are listed in Table 4–7. These communication methods are used in the interview during assessment, goal setting, and intervention with a family or individual client,

TABLE 4–7. EFFECTIVE COMMUNICATION METHODS AND THEIR RATIONALE

Communication Method	Rationale
Be accepting in nonverbal and verbal behavior. (does not mean agreement with person's words or behavior)	All behavior is motivated and purposeful. Promotes climate in which person feels safe and respected. Indicates that you are following the person's trend of thought and encourages further talking while you remain nonjudgmental.
Use thoughtful silence at intervals, while continuing to look at and focus on person.	Indicates accessibility to mute, withdrawn, or depressed person. Encourages person to talk and set own pace. Gives both you and client time to organize thoughts. Aids consideration of alternate courses of action; provides opportunity for explanation of feelings; gives time for contemplation. Conserves energy and promotes relaxation in physically ill person.
Use "I" and "We" in proper context; **call person by name and title, as preferred.**	Strengthens identity of person in relation to others.
State **open-ended, general, leading statements or questions;** "Tell me about it." "What are you feeling?"	Encourages person to take the initiative in introducing topics and to think through problems. May gain pertinent information that you would not think to ask about because client has freedom to pursue feelings and ideas important to him/her.
Ask **related or peripheral questions** when indicated: "And what else happened?" "You have four children. What are their ages?"	Explores or clarifies pertinent topic. Adds to database. Encourages person to work through larger or related issues and to engage in problem solving. Explores subject in depth without appearing to pry. Helps person see implications, relationships, or consequences. Helps keep communication flowing and person talking.
Encourage description of feelings: "Tell what you feel."	Helps person identify, face, and resolve own feelings. Validates your observation. Deepens your empathy and insight.
Place described events in time sequence: "What happened then?" "What did you do after that?" "And then what?"	Clarifies how event occurred or explains relationships associated with given event. Places event in context or manageable perspective. Helps identify recurrent patterns or difficulties or significant cause–effect relationships.

(continued)

TABLE 4–7. EFFECTIVE COMMUNICATION METHODS AND THEIR RATIONALE (continued)

Communication Method	Rationale
State your observations about the person: "You appear . . . ," " "I sense that you . . . , " "I notice that you . . . . "	Acknowledges client's feelings, needs, behavior, or efforts at a task. Offers content to which person can respond. Encourages comparisons or mutual understanding of client's behavior. Validates your impressions. Helps person notice own behavior and its effects; encourages self-awareness. Reinforces behavior. Adds to person's self-esteem.
State the implied, what client has hinted, or a feeling that you sense may be a consequence of an event.	Expresses acceptability of feeling or idea. Clarifies information. Conveys your attention, interest, and empathy. May be used as subtle form of suggestion for action.
Paraphrase; translate into your own words the feelings, questions, ideas, key words of other person: "I hear you saying . . . , " "You feel . . . . "	Indicates careful listening and focus on client. Encourages further talking. Validates and summarizes what you think client has said. Conveys empathy and understanding. Indicates that person's words, ideas, feelings, opinions, or decisions are important. Promotes integration of feelings with content being discussed.
Restate or repeat main idea expressed by client.	Conveys interest and careful listening or desire to clarify a vague point. Helps to reformulate certain statements or to emphasize key words to help client recognize less obvious meanings or associations.
Clarify: "Could you explain that further?" "Explain that to me again."	Indicates interest and desire to understand. Helps the person become clearer to him- or herself. Encourages exploration of subject in depth or of meaning behind what is being said.
Make reflective statement, integrating feelings and content.	Indicates active listening and empathy. Synthesizes your perceptions and provides feedback to client. Shares your perception of congruity between person's statements and other behavior. Provides client with new ways of considering ideas, behavior, or a situation. Identifies and encourages understanding of latent meanings.
Suggest collaboration and a cooperative relationship.	Offers to do activities **with, not for or to** person. Encourages person to participate in identifying and appraising problems. Involves person as active partner in care. Tells person you are available and interested. Provides reassurance.
Offer information; self-disclose by sharing own thoughts and feelings briefly, if appropriate.	Makes facts available whenever client needs or asks for them. Builds trust; orients; enables decision making. Reduces client's anxiety, frustration, or other distressing feelings that hinder comfort, recovery, or realistic action. Helps client focus on deeper concerns.
Encourage evaluation of situation.	Helps client appraise quality of his or her experience and consider people and events in relation to own and others' experience and values. Assists person in determining how others affect him or her, and personal effect on others. Promotes understanding of own situation and avoidance of uncritically adopting opinions, values, or behavior of others.
Encourage formulation of plan of action.	Conveys that person is expected to be active participant in own care. Helps person consider alternate courses of action. Helps person plan how to handle future problems.
Voice doubt; present own perceptions or facts; **suggest alternate line of reasoning:** "What gives you that impression?" "Isn't that unusual?" "I find that hard to believe." Respond to underlying feeling.	Promotes realistic thinking. Helps person consider that others do not perceive events as he does nor draw the same conclusions. May reinforce doubts person already has about an idea or course of action. Avoids argument. May help to gradually reduce delusion. Conveys acceptance that delusion is the client's reality; acknowledges the communication.
Seek consensual validation of words; give definition or meaning when indicated.	Ensures that words being used mean the same to both you and client. Clarifies ideas for you and client as client defines meaning for self. Avoids misunderstanding. May help to gradually reduce autistic thinking.
Summarize; condense what speaker said, using speaker's own words.	Synthesizes and emphasizes important points of dialogue. Helps both you and client leave session with same ideas in mind. Emphasizes progress made toward self-awareness, problem solving, and personal development. Provides sense of closure.

Source: Ref # 81.

well or ill, in any setting. Table 4–8 lists *guidelines for an effective interview*. Table 4–9 lists *barriers to effective communication* and interviewing (81, 85–87, 113, 114).

The quality of any response depends on the degree of mutual trust in the relationship. Techniques can be highly successful, or they can misfire or be abused, depending on how they are used, on your attitude at the time, and on the other person's interpretation. Techniques are steppingstones to better understanding, an understanding that nurtures the trust, relationship, and expression of feeling. There must be a feeling of caring, or safety and security in your company, and a feeling that you want to help the person help himself or herself. The more important or highly personal a feeling or idea is, the more difficult it is to say. The situation causes hesitancy in revealing thoughts, feelings, or intimate needs. By using therapeutic principles you will help the person and family identify you as someone to whom ideas and feelings can be safely and productively revealed.

You may find the following *guidelines helpful in evaluating your communication methods.* Do you

- Examine the purpose of your communications?
- Consider the total physical and human setting?
- Plan your communication, clarifying ideas and seeking consultation?
- Analyze the methods used and their effectiveness?
- Identify hidden meanings as well as basic content of message you conveyed?
- Support communication with actions?
- Follow up communication to determine if purpose was accomplished?

The **therapeutic or helping relationship/alliance,** or therapeutic nurse–client relationship, is a *purposeful interaction over time between an authority in*

TABLE 4–8. GUIDELINES FOR AN EFFECTIVE INTERVIEW

Method	Rationale
1. **Wear clothing that conveys the image of a professional and is appropriate for the situation.** Consider wearing casual clothing without excessive adornment instead of a uniform when working in the school, home, occupational setting, or community clinic.	1. Consider expectations the interviewee may have of you. In some cases he/she will respond more readily to your casual dress; at other times the person may need your professional dress as part of the image to help him or her talk confidentially.
2. **Avoid preconceived ideas, prejudices, or biases.** Avoid imposing personal values on others.	2. Acceptance of client promotes feeling of self-respect and security and promotes more accurate assessment.
3. **Control the external environment** as much as possible. This is sometimes difficult or impossible to do, but try to minimize external distractions or noise, regulate ventilation and lighting, and arrange the setting.	3. Minimize discomfort, external distractions, and sense of distance. Comfort factors show respect to client and promote expression of feelings.
4. **Arrange comfortable positions** for yourself and the client.	4. Full attention can be given to the interview.
5. **Establish rapport.** Create a warm, accepting climate and a feeling of security and confidentiality.	5. The person feels free to talk about what is important to her or him.
6. **Use a vocabulary on the level of awareness or understanding of the person.** Avoid professional jargon or abstract words. **Be precise in what you say.**	6. Convey respect for and respond to the interviewee's level of understanding or health condition. Convey that you want client to understand the meaning of what you say and that you consider the client as part of the health care team.
7. **Begin by stating and validating with the client the purpose of the interview.** Either you or the interviewee may introduce the theme. You may start the session by briefly expressing friendly interest in the everyday affairs of the person, but avoid continuing trivial conversation. Maintain the proposed structure.	7. The client realizes the importance of the interview, that she or he is taken seriously and will be listened to. Client does not confuse interview with social event.
8. **Say as little as possible to keep the interview moving.** Ask questions that are well-timed, open-ended, and pertinent to the situation.	8. This pattern allows the person to place his or her own style, organization, and personality on the answers and on the interview. Getting unanticipated data can be useful in assessment. Questions that bombard the person produce unreliable information. Open-ended sentences usually keep the person talking at her or his own pace. Careful timing of your messages, verbal and nonverbal, allows time for the interviewee to understand and respond and increase accuracy and meaning of response.

(continued)

TABLE 4–8. GUIDELINES FOR AN EFFECTIVE INTERVIEW (continued)

Method	Rationale
9. **Avoid asking questions in ways that elicit socially acceptable answers.**	9. The interviewee often responds to questions with what he or she thinks the interviewer wants to hear, either to be well thought of, to gain status, or to show that she or he knows what other people do and what is considered socially acceptable.
10. **Ask questions beginning with "What . . . ?" "Who . . . ?" and "When . . . ?" to gain factual information.**	10. Words connoting moral judgments are not conducive to a feeling of neutrality, acceptance, or freedom of expression. The "How" question may be difficult for the person to answer because it asks, "In what manner . . . ?" or "For what reason . . . ?" and the individual may lack sufficient knowledge to answer. The "Why" question asks for insights that the person should not be expected to give.
11. **Be gentle and tactful when asking about home life or personal matters.** If a subject meets resistance, change the topic; when the anxiety is reduced, return to the matter for further discussion. Be alert to what the person omits or avoids, "forgets" to mention, or deliberately refuses to discuss.	11. What you consider common or usual information may be considered very private by some. Matters about which it would be tactless to inquire directly can often be arrived at indirectly by peripheral questions. Remember, what the person does not say is as important as what is said.
12. **Be an attentive listener.** Show interest by nodding, responding with, "I see," etc. Remain silent and control your responses when another's comments evoke a personal meaning and thus trigger an emotional response in you. While the person is talking, find the nonverbal answers to the following: What does this experience mean? Why is this content being told at this time? What is the meaning of the choice of words, the repetition of key words, the inflection of voice, the hesitant or aggressive expression of words, the topic chosen? Listen for feelings, needs, and goals. Listen for what is not discussed. Do not answer too fast or ask a question too soon. If necessary, learn if the words mean the same to you as to the interviewee. Explore each clue as you let the person tell his/her story.	12. Careful listening conveys respect, promotes self-esteem and a sense of security and safety, and aids assessment. It is an important intervention tool.
13. **Carefully observe nonverbal messages for signs of anxiety, frustration, anger, loneliness, or guilt.** Look for feelings of pressure hidden by the person's attempts to be calm. Encourage the free expression of feelings, for feelings often bring facts with them. Focus on emotionally charged topics when the person is able to share deep feelings.	13. Nonverbal behavior is often the key to the message and is usually not under the client's voluntary control or in his or her awareness. Nonverbal behavior often conveys more directly the feelings. Ventilation of feeling is the key resolution of many emotional difficulties and opens the door to new data as well as increased understanding and insight in the client.
14. **Encourage spontaneity.** Provide movement in the interview by picking up verbal leads, clues, bits of seemingly unrelated information, and nonverbal signals from the client. If the person asks you a personal question, redirect it to him or her; it may be the topic he or she unconsciously (or even consciously), wishes to speak about.	14. Movement of the interview gives you understanding about the person, her or his behavior, needs, health, illness, and relationships. Only occasionally will it be pertinent for you to answer personal questions. Sometimes brief self-disclosure will help the interviewee feel comfortable and elicit additional data. Be sure to disclose such information for the benefit of the client, not yourself.
15. **Indicate when the interview is terminated,** and terminate it graciously if the interviewee does not do so first. Make a transition in interviewing or use a natural stopping point if the problem has been resolved, if the information has been obtained or given, or if the person changes the topic. You may say, "There is one more question I'd like to ask," or "Just two more points I want to clarify," or "Before I leave, do you have any other questions, comments, or ideas to share?"	15. The client feels more secure with structure. Avoid social conversation or a feeling in the client that you lack skill. Skillful and distinct termination prevents you from feeling manipulated by the client's prolonging of the interview.
16. **Keep data obtained in the interview confidential and share this information only with the appropriate and necessary health team members,** leaving out personal assumptions. If you are sharing an opinion or interpretation, state it as such, rather than have it appear to be what the other person said or did. The person should be told what information will be shared and with whom and the reason for sharing.	16. Show respect for the individual. Confidentiality is the client's right and your responsibility.
17. **Evaluate the interview.** Were the purposes accomplished?	17. Evaluate yourself in each situation. Recognize that not everyone can successfully interview everyone. Others may see you differently from the way you see yourself. Validation with someone who is a skilled interviewer is helpful.

Source: Ref # 81.

TABLE 4–9. BARRIERS TO EFFECTIVE COMMUNICATION

1. **Conveying your feelings of anxiety, anger, judgment, blame, ambivalence, condescension, placating approach, denial, isolation, lack of control, or lack of physical or emotional health.**

2. **The appearance of being too busy, of not having time or desire to listen, of not giving sufficient time for an answer, or of not really wanting to hear.**

3. **Not paying attention to what is being said verbally and nonverbally; rehearsing** what you plan to say as the other is talking; **filtering** (listening selectively); **trying to second-guess the other person (mind-reading);** daydreaming while the other talks.

4. **Using the wrong vocabulary**—vocabulary that is abstract or intangible, or full of jargon, slang, or implied status; talking too much; or using unnecessarily long sentences or words out of context.

5. **Failing to understand the reason for the person's reluctance to make a message clear.**

6. **Making inappropriate use of facts, twisting facts, introducing unrelated information, offering premature interpretation, wrong timing, saying something important when the person is upset or not feeling well and thus unable to hear what is really said.**

7. **Making glib statements, offering false reassurance** by saying, "Everything is OK."

8. **Using cliches, stereotyped responses, trite expressions, and empty or patronizing verbalisms** stated without thought, such as "It's always worse at night." I know," "You'll be OK," or "Who is to say?"

9. **Expressing unnecessary approval,** stating that something the person does or feels is particularly good, implies that the opposite is bad.

10. **Expressing undue disapproval,** denouncing another's behavior or ideas, implies that you have the right to pass judgment, and that he or she must please you.

11. **Giving advice; stating personal experiences, opinions, or value judgments; giving pep talks; telling another what should be done.**

12. **Requiring explanations, demanding proof, challenging or asking "Why . . . ?"**—when the person cannot provide a reason for thoughts, feelings, and behavior and for events.

13. **Belittling the person's feelings** (equating intense and overwhelming feelings expressed by the client with those felt by everyone or yourself) implies that such feelings are not valid; that he or she is bad; or that the discomfort is mild, temporary, unimportant.

Source: Ref. 81.

health care and a person, family, or group with health care needs, with the focus on needs of the client, being empathic, and using knowledge. The therapeutic relationship/alliance must be differentiated from mere association. Social contact with another individual, verbal or nonverbal, may exercise some influence on one of the participants and needs may be met. But inconsistency, nonpredictability, or partial fulfillment of expectations often results. *Characteristics of social relationships* are as follows:

- The contact is primarily for pleasure and companionship.
- Neither person is in a position of responsibility for helping the other.
- No specific skill or knowledge is required.
- The interaction is between peers, often of the same social status.
- The people involved can, and often do, pursue an encounter for the satisfaction of personal or selfish interests.
- There is no explicit formulation of goals.
- There is no sense of accountability for the other person.
- Evaluation of interactions does not concern personal effectiveness in the interaction.

Phases of the therapeutic relationship/alliance were first researched and formulated by a nurse, Hildegard Peplau (85). The phases are: (1) orientation, establishment, or initial phase, (2) identification phase, (3) working or exploitation phase, and (4) termination or resolution phase. Certain behaviors and feelings, for both the nurse/helper and client/patient are typical of these phases (Table 4–10). Because of the nature of mutual participation in a therapeutic relationship, mutual behaviors are also noted in Table 4–10 (41, 42, 81, 85–87).

The relationship will be therapeutic when the nurse or helper uses a *caring, client-centered approach.* Establishing and maintaining a relationship or counseling another does not involve putting on a facade of behavior to match a list of characteristics. Rather, both you and the client will change and continue to mature. As the helper, you are present as a total person, blending potentials, talents, and skills while assisting the client to come to grips with needs, conflicts, and yourself. The capacity to be a helping person is strengthened by a genuine desire to be responsible and sensitive to another person. In addition, experience with a variety of people will increase your awareness of others' reactions and feelings, and the feedback you receive from others will teach you a great deal on both the emotional and cognitive levels.

Characteristics of a helping person in a humanistic approach with a client are described in Table 4–11 (81, 93). These characteristics were first combined into a total approach by Carl Rogers, and they are considered basic to a professional therapeutic relationship or alliance, and to any counseling or educational role.

Your use of therapeutic communication and a client-centered approach will move you through the relationship; however, *certain constraints* may be experienced if you are not careful about your feelings and behaviors. Table 4–12 describes problems commonly

TABLE 4–10. PHASES OF THE HELPING RELATIONSHIP

Orientation Phase
(Problem-defining phase)

Nurse Behaviors

_____ Initiates interaction:
     _____ Introduces self
     _____ Meets client as a stranger
     _____ Know client from prior admission/contact
     _____ Listens to client's/family's perception of problem or expectations
     _____ Responds to client's expressed need or emergency
     _____ Establishes rapport with client
     _____ Demonstrates acceptance
     _____ Explains own role to person/family
_____ Establishes contract (verbal or written):
     _____ Explains nature of relationship
     _____ Schedules time, duration and place of interview
     _____ Discusses goals of relationship/expectations of relationship
     _____ Explains commitment of nurse to client
     _____ Discusses issues of confidentiality
     _____ Discusses parameters of relationship and termination
     _____ Gathers information from person or family
     _____ Becomes better acquainted with person/family
_____ Collaborates with patient to analyze situation and establish goals:
     _____ Validates whether care plan matches client's impression of problem
     _____ Focuses client's energy on the task/responsibilities to be accomplished
     _____ Acts as a resource to person and/or family
     _____ Refers person and/or family to services within the agency
     _____ Continues assessment
_____ Demonstrates therapeutic emotional response:
     _____ Demonstrates empathy
     _____ Demonstrates unconditional positive regard
     _____ Demonstrates trustworthiness to client

_____ Examines own thoughts, feelings, expectations, and actions
_____ Describes and clarifies personal attitudes about caring for client
_____ Describes and clarifies client's reactions to nurse
_____ Identifies person's transference and own countertransference feelings and behaviors
_____ Demonstrates ability to control countertransference behavior
_____ Reduces anxiety/tension in the relationship through use of communication and relationship principles

Patient/Client Behaviors

_____ Meets nurse as a stranger
_____ Describes perceived need(s)
_____ Unable to identify need for assistance
_____ Seeks assistance
_____ Describes expectations of nurse and/or reactions due to prior experiences
_____ Asks questions about role, care plan, agency
_____ Tests parameters of relationship with a variety of behaviors or questions
_____ Demonstrates comfort with nurse
_____ Responds to trust demonstrated by nurse behavior
_____ Demonstrates trust in the nurse
_____ Settles into helping environment
_____ Identifies specific problems to be explored within context of relationship (indicates end of phase)

Mutual Behaviors

_____ Identify and define existing problems
_____ Clarify facts
_____ Make decisions about assistance needed
_____ Develop goals and care plan
_____ Validate that implementation of a care plan meets expectations

Identification Phase

Nurse Behaviors

_____ Promotes sense of security in person/family
_____ Continues assessment; becomes better acquainted with client
_____ Listens attentively and on deeper level
_____ Discusses confidentiality issues with person/family
_____ Provides opportunities for increasing self-care and independence in client and decreasing helplessness
_____ Continues interventions as indicated
_____ Provides suggestions, information, and educational materials
_____ Provides experiences for client to release anxiety and tension feelings
_____ Assists client to focus on goals, coping with problems, and treatment
_____ Demonstrates therapeutic emotional response:
     _____ Demonstrates deeper level of empathy
     _____ Demonstrates unconditional acceptance
     _____ Maintains separate identity
     _____ Identifies patient's transference and own countertransference feelings/behavior

_____ Demonstrates ability to control countertransference behavior
_____ Identifies discomfort with patient's dependency on nurse
_____ Accepts patient's dependency behavior

Patient/Client Behaviors

_____ Responds selectively to nurse who is perceived as most helpful:
     _____ Describes nurse as significant, own nurse, or capabilities of nurse
     _____ Imitates selected nurse's behaviors, behavioral or verbal patterns
     _____ Describes or demonstrates positive transference feelings/behavior
     _____ Demonstrates dependency on and identification with nurse
_____ Participates in clarifying problem(s)
_____ Demonstrates diminishing testing behavior
_____ Responds to nurse's care, interventions
     _____ Follows nurse's suggestions, teaching
     _____ Works closely (participates) with nurse in interventions
     _____ Demonstrates increased attention to goals or treatment tasks
_____ Maintains continuity between sessions by following assignments, tasks, attending to process

(continued)

TABLE 4–10. PHASES OF THE HELPING RELATIONSHIP (*continued*)

_____ Describes understanding of purpose of interview sessions

_____ Changes appearance, self-care behavior in a positive direction

_____ Discloses and explores deeper feelings, more intimate behavior, or information about self/family:

    _____ Describes feeling of belonging in care setting

    _____ Describes diminishing feelings of helplessness and hopelessness

    _____ Describes increasing self-esteem and optimism about ability to deal with problems

Mutual Behaviors

_____ Explore mutually deeper feelings, needs, and goals

_____ Describe feelings of trust in each other

_____ Move emotionally closer to each other

_____ Clarify each other's perceptions and expectations, depending on past experiences

_____ Continue development of care plan

Working Phase

Nurse Behaviors

_____ Continues assessment:

    _____ Encourages client to express feelings and thoughts

    _____ Gains deeper understanding of person/family

    _____ Listens carefully; client does more talking than nurse

    _____ Evaluates problems and goals and redefines as necessary

_____ Helps client overcome resistance to change

_____ Assists client, as necessary, with tasks and meeting goals

_____ Intervenes, using communication principles:

    _____ Offers support, as patient works on problems at his/her own pace

    _____ Reflects and gives feedback to client

    _____ Explores areas of client's life that causes problems, underlying needs, and dysfunctional behavior patterns

    _____ Confronts incongruities in client's verbal and/or nonverbal behavior and life patterns in a way that does not threaten client

    _____ Explores possible causes for client's behavior

    _____ Clarifies possible solutions, resources, options with client

    _____ Discusses the meaning of changes in client's behavior

    _____ Interprets meaning of client's behavior in a way that client can accept and use the information to change behavior, gain new self-view

_____ Promotes client's development: emotional, interpersonal, and behavioral:

    _____ Assists client in developing healthy methods to reduce anxiety

    _____ Provides opportunities for client to become more independent and interdependent

    _____ Facilitates behavioral change in person/family

    _____ Deals with particular behavior that is presented by the person/family

    _____ Deals with therapeutic impasse when it occurs

    _____ Discusses strengths and positive factors in person/family

_____ Supports, instills optimism, conveys hope, and reinforces positive directions in client's behavior

_____ Teaches client as needs emerge, pertinent to life situation and illness:

    _____ Teaches effective interpersonal behavior patterns

    _____ Teaches problem-solving skills

    _____ Teaches about medication regimen and other aspects of illness/treatment

    _____ Accepts that client may not follow nurse's suggestions/teaching

_____ Discusses approaching discharge and rehabilitation plans:

    _____ Initiates discharge and rehabilitation plans and specific measures

    _____ Involves family in treatment and rehabilitation

    _____ Teaches patient's family about their role in rehabilitation and recovery of patient

    _____ Accepts that patient's family may not consider or follow nurse's suggestions or teaching

_____ Demonstrates therapeutic emotional response:

    _____ Demonstrates deeper empathy

    _____ Continues to convey attitudes of acceptance, concern, and trust

    _____ Controls countertransference feelings

Patient/Client Behaviors

_____ Maintains relationship with nurse

_____ Describes feeling of trust in and acceptance by nurse

_____ Fluctuates between dependency and independency

_____ Demonstrates increasing ability to establish own goals:

    _____ Demonstrates increasing assertiveness and self-reliance in self-care and goal attainment

    _____ Insists on doing tasks in his/her own way

    _____ Appears manipulative at times

    _____ Demonstrates attention-seeking and self-centered behavior at times

_____ Participates increasingly in decision-making about own welfare, treatment, rehabilitation, and post-discharge plans

_____ Demonstrates progressive responsibility for self, self-reliance, and independence

_____ Utilizes services and resources offered by the nurse and health team that meet his/her needs:

    _____ Makes demands on nurse and other health care members

    _____ Pursues helpful resources

    _____ Demonstrates taking advantage of all available resources, based on personal needs and interests

    _____ Carries out assignments between sessions

_____ Demonstrates increasingly more open and effective communication skills:

    _____ Describes willingness to accept help while recognizing own strengths, abilities, and limits

    _____ Describes sense of hope and self-confidence about own potential

    _____ Discusses belief that what is explored in sessions can be applied to life situations

    _____ Considers, integrates, and acts on interpretations given by nurse

    _____ Describes feeling of being integral part of helping environment

    _____ Describes some control over situation as services are given by others

    _____ Describes a progressively developing sense of identity

(continued)

TABLE 4–10. PHASES OF THE HELPING RELATIONSHIP (continued)

_____ Demonstrates increasingly the signs of physical and emotional health or a higher level of functioning:

    _____ Demonstrates increasing ability to cope with situations

    _____ Functions optimally in more situations

    _____ Demonstrates increasing self-initiation and self-direction in behavior

    _____ Demonstrates increasing skills in interpersonal relationships and problem-solving

    _____ Changes behavior patterns with significant people in a positive direction

    _____ Demonstrates sources of inner strength or new problems as new problems or challenges arise

    _____ Describes feelings of wellness and readiness for approaching discharge

Mutual Behaviors

_____ Examine together the relationship and its meaning

_____ Collaborate as partners in meeting health care goals

_____ Utilize multidisciplinary team members in various facets of intervention and rehabilitation plans

_____ Demonstrate progression toward resolution/termination phase

_____ Formulate discharge and rehabilitation plans/goals

Termination Phase

Nurse Behaviors

_____ Continues to demonstrate empathy and caring for the client

_____ Sustains relationship as long as client demonstrates need

_____ Plans for discharge and termination of relationship with client:

    _____ Validates client's strengths and progressively positive coping mechanisms

    _____ Explores impending separation and discharge

    _____ Discusses anticipation of client developing and maintaining new relationships

    _____ Shares feelings about separation and termination in an appropriate way with person/family

_____ Teaches measures to help person prevent further illness and maintain self-care

_____ Promotes interaction between person and family

_____ Discusses community resources or networks that could be utilized by person/family

_____ Resolves feelings of separation, guilt, or uncertainty related to client's progress or ability to function, misplaced sense of responsibility, countertransference

Patient/Client Behaviors

_____ Demonstrates fewer or diminished symptoms

_____ Demonstrates defensive maneuvers that are meant to delay discharge and termination:

    _____ Does not keep interview appointments

    _____ Is sarcastic or hostile to nurse

    _____ Accuses nurse of using client as a guinea pig to deflect awakening pain of past separations

    _____ Denies relationship had any impact

    _____ Demonstrates regressive behavior

    _____ Demonstrates increasing dependency

    _____ Describes lack of confidence in ability to manage post-discharge

    _____ Describes feelings of being pushed out by nurse or health care system

    _____ Does not meet nurse at final established session

_____ Demonstrates or describes that needs have been met and goals accomplished:

    _____ Demonstrates improved social functioning

    _____ Demonstrates being independent of helping person

_____ Explores feelings about impending separation and discharge:

    _____ Explores past unresolved separations

    _____ Describes feelings about being cared for and cared about

_____ Indicates verbally and/or behaviorally that he/she is ready for discharge:

    _____ Demonstrates more adaptive mechanisms of behavior

    _____ Describes increased self-esteem, self-confidence, and significance to others

    _____ Describes hope for the future

    _____ Demonstrates or describes an integration of behavior and ability to live independently

_____ Maintains behavioral and communication changes

Mutual Behaviors

_____ Discuss what was accomplished in therapy, goals set and accomplished

_____ Examine uncertainty about patient's ability to manage after discharge

_____ Explore resolution of illness and treatment

_____ Plan together how the client will continue to interact and manage life's patterns and stresses

_____ Utilize community resources as necessary

_____ Discuss feelings to each other and about separation

_____ Resolve issue of gift giving if client gives gift to nurse

_____ Resolve mourning process that is part of separation and termination

_____ Demonstrate more mature behavior as result of relationship

_____ Terminate relationship; links are dissolved, each feeling other phases have been successfully completed

TABLE 4–11. CHARACTERISTICS OF A HELPING RELATIONSHIP

Respectful—Feeling and communicating an attitude of seeing the client as a unique human being, filled with dignity, worth, and strengths, regardless of outward appearance or behavior; being willing to *work* at communicating with and understanding the client because he/she is in need of emotional care

Genuine—Communicating spontaneously, yet tactfully, what is felt and thought, with proper timing and without disturbing the client, rather than using professional jargon, facade, or rigid counselor or nurse role behaviors

Attentive—Conveying an active listening to verbal and nonverbal messages and an attitude of working with the person

Accepting—Conveying that the person does not have to put on a facade and that the person will not shock you with his/her statements; enabling the client to change at his/her own pace; acknowledging personal and client's feelings aroused in the encounter; to "be for" the client in a nonsentimental, caring way

Positive—Showing warmth, caring, respect, and agape love; being able to reinforce the client for what he/she does well

Strong—Maintaining a separate identity from the client; withstanding the testing

Secure—Permitting the client to remain separate and unique; respecting his/her needs and your own; feeling safe as the client moves emotionally close; feeling no need to exploit the other person

Knowledgeable—Having an expertise based on study, experience, and supervision

Sensitive—Being perceptive to feelings; avoiding threatening behavior, responding to cultural values, customs, norms as they affect behavior; using knowledge that is pertinent to the client's situation, being kind and gentle

Empathic—Looking at the client's world from his/her viewpoint; being open to his/her values, feelings, beliefs, and verbal statements; stating your understanding of his/her verbal or nonverbal expressions of feelings and experiences

Nonjudgmental—Refraining from evaluating the client moralistically, or telling the client what to do

Congruent—Being natural, relaxed, honest, trustworthy, and dependable, and demonstrating consistency in behavior and between verbal and nonverbal messages

Unambiguous—Avoiding contradictory messages

Creative—Viewing the client as a person in the process of becoming, not being bound by the past, and viewing yourself in the process of becoming or maturing

Source: Ref. 81.

encountered as you work closely with a family member or unit (8, 85–87, 93, 113).

Family Assessment

In doing a family assessment, ask questions related to family structure and develop a **genogram,** *a diagram of family members and their characteristics and processes* (see Fig. 4–1). Also, determine communication patterns and relationships, family health, access to health care, occupational demands and hazards, religious beliefs and practices, childrearing practices, participation in the community, and support systems. When you work

► **CRITERIA FOR ASSESSING HEALTHY FAMILIES**

- Ability to provide for the physical, emotional, social, and spiritual needs of the family
- Ability to be sensitive to the needs of family members
- Ability to listen and communicate effectively
- Ability to provide trust, support, security, affirmation, and encouragement
- Ability to initiate and maintain growth-producing relationships and experiences within and without the family
- Demonstration of mutual respect, for family and others
- Commitment to teach and demonstrate moral code
- Concern for family unity, loyalty, and interfamily cooperation
- Capacity to use humor and to share leisure time with each other, to enjoy each other
- Commitment to strong sense of family where rituals and traditions abound
- Ability to perform roles flexibly and sense of shared responsibility
- Ability to maintain balance of interaction and sense of privacy among the members
- Ability for self-help and to accept help, when appropriate
- Ability to use crisis or seemingly injurious experience as a means of growth
- Ability to grow with and through children
- Capacity to maintain and create constructive and responsible community relationships in the neighborhood, school, town, local and state governments, and to value service to others

Taken from References (1, 6, 9, 34, 44, 65, 75, and 83).

with the family unit the information in Fig. 4–2 will help you assess the family's lifestyle and needs. Other criteria for assessment are listed above in Criteria for Assessing Healthy Families.

Formulation of Nursing Diagnoses

In a general hospital setting, where you are including the family unit as part of your care of the client, your nursing diagnoses may be general, or family issues may be included in the client's nursing diagnoses. For example, you may state your nursing diagnoses as follows:

- Anxiety in client related to lack of family contact
- Family's denial of client's disease and of need for special diet and hygiene measures related to lack of understanding on the part of the family

Examples of a nursing diagnosis may be derived from some of the material presented earlier in the chapter. Using family systems theory, you may state your nursing diagnoses in the following manner:

TABLE 4–12. CONSTRAINTS IN THE HELPING RELATIONSHIP

- **Certain limits exist for you, the helper, and the client. Relationship means involvement and commitment;** it takes time. The client's dependency may create demands for extra time or responsibility. You will have to consider feelings and needs, meet important demands, and set limits whenever necessary.
- **The client may not be willing to change sufficiently to resolve the problem.** The person may not be able to give up his or her discomforts because these may be a core part of his or her identity.
- **As the helper, you may experience the phenomenon of countertransference** — *an unconscious, inappropriate emotional response to the client as if he or she were an important figure in your life, or unconsciously based in past unresolved experiences with key people in your life.* The helpful measure in this situation would be to respond to the client realistically as he/she really is. Countertransference works in much the same ways as transference does for the client. You relate to the client based on your feelings toward someone from the past.

If you are *experiencing countertransference,* you may have *any of the following reactions.*

1. Overidentify with the client; you exert pressure on the person to act a certain way or to improve.
2. Attempt to make the person over in your own image.
3. Invite gifts or favors, dependence on the client's praise or affection.
4. Offer excessive reassurance or help that is not really necessary.
5. Feel a need to impress the client.
6. Wish to be the client's child, grandchild, or younger sibling may occur with older people, especially if they actually resemble your parents, grandparents, or siblings.
7. Realize thoughts wander from the client, or the client's words trigger unrelated thoughts.
8. Focus repetitively on one aspect or way of looking at the person's behavior or statements. Be attentive to the client's verbal and nonverbal behavior.
9. Defend interactions with the patient to others. Ignore behavior; show lack of objectivity about the behavior or focus on one aspect of behavior.
10. Be impatient with or have guilt about the client's lack of progress, insensitivity to or lack of empathy for his or her needs, or feelings of being unable to help.

11. Experience conflicting feelings of intense affection, dislike, defensiveness, indifference, fear, or angry sympathy with the person.
12. Feel overconcern about the person between sessions or overemotional reaction to the client's troubles, believing no one else can care for the person as well as you can.
13. Experience sexual or aggressive fantasies about the client.
14. Experience dreams about the client; be preoccupied with the client when awake.

Countertransference can be overcome through guidance from a supervisor and a willingness to examine your personal behavior and comments.

- **You may feel anger toward the client.** Your anger may be a reaction to his or her overt behavior and your fear of acting that way. Your anger may be a counter-reaction to the client's anger that is related to something else but is directed toward you. You can stop the cycle by recognizing your own feelings as well as the helplessness felt by the client, by talking with him or her to determine possible sources of anger, and by avoiding either a hostile or too sweet response. Do not joke about anger in yourself or the client and do not reject or punish the client for anger. Make sure that you are not the cause of anger because of actions that demean, aggravate, or neglect him or her. If the person arouses anger in you, seek help from a skilled colleague to work through possible reasons for your anger, to talk about how you demonstrate anger in your behavior, and to explore how to handle such feelings.
- **You may think you are the only person who can care for the client** or that you can solve all of the problems. Such a feeling of omnipotence is unfounded.
- **You may have difficulty with dependence and independence within a relationship.** You may want to have others depend on you. Therefore, you do things for the client that he or she can do. Such smothering discourages independent behavior. On the other hand, you may not be able to tolerate the person's dependency, clinging, helplessness, or need for total assistance. Seek help to work through your own feelings.
- **If you joke or tease in a harsh or belittling manner, if you use jestful sarcasm, if you laugh at the client's appearance or behavior, if you play childish games to get him or her to cooperate or be pleasant, or if you use her or him as a scapegoat,** you will be the cause of the client's anger, hate, despair, hopelessness, and finally complete withdrawal and regression.

Source: Ref. 81.

- Family system insufficiently open to internal (or external) environment related to inability of members to express feelings (or impaired ability to interact with neighbors)
- Impaired communication processes in family system related to power struggles
- Family goals and functions unmet related to disorganized lifestyle patterns of members
- Dysfunctional family system related to limited communication between family members, including extended family

Or you may state your nursing diagnoses as follows:

- Impairment in fulfilling family functions and activities related to inadequate material resources
- Impaired intrafamily interactions and lack of communication related to abusive behavior between spouses
- Disruptive family interpersonal relationships related to power conflicts and lack of closeness

Using a genogram, you may state your nursing diagnoses as follows:

- Altered family relationships related to mourning of death of parent (or divorce, remarriage, or coalitions between stepchildren against wife, children, or death of another family member)

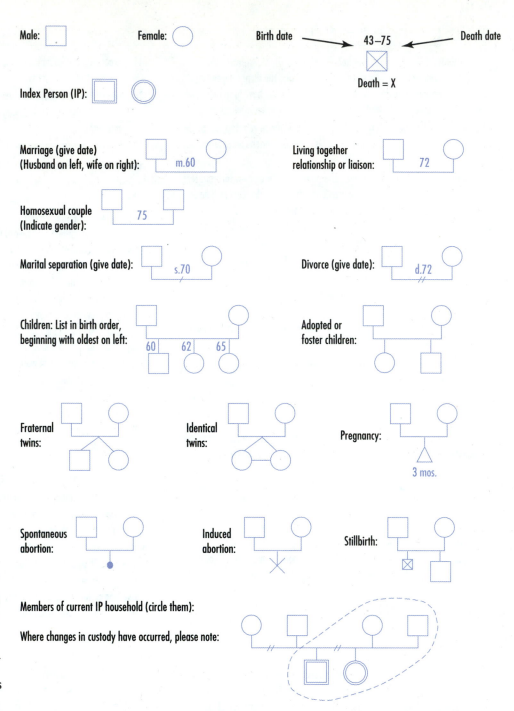

Figure 4–1. Genogram format. Symbols to describe basic family membership and structure (include on genogram significant others who lived with or cared for family members — place them on the right side of the genogram with a notation about who they are). Religion, education, or ethnic origin can be written in by oldest generation or other units. Health problems noted by person.

- Unachieved family goals related to inability of family to use environmental resources

You will think of other ways to formulate nursing diagnoses so that the statements are meaningful to you and to other nurses. Refer also to Selected Nursing Diagnoses Related to Family Nursing on page 185 for other statements of nursing diagnoses that may apply to the family.

Formulation of Goals and a Plan of Care

The primary *goal* in working with families is to use yourself and your assessment in a way that allows the family to: (1) bring issues into the open, (2) gain a new awareness, (3) learn new ways to facilitate balance in the family system, and (4) fulfill family functions in more healthful way. Having diagnosed a dysfunctional pattern(s) within a family system, your specific goal(s)

Meeting of Physical, Emotional, and Spiritual Needs of Members
Ability to provide food and shelter
  Space management as regards living, sleeping, recreation, privacy
  Crowding if over 1.5 persons per room
  Territoriality or control of each member over lifespace
  Access to laundry, grocery, recreation facilities
  Sanitation including disposal methods, source of water supply, control
    of rodents and insects
  Storage and refrigeration
  Available food supply
  Food preparation, including preserving and cooking methods,
    (stove, hotplate, oven)
  Use of food stamps and donated foods as well as eligibility for
    food stamps
  Education of each member as to food composition, balanced
    menus, special preparations or diets if required for a specific
    member
Access to health care
  Regularity of health care
  Continuity of caregivers
  Closeness of facility and means of access such as car, bus, cab
  Access to helpful neighbors
  Access to phone
Family health
  Longevity
  Major or chronic illnesses
  Familial or hereditary illnesses such as rheumatic fever, gout, allergy,
    tuberculosis, renal disease, diabetes mellitus, cancer, emotional illness,
    epilepsy, migraine, other nervous disorders, hypertension, blood diseases,
    obesity, frequent accidents, drug intake, pica
  Emotional or stress-related illnesses
  Pollutants that members are chronically exposed to such as air, water,
    soil, noise, or chemicals that are unsafe to health
Neighborhood pride and loyalty
Job access, energy output, shift changes
Sensitivity, warmth, understanding between family members
  Demonstration of emotion
  Enjoyment of sexual relations
    Male: Impotence, premature or retarded ejaculation, hypersexuality
    Female: Frigidity (inability to achieve orgasm), enjoyment of sexual
      relations, feelings of disgust, shame, self-devaluation; fear of injury,
      painful coitus
      Menstrual history, including onset, duration, flow, missed periods and
      life situation at the time, pain, euphoria, depression, other difficulties
Sharing of religious beliefs, values, doubts
  Formal membership in church and organizations
  Ethical framework and honesty
  Adaptability, response to reality
  Satisfaction with life
  Self-esteem

Childrearing Practices and Discipline
Mutual responsibility
  Joint parenting
  Mutual respect for decision making
  Means of discipline and consistency
Respect for individuality
Fostering of self-discipline
Attitudes toward education, reading, scholarly pursuit
Attitudes toward imaginative play
Attitudes toward involvement in sports
Promotion of gender stereotypes

Communication
Expression of a wide range of emotion and feeling
Expression of ideas, concepts, beliefs, values, interests
Openness
Verbal expression and sensitive listening
Consensual decision making

Support, Security, Encouragement
Balance in activity
Humor
Dependency and dominance patterns
Life support groups of each member
Social relationship of couple: go out together or separately; change
  since marriage mutually satisfying; effect of sociability
  patterns on children

**Growth-Producing Relationships and Experiences Within and
Without the Family**
Creative play activities
Planned growth experiences
Focus of life and activity of each member
Friendships

Responsible Community Relationships
Organizations, including involvement, membership, active participation
Knowledge of and friendship with neighbors

Growing with and Through Children
Hope and plans for children
Emulation of own parents and its influence on relationship with children
Relationship patterns: authoritarian, patriarchal, matriarchal
Necessity to relive (make up for) own childhood through children

Unity, Loyalty, and Cooperation
Positive interacting of members toward each other

Self-Help and Acceptance of Outside Help in Family Crisis

Figure 4–2. Family assessment tool.

in conjunction with the family is to determine what changes can be effected to create a more constructive pattern(s).

Short-term goals could be stated as follows:

- Family system will convey support to the ill member through daily visits and empathic conversation.
- Family members will be able to describe special dietary needs and other self-care measures essential to client recovery.
- Family member (specific person) will demonstrate correct techniques for rehabilitative care of client.
- Family members will admit each person's contribution to disruptive communication and lifestyle patterns.
- Family members will formulate a contract for 20 minutes of conversation each day where feelings can be expressed honestly and without argument (or fear, blame, scapegoating, derision, etc.).
- Husband and wife will discuss dominance/submission patterns and ways to share in decision making.
- Family system will use community agency (name specific one) as a support while adjusting to changes produced by _____.

Long-term goals are appropriate if you will be working with a family over time. Such goals could include the following:

- Family system will accurately identify key issues that contribute to hostile communication and withdrawal of members from participation in family life.
- Family members will practice daily (for an increasing amount of time) communication methods that promote cohesion.
- Parents will discuss and adhere consistently to effective disciplinary measures of child(ren).
- Nuclear family will reestablish harmonious relationships with extended family.
- Spouse will be less authoritarian in interactions with partner and child(ren).
- Husband/wife will contribute toward completion of daily activities related to homemaking, instead of using illness to escape these family functions.
- Husband will avoid seductive behavior toward his daughter and relate affectionately toward his wife.

You will write goals specific to the family systems with which you are working. Perhaps the above examples will stimulate your thinking.

Intervention

You can help families understand some processes and dynamics underlying interaction so that they, in turn, learn to respect the uniqueness of the self and of each other. Certainly members in the family need not always agree with each other. Instead, they can learn to listen to the other person, about how he or she feels and why, accepting each person's impression as real for self. This attitude becomes the basis for mutual respect, honest communication, encouragement of individual fulfillment, and freedom to be. There is then no need to prove or defend the self.

Once the attitude "We are all important people in this family" is established, conflicts can be dealt with openly and constructively. Name calling and belittling are out of place. Families need to structure time together; otherwise individual schedules will allow them less and less time to meet. Parents need to send consistent messages to their children. To say "Don't smoke" while immediately lighting a cigarette is hardly effective.

Times of communication are especially necessary when children are feeling peer pressure; children, moreover, should be praised for what they do right rather than reprimanded for what they do wrong. Children need structure but should be told the reason for the structure if old enough to comprehend. As you help the family achieve positive feelings toward and interaction with one another, you are also helping them to fulfill their tasks, roles, and functions. Review the adaptive mechanisms of families described in this chapter.

The person's health problems, especially emotional ones, may well be the result of the interaction patterns in childhood or in the present family. Knowledge of the variables influencing family interaction—parents' self-esteem and upbringing, number of siblings, person's ordinal position in the family, cultural norms, family rituals—will help you assist the person in talking through feelings related to past and present conflicts. Sometimes helping the person understand these variables in relation to the spouse's upbringing and behavior can be the first step in overcoming current marital problems.

You may assist families to cope with crises or various unexpected disorganizing events, such as illness and natural disasters. Table 4–13 summarizes steps in *crisis intervention* or *brief therapy.*

You may help families explore and resolve *ethical dilemmas* related to their decisions whether their plans

► SELECTED NURSING DIAGNOSES RELATED
TO FAMILY NURSING*

Pattern 2: Communicating

Impaired Verbal Communication

Pattern 3: Relating

Impaired Social Interaction
Social Isolation
Altered Role Performance
Altered Parenting
Risk for Altered Parenting/Infant/Child Attachment
Sexual Dysfunction
Altered Family Processes
Parental Role Conflict
Altered Sexuality Patterns

Pattern 4: Valuing

Spiritual Distress

Pattern 5: Choosing

Ineffective Individual Coping
Impaired Adjustment
Defensive Coping
Ineffective Denial
Ineffective Family Coping: Disabling
Ineffective Family Coping: Compromised
Family Coping: Potential for Growth
Decisional Conflict
Health-Seeking Behaviors

Pattern 6: Moving

Diversional Activity Deficit
Impaired Home Maintenance Management
Altered Health Maintenance
Ineffective Breastfeeding
Altered Growth and Development

Pattern 7: Perceiving

Chronic Low Self-Esteem
Situational Low Self-Esteem
Personal Identity Disturbance
Unilateral Neglect
Hopelessness
Powerlessness

Pattern 8: Knowing

Knowledge Deficit

Pattern 9: Feeling

Dysfunctional Grieving
Anticipatory Grieving
Risk for Violence: Self-Directed or Directed at Others
Post-Trauma Response
Anxiety
Fear

*Many of the NANDA nursing diagnoses are applicable to the ill individual in the family unit.
From North American Nursing Diagnosis Association, NANDA Nursing Diagnoses Definitions & Classification 1995–1996. Philadelphia: North American Nursing Diagnosis Association, 1994.

involve use of newer technology for getting pregnant or dealing with an adoptive child. Technology that allows infertile couples to become pregnant with in vitro fertilization may also cause parents to face major ethical dilemmas as they determine which of the fertilized embryos should be transplanted into the uterus and which should be frozen for future use. Exploration of feelings and implications is essential.

You may explore with the family the decision to use sperm donors for artificial insemination who are paid for their service. The donor should be carefully screened for a family history of inherited diseases and for current pathogens such as human immunodeficiency virus (HIV). Because some infections such as HIV are present long before they may be detected (as long as 10 years), transmission of this disease via insemination may become known in the future. The donor is also screened in terms of race, intelligence quotient, physical characteristics, and health. Recipients may choose the baby's gender. Some women become pregnant after the first insemination; others require several inseminations (80).

TABLE 4–13. FAMILY CRISIS INTERVENTION TO ASSIST FAMILIES WITH COPING

1. Encourage family to identify the stressor or hazardous life event.
2. Assess family's interpretation of event and its actual impact.
3. Determine family's usual and current coping abilities and resources to handle the event.
4. Assess family's level of functioning as a whole, as well as function of individual members.
5. Assist family members in communicating with each other.
6. Encourage all family members to be involved in finding a solution(s) or resources.
7. Be supportive but encourage the family to mobilize its own resources and resources that exist in the extended family or community.
8. Empower families by indicating their strengths, reinforcing positive behavior, helping them make sense of the event, and promoting a sense of being normal.
9. Explore how to prevent and cope with future stressful experiences.
10. Teach coping strategies, ways to prevent or minimize future stressors, stress management, and lifestyle alterations.
11. Recognize members at risk for violence and intervene as necessary.
12. Either continue longer-term therapy, if needed, with the family unit or members or refer them to ongoing therapy as necessary.

Hiring a surrogate mother—a woman to become pregnant and bear the baby for the family—must also be carefully explored because of implications for the surrogate mother and her feelings, consequent feelings of the childrearing family, and legal issues (80).

Other decisions may not be as difficult but are key to future family development and relationships, for example, helping adoptive parents relate with their child (7) or the homosexual family explain "coming out" to the children from an earlier marriage (46). These parents must be prepared to explain the child's origins when the child asks and to help the child understand that there are many kinds of families in the United States. We do not yet know the consequences, developmentally and emotionally, for children who are raised without guidance from the opposite sex or who are raised by only one parent. Your assessment, exploration, and teaching with such families are important.

More research is needed in all of these areas. To help families explore values and ethical principles, you must *first* explore and resolve these issues within yourself. You cannot give another *the* answer; you can use therapeutic communication skills to enable clients to find their own answers.

You are not a specialized family counselor, although with advanced preparation you could do family therapy. But you can often sense lack of communication in a family. Through use of an empathic relationship and effective communication, teaching, and crisis therapy, you can encourage family members to talk about their feelings with one another and assist in the resolution of their conflicts. Help them become aware of the need to work for family cohesiveness just as they would work at a job or important project. Refer them to a family counseling service if the problems are beyond your scope. Your work with them should also help them better use other community resources such as private family or psychiatric counseling or family and children's services.

One family self-help resource can be the formation of a group of four or five complete family units (including stepfamily, single-parent, cohabitation, or the traditional unit) who contract to meet together over an extended period for shared educational experiences that concern relationships within their families. This setting provides a positive approach and affirms family members because a commitment is made for all persons—no matter what their age—to have both power and input into the group.

Table 4–14 summarizes *intervention measures for counseling or educating families* to promote their health.

Role of the Nurse in Well-Baby Care

You may care for well babies and mothers in a variety of settings—clinic, hospital, home, or doctor's office. Your actions contribute significantly to their health.

Prenatal Care

Prenatal care for the mother and her partner may include physical assessment, teaching healthful practices for mother and baby, listening to mother vent frustrations or share fears, counseling her during periods of depression or uncertainty, and sharing her happy feelings about becoming a mother. You may conduct childbirth classes for mother and father so that they can better understand changes occurring in the mother and the nutrition and hygiene necessary during pregnancy; know what to expect during labor, delivery, and postpartum; and prepare for an active role during birth. A maternity nursing book will give adequate detail to help you do prenatal assessment and care and intrapartum and postpartum assessment and intervention.

If the mother-to-be is unwed, you may also try to work with the father-to-be if both are willing. The father-to-be needs help in talking about his feelings and needs to support her, if they are compatible. He may also seek sex education.

TABLE 4–14.   SUMMARY OF INTERVENTION MEASURES

1. **Develop a therapeutic relationship.** Establish rapport and trust between yourself and the family by being open to the family structure or system and the cultural values and norms that are manifested. Use therapeutic communication principles. Use the family's language, but be a model for clear, effective communication. Remember the trust, influence, and impact that you have on the family unit. Be empathic, supportive, and impartial as you give feedback to the family. Thus you will enable the family members to identify and modify patterns that cause dysfunction and discomfort.

2. **Identify issues with the family.** Subjective issues are what the family members perceive as problem areas. Objective issues are what you see as limits or problems. Have each family member list or identify problems and areas for change. Refrain from challenging or questioning the accuracy of anyone's values or statements of problem areas. Do not side with any one particular member. Encourage family members also to explore those areas that you see as dysfunctional.

3. **Encourage and assist members in their communication skills,** to listen to one another, to talk kindly, and to clarify their own perceptions and the feelings, thoughts, and behaviors of the others. You gently confront and are a mirror for the family members so that they can gain increased understanding of themselves as a unit. As they learn to talk honestly to one another, members will have less need to deny the pain they feel or deny hurtful behaviors practiced in family living.

4. **Establish a teaching plan for the family unit if it is appropriate,** either for the client as a member of the family or for the family as a whole. Help each one to find appropriate resources in the external environment as well as to identify personal strengths for managing a situation. Encourage the family to find ways to adapt the life style or home situation to manage better an illness or crisis.

5. **Determine willingness of family members to participate in counseling and change.** Keep in mind that families, according to Systems Theory, strive to maintain their balance and are frightened and ambivalent about negotiating

and enacting change. Have each member participate in defining the problem and in making the decision for change to enable family members to feel more in control of what is occurring and more willing to participate. Even so, some members may continue to be resistant to change during counseling or may choose not to participate at all. It is essential for you to remain objective, reassuring, and supportive. Considerable theoretical knowledge, communication skill, and supervised practice are necessary before you will be able to work with deep, long-term, or complex problems; resistant behavior; power struggles; or coalitions.

6. **Negotiate a contract as to the goals for treatment.** (See Chapter 5 for guidelines for contracting.) Identify with the family one or two goals that are crucial to work toward to begin to achieve some happiness and smoother function. Later, other goals may be added to the list. It is better to set small achievable goals that the family perceives as worthwhile than to inhibit family change through an extensive list of statements. Remember that the behavior of any one family member is a symptom of a problem in the family system.

7. **Negotiate a contract about specific behavioral changes that can be accomplished** and that will encourage family members to interact or behave in ways that break dysfunctional patterns or rigid structures. Assist members to disagree constructively and to contract with one another for change. Help the family to anticipate problem areas, work through alternatives, and explore consequences of the alternatives. P. Coleman's book, *The Forgiving Marriage,* is an example of literature that can be useful in helping the family work at change (33).

8. **Be patient.** Do not expect great change. The family may change its behavior, but only to the point that is comfortable and tolerable to all. Regression to previous patterns will occur. Your consistent kindness and encouragement may be the main factors in the family coping with stressors or crises, adjusting daily routines to the needs of an ill member, or staying with therapy and trying to modify behavior.

To help the unwed parents and break the cycle for future generations, we must gain a better understanding of the unwed father. Do not perceive him as irresponsible or having taken advantage of an innocent girl. The relationship between the unwed mother and the father is not necessarily a hit-and-miss affair but often meaningful to both. If the parents-to-be are adolescents, they realize that a new life has been created as a result of their actions. They want to act in a responsible way. They are concerned about the child's well-being (73, 115).

The unwed father can be encouraged to stand by the unmarried mother. Often he feels proud of fathering; he has proved his masculinity. The long-term consequences of having a child are such, however, that alternate solutions regarding the future of the child should be thoroughly explored with and by both partners. Alternatives include marriage, placing the child for adoption, or assumption by either parent or the grandparents of the responsibility for caring for and

rearing the child. The man needs help in understanding how and why he became a father and the serious implications for the mother, the child, and himself.

Adolescents may admit that their sexual experiences were unsatisfactory, leaving them depressed, guilty, and scared. The good relationship with the girlfriend may have begun to deteriorate when sexual relations were started. Pregnancy comes as a shock to both. They know about contraceptives, but their use may have been sporadic, if at all, for some people believe that the spontaneity and sincerity of the sexual act are lessened when prepared for (73, 115).

Sex education must relate to the values of interpersonal relations and concern for others if it is to be successful. The implications and responsibilities of sexual behavior must be discussed with the teenagers. The difference between teenage love and a more mature relationship between people who are ready to meet the problems and responsibilities of adulthood should be discussed (73, 115).

Parents of the unwed father must be involved in helping their son; communication between the boy and parents should be reestablished. In addition, parents should assert themselves in helping the boy take responsibility for his actions and assist the boy in the case of marriage.

Efforts to prevent unwed pregnancies must be directed to improving and strengthening family life and developing a better respect for the father's role in the family. Many unwed fathers come from female-dominated homes or from homes in which the father is absent or inadequate in his role (73, 115).

Fathers can help adolescent sons by talking with and listening to them, by being slow to judge, by taking them to the job so the youth can see how the father earns a living, and by being a role model in relating maturely to the spouse and other women. Fathers can create an atmosphere in which the sons will want to talk about emerging sexual feelings and experiences (73, 115). If the adolescent son comes from a home where no father is present, the mother can work at listening to and discussing problems and feelings with the son. She may also be able to foster a bond between the son and another male member of the family.

Childbirth Education Classes

If you conduct childbirth and parenting education classes, try to interview each couple in their home early in the pregnancy, by the fourth month if possible, to observe their relationship and determine their response to pregnancy. Their response may be different and more honest in their own home than in class. During the classes include opportunities for both men and women to talk about the problems they feel are uniquely theirs, their feelings, or the commonality of the couvade syndrome. Provide anticipatory guidance about the couvade syndrome. Avoid pushing the father into participation and provide support for him. Focus childbirth education on the known benefits to the baby and parents and not on overromanticized and dramatic statements about improved marital relationships. Educate both parents about family planning so that future pregnancies can be mutually planned. Refer either partner, or both, to psychological counseling when necessary, especially if antisocial behavior is seen or if there has been fetal loss.

Labor and Delivery

During labor and delivery, the nurse gives necessary physical care, may act as a coach for the mother, or may support the father as he assists his wife. Flexibility in hospital routines for obstetric patients is usually possible and contributes to the parents' sense of control. In fact, negative feelings about traditional hospital deliveries have become so widespread that home deliveries are increasing in many cities, often attended by a nurse-midwife instead of a professional doctor.

The physician and nurse or nurse-midwife can work as a team with the expectant couple. In some facilities the nurse-midwife assumes primary responsibility for the family unit. Whenever a mother delivers, she has the right to capable, safe care by qualified caretakers. Home deliveries can be carefully planned and safe. Hospital deliveries can be more homelike. Maternity centers now provide families anticipating a normal childbearing experience with antepartum care that is educational in nature; labor and delivery in a homelike setting (but with adequate equipment) and discharge to home whenever it is safe for mother and baby; and follow-up care by public health nurses in the home during the postpartum course. The labor and delivery rooms can be designed to accommodate the presence of the father or family during delivery and be less traumatic (cold, with intense lights) for the newborn. After the birth, the infant can remain with the mother, and the newborn's physical examination can be done in her presence with the father present. Childbirth should be a positive, maturing experience for the couple. Expectant parents have the right and responsibility to be involved in planning their care with the health team and to know what is happening. Cultural beliefs should be recognized, respected, and accommodated whenever possible. A positive childbearing experience contributes to a healthy family unit.

Postpartum Period

Because of short hospital stays following delivery of the baby (6–48 hours), you may not be able to give the traditional essential physical or emotional postpartum care. Instead, the care will be delivered in the home by the family, with the continuing support and assistance from a home health nurse or maternal–child advanced practice nurse who is a consultant. The following guidelines must be taught to the family member(s) who will be caring for the new mother and baby or carried out by the nurse in the home.

Realize that various cultural groups may have specific traditions that will be done in addition. Some populations, such as Mexican-Americans and Asian-Americans, carry out practices related to the hot–cold theory of concepts of yin and yang (see Chapter 1). The postpartum period is considered a cold or yin period. Practices related to balance of heat and cold, such as avoiding cold and contact with water, avoiding conflict in relationships, ambulation, dietary norms, and rituals to overcome what is considered the state of pollution of mother and baby after birth are described by Horn (61).

In the early postpartum period, assess mother and baby. Give the mother physical care and assist her as necessary, even if she looks well and able. Mother needs to be mothered to enhance bonding between mother and baby. Listen to the mother's (and father's) concerns; answer questions; support maternal and paternal behavior. In a nonthreatening way, teach the parents how to handle baby. Help them begin to unlearn preconceived ideas about the baby and to perceive self and the baby positively. If the mother is breastfeeding, teaching and assistance are necessary. After the initial "taking in" period of having received special care and attention, the mother moves to the "taking hold" stage where she is able to care for the child (18, 94, 95, 102, 115).

The interaction between the infant and primary caretaker is crucial. The mothering person helps the baby feel secure and loved, fosters a sense of trust, provides stimulation, reinforces certain behavior, acts as a model for language development, and trains the baby in basic learning strategies. In turn, maternal behavior is influenced by baby's cries, coos, smiles, activity, and gazes and by how well baby's behavior meets the mother's expectations.

Your significant contribution to the family unit is to promote attachment between parents and baby, encourage continuing contacts between the family and health professionals so that adequate health and illness care are received, and encourage parents to meet the baby's needs adequately. You can help the parents feel good about themselves and the baby.

You can be instrumental in continuing new trends in care to make the hospital or clinic environment more homelike while providing safe, modern care.

Continued Care in the Postpartum Period

During the *6 or 8 weeks after delivery*, the mother needs assistance with child care and an opportunity to regain her former self physically and emotionally. Father also needs support as he becomes involved in child-care responsibilities. In the nuclear or single-parent family the parent(s) may struggle alone. Continued visits by a home health nurse may be useful. Some communities have a crisis line for new parents. You may be able to suggest services or help the parent(s) think of people who could be helpful.

As you assess the mother's functioning, consider her physical and emotional energy, support systems,

and current level of parenting activity. If she apparently is not caring adequately for the child, assess for anemia, pain, bleeding, infections, lack of food or sleep, drug use, or other medical conditions that would interfere with her activity level and feelings of caring. Depression and postpartum blues are difficult to differentiate. In depression the mother is immobilized and forgets basic care, but with postpartum blues she may cry but care for the baby's physical needs.

The new mother usually has enough energy to do only top-priority tasks: eating, sleeping, baby care, and essentials for other family members. A house that is too clean is a danger signal that she is neglecting the baby, herself, or both.

The mother's support system is crucial for her energy maintenance, both physical and emotional. She needs direct support and assistance with daily tasks, plus moral support, a listener, a confidant. Support comes from personal and professional sources—the partner, parents, friends, other relatives, and the nurse, doctor, social worker, or pastor. Negative attitudes from others can drain emotional energy. Actual parenting skills can be manifested in various ways: touching, cuddling, a tender, soft voice tone, and loving gazes. Additional information about parents' feelings and the parenting process are described in Chapter 7.

If the baby is progressing in normal fashion, focus on the mother's needs and concerns. Help her find nonprofessional support systems that can assist her when the professional is unavailable or that can help with child care. In addition to concern over child care, we must help the mother grow developmentally. Helping her stay in good physical and emotional health ensures better parenting.

Care of Families Who Have a Child Born Prematurely or With Disability

Prematurity accounts for 50% of neonatal mortality, and premature infants who survive contribute significantly to the number of physically, intellectually, and emotionally disabled children in the United States. Complications of prematurity include major and minor physical abnormalities, general motor incoordination, short attention span, distractibility and hyperactivity, difficulty separating from parents, preoccupation with the body, and scholastic underachievement (102, 115).

The last complications may be related more to an early disturbed mother–child relationship than to prematurity, perinatal complications, or the child's birth defects. Typically the infant is rushed to the nursery after birth, thereby preventing physical or eye contact between mother and baby. The mother is often isolated from other mothers; professionals and family may avoid conversation about the baby. Mother often sees the baby in the premature or intensive care nursery at a distance and only indistinctly; or the baby may have been transported to a children's hospital at some distance so that visiting the baby after her discharge is difficult. The mother may have no opportunity to form any attachment feelings unless nursing staff foster the involvement in child care to the extent possible and keep her informed of baby's condition and progress. The baby who finally comes home to the parents may be a stranger for whom the parents have little response or commitment. Additionally, the mother has developed little confidence in her mothering abilities and no caretaking regimen.

Certain *behavior patterns in parents strongly suggest a disturbed parent–child relationship and future problems in parenting the premature or defective child,* for example, if the parent:

- Is unable to talk about guilt feelings, fears, and their sense of responsibility for the child's early arrival with each other or others
- Demonstrates no visible anxiety about the baby's condition, denies the reality, or displaces anxiety onto less-threatening matters
- Makes little effort to secure information about the baby's condition
- Consistently misinterprets or exaggerates either positive or negative information about the baby and displays no signs of hope as baby's condition improves
- Receives no practical support or help from family or friends, and community resources are lacking
- 6. Is unable to accept and use help offered

You may be instrumental in promoting *certain procedures that can be used to promote the parent–child relationship:*

- Permit the mother to see and touch the baby as soon as possible, preferably in the delivery room; or transfer the baby to the mother's room in a portable incubator if the baby remains in the same hospital.
- Permit the mother's involvement in baby's care as soon as possible. Take the mother to the premature care unit, teaching her to use the aseptic technique needed to touch, care for, and visit with the baby.
- Provide an atmosphere that encourages questions.

- Encourage parents to talk with each other, family members, and friends, using others for support.
- Recognize that parent's excessive questions, demands, and criticisms are a reaction to stress and not personal attacks on the professional worker or hospital.
- Do not offer reassuring cliches or comforting statements too quickly. Encourage parents to cry, to face the reality of the situation.
- Do not pressure parents to talk about their feelings all at once, but avoid using the excuse of "not wanting to probe" to avoid talking with them.
- Encourage the mother to express breast milk if she wishes; the breast milk can be taken to a breast-milk bank and used for the infant. When the baby is sucking well, the mother can help bottlefeed the baby until the baby is strong enough to breastfeed.
- Arrange for father to visit the baby before discharge, calling him about baby's progress at intervals when he is unable to visit.
- Encourage the parents to handle the baby and do baby's care before discharge; teach about baby care as necessary while the parents are engaged in care of their baby.

Refer also to Chapter 7 for additional information. The book by Featherstone (40) is a useful reference. It was one of the first books written that focuses on family issues that arise when there is a developmentally disabled child, on the system as a whole, on the marital subsystem, and on the sibling subsystem. Because of the chronicity of developmental disability or some congenital defects, the article by Woods, Yates, and Primomo (126) is a helpful reference.

Care of Families with Chronically Ill or Special-Needs Child

Families who have a *child with chronic illness or a special-needs child with developmental disabilities or chronic physical or emotional illness* experience a number of stressors in addition to the physical, emotional, and social burdens and financial costs of continuing care. Parents may feel like they want collaboration and control, but have no control over the care of and treatment consequences for their child, depending on the health care providers' approaches to the child and family. Some families passively depend on the professional providers for all directions. Parents experience a sense of loss, chronic sorrow, and ongoing grief and mourning process related to the ideal or normal child they expected, as they adapt their expectations to fit the real child they have. Ongoing physical care and guidance problems are constant reminders of developmental lag, that the child will not achieve certain developmental tasks and will remain dependent on someone, perhaps for life. There are continual, lifelong adjustments to the child and care. Parents worry about the child's care and quality of life in the future when they are unable to continue care. All family members react to the time and energy demands of a special-needs child, realizing that means less time and energy for each other or themselves. All family members will realize the effects of the financial drain on the previous standard of living. Financial stress includes more than cost of care; it also includes loss of employment or educational opportunities when a parent must either stop or reduce these activities because of child-care demands.

Marital stress occurs as parents negotiate parental roles and responsibilities, time, energy, and finances and reconcile career-versus-family demands. Career mobility, especially related to geographic moves, may occur because of dependence on a specific treatment agency or team or the employer's insurance plan. Divorce in families with special-needs children is not unusual.

Families with special-needs children need a social support system to maintain family stability and care adequately for the child. Social support may include an extended family, close friends, religious affiliation, parents of other children with special needs, and access to empathetic professionals. Extra effort is often needed to encourage these parents to participate in self-help or other groups, as they often do not develop or maintain social contacts, becoming more isolated. A family with adequate finances, who has lived in a community long enough to have developed contacts and friendships, who has a car and telephone, and who has a good understanding of and collaboration with the health care system will fare better than a family without any or all of these characteristics.

Health care professionals can develop family support groups to provide:

- Education about the diagnosis and how to cope with and treat it
- A place where parents can discuss their feelings and concerns and receive acceptance and empathy as they grieve losses in the situation
- Information about available services and resources in the community
- Assistance with fulfilling role responsibility and demand

- Assistance to parents to become advocates for their children in negotiating for services, education, and favorable legislation
- Social functions to reduce the sense of isolation the families may feel

Table 4–15 lists toll-free telephone numbers of organizations that can provide information for families with special needs children (127).

Parent Education

To combat the problems associated with the high adolescent birth rate, some junior and senior high schools are establishing creative programs in parenthood education. Some hospitals and health clinics are initiating

TABLE 4–15. TOLL-FREE TELEPHONE NUMBERS FOR SPECIAL-NEEDS INFORMATION

American Cancer Society	800–227–2345
American Cleft Palate Educational Foundation Cleftline	800–24–CLEFT
American Council for the Blind	800–424–8666
American Diabetes Association	800–682–9692
American Foundation for Liver	800-223–0179
American Kidney Fund	800–638–8299
Association for Retarded Citizens	800–433–5255
Beginnings (Hearing)	800–541–HEAR
Child Abuse/Parents Anonymous	800–421–0353
Cystic Fibrosis Foundation	800–344–4823
Epilepsy	800–642–0500
Fetal Alcohol Syndrome	800–532–6302
Lung Disease/Asthma Hotline	800–222–5864
National Association for Hearing and Speech Action (Voice or TDD)	800–638–TALK
National Down Syndrome Society	800–221–4602
National Hearing Aid Society	800–521–5247
National Information Center for Children and Youth	800–999–5599
National Organization for Rare Disorders	800–477–6673
National Reye's Syndrome Foundation	800–233–7393
National Spinal Cord Injury Hotline	800–526–3456
National Tuberous Sclerosis Association, Inc.	800–CAL–NTSA
Orton Dyslexia Society	800–222–3123
Shriners Hospitals for Crippled Children	800–237–5055
Sickle Cell Disease	800–421–8453
Spina Bifida Hotline	800–621–3141
Stuttering Hotline	800–221–2483
Sudden Infant Death Syndrome	800–232–7437

specialized prenatal and postnatal services for the adolescent mother and her at-risk infant. You can initiate nontraditional programs in your own community.

Some hospitals have established programs to help adolescent mothers become more effective parents. The adolescent mother who decides to keep her baby needs all the family and outside help she can get. She fears that whatever personal ambitions she has will be thwarted by the baby. Unmarried and unprepared for employment, she finds it almost impossible to make her own way in the world. Anger, frustration, and ignorance hamper her ability to attach to and appropriately care for the baby. Repeated pregnancies, child neglect and abuse, and welfare dependency often occur.

Formation of a mother's group, including women of various ethnic origins and income brackets, can provide parent education and support and foster talking about feelings. You should also educate parents about using community resources.

Your work with the mother may prevent maternal deprivation, insufficient interaction between mother and child, conditions under which deprivation or even abuse develops, and negative effects on the child's development.

Working With Adoptive Families

You can help the adoptive parents in their adjustment. Assure them that attachment develops over time. Help them think through how and when to tell the child that he or she is adopted so that the child understands and is not traumatized. Help the parents anticipate how they will help the child cope when the child is taunted by peers about being adopted. Help them realize that the adopted child will probably seek answers to many questions when he or she gets older. Who were the parents? Their cultural, racial, or ethnic background? Their ages, occupations, interests, appearance? Why was he or she relinquished? What are the medical facts surrounding heredity and birth? Help parents realize that these questions do not mean that the child does not love them. Various articles supply information on adoption procedures, stresses encountered, and how to make adoption a success (24, 25, 26, 36, 50, 67, 71, 91, 99, 120, 122).

Working With Stepfamilies

The guidelines already discussed will be useful to you as you help the single-parent family or stepfamily adjust to its situation. The single-parent family can be referred to a local chapter of Parents Without Partners if the person seeks support from peers. Do not rush in with answers for these families until you have heard their unique problems. Acknowledge their strengths; help them formulate their own solutions. Often a few sessions of crisis therapy will be sufficient. Several references give further information (47, 67, 90, 97, 116, 117, 124).

Family Care Throughout the Life Cycle

You may be called on to assist families as they meet various developmental crises throughout the life cycle: school entry of the child, the adolescent period, children leaving home, divorce, retirement, death of a member. Your goal is health promotion and primary prevention. Your intervention early in the family life cycle may help establish a positive health trend in place of its negative counterpart. The care you give to young parents lays the foundation for their children's health. You may also find yourself becoming an advocate for families in relation to state or federal legislation that affects families and child care.

Another way to improve the family as an institution is from within. Parents should teach their children not just to get ahead but to serve, to cooperate, to be kind. We should be teaching our children to believe that family ties are the most rewarding values, that social, cultural and community activities can be deeply satisfying, and that the gratification from income and jobs is not the main priority (14, 18, 37, 68, 75, 115).

Our excessive competitiveness is being passed on to our children as parents try to produce "superkids." Misplaced educational pressure is likely to produce lopsided development and an aversion to schooling. To diminish the competitive atmosphere in schools, grades and examination could be dropped. Excessive competiveness overlaps with excessive materialism. In most parts of the world materialism is balanced by spiritual values (e.g., dedication to God in Islamic countries, dedication to the nation in Israel, dedication to the family in Greece). By contrast, in the United States many children get their values—materialism, competitiveness, and brutality—from television. In turn, rates for violent crime are shockingly high. Parents should demand good programs from television producers and forbid their children's watching the violence and sordid sex. It is no wonder some youths panic at finding they have no supporting beliefs and turn to extremist cults and lifestyles and that the rate of teenage suicide has tripled in the past 20 years (14, 18, 37, 68, 75, 115).

Parents can make a profound difference by teaching spiritual values—helpfulness, cooperation, generosity, love—throughout childhood. Two-year-old children can be encouraged to help set the table and then be thanked and praised. Teenagers can be expected to work in hospitals and to tutor younger children. Such jobs should not be presented as distasteful. Children enjoy taking on adult jobs when they are presented as opportunities and efforts are appreciated (14).

Just as vital is a family atmosphere in which parents treat each other and their children with respect and affection and smile. The best forum is still mealtime and the family meeting. When teenagers first give excuses why they cannot make it to a meal, parents should say very positively, "We like to have the whole family get together." Parents should avoid talking down to children and the attitude that being older makes them right but they can still be very clear about their beliefs and expectations (14, 18, 37, 75).

Parents must give careful attention to the topic of sex. We have done well to overcome the shame that used to surround sex; but in declaring sex more wholesome and natural, we have mistakenly ignored its tenderness, generosity, and intensely spiritual aspects. We have failed to instill that the impulse in idealistic youths to save intimacy for the ultimate partner has existed for centuries and has contributed to creativity in all the arts (23).

When parents are asked questions about sexual matters by 2-, 3-, and 4-year-old children, they should advance from anatomy and physiology to emphasize the loving and caring aspects of sex and marriage. An even greater influence on children is their parents' behavior toward and commitment to a partner and their admiration and respect for one another. Joking and disparaging remarks about marriage should be avoided. Parents can suggest that if young people want to claim the right to sexual freedom, they should be aware of the responsibilities. If a youthful marriage soon ends in divorce, parents can point out that no marriage succeeds by itself but must be continually cultivated, like a garden. It is wise to look for openings to discuss these topics when children are 9, 10, or 11 years of age. When they are 13 years old and beyond, they think their parents are hopelessly old-fashioned and consider peer opinions as the only truth (14, 75).

If we allow the strains of our society to worsen, then living here will be ever more painful. In our democracy we can control our society by guiding our children and using our political power. We need to move from an emphasis on ambitious individualism and self-centeredness into cooperation for the common good. We need leaders who have vision and courage, and we need mature parents who present a positive model for the future of the family and society.

SUMMARY

- There are various types of family structures and systems.
- You will care for clients who may come from a family background quite different from your own family system in structure and dynamic relationships.
- People who come from the same type of family structure, for example, matrifocal, homosexual, will be different from each other.
- All families, regardless of structure, share similar developmental tasks.
- Family relationships and dynamic processes and the extent to which developmental tasks are met within the family are a major influence on development and health.
- You will practice principles of family-centered care, based on concepts in this chapter, in every health care setting.
- Engage in life-long learning about your own and other family systems to assess, plan, and provide comprehensive care to the client and family.

► REFERENCES

1. Ackerman, N., *Diagnosis and Treatment of Family Relations*. New York: Basic Books, 1972.
2. Allen, M., Primary care nursing: Research in action. In L. Hockey, ed., *Recent Advances in Nursing: Primary Care Nursing*. Edinburgh: Churchill-Livingstone, 1983, pp. 32–77.
3. American Nurses' Association, *Nursing's Agenda for Health Care Reform*. Kansas City, MO: American Nurses' Association, 1991.
4. Ames, K., S. Lewis, P. Kaudell, D. Rosenberg, and F. Chideya, Cheaper by the Dozen, *Newsweek*, September 14 (1992), 52–53.
5. Anderson, M., The Mental Health Advantages of Twinship, *Perspectives of Psychiatric Care*, 23, no. 3 (1985), 114–116.
6. Barnhill, L.R., Healthy Family Systems. *The Family Coordinator*, 28 (1979), 94–100.
7. Barth, R., and M. Berry, *Adoption and Disruption: Rates, Risks, and Responses*. Hawthorne, NY: Aldine de Gruyter, 1988.
8. Bauer, G., American Family Life Worth Expecting, *Focus on the Family*, July (1994), 2–3.
9. Beavers, R., and R. Hampson, *Successful Families: Assessment and Intervention*. New York: W.W. Norton, 1990.
10. Bell, A., M. Weinberg, and S. Hammersmith, *Sexual Preference: Its Development in Men and Women*. Bloomington, IN: Indiana University Press, 1981.
11. Bell, J.M., The Dysfunction of "Dysfunctional," *Journal of Family Nursing, 1*, no. 3 (1995), 235–237.
12. Benedek, T., Parenthood During the Life Cycle. In Anthony, E.J., and Benedek, T. eds., *Parenthood: Its Psychology and Psychopathology*. Boston: Little, Brown, 1970, pp. 185–206.

13. Betta, R., and Musi, D., Families South of the Border: Mexico—Trading Its Values, *Focus on the Family,* July (1995), 6.

14. Bettelheim, B., *A Good Enough Parent: A Book on Child-Rearing.* New York: Alfred A. Knopf, 1987.

15. Blankenhorn, D., *Fatherless America: Confronting Our Most Urgent Social Problem.* New York: Basic Books, 1995.

16. Booth, J., British Families: Loss of a Stiff Upper Lip? *Focus on the Family,* July (1995), 5.

17. Borisov, B., Russian Families Caught in a Wave of Changes, *Focus on the Family,* July (1994), 11.

18. Bossard, J., and E. Boll, *Sociology of Child Development* (4th ed.). New York: Harper & Row, 1960.

19. Bowen, M., *Family Therapy in Clinical Practice.* New York: Jason Aronson, 1978.

20. Bowlby, J., The Making and Breaking of Affectional Bonds, *British Journal of Psychiatry,* 130 (March 1977), 201–210.

21. Bozett, F., ed., *Gay and Lesbian Parents.* New York: Preager, 1987.

22. ———, Social Control of Identity by Children of Gay Fathers, *Western Journal of Nursing Research,* 10, no. 5 (1988), 550–565.

23. Bozett, F., and S. Hanson, eds. *Fatherhood and Families in Cultural Context.* New York: Springer, 1991.

24. Brockhaus, J., and R. Brockhaus, Adopting an Older Child—The Emotional Process, *American Journal of Nursing,* 82, no. 2 (1982), 288–291.

25. ———, Adopting a Child With Special Needs: The Legal Process, *American Journal of Nursing,* 82, no. 2 (1982), 291–294.

26. ———, Foster Care, Adoption, and the Grief Process, *Journal of Psychiatric Nursing and Mental Health Services,* 20, no. 9 (1982), 9–16.

27. Broderick, C.B., *Understanding Family Process: Basics of Family Systems Theory.* Newbury Park, CA: Sage, 1993.

28. Carlson, G., When Grandmothers Take Care of Grandchildren, *MCN: American Journal of Maternal–Child Nursing,* 18 (1993), 206–207.

29. Carmichael, C., *Nonsexist Childraising.* Boston: Beacon Press, 1977.

30. Cass, V., Homosexual Identity Formation: A Theoretical Model, *Journal of Homosexuality,* 4, no. 3 (1985), 219–235.

31. Center for the Future of Children, *The Future of Children: Children and Divorce,* 4, no. 1 (1994), 1–247.

32. Clinton, J., Expectant Fathers at Risk for Couvade, *Nursing Research,* 35, no. 5 (1986), 290–294.

33. Coleman, P., *The Forgiving Marriage.* Chicago, Contemporary Books, 1989.

34. Curran, D., *Traits of a Healthy Family,* New York: Balantine, 1983.

35. Dugan, A., Compadrazgo: A Caring Phenomenon Among Urban Latinos and Its Relationship to Health. In Leininger, M., ed., *Care: The Essence of Nursing and Health,* Detroit: Wayne State University Press, 1988, pp. 183–194.

36. Dunn, L., ed., *Adopting Children with Special Needs: A Sequel,* Washington, DC: North American Council on Adoptable Children, 1983.

37. Duvall, E., and B. Miller, *Marriage and Family Development* (6th ed.), New York: Harper & Row, 1984.

38. Erikson, E., *Childhood and Society* (2nd ed.), New York: W.W. Norton, 1963.

39. Family Aggression May Compound Hyperactivity in Children, *The Menninger Letter,* 3, no. 11 (1995), 6–7.

40. Featherstone, H., *A Difference in the Family.* New York: Penguin Books, 1981.

41. Forchuk, C., Peplau's Theory: Concepts and Their Relations, *Nursing Science Quarterly,* 4, no. 2 (1991), 54–59.

42. ———, and B. Brown, Establishing a Nurse–Client Relationship, *Journal of Psychosocial Nursing,* 27, no. 2 (1989), 30–34.

43. Ford-Gilboe, M., Family Strengths, Motivation, and Resources as Predictors of Health Promotion Behavior in Single-parent and Two-parent Families. Unpublished dissertation. Detroit: Wayne State University, 1994.

44. Friedman, M., *Family Nursing: Theory and Assessment* (2nd ed.). Norwalk, CT: Appleton-Century-Crofts, 1985.

45. Furstenberg, F., History and Current Status of Divorce in the United States, *The Future of Children: Children and Divorce,* 4, no. 1 (1994), 37–40.

46. Gantz, J., *Whose Child Cries: Children of Gay Parents Talk About Their Lives.* Rolling Hills Estates, CA: View Press, 1983.

47. Gardner, R., *Psychotherapy With Children of Divorce.* New York: Jason Aronson, 1976.

48. Garrison, J., Part 7: Gay in America, A Special Report: Creating New Families. *San Francisco Examiner,* June 12 (1989), Sect. A, p 17.

49. Gieleghem, P., Discovery of the Couvade Phenomenon: Theory and Clinical Uses. In Leininger, M., ed., *Care: Discovery and Uses in Clinical and Community Nursing.* Detroit: Wayne State University Press, 1988.

50. Gil, O., and B. Jackson, *Adoption and Race: Black, Asian, and Mixed-Race Children in White Families.* New York: St. Martin's Press, 1983.

51. Goodrich, T., et al: *Feminist Family Therapy.* New York: W.W. Norton, 1988.

52. Gordon, T., *Parent Effectiveness Training.* New York: Peter H. Wyden, 1970.

53. Greenberg, M., and N. Morris, Engrossment: The Newborn's Impact Upon the Father, *American Journal of Orthopsychiatry,* 44, no. 4 (1974), 520–531.

54. Hall, L., Family Life in Canada, *Focus on the Family,* July (1994), 4.

55. Hammond, T., and C. Deans, A Phenomenological Study of Families and Psychoeducation Support Groups, *Journal of Psychosocial Nursing,* 33, no. 10 (1995), 7–12.

56. Hanson, S., Healthy single-parent families. *Family Relations,* 35 (1986), 125–132.

57. Harris, M., and P. Turner, Gay and Lesbian Parents, *Journal of Homosexuality,* 12, no. 2 (1986), 101–113.

58. Hartrick, G., A.E. Lindsey, and A. Hills, Family Nursing Assessment: Meeting the Challenge of Health Promotion, *Journal of Advanced Nursing,* 20, no. 1 (1995), 85–91.

59. Holtzworth-Monroe, A., Marital Violence, *The Harvard Mental Health Letter,* 12, no. 2 (1995), 4–6.

60. Hoopes, M., and J. Harper, *Birth Order Roles and Sibling Patterns in Individual and Family Therapy.* Rockville, MD: Aspen, 1987.

61. Horn, B., Cultural Concepts and Postpartal Care, *Journal of Transcultural Nursing,* 2, no. 1 (1990), 48–51.

62. Hott, J., The Crisis of Expectant Fatherhood, *American Journal of Nursing,* 76, no. 9 (1976), 1436–1440.

63. Hutchins, D., and C. Cole, *Helping Relationships and Strategies* (2nd ed.). Belmont, CA: Brooks/Cole, 1992.

64. Iida, C., Is the Sun Setting on the Family, *Focus on the Family,* June (1994), 14.

65. Jansen, L.T., Measuring Family Solidarity. *American Sociological Review,* 17 (1952), 727–733.

66. Jendrek, M., Grandparents Who Parent Their Grandchildren: Circumstances and Decisions, *Gerontologist,* 34 (1994), 206–216.

67. Jolley, J., and M. Mitchell, *Lifespan Development: A Topical Approach.* Madison, WI: Brown & Benchmark, 1996.

68. Kahana, E., D. Biegel, and M. Wykle, *Family Caregiving Across the Lifespan.* Thousand Oaks, CA: Sage, 1994.

69. Kirkpatrick, M., C. Smith, and R. Roy, Lesbian Mothers and Their Children: A Comparative Survey, *Journal of Orthospsychiatry,* 51, no. 3 (1981), 545–557.

70. Kramer, J., *Family Interfaces: Transgenerational Patterns.* New York: Brunner/Mazel, 1987.

71. Krementz, J., *How It Feels to Be Adopted.* New York: Alfred Knopf, 1982.

72. Lamb, M., *The Father's Role.* New York: John Wiley & Sons, 1986.

73. Lamb, M., The Emergent American Father. In Lamb,M. ed., *The Father's Role: Cross Cultural Perspectives.* Hillsdale, NJ: Erlbaum, 1987.

74. LaRossa, R., Fatherhood and Social Change, *Family Relations,* 37, 451–457.

75. Lidz, T., *The Person: His and Her Development Throughout the Life Cycle* (2nd ed.). New York: Basic Books, 1983.

76. McFarlane, A., A Nursing Reformulation of Bowen's Family Systems Theory, *Archives of Psychiatric Nursing,* 2 (1988), 319–324.

77. McLanahan, S., and G. Sandefur, *Growing up With a Single Parent.* Cambridge, MA: Harvard University Press, 1994.

78. Messer, A., *The Individual in His Family: An Adaptational Study.* Springfield, IL: Charles C Thomas, 1970.

79. Minuchin, S., *Family Kaleidoscope.* Cambridge, MA: Harvard University Press, 1984.

80. Montgomery, P., Should Surrogate Motherhood Be Banned? *Common Cause Magazine,* May/June (1988), 36–38.

81. Murray, R., and M. Huelskoetter, *Psychiatric/Mental Health Nursing: Giving Emotional Care* (3rd ed.). Norwalk, CT: Appleton & Lange, 1991.

82. Olson, D., *2001: Preparing Families For the Future.* Minneapolis, MN: Bolger Publications/Creative Printing, 1990.

83. Otto, H.A., Criteria for Assessing Family Strengths, *Canada's Mental Health,* 6 (1966), 257.

84. Parental Work Load Affects Adolescents, *The Menninger Letter,* 3, no. 11 (1995), 6.

85. Peplau, H., *Interpersonal Relations in Nursing.* New York: G.P. Putnam's Sons, 1952.

86. ———, *Basic Principles of Patient Counseling* (2nd ed.). Philadelphia: Smith, Kline & French Laboratories, 1969.

87. ———, Talking With Patients, *American Journal of Nursing,* 70, no. 7 (1970), 964–966.

88. Petze, C., Health Promotion for the Well Family, *Nursing Clinics of North America,* 19, no. 2 (1984), 229–237.

89. Poponoe, D., The Controversial Truth, *New York Times,* December 26 (1992), A-21.

90. Reder, N., Single Parents/Dual Responsibilities, *The National Voter,* 39, no. 1 (1989), 9–11.

91. Ritchie, C., Adoption: An Option Often Overlooked, *American Journal of Nursing,* 89, no. 9 (1989), 1156–1157.

92. Rodriguez, R., Families South of the Border: Costa Rica—Paradise Lost? *Focus on the Family,* July (1995), 6–7.

93. Rogers, C., *Client-Centered Therapy.* Boston: Houghton Mifflin, 1951.

94. Rubin, R., Attainment of the Maternal Role. Part 1: Processes, *Nursing Research,* 16, no. 3 (1967), 237–245.

95. ———, Attainment of the Maternal Role. Part II: Models and Referrants, *Nursing Research,* 16, no. 4 (1967), 342–346.

96. Sagan, L., Family Ties: The Real Reason That People Are Living Longer. *Annual Editions: Health, 89/90.* Norwalk, CT: Dushkin Press, 1989.

97. Sager, C., et al., *Treating the Remarried Family.* New York: Brunner/Mazel, 1983.

98. Satir, V., Love, Understanding, Communication Are Vital Elements of Family Health, *Parameters,* 4, no. 3 (1979), 8–10.

99. Schaffer, J., and C. Londstrum, *How to Raise an Adopted Child.* New York: Crown, 1989.

100. Shavelson, E., et al., Lesbian Women's Perception of Their Parent–Child Relationships, *Journal of Homosexuality,* 5, no. 3 (1980), 205–215.

101. Shepherd, E., The Multicultural Families Down Under, *Focus on the Family,* July (1994), 13.

102. Sherwen, L., M. Scoloreno, and C. Wengerten, *Nursing Care of the Childbearing Family* (2nd ed). Norwalk, CT: Appleton-Lange, 1991.

103. Smilkstein, G., The Cycle of Family Function: A Conceptual Model for Family Medicine, *Family Practitioner,* 11 (1980), 223.

104. Smith, S., Big Families Can Be Happy, Too, *Newsweek,* January 14 (1985), 12–13.

105. Smoyak, S.A., General Systems Model: Principles and General Applications. In Reynolds, W., and Cormack, D. eds., *Psychiatric and Mental Health Nursing: Theory and Practice.* New York: Chapman & Hall, 1990, pp. 133–152.

106. ———, Changing American Families. In Hoekelman, R., S. Friedman, N. Nelson, and Seidel, H. eds., *Primary Pediatric Care* (2nd ed.). St. Louis: Mosby, 1992.

107. Soloman, J., and J. Marx, To Grandmother's House We Go: Health and School Adjustment of Children Raised Solely by Grandparents, *The Gerontologist,* 35 (1995), 386–394.

108. Starkey, P., Genograms: A Guide to Understanding One's Own Family System, *Perspectives of Psychiatric Care,* 14, nos. 5 and 6 (1987), 164–173.

109. Stuart, W., European Families: Old Customs, New Morality, *Focus on the Family,* July (1995), 10.

110. Taylor, M., and J. Gardner, African Families: Turbulent Times Ahead, *Focus on the Family,* July (1994), 12.

111. Terkelson, K., Toward a Theory of the Family Life Cycle. In Carter, E., and McGoldrich, M. eds., *The Family Life Cycle: A Framework for Family Therapy.* New York: Gardner Press, 1980, pp. 21–52.

112. Toman, W., *Family Constellation* (3rd ed.). New York: Springer, 1976.

113. Travelbee, J., *Interpersonal Aspects of Nursing.* Philadelphia: F.A. Davis, 1967.

114. ———, *Intervention in Psychiatric Nursing.* Philadelphia: F.A. Davis, 1969.

115. Turner, J., and D. Helms, *Lifespan Development* (5th ed.). Ft. Worth, TX: Harcourt Brace College, 1995.

116. Visher, E., and J. Visher, *Step Families: A Guide to Working With Step Parents and Step Children.* New York: Brunner/Mazel, 1979.

117. ———, *Old Loyalties, New Ties: Therapeutic Strategies with Stepfamilies.* New York: Brunner/Mazel, 1988.

118. Von Bertalanffy, L. (1968). *General System Theory.* New York: Braziller, 1968.

119. Wachtel, E., and P. Wachtel, *Family Dynamics in Individual Psychotherapy: A Guide to Clinical Strategies.* New York: Guilford Press, 1986.

120. Ward, M., Parental Bonding in Older Child Adoptions, *Child Welfare,* 40, no. 1 (1981), 24–34.

121. Warda, M., The Family and Chronic Sorrow: Role Theory Approach. *Journal of Pediatric Nursing,* 7 (1992), 205–206.

122. Warren, A., Adopting a Foreign Child, *Better Homes and Gardens,* 63, no. 10 (1985), 25–27.

123. Warshaw, R., Can Grandparent Caregivers Find Help? *Modern Maturity,* July–August (1995), 28.

124. Whall, A., *Nursing Approach to Family Therapy.* New York: Brady, 1994.

125. Willie, C., *A New Look at the Black Family.* Bayside, NY: Bayside Press, 1976.

126. Woods, N., B. Yates, and J. Primomo, Supporting Families During Chronic Illness, *IMAGE: Journal of Nursing Scholarship,* 21, no. 1 (1989), 46–50.

127. Worthington, R., Family Support Networks: Help for Families of Children with Special Needs, *Family Medicine,* 24, no. 1 (1992), 141–144.

128. Wright, L., and M. Leahey, *Nursing Families: A Guide to Family Assessment and Intervention* (2nd ed.). Philadelphia: F.A Davis, 1994.

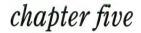

chapter five

Overview: Theories Related to Human Development

No theory explains everything about the person.

—*Ruth Beckmann Murray*

Key Terms

Psychology

Heterozygous

Homozygous

Monozygotic twins

Dizygotic twins

Polygenic inheritance

Principle of differential susceptibility

Principle of differential exposure

Neurotransmitters

Localization of brain function

Biorhythms

Ecology

Anomie

System

Social system

Open system

Closed system

Linkage

Behaviorists

Neo-Behaviorists

Learning

Shaping

Classical conditioning

Behaviorism

Instrumental conditioning

Operant conditioning

Transfer

Positive reinforcement

Negative reinforcement

Reinforcement schedule

Punishment

Extinction

Behavior modification

Shaping

Contract

Psychoanalytic theory

Psychodynamic perspective

Id

Tension

Primary process thinking

Ego

Reality principle

Secondary process thinking

Superego

Ego ideal

Conscience

Conscious

Preconscious

Unconscious

Anxiety

One Genus Postulate

Prototaxic mode of experiencing

Parataxic mode of experiencing

Syntaxic mode of experiencing

Concept of anxiety

Self-system

Consciousness

Persona

Shadow

Anima/animus

Personal unconscious

Collective unconscious

Mandalas

Individuation

Introversion

Extrovert

Cognitive psychology

Modeling

Maturational	Decenter	Distress	Psychosomatic or
Learning	Existentialism	Local adaptation syndrome	psychophysiologic
Equilibration	Humanism	General adaptation syndrome	Somatopsychic
Assimilation	Phenomenal field	Alarm stage	Psychoneuroimmunology
Accommodation	Self-actualization	Stage of resistance	Crisis
Adaptation	Stress	Protective factors	Transition
Schema	Stressors	Stage of exhaustion	Developmental crises
Egocentric	Eustress	Mind–body relationship	Situational crisis
Anthropomorphic	Daily hassles		

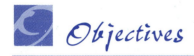

Objectives

Study of this chapter will enable you to:

1. Identify major theoretic perspectives for understanding the developing person.

2. Describe some physiologic theories about aspects of the developing person.

3. Discuss Ecologic Theory as it applies to the developing person.

4. Identify major psychological developmental theorists, according to their views about the developing person.

5. Compare major concepts of Behavioral, Psychoanalytic and Neo-Analytic, Cognitive, Existential, and Humanistic theories.

6. Describe and relate major concepts of Stress and Crisis theories.

7. Apply concepts from at least three theories of development in care of the client.

PROGRESSION OF STUDY OF HUMAN DEVELOPMENT

In the past, human development was considered something that just happened. Children at first were seen as little adults, only weaker and less capable. Gradually children were seen as different, not only in proportion, but in needs and characteristics. Until the 20th century, the study of child development and advice on how to care for children was not based on the scientific method but on biases and folklore.

During the 18th century scientific, religious, economic, and social trends combined to foster the study of child development. The "nature versus nurture" argument began. The child was considered the product of either heredity or environment. With the rise of Protestantism, which emphasized self-reliance, independence, and responsibility for self and others, adults began to feel more responsible for how the child developed into an adult. With the Industrial Revolution, the family changed from a clanlike group to the nuclear family, and children became more visible and more important to their parents. In turn, parents concentrated more intensely on their offspring. Education was provided for children, and teachers became important in the child's development. As the spirit of democracy filtered into the home, parents became more uncomfortable about autocratic attitudes toward and discipline of children. Eventually the science of **psychology,** *the study of human behavior,* led people to understand themselves better by learning more about child behavior. By the 19th century all these forces had come together, and the study of the child was more common and systematic. Yet the study of child development was not based on the variety or sophistication of theory that was to evolve during the 20th century (121).

The study of development, which began with study of the child, expanded in the beginning of the 20th century to include adolescence as a transitional period of life. In the early 20th century the study of the aged person began. By the mid-20th century, as more people were living longer, the study of aging and the aged person became popular. The study of young adulthood and middle age as developmental periods is a phenomenon of the past two or three decades. In the last quarter of the 20th century, the focus is on the study of human development through the life span.

Persons continue to develop or undergo change—physically, emotionally, cognitively, spiritually, and socially—throughout the life span. Dying is seen as the last developmental phase, the final attempt to come to terms with self, others, and life in general. The study of the changes made by the individual and the family unit throughout the life span is the focus of this book. By learning more about ourselves and others, including how people respond to surrounding influences to meet basic needs, we hope to help people become better able to meet their individual potential and, in turn, create a better world.

Theories that are used to explain the developing person and the person's behavior use either a biological, ecologic–social, or psychological basis. Although we focus on the psychological theories, a brief explanation of biological and ecologic–social theories is given. The psychological theories are divided according to their emphases: behaviorism, analytic, cognitive, and humanistic. Theorists who focus on these various psychological theories have been grouped according to similarity of theories.

Keep in mind that any theory explains an aspect of the person. *The whole person is best understood when several theories are combined to explain the person's total development.* The theories have been developed by one or several methods for studying people.

BIOLOGICAL THEORIES

Basic to the person is his or her anatomic and physiologic structure and function. Various areas of the brain control certain functions and influence development and behavior. The concept that behavior is an expression of neural activity is central to the philosophy of modern neuroscience. The mind represents a range of brain functions—simple to complex, including motion, sensory, cognitive and affective functions. The brain controls behavior—how we perceive, think, feel, behave, act, and interact. The two halves of the brain are mutually involved in all high levels of psychological functioning. Each hemisphere functions independently in perception, learning, and memory (see Table 5–1); however, consciousness and the conscious self are single and unified, mediated by brain processes that span both hemispheres. Consciousness is a dynamic result of brain activity, neither identical with, nor reducible to, the neural events of which it is composed. Consciousness is an active integral part of the cerebral process; it exerts control over the biophysical and chemical activities at subordinate levels (180).

The huge quantity and vast range of sensory information that is transmitted to the cerebral cortex and the way in which the brain sorts, classifies, organizes, and interprets sensory information; handles input and output; considers expectations, past experiences, and other sources of information; and sends messages throughout the body are beyond the capability of any computer system. In many ways the human brain may be like that of other animals, but it differs in its capacity to think, make judgments, remember, use symbols, store maps of the body and the world, and create.

Research on the physiologic basis for behavior has gained sophistication with advancing technology in studying the brain and nervous system, endocrine and immune functions, and physiologic responses in a variety of situations. These findings affect current beliefs about health, normality, and development. In the following discussion, theories related to genetic, biochemical, and neurophysiologic factors are covered briefly. For comprehensive study, refer to references listed at the end of the chapter (67, 89, 91, 121). Also, Chapters 6 and 7 through 14 present physiologic factors that affect the person.

Genetic Factors

Understanding of the role of genetic factors has been derived historically from studies focusing on pedigree descriptions, incidence of abnormalities in generations of families, and more recently in direct visual examination of chromosomes and biochemical analyses of genetic material and enzymatic processes (105).

The Mendelian Law of Inheritance states that a dominant gene for a trait or characteristic in at least one parent will cause, on the average, one-half of the children to inherit it. If both parents have the dominant gene, three-fourths of their children will inherit the trait. When the trait is attributed to a recessive gene, the offspring does not inherit it unless the gene was received from both parents. If the gene was received from only one parent, the offspring is not affected but will probably pass on the gene to the child (the grandchild). If the spouses are **heterozygous** for a recessive gene (*both received the same gene type from only one of their parents*), one-fourth of the children probably will be affected. If the spouses are **homozygous** for the recessive gene (the *same gene type was received from both of*

TABLE 5–1. RIGHT BRAIN–LEFT BRAIN INFORMATION PROCESSING DIFFERENCES

Mode	Left Brain (Controls Right Side of Body)	Right Brain (Controls Left Side of Body)
Thinking	Time bound Rational, logical, sequential or linear, analytical, interpretive Synthesis of sensory input	Space bound Concrete, appears irrational Artistic Intuitive; holistic Spirituality
Language	Hearing words Writing words Voice recognition Reading Speech comprehension Verbal memory	Metaphoric Singing songs Face and form recognition Draw figures Body image
Mathematics	Algebraic functions, adding, subtracting, multiplying, dividing	Geometric, spatial, relational
Problem solving	Focus on specifics Breaks problems into parts, linear, sequential Details	Focus on generalities Grasps problem in totality Grasps relational dimensions Patterns
Organizational	Action mode-primed to manipulate environment Focal attention Heightened boundary perception Object oriented Dominance of formal over sensory	Receptive mode-primed to take in environment Diffuse attention Boundary fusion Dominance of sensory over formal
Interactional	Controlled, consistent Explicit, directed, objective, judgmental, evaluative	Emotive Affect-laden Tacit Tolerant of ambiguity, subjective Nonjudgmental, noncritical
Operational	Figures things out in stepwise order One idea follows another Comfortable with precise connotations, right/wrong Computer-like functions Memory for verbal and auditory stimuli	Makes leaps of intuition Creativity Pattern recognition and relationships form basis of ideas Comfortable with alternatives and multiple explanations, nonlinguistic stimuli

their parents), all the children probably will inherit the trait or characteristic (67, 121).

To isolate environmental factors from genetic effects, researchers have used several methodologic designs, such as the family resemblance method, the twin study method, and a combination of the two. The family resemblance method looks for similarity between a person with a disorder and his or her relatives. The twin study method relies on differences between **monozygotic twins** (*from a single ovum and therefore identical*) and between **dizygotic twins** (*from two ova fertilized by two sperm and therefore not identical, i.e., fraternal twins.*) For example, one study indicates the correlation for depressive symptoms is highest among identical twins. Twin studies indicate that there is a stable predis-

position to temperament and that environment of the child contributes little to adult depression (91); however, recent stressful events were a powerful predictor for onset of illness in those genetically predisposed. Genetic factors may alter the person's response to the depression-inducing effect of stressors such as death of a close relative, assault, severe marital problems, and divorce (92). Monozygotic twins have been found to resemble each other more in mood level and lability than dizygotic twins. Research is also being done on identical and fraternal twins reared apart (67, 123).

The Mendelian law explains the occurrence of many physical traits such as eye color and height and may explain certain physiologic characteristics; *however, the Mendelian law does not fully explain emotional or mental development and does not include social, moral, or spiritual development.*

Genes determine a foundation for reaction or predisposition; the exact behavioral expression depends on many prenatal, parental, and postnatal influencing factors. For example, a specific chromosomal aberration such as the presence of an extra chromosome is directly related to Down syndrome, with resultant limited intellectual function. Yet the intellectual achievement may be lower than the inherited capacity if the person receives inadequate education, and the achievement may be somewhat higher than indicated by early testing when a loving family and appropriate education coexist to develop fully the inherited potential (123).

Deoxyribonucleic acid (DNA) is the genetic command center of every human cell. When DNA strands have defects, disease occurs. Some of the mutations may be inherited. Research is currently underway to develop a test to reveal risk for certain diseases based on genetic defects, which would enable us to determine ways to prevent illness related to risk factors (123).

Further, **polygenic inheritance,** the *combination of many genes acting together to produce a behavioral characteristic,* is believed to be a factor if certain characteristics or behavioral defects occur. Environmental effects contribute to the person's development of genetic potential from the moment of conception (82, 88, 121). For example, three factors determine cholesterol levels: presence of a single gene, polygenetic inheritance, and environment. One gene plays a key role in determining serum cholesterol levels and subsequent risk for coronary artery disease. This gene causes blood cholesterol levels of 300 mg/dL and results in heart attacks between 30 and 39 years of age for men and in the sixties for women; however, it is found in only 3% of the population. Polygenetic inheritance determines blood cholesterol levels (120–300 mg/dL). Environmental factors that increase risk include cigarette smoking, inactivity, stress, and diet.

Cholesterol levels below 160 mg/dL are at a preventive level; 10% of the population fall into this category. These individuals need not worry about coronary artery disease, regardless of environmental factors or diet. People with levels above 180 mg/dL should have the ratio of high-density lipoproteins to low-density lipoproteins measured. Low-density lipoproteins carry most of the cholesterol in the blood, whereas high-density lipoproteins (the so-called "good lipoproteins") carry cholesterol to the liver for metabolism or removal from the body (184).

Practice applications are apparent because of the rapidly advancing knowledge about genetics and health care, and requests for genetic services will be affected. A 2-year grant project, "Managing Genetic Information: Policies for U.S. Nurses," was funded by the Center for Human Genome Research at the National Institutes for Health and was coordinated by the American Nurses Association's Center for Ethics and Human Rights. The purpose of the project was to collect data about how genetic information can be used in practice and ethical, legal, and social concerns related to genetic engineering and services. There are a number of practice implications, including the need to (80, 125, 183):

- Obtain a genetic history as part of assessment.
- Explain diagnostic tests related to genetic-based disease and the meaning of positive and negative results.
- Provide emotional support to persons with genetic disorders and to their families.
- Offer genetic screening and testing to those who do not request it.
- Address ethical issues related to expansion of genetic information, such as reproductive issues, individual rights, confidentiality, and treatment issues.
- Learn about gene therapy, gene transfer, rationale, and constraints.
- Realize that genetic tests can tell the client if she or he carries the disease but do not predict if the person will eventually be diagnosed with the disease.
- Teach that with positive genetic findings, environmental or other events may have to occur before a disease, such as cancer or depression, is manifested.
- Teach that with negative genetic findings, not having a gene for a disease does not mean that the disease will not occur, for other reasons.
- Explain that knowledge that the client has a defective gene does not mean prevention or treatment is available related to the disease or that the disease course can be altered.
- Counsel the client if he or she feels guilt about having the flawed gene.
- Advocate for the client with genetic predisposition to disease in relation to employment and health insurance coverage.
- Teach that the person may not want, and has a right not to have, genetic testing.

In summary, two principles explain how differences in heredity may exert influence. The **Principle of Differential Susceptibility** suggests that *individual differences in heredity exist that make people susceptible to the influence of certain environments.* Given different experiences, a person with certain hereditary potential would develop in different ways. For example, the person with hereditary predisposition to schizophrenia would be likely to develop the disease if raised in a certain kind of environment. The **Principle of Differential Exposure** suggests that *inherited characteristics cause differing reactions from people, which in turn affect or shape the personality of the individual.* For example, body build, facial structure, and presence or absence of overall physical attractiveness result primarily from inheritance. People perceive, judge the actions of, and react more favorably to physically attractive children than to less attractive children. Over time, reactions of others contribute to formation of the self-concept, positive or negative feelings about self, and a sense of competency or incompetency that may affect behavior toward others or general performance. Excessive negative reaction from others may predispose to abnormal behavior and even mental illness if the stress is great enough (123).

Much remains unknown about the manner and extent to which early individual differences result in later personality differences, and the extent to which early transactions between parents and child obscure genetic characteristics. Intellect, emotions, societal factors, values, and learned life patterns are crucial to consider in health promotion (28).

Biochemical Factors

Research on the relationship between biochemical factors and behavior involves the areas of neurochemistry and hormones.

Neurochemistry is implicated in some behavioral development. The amount of biogenic amines, especially the **neurotransmitters,** *chemicals involved in transfer or modulation of nerve impulses from one cell to another,* apparently is related to mood. Catecholamines, including adrenaline, noradrenaline, dopamine, and serotonin, are important neurotransmitters in the brain and are involved in such emotional states as arousal, fear, rage, pleasure, motivation, exhilaration, sleep, and wakefulness (67). Such behavior, in turn, affects reactions of others, especially parents, to the child, and the child's moods may affect childrearing behavior.

Hormonal factors, based on changes in the endocrine system during stress or endocrine system disorders, may contribute to certain behaviors. Steroid hormones are increased during stress behavior, which in turn may interfere with normal developmental processes physically and cognitively (105). Excess steroid hormone intake (prescribed for illness or to build muscles and strength in athletes) causes mental as well as physical problems. The person may develop depression, elation, aggression, paranoia, hallucinations, delusions, or psychosis. The mental disorders dis-

appear after discontinuation of the drug, although it may take some time (67, 123). The pineal gland secretes the hormone melatonin, which increases when darkness falls and appears to keep the mind synchronized with the outside world. An imbalance may be linked to inducing sleep and melancholia. Various benefits attributed to melatonin, such as protecting cells from damage, boosting the immune system, preventing aging, and extending life, have been claimed but are unproven (26).

Thyroid dysfunction such as hypothyroidism or autoimmune thyroiditis, which results in thyroid atrophy, may cause signs and symptoms that match the criteria for depression: fatigue, constipation, vague aches and pains, feeling cold, poor memory, anxiety, and low mood. Eventually, the person may manifest confusion, cognitive impairment, and psychosis. Hyperthyroidism may manifest as anxiety, irritability, restlessness, euphoria, or mild manic disorder (67, 123).

Excess cortisol production may manifest as depression or mania, confusion, and eventually psychosis. Hypocortisolism may result in apathy, fatigue, and depression (67, 123).

Biochemical differences exist between persons and can be identified. What is not clear is whether the biochemical changes precede—and thus contribute to—abnormal behavior or result from changes that occur interpersonally or socially as a result of the person's abnormal behavior. The person in acute or short-term stress or crisis may have an abnormal level of a neurotransmitter as a result of normal feelings precipitated by and related to the event, yet that person is not determined to be, or does not become, mentally ill (123).

The relationships need to be clarified by further research. Chemical imbalances, however, appear to be improved by various medications. Pharmacology texts explain these drug actions in detail (123).

Neurophysiologic Factors

Neurophysiologic factors mediate all physiologic processes and behavior via the nervous system; however, neurophysiologic factors in behavior and personality development are inconclusive. Some specific motor and speech functions and various sensations in different body parts can be traced to specific brain areas.

Localization of brain function means that *certain areas of the brain are more concerned with one kind of function than another.* It does not imply that a specific function is mediated by only one brain region. Specific brain function requires the integrated action of neurons located in many different brain regions.

Specialized functions of brain regions are as follows (53, 67, 78, 89, 90, 99):

I. Cerebral cortical lobes
   A. Frontal—planning and movement: aggression
   B. Parietal—somatic sensation
   C. Temporal—hearing, memory, learning, and emotion
   D. Occipital—vision
   E. Major association cortices
      1. Prefrontal cortex—highest brain functions
      2. Limbic cortex—memory, emotion, motivation of behavior
      3. Parietal-temporal-occipital—higher sensory function, language
      4. Premotor association cortex—planning of action and initiation of movement (Damage effects execution of movement.)
      5. Parietal-temporal-occipital association cortex—links information from the senses which is necessary for perception. (Damage causes deficit in body image and spatial relations, aphasia, agnosia, and astereognosia.)
      6. Limbic association cortex, composed of the medial and ventral surfaces of the frontal lobe, the medial surface of the parietal lobe, portions of the temporal lobe, the orbitofrontal cortex, the cingulate region, the anterior tip of the temporal lobe, and the parahippocampal region—receives from higher-order sensory areas and projects to other critical regions and the prefrontal cortex; orbitofrontal portion concerned with motivation and emotional behavior; temporal lobe concerned with memory (90); basal ganglia involved in how we handle habits and physical skills (53, 78); amygdala associated with fear and anxiety

Linkage of the hypothalamus, limbic system, and cerebral cortex maintains homeostasis directly by regulating the endocrine and autonomic nervous systems and indirectly by regulating emotions and drives, including sexual preference, and any pleasure, by acting through the external environment. The hypothalamus and cerebral cortex mediate arousal. Hypothalamic integration of cardiovascular and respiratory function, motor and endocrine responses, combined with forebrain suppression of emotional responses, mediates emotional behavior. The forebrain delays responses to external events, which allows for planning, and is crucial to conscious experiences of emotion (99).

The limbic system is the seat of emotion and is involved in affective and cognitive function and motivation, feelings, and behavioral homeostasis. The limbic structures are all involved in comparison of external stimuli with internal states; all are involved in learning, memory, and motivation. The limbic system is especially prone to pathology because neurotransmitter effects are rapid and the neuromodulatory effects are slow (99).

Motivated behavior can be regulated by factors other than tissue needs, including learned habits and subjective pleasurable feelings. Central reward circuitry or the central reward system (CRS) is located within the limbic system. It is not fully known how the CRS mediates and registers reward or reinforcement, but it is responsible for the pleasure response. A neuromodulator reward cascade model depicts interactions involved in the CRS. The reward cascade begins in the hypothalamus and affects the opioid peptide methionine enkephalin, which is released in the substantia nigra, where enkephalin inhibits release of γ-aminobutyric acid (GABA). GABA is inhibited; dopamine supply is increased and acts to give a feeling of reward, pleasure, or elation (90).

Children apparently are born with a predisposition to be outgoing or quiet, and there may be a chemical predisposition to seeking danger or high risk. Yet neurophysiology does not supply all the answers. A supportive environment may cause further development of certain neurophysiologic rudiments and promote further development of the neurophysiologic processes that are manifested: thus environment helps to produce a well-adjusted child. A hostile home environment, especially in early life, produces the opposite result.

Immunologic Factors

The *immune system* functions to protect the body against disease; it recognizes and distinguishes foreign substances, such as bacteria, toxins, and cancer, from the body's own tissue. Immune suppression and stimulation are both necessary at different times to maintain health. At times the system responds excessively and destroys normal tissues. The system's function is closely interrelated with the central nervous system, endocrine system, perceptions, and behavior. Inordinate stress affects the immune system adversely, causing a variety of physical illnesses (e.g., musculoskeletal disease, cancer, asthma, thyroid and heart disease, colitis) with concomitant emotional effects (67, 169). The field of psychoneuroimmunology has shown the connections between stress in the environment and physical and emotional health. Certain mechanisms, not yet fully understood, produce greater physical health when there is emotional well-being. The stress of rapid or unexpected change can negatively affect health (169).

Maturational Factors

The maturational view emphasizes the emergence of patterns of development of organic systems, physical structures, and motor capabilities under the influence of genetic and maturational forces. Because of an inherent predisposition of the neurologic, hormonal, and skeletal-muscular systems to develop spontaneously, *physiologic and motor development occurs in an inevitable and sequential pattern in children throughout the world.* The growth of the nervous system is critical in this maturation unless the normal process is inhibited by severe environmental, physiologic, and emotional deprivation. Gesell, Ilg, and Ames (51) did extensive longitudinal studies in a large number of individuals from birth to 16 years of age from 1922 to 1946 that were instrumental in determining developmental sequences. Research by others since then has confirmed and added to their studies (52, 82, 88, 105, 121).

Sex differences may be inherent for some characteristics. For example, women generally have a greater response to the intuitive and analytic side of the brain, whereas men have a greater response to the spatial side of the brain. Yet many characteristics are the result of sociocultural influences; women from certain cultures may demonstrate characteristics common to men in other cultures. Sex differences are described in Chapters 10 to 14.

Biological Rhythms

Biorhythms are *self-sustaining, repetitive, rhythmic patterns established in plants, animals, people, and seasonal environmental events.* These daily or monthly biological cycles affect a number of physical functions, such as blood cell, blood glucose, and hormone levels; body temperature; heartbeat; blood pressure; renal and gastrointestinal function; sleep; and muscular strength and coordination (67). Mental skills and emotional changes are also apparently affected. Biological rhythm is unique to the individual and may be recorded through (1) interview, (2) a detailed diary recording quantitative information about body process and subjective experiences, and (3) autorhythmometry, in which the person records and rates physiologic processes and mood (123). Biological rhythms are discussed in Chapter 12.

Biological Deficiencies

Biological stressors such as certain kinds of foods, lack of food or malnutrition, medications, and lack of sleep may change behavior and the course of development. These factors are discussed further in Chapters 6 and 14.

ECOLOGIC THEORIES

Ecology is a *science that is concerned with the community and the total setting in which life and behavior occur.* A basic ecologic principle is that the continuity and survival of a person depend on a deliberate balance of factors influencing the interactions between the family or person and the environment.

Family is dependent on the resources and groups in the community to survive and continue its own development and to nurture adequately development of offspring. Further, climate, terrain, and natural resources affect family lifestyle and development and behavior of family members. The neighborhood may adversely affect development, especially if the person is reared in a family that lives in a deteriorating neighborhood or in an area with poor schools, inadequate housing, and a high crime rate. Excessively crowded housing may create stresses within the family that contribute to sleep deprivation, bickering, incest, or other abuse, which, in turn, affects developmental progress in all spheres of the person. Job loss because of a changing community and the resultant financial problems may affect health care practices and nutrition and, in turn, physical growth and emotional security.

Urbanization, rapid social changes, social stressors, discrimination, unemployment, poor housing, inadequate diet and health care, poverty, feelings of **anomie** (*not being part of society*), and negative self-image all contribute to stress and developmental difficulties in the vulnerable, immature person or in one without an adequate support system (121).

There are four theories about how neighborhoods affect behavior:

1. *Contagion Model:* People follow the example of others in their neighborhood or immediate community. Part of this Model includes the Social Control Model, where adults are enforcers who keep children off the streets and out of trouble; police help maintain order, high-socioeconomic-status adults act as behavioral role models because they show that success is possible if one works hard and behaves appropriately.

2. *Relative Deprivation Model:* High-socioeconomic-level neighbors and affluence shown in mass media provoke resentment in the poor; the poor feel a greater need to create a deviant subculture if they live nearer to the affluent than the poor.

3. *Neighbors Are Irrelevant Model:* People base their decisions and actions on their own circumstances and long-term interests, not on what neighbors consider acceptable; however, rational behaviors are usually restricted to choosing among familiar alternatives. Even in the poorest neighborhoods, a youth can find a friend who stays out of trouble and stays in school. In affluent neighborhoods, some youth get into trouble.

4. *Neighbors Do Not Matter But Neighborhoods Do Model:* Individuals in the neighborhood may not matter, but institutions such as schools and resources such as health care facilities do matter. Authorities often treat youth differently based on where they live (117).

Sociologic variables, including family socioeconomic level and position in the community, and the prestige related to birth, race, age, cultural ties, and power roles affect development, behavior, and adaptation of the person and family. Certain behaviors may be expected from a person because of age, sex, race, religion, or occupation. The individual may experience role conflicts and developmental problems when there are discrepancies between norms and values and the demands of age, sex, occupation, or religion (105).

Cultures vary in their definitions of normal and abnormal behavior; cross-cultural comparisons of developmental norms are difficult. Theorists in each culture describe their research findings about normal child or adult characteristics or behavior based on norms of their culture and their cultural bias. For example, cognitive impairment in the elderly is rare in cultures that revere their elderly or in which people live only 20 or 30 years. What might be associated with homosexuality in our culture, such as men embracing, is considered normal male heterosexual behavior in the Arab world.

Some authors believe that minorities must be evaluated by psychological criteria different from those used for Caucasians. They cite adaptive personality traits that African-Americans have adopted to survive in American society (105).

Geographic moves may create many adjustments for the person as he or she attempts to meet norms of the new community. Developmental problems and dysfunctional behavior may occur among those who migrate (105). Persons who move often as children may

never form chumships or close relationships later in adulthood; however, the mobile family and individual do learn coping skills that help them adjust to unfamiliar or stressful situations.

Some professionals and some lay people think abnormal behavior results from individual failure. In this view an individual's psychological problems are the result of some personal circumstance such as deficient achievement of developmental tasks, immaturity, character defect, or maladjustment (105). An alternate view is to see the individual problems as stemming from social causes. The broad economic, political, cultural, and social patterns of the nation and particular subcultures can be viewed as determinants of individual developmental responses. Then the community is the place to begin making changes if individual dysfunction is to be decreased (105). Chapters 1, 2, 3, and 4 discuss cultural, environmental, religious/spiritual, and family variables, and Chapters 7 through 14 present the interrelationship of these variables on the person.

Systems Perspective: General Systems Theory Applied to Behavior

First proposed by von Bertalanffy (189), General Systems Theory presents a comprehensive, holistic, and interdisciplinary view. This theory proposes that the family, individual, various social groups, and cultures are systems. Nothing is determined by a single cause or explained by a single factor. Nothing can be studied as a lone entity, be it the environment; various sociocultural components; political-legal, religious, educational, and other social institutions or organizations; the person, family, group, or community; or the health care delivery organization. All have interrelating parts, and all components interact with each other (1, 15, 179). An interconnectedness or interrelationship exists at and between every system level. A complementarity exists between parts of a system.

A **system** is an *assemblage, unit, or organism of interrelated, interdependent parts, persons, or objects that are united by some form or order into a recognizable unit and that are in equilibrium* (1, 15, 107, 179, 189).

People satisfy their needs within social systems. The **social system** is a *group of people joined cooperatively to achieve common goals, using an organized set of practices to regulate behavior* (15). The person occupies various positions and has defined roles in the social system. The person's development is shaped by the system; in turn, people create and change social systems (1, 107). The elements or components that are common to all systems are listed in Table 5–2. A given

TABLE 5–2. ELEMENTS AND CHARACTERISTICS OF A SYSTEM

Element	Definition/Example
Parts	*The system's components that are interdependent units.* None can operate without the other. Change in one part affects the entire unit.
	The person as a whole system is composed of physical, emotional, mental, spiritual, cultural, and social aspects. Physically, he or she is composed of the body systems—neurologic, cardiovascular, and so on. The health agency is one part of the health care system, and it, in turn, is composed of parts: physical plant, employees, clients, departments that give services.
Attributes	*Characteristics of the parts* such as temperament, roles, education, age, or health of the person or family members.
Information/communication	*Sending of messages and feedback, the exchange of energy,* which varies with the system but is essential to achieve goals. A system has input and output with the environment.
Boundary	*A barrier or area of demarcation that limits or keeps a system distinct from its environment and within which information is exchanged.*
	The skin of the person, home of the family, or walls of the health agency are boundaries. The boundary is not always rigid. Relatives outside the home are part of the family. The boundary may be an imaginary line such as the feeling that comes from belonging to a certain racial or ethnic group.
Organization	The *formal or informal arrangement of parts to form a whole entity so that the organism or institution has a working order that results in established hierarchy, rules, or customs.*
	The person is organized into a physical structure, basic needs, cognitive stages, and achievement of developmental tasks. Hierarchy in the family or health agency provides organization that is based on power (ability to control others) and responsibility. Nursing care may be organized into primary or team nursing, which is a way of differentiating services. The specialization of medical practice is also a way of organizing care. Organization in an institution is also maintained by norms, roles, and customs that each member must follow.
Goals	*Purposes of or reasons for the system to exist.* Goals may be long-term or short-term. Goals include survival, development, and socialization of the individual member of the family, or contributions to society.
Environment	The *social and physical world outside the system, boundaries, or the community in which the system exists.* The person's or family's environment may be a tribal enclave, farm, small town and surrounding area, or an urban neighborhood and surrounding city. Environment of a health care system may be the city in which the agency is located or may extend to other states and countries for a major urban medical center.
Evolutionary processes	*Changes within the person and the environment, proceeding from simple to complex,* occur at all times, in all systems. The person undergoes changes in physical, psychological, and social growth throughout the life span, within certain parameters.

Data from References 1, 15, 107, and 189.

entity is not a system unless these characteristics are present (1, 15, 107, 189).

All living organisms (i.e., every person) comprise an open social system. Change occurs constantly within and between the system and other systems. An **open system** is *characterized by the ability to exchange energy, matter, and information with the environment to evolve into higher levels of heterogeneity, organization, order, and development* (1). Physically, there is a *hierarchy of components* such as cells and organ systems. Emotionally, there are levels of needs and feelings. Cognitively, a person has memories, knowledge, and cognitive strategies. Socially, the person is in a relative rank in a hierarchy of prestige roles such as boss, worker, adult, or child. Although internal stimuli such as those governed by the nervous and endocrine systems are at work, outer stimuli also affect the person. The *boundaries or environment,* such as one's skin, the limits set by others, social status, home, and community, influence the person's *needs* and *goal achievement.* To re-

main healthy, the person must be able to *communicate* and must have *feedback:* the condition of the skin tells about temperature control; an emotional reaction signifies a sense of security, a job well done, or a failure; a pain signifies malfunction or injury. In turn, the person influences the external world through his or her developmental behavior. A constant *exchange of energy and information* must exist with the surrounding specified environment if the system is to be open, useful, and creative. If this *information or energy exchange does not occur,* the system becomes a **closed system** and ineffective, and disorganization, disease, and sometimes death result.

Other social systems are the family, church, economic systems; politico-legal and educational institutions; and health care agencies.

Linkage *occurs when two systems exchange energy across their boundaries* (1). Industry, the church, or the health agency, for example, draws energy from its linkage to the family. In return, industry is willing to contribute to family welfare funds, United Fund, mental health campaigns, or ecologic improvements. The church maintains its role as prime defender of family stability. The health agency sets standards of health care.

Each person and family you care for is a system interacting with other systems in the community. Development and function are greatly affected by the interdependence and interrelationships of each component part and by all other surrounding systems.

Family Systems Theory has been derived from General Systems Theory. Relationships that exist between family members constitute a system, and a reaction in one family member is followed by a predictable reaction in others. The smallest stable relationship system within a family or social system is the *three-person system* or *triangle*. Within this triangle, predictable relationships recur in times of calm and stress. During calm periods, there is a comfortable twosome and a less comfortable outsider who attempts to get closer to the other two; however, tension exists between the twosome and the threesome. If tension is sufficiently high, the most comfortable position for a member of the threesome or triangle is to be outside the system. In that case, the twosome will try to maneuver or "triangulate in" someone new into the threesome. The same emotional patterns are then repeated, so that family members develop fixed, often unchanging, roles in relation to each other (16, 17, 118).

For example, if parents are under a great deal of stress but cannot cope with the tension between them, the mother or father may become overly involved with the child, leaving the other parent outside the interaction. Eventually the parent on the outside of the twosome again displaces the child in the interaction with mate, but with stress the pattern is repeated. One child may unconsciously be assigned the role of "saving the marriage." Another child may unconsciously be assigned the role of wife to the father or the role of husband to the mother, with the respective spouse being displaced in relationships when stress is high. Or the wife may continue to rely heavily on her mother after marriage, or the husband on his father, so that the spouse is never quite so closely related to unless there is tension between the adult offspring and her or his parent. Or the family routines about attending family gatherings or rearing children are never changed by one spouse because of fear of what parents, inlaws, or others will say (16, 17, 118).

Dependence on the family members may be great; the self-concept of one person may fuse with the self or personality of another so little independence is left. Family members have as a result little degree of differentiation, and the more the members are undifferenti-

ated, the less they can change or think objectively under stress. At first in a marriage it may appear that one person is functioning at a much higher level than the other; however, this arrangement is usually with consent of and at the expense of the spouse. The relationship may become distant between the two, so that the neediest of the two seeks an extramarital companion. The other spouse seems unaware of the affair and will be surprised when divorce is sought. Or the couple may remain together but have a distant relationship, perhaps neither really being genuine, maturing, or self-actualizing. Or one will continue to define the personhood of the other; the submissive partner will never have a solid sense of self-awareness. But the dominant member may actually be the more immature, being a child inside who manipulates nurturance or mothering from the submissive spouse. The submissive spouse may get inner satisfaction from knowing that he or she holds the unit together and that the spouse cannot get along otherwise. Both are likely to feel very lonely (16, 17, 118).

PSYCHOLOGICAL THEORIES

A number of psychological theories have been formulated to explain human development, behavior, and personality. Theorists from different perspectives are discussed. A theorist who follows one perspective may disagree with another theorist from the same perspective. For example, some behaviorists would disagree with B.F. Skinner on some points. Further, no theorist or group of theorists has all the answers about human behavior, development, or learning. Realize that often theorists who sound very different in their theory may be stating basically similar concepts.

BEHAVIORAL THEORY

Overview

Behaviorists *adhere to stimulus–response conditioning theories.* This scientific approach to the study of the person generalizes results from animal experiments to people. The **Neo-Behaviorists**—*contemporary behavioral theorists and the theorists in this school who have changed their ideas*—obtain data for laws of behavior by observing the human's behavioral response to stimuli. The person is considered in terms of component parts. The focus is on isolated, small units of behavior or parts of behavioral patterns that are objectively observed and analyzed from the perspective of nonmental, physiologic associations.

View of the Human

Behavioral theorists view the living organism as a self-maintaining mechanism. The essence of a human machine is a system of receptors (sense organs), conductors (neurons), switching organs, (brain and spinal cord), and effectors (muscles) attached to levers (bones), along with fueling and controlling organs, for example, stomach and glands. The person is seen as an object, a reactive organism responding mechanically, automatically, involuntarily, overtly, and quantitatively to past conditioning and present situations. The person is regarded as a product of learning. The person has sensory input and, in turn, acts to reduce a need; there is a natural tendency and drive to satisfaction. The person is seen as neither inherently good nor evil, acted on or reinforced by the environment, which causes learning and predictable behavior (20, 74).

Because the focus is on physiologic processes and identifiable aspects of the person, subjective, unobservable, unique, and inner aspects of the human are denied or dismissed as illusory. There are no concepts that explain self-concept; ideas; emotions such as love, joy, sadness, and anger; the meaning in a situation; memory; understanding; insight; empathy; the person initiating and being an active agency in his or her behalf; or variety in human behavior. The person has sensory input; she or he does not perceive. There are no biases except for past conditioning. The person simply acts to reduce a need; there is a natural tendency and drive to satisfaction. The learner or the client is considered deficient, which results in activity or behavior called **learning.** Rest or cessation of behavior follows reward (123, 128).

View of Education and Therapy

The goals of education and psychiatric treatment are to (1) control the person's behavior; (2) help the person become more efficient and realistic, as defined by others in the environment; (3) move toward a goal set by external standards; and (4) create learning by forming bonds, connections, or associations. Responses that are appropriate are rewarded and therefore are stamped in to form habits (20, 68, 123, 128).

The teacher or therapist is at the center of and in control of the educational or treatment process. The learner or client is passive. Programmed or computer-

ized instruction is considered efficient education, with the teacher functioning as a reinforcement machine to help the learner achieve behavioral objectives. The teacher sets up the external situation to elicit the desired response and creates organized sequential steps so that the person achieves a goal and receives a reward. The therapist looks on the treatment process from the outside, controlling interchanges and diagnosing and interpreting the client's statements and problems. That which is predetermined will be accomplished. Intent or insight is not considered. Bad, superstitious, or inefficient behavior is removed from the person by **shaping,** *setting up the situation so that the person acts in a desired way, and then rewarding the desired behavior.* If education or treatment is individualized, it is as a means to an end, as the emphasis is on the preconceived end product rather than on the process (68, 123, 128).

Behavioral theorists propose that maladaptive behaviors are reinforced and learned. A treatment approach is to identify factors in the environment or in prior learning that must be modified to change the problem behavior. A problem with this approach is that the person who is elderly or of a minority group and feels powerless may feel he or she is being manipulated, that something is being done to rather than with the person or being done for rather than allowing the person to do for self. Further, who defines which behavior is maladaptive, the client or therapist? What the therapist considers maladaptive, such as hypervigilance, may be adaptive for the client's life situation. To change that behavior would make the client more vulnerable to harm. Also, the approach may seem too superficial or simplistic. The person may develop different symptoms to express the underlying problem or pathology, the person may resist behavior change, or the person may not return to the therapist after the initial visit because he or she felt misunderstood.

Behavioral Theorists

Early Theorists. Ivan Pavlov laid the foundations for the Behavioral School. He was a Russian physiologist and pharmacologist of the mid-19th century who wrote about psychic processes during his study of salivation and flow of digestive juices in dogs. His experiments established **classical conditioning:** *An unconditioned or new stimulus is presented with a stimulus that is already known just before the response to the conditioned familiar stimulus. The organism learns to respond to a new stimulus in the same way it responded to a familiar stimulus.* Associations are shifted from one stimulus to another, with the same response being made to the substituted stimuli (73, 121).

John B. Watson is considered the founder of **Behaviorism.** His experiments showed that fears and phobias could result from classical conditioning in childhood and could, in turn, be unlearned in adulthood (82). He emphasized physiologic associations and connections in understanding physiological processes.

Some present-day relaxation methods used by health care providers are based on classical conditioning. The client is trained to respond to a therapist's direction by relaxing a muscle group; music is then played while the therapist gives directions for relaxing. Later the person is able to respond automatically by relaxing when music plays (82). Classical conditioning is also used in the Lamaze preparation for childbirth or other kinds of childbirth education classes. Behaviorists believe emotions arise from body changes or are learned through classical conditioning. Emotions arise in the present situation based on past learning that is associated with the present event. For example, a person likes men with beards because he or she learned this response during childhood as a result of associating beards with a kindly bearded grandfather.

Thorndike: S-R Bond Theory or Connectionism

E. Thorndike was the most dominant figure in American psychology for much of the 20th century. From experiments with cats, he formulated a theory of learning called **S-R Bond Theory** or **Connectionism,** which affected every educational facility directly and many psychiatrists and mental health facilities at least indirectly. Thorndike's theory implies that, through **instrumental conditioning,** *a specific response is linked with a specific stimulus, and the response is followed by a reward or is instrumental in bringing about reinforcement.* The reward increases the likelihood of the response recurring, thereby causing a behavioral change. These links, bonds, or connections are products of biological, synaptic changes in the nervous system. Thorndike thought that trial and error (selecting and connecting) was primarily responsible for S-R connections but that learning was a process of "stamping in" connections in the nervous system that had nothing to do with insight or understanding. Transfer of learning was facilitated when the second situation was identical to the first.

Thorndike is best known for three laws, which are paraphrased and applied as follows (74, 123):

1. **Law of Readiness:** When the person is ready to perform or learn, it is satisfying to do so. It is annoying not to be able to act when a state of readiness exists or when action is demanded but there is no readiness. In education and therapy, the readiness level of the person toward action, learning, or behavioral change must be assessed and is considered essential for results.

2. **Law of Effect:** When a connection is made between a stimulus and response and is accompanied by a satisfying state of affairs, the connection is increased. If a person is ready to respond, the response is itself pleasurable, and the response will be fixed or learned. When working with the client, the teaching–learning situation should be satisfying, pleasurable, or harmonious, rather than boring, harsh, or conflictual, in order for the person to follow through with directions or suggestions.

3. **Law of Exercise (Repetition).** Whenever a connection is made between a stimulus and a response, the connection's strength is increased. The more times a stimulus-induced response is repeated or the person performs an activity, the longer it will be retained in behavior.

Thorndike later claimed that exercise and repetition were not important other than to provide an opportunity to give reinforcement. Behavior that is not rewarded would become boring and be discontinued. Yet most people continue to apply the Law of Exercise because repetition is used in education. Repetition, however, may be considered excessive by the learner, and too much repetition of an idea in therapy may cause resistance to carrying out directions.

One of Thorndike's secondary laws, **Associative Shifting,** or **Stimulus Substitution,** is now considered important by all Behaviorists. The law states that any response can be linked with any stimulus; the person's purposes or thoughts have nothing to do with learning. This is an example of automatic behavior, which all people use in certain situations, although such behavior would be inappropriate elsewhere. The social courtesies are an example. If too much behavior undergoes associative shifting, the behavior may be inappropriate; the person may be considered emotionally ill (68, 123).

Other ideas and principles proposed by Thorndike remain in use today. He advocated reward of acceptable behavior (strengthening a connection) rather than punishment of undesirable behavior. The **Principle of Set or Attitude** states that the person's attitude or mental set guides learning and behavior change; the response is set or determined by enduring adjustment patterns that result from being reared in a certain environment or culture. The mind set or attitude will determine what will be satisfying or annoying to the person. Certainly the client who has an attitudinal set against counseling is unlikely to benefit by it.

Skinner: Operant Conditioning Theory

Skinner is well known for his Operant Conditioning Theory, which used animal studies and built on the theories of Watson and Thorndike. According to Skinner, **behavior** is an *overt response that is externally caused and is controlled primarily by its consequences.* The environmental stimuli determine how a person alters behavior and responds to people or objects in the environment. Feelings or emotions are the accompaniments or result, not the cause of behavior. Innate or hereditary reflexes activate the internal glands and smooth muscles, but reflexive behavior accounts for little of human behavior (74, 171, 177).

Learning is a *change in the form or probability of response as a result of conditioning.* **Operant conditioning** is the *learning process whereby a response (operant) is shaped and is made more probable or frequent by reinforcement.* **Transfer** is an *increased probability of response in the future.* A set of acts are called *operant responses* because *they operate on the environment and generate consequences.* The important stimulus is the one immediately *following* the response, not the one preceding it.

According to Operant Conditioning Theory, certain kinds of events are reinforcers; when such an event follows a response, similar responses are more likely to occur. The reinforcing events can be identified, and responses can be planned. Operant reinforcement strengthens a given response and brings the response under the control of a stimulus. The stimulus does not elicit a reflexive response; it sets the occasion in which the response is likely to occur. Stimulus control can be programmed to maintain behaviors in spite of infrequent or intermittent reinforcement. Different reinforcement schedules generate different patterns of behavioral changes. Behavior may continue as the result of more than one reinforcer. Certain behaviors that have a genetic basis are more likely to respond to reinforcers. When there is no reinforcement, the behavior is extinguished or no longer occurs. Certain concepts, such as need, drive, emotion, and traits, are not used; only that which is observable, measurable behavior is included in this theory (174).

Operant conditioning occurs in most everyday activities, according to Skinner. People constantly cause others to modify their behavior by reinforcing certain behavior and ignoring other behavior. During development people learn to balance, walk, talk, play games, and handle instruments and tools because they are reinforced after performing a set of motions, thereby increasing the repetition of these motions. Social and ethical behaviors are learned as people are reinforced to continue them through their reinforcing of others for the same behaviors. Operant reinforcement improves the efficiency of behavior, whether the behavior is appropriate or inappropriate. Any attention, even if negative, reinforces response to a stimuli (74, 123, 170–177).

Positive reinforcement occurs when the *presence of a stimulus strengthens a response;* **negative reinforcement** occurs when *withdrawal of a stimulus strengthens the tendency to behave in a certain way.* A positive reinforcer is food, water, or a smile. A negative reinforcer consists of removing painful stimuli. Skinner's theory emphasizes positive reinforcement (74, 177). He rejected use of negative reinforcement or aversive control, contending that this merely produces escape and/or avoidance behavior. A **reinforcement schedule** is a *pattern of rewarding behavior at fixed time intervals, with a fixed number of responses between reinforcements.* Reinforcement does not strengthen a specific response, but rather it tends to strengthen a general tendency to make the response, or a class of responses, in the future. Thus trial-and-error learning does not exist (123, 170–177).

Punishment *consists of presenting a negative stimulus or removing a positive one.* Experiments show that punishment does not reduce a tendency to respond. Apparently, reward strengthens behavior because the response is stamped in. Punishment does not weaken behavior, however, because the response cannot be stamped out. **Extinction,** *letting a behavioral response die by not reinforcing it,* is preferred instead of punishment for breaking habits. Extinction is a slower process than reinforcement in modifying behavior (123, 170–177).

Two types of operant reinforcement cover most human behavior, along with reflex conditioning: stimulus discrimination and response differentiation. Discrimination of stimuli involves establishing a certain behavior as a result of a given stimulus preceding or accompanying the behavior and then reinforcing the behavior. Imitative behavior is an example. It arises over time because of discriminative reinforcement. A person waves to someone because of the reinforcement, not because of the stimulus of the other person's hand waving. Differentiation of responses improves motor skills. The person selects a motion because it was reinforced. In this process, reinforcement must be immediate (123, 170–177).

Application of Skinner's theory is threefold. His theory, when applied to clinical and classroom problems, is called *behavior modification.* When applied to courses of study, it is called *programmed learning*. When applied to correction of physiologic problems, it is called *biofeedback* (88, 177). As a nurse, you may use each of these applications in client care and teaching.

Behavior modification is the *deliberate application of learning theory and conditioning, thereby structuring different social environments to teach alternate behaviors and to help the person gain control over behavior and environment*. Shaping also achieves behavioral change (see Table 5–3) (123, 170–177). **Shaping** is the *gradual modification of behavior by breaking complex behavior into small steps and reinforcing each small step that is a closer approximation to the final desired behavior* (149).

In behavior modification the behavior first must be reinforced each time it occurs. Once the desired response has been established and maintained by a continuous reinforcement schedule (i.e., each time the desired response is seen, it is reinforced), the next step is to switch to an **intermittent schedule of reinforcement,** *whereupon reinforcement is contingent on increasingly multiple emissions of the desired behavior*. After this, occasional reinforcement will keep the desired behavior going. Behavior that has been maintained by an intermittent schedule of reinforcement or partial reinforcement is highly resistant to extinction (123, 149, 170–177, 195). For example, the child learns to talk not only through imitation of others but because of parental approval, love, and verbal responses that serve as rewards or reinforcement. To teach a client to talk, you would first reward him or her, possibly with food, every time there was the slightest movement of lips. Later, the reward would be given only for an utterance. Even-

tually, food would be given only for sounds or words, then phrases, and then meaningful sentences.

The aim of behavioral therapy is maximum benefit for the client and society, but behavior therapy is exclusively reliant on the therapist's judgment and goals for the client.

Sometimes aversive methods (e.g., seclusion) are used to change behavior. The purpose is not punishment but time-out, as in allowing a tantrum to run its course without accidental reinforcement and without triggering similar behavior in other people. Strategies of punishment and deprivation, which are standard techniques in childrearing, are examples of using Skinner's principles of behavior modification. Some parents do not question sending a child to bed without a meal as punishment, and parents may even be criticized by other parents if they do not spank their children for naughty behavior.

Operant techniques include the following (123, 170–177):

- *Time-out:* seclusion for extinction of behaviors
- *Assertion training:* using role playing, modeling, feedback, and social reinforces to change communication patterns
- *Token economies:* rewards, payments for behavior improvement that is applied to entire unit of patients
- *Social skills training:* rehearsal of appropriate social behaviors

Operant conditioning is used in many situations, including to:

- Replace undesirable behaviors of normal or developmentally disabled children
- Reduce abnormal or self-destructive behavior
- Train parents, teachers, probation officers, and nurses to be more efficient in their roles
- Reduce specific maladaptive behaviors such as stuttering, tics, poor hygiene, and messy eating habits
- Control physical symptoms through biofeedback

Figure 5–1 illustrates how development is viewed by learning theorists. Table 5–4 lists key terms and definitions, with examples (170–177, 195).

Wolpe: Desensitization Theory

Joseph Wolpe uses Skinner's principles in deconditioning of anxiety or desensitization of phobias or other neurotic behaviors. When treating symptoms of fear by desensitization, the person is helped to relax com-

---

TABLE 5–3. FACTORS TO BE ANALYZED BY THERAPIST BEFORE BEGINNING A BEHAVIOR MODIFICATION PROGRAM

1. Maladaptive behavior, or the behavior to be decreased
2. Target or desired observable outcome
3. Current repertoire of behaviors, which is a starting point to get to desired behaviors
4. Environmental factors supporting present behavior
5. Specific steps to lead client from current to desired behaviors
6. Consequences considered as rewards and punishments by the client that can be manipulated to alter the client's behavior, for example:
   - Material rewards (money, food, trinkets)
   - Surrogate rewards (tokens, stars, points on a chart)
   - Social rewards (approval or joining in group activities)
   - Behavioral rewards (opportunity to do special activities)

Presentation of each new program step or behavioral unit is contingent on meeting the requirements of the preceding one. Behavior therapy deals with a specific problem at a time, rather than with a combination of all the perceived behavioral problems.

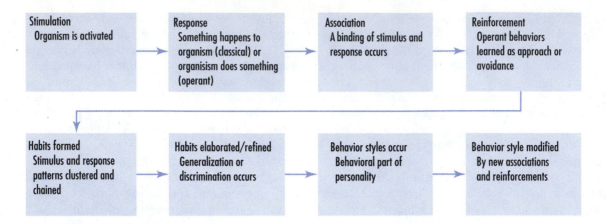

Figure 5–1. Development as viewed by learning theorists. Stimuli from inside or outside the organism are reinforced (positively or negatively) and on a particular schedule that determines their force and strength. Habits develop. The response processes of generalization and discrimination elaborate these habits and modify them. Effective habits are equated with effective development. This force rarely speaks about the whole organism but rather about situationally determined behaviors.

pletely. Then, over many sessions, the person is presented with progressively more threatening situations and is instructed to remain simultaneously relaxed. Then the person is asked to think of the feared object but to stop thinking about it if he or she feels uneasy. Step by step the person is helped to remain relaxed while thinking about all the factors that have previously been frightening. After a number of treatments, the person can face directly, with feelings of relaxation, what was frightening (123, 195).

The major criticism of Wolpe's therapy is that only the symptom and not the underlying problem is treated. Therefore, symptom substitution, another maladaptive behavior replacing the extinguished behavior, will occur. Wolpe states that the behavior, not the symptom, is the problem. He denies symptom substitution (123, 195).

Behavioral Contract

Use a contract with your client in your practice. A **verbal or written contract** is an *explicit mutual agreement between you and the client that defines the nature of your relationship, your mutual expectations, the different but equal responsibilities toward a common goal(s), and accountability for the outcome.* Terms in the contract include appointment time and place, or the specific care activities and their timing that are involved for the person. Tentative duration of treatment, specific contributions of other professionals, and fees, if any, are included in the contract. The contract should be evaluated periodically by nurse and client to be sure that each is meeting the contract terms and goals, and the terms should be changed when necessary. If an aspect

of a contract is broken by the client, do not become judgmental. Renegotiate the terms (123).

PSYCHOANALYTIC AND NEO-ANALYTIC THEORIES

Overview

Psychoanalytic theorists include those who adhere to Psychoanalytic and Neo-Analytic theories. These theorists generally believe data for study about the person come from within the developing person, observation of interpersonal relationships, and knowledge of the impact of social units, norms, and laws on the person. Data from early development are used to understand present behavior and goal direction. This group of theorists studies the person more comprehensively and as a social being, using experimentation, objective observation, and self-report methods. These theorists give us a helpful view of causation and provide a way of dealing with developmental and behavioral problems (105).

View of the Human

Knowledge of genetics, developmental levels, effects of internal stimuli, unconscious processes, social relationships, and environmental context are all used to understand the person.

Reality is external and interpersonal—what people agree on. The person is a social organism with a developmental past on which to build and a level of readiness that influences or contributes to learning and behavior.

TABLE 5–4. SELECTED TERMINOLOGY PERTAINING TO APPLICATION OF BEHAVIORAL THEORY

Term	Definition	Example
Respondent conditioning	Pairing a neutral stimulus with a nonneutral stimulus until the person learns to respond to the neutral stimulus as to the nonneutral stimulus	Baby learns to "love" a sibling (nonneutral stimulus) because the sibling shakes a rattle and offers other toys (neutral stimulus) while cooing, touching, and smiling to baby.
Operant conditioning	Rewarding or punishing a response until the person learns to repeat or avoid that response in anticipation of positive or negative consequences	Preschooler returns toys to the toy box at the end of the day because he remembers the consequences: doing so is followed by 10 minutes of time with the parent; failure to do so results in sitting alone in his room for 5 minutes.
Positive reinforcement	Rewarding desired behavior to maintain that behavior	Parent buys a desired item for the child who earns an A in a course.
Negative reinforcement	Removing an aversive stimulus in response to behavior, which maintains that behavior	Parent allows the child to forego household tasks if he complains when asked to do them, yet the child receives an allowance weekly.
Extinction	Suppressing a behavior by removing reinforcers that are maintaining the behavior	Parent does not give the child who complains about doing household tasks the allowance at the end of the week and explains why.
Punishment	Suppressing an undesirable behavior by using an aversive stimulus in response to the person's behavior	Parent spanks the child for running into the street.
Time-out	Suppressing maladaptive behavior by removing the subject to a neutral environment, void of reinforcements, when the behavior is manifested	Parent makes the 4-year-old child sit facing a corner for 5 minutes after hitting a sibling.
Generalization	Transferring a conditioned response from the conditional stimulus to another stimulus	Child who is bitten by a dog fears all animals.
Systematic desensitization	Pairing an anxiety-causing stimulus with an induced state of relaxation to extinguish fearful behavior	Parent remains with the child who has been bitten by a dog when the child is in the vicinity of animals, gradually helps the child to relax, and eventually pet a very friendly dog.
Discrimination	Responding only to a specific stimulus	Toddler learns via punishing encounters with mother that playing in water in the bathtub is acceptable and playing in the water in the toilet is not.
Escape behavior	Initiating a response to escape an unpleasant or aversive stimulus	Adolescent brings the parents a gift when returning late from a weekend with a friend.
Avoidance learning	Arranging responses to avoid exposure to an aversive stimulus	Adolescent verbally refuses the offer and walks away from the person offering a marijuana joint after a bad experience with it.
Chaining	Developing complex behavior by focusing on the individual components of the behavior; this is done in a backward fashion	Schoolchild learns to clean his room with the parent instructing and assisting with each step of the task and then verbally repeating in reverse order the steps after the task is finished.
Shaping	Reinforcing successive approximations or small units of a desired response until that behavior is gradually achieved	Parent teaches the child to clean his room by praising him for doing every step of the process—vacuuming the rug, dusting each piece of furniture.
Fading	Removing gradually the reinforcement given to the person	Parent gives less and less verbal approval to the schoolchild for doing assigned household tasks.

The person has maturational and social needs that affect development, learning, and behavior; he or she seeks social role satisfaction and reacts to social values and symbolic processes. The person internalizes societal rules to gain approval, can understand cause-and-effect relationships and complex abstract issues, is capable of insight and emotions, and initiates action and makes choices. The person is seen as a reactive being responding to stimuli that are usually sociosexual in nature. The goal of behavior is seen as reduction of symbolic or internal needs or tension (105).

View of Education and Therapy

The goal of developmental guidance and discipline is to help the person become an adaptive, effective social being, aware of and responsive to social reality and patterns. The person has to learn and follow socially prescribed values, customs, and norms to fit into society as an effective and well citizen. Development, learning, and behavior are also influenced strongly by the person's developmental level, personal history, cognitive processes and intellect, and intrapsychic processes (105, 123, 128).

The teacher or therapist is the central figure, a social role model who directs the client. Emphasis is on the person, even in the younger years, understanding self and his or her behavior. Increased insight promotes development and maturation. If the person is not ready to learn or change behavior, the parent, teacher, or another acts as an external motivator or facilitator of readiness to change. Rewards are given through approval, affiliation, and various verbal and nonverbal methods. Learning and behavior change also are self-reinforcing to the person (105).

Psychoanalytic and Neo-Analytic Theorists

The **Psychoanalytic Theory** or perspective is divided into two groups: Psychoanalytic (Freud [40–45]) and Neo-Analytic (Jung [85], Adler [122], Rank [122], Horney [79, 144], Fromm [47], Sullivan [182], Erikson [35], and Berne [2, 14]). The writings of Freud, Sullivan, Erikson, and Jung are discussed in this chapter. They are known as "stage theorists" because they emphasize that people develop in sequential stages. Other current stage theorists are George Vaillant (188), Roger Gould (62), Gail Sheehy (167), and Daniel Levinson (104). Their concepts and theories are referred to in Chapters 12 and 13 on young adulthood and middle age. The Neo-Analytic theorists reinterpreted Freud's Psychoanalytic Theory in formulating their theories. Sullivan further developed new emphases in his Interpersonal Theory: causation of behavior was seen as the result of dyad (mother–child) relationships and development continued into adulthood. Erikson, in his Epigenetic Theory, expanded understanding of normal developmental stages and tasks through the life span, emphasized sociocultural influences to a greater degree, and saw the person as capable of emotional growth throughout life.

Psychodynamic Perspective

The **psychodynamic perspective** is concerned with the *inner and unconscious processes of the person— drives, needs, motivations, feelings, and conflicts.* Past developmental experiences are important in the causation of behavior and for achieving present developmental tasks and maturity. Most of the Neo-Analytic theorists have paid little attention to biology. Because thoughts and feelings are not directly observable, these theorists infer them from overt behavior (105).

Freud: Psychoanalytic Theory. Sigmund Freud, a Viennese neurologist, developed Psychoanalytic Theory; the first psychological theory to include a fully developed explanation of abnormal behavior. He gave biological factors little emphasis but used the medical model of emphasizing pathology and symptoms.

Freud's theory of personality seems complicated because it incorporates many interlocking factors. Major components are psychic determinism; psychic structures of id, ego, and superego; primary and secondary process thinking; the conscious–unconscious continuum; libido or psychic energy; behavior; anxiety and defense mechanisms; transference; and psychosexual development. Some of his theory is discussed here and referred to in the chapters on childhood. Table 5–5 summarizes these concepts (40–45, 123).

Anxiety is the *response of tension or dread to perceived or anticipated danger or stress and is the primary motivation for behavior.* There are two types of anxiety-provoking situations. Anxiety may be caused by excessive stimulation that the person cannot handle, of which birth is the prototype experience. Anxiety may also rise from intrapsychic or unconscious conflicts, unacceptable wishes, unknown or anticipated events, superego inhibitions and taboos, and threatened loss of self-image. Anxiety at the mild level is probably always present in the awake state but can escalate to panic levels. Table 5–6 summarizes the level of anxiety and manifestations of each level. If anxiety cannot be managed by direct action or coping strategies, the ego initiates unconscious defenses by warding off awareness of the conflict to keep the material unconscious, to lessen discomfort, and to maintain the self-image. Because everyone experiences psychological danger, the use of defense mechanisms clearly is not a special characteristic of maladaptive behavior. Such mechanisms are used by all people, either singly or in combination, at one time or another, and are considered adaptive (41, 42, 44, 105, 129). Commonly used ego adaptive (defense) mechanisms are summarized in Table 5–7 and described throughout the text in relation to the developmental era during which they arise.

Freud proposed five stages of psychosexual development and contended that personality was formed by age 5 (40, 105). The stages in psychosexual development, each resolved in turn, are summarized in Table 5–8 and are referred to throughout the text.

TABLE 5–5. SUMMARY OF FREUD'S THEORY OF PERSONALITY

Psychic determination	All behavior determined by prior thoughts and mental processes

Psychic structures of the personality	**Id** — *Unorganized reservoir of psychic energy;* furnishes energy for ego and superego
	   Consists of instinctual forces, primitive biological drives, and impulses necessary for survival
	   Operates on **pleasure principle** (*seeking of immediate gratification and avoidance of discomfort*)
	   Discharges **tension** (*increased energy*) through reflex physiologic activity and **primary process thinking** (*image formation, drive-oriented behavior, free expression of feelings and impulses, inability to distinguish between reality and nonreality; dream-like state*)
	Ego — *Establishes relations with environment through conscious perception, feeling, action*
	   Controls impulses from id and demands of superego
	   Operates on **reality principle** (*external conditions considered and immediate gratification delayed for future gains that can be realistically achieved*)
	   Controls access of ideas to conscious
	   Appraises environment and reality
	   Uses various mechanisms to help person feel emotionally safe
	   Guides person to acceptable behavior
	   Directs motor and all cognitive functions
	   Assists with **secondary process thinking** (*delayed or substitutive gratification; realistic thoughts; conscious processes; cognitive strategies*)
	Superego — *Represents internalized moral code based on perceived social rules and norms; restrains expression of instinctual drives; prevents disruption of society*
	   Active and concrete in directing person's thoughts, feelings, actions
	   Made up of two systems:
	      Ego Ideal — *Perfection to which person aspires; corresponds to what parents taught was good*
	      Conscience — *Responsible for guilt feelings; corresponds to those things parents taught were bad*

Conscious–unconscious continuum	**Conscious** — *All aspects of mental life currently in awareness or easily remembered* **Preconscious** — *Aspects of mental life remembered with help; not currently in awareness* **Unconscious** — *Thoughts, feelings, actions, experiences, dreams not remembered; difficult to bring to awareness; not recognized* Existence inferred from effects on behavior

Instincts (drives)	Basic force in personality and behavior
	   Inborn psychological representation or wish of inner somatic source of excitation
	   Kinds of instincts: self-preservation, preservation of species, life, death; life and death instincts in conflict

Libido (sexuality)	*Sexual or psychic energy arising from hidden drives or impulses involved in conflict*
	   Desire for pleasure, sexual gratification
	   Not limited to biology or genital areas; includes capacity for loving another, parental love, and preservation of species

Anxiety	*Response to presence of unconscious conflict, tension, or dread; perceived or anticipated danger; and stress — primary motivation for behavior*
	   Basic source is the unconscious, related to loss of self-image
	   Psychic energy accumulates if anxiety not expressed; many overwhelm ego controls; panic may result
	   Kinds of anxiety: (1) neurotic — id–ego conflict; (2) realistic — in response to real dangers in world; (3) moral anxiety — id–superego conflict
	   Managed by direct action, coping strategies, or unconscious defense mechanisms

Transference	*Phenomenon of investing libido in another object, projection of feelings, thoughts, and wishes onto therapist, who represents significant person from the past (usually the parent), and which is based on unconscious and repressed material and is therefore not realistic or appropriate to the situation*
Primary process	*Thought processes based in the id and unconscious; thought processes are drive-oriented, unable to distinguish between reality and nonreality, primitive, illogical, labile, and without synthesis; thought processes are related to instinctual impulses, obtaining self-pleasure, and to free expression of feelings and impulses; opposite thought processes may coincide; process carried out through pictoral, concrete images or dreams*
Secondary process	*Realistic, conscious thought processes based in the ego and occurring in normal waking life; association of ideas subject to reality conditions and conform to ethical and moral laws; instinctual impulses cannot obtain gratification because of ego and superego constraints; process based on use of words, cognitive strategies, and delayed or substitutive gratification*
Cathexis	*Energy responsible for behavior*

TABLE 5–6. MANIFESTATIONS AND LEVELS OF ANXIETY

Level	Type	Effect
Mild	Physiologic	Tension of needs motivates behavior
		Adaptive to variety of internal and external stimuli
	Cognitive	Attentive, alert, perceptive to variety of stimuli, effective problem solving
	Emotional	No intense feelings; self-concept not threatened
		Use of ego adaptive mechanisms minimal, flexible
		Behavior appropriate to situation
Moderate	Physiologic	Some symptoms may be present
		Accelerated rate of speech; change in pitch of voice
	Cognitive	Perceptual field narrows; responds to directions; repetitive questioning
		Tangible problems solved fairly effectively, at least with direction and support
		Selective inattention—focus is on stimuli that do not add to anxiety
	Emotional	Impatient, irritable, forgetful, demanding, crying, angry
		Uses any adaptive mechanism (e.g., rationalization, denial, displacement) to protect from feelings and meaning of behavior (Physiologic, cognitive, and emotional changes of Alarm and Resistance Stages of stress response. Individual functions in normal pattern but may not feel as healthy physically or emotionally as usual. Illness may result if feeling persists.)
Severe	Physiologic	Alarm stage changes intensify, and stage of resistance may progress to stage of exhaustion stress response
	Cognitive	Perceptual field narrows; stimuli distorted, focus is on scattered details
		Selective inattention prevails
		Learning and problem solving ineffective
		Clarification of restatement needed repeatedly
		Misinterprets statements
		Unable to follow directions or remember main points
		Unable to plan or make decisions; needs assistance with details
		Disorganized; unable to see connection between events
		Consciousness and lucidity reduced
	Emotional	Self-concept threatened; sense of helplessness or impending doom; mood changes
		Behavior erratic, inappropriate, regressive, inefficient; may be aware of inappropriate behavior but unable to improve
		Many ego defense mechanisms used; dissociation and amnesia may be used
		Disorientation, confusion, suspicion, hallucinations, and delusions may be present (Psychoses or physical illness or injury may result.)
Panic	Physiologic	Severe symptoms of exhaustion stage may be ignored
	Cognitive	Sensory ability and attention reduced so that only object of anxiety noticed
		May fail to notice specific object of concern or disastrous event but will be preoccupied with trivial detail
	Emotional	Self-concept overwhelmed; feeling of personality disintegration
		Ego defense mechanism used, often inappropriately and uncontrollably
		Behavior focused on finding relief; may scream, cry, pray, thrash limbs, run, hit others, hurt self
		Often easily distracted; cannot attend or concentrate
		No learning, problem solving, decision making, or realistic judgments
		May become immobilized, assume fetal position, become mute, or be unresponsive to directions
		Needs protection (Psychoses may occur.)

Freud's ideas about psychosexual development are undoubtedly the most controversial aspects of his theory. Although many theorists agree that childhood experiences are very important in personality development, many reject Freud's assertions about childhood sexuality and the Victorian and stereotyped ideas about men and women (105).

Psychoanalytic Theory has been criticized for many reasons (see an objective critique by Graves [63]). In contrast, Greenberg and Fisher (64) have reviewed the thousands of scientific studies done worldwide to check the validity of Freud's ideas and have found that Freud's model of personality development and behavior is supported by other studies. His theory

TABLE 5–7. EGO ADAPTIVE OR DEFENSE MECHANISMS

Mechanism	Definition/Example
Compartmentalization	Separation of two incompatible aspects of the psyche from each other to maintain psychological comfort; behavioral manifestations show the inconsistency. **Example:** The person who attends church regularly and is overtly religious conducts a business that includes handling stolen goods.
Compensation	Overachievement in one area to offset deficiencies, real or imagined, or to overcome failure or frustration in another area. **Example:** The student who makes poor grades devotes much time and energy to succeed in music or sports.
Condensation	Reacting to a single idea with all of the emotions associated with a group of ideas; expressing a complex group of ideas with a single word or phrase. **Example:** The person says the word *crazy* as a shorthand expression for many types of mental illness and for feelings of fear and shame.
Conversion	Unconscious conflicts are disguised and expressed symbolically by physical symptoms involving portions of the body, especially the five senses and motor areas. Symptoms are frequently not related to innervation by sensory or motor nerves. **Example:** The person is under great pressure on the job; awakes at 6 AM and is unable to walk but is unconcerned about the symptom.
Denial	Failure to recognize an unacceptable impulse or undesirable, but obvious thought, fact, behavior, conflict, or situation, or its consequences or implications. **Example:** The alcoholic person believes that he or she has no problem with drinking even though family and work colleagues observe the classic signs.
Displacement	Release or redirection of feelings and impulses on a safe object or person as a substitute for that which aroused the feeling. **Example:** The person punches a punching bag after an argument with the boss.
Dissociation	Repression or splitting off from awareness of a portion of a personality or of consciousness; however, repressed material continues to affect behavior (compartmentalization). **Example:** A client discusses a conflict-laden subject and goes into a trance.
Emotional isolation	Repression of the emotional component of a situation, although the person is able to remember the thought, memory, or event, dealing with problems as interesting events that can be rationally explained but have no feelings attached. **Example:** The person talks about the spouse's death and details of the accident that caused it with an apathetic expression and without crying or signs of grieving.
Identification	Similar to and the result of introjection; unconscious modeling of another person so that basic values, attitudes, and behavior are similar to those of a significant person or group, but overt behavior is manifested in an individual manner. (Imitation is not considered a defense mechanism per se, but imitation usually precedes identification. Imitation is consciously copying another's values, attitudes, movements, etc.). **Example:** The adolescent over time manifests the assertive behavior and states ideas similar to those that she admires in one of her instructors, although she is unaware that her behavior is similar.
Introjection	Symbolic assimilation of or process of taking in attitudes, behavior, wishes, ideals, or values of significant person into the ego and/or superego (a part of identification). **Example:** The client talks about how much she or he helps other people with their problems.
Projection	Attributing one's unacceptable or anxiety-provoking feelings, thoughts, impulses, wishes, or characteristics to another person. **Example:** The person declares that the supervisor is lazy and prejudiced; work colleagues note that this person often needs help at work and frequently makes derogatory remarks about others.
Rationalization	Justification of behavior or offering a socially acceptable, intellectual, and apparently logical explanation for an act or decision actually caused by unconscious or verbalized impulses. Behavior in response to unrecognized motives precedes reasons for it. **Example:** A student fails a course but maintains that the course was not important and that the grade can be made up in another course.
Reaction formation	Unacceptable impulses repressed, denied, and reacted to by opposite overt behavior. **Example:** A married woman who is unconsciously disturbed by feeling sexually attracted to one of her husband's friends treats him rudely and keeps him at a safe distance.
Regression	Adopting behavior characteristic of a previous developmental level; the ego returns to an immature but more gratifying state of development in thought, feeling, or behavior. **Example:** The person takes a nap, curled in a fetal position, on arriving home after a stressful day at work.
Repression	Automatic, involuntary exclusion of a painful or conflictual feeling, thought, impulse, experience, or memory from awareness. The thought or memory of the event is not consciously perceived. **Example:** The mother seems unaware of the date or events surrounding her child's death and shows no emotion when the death is discussed.
Sublimation	Substitution of a socially acceptable behavior for an unacceptable sexual or aggressive drive or impulse. **Example:** The adolescent is forbidden by her parents to have a date until she graduates from high school. She gives much time and energy to editorial work and writing for the school paper. The editor of the school paper and the faculty advisor are males.

(continued)

TABLE 5–7. EGO ADAPTIVE OR DEFENSE MECHANISMS (continued)

Mechanism	Definition/Example
Suppression	*Intentional exclusion of material from consciousness.* **Example:** The husband carries the bills in his pocket for a week before remembering to mail in the payments.
Symbolization	*One object or act unconsciously represents a complex group of objects and acts,* some of which may be in conflict or unacceptable to the ego; external objects or acts stand for any internal or repressed desire, idea, attitude, or feeling. The symbol may not overtly appear to be related to the repressed ideas or feelings. **Example:** The husband sends his wife a bouquet of roses, which ordinarily represents love and beauty. But roses have thorns; his beautiful wife is hard to live with, but he consciously focuses on her beauty.
Undoing	*An act, communication, or thought that cancels the significance or partially negates a previous one;* treating an experience as if it had never occurred. **Example:** The husband purchases a gift for his wife after a quarrel the previous evening.

TABLE 5–8 FREUD'S STAGES OF PSYCHOSEXUAL DEVELOPMENT: LIBIDINAL EXTENSION

Stage (years)	Major Body Zone	Activities	Extension to Others
Oral (0–1½)	Mouth (major source of gratification and exploration)	Security—primary need Pleasure from eating and sucking Major conflict—weaning Incorporation (suck, consume, chew, bite, receive)	Sense of *We*—no differentiation or extension Sense of *I* and *Other*—minimum differentiation and total incorporation Beginning of ego development at 4–5 months
Anal (1½–3)	Bowel (anus) and bladder source of sensual satisfaction, self-control, and conflict (mouth continues in importance)	Expulsion and retention (differentiation, expelling, controlling, pushing away) (Incorporation still is used.) Major conflict—toilet training	Sense of *I* and *Other*—separation from other and increasing sense of *I* Beginning control over impulses
Phallic (4–6)	Genital region—penis, clitoris (mouth, bowel, and bladder sphincters continue in importance)	Masturbation Fantasy Play activities Experimentation with peers Questioning of adults about sexual topics Major conflict—Oedipus complex, which resolves when child identifies with parent of same sex (Mastery, incorporation, expulsion, and retention continue.)	Sense of *I* and *Other*—fear of castration in boy Sense of *I* and *Other*—strengthened with identification process with parents Sense of *Other*—extends to other adults
Latency (6–puberty)	None (penis, clitoris, mouth, anus)	Diffuse activity and relationships (Mastery, incorporation, expulsion, and retention continue.)	Sense of *I* and *Other*—extends out of nuclear family and includes peers of same sex
Genital (puberty and thereafter)	Penis, vagina (mouth, anus, clitoris)	Develop skills needed to cope with the environment Full sexual maturity and function (Mastery, incorporation, expulsion, and retention continue.) Addition of new assets with each stage for gratification Realistic heterosexual expression Creativity and pleasure in love and work	Sense of *I* and *Other*—extends to other adults and peers of opposite sex

continues to influence 20th-century thought and research, especially in Western cultures, in relation to development and therapy of the ill person (72). Recently, feminist scholars have begun to reassess Freud's theory, recognizing the value of his ideas and their applicability to understanding men and women, boys and girls (23).

You will find Freud's concepts pertinent to your understanding of the developing person and to nursing and health care.

Major Neo-Analytic Theorists

Neo-Freudians or Neo-Analysts follow Freud's theory in general but disagree with or have modified some of the original propositions. They maintain the medical model and share the view of intrapsychic determinism as the basis for external behavior. Some take into account the social and cultural context in which the person lives. Harry Stack Sullivan (182), Erik Erikson (35), and Carl Jung (85–87) are described briefly; Sullivan and Erikson are referred to throughout the text.

Sullivan: Interpersonal Theory of Psychiatry. Harry Stack Sullivan (182) formulated the Interpersonal Theory of Psychiatry. The theory focuses on relationships between and among people, in contrast to Freud's emphasis on the intrapsychic sexual phenomena and Erikson's focus on social aspects. Experiences in major life events are the result of either positive or negative interpersonal relationships. Personality development is largely the result of the mother–child relationship, childhood experiences, and interpersonal encounters. There are two basic needs: satisfaction (biological needs) and security (emotional and social needs). Biological and interpersonal needs are interrelated. How biological needs are met in the interpersonal situation determines sense of satisfaction and security and provides avoidance of anxiety.

Sullivan used the following biological principles to understand the person's development (182):

- **Principle of communal existence:** *A living organism cannot survive if separated from the necessary environment for survival.* For example, the embryo must have the correct intrauterine environment to live, and the baby must have love and human contact to become socialized or human.
- **Principle of functional activity:** *Functional or physiologic activities and processes affect the person's interaction with the environment.*
- **Principle of organization:** *The person is systematically arranged physically and emotionally and*

within societies, and this organization enables function.

An important principle for the study and care of people is the **One Genus Postulate,** which states *we are all more simply human than otherwise, hence more similar than different in basic needs, development, and in the meaning of our behavior* (182).

Sullivan postulated that people experience events in the following three modes (182):

1. **Prototaxic mode of experiencing:** *Experiences that occur in infancy before language symbols are acquired or the first time a person experiences an event that is difficult to describe in words.*
2. **Parataxic mode of experiencing:** *Experiences characterized by symbols used in a private (autistic) way; encompasses fantasy, magical thinking, and lack of cause-and-effect thinking that is seen in children and adults.*
3. **Syntaxic mode of experiencing:** *Experiences of preadolescence, adolescence, and adulthood characterized by consensual validation, whereby persons communicate with each other using language or symbols that are mutually understood.* This mode of experiencing begins during the chum stage in the school-age child or thereafter. The differences between these models are due to the crucial role of language in experience and development and are described further in Chapters 7, 9, and 10.

Sullivan implied that the need to avoid anxiety and the need to gratify basic needs are the primary motivations for behavior. His **concept of anxiety** states that *anxiety has its origin in the prolonged dependency of infancy, urgency of biological and emotional needs, and how the mothering person meets those needs. Anxiety is the result of uncomfortable interpersonal relationships, is the chief disruptive force in interpersonal relationships, is contagious through empathic feelings, and can be relieved by being in a secure interpersonal relationship* (182).

The **self-system** is the *internal organization of experiences that exists to defend against anxiety and to secure necessary security.* One aspect of the self-system is known as *good-me, bad-me,* and *not-me,* which refers to feelings about the self that begin to form in infancy (182).

Sullivan's developmental stages and concepts are summarized in Table 5–9 and described in Chapters 7 through 14 in relation to each developmental era. These concepts are pertinent to the understanding and care of the developing person and family unit (22, 182).

TABLE 5–9. SUMMARY OF SULLIVAN'S STAGES OF DEVELOPMENT

Stage/Chronological Age Period	Developmental Tools	Mode of Experience	Emotional Manifestations	Developmental Task
Birth to emergence of speech: 1–1½ years	Mouth Ability to cry, babble, coo Satisfaction response (pleasure principle) Empathic observation and response Exploration of environment Autistic invention (infant feels master of all that is seen)	Prototaxic	Fear, rage, anxiety during times of discomfort	Learns to rely on others to gratify needs; infant cannot be spoiled; needs must be met promptly, tenderly, and consistently to lay firm foundation for trust and to avoid anxiety of needs
Childhood 1½ years to emergence of need for peers (up to 6 years of age)	Language Anus Self-system and self-concept Experimentation with self and environment Motor skills Peer associations Identification	Parataxic	Anxiety, anger, shame, guilt, and doubt when distress is felt Good-me, positive self-concept, self-esteem and sense of reality about environment when needs for satisfaction and security are met and realistic limits are set consistently	Learns to delay gratification and accept interference with wish fulfillment
Juvenile 6 years to emergence of capacity to care for another (9–12 years, approximately)	Increasing intellectual ability Internal control over behavior Competition Compromise Collaboration Experimentation and exploration Motor skills Use of family allegiance and rules	Parataxic Beginning syntaxic	Wide variety of emotions in response to needs met or not met	Attends to peers' wishes and forms satisfactory relationship with peers of both sexes in order to have personal needs met, sometimes in opposition to parental rules
Preadolescence (chum stage) (9 years to puberty, approximately)	Collaboration Experimentation Exploration Manipulation of people and environment Use of communication and consensual validation with peers Use of family rules	Syntaxic May revert to parataxic	Capacity to care emotionally and unselfishly for another person of same sex Wide range of emotions Allegiance to peers increases	Becomes interested in and relates closely to friend of same sex (chum) and cares about chum as fully as for oneself Corrects previously encountered deprivation of needs or high anxiety through sharing with chum secrets, dreams, fantasies, and reality aspects of life
Early adolescence Onset of puberty until completion of primary and secondary sexual changes (12–14 years, approximately)	Sexual feelings Fantasies Experimentation Exploration Motor skills Interpersonal skills Heightened anxiety in interpersonal contacts Use of peer relations and mores instead of family rules	Syntaxic May revert to parataxic	Variety of emotions Rebellion and dependence may be present alternately with cooperation, collaboration, and independent behavior	Masters independence Establishes satisfactory relationships with peers of opposite sex
Late adolescence Completion of sexual changes (about 14 years) until establishment of durable relationship	Sense of self as integrated and sexual being Ability to use logic and abstractions Exploration Experimentation Interpersonal skills	Syntaxic May revert to parataxic	Initial feelings of love for member of opposite sex	Learns to maintain enduring relationship with member of opposite sex, which may eventuate in marriage or cohabitation

(continued)

TABLE 5–9. SUMMARY OF SULLIVAN'S STAGES OF DEVELOPMENT (continued)

Stage/Chronological Age Period	Developmental Tools	Mode of Experience	Emotional Manifestations	Developmental Task
Adulthood Biological maturity	Collaboration (ability to adjust own behavior and needs in pursuit of mutual gratification of needs with another) Feelings of lust Genital organs Feelings of responsibility and caring Assumption of vocation Reaffirmation of values	Syntaxic May revert to parataxic	Interdependent and permanent love for another Responsible and creative Balanced involvement with family, friends, vocation, and community	Achieves feelings of love and intimacy (situation where two people both accept all aspects of other, and physical and psychological needs of the other are more important than one's own needs; person's sense of identity firm so able to give self to another without fear of loss of own identity)

Erikson: Epigenetic Theory of Personality Development. Erik Erikson (35) formulated the Epigenetic Theory based on the principle of the unfolding embryo: anything that grows has a ground plan out of which parts arise. Each part has its time of special ascendancy until all parts have arisen to form a functional whole. Thus each stage of development is the base for the next stage. A result of mastering the developmental tasks of each stage is virtue or a feeling of competence, or direction.

His theory explains step-by-step unfolding of emotional development and social characteristics during encounters with the environment. Erikson's psychosexual theory enlarges on Psychoanalytic Theory because it is not limited to historical era, specific culture, or personality types; encompasses development through the life span and is universal to all people; and acknowledges that society, heredity, and childhood experiences all influence the person's development (35).

The following are basic principles of his theory, based on cross-cultural studies (35):

- Each phase has a specific developmental task to achieve or solve. These tasks describe the order and sequence of human development and the conditions necessary to accomplish them, but actual accomplishment is done at an individual pace, tempo, and intensity.
- Each psychosexual stage of development is a developmental crisis because there is a radical change in the person's perspective, a shift in energy, and an increased emotional vulnerability. During this peak time the potential in the personality comes in contact with the whole environment, and the person has some degree of success in solving the crucial developmental task of the specific era. How the person copes

with the task and crisis depends on previous developmental strengths and weaknesses.
- The potential inherent in each person evolves if given adequate chance to survive and grow. Anything that distorts the environment essential for development interferes with evolvement of the person. Society attempts to safeguard and encourage the proper rate and sequence of the unfolding of human potential so that humanity is maintained.
- Each developmental task is redeveloped, reworked, and redefined in subsequent stages. Potential for further development always exists.
- Internal organization is central to development. Maturity increases as the tasks of each era are accomplished, at least in part, in proper order.

Erikson proposed eight stages of development and described the developmental task of crisis for each stage (see Fig. 5–2). They are described in Chapters 7 through 14 in relation to each developmental era. His theory is widely accepted and used in understanding the developing person and in administering nursing care.

Jung's Theory. Carl Jung (37, 85–87, 181), another Neo-Analytic theorist, proposed the following assumptions about personality structure:

1. The ego or **consciousness** includes *awareness of self and the external world.*
2. The **persona** is the *image or mask presented to the outer world,* depending on the roles of the person.
3. The **shadow** consists of *traits and feelings that cannot be admitted to the self;* it is the opposite of ego or self-image.

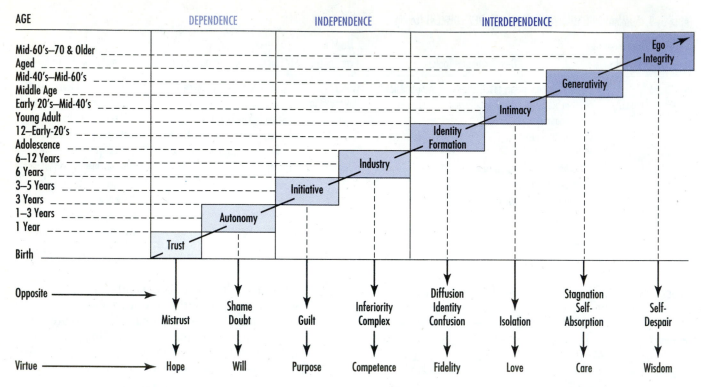

Figure 5–2. Erikson's Eight Stages of the Person.

4. The **anima** and **animus** in the personality refer to the *characteristics traditionally considered feminine and masculine.* Each person has both characteristics or is androgynous or bisexual with the feminine, nurturing, feeling side and the masculine, logical, assertive side. Socialization forces the person to overemphasize gender characteristics so that the opposite aspect of the person is not usually fully developed.

5. The unconscious is composed of two layers:

   a. The **personal unconscious** is unique, *contains all the repressed tendencies and feelings that build over the lifetime,* and *includes the shadow and some of the anima or animus.*

   b. The **collective unconscious** is *inherited and shared by all humankind and is composed of archetypes, or innate energy forces and organizing tendencies.* Archetype images are unknowable and are found in myths, art, dreams, and fantasies throughout the world and include the image of Earth Mother, Wise Old Man, death, the witch, rebirth, and God. The archetypes influence the nature and growth of other parts of the personality.

They are essentially unknowable, like instincts or innate perceptual tendencies.

6. Self is the most important archetype, our unconscious centeredness, wholeness, and meaning. It is an inner urge to balance and reconcile the opposing aspects of our personalities, represented in drawings of **mandalas,** *figures in which all sides are perfectly balanced around a center point.*

7. **Individuation** is the unattainable goal pursued by the self, which *involves finding the unique way, achieving a measure of psychic balance while separating self from societal conformity to goals and values.*

8. There are two basic personality types or tendencies:

   a. **Introversion** refers to being *inner-reflective, caught up in one's inner state, fears, hopes and feelings.* The introvert hesitates in relationships, is more secure in his or her inner world, and takes pleasure in activities that can be done alone.

   b. The **extrovert** confidently *engages in direct action and starts interactions with others.* The extrovert moves outward toward the world and prefers activities with people.

Research Abstract

Zerhusen, J., K. Boyle, and W. Wilson, Out of the Darkness: Group Cognitive Therapy for Depressed Elderly, Journal of Psychosocial Nursing, 29, no. 9 (1991), 16–21.

Depression affects approximately 50% of people over 65 years of age. With the current expansion of elderly in the United States, the problem is likely to increase. The depressed person perceives situations negatively when more positive interpretations are equally valid and misinterprets interactions in the environment. Cognitive therapy is intended to focus on cognitive distortions and the relearning of thought processes as a way to alter negative emotions such as depression, to raise self-esteem, and to gain hope for the future. Cognitive therapy can be used with groups as well as individuals. The purpose of this study was to determine if nursing home personnel could become effective cognitive therapy group leaders and if nursing home residents would be receptive to such a program.

The samples were 60 residents in a 100-bed intermediate-care nursing home in a Midwestern state. The samples were mostly Caucasian women; age ranged from 70 to 82. Four professional nurses and one social worker at the facility completed training to be cognitive group therapy leaders.

To determine effectiveness of cognitive therapy, the sample or treatment group was compared with two central groups matched for depression score on the Beck Depression Inventory, race, and sex. One control group received music therapy for 1 hour twice weekly. The second control group received the nursing care and rehabilitation services normally provided. The experimental group was divided into three smaller groups, and each received a 10-week program of cognitive therapy; each session met 1½ hours twice weekly. Sessions for the sample were divided into four phases: (1) preparation for cognitive therapy, (2) basis techniques for changing behavior, (3) basic techniques for changing cognition, and (4) preparation for termination of treatment.

Results indicated that resident attendance at the cognitive therapy group was significantly higher than at the music group. Ratings of the group leaders by the residents showed that in all three experimental groups the leaders were conducting cognitive therapy as conceived by Beck. The improvement in depression scores in the cognitive therapy groups was significantly higher than in the control groups. All outcomes of the study were positive, including those in physical function as well as in thought processes. Residents in the experimental group were pleased with the sessions and wanted more sessions.

Implications of this study are that cognitive group therapy is effective with depressed elders and is one way to help elders feel more satisfied about their life.

To Jung, life is a series of periods identified by different energy uses. Early childhood years were not emphasized in this developmental theory. The first period, until age 35 or 40, is a time of outward expansion. Maturational forces direct the growth of the ego and unfolding of capacities. After age 40, the person undergoes a transformation and looks for meaning in personal activities. With increasing age, there is increasing reflection. Late thirties and early forties were seen as important in life transition: this was seen as a time when energy from youthful interests was channeled to cultural and spiritual pursuits (87). Jung's theory is referred to again in the chapters on adulthood. His theory is gaining wider acceptance in the understanding of the developing adult.

COGNITIVE THEORY AND THEORISTS

Cognitive theorists can be divided into four groups:

1. Beck's Cognitive Theory (9, 10)
2. Behavioral-cognitive theorists (30, 34, 59, 61)
3. Social learning theorists (3, 4)
4. Cognitive development theorists (134, 136, 142)

Several theorists are discussed in this section.

Cognitive psychology *deals with the person as an information processor and problem solver.* The cognitive perspective is concerned with internal processes but emphasizes how people attempt to acquire, interpret, and use information to solve life's problems and to remain normal or healthy. It emphasizes conscious processes, present thoughts, and problem-solving strategies. The cognitive perspective has grown out of new directions in learning and psychodynamic theories. Some present-day learning theorists are becoming increasingly interested in what goes on within the person between the application of a stimulus and the response, and some current psychodynamic theorists are focusing on thinking and problem solving and on feelings and emotions. Relationships among emotions, motivations, and cognitive processes are being studied. Overlap between the cognitive perspective and other approaches is becoming more evident (88, 121).

Cognitive Theory of Beck

Aaron Beck originated Cognitive Theory and therapy. His premise was that psychological problems may result from repetitive automatic distorted or dysfunctional patterns of thinking, which have evolved from faulty learning, making incorrect inferences on the basis of inadequate or incorrect information, and not distinguishing adequately between imagination and reality. Unrealistic thinking may be attributed to enduring negative attitudes (low self-esteem, hopelessness, and helplessness) about self, the world, and the future (see Table 5–10). Dysfunctional thoughts represent the person's personal view of reality but may appear illogical to others. The idiosyncratic, angry, or distorted thought patterns may become activated by life stresses, yet the responses are automatic or based on past experiences, usually developed early in life and formed by relevant experience (10, 123, 128).

Cognitive therapy is a short-term, structured therapy involving an active collaboration between the patient and therapist toward achieving the therapy goals. It is usually conducted on an individual basis but may also be used with groups. The goals of therapy are to (1) help the person identify erroneous beliefs in relation to stressful events or behaviors; (2) help the person look at these thoughts, compare them with objective evidence, and correct distortions; (3) give feedback to the person about the accuracy of the new thoughts; and (4) allow and encourage the person to rehearse new cognitions in therapy and at home. Cognitive therapy helps the patient to use problem-solving techniques to identify distorted thoughts, to correct the dysfunctional thoughts, and to learn more realistic ways to formulate the experiences. The therapist serves as a teacher or

TABLE 5–10. DEFINITIONS OF COGNITIVE DISTORTIONS

Distortion	Definition
All-or-nothing thinking or dichotomous thinking	*Seeing events in black-and-white categories; if performance falls short of perfect, the self is a total failure.*
Overgeneralization	*Seeing a single negative event as a never-ending pattern of defeat.*
Mental filter or selective inattention	*Focusing on a single negative detail and exclusively so that vision of all reality becomes darkened; interpreting situation or life on basis of one incident.*
Disqualifying the positive	*Rejecting positive experiences by insisting they "don't count" for some reason or other. In this way a negative belief that is contradicted by everyday experiences is maintained.*
Jumping to conclusions or arbitrary inference	*Making a negative interpretation even though there are no definite facts that convincingly support the conclusion; holding to beliefs without supporting evidence.*
Mind reading	*Arbitrarily concluding that someone is reacting negatively to the self and not checking this out.*
The fortune teller error	*Anticipating that things will turn out badly, and feeling convinced that prediction is an already established fact.*
Magnification (catastrophizing) or minimization	*Exaggerating the importance of things (such as a goof-up or someone else's achievement), or inappropriately shrinking things until they appear tiny (own desirable qualities or the other person's imperfections). This is also called the "binocular trick."*
Emotional reasoning	*Assuming that negative emotions necessarily reflect the way things really are: "I feel it, therefore it must be true."*
Should statements	*Trying to motivate self with "shoulds" and "should nots." "Musts" and "oughts" are also offenders. The emotional consequence is guilt. Directing should statements toward others creates feelings of anger, frustration, and resentment.*
Labeling and mislabeling	*An extreme form of overgeneralization. Instead of describing the error, a negative label is attached to self: "I'm a loser." When someone else's behavior rubs the wrong way, attaching a negative label to him: "He's a louse." Mislabeling involves describing an event with language that is highly colored and emotionally loaded.*
Personalization	*Seeing self as the cause of some negative external event for which there was no responsibility.*

guide in the process and is nonjudgmental, objective, and empathetic. Questioning rigid beliefs and attitudes guide the person to refocus problems, alter errors in thinking, and rehearse new behavior patterns (10–13, 123, 128).

Behavioral-Cognitive Theorists

Two theorists, Albert Ellis and William Glasser, are a part of this group, and each have formulated a therapy approach based on their beliefs about people's needs and behavior.

Ellis: Rational-Emotive Therapy. Ellis developed Rational-Emotive Therapy (RET), a cognitive-behavioral therapy that includes a here-and-now or existential focus. The basic premises of RET are:

- The person is the center of his universe and has an enormous amount of potential control over what he or she feels and does, and can change behavior.
- All people have a basic set of values and assumptions that govern much of life. After assumptions are made, subsequent rational and irrational thinking and behaving can be specified, understood, and worked with. Negative self-talk about these values and assumptions is the cause of much misery.
- All people want to be happy and free from unnecessary pain and can learn to overcome biological handicaps and various idiosyncrasies.
- People want to live in and get along with members of a social group and can learn to overcome manifestations of hurt, self-depreciation, rejection, and depression.
- People want to relate closely with a few selected members of the group.
- People are not disturbed by the things that happen to them but by their view of these things.

Behaviors that support these basic values are rational; those that interfere with achieving happiness and value achievement are irrational (29–33, 123).

Ellis considers the ABCDE theory of personality in health and illness as central to his therapy (29–33, 123):

A Activating event
B Belief system or attitudes, values, beliefs about A, which may be irrational (negative)
C Emotional consequence—appropriate or inappropriate

D Disputing the irrational thought through logical examination and interrupting the learned patterns
E Effects of disputing—new emotional effect or consequences, new feelings and ways of thinking, as a result of various methods and exercises that direct the person to test different ways of interpreting the environment.

The goal of RET is creation of personal autonomy through a philosophic and educative approach. The person must understand that the universe is neither for or against him or her and that there are no absolute values by which to live. There are five criteria for rational thinking that are guides for determining whether a thought is rational or irrational and should be accepted by the self (29–33, 123):

1. **Objective reality:** This really happens; it is a fact.
2. **Life preserving:** What is rational will not take life.
3. **Goal producing:** Action and thoughts that assist in meeting personal goals.
4. **Significant personal conflict:** Person must determine how much conflict he or she will take and how to prevent this conflict.
5. **Significant environmental conflict:** Person must determine if his or her behavior will cause great problems with others (e.g., rejection or punishment). If problems with others are prevented, conflict is prevented.

The therapist is active and collaborates with the client in a carefully structured, time-limited therapy that focuses on specific problem areas or issues. The therapist may use a combination of behavioral and cognitive techniques, such as relaxation, thought stopping, assertiveness training, self-instruction, internal dialogues, and problem solving related to perceptions.

The person is taught to state the problem and feelings in response to the problem, challenge the thoughts through self-talk, and apply the five criteria for rational thinking. If the thought does not meet four out of the five criteria, it is irrational. The person then imagines self in a real situation that is positive and continues to hold that image until he or she can think and act in a more positive way, and thus feel more positive (29–33, 123).

Albert Ellis (85, 86, 123) developed a system to attack irrational ideas or beliefs and replace them with more realistic interpretations and self-talk. Irrational self-talk includes statements that "awfulize" experience, that is, make catastrophic, nightmarish interpretations of events. An irrational self-thought leads to unpleasant emotions. Rational self-talk leads to pleasant feelings and a positive interpretation of experiences. Rational thought is based on the idea that events occur and people experience these events (29–33, 40, 85, 86, 123).

The kinds of statements that Ellis (29–33, 85, 123) considers irrational include the following:

- External events cause most human misery; people simply react as events trigger their emotions.
- People must always be competent and perfect in all endeavors.
- Happiness can be achieved by inaction, passivity, and endless leisure.
- It is easier to avoid than to face life's difficulties and responsibilities.
- The past determines the present.
- It is horrible when people and things are not the way you want them to be.
- Unfamiliar or potentially dangerous situations always lead to fear and anxiety.
- People are helpless and have no control over what they experience or feel.
- People are fragile and cannot be told the truth.
- Rejection and abandonment are the result if one does not always try to please others.
- There are perfect loves and perfect relationships.
- A person's worth is dependent on achievement and production.
- Anger is bad and destructive.
- It is bad and wrong to go after what you want and need.

Refuting irrational ideas is a skill and requires practice in the following nine steps (29–33, 85, 123):

1. Write down the facts of the event, including only the observable behaviors.
2. Write down self-talk about the event, including all subjective value judgments, assumptions, beliefs, predictions, and worries.
3. Note which statements are classified by Ellis as irrational.
4. Focus on the emotional response to the event, using one or two words such as angry, hopeless, worthless, and afraid.
5. Select one irrational idea to refute.
6. Write down all evidence that the idea is false.
7. Write down the worst outcome that could happen if what is feared happens or what is desired is not attained.
8. Write down positive results that might occur if what is feared happens or if what is desired is not attained.
9. Substitute alternative self-talk to focus on positive statements.

Glasser: Reality Therapy. William Glasser is the founder of Reality Therapy, which derives its name from the insistence on dealing with behavior in the real world rather than with a client's subjective interpretation of feelings and thoughts. Reality Therapy can be used with people of any age and with any problem. Like problems are handled in the same manner (58–61, 123).

Glasser believes that all humans, in addition to survival, have a need to:

- Be loved, accepted, and belong
- Feel respect and worthwhile to self and others
- Be competent, achieve, and gain status, recognition, and power
- Have fun and enjoyment
- Have freedom, independence, and autonomy

Behavior is the attempt to reduce the difference between what we want and what we have. When needs are not met, the person acts differently, irresponsibly, or in a way that is called mental illness. The person's behavior will get him or her into trouble, and behavior, not feelings, is the key. It is the person's choice whether or not to act responsibly or to feel miserable. Yet the person is suffering because she or he cannot meet her or his needs and wants involvement with another person. The caring, involvement, and responsible behavior of the therapist will help the person face the unresponsible behavior and work toward or relearn more realistic, acceptable, or responsible behavior (58–61).

The reality therapist helps the client to meet these needs in the following ways (58–61, 123, 196, 197):

- Teaching what is realistic, responsible, and right behavior.
- Focusing on present behavior rather than on interpretations of past events, feelings, attitudes, insights, or reasons. The past is discussed only if it pertains to the present. The person is taught to accept her or his history and that it cannot be changed. All that can be changed is the present.
- Discussing the client's strengths and capacities as well as problems.
- Helping the person to evaluate his or her behavior and what is contributing to failure to meet needs.
- Eliciting a commitment from the client to change behavior without imposing values on the client.
- Supporting the client with personal involvement, enabling the client to face that he or she is responsible for personal behavior and change.
- Presenting specific alternatives and teaching the client better ways to fulfill needs.

- Encouraging the client to make a plan aimed at a desired goal and writing a specific plan.
- Encouraging the person to make choices and live responsibly from day to day, taking into consideration consequences to self and others.
- Not permitting the person to make excuses or place blame if the plan fails or if the commitment is not kept; reassessing the plan.
- Believing in the client's integrity, avoiding rejection or punishment if the person is not successful in changing behavior.
- Avoiding punishment and continuing to rework plans.

The most effective ways for the therapist to use the involvement–commitment process is to remember the following points: (1) A single experience with definition of a problem, involvement, and satisfaction of the person's needs does not guarantee responsible behavior in the next experience of a similar nature. (2) Responsible behavior is not necessarily generalized by the client and applied in a cognitive way. (3) The therapist's demands for behavioral standards may be unrealistic for the client. (4) The client may find ways of satisfying his or her psychological needs without using responsible behavior. (5) Behavior changes slowly; thus, the therapist or client should never give up (58–61, 123).

The goal of therapy is to develop a sense of responsibility defined as the ability to satisfy one's own needs without interfering with the needs of others, while behaving responsibly. The therapeutic problem is to get the client to abandon what may be called the "primitive pleasure principle" and to adopt long-term, wise pursuit of pleasure, satisfaction, joy, and happiness, which the reality principle implies (58–61, 123).

Advocates of Reality Therapy differ from advocates of conventional psychiatry and clinical psychology in the following ways (58–61, 123):

- They do not believe in a concept of mental illness and its associated concepts of classification and diagnosis. Such labeling tends to relieve the individual of responsibility for behavior.
- They work in the present and future, and do not get involved with the past, which is unchangeable.
- They relate to clients as people, not as transference figures.
- Unconscious conflicts are considered excuses for undesirable behavior.
- Morality of behavior is emphasized; that is, it is important for a person to know if behavior is right or wrong.

- Reality Therapy stresses teaching people behaviors that will help fulfill their needs rather than teaching an understanding of historical or unconscious conflicts or motivations.

Social Learning Theorist: Bandura

Albert Bandura's Social Learning Theory (3) states that learning occurs without reinforcement, conditioning, or trial-and-error behavior because people can think and anticipate consequences of behavior and act accordingly. This theory emphasizes (1) that cognitive processes, modeling, environmental influences, and the person's self-directed capacity all contribute to development, learning, and behavior; (2) the importance of vicarious, symbolic, and self-regulatory processes in psychological functioning; and (3) the capacity of the person to use symbols, represent events, analyze conscious experience, communicate with others at any distance in time and space, and plan, create, imagine, and engage in foresightful action. The person does not simply react to external forces: he or she selects, organizes, and transforms impinging stimuli and thus exercises some influence over personal behavior (3–8). Bandura's model of causation involves the interaction of three components: (1) the person, with cognitive, biological, and other internal events that affect perceptions and actions, (2) the external environment, and (3) behavior (5, 6).

Human nature is characterized as a vast potentiality that can be fashioned by direct and vicarious experience into a variety of forms of development and behavior within biological limits. The level of psychological and physiologic development restricts what can be acquired at any given time (3).

The person may be motivated by ideas or fantasies of future consequences or by personal goal-setting behavior. If the person wants to accomplish a certain goal and there are distractions from the task, the person visualizes how he or she will feel when the goal is attained. People respond evaluatively to their own behavior and tend to persist until the behavior or performance meets the goal (3).

Bandura (3) proposes that learning occurs through **modeling,** *imitation of another's behavior.* According to his theory, much of our daily behavior is learned by modeling and the perceptions that form in the process. Imitation is one of the most effective forms of learning. Babies learn to speak by imitating the sounds of their parents; older children learn a number of behaviors by watching teacher, parent, or peers. People learn how to be normal or abnormal. Maladaptive behavior arises from modeling when the child imitates abnormal parental behavior. Bandura's research also shows the power of watching television on people's behavior and that for some people the model of aggressive behavior will cause later acting-out behavior. This research is discussed further in Chapter 10.

Bandura's research combines aspects of Behavioral and Psychodynamic theories and is pertinent to understanding certain aspects of the developing person. His theory is also pertinent to nursing care, especially the educational role (4–8, 68, 128).

Cognitive Development Theorist: Piaget

Jean Piaget (131–142) formulated the Theory of Cognitive Development. The bulk of his research was concerned with the child's thinking at particular periods of life and with studying differences among well children of a specific age. A great amount of empirical data was used in developing the theory. He believed that development is neither **maturational,** an *unfolding of the innate growth process,* nor **learning,** an *accumulation of experiences.* Rather, development is an active process resulting from **equilibration,** an *internal force that is set in motion to organize thinking when the child's belief system develops sufficiently to contain self-contradictions.*

Four factors interact within the person to stimulate mental development (142):

1. Maturation of the nervous and endocrine systems, which provides physical capabilities
2. Experience involving action, with a consequent discovery of properties of objects
3. Social interaction with opportunity to observe a wide variety of behaviors and gain direct instruction and to receive feedback about individual performance
4. An internal self-regulation mechanism that responds to environmental stimuli

Intelligence is an adaptive process by which the person modifies and structures the environment to fit personal needs and also modifies self in response to environmental demands.

By interaction with the environment, the person constructs reality by assimilation, accommodation, and adaptation. **Assimilation** is *taking new and content experiences into the mind or cognitive structure.* **Accommodation** is the *revising, realigning, and readjusting of cognitive structure to take into account the new content.* **Adaptation** is the *change that results from the first two processes.* Piaget emphasizes the innate, inborn processes of the person as the essential force to start

the process of equilibration or cognitive growth. Cognitive development proceeds from motor activity to interaction with the wider social world and, finally, to abstract ideas. Development is seen as solidly rooted in what already exists, and it displays a continuity with the past. Adaptations do not develop in isolation; all form a coherent pattern so that the totality of biological life is adapted to its environment. The theory focuses on development of intellectual capacities with little reference to emotional or social development (131–143, 190).

The thinking process is explained by schematic mental structures of pictures formed in response to stimuli. A **schema** is a *cognitive structure, a complex concept encompassing both motor behavior and internalized thought processes.* A schema *involves movement of the eyeballs, paying attention, and the mental picture that is formed as a result of the sensory process.* Thinking eventually involves using combinations of mental pictures, forming concepts, internalizing use of language or subvocal speech, drawing implications, and making judgments. When these internal actions become integrated into a coherent, logical system, they are considered logical operations. The schemata that are developed and the specific levels of function are unique to each person and, in turn, structure future learning. Learning is determined by (1) what is observed, (2) whether new information is fit into old schemata accurately or in a distorted way, and (3) how much increase in competence results from the encounter or experience (131–143).

Piaget divided human development into four periods: sensorimotor, preoperational, concrete operations, and formal operations. See Table 5–11 for a summary of the periods. In each stage the person demonstrates interpretation and use of the environment through certain behavior patterns. He or she incorporates and restructures the previous stage and refines ability to perceive and understand. Suggested ages for each stage are indicated, but innate intellectual ability and environmental factors may cause variation. These periods are discussed with development of the infant, toddler, preschooler, schoolchild, and adolescent. You will find these stages pertinent to determining mental development of the person and corresponding educational approaches and activities (48, 131–143, 190).

Moral Development Theorists

Kohlberg's Theory of Moral Development. Lawrence Kohlberg formulated a Theory of Moral Development. Moral development is related to cognitive and emotional devel-

TABLE 5–11 SUMMARY OF PIAGET'S THEORY OF COGNITIVE DEVELOPMENT

Period	Age	Characteristics
Sensorimotor Period		
Stage 1: Use of reflexes	0–1 month	Behavior innate, reflexive, specific, predictable to specific stimuli *Example:* sucking, grasping, eye movements, startle (Moro reflex)
Stage 2: First acquired adaptations and primary circular reactions	1–4 months	Initiates, prolongs, and repeats behavior not previously occurring Acquires response to stimulus that creates another stimulus and response Modifies innate reflexes to mroe purposeful behavior; repeated if satisfying Learns feel of own body as physiologic stabilization occurs *Example:* Looks at object, reaches for it, and continues to repeat until vision, reaching, and mouthing are coordinated
Stage 3: Secondary circular reactions	4–8 months	Learns from unintentional behavior Motor skills and vision further coordinated as infant learns to prolong or repeat interesting act Interest in environment around self Explores world from sitting position Assimilates new objects into old behavior pattern Behavior increasingly intentional *Example:* looks for object that disappears from sight; continues to drop object from different locations, which adult continues to pick up
Stage 4: Coordination of secondary schema: acquisition of instrumental behavior, active search for vanished objects	8–12 months	Uses familiar behavior patterns in new situation to accomplish goal Differentiates objects, including mother from stranger (stranger anxiety) Retains memory of object hidden from view Combines actions to obtain desired, hidden object; explores object Imitates others when behavior finished Develops individual habits Cognitive development enhanced by increasing motor and language skills
Stage 5: Tertiary circular reactions and discovery of new means by active experimentation	12–18 months	Invents new behavior not previously performed Uses fewer previous behaviors Repeats action without random movements Explores variations that occur when same act accomplished Varies action deliberately as repeats behavior Uses trial-and-error behavior to discover solution to problem Differentiates self from object and object from action performed by self; increasing exploration of how objects function Invents new means to solve problems and variation in behavior essential to later symbolic behavior and concept formation
Stage 6: Internal representation of action in external world	18–24 months	Pictures events to self; follows through mentally to some degree Imitates when model out of sight Forms mental picture of external body, of body in same space with another object, and of space in limited way Uses deliberate trial and error in solving problems
Preoperational Period	2–7 years	Internalizes schemata of more and more of the environment, rules, and relationships Forms memories to greater extent Uses fantasy or imitation of others in behavior and play Intermingles fantasy and reality Uses words to represent objects and events more accurately; symbolic behavior increases **Egocentric** *(self-centered in thought)*—focuses on single aspect of object and neglects other attributes because of lack of experience and reference systems, which results in false logic Follows rules in egocentric way; rules external to self Is static and irreversible in thinking; cannot transform from one state to another (e.g., ice to water) Develops story or idea while forgetting original idea so that final statements disconnected, disorganized; answer not connected to original idea in monologue Tries logical thinking; at times sounds logical but lacks perspective so that false logic and inconsistent, unorganized thinking result Is magical, global, primitive in reasoning Begins to connect past to present events, not necessarily accurate Links events by sequence rather than causality

(continued)

TABLE 5–11 SUMMARY OF PIAGET'S THEORY OF COGNITIVE DEVELOPMENT (continued)

Period	Age	Characteristics
		Deals with information by recall; begins to categorize
		Is **anthropomorphic** *(attributes human characteristics to animals and objects)*
		Unable to integrate events separated by time, past to present
		Lacks reversibility in thinking
		Unable to anticipate how situation looks from another viewpoint
Preconceptual stage	2–4 years	Forms images or preconcepts on basis of thinking just described
		Lacks ability to define property or to denote hierarchy or relationships of objects
		Constructs concepts in global way
		Unable to use time, space, equivalence, and class inclusion in concept formation
Intuitive stage	4–7 years	Forms concepts increasingly; some limitations
		Defines one property at a time
		Has difficulty starting definition but knows how to use object
		Uses transductive logic (from general to specific) rather than deductive or inductive logic
		Begins to classify in ascending or descending order; labels
		Begins to do seriation; reverses processes and ordinality
		Begins to note cause–effect relationships
Concrete Operations Period	7–11 years (or beyond)	Organizes and stabilizes thinking; more rational
		See interrelationships increasingly
		Does mental operations using tangible, visible references
		Able to **decenter** *(sees other perspectives; associates or combines events;* understands reversibility [e.g., add–subtract, ice–water transformation])
		Recognizes number, length, volume, area, weight as the same even when perception of object changes
		Develops conservation as experience is gained with physical properties of objects
		Arranges objects in order of size and other characteristics
		Fits new objects into series
		Understands simpler relationships between classes of objects
		Distinguishes between distances
		Understands observable world, tangible situations, time, and tangible space
		Retains essential idea when perceiving conflicting or unorganized data
		Recognizes rules as essential; perceives mutually agreed on standards
		Is less egocentric except in social relationships
Formal Operations Period	12 years and beyond	Manifests adultlike thinking
		Not limited by own perception or concrete references for ideas
		Combines various ideas into concepts
		Coordinates two or more reference systems
		Develops morality of restraint and cooperation in behavior
		Uses rules to structure interaction in socially acceptable way
		Uses probability concept
		Works from definition or concept only to solve problem
		Solves problem mentally and considers alternatives before acting
		Considers number of variables at one time
		Links variables to formulate hypotheses
		Begins to reason deductively and inductively instead of solving problem by action
		Relates concepts or constructs not readily evident in external world
		Formulates advanced concepts of proportions, space, destiny, momentum
		Increases intellectual ability to include art, science, humanities, religion, philosophy
		Is increasingly less egocentric

opment and to societal values and norms and is divided into stages by Kohlberg (94–98).

Moral reasoning focuses on 10 universal values: punishment, property, roles and concerns related to affection, roles and concerns related to authority, law, life, liberty, distribution of justice, truth, and sexual behavior. A conflict between two or more of these universal values necessitates a moral choice and its subsequent justification by the individual, requiring systematic problem solving and other cognitive capabilities (94–98, 147).

Kohlberg theorized that a person's moral reasoning process and behavior develop through six stages over varying lengths of time. Each stage is derived from a prior stage and is the basis for the next stage. *Each moral stage is based or dependent on the reason for behavior and shows an organized system of thought by which the person is consistent in the level of moral judgment.* The person is considered in a specific stage when the same level of reason for action is given at least half the time. More advanced logical thinking is needed for each successive moral stage. One criterion of moral maturity, the ability to decide autonomously what is right and caring, is lacking in the Preconventional and Conventional levels because in each level the person is following the commands of authority figures. If the person's cognitive stage is at Concrete Operations, according to Piaget, the person is limited to the Preconventional or Conventional Levels of moral reasoning. Even the person in Formal Operations may not be beyond the Conventional Level of moral maturity. Kohlberg found that 50% of late adolescents and adults are capable of formal operations thinking, but only 10% of these adults demonstrated the Postconventional Level in stages 5 and 6. Thus the person moves through stages, but few people progress through all six stages. Table 5–12 shows the three levels and six stages. Moral development is discussed in relation to each developmental era in Chapters 7 through 14 (94–98).

Development of moral judgment is stimulated whenever (1) the educational process intentionally creates cognitive conflict and disequilibrium so that the person can work through inadequate modes of thinking, (2) when the person has opportunity for group discussion of values and can participate in group decision making about moral issues, and (3) the person has opportunity to assume responsibility for the consequences of behavior (97). Walker found that Kohlberg's moral stages were revealed over a 2-year interval in 233 subjects aged 5 to 63 years (191). Kohlberg's theory has application to nursing, education (97, 191, 192), and family counseling (147). Studies show that moral development continues as he describes through adulthood (108, 147).

Gilligan's Theory of Moral Development. Gilligan's research on moral development has focused on women, in contrast to Kohlberg's focus on men. Gilligan found that moral development proceeds through three levels and two transitions, with each level representing a more complex understanding of the relationship of self and others and each transition resulting in a crucial reevaluation of the conflict between selfishness and responsibility. Women define the moral problem in context of human relationships, exercising care and avoiding hurt. In her studies women's moral judgment proceeded from initial concern with survival, to a focus on goodness, to a principled understanding of others' need for care. Table 5–13 summarizes the three levels and two transitions of moral development proposed by Gilligan (54–56).

The focus on justice by Kohlberg is concerned with issues of inequality and oppression, and the theory values reciprocal rights and equal respect for individuals. The care focus proposed by Gilligan is concerned with issues of abandonment, and the theory values ideals of attention and response to need (54–56). Cooper describes how the value of caring makes it pertinent to nursing (25).

Some people may combine both perspectives and incorporate them into their moral development—such values as honesty, courage, and community, which are implied in Kohlberg's Postconventional Level. More research in all age groups, men and women, and all races and ethnic groups is needed to understand moral development fully.

Friedman (46) tested Gilligan's claim that men and women differ in moral judgments. College students read four traditional moral dilemmas and rated the importance of 12 considerations for deciding how the protagonist should respond. There were no reliable sex differences on moral reasoning. Sex-typed personality measures also failed to predict individual differences in moral judgments.

EXISTENTIAL AND HUMANISTIC THEORIES

Overview

Existential and humanistic psychologies acknowledge the dynamic aspect of the person but emphasize the impact of environment to a greater degree.

Existentialism has its roots in philosophy, theology, literature, and psychology and *addresses the person's existence in a hostile or indifferent world and within the context of history.* It is phenomenologic in nature; the context, uniqueness, and ever-changing aspects of events are considered. Existentialism regards human

TABLE 5–12 PROGRESSION OF MORAL DEVELOPMENT

Level	Stage
Preconventional Person is responsive to cultural rules of labels of good and bad, right or wrong. Externally established rules determine right or wrong actions. Person reasons in terms of punishment, reward, or exchange of favors. Egocentric focus	I. *Punishment and Obedient Orientation* Fear of punishment, not respect for authority, is the reason for decisions, behavior, and conformity. *Good* and *bad* are defined in terms of physical consequences to the self from parental, adult, or authority figures. The person defers to superior power or prestige of the person who dictates rules ("I'll do something because you tell me, and to avoid getting punished"). Average age: toddler to 7 years II. *Instrumental Relativist Orientation* Conformity is based on egocentricity and narcissistic needs. The person's decisions and behavior are usually based on what provides satisfaction out of concern for self: something is done to get something in return. Occasionally the person does something to please another for pragmatic reasons. There is no feeling of justice, loyalty, or gratitude. These concepts are expressed physically ("I'll do something if I get something for it or because it pleases you"). Average age: preschooler through school age.
Conventional Person is concerned with maintaining expectations and rules of the family, group, nation, or society. A sense of guilt has developed and affects behavior. The person values conformity, loyalty, and active maintenance of social order and control. Conformity means good behavior or what pleases or helps another and is approved. Societal focus	III. *Interpersonal Concordance Orientation* A. Decisions and behavior are based on concerns about others' reactions; the person wants others' approval or a reward. The person has moved from egocentricity to consideration of others as a basis for behavior. Behavior is judged by the person's intentions ("I'll do something because it will please you or because it is expected"). B. An empathic response, based on understanding of how another person feels, is a determinant for decisions and behavior ("I'll do something because I know how it feels to be without; I can put myself in your shoes"). Average age: school age through adulthood. (Most American women are in this stage.) IV. *Law-and-Order Orientation* The person wants established rules from authorities, and the reason for decisions and behavior is that social and sexual rules and traditions demand the response. The person obeys the law just because it is the law or out of respect for authority and underlying morality of the law. The law takes precedence over personal wishes, good intentions, and conformity to group stereotypes ("I'll do something because it's the law and my duty"). Average age: adolescence and adulthood (Most men are in this stage; 80% of adults do not move past this stage.)
Postconventional The person lives autonomously and defines moral values and principles that are distinct from personal identification with group values. He or she lives according to principles that are universally agreed on and that the person considers appropriate for life. Universal focus	V. *Social Contract Legalistic Orientation* The social rules are not the sole basis for decisions and behavior because the person believes a higher moral principle applies such as equality, justice, or due process. The person defines right actions in terms of general individual rights and standards that have been agreed on by the whole society but is aware of relativistic nature of values and opinions. The person believes laws can be changed as people's needs change. The person uses freedom of choice in living up to higher principles but believes the way to make changes is through the system. Outside the legal realm, free agreement and contract are the binding elements of obligation ("I'll do something because it is morally and legally right, even if it isn't popular with the group"). Average age: middle-age or older adult. Only 20% or less of Americans achieve this stage. VI. *Universal Ethical Principle Orientation* Decisions and behavior are based on internalized rules, on conscience rather than on social laws, and on self-chosen ethical and abstract principles that are universal, comprehensive, and consistent. The rules are not concrete moral rules but instead encompass the Golden Rule, justice, reciprocity, and equality of human rights, and respect for the dignity of human beings as individual persons. Human life is inviolable. The person believes there is a higher order than social order, has a clear concept of civil disobedience, and will use self as an example to right a wrong. The person accepts injustice, pain, and death as an integral part of existence but works to minimize injustice and pain for others ("I'll do something because it is morally, ethically, and spiritually right, even if it is illegal and I get punished and even if no one else participates in the act"). Average age: middle-age or older adult. (Few people attain or maintain this stage. Examples of this stage are seen in times of crisis or extreme situations.)

Data from References 94–97.

TABLE 5–13. GILLIGAN'S THEORY OF MORAL DEVELOPMENT

Level	Characteristics
I. Orientation of Individual Survival	*Concentrates on what is practical and best for self; selfish; dependent on others*
Transition 1: **From Selfishness to Responsibility**	Realizes connection to others; thinks of responsible choice in terms of another as well as self
II. Goodness as Self-Sacrifice	*Sacrifices personal wishes and needs to fulfill others' wants* and to have others think well of her; feels responsible for others' actions; holds others responsible for her choices; dependent position; indirect efforts to control others often turn into manipulation through use of guilt; aware of connectedness with others.
Transition 2: **From Goodness to Truth**	*Makes decisions on personal intentions and consequences of actions rather than on how she thinks others will react; takes into account needs of self and others; wants to be good to others but also honest by being responsible to self; increased social participation; assumes more responsibilities.*
III. Morality of Nonviolence	*Establishes moral equality between self and others; assumes responsibility for choice in moral dilemmas; follows injunction to hurt no one, including self, in all situations; conflict between selfishness and selflessness; judgment based on view of consequences and intentions instead of appearance in the eyes of others.*

Data from References 54–56.

nature as unexplainable but emphasizes freedom of choice, responsibility, satisfaction of ideals, the burden of freedom, discovery of inner self, and consequences of action. Themes addressed include suffering, death, despair, meaninglessness, nothingness, vacuum, isolation, anxiety, hope, self-transcendence, and finding spiritual meaning. The transcendence of inevitable suffering, anxiety, and alienation is emphasized (38, 39, 186).

Humanism *emphasizes self-actualization, satisfaction of needs, the individual as a rule unto himself or herself, the pleasure of freedom, and realization of innate goodness and creativity* (187). Humanism shares the following assumptions with existentialism: uniqueness of the person, potential of the person, and necessity of listening to or studying the person's perceptions, called the *phenomenologic approach.*

Both existentialists and humanists seek to answer the following questions: What are the possibilities of the person? From these possibilities, what is an optimum state for the person? Under what conditions is this state most likely to be reached? These disciplines strive to maximize the individuality and developmental potential of the person (110, 114, 119, 187).

Because all behavior is considered a function of the person's perceptions, data for study of the person are subjective and come from self-reports, including (1) feelings at the moment about self and the experience, (2) meaning of the experience, and (3) personal values, needs, attitudes, beliefs, behavioral norms, and expectations. Perception is synonymous with reality and meaning. The person has many components—physical, physiologic, cognitive, emotional, spiritual, cultural, social, and familial—and cannot be adequately understood if studied by individual components. The person is also affected by many variables, both objective and subjective.

All behavior is pertinent to and a product of the phenomenal or perceptual field of the person at the moment of action. The **phenomenal field** is the *frame of reference and the universe as experienced by the person at the specific moment (the existential condition)* (20, 111, 187).

View of the Human

The person is viewed as a significant and unique whole individual in dynamic interaction with the environment and in the process of becoming. In addition, the person is seen as holistic, with organizational complexity, more than the sum of the parts. The person is constantly growing, changing, expanding perceptual processes, learning, developing potential, and gaining insights. Every experience affects the person, depending on the perceptions. The person is never quite the same as he or she was even an hour or day earlier. The goals of the creative being are growth, feeling adequate, and reaching the potential. The person is active in pursuing these goals. Basic needs are the maintenance and enhancement of the self-concept and a sense of adequacy and self-actualization (20, 109, 111, 187).

Reality is internal; the person's reality is the perception of the event rather than the actual event itself. No two people will view a situation in exactly the same way. Various factors affect perception: (1) the sensory apparatus and central nervous system of the person; (2) time for observation; (3) opportunities available to experience events; (4) the external environment; (5) interpersonal relationships; and (6) self-concept. What is most important to the person is conscious experience, what is happening to the self at a given time. The person is aware of social values and norms but lives out those values and norms in a way that has been uniquely and personally defined (111).

Perceptions are crucial in influencing behavior. Of all the perceptions that exist for the person, none is more important than those held about the self and the personal meaning and belief related to a situation. Self-concept is learned as a consequence of meaningful interactions with others and the world and has a high degree of stability at its core, changing only with time and opportunity to try new perceptions of self.

The truly adequate person sees self (and others) as having dignity, integrity, worth, and importance. Only with a positive view of self can the person risk trying the untried or accepting the undefined situation. The person can become self-actualized only through the experience of being treated as an adequate person by significant others. This person is open to all experiences, develops trust in self, and dares to recognize feelings, live life fully, and express uniqueness. The person feels a sense of oneness with other people, depending on the nature of previous contacts.

View of Education and Therapy

Education and therapy are (1) growth-oriented rather than controlling, (2) rooted in perceptual meaning rather than facts, (3) concerned with people rather than things, (4) focused on the immediate rather than the historical view of people, and (5) hopeful rather than despairing. The goals of education and therapy are the same goals as those of the person: full functioning of the person, ongoing development, meeting the individual's potential, and movement toward self-actualization. Education and therapy are a process, not a condition or institution, and through the process the person achieves effective behavior. The basic tenets of freedom and responsibility are essential focal points in this approach (20, 123, 151–156).

The learner or client brings to the learning or counseling situation a cluster of understandings, skills, values, and attitudes that have personal meaning and are the sum of reactions to previous experiences. The learner or client is unique, with a unique heredity and cultural and home background. He or she wants to learn that which has personal meaning and which will contribute to making a more adequate person. Therefore, the person must be fully involved, and learning involves all dimensions of the person. Learning results from experiencing. Facts are not as important as developing the perceptual field and finding the self. The

learning that occurs depends on the meaning given by the person to the situation (20, 123, 151–156).

The teacher or therapist is also a unique, whole person with a self-concept that directly affects the philosophy and style of teaching or counseling. He or she does not consider self as central, but instead is learner- or client-centered. Each sees the self as using the personality as an instrument, acting as a permissive facilitator, and providing a warm, accepting, supportive environment that is as free from threat and obstacles as possible. The teacher or therapist provides an enriched environment and a variety of ways for the person to perceive new experiences and to learn. The teacher/therapist realizes that all people need to be perceived and related to as empathic, cooperative, forward-looking, trustworthy, and responsible. These theorists reject the traditional, pessimistic, or mechanical view of people (123, 151–156).

One of the most positive contributions of this viewpoint is its focus on human consciousness. The Behaviorists rejected the idea of a conscious mind. Psychodynamic writers agreed that conscious mental activity was important but only as much as it reflected what was going on in the unconscious. These theorists are very much interested in consciousness as the vehicle by which we solve personal problems (123).

Humanistic psychology emphasizes the natural tendency of all people, regardless of age or stage of life, to strive for self-actualization. Treatment approaches promote increased self-esteem and positive self-concept, problem solving to achieve goals, and helping the person achieve optimal functioning through a supportive therapeutic relationship characterized by warmth, nonpossessive caring, and validation of the person's worth and dignity. This approach of emphasizing the person's worth, achievement, and goals is ineffective and unacceptably narcissistic if the cultural value adhered to emphasizes the group or collective gain. If realistic environmental stressors are not acknowledged in relation to the self, the approach may be considered irrelevant, inappropriate, or ineffective (123).

Existential and Humanistic Theorists

Theorists in this group include the humanist Abraham Maslow (Theory of Motivation and Hierarchy of Needs [109–111]) and the humanist–existentialist Carl Rogers (Theory on Self-concept and Client-centered Therapy [151–156]). Other humanist–existentialists are Sidney Jourard (84) and Rollo May (112–116). Humanistic nursing as a framework has been developed by Josephine Paterson and Loretta Zderad (127) and Joyce

Travelbee (186). Although found as a thread in other nursing models, including Neuman's Health Care Systems Model (124), humanism is the basis for the views of Hildegard Peplau (129), Dorothy Johnson (148), and Martha Rogers (157). Maslow and Carl Rogers are discussed in this chapter. References at the end of the chapter give information on other theorists who have contributed to nursing.

Maslow: Theory of Motivation and Hierarchy of Needs

Maslow studied normal people and mental health in contrast to other developmental and personality theorists. One of his most important concepts is **self-actualization,** the *tendency to develop potentialities and become a better person,* and the need to help the person achieve the sense of self-direction implicit in self-actualization. Implicit in this concept is that people are not static but are always in the process of becoming different and better (109–111).

The needs that motivate self-actualization can be represented in a hierarchy of relative order and predominance. The basic needs, always a consideration in client care, are listed in Table 5–14.

Maslow's study of self-actualizing people refutes Freudian theory that the human unconscious, or id, is only bad or dangerous. In self-actualizing people the unconscious is creative, loving, and positive.

Although Maslow ranked these basic human needs from lowest to highest, they do not necessarily occur in a fixed order. The physiologic and safety needs (deficiency needs), however, are dominant and must be met before higher needs can be secured. Personal growth needs are those for love and belonging, self-esteem and recognition, and self-actualization. The highest needs of self-actualization, knowledge, and aesthetic expression may never be as fully gratified as those at lower levels. Individual growth and self-fulfillment are a continuing, lifelong process of becoming (110).

To motivate the person toward self-actualization, there must be freedom to speak, to pursue creative potential, and to inquire; an atmosphere of justice, honesty, fairness, and order; and environmental stimulation and challenge. Many have trouble moving toward self-actualization because of the environment in which they live. For example, socialization practices may hinder women in using fully their intellectual abilities. Men may be inhibited from expressing emotions of tenderness, love, or need of others by cultural norms. Deprivation of growth needs results in feelings of despair and depression and a sense that life is meaningless (109–111).

TABLE 5–14. MASLOW'S THEORY OF HIERARCHY OF NEEDS

Needs*	Characteristics
Physiologic	Requirements for oxygen, water, food, temperature control, elimination, shelter, exercise, sleep, sensory stimulation, and sexual activity met
	Needs cease to exist as means of determining behavior when satisfied, re-emerging only if blocked or frustrated
Safety	Able to secure shelter
	Sense of security, dependency, consistency, stability
	Maintenance of predictable environment, structure, order, fairness, limits
	Protection from immediate or future danger to physical well-being
	Freedom from fear, anxiety, chaos, and certain amount of routine
Love and belonging	Sense of affection, love, and acceptance from others
	Sense of companionship and affiliation with others
	Identification with significant others
	Recognition and approval from others
	Group interaction
	Not synonymous with sexual needs, but sexual needs may be motivated by this need
Esteem from others	Awareness of own individuality, uniqueness
	Feelings of self-respect and worth and respect from others
	Sense of confidence, independence, dignity
	Sense of competence, achievement, success, prestige, status
	Recognition from others for accomplishments
Self-actualization	Acceptance of self and others
	Empathetic with others
	Self-fulfillment
	Ongoing emotional and spiritual development
	Desire to attain standards of excellence and individual potential
	Use of talents, being productive and creative
	Experiencing fully, vividly, without self-consciousness
	Having peak experiences
Aesthetic	Desire for beauty, harmony, order, attractive surroundings
	Interest in art, music, literature, dance, creative forms
Knowledge and understanding	Desire to understand, systematize, organize, analyze, look for relations and meanings
	Curiosity; desire to know as much as possible
	Attraction to the unknown or mysterious

*Needs are listed in descending order. Physiologic needs are most basic; self-actualization is highest level of needs.
Data from References 109–111.

Carl Rogers: Theory on Self-concept and Client-centered Therapy

Carl Rogers is, along with Maslow, one of the leaders of humanistic–existentialist psychology. He has questioned several traditional concepts of science and has developed a perspective on personality with a focus on self-concept. Self-actualization is also a key concept in his theory. Rogers assumed that the person sees self as the center of a continually changing world and that he or she responds to the world as it is perceived. The person responds as a whole in the direction of self-actualization. The ability to achieve self-understanding, self-actualization, self-regard, and perception of social acceptance by others is based on experience and interaction with other people. The person who, as a child, felt wanted and highly valued is likely to have a positive self-image, be thought well of by others, and have the capacity to achieve self-actualization. Optimal adjustment results in what Rogers calls the fully functioning person. The fully functioning person accepts self, avoids a personality facade, is genuine and honest, is increasingly self-directive and autonomous, is open to new experiences, avoids being driven by other people's expectations or the cultural norms, and has a low level of anxiety (123, 151–156).

The person also has an ideal self, an idea of what he or she wishes to be, which may or may not be congruent with the "real" self. When a discrepancy develops between the "ideal" self and the "real" self, a state of tension and confusion results. For example, interactions with the environment may present an unfavorable picture of the self, which will result in internal conflict. Feelings of unworthiness may produce anxiety and defensive psychological reactions (123, 151).

Although the ways in which they have talked about behavior contrast sharply, both Rogers and Freud have developed their theoretical positions on the basis of similar observational data: the behavior of clients and therapists in psychotherapy. Rogers rejects, however, the psychoanalytic notion that the individual is by nature irrational and unsocialized. He asserts, on the contrary, that each person is basically rational, socialized, and constructive (154). Behavior is goal-directed and motivated by needs. Unlike the intrapsychic and interpersonal theorists. Rogers states that current needs are the only ones the person endeavors to satisfy (123, 151, 152).

Rogers identifies neurotic and psychotic people as those whose self-concept and experiences do not match up. They are afraid to accept their own experiences as valid, so they distort them, either to protect themselves or to win approval from others. A therapist can help them give up the false self that has been formulated (123, 151).

Rogers's technique of client-centered therapy brings about behavioral change by conveying complete acceptance, respect, and empathy for the client. The therapist neither provides interpretations nor gives advice. Providing this high degree of acceptance allows the person to meet basic needs that should have been met in childhood by significant people, to incorporate into the self-structure threatening feelings that were previously excluded, and to become aware of unconscious material that is controlling life. Perceptions and behavior change. The person may then continue the self-actualizing process. Recently Rogers has given the therapist a more active role that includes sharing emotions and feelings in an interchange with the client. Chapter 6 discusses use of Rogers's technique as it can be applied to the nurse–client relationship (123, 151).

STRESS AND CRISIS THEORIES

Two theories describe how a person responds to stressors, both routine and severe, and to overwhelming events. The Theory of Stress and General Adaptation Syndrome, as formulated by Seyle, described the physiologic adaptive response to stress, the everyday wear and tear on the person (160–166); however, continued studies show that the stress response has emotional, cognitive, and sometimes social effects as well. Crisis Theory was formulated to explain how people respond psychologically and behaviorally when they cannot cope adequately with stressors, but crises or overwhelming events also have physical effects. The two theories together explain a range of adaptive responses, for stress response always occurs in crisis to some extent, although not every stressor constitutes a crisis. Stressors and crises are a part of development throughout the life span and do affect health. An understanding of the theories is essential for health promotion.

Theory of Stress Response and Adaptation

Stress Response and Adaptation Syndrome

Stress is a *physical and emotional state always present in the person, one influenced by various environmental, psychological, and social factors but uniquely perceived by the person and intensified in response when environmental change or threat occurs internally or externally and the person must respond.* The manifestations of stress are both overt and covert, purposeful, initially protective, maintaining equilibrium, productivity, and satisfaction to the extent possible (123, 160–166).

The person's survival depends on constant mediation between environmental demands and adaptive capacities. Various self-regulatory physical and emotional mechanisms are in constant operation, adjusting the body to a changing number and nature of internal and external stressors, agents, or factors causing intensification of the stress state. **Stressors** (*stress agents*) encompass a number of types of stimuli (see Table 5–15) (123). **Eustress** is the *stress that comes with successful adaptation and that is beneficial or promotes emotional development and self-actualization.* It is *positive stress,* an optimum orientation to life's challenges coupled with the person's ability to regulate life and maintain optimum levels of stress for a growth-promoting lifestyle (161, 165). A moderate amount of stress, when regulatory mechanisms act within limits and few symptoms are observable, is constructive. **Daily hassles** are the *repeated and chronic strains of everyday life.* Daily hassles have a negative effect on both somatic health and psychological status (28). The exaggerated stress state occurs when stressors are excessive or intense, limits of the steady state are exceeded, and the person cannot cope with the stressor's demands. **Distress** is *negative, noxious, unpleasant, damaging stress* that results when adaptive capacity is decreased or exhausted.

What is considered a stressor by one person may be considered pleasurable by another. The amount of stress in the immediate environment cannot be determined by examining only the stressor or source of stress. Certain principles, however, apply to most people (123, 160–166).

- **The primary response to stressor is behavioral.** When an event or situation is perceived as threatening, the person reacts in intensity and scope to meet the threat; physiologic impact is secondary.
- **The impact is cumulative.** Most stressors in the environment occur at levels below that which would cause immediate physical or emotional damage.
- **Circumstances alter the impact or harm done by a stressor.** The social and emotional context of an event and the attitude and previous experiences of the person are as important as physical properties of the stimuli.
- **People are remarkably adaptable.** Each person has evolved a normal range of response or a unique pattern of defense. What may at first be considered uncomfortable or intolerable may eventually be perceived as normal routine. The immediate impact of a stressor is apparently different from long-term or indirect consequences, which are more difficult to detect.
- **Various psychological or social factors can ease or exaggerate the effects of a stressor.** If a stressor is predictable, it will not be as harmful as an unpredictable one. If the person feels in control of the situation or can relate positively or directly to the stressor, the effects are less negative. For example, the person in a noisy environment suffers less startle reaction if sudden noises come regularly and are anticipated. Those who work in a noisy environment without the ability to control the noise show low frustration tolerance, uncooperative behavior, and more errors on reading and arithmetic problems. Studies also show less stress response when people feel control and actually have control over a stressful environment.
- **There are definite low points when stressors are poorly tolerated. Time of day** affects stress response. For example, in most people, hydrocortisone secretion normally peaks in the early morning and decreases through the day, until it is almost undetectable at night. Although diurnal rhythms vary from person to person, stressors may be better tolerated early in the day.
- **Conditioning is an important protection.** The person whose heart, lungs, and skeletal muscles are conditioned by exercise can with-

TABLE 5–15. STIMULI THAT ARE STRESSORS

Physical: excessive or intense cold or heat, sound, light, motion, gravity, or electrical current

Chemical: alkalines, acids, drugs, toxic substances, hormones, gases, or food and water pollutants

Microbiologic: viruses, bacteria, molds, parasites, or other infectious organisms

Physiologic: disease processes, surgery, immobilization, mechanical trauma, fever, organ hypo- or hyperfunction, or pain

Psychological: anticipated marriage or death, imagined events, intense emotional involvement, anxiety or other unpleasant feelings, distortions of body image, threats to self-concept, others' expectations of behavior, rejection by or separation from loved ones, role changes, memory of negative past experiences, actual or perceived failures

Developmental: genetic endowment, prematurity, immaturity, maturational impairment, or the aging process

Sociocultural: sociocultural background and pressures, unharmonious interpersonal relationships, demands of our technologic society, social mobility, changing social mores, job pressures, economic worries, childrearing practices, redefinition of sex roles, or minority status

Environmental: unemployment, air and water pollution, overcrowding, disasters, war, or crime

stand cardiovascular and respiratory effects of the alarm stage better than someone who leads a sedentary life.

- **Responses to stress throughout life are both local and general.**

The **local adaptation syndrome,** typified by the inflammatory response, is the *method used to wall off and control effects of physical stressors locally.* When the stressor cannot be handled locally, the *whole body responds to protect itself and ensure survival in the best way possible through the* **general adaptation syndrome.** The general body response augments body functions that protect the organism from injury, psychological and physical, and suppresses those functions nonessential to life. The general adaptation syndrome is characterized by alarm and resistance stages and, when body resistance is not maintained, an end stage, exhaustion (160–166).

General Adaptation Syndrome

The **alarm stage** is an *instantaneous, short-term, life-preserving, and total sympathetic nervous system response* when the person consciously or unconsciously perceives

a stressor and feels helpless, insecure, or biologically uncomfortable. This stage is typified by a "fight-or-flight" reaction (160, 166). Perception of the stressor—the alarm reaction—stimulates the anterior pituitary to increase production of adrenocorticotropic hormone (ACTH). The adrenal cortex is stimulated by ACTH to increase production of glucocorticoids, primarily hydrocortisone or cortisol, and mineralocorticoids, primarily aldosterone. Catecholamine release triggers increased sympathetic nervous system activity, which stimulates production of epinephrine and norepinephrine by the adrenal medulla and release at the adrenergic nerve endings. The alarm reaction also stimulates the posterior pituitary to release increased antidiuretic hormone (123, 160–166). Generally the person is prepared to act, is more alert, and is able to adapt (Figs. 5–3 and 5–4).

Physiologically, the responses that occur when the sympathetic nervous system is stimulated are shown in Figure 5–5 (123, 160–166).

To complicate assessment, there are times when *parts* of the parasympathetic division of the autonomic nervous system are inadvertently stimulated during a stressful state because of the proximity of sympathetic and parasympathetic nerve fibers. With intensification of stress, opposite behaviors are then observed. They are shown in Figure 5–6 (123, 163).

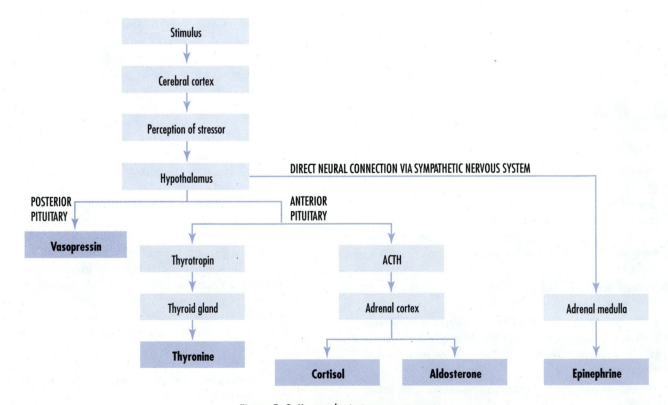

Figure 5–3. Neuroendocrine response to stress.

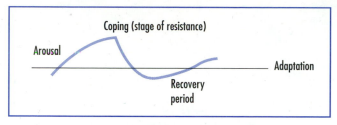

Figure 5–4. Reaction pattern in acute stress.

Lazarus identified three psychological stages that occur during the alarm stage: threat, warning, and impact. The psychological processes that occur when the stress stage is intensified begin with appraisal of the **threat** or potential degree of harm (**warning**). This process is cognitive and affective and involves perception, memory, thought, and a feeling response to the **meaning of the impact** of the threat, such as anxiety, fear, anger, guilt, or shame (100).

Headache from neck & shoulder tense muscles.

Anti-inflammatory responses increase from glucocorticoid production. Defenses against inflammation/infection high for short time.

Thymus and lymph nodes atrophy if stage prolonged.

Respiratory rate/depth increased as bronchi dilate, due to increased epinephrine; allows adequate oxygenation.

Hyperglycemia from glucagon secretion in pancreas causing glycogenolysis; for energy demands after initial hypoglycemia. Increased glucocorticoid production results in gluconeogenesis in liver; body cells have sufficient glucose for stress response. Protein catabolism due to conversion of protein to glucose.

Gastric glandular acid and volume secretion increased; less essential functions such as digestion and excretion reduced. Intestinal smooth muscle relax, reducing motility. Sphincters contract. Anorexia, constipation, or flatulece may occur.

Adrenals enlarge, hyperactive, discolor. Salt and water retained by kidneys bolster intravascular blood volume due to increased antidiuretic hormone and aldosterone production and peripheral vasoconstriction; fuller blood pressure, less urinary output, and hemoconcentration result. Sodium chloride in extracellular fluid reduced; potassium levels rise. Hypochloremic.

Muscle tonus increased by epinephrine production; activities may be better coordinated, or rigidity and tremors may occur. Metabolic alterations in muscles with glycogenolysis and reduced use of glucose. Blood lactate and glucose increase.

Metabolic changes in adipose tissue; lipolysis and release of free fatty acids for use by muscles. Glycerol converted to glucose. Depletion of corticolipids in adrenal cortex.

Pupils dilate, use maximum light for vision. Vision initially sharp, later blurred.

Myocardial rate, strength, and output increased by greater epinephrine production; more blood available throughout body as pulse rate and strength increase. Palpitations of arrhythmias may occur.

Blood pressure rises when increased norepinephrine produces peripheral vasoconstriction.

Increased blood clotting due to catecholamine stimulation of increased production of clotting factors. Increased blood viscosity may result in stasis and thrombosis if Alarm Stage persists.

Disappearance of blood eosinophiles.

In urinary bladder, detrusor muscle relaxes and trigone sphincter contracts; micturition inhibited. Or person voids only small amounts but feels urgency.

Blood supply shunted to brain, heart, and skeletal muscles rather than to periphery due to peripheral vasoconstriction. Skin pale, ashen, cool. Vasoconstriction stimulated by increased secretion of renin by kidney with reduced blood supply to kidney. Renin secretion stimulates production of plasma angiotensinogen; in turn, production of angiotension I and II causes vasoconstriction and increased blood pressure in vital organs.

Tissue Catabolism.

Metabolism increased up to 150%, providing immediate energy and producing more heat due to catecholamine release. Body temperature may rise. Perspiration. Mild dehydration from increased insensible fluid loss. (Dry lips and mouth occur.) If metabolism remains high, tissue catabolism, insomnia, fatigue, and signs of dehydration such as dry skin, weight loss, and decreased urinary output occur.

Immune responses initially suppressed.

Figure 5–5. Alarm stage, general adaptation syndrome: physiologic responses to sympathetic nervous system stimulation. *(From Murray, R., and M. M. Huelskoetter, Psychiatric/Mental Health Nursing: Giving Emotional Care (3rd ed.). Stamford, CT: Appleton & Lange, 1991, p. 336.)*

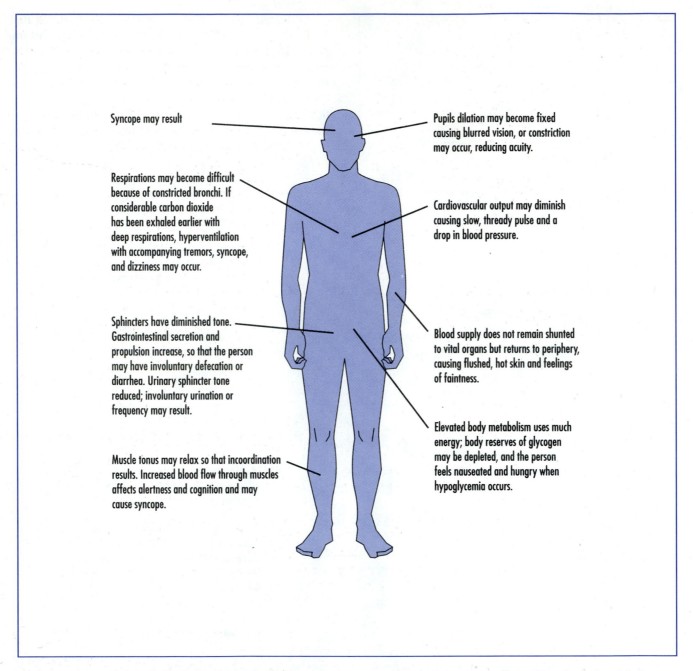

Figure 5–6. Alarm stage, general adaptation syndrome: physiologic responses to parasympathetic nervous system stimulation. *(From Murray, R., and M. M. Huelskoetter, Psychiatric/Mental Health Nursing: Giving Emotional Care (3rd ed.). Stamford, CT: Appleton & Lange, 1991, p. 337.)*

The **stage of resistance** is the *body's way of adapting, through an adrenocortical response, to the disequilibrium caused by the stressors of life.* Because of the adrenocortical response, increased use of body resources, endurance and strength, tissue anabolism, antibody production, hormonal secretion, and changes in blood sugar levels and blood volume sustain the body's fight for preservation. Body response eventually returns to normal.

The tissue tranquilizers released help us adapt passively to stimuli, and the enzymes and blood cells released attack pathogens. Moderate anxiety is felt; habitual ego defenses are unconsciously used. Responses eventually return to normal when stressors diminish or when the person has found adaptive mechanisms that meet emotional needs and physical demands (123, 160–166).

If biological, psychological, or social stresses, alone or in combination, occur over a long period without adequate relief, the stage of resistance is maintained. With continued stressors, the person becomes distressed and manifests objective and subjective emotional, intellectual, and physiologic responses, as shown in Figures 5–7 and 5–8 (123, 160–166).

Protective factors *modify, ameliorate, or alter the person's response to stressors and to a potentially maladaptive outcome.* They include such factors as positive temperament; intelligence; ability to relate well to others; participation in achievements; success in school or the job; family support, closeness, and safe family environment; and extended family, friends, and teachers (123).

The **Stage of Exhaustion** occurs when the *person is unable to continue to adapt to internal and external environmental demands.* Physical or psychic disease or

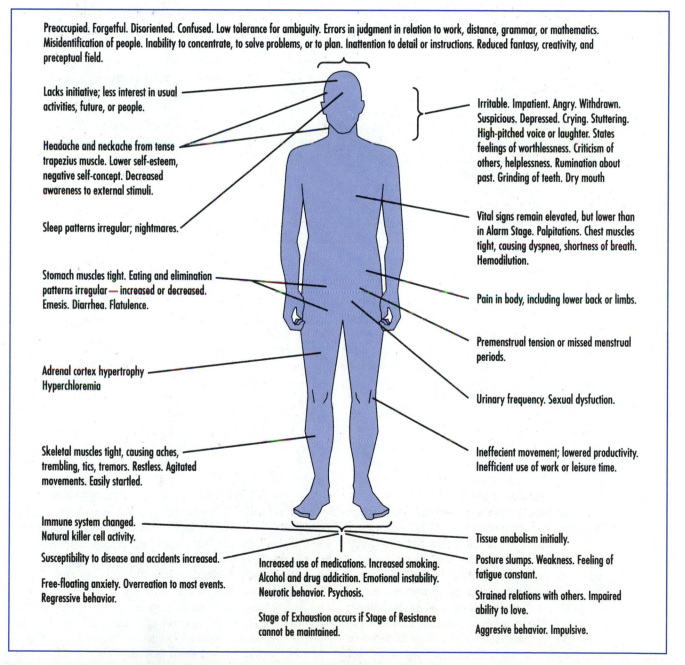

Preoccupied. Forgetful. Disoriented. Confused. Low tolerance for ambiguity. Errors in judgment in relation to work, distance, grammar, or mathematics. Misidentification of people. Inability to concentrate, to solve problems, or to plan. Inattention to detail or instructions. Reduced fantasy, creativity, and preceptual field.

Lacks initiative; less interest in usual activities, future, or people.

Headache and neckache from tense trapezius muscle. Lower self-esteem, negative self-concept. Decreased awareness to external stimuli.

Sleep patterns irregular; nightmares.

Stomach muscles tight. Eating and elimination patterns irregular — increased or decreased. Emesis. Diarrhea. Flatulence.

Adrenal cortex hypertrophy Hyperchloremia

Skeletal muscles tight, causing aches, trembling, tics, tremors. Restless. Agitated movements. Easily startled.

Immune system changed. Natural killer cell activity.

Susceptibility to disease and accidents increased.

Free-floating anxiety. Overreation to most events. Regressive behavior.

Irritable. Impatient. Angry. Withdrawn. Suspicious. Depressed. Crying. Stuttering. High-pitched voice or laughter. States feelings of worthlessness. Criticism of others, helplessness. Rumination about past. Grinding of teeth. Dry mouth

Vital signs remain elevated, but lower than in Alarm Stage. Palpitations. Chest muscles tight, causing dyspnea, shortness of breath. Hemodilution.

Pain in body, including lower back or limbs.

Premenstrual tension or missed menstrual periods.

Urinary frequency. Sexual dysfuction.

Ineffecient movement; lowered productivity. Inefficient use of work or leisure time.

Increased use of medications. Increased smoking. Alcohol and drug addiction. Emotional instability. Neurotic behavior. Psychosis.

Stage of Exhaustion occurs if Stage of Resistance cannot be maintained.

Tissue anabolism initially.

Posture slumps. Weakness. Feeling of fatigue constant.

Strained relations with others. Impaired ability to love.

Aggresive behavior. Impulsive.

Figure 5–7. Stage of resistance, general adaptation syndrome: signs of emotional, intellectual, and physiologic distress. *(From Murray, R., and M. M. Huelskoetter, Psychiatric/Mental Health Nursing: Giving Emotional Care (3rd ed.). Stamford, CT: Appleton & Lange, 1991, p. 338.)*

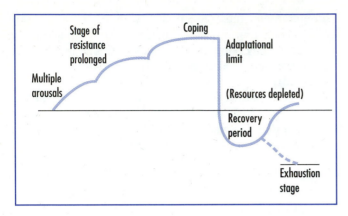

Figure 5–8. Reaction pattern in chronic stress. *(Data from M. Horowitz and H. Selye.) Source: Ref. #123.*

death results because the body can no longer compensate for or correct homeostatic imbalances. Manifestations of this stage are similar to those of the Alarm Stage except that all reactions first intensify and then diminish in response and show no ability to return to an effective level of function. Frequent or prolonged General Adaptation Syndrome response triggers disease through adrenocortical hypertrophy, thymolymphatic atrophy, elevated blood glucose, ulceration of the gastrointestinal tract, reduced tone and fibrosis of tissues, and vasoconstriction (161, 162).

Health care providers are concerned with promoting the Resistance Stage and preventing or reversing the Exhaustion Stage, whether through drugs, bed rest, medical treatments, crisis intervention, psychotherapy, or social action. Ideally you should identify potential stressors that the person might encounter and determine how to alter the stressors or best support the person's adaptive mechanisms and resources physically, emotionally, and socially, for the person will respond as an entity to the stressors. The relationship of stress to life crises or changes must be considered whenever you are doing health promotion measures or intervening with the ill person (123).

Although responses to stressful situations vary, anxiety is a common one (see Table 5–6). Other responses include the adaptive mechanisms described in Table 5–7.

The **mind–body relationship,** the *effect of emotional responses to stress on body function and the emotional reactions to body conditions,* has been established through research and experience. Emotional factors are important in the precipitation or exacerbation of nearly every organic disease and may increase susceptibility to infections. Stress and emotional distress, including depression, may influence function of the immune system via central nervous system and endocrine mediation. Apparently adrenocortical steroid hormones are immunosuppressive. Recurring or chronic emotional stress has a cumulative physiologic effect and eventually may produce chronic dysfunction such as hypertension or gastric ulcers (67). The dynamics involves repression of certain feelings such as rage or guilt, fooling the mind into thinking the feelings have disappeared. But the body's physiologic functions respond to the feelings or perception of the effect (stressor) (65, 120, 123, 150, 160–166, 169, 182). *When physical or organic symptoms or disease result from feeling states, the process is called* **psychosomatic** *or* **psychophysiologic.** *The opposite process, feeling states of depression or worry in response to physical states, is called* **somatopsychic.**

The field of **psychoneuroimmunology** *focuses on the links between the mind, brain, and immune system.* This is a newer perspective of the mind–body relationship in psychophysiologic causation of illness. Research shows that the immune system responds to the mind (65).

Crisis Theory

Definitions and Characteristics

Crisis is *any temporary situation that threatens the person's self-concept, necessitates reorganization of the psychological structure and behavior, causes a sudden alteration in the person's expectation of self, and cannot be handled with the person's usual coping mechanisms* (19, 36). Crises always involve change and loss. Either the changes or losses that occur result in the person's inability to cope, or as a result of the crisis the person is no longer the same. He or she will have to change behavior to remain adaptive and functional, and in the process, loss will be felt. Resolution of the crisis and growth mean that something is lost even while something else is gained.

During crisis, the person's ordinary behavior is no longer successful—emotionally, intellectually, or physically. The person may refer to a crisis as a "tough time" or speak of the lack of coping ability by saying, "I'm at the end of my rope. I can't manage anymore." The usual coping skills or adaptive mechanisms do not work in the situation; old habits and daily patterns are disturbed. Thus, the person feels motivated to try new behavior to cope with the new situation. Although behavior during crisis is inadequate or inappropriate to the present situation and may be different from normal, it should not be considered pathologic. For example, rage or bitterness or prolonged crying by a usually jovial person may be an emotional release that paves the way for problem solving (123).

The crisis may also reactivate old, unresolved crises or conflicts, which can impose an additional burden to be handled at the present time. The crisis is a turning point, however; it operates as a second chance for resolving earlier crises or for correcting faulty problem solving. The time of crisis serves as a catalyst or opportunity for growth emotionally. Readjustment of behavior occurs; if all goes well, a state of equilibrium or behavior that is more mature than the previous status results. On the other hand, because of the stress involved and the felt threat to the equilibrium, the person is also more vulnerable to regression and emotional or physical illness. The outcome—either increased, the same level of, or decreased maturity, or illness—depends on how the person handles the situation and on the help others give. Encountering and resolving crisis is a normal process that each person or family faces many times during a lifetime (123).

Not all persons facing the same hazardous event will be in a state of crisis, but some events or situations are viewed as a crisis by all persons, of any age, in that some behavioral adjustment must be made by anyone facing that situation. Research by Holmes and Rahe has shown that the number and seriousness of certain kinds of life changes or crises, ranging from death of a loved one to receiving a parking ticket, that are encountered within a year will increase the person's chance of facing other crises, including illness or accidental injury (Table 5–16) (77). Crises also vary in degree; a situation may be perceived as major, moderate, or minimal in the degree of discomfort caused and in the amount of behavioral change demanded. A person may view minimal crises as stressful life situations, but the objective observer would see that the individual is ineffective in coping.

Crisis differs from transition. **Transition** refers to a *passage or movement from one state or place to another that occurs over time, involving changes that can be managed* (159).

Types of Crises

Crises are divided into two categories: (1) developmental, maturational, or normative, and (2) situational, accidental, or catastrophic (12, 123). **Developmental crises** *occur during transition points, those periods that every person and family experience in the process of biopsychosocial maturation.* Examples are school entry, puberty, graduation, marriage, pregnancy, childbirth, menopause, retirement, and death. These are times in development when new relationships are formed and old re-

TABLE 5–16. SOCIAL READJUSTMENT RATING SCALE

Rank	Life Event	Mean Value
1	Death of spouse	100
2	Divorce	73
3	Marital separation	65
4	Jail term	63
5	Death of close family member	63
6	Personal injury or illness	53
7	Marriage	50
8	Fired at work	47
9	Marital reconciliation	45
10	Retirement	45
11	Change in health of family member	44
12	Pregnancy	40
13	Sex difficulties	39
14	Gain of new family member	39
15	Business readjustment	39
16	Change in financial state	38
17	Death of close friend	37
18	Change to different line of work	36
19	Change in number of arguments with spouse	35
20	Mortgage over $10,000	31
21	Foreclosure on mortgage or loan	30
22	Change in responsibilities at work	29
23	Son or daughter leaving home	29
24	Trouble with inlaws	29
25	Outstanding personal achievement	28
26	Wife begins or stops work	26
27	Begin or end school	26
28	Change in living conditions	25
29	Change in personal habits	24
30	Trouble with boss	23
31	Change in work hours or conditions	20
32	Change in residence	20
33	Change in schools	20
34	Change in recreation	19
35	Change in church activities	19
36	Change in social activities	18
37	Mortgage or loan less than $10,000	17
38	Change in sleeping habits	16
39	Change in number of family get-togethers	15
40	Change in eating habits	15
41	Vacation	13
42	Christmas	12
43	Minor violations of the law	11

Life Crisis Categories and LCU Scores*

No life crisis	0–149
Mild life crisis	150–199
Moderate life crisis	200–299
Major life crisis	300–or more

*The LCU score includes those life event items experienced during a 1-year period.

From Holmes, T. H., and R. H. Rahe, The Social Readjustment Rating Scale, Journal of Psychosomatic Research, 11, no. 8(1967), 213–217.

lationships take on new aspects. There are new expectations of the person, and certain emotional tasks must be accomplished to move on to the next phase of development. The onset of the developmental or maturational crisis is gradual because it occurs as the person moves from one stage of development to another. The crisis resolves when the individual succeeds in new age-level behaviors; disruption does not last for the entire developmental phase (123).

There are three main reasons why someone may be unable to make role changes necessary to prevent a maturational crisis (69, 123):

1. The person may be unable to picture self in a new role. Roles are learned, and adequate role models may not exist.
2. The person may be unable to make role changes because of a lack of intrapersonal resources, for example, inadequate communication skills; the realization that, with life passing, certain goals will not be achieved; or the lack of past opportunities to learn how to cope with crises because of overprotection.
3. Others in the social system may refuse to see the person in a different role. For example, when the adolescent tries to move from childhood to the adult role, the parent may persist in keeping him or her in the child role.

Several factors help the person adjust to a new life era: (1) desire for a change and boredom with present experiences, (2) agenda for a life course—present versus future plans, (3) accomplishments in the present era, (4) past success in coping with turning points, (5) group support in meeting turning points, and (6) examples of how peers have coped with similar situations. The more clear-cut the cultural definitions, the less frightening is the future situation because the person has models of behavior and can prepare in advance for change.

Situational crisis *is an external event or situation, not necessarily a part of normal living, often sudden, unexpected, and unfortunate, that looms larger than the person's immediate resources or ability to cope and thereby demands a change in behavior.* Life goals are threatened; tension and anxiety are evoked; unresolved problems and crises from the past are reawakened. The amount of time taken for healthy or unhealthy adaptation to occur usually ranges from 1 to 6 weeks, although resolution may take longer. A situational crisis may occur at the same time as a developmental crisis.

Situational crises include natural disasters, such as hurricane, tornado, earthquake, and flood; loss through separation, divorce, or death of a loved one; loss of one's job, money, or valued possessions; and a job

change. Additions to the family such as an unwanted pregnancy; return of a prisoner of war, a deserter, or someone taken as a hostage; adoption of a child; and remarriage resulting in a stepparent and stepsiblings also can cause a change in lifestyle and are potential crises. Illness, hospitalization, or institutionalization; a power struggle on the job; a sudden change in role responsibilities; and a forced geographic relocation are other examples. Rape, suicide, homicide, and imprisonment can also be classified as this type of crisis.

Crisis always involves a sense of loss. Developmental and situational events that involve loss, in reality or symbolically, are listed in Table 5–17 (19, 75, 123).

Phases of Crisis

All crises require a sudden and then a later restructuring of biopsychosocial integration before normal function can be restored. The phases involved are (1) shock, followed closely by general realization of the crisis; (2) defensive retreat; (3) acknowledgment and mourning; and, finally, (4) adaptation or resolution (36, 101, 123).

Table 5–18 presents the feelings and behaviors that may be experienced by the person during the phases of crisis. These behaviors are normal when a crisis is en-

TABLE 5–17. LOSS SITUATIONS THAT CONTRIBUTE TO CRISES

1. Period of weaning in infancy; learning to wait
2. First haircut, even when it involves pride and anticipation
3. Period of increasing locomotion, exploration, and bowel and bladder control and resultant loss of dependency
4. Loss of baby teeth, baby possessions, toys, clothes, or pets
5. Change in the body, body image, self-concept, and self-attitude with ongoing growth and development
6. Change in body size and shape and in feelings accompanying pregnancy and childbirth; loss of body part or function, external or internal, through accident, illness, or aging
7. Departure of children from the home when they go to school or marry
8. Menopause and loss of childbearing functions
9. Loss of hearing, vision, memory, strength, and other changes and losses associated with old age
10. Changes and losses in relationships with others as the person moves from childhood to adulthood—loss of friends and lovers; separation from or death of family members; changes in residence, occupation, or place of business; promotions and graduations
11. Losses with symbolic meanings, such as the loss of a symptom that attracted others' attention; a loss or change that necessitates a change in body image; or "loss of face", honor, prestige, or status
12. Loss of home due to natural disaster or relocation projects; loss of possessions or money
13. Loss experienced with divorce or incapacitation of a loved one

TABLE 5–18. INDIVIDUAL REACTIONS IN THE CRISIS PHASES

Phase and Duration	Feelings	Cognitive Manifestations	Physical Symptoms	Interpersonal/Social Behavior
Initial Impact; Shock (duration of 1 to 24–48 hours)	Anxiety. Helplessness. Chaos. Overwhelmed. Hopeless. Incomplete. Detached. Despair. Depersonalized. Panic. Self-concept threatened. Self-esteem low. Anguish may be expressed by silent, audible, or uncontrollable crying *Developmental Crisis* Response more gradual. Feelings less intense. May feel anxiety, frustration, lack of confidence, discouragement, imperfection, unfamiliarity with self, loss of self-control as realizes new responsibilities. Cannot move emotionally into next stage or change life perception	Altered sensorium. Disorganized thinking. Unable to plan, reason logically, or understand situation. Impaired judgment. Preoccupation with image or hallucination of lost object/person	Somatic distress. May suffer physical illness or injury and ignore symptoms. Shortness of breath. Choking. Sighing. Hyperventilation. Weakness. Fatigue. Tremors. Anorexia. Lump in throat or abdomen. Respiratory or other infection may develop	Disorganized behavior. Habitual or automatic behaviors used unsuccessfully. Withdrawn. Docile. Hyperactive. May appear overtly as if nothing happened or may be unable to carry out routine behavior. Lacks initiative for daily tasks. May need assistance meeting basic needs. Very suggestible, even if contrary to values or well-being *Developmental Crisis* May try to do more than is biologically or emotionally realistic. Unable to achieve behavior or appropriate to role or to change inappropriate behavior in relationships
Defensive Retreat (duration of hours to weeks)	May feel tense and inadequate, but usually feels as if nothing is wrong because of use of repression and defense mechanisms. Apathetic or euphoric. Feelings displaced onto other objects	Tries habitual coping mechanisms unsuccessfully. States nothing is wrong. May try to redefine problem unrealistically. Fantasizes about what could be done, how well past problems handled. Avoids thinking about event. May be disoriented. Maintains rigid thinking. States same ideas over and over. May be unable to devise alternate courses of action or predict effects of behavior. Denies through rationalization cause for situation *Developmental Crisis* Denies that physical, emotional, or role changes are occurring or that different behavior is expected; behavior reflects earlier developmental stage; developmental tasks not worked at or met	Denies symptoms including presence of physical illness	Tries habitual behaviors and defense mechanisms unsuccessfully. May seek support of others indirectly. Usually withdraws from others. Superficial response. May avoid reality with overactivity. Resistant to change suggested by others. Unwilling to initiate new behavior. Ineffective, disorganized behavior. May be unable to maintain daily activities, work performance, or social roles. Denies through demands, complaints, or projections of inadequacy

(continued)

TABLE 5–18 INDIVIDUAL REACTIONS IN THE CRISIS PHASES (continued)

Phase and Duration	Feelings	Cognitive Manifestations	Physical Symptoms	Interpersonal/Social Behavior
(*Note:* Temporary retreat emotionally, mentally, and socially is adaptive and protective from perceived stress and loss and overwhelming anxiety. Allows time to gradually realize what has happened; avoids debilitating effects of high anxiety or panic. Initially person fluctuates between the phases of Defensive Retreat and Acknowledgment of Reality.)				
Acknowledgment of Reality (duration varies)	Tension and anxiety rise. Loneliness. Irritable. Depressed. Agitated. Apathetic. Self-hate. Low self-esteem. Grief—mourning occurs. Gradually self-satisfaction increased. Self-concept becomes more positive. Gains self-confidence in ability to cope	Becomes aware of facts about change, loss, event. Asks questions about situation. Slowly redefines situation. Attempts problem solving. May be disorganized in thinking. Trial-and-error approach to problems. Gradually perceives alternatives. Makes appropriate plans. Gives up unattainable goals. Validates personal experiences and feelings. Coping skills improved	Symptoms may reappear or intensify. New symptoms may occur. May somatize feelings. Gradually regains physical health	Exhibits mourning behaviors. Gradually demonstrates appropriate behaviors and resumes roles. Uses suggestions. Tries new approaches. Greater maturity demonstrated
Resolution; Adaptation; Change (duration of mourning and crisis work may be 6–12 months)	Painful feelings integrated into self-concept and sense of worth. New sense of maturity. Firm identity. Gradual increase in self-satisfaction about mastery of situation. Gradual lowering of anxiety. Does not feel bitter, guilty, or ashamed	Perceives crisis situation in positive way. Integrates crisis event into self. Problem solving successful. Discusses feelings about event. Organizes thinking and planning. Redefines thinking and priorities. Does not blame self or others. Remembers comfortably and realistically pleasures and disappointments of lost relationship	Functions at optimum level	Discovers new resources. Uses support systems and resources appropriately. Resumes status and roles. Strengthens relations with others. Adaptive in relationships. Lifestyle may be changed. Initiates measures to prevent similar crisis if at all possible

countered and you must be aware of that fact in your assessment (36, 57, 123). Grief and mourning processes are discussed further in Chapter 13.

Table 5–19 summarizes factors that influence how the person, family, or community will react to and cope with crisis and, thereby, the crisis outcome (19, 36, 75, 77, 123).

The family unit undergoes essentially the same phases of crisis and manifests similar reactions as the designated client, although the intensity and timing may be different for each person. Furthermore, members of the family in crisis interact with each other, compounding the crisis reaction and creating more intense or complex behavioral responses. Roles are disorganized; expectations of self, other family members, and outsiders change, and individual needs intensify (123). All families have problems, and all families have ways of managing them, successfully or otherwise.

Crisis events for the family include the developmental and situational crises previously discussed, which can also be categorized as follows (75, 123):

- **Dismemberment**: *medical emergencies; loss of family member through death, divorce, separation, marriage, or geographic mobility*
- **Accession**: *addition of family member through birth, adoption, marriage, or foster placement, or older relative moving into the home*
- **Demoralization**: *loss of morale in the family unit* through delinquency, legal problems, economic problems, job loss, child or spouse abuse, certain illnesses such as AIDS, crimes, or events that cause alienation from the community or carry a social stigma
- **A combination of the above.**

Various factors influence the crisis proneness of a group or community (75, 123):

1. Personal strengths, characteristics, and level of need satisfaction of its members
2. Social and economic stability of family units or groups versus social and economic inequities among ethnic, racial, or socioeconomic groups
3. Adherence to versus rebellion against social norms by families and groups
4. Adequacy of community resources to meet social, economic, health, welfare, and recreational needs of individuals and families
5. Geographic, environmental, and climatic resources and characteristics that surround the group or community

The community is also affected by natural disasters, such as flood, tornado, hurricane, earthquake, vol-

TABLE 5–19 FACTORS INFLUENCING THE OUTCOME OF CRISIS

1. **Perception of the event.** If the event (or the implications or consequences of it) threatens the self-concept; conflicts with the value system, self-expectations, or wishes for the future; contributes to a sense of shame or guilt; or is demoralizing or damaging to self, family, or personal objects, the situation is defined as **hazardous.** The perception of the event is reality for the person or family, regardless of how others might define reality. How the event is perceived depends in large measure on past experience.

2. **Degree of perceived dependency on a lost object.** This is also crucial; the greater the dependency, the more difficult the resolution of loss.

3. **Physical and emotional status.** This includes level of health, amount of energy present, age, genetic endowment, and biological rhythms of the person or family, or the general well-being of the community. Working through crisis takes considerable energy.

4. **Coping techniques or mechanisms and level of personal maturity.** If adaptive capacities are already strained, or if the stress is overwhelming, the person will cling to old habits or existing defenses, and behavior will very likely be inappropriate to the task at hand. The person or family who has met developmental tasks all along and who perceives self as able to cope will adapt more easily in any crisis. The group or community that has mechanisms, policies, or procedures defined and in operation to cope with the unexpected event or disaster can better meet the crisis.

5. **Previous experiences with similar situations.** The person, family, or group needs to learn to cope with stress, change, and loss. If past crises were handled by distorting reality or by withdrawing, when similar crises arise, burdens of the prior failure will be added to the problem of coping with the new situation. Unresolved crises are cumulative in effect. The most recent crisis revives the denial, depression, anger, or maladaptation that was left unsettled from past crises. If the person, family, or group successfully deals with crises, self-confidence and self-esteem will thereby be increased, and future crises will be handled more effectively.

6. **Realistic aspects of the current situation.** These include personal, material, or economic losses, the extent to which group ties or community services are interrupted, and changes in living pattern or family life necessitated by the loss.

7. **Cultural influences.** How the person is trained and socialized in the home to solve problems and meet crisis situations; the use of religious, cultural, or legal ceremonies or rituals to handle separation or loss and facilitate mourning; expectations of how the social group will support the person or family during crisis; and the method established by the community to provide help—all influence present behavior.

8. **Availability and response of family and close friends, community groups, or other helping resources, including professional persons.** The less available the environmental or emotional support systems are to decrease stress or buttress the coping response, the more hazardous the event will be. The family system, by its influence on development of self-concept and maturity, can increase or decrease the person's vulnerability to crisis.

canic eruptions, and blizzard; by disasters resulting from advances in our civilization, such as chemical or radiation spills and electrical blackouts; and by disasters for which humans are responsible, such as snipings in a schoolyard or restaurant, fire, and war. Reactions of a community to any of these disasters will be influenced by the factors listed in Table 5–20 (21, 24, 70, 71, 75, 83, 103, 106, 123, 130, 168).

A group in crisis demonstrates:

- Acute unmanageable anxiety that interferes with daily function
- Sudden alteration in perceptions of meaning, purpose, and goals—a turning point
- Sudden disruption in cognitive, emotional, or physical alterations

TABLE 5–20. FACTORS THAT INFLUENCE COMMUNITY RESPONSE TO DISASTERS

1. **Element of surprise versus preparedness.** If warnings are not given about an impending crisis—or if warnings are given without an action plan—panic, shock, denial, and defensive retreat are more likely to occur.
2. **Separation of family members.** Children are especially affected by separation; the family should be evacuated from a disaster area as a unit.
3. **Availability of outside help,** for example, the sending of food, shelter, and workers.
4. **Leadership.** Someone must make decisions and give directions. Usually the police, Red Cross and Civil Defense workers, National Guard, military, or professionals in a community are seen as authoritative persons. Coordination of the activities of all of these groups is essential to deliver services and avoid chaos.
5. **Communication.** Public information centers have to be established to avoid rumor, provide reassurance and direction, and ensure that all citizens get information about coping measures, evacuation, reconstruction, rehabilitation, and available financial aid. Otherwise citizens will later be bitter and suspicious when some learn that others benefited more than they did.
6. **Measures taken to help reorientation.** Communication networks lay the foundation for reidentification of individuals into family and social groups and for registration of survivors.
7. **Presence of plans for individuals and social institutions to cope with disaster,** including evacuation of a population from a stricken area if necessary. Emergency plans focus on the following concerns:
   a. Preservation of life and health through rescue, triage, inoculation, and treatment of the injured
   b. Conservation and distribution of resources, such as shelter, water, food, and blankets
   c. Conservation of public order by police surveillance to prevent looting and further accidents or injuries
   d. Maintenance of morale through dispatching of health and welfare workers to the disaster scene
   e. Administration of health services

Communities in crisis have characteristics in common with individuals and groups in crisis. The most immediate social consequence of a disaster is disruption of normal social patterns and services; the community is socially paralyzed. Furthermore, one disaster such as a chemical spill may contribute to another disaster, such as an explosion or fire (70, 71, 168).

In a major disaster, about 75 to 90% of the victims will be in shock; this is followed by the phase of defensive retreat, in response to warnings of disaster, orders of evacuation, destruction of homes, and disruption of water, electricity, heat, food supplies, communication, traffic, and transportation. Furthermore, there is potential inability of the health agencies to care for the injured and ill because of manpower and supply shortages or damage. In addition to individual reactions, an atmosphere of tension, fear, confusion, and suspicion exists; facts are distorted and rumors are rampant. Normal functioning is reduced as businesses, vital services, schools, and recreational areas may be closed. Yet, one may see all available community service providers, such as policemen, firemen, construction workers, city planners, Red Cross volunteers, medical personnel, and corporation executives, cooperating to assist in rescue, cleanup, and restoration of services and a sense of normality. Although some people are in shock or denial, a proportionate few will display altruism and heroic behavior. There will be a few who take advantage of the chaos to loot and steal, and a few businesses may profiteer (70, 71, 168).

Response to external emergencies is often quicker than the response to internal stresses or crises. About 10 to 25% of the victims remain reality oriented, calm, and able to develop and implement a plan of action. These people often are those with advanced training; however, these people may experience the crisis phases later.

► HEALTH CARE AND NURSING APPLICATIONS

Table 5–21 summarizes how the theories discussed in this chapter can be applied in nursing and health care practice (123).

SUMMARY

1. Various theories describe aspects of the developing person; no theory describes all dimensions (physiologic, emotional, cognitive, cultural, social, moral, spiritual) of development.

TABLE 5–21. NURSING IMPLICATIONS OF SELECTED THEORIES

Theorist/Theory	Practice Implications
General Systems Theory	1. Consider self as an individual system as well as part of other systems. 2. Consider client (individual, family, group, or community) as part of a system in implementing nursing process. 3. Consider client in totality and the relationships and interactions between parts: physiologic, psychological, spiritual, and sociocultural. Dysfunction in one part affects all parts. 4. Client, as a system, has definite range for absorption, processing, and retention of stimuli. Avoid overstimulation or deprivation of stimuli. Assess needs and intervene accordingly. 5. Help client determine resources and supportive systems that will maintain or return function and wellness.

Skinner's Operant Conditioning Theory	1. In teaching or therapy, follow the guidelines previously described for a behavior modification program.
	2. The general procedure for behavior modification is to:
	  a. Plan what behavior is to be established; plan what is to be taught and at what specific time. Objectives are specific. Follow the teaching or treatment plan explicitly.
	  b. Determine available reinforcers. Feedback from physical sensations, excelling over others, or the teacher's affection—all may reinforce. The only way to determine whether a consequence is rewarding is to observe its effect on the behavior associated with it.
	  c. Identify the responses that can be made by the person.
	  d. Plan how reinforcements can be efficiently scheduled so the behavior will be repeated. Reinforcements must immediately follow the desired behavior.

Freud's Psychoanalytic Theory	1. Insight into own behavior can add to personal maturity and understanding of others. 2. Constructs of id, ego, superego, conscious–unconscious continuum, manifestations of anxiety and defense mechanisms, and psychosexual development are useful in assessment and therapy. 3. All behavior is meaningful; outer behavior may hide inner need or conflict. 4. Use knowledge of psychosexual development to teach parents about norms and meaning of child's behavior. 5. Transference and resistance must be worked through in therapy.
Sullivan's Interpersonal Theory	1. One Genus Postulate basic to nursing practice with clients from all settings and backgrounds. 2. Assess developmental stage and task; teach family about normal development and development of self-system. 3. Promote syntaxic rather than parataxic mode of experiencing through intervention. 4. Promote positive experiences for client so that "good-me" or positive self-concept can develop.
Erikson's Epigenetic Theory	1. Assessment of and insight into own stage of development. 2. Use knowledge of eight stages and psychosexual tasks in assessment, therapy, and teaching parents about child development. 3. Help clients and staff realize that emotional development is lifelong process and that society influences health and behavior.
Jung's Theory	1. Assessment of personality tendencies. 2. Promote self-acceptance, including masculine and feminine characteristics. 3. Assist person in finding unique self, balance spirituality. 4. Promote reflection, finding meaning of life.

Beck's Cognitive Therapy	1. Facilitate person's recognition of how thoughts influence emotions through questions, examples, examination of person's self-conversation.
	2. Facilitate person's recognition of irrational beliefs by having person tell what would happen if belief actually was true; enumerate reasons for problems created by the belief.
	3. Facilitate person's recognition that rational beliefs influence emotional or physical distress by systematically exploring situations related to feelings of inadequacy, helplessness, aloneness, depression, or anger. Sort out facts in a supportive way.
	4. Facilitate person's efforts to revise and contradict irrational beliefs through alternative self-messages, homework assignments, role play, rehearsal, and invalidation of distorted belief.
	5. Restructuring experience with person helps him or her recognize and revise unrealistic expectations and negative self-conversations, reduce sensitivity to other's response, and interact more flexibly and effectively.
	6. Therapy lasts about 6 months and is divided into stages:
	  a. Eliciting and answering automatic thoughts
	  b. Discovering and testing underlying assumptions
	  c. Cognitive restructuring
	7. Basis for improvement is in change of basic philosophy of the person, not necessarily in removal of present symptoms.
	8. Therapist is active in confronting person; person is expected to do homework assignments.
	9. Therapist is to act as role model for person; as an authoritative, scientific helper who is highly trained and rational, and to show unconditional positive regard for the person.

(continued)

TABLE 5–21. NURSING IMPLICATIONS OF SELECTED THEORIES (continued)

Theorist/Theory	Practice Implications
Ellis' Rational Emotive Therapy	1. Facilitate person's recognition of how thoughts influence emotions and how the person can control own behavior.
	2. Facilitate person's recognition of basic values and assumptions that govern life.
	3. Facilitate person's recognition of irrational thoughts and negative self-talk, and how these contribute to emotional pain.
	4. Facilitate person's ability to identify the ABCDE of situation and personal feelings and five criteria for rational thinking.
	5. Facilitate person's efforts to revise and contradict irrational beliefs and perceptions of events.
	6. Teach relaxation techniques, control of thoughts, assertive communication, self-instruction, internal self-talk, and problem-solving methods to strengthen realistic perceptions, rational thoughts, and personal autonomy.
	7. Teach person to hold a positive image and act on that image until the person feels more positive.
	8. Therapy is weekly and short-term, but may last 2 years, and focuses on specific current problem.
Glasser's Reality Therapy	1. Assess current needs, problems, and unrealistic behavior.
	2. Assess strengths and capacity for change.
	3. Explore discrepancy between needs and wants of client.
	4. Develop specific plan for client to meet needs.
	5. Elicit commitment from client to follow plan.
	6. Determine if plan works.
	7. Revise plan if unable to achieve prior plan; avoid negative reaction or blame.
	8. Continue encouragement and plan revision until behavior changes, needs are met, and person acts realistically and responsibly.
Bandura's Social Learning Theory	1. Your appearance and behavior are a model for client.
	2. Determine who significant adults were in the person's life and who role models were.
	3. In teaching, demonstrate desired self-care behavior.
	4. Recovered person visiting an ill client can serve as model for rehabilitation and a normal life, e.g., person with mastectomy, colostomy, amputation, alcoholism.
	5. Demonstrate nurturing approaches or discipline methods to child client so that parents can learn effective childrearing methods.
	6. Nurse–client relationship is a behavioral model of trust and interpersonal relations for the client.
Piaget's Theory of Cognitive Development	1. Teach parents about process of child's cognitive development and the implications for education, purchase of toys, and interactions.
	2. Assess cognitive stage of client as basis for planning content and presentation in teaching sessions.
	3. Assess cognitive development to determine language and abstraction level to use in therapy.
	4. Use knowledge of cognitive development in play therapy.
Kohlberg's Theory of Moral Development/Gilligan's Theory of Moral Development	1. Assess own level of moral development.
	2. Assess client's level of moral development when working with children, adolescents, or adults.
	3. Through your modeling, clarification, explanation, and validation, contribute to client's moral development.
Existential Theory	1. Each person is in charge of own destiny; each person is primary agent of change and is responsible for own future. Destiny is not in hands of others.
	2. In therapy, be concerned with basic conflicts that are outgrowths of confrontation with existence—death, freedom, helplessness, loss, isolation, aloneness, anxiety, and meaninglessness—and promote reflection about these life issues.
	3. Nurse is facilitator who understands and accepts the person as being and becoming. Main themes of therapy are self-awareness, self-determination, search for meaning, and relatedness.
	4. In therapy, assist person in learning how to confront self, how behavior is viewed by others, how others feel about own behavior, and how behavior contributes to opinions about self.
	5. In therapy, assist person to learn how to change; give support to reduce anxiety, low self-esteem, and loneliness.
	6. Help person move to self-actualization and achieve maximum potential.
Maslow's Theory of Motivation and Hierarchy of Needs	1. Assessment can be done around hierarchy of needs. Planning and intervention must consider need hierarchy and priorities in care.
	2. Person is a unified whole, not divided into components of needs.
	3. Higher-level needs can be met simultaneously with some lower-level needs.
	4. Concepts of needs and motivation can be used in teaching and therapy. By meeting needs of client on one level, you can help client mature and feel motivated to meet growth needs.
Carl Rogers' Theory on Self-Concept and Client-Centered Therapy	1. Assess own self-concept and self-actualization needs prior to counseling clients.
	2. Assess client's self-concept; promote positive experiences and contribute to development of positive self-concept.
	3. In therapy, assume as much as possible client's frame of reference to perceive world as she or he does.
	4. Be accepting, warm, genuine, and empathic to help client discover self and mature.

(continued)

TABLE 5–21 NURSING IMPLICATIONS OF SELECTED THEORIES (continued)

Theorist/Theory	Practice Implications
Stress and Adaptation Theory	1. Assess physical, emotional, and cognitive manifestations of stress response. 2. Assess level of anxiety. 3. Determine stage of adaptation. 4. Teach stress management methods. 5. Counsel as necessary. 6. Intervene as necessary to prevent exhaustion stage.
Crisis Theory/Crisis Intervention (Brief Therapy)	1. Assess anxiety level, feelings, and perceptions of client. 2. Assess presence of emotional and physical symptoms. 3. Determine whether person is suicidal or homicidal. 4. Explore support system and usual coping patterns. 5. Clarify crisis event, its onset and impact. 6. Provide comfort measures for client. 7. Help client work through feelings about situation. 8. Develop plan with client to resolve crisis; develop alternative options to achieve goal. 9. Reinforce strengths and healthy adaptive patterns. 10. Involve client in decisions and working on specific tasks. 11. Help person establish necessary social relationships; assist person in seeking and accepting help. 12. Refer as necessary for additional services.

2. Biological theories include study of genetics, biochemistry, neurophysiology, immunology, maturational factors, biological rhythms, and biological deficiencies.

3. Ecologic theories include study of sociologic variables, culture, geographic environments, and systems such as the family, school, community, and organization.

4. Behavioral theories study behavior that is learned or modified through various kinds of conditioning and shows a measurable outcome.

5. Psychoanalytic and Neo-Analytic theories include study of the intrapsychic processes; emotional life stage, and interpersonal development of the person, and the effect of these dimensions on behavior of the person, family unit, or the broader society.

6. Cognitive theories include study of the stages of the person's cognitive development, the person as an information processor and problem solver, and effects of modeling or imitation on behavior.

7. Moral theories study how the person learns to incorporate societal and philosophic norms into behavior and the relationship of moral to cognitive and emotional behavior.

8. Existential and Humanistic theories study the needs, self-concept, and dynamic aspects of the person's existence and development within the self and in relation to the environment or society.

9. Stress and Crisis theories study the person's responses to routine, severe, and overwhelming events; the local and general adaptation syndromes and phases of response to various types of crisis explain the reactions of the person to unexpected, situational, or developmental events.

10. The theories presented in this chapter form the basis for various approaches for therapy, nursing, and health care.

► REFERENCES

1. Anderson, R., and I. Carter, *Human Behavior in the Social Environment*. Chicago: Aldine, 1974.
2. Babcock, D., Transactional Analysis, *American Journal of Nursing*, 76, no. 7 (1976), 1152–1155.
3. Bandura, A., *Social Learning Theory*. Morristown, NJ: General Learning Press, 1977.
4. Bandura, A., *Social Foundations of Thought and Action: A Social Cognitive Theory*. Englewood Cliffs, NJ: Prentice-Hall, 1986.
5. Bandura, A., Regulation of Cognitive Processes Through Perceived Self-efficacy. *Developmental Psychology*, 25 (1989), 729–735.
6. Bandura, A., Social Cognitive Theory. In Vasta, R., ed., *Annals of Child Development: Six Theories of Child Development: Revised Formulations and Current Issues*. Greenwich, CT: Jai Press, 1989, pp. 1–60.

7. Bandura, A., Social Cognitive Theory of Moral Thought and Action. In Kurtines, W., and Gerwitz J., eds., *Handbook of Moral Behavior and Development*. Hillsdale, NJ: Lawrence Erlbaum, 1991, pp. 45–103.

8. Bandura, A., Social Cognitive Theory of Self-Regulation, *Organizational Behavior and Human Decision Processes,* 50 (1991), 248–287.

9. Beck, A.T., *Depression: Causes and Treatment.* Philadelphia: University of Pennsylvania Press, 1967.

10. Beck, A. Cognitive Therapy, in Kaplan, H., and Sadock, B. eds., *Comprehensive Textbook of Psychiatry* (4th ed.) Baltimore: Williams & Wilkins, 1985.

11. Beck, A.T., G. Brown, and R.A. Steer, Sex Differences on the Revised Beck Depression Inventory for Outpatients with Affective Disorders. *Journal of Personality Assessment,* 53 (1989), 693–702.

12. Beck, A.T., N. Epstein, R.A. Steer, and G. Brown, Beck Self-Concept Test, *Psychological Assessment: A Journal of Consulting and Clinical Psychology,* 2 (1990), 191–197.

13. Beck, A.T., and M.E. Weisharr, *Suicide Risk Assessment and Prediction.* Philadelphia: Hogrefe & Huber, 1990.

14. Berne, E., *Transactional Analysis in Psychotherapy: A Systematic Individual and Social Psychiatry.* New York: Grove Press, 1986.

15. Berrien, K., *General and Social Systems.* New Brunswick, NJ: Rutgers University Press, 1968.

16. Bowen, M., "The Family as a Unit of Study and Treatment," *American Journal of Orthopsychiatry,* 31, no. 1 (1961), 40–60.

17. Bowen, M., *Family Therapy in Clinical Practice.* New York: Jason Aronson, 1978.

18. Burnard, P., Existentialism as a Theoretical Basis for Counseling in Psychiatric Nursing, *Archives of Psychiatric Nursing,* 3, no. 3 (1989), 142–147.

19. Caplan, G., *Principles of Preventive Psychiatry.* New York: Basic Books, 1964.

20. Carter, S., The Nurse Educator: Humanist or Behaviorist? *Nursing Outlook,* 26, no. 9 (1978), 554–557.

21. Cassetta, R., Natural Disasters Stress Providers and Victims, *The American Nurse,* September (1994), 24.

22. Chapman, A., *The Treatment Techniques of Harry Stack Sullivan,* New York: Brunner/Mazel, 1978.

23. Chodoran, N., *Feminism and Psychoanalytic Theory.* New Haven, CT: Yale University Press, 1991.

24. Controlling Rumors as Well as Disease Is Disaster Response Priority. *The Nation's Health,* March (1994), 1, 6–7.

25. Cooper, M., Gilligan's Different Voice: A Perspective for Nursing. *Journal of Professional Nursing,* 5, no. 1 (1989), 10–16.

26. Cowley, G., Melantonin, *Newsweek,* August 7 (1995), 46–48.

27. Dawson, P., Philosophy, Biology, and Mental Disorders, *Journal of Advanced Nursing,* 20 (1994), 587–596.

28. De Longis, A., S. Folkman, and R. Lazarus, The Impact of Daily Stress on Health & Mood: Psychological and Social Resources as Mediators, *Journal of Personality and Social Psychology,* 54 (1988), 486–495.

29. Ellis, A., *Reason and Emotion in Psychotherapy.* New York: Lyle Stuart, 1962.

30. ———, *A New Guide to Rational Living.* Englewood Cliffs, NJ: Prentice-Hall, 1975.

31. ———, The Rational-Emotive Approach to Counseling, in Burks, H., and Stefflre, B. eds., *Theories of Counseling* (3rd ed.). New York: McGraw-Hill, 1979, pp. 172–219.

32. ———, *Humanistic Psychotherapy: The Rational Emotive Approach.* New York: Julian Press, 1978.

33. ———, *The Practice of Rational-Emotive Therapy (RET).* New York: Springer, 1987.

34. ———, The Revised ABC's of Rational-Emotive Therapy. *Journal of Rational-Emotive & Cognitive-Behavior Therapy.* 9 (1991), 139–167.

35. Erikson, E., *Childhood and Society* (2nd ed.). New York: W. W. Norton, 1963.

36. Fink, S., Crisis and Motivation: A Theoretical Model, *Archives of Physical Medicine and Rehabilitation,* 48, no. 11 (1967), 592–597.

37. Fordham, F., *An Introduction to Jung's Psychology.* Baltimore: Penguin Books, 1966.

38. Frankl, V., *Man's Search for Meaning.* New York: Washington Square Press, 1967.

39. ———, *The Unheard Cry for Meaning.* New York: Washington Square Press, 1978.

40. Freud, S., *A General Introduction to Psychoanalysis.* New York: Simon & Schuster, 1935.

41. ———, *The Problem of Anxiety.* New York: W. W. Norton, 1936.

42. ———, *The Ego and the Mechanisms of Defense.* London: Hogarth Press, 1937.

43. ———, *Ego and the Id.* London: Hogarth Press, 1947.

44. ———, *Inhibitions, Symptoms, and Anxiety.* London: Hogarth Press, 1948.

45. ———, *Outline of Psychoanalysis.* New York: W. W. Norton, 1949.

46. Friedman, W., et al., Sex Differences in Moral Judgments: A Test of Gilligan's Theory, *Psychology of Women Quarterly,* 7, no. 1 (1987), 87.

47. Fromm, E., *The Art of Loving.* New York: Harper & Row, 1963.

48. Furth, H.G., and H. Wachs, *Thinking Goes to School: Piaget's Theory in Practice.* New York: Oxford University Press, 1975.

50. Gavin, F., Cocaine Addiction: Physiology and Neurophysiology, *Science,* 251 (1991), 1580–1586.

51. Gesell, A., F. Ilg, and L. Ames, *Youth: The Years From 10 to 16.* New York: Harper & Brothers, 1956.

52. ———, et al., *Infant and Child in the Culture of Today: The Guidance of Development in Home and Nursery School.* New York: Harper Collins, 1974.

53. Giancola, P., and A. Zeichner, Neuropsychological Performance on Tests of Frontal Lobe Functioning and Aggressive Behavior in Men, *Journal of Abnormal Psychology,* 103 (1994), 832–835.

54. Gilligan, C., In a Different Voice: Women's Conceptualization of Self and of Mortality, *Harvard Educational Review,* 47, no. 4 (1977), 481–517.

55. ———, *In A Different Voice: Psychological Theory and Women's Development.* Cambridge, MA: Harvard University Press, 1982.

56. ———, and D. Attanucci, Two Moral Orientations: Gender Differences and Similarities, *Merrill-Palmer Quarterly,* 34, no. 3 (1988), 332–333.

57. Gist, R., and Lubin, B., eds., *Psychosocial Aspects of Disaster.* New York: John Wiley and Sons, 1989.

58. Glasser, W., *Mental Health or Mental Illness.* New York: Harper & Row, 1961.

59. ———, *Reality Therapy: A New Approach to Psychiatry.* New York: Harper & Row, 1965.

60. ———, *The Identity Society.* New York: Harper & Row, 1975.

61. ———, *Take Effective Control of Your Life.* New York: Harper & Row, 1984.

62. Gould, R., The Phases of Adult Life: A Study in Developmental Psychology, *American Journal of Psychiatry,* 129, no. 5 (1972), 521–531.

63. Graves, J., Psychoanalytic Theory. A Critique, *Perspectives in Psychiatric Care,* 11, no. 3 (1973), 114–120.
64. Greenberg, R., and S. Fisher, Testing Dr. Freud, *Human Behavior,* 7, no. 9 (1978), 28–33.
65. Groër, M., Psychoneuroimmunology, *American Journal of Nursing,* 91, no. 8 (1991), 33.
66. Gulino, C., Entering the Mysterious Dimension of Other: An Existential Approach to Nursing Care, *Nursing Outlook,* no. 6 (1982), 352–357.
67. Guyton, A., *Textbook of Medical Physiology* (9th ed.). Philadelphia: W. B. Saunders, 1995.
68. Hall, C., and G. Lindzey, *Theories of Personality* (3rd ed.). New York: John Wiley & Sons, 1978.
69. Hardy, M., and Conley, M., *Role Theory: Perspectives for Health Professionals.* New York: Appleton-Century-Crofts, 1978.
70. Hargreaves, A. Coping with Disaster, *American Journal of Nursing,* 80, no. 4 (1980), 683.
71. Hargreaves, A., et al. Blizzard '78: Dealing with Disaster, *American Journal of Nursing,* 79, no. 2 (1979), 268–271.
72. Hartmann, H., *Essays on Ego Psychology.* New York: International Universities Press, 1964.
73. Heidbreder, E., *Seven Psychologies.* Englewood Cliffs, NJ: Prentice-Hall, 1963.
74. Hilgard, E., and G. Bower, *Theories of Learning* (5th ed.). Englewood Cliffs, NJ: Prentice-Hall, 1981.
75. Hoff, L.A., *People in Crisis: Understanding and Helping.* (3rd ed.). Redwood City, CA: Addison-Wesley, 1987.
76. Holloway, M., Trends in Pharmacology: Rx for Addiction, *Scientific American,* 264, no. 3 (1991), 94–103.
77. Holmes, T., and R., Rahe. The Social Readjustment Rating Scale, *Journal of Psychosomatic Research,* 11, no. 8 (1967), 213–217.
78. Horker, F., Mapping the Brain, *Washington University School of Medicine Outlook,* 29, no. 1 (1992), 10–14.
79. Horney, K., *The Neurotic Personality in Our Time.* New York: W. W. Norton, 1937.
80. Is DNA Destiny? Genetic Discoveries Raise Women's Expectations—and Tougher Questions, *Women's Health Advocate Newsletter,* 2, no. 9 (1995), 1, 7–8.
81. Jones, A., Existential Psychotherapy, *Nursing Standard,* 4, no. 25 (March 14, 1990), 32–34.
82. Jones, F., K. Garrison, and R. Morgan, *The Psychology of Human Development* (2nd ed.). New York: Harper & Row, 1985.
83. Jones, M., "Fire!" *American Journal of Nursing,* 84, no. 11 (1984), 1368–1371.
84. Jourard, S., *Disclosing Man to Himself.* New York: D. Van Nostrand, 1968.
85. Jung, C., *Modern Man In Search of a Soul.* New York: Harcourt, Brace, & World, 1933.
86. ———, *The Undiscovered Self* (transl. by R. F. C. Hall). New York: Mentor Books, 1958.
87. ———, Psychological Types. In Adler, G., et al., eds. *Collected Works of Carl G. Jung.* Vol. 6. Princeton. NJ: Princeton University Press, 1971.
88. Kaluger, G., and M. Kaluger, *Human Development: The Span of Life* (3rd ed.). St. Louis: Times Mirror/Mosby, 1984.
89. Kandel, E., J. Schwartz, and T. Jessell, eds., *Principles of Neural Science* (3rd ed.). New York: Elsevier, 1991.
90. Kelly, J., and J. Dodd, Anatomical Organization of the Nervous System, in Kandel, E., Schwartz J., and Jessell, T. eds., *Principles of Neural Science.* New York: Elsevier, 1991, pp. 273–282.
91. Kendler, K., E. Walters, K. Truett, et al., Sources of Individual Differences in Depressive Symptoms: Analysis of Two Samples of Twins and Their Families. *American Journal of Psychiatry,* 51 (1994), 1605–1614.
92. Kendler, K., et al., Stressful Life Events, Genetic Liability, and Onset of an Episode of Major Depression in Women, *American Journal of Psychiatry,* 152 (1995), 833–842.
93. Kirschenbaum, H., and V. Henderson, eds., *A Carl Roger's Reader.* Boston: Houghton Mifflin, 1989.
94. Kohlberg, L., ed., *Collected Papers on Moral Development and Moral Education,* Cambridge, MA: Moral Educational Research Foundation, 1973.
95. ———, Moral Stages and Moralization: The Cognitive Developmental Approach, in Lickona, T., ed., *Moral Development and Behavior.* New York: Holt, Rinehart, & Winston, 1976, pp. 31–53.
96. ———, *Recent Research in Moral Development.* New York: Holt, Rinehart, & Winston, 1977.
97. ———, The Cognitive-Developmental Approach to Moral Education, in Scharf, P., ed., *Readings in Moral Education.* Minneapolis: Winston Press, 1978, pp. 36–51.
98. ———, and E. Turiel, Moral Development and Moral Education, in Lesser, G.S., ed., *Psychology and Education Practice.* Chicago: Scott, Foresman, 1971.
99. Kupferman, I., Hypothalamus and Limbic Systems: Motivation, in Kandel, E., J. Schwartz, and Jessell, T. eds., *Principles of Neural Science* (3rd ed.). New York: Elsevier, 1991, pp. 750–760.
100. Lazarus, R., *Psychological Stress and the Coping Process.* New York: McGraw-Hill, 1966.
101. Lee, J. Emotional Reactions to Trauma, *Nursing Clinics of North America,* 5, no. 4 (1970), 577–587.
102. Lemenick, M., Glimpses of the Mind, *Time,* July 17 (1995), 44–48.
103. Lesher, D., and A. Bomberger, Experience at Three-Mile Island, *American Journal of Nursing,* 79, no. 8 (August 1979), 1403–1408.
104. Levinson, D., *The Seasons of a Man's Life.* New York: Ballantine Books, 1978.
105. Lidz, T., *The Person: His and Her Development Throughout the Life Cycle* (2nd ed.). New York: Basic Books, 1983.
106. Lindemann, E. Symptomology and Management of Acute Grief, *American Journal of Psychiatry,* 101 (1944), 141–148.
107. Loomis, C.P., *Social Systems.* New York: D. Van Nostrand, 1960.
108. Marchand, J.L., and J. Samson, Kohlberg's Theory Applied to the Moral and Sexual Development of Adults, *Journal of Moral Education,* 7, no. 4 (1982), 247–258.
109. Maslow, A., *Towards a Psychology of Being* (2nd ed.). New York: D. Van Nostrand, 1968.
110. ———, *Motivation and Personality* (2nd ed.). New York: Harper & Row, 1970.
111. ———, *The Farther Reaches of Human Nature.* New York: Viking Press, 1971.
112. May, R., *Existential Psychology.* New York: Random House, 1960.
113. ———, *Man's Search for Himself.* New York: Signet Books, 1967.
114. ———, *Psychology and the Human Dilemma.* New York: D. Van Nostrand, 1967.
115. ———, *Love and Will.* New York: W. W. Norton, 1969.
116. ———, Angel, and H. Ellenberg, *Existence: A New Dimension in Psychiatry and Psychology.* New York: Basic Books, 1958.
117. Mayer, S., and C. Sencks, Growing Up in Poor Neighborhoods: How Much Does It Matter? *Science,* 243 (March 17, 1989), 1441–1445.

118. McFarlane, A., A Nursing Reformulation of Bowen's Family Systems Theory, *Archives of Psychiatric Nursing,* 2 (1988), 319–324.

119. Middleton, J., Existentialist as Helper? *Canadian Psychiatric Nursing,* 20, no. 3 (1979), 7–8.

120. Miller, T., Advances in Understanding the Impact of Stressful Life Events on Health, *Hospital and Community Psychiatry,* 39 (1988), 625.

121. Moshman, D., J. Glover, and R. Bruning, *Developmental Psychology: A Topical Approach.* Boston: Little, Brown, 1987.

122. Munroe, R., *Schools of Psychoanalytic Thought.* New York: Holt, Rinehart & Winston, 1955.

123. Murray, R.B., and M. Huelskoetter, *Psychiatric/Mental Health Nursing: Giving Emotional Care* (3rd ed.). Norwalk, CT: Appleton-Lange, 1991.

124. Neuman, B., The Betty Neuman Health-Care Systems Model: A Total Person Approach to Patient Problems, in Riehl, J.P., and Roy, C. eds., *Conceptual Models for Nursing Practice* (3rd ed.). New York: Appleton-Century-Crofts, 1988.

125. O'Rourke, K., Genetic Testing: Ethical Issues, *Ethical Issues in Health Issues in Health Care,* 16, no. 9 (1995), 1–2.

126. Patel, P., Identification of Disease Genes and Somatic Gene Therapy: An Overview and Prospects for the Aged, *Journal of Gerontology: Biological Sciences,* 48, no. 3 (1993), B80–B85.

127. Paterson, J., and L. Zderad, *Humanistic Nursing.* New York: John Wiley & Sons, 1976.

128. Patterson, C., *Theories of Counseling and Psychotherapy* (4th ed.). New York: Harper Collins, 1986.

129. Peplau, H., *Interpersonal Relations in Nursing.* New York: G.P. Putnam's Sons, 1952.

130. Petersen, R., and S. LaVone, Plane Crash, *American Journal of Nursing,* 89, no. 10 (1989), 1258–1289.

131. Piaget, J., *The Child's Conception of Physical Causality.* London: Kegan Paul, 1930.

132. ———, *The Moral Judgment of the Child.* New York: Free Press of Glencoe, 1948.

133. ———, *Play, Dreams, and Imitation in Childhood.* New York: W. W. Norton, 1951.

134. ———, *The Child's Conception of the World.* London: Routledge and Kegan Paul, 1951.

135. ———, *Judgment and Reasoning in the Child.* London: Routledge and Kegan Paul, 1951.

136. ———, *The Origins of Intelligence in Children.* New York: W. W. Norton, 1963.

137. ———, *Six Psychological Studies.* New York: Random House, 1967.

138. ———, *Biology and Knowledge.* Chicago: University of Chicago Press, 1971.

139. ———, *Psychology and Epistemology.* New York: Orion Press, 1971.

140. ———, *Understanding Causality.* New York: W. W. Norton, 1974.

141. ———, *The Grasp of Consciousness.* Cambridge, MA: Harvard University Press, 1976.

142. ———, and B. Inhelder, *The Psychology of the Child.* New York: Basic Books, 1969.

143. ———, and Inhelder, B., *The Origin of the Idea of Chance in Children.* New York: W. W. Norton, 1975.

144. Quinn, S., *A Mind of Her Own: The Life of Karen Horney.* New York: Summit Books, 1987.

145. Rabinowitz, F., G. Good, and L. Cozad, Rollo May: A Man of Meaning and Myth. *Journal of Counseling and Development,* 67 (1989), 436–441.

146. Rahe, R., and R. Arthur, Life Change Patterns Surrounding Illness Perception, *Journal of Psychosomatic Research,* 11, no. 3 (1968), 341–345.

147. Rest, J., The Legacy of Lawrence Kohlberg, *Counseling and Values,* 32, no. 3 (1988), 156–162.

148. Riehl, J., and C. Roy, Theory and Models, in *Conceptual Models for Nursing Practice* (3rd ed.). New York: Appleton-Century-Crofts, 1988.

149. Rimm, R.C., and J.C. Masters, *Behavior Therapy Techniques and Empirical Findings.* New York: Academic Press, 1979.

150. Robinson, L., Stress and Anxiety, *Nursing Clinics of North America,* 25, no. 4 (1990), 935–943.

151. Rogers, C., *Client-Centered Therapy.* Boston: Houghton-Mifflin, 1951.

152. ———, *On Becoming a Person.* Boston: Houghton-Mifflin, 1961.

153. ———, *Freedom to Learn.* Columbus, OH: Charles E. Merrill, 1969.

154. ———, *On Encounter Groups.* New York: Harper & Row, 1970.

155. ———, A Theory of Personality, in Millan, T., ed. *Theories of Psychopathology.* Philadelphia: W.B. Saunders, 1973.

156. ———, *Way of Being.* Boston: Houghton Mifflin, 1980.

157. Rogers, M., *An Introduction to the Theoretical Basis of Nursing.* Philadelphia: F.A. Davis, 1970.

158. San Blise, M., Crisis Intervention: Aftershocks in the Quake Zone, *Journal of Psychosocial Nursing,* 32, no. 5 (1994), 29–32.

159. Schumacher, K., and A. Meleis, Transitions: A Central Concept in Nursing, *IMAGE: Journal of Nursing Scholarship,* 26, no. 2 (1994), 119–127.

160. Seyle, H., Stress Syndrome, *American Journal of Nursing,* 65, no. 3 (1965), 97–99.

161. ———, *Stress Without Distress.* Philadelphia: J.B. Lippincott, 1974.

162. ———, Implications of Stress Concept, *New York State Journal of Medicine,* October (1975), 2139–2145.

163. ———, Forty Years of Stress Research: Principal Remaining Problems and Misconceptions, *Canadian Medical Association Journal,* 115 (July 3, 1976), 53–56.

164. ———, *The Stress of Life* (rev.). New York: McGraw-Hill, 1976.

165. ———, Stress and the Reduction of Distress, *Primary Cardiology,* 5, no. 8 (1979), 22–30.

166. ———, The Stress Concept Today, in Kutash, I.C., and Schlesinger, L.B. eds., *Handbook on Stress and Anxiety.* New York: Jossey-Bass, 1980, pp. 127–144.

167. Sheehy, G., *Passages.* New York: Bantam Books, 1984.

168. Shore, J., E. Tatum, and W. Vollmer, Evaluation of Mental Effects of Disaster, Mount St. Helens Eruption, *American Journal of Public Health,* 76, no. 3, suppl. (1986), 76–83.

169. Simonton, O.C., et al., *Getting Well Again: A Step-by-Step Self-Help Guide to Overcoming Cancer for Patients and Their Families.* New York: Bantam, 1982.

170. Skinner, B.F., *The Behavior of Organisms.* New York: Appleton-Century-Crofts, 1938.

171. ———, *Walden Two.* New York: Macmillan, 1948.

172. ———, *Science and Human Behavior.* New York: Macmillan, 1953.

173. ———, Behaviorism at Fifty. *Science,* 140 (1963), 951–958.

174. ———, The Phylogeny and Ontogeny of Behavior, *Science,* 153 (September 1966), 1205–1213.

175. ———, *Contingencies of Reinforcement: A Theoretical Analysis.* New York: Appleton-Century-Crofts, 1969.

176. ———, *Beyond Freedom and Dignity.* New York: Alfred A. Knopf, 1971.

177. ———, *Cumulative Record* (3rd ed.). New York: Appleton-Century-Crofts, 1972.

178. Smith, M., Existential-Phenomenological Foundations in Nursing: A Discussion of Differences, *Nursing Science Quarterly,* 4, no. 1 (1991), 5–6.

179. Smoyak, S., Changing American Families, in Hoekelman, R., S. Friedman, N. Nelson, and H. Seidel, eds., *Primary Pediatric Care* (2nd ed.). St. Louis: Mosby, 1992.

180. Sperry, R., Forebrain Commissurotomy and Conscious Awareness, in Travarthen, C., ed., *Brain Circuits and Functions on the Mind.* New York: Cambridge University Press, 1990, pp. 371–388.

181. Storr, A., *The Essential Jung.* Princeton, NJ: Princeton University Press, 1983.

182. Sullivan, H.S., *The Interpersonal Theory of Psychiatry.* New York: W.W. Norton, 1953.

183. Survey Assesses RN Management of Genetic Information, *The American Nurse,* January–February (1995), 27.

184. Taylor, R., *Distinguishing Psychological From Organic Disorders.* New York: Springer, 1990.

185. The Cruelest Kind of Grief, *Newsweek,* January 2 (1989), 21–23.

186. Travelbee, J., *Interpersonal Aspects of Nursing.* Philadelphia: F.A. Davis, 1971.

187. Urban, H., Humanist, Phenomenological, and Existential Approaches, in Hersen, M., Kadzin A., and Bellak, A. eds., *The Clinical Psychology Handbook* (2nd ed.). New York: Pergamon Press, 1991, pp. 200–219.

188. Vaillant, G., The Normal Body in Later Life: How Adaptation Fosters Growth, *Harvard Magazine,* 6 (1977), 234–239.

189. Von Bertalanffy, L., *General System Theory.* New York: George Braziller, 1968.

190. Wadsworth, B., *Piaget's Theory of Cognitive and Affective Development* (5th ed.). New York: Longman, 1996.

191. Walker, L., A Longitudinal Study of Moral Reasoning, *Child Development,* 60, no. 1 (1989), 157–166.

192. Weinrich, H., Some Consequences of Replicating Kohlberg's Original Moral Development Study in a British Sample, *Journal of Moral Education,* 7, no. 1 (1977), 32–39.

193. Wolpe, J. *Theme and Variations: A Behavioral Therapy Case Book.* New York: Pergamon Press, 1976.

194. ———, Individualization: The Categorical Imperative Behavior Therapy Practice, *Journal of Behavior Therapy and Experimental Psychiatry,* 17, no. 3 (1986), 145–153.

195. ———, *Practice of Behavior Therapy* (3rd ed.). New York: Pergamon Press, 1991.

196. Wubbolding, R., *Understanding Reality Therapy.* New York: Harper Collins, 1991.

197. ———, *Using Reality Therapy.* New York: Harper & Row, 1988.

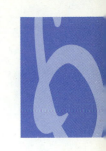

chapter six

The Developing Person: Principles of Growth and Development

Nothing has a stronger influence on their children than the unlived lives of their parents.

—Carl Jung

Key Terms

Social time
Historical time
Cohort
Norms
Growth
 Incremental growth
 Replacement growth
 Hypertrophy
 Hyperplasia
Development
Developmental task
Maturation
Biological age
Psychological age
Social age
Chronologic age
Learning
One Genus Postulate

Critical periods
Physical competency
Cognitive competency
Emotional competency
Social competency
Principle of Development Toward
 Self-Knowledge and Autonomy
Principle of Readiness
Principle of Differentiation
Cephalocaudal Principle
Proximodistal Principle
Bilateral Principle
Principle of Asynchronous Growth
Principle of Discontinuity
 of Growth Rate
Chromosomes
Genes
Ovum

Zygote
Gametes
Meiosis
Follicle
Ovulation
Orgasm
Cervix
Fraternal twins
Identical twins
Germinal stage
Embryonic stage
Fetal stage
Conceptus
Anemia
Pica
Teratogen
Teratogenesis
Folklore

Anoxia
Prematurity
Low-birth-weight infant
Hormone
Integration
Regulation
Morphogenesis
Socialization
Resilient children
Vulnerable Children
Child abuse
Sexual molestation
Emotional abuse
Neglect
Maternal deprivation
Failure to thrive
Perceptual deprivation

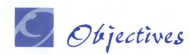

Objectives

Study of this chapter will enable you to:

1. **Define** growth, development, and related terms.

2. **Explore** general insights into and principles of human behavior.

3. **Discuss** various influences that have an effect on the developing person: prenatal variables involving father, mother, and fetus; variables related to childbirth; early childhood variables, including child abuse; sociocultural experiences; and environmental factors.

4. **Relate** information in this chapter to yourself as a developing person.

5. **Use** information from this chapter when assessing the person through the life span.

6. **Teach** the person and family about factors that influence development of self or offspring, when appropriate.

Developmental theory, which discusses the person throughout the life span, centers around certain principles of and influences on the person's growth and development. Although growth and development are usually thought of as a forward movement of a kind of adding on such as increase in height and weight or the self-actualizing personality, the model can also apply to reversal, decay, deterioration, or death. Three kinds of reversals occur: (1) loss of some part such as occurs with **catabolism** (changing of living tissue into wastes or destructive metabolism), (2) purposefully changing behavior when it is no longer useful, and (3) death (66).

Growth and development are generally characterized by the following (66, 134):

- Direction, goal, or end state
- Identifiable stage or era
- Forward progression, so that once a stage is worked through, the person does not return to the same position
- Increasing specialization
- Causal forces that are either genetic or environmental
- Potentialities and capabilities for various behaviors and achievements

DIMENSIONS OF TIME

Lifetime or chronologic age is frequently used as an **index** of maturation and development but is only a **rough** indicator of the person's position on any one of **the** numerous physical or psychological dimensions. **Further,** the society is a reference point for understand**ing** the behavior; what is appropriate for a 14-year-old **individual** in one society is not in a different society (66, **134).**

Social time, or *social expectations of behavior for each age era,* is not necessarily synchronous with biological timing. Neither chronologic age nor maturational stage is itself a determinant of aging status but only signifies the biological potentiality on which a system of age norms and age grading can operate to shape the life cycle (66, 134).

Historical time shapes the social system, and the social system creates a changing set of age norms and a changing age-grade system that shapes the person's life cycle. **Historical time** refers to a *series of economic, political, and social events that directly shape the life course of the person and long-term processes* such as industrialization and urbanization that create the social cultural context and changing definitions of the phases of the life cycle (66, 134).

A group of people born at a certain calendar time **(cohort)** has, as a group, a particular background and demographic composition so that most of the people of that specific age or generation will have similar experiences, level of education, fertility and childrearing patterns, sexual mores, work and labor force participation patterns, value systems, leisure patterns, religious behavior, consumer behavior, and ideas about life generally (66, 134).

Social time is prescribed by each society in that all societies rationalize the passage of lifetime, divide life into socially relevant units, and transform calendar or biological time into social time. Thus age grading occurs; the life cycle consists of a succession of formally age-graded, descriptive norms. Duties, rights, and rewards are differentially distributed to age groups. In societies in which division of labor is simple and social change is slow, a single age-grade system becomes formalized, and family, work, religious, and political roles are allocated. A modern, complex, rapidly changing society, which has several or overlapping systems of age status, has some tasks and roles that are tied to chronologic age and some that are more fluid or less defined. In every society there is a time to be a child and dependent, a time to be educated to whatever level is needed, a time to go to work, to marry, to have a family, to retire, and to die. The members of the society have a general consensus about these age expectations and norms, although perceptions may vary somewhat by age, sex, or social class. Thus there is some pressure to conform. If the person engages in the tasks earlier or later than others in the society, he or she is considered deviant. Patterns of timing can play an important role with respect to self-concept and self-esteem, depending on the person's level of awareness about his or her fit to social age norms and the rigidity in the culture. The young are more likely to deny that age is a valid criterion by which to judge behavior. Middle-aged and old adults, who see greater constraints in the age-norm system than do the young, have learned that to be off time involves negative consequences. Many of the major marks in the life cycle are ordered and sequential and are social rather than biological, and their time is socially regulated (66, 134).

The life course dimension is indexed by chronologic age, which serves as an indicator of the person's experience, including age-related organic changes affecting physical and mental functioning and including the probability of certain psychological and social experiences (66, 134).

This book is organized along chronologic lines, with the life cycle divided into different periods rather than having content organized around a topical approach. The person's life is divided into the following chronologic stages; the prenatal period (from the moment of conception to birth); infancy (birth to 1 year); toddlerhood (1 to 3 years); preschool (3 to 6 years); school years (6 to 12 years); adolescence (12 to 20 or 25 years); young adulthood (20 or 25 to 45 years); middle age (45 or 50 to 65 or 70 years); and late maturity (65 or 70 years and over). The divisions are somewhat arbitrary because it is difficult to assign definite ages as individual lives are not marked off so precisely. In discussion of stage theories such as those of Freud, Erikson, and Piaget, we use the theorists' own age ranges, and the same reservations apply to them.

The study of development is not merely a search for facts about people at certain ages. The study involves finding *patterns* or *general principles* that apply to most people most of the time.

People are often at one level in one area of development and at another level in another area. For example, an 11-year-old girl may have begun to menstruate—an activity that marks her physical transition from childbirth to puberty—before she has outgrown many child-

ish feelings and thoughts. A 48-year-old man who took several years to find his career direction, who married in his thirties, and who became a father in his forties may in many important psychological ways be in the young adulthood period. On the other hand, his 49-year-old neighbor who settled early on a professional direction and into family life may already be a grandfather and may act and feel more like a middle-aged man. Furthermore, individual differences among people are so great that they enter and leave these age periods at different times of life. People are aware of their own timing and are quick to describe themselves as "early," "late," or "on time" regarding developmental tasks.

Ideal **norms,** *standards* or *expectancies,* for different behaviors vary among different groups of people. The entire life cycle is speeded up for the poor and working classes, who tend to finish their education earlier than middle- or upper-class people, to take their first jobs sooner, marry younger, have children earlier, reach the peak of their careers earlier, and become grandparents earlier. These differences are related to financial needs that make it imperative for poor and working-class people to get paying jobs earlier in life. People from more affluent backgrounds can pursue their educations for a longer time, can use young adulthood to explore options, and then delay becoming financially independent and beginning a family (42, 66).

PRINCIPLES OF GROWTH AND DEVELOPMENT

Definitions

Certain words are basic to understanding the person and are used repeatedly. They are defined below for the purpose of this book.

Growth refers to *increase in body size or changes in structure, function, and complexity of body cell content and metabolic and biochemical processes up to some point of optimum maturity* (66). Growth changes occur through incremental or replacement growth. **Incremental growth** refers to *maintaining an excess in growth over normal daily losses from catabolism, seen in urine, feces, perspiration, and oxidation in the lungs.* Incremental growth is observed as increases in weight or height as the child matures. **Replacement growth** refers to *normal refills of essential body components* necessary for survival (53). For example, once a red blood cell (erythrocyte) has entered the cardiovascular system, it circulates an average of 120 days before disintegrating, when another red blood cell takes its place (53). Growth occurs through **hypertrophy,** *increase in the size of cellular structures,* and **hyperplasia,** *an increase in the num-*

ber of cells (53). Growth during the fetal and infancy periods is achieved primarily through hyperplasia, which is gradually replaced by hypertrophic growth. Each body organ has its own optimum period of growth. Body tissues are most sensitive to permanent damage during periods of the most rapid hyperplastic growth.

Development is the *patterned, orderly, lifelong changes in structure, thought, or behavior that evolve as a result of maturation of physical and mental capacity, experiences, and learning and result in a new level of maturity and integration* (66, 134). Development should permit the person to adapt to the environment by either controlling the environment or controlling responses to the environment. Developmental processes involve interplay among the physiologic characteristics that define the person; the environmental forces, including culture, that act on him or her; and the psychological mechanisms that mediate between them. Psychological processes include the person's perception of self, others, and the environment, and the behaviors he or she acquires in coping with needs and the environment. Development combines growth, maturation, and learning and involves organizing behavior (32).

Developmental task is a *growth responsibility that arises at a certain time in the course of development, successful achievement of which leads to satisfaction and success with later tasks.* Failure leads to unhappiness, disapproval by society, and difficulty with later developmental tasks and functions (27, 32, 66).

Maturation refers to the *emergence of genetic potential for changes in form, structure, complexity, integration, organization, and function, physically and mentally* (27).

Biological age is the *level of physical growth and development and how the body functions over time.* **Psychological age** *is the person's perception of aging processes.* **Social age** *refers to society's expectations of the person at a specific age or stage* (134). **Chronologic age** is the *time since birth* and is not always identical to the other ages.

Learning is the *process of gaining specific knowledge or skill and acquiring habits and attitudes as a result of experience, training, and behavioral changes.* Maturation and learning are interrelated. No learning occurs unless the person is mature enough to be able to understand and change his or her behavior (134).

GENERAL ASSUMPTIONS ABOUT BEHAVIOR

C. Buhler is a developmental theorist whose thinking in the early 1900s influenced a number of present well-known personality and developmental theorists.

Buhler described the person's life course as having a definite basic structure and direction or goals (14). These structures and goals are evidence in the biological life cycle and in psychological development. The structure and phasic organization of the person's life, with its properties and potentials, determine the person's goals and are influenced by environmental circumstances, time limits, personal characteristics, and society's assignment of roles.

In Buhler's theory life is divided biologically into a nonreproductive phase (first 15 years, approximately), a reproductive phase from approximately 15 to 45 years, and then a decline and loss in the reproductive ability, first in the female and then in the male (after middle age for a woman and in old age for the man). Onset of reproductive ability, from puberty to 25 years, is followed by a peak period for reproductive ability and stationary growth (25–45 years). A period of gradual decline follows (14).

Psychological development is not parallel to biological development because (1) psychological development is continuous, and (2) there is no exact parallel between the two aspects of life so far as tasks or goals are concerned. Psychological and mental development may be behind biological development, is generally independent of physical or biological factors, and extends beyond reproductive abilities. The psychological system develops in a maturational order and is influenced by learning and the impact of emotional experiences. Abilities, aptitudes, motives, and goals contribute to personality development (14).

The following statements have not been proved by strict scientific study, but they have been observed so regularly that they seem to be true.

The person is a unified but open system composed of the components of body, mind, feelings, and spirit, which are, in turn, continually influenced by the environment. The person, in turn, influences the environment (130). Change in one part produces change in all parts of the system (11, 139).

All persons are similar and have the same basic needs, but they are also unique in following and expressing their own developmental patterns. The **One Genus Postulate** states that *people are more similar than different simply because they are all Homo sapiens* (130).

The person is a unified whole. Thus understanding the whole person is not possible through study of isolated components of the person (108).

The person's life process evolves irreversibly; the person cannot totally return to something he or she was developmentally (67, 108). Nevertheless, the past influences the person to some degree whether or not he or she is aware of the influence, and it sets the direction for present and future patterns of behavior (67, 129).

The person responds as a total organism at any given moment to events, persons, or objects in terms of personal perception, needs, and expectations (27, 67).

Each person is a social being who has the capacity to communicate and react to other people and the environment. Thus the person can function in the social system and its various institutions such as family, school, and church (67).

The person cannot understand the self without understanding others, and he or she cannot understand others without understanding the self. Understanding the past and the parents helps to understand the self, as developmental patterns of the parents are repeated in the child (129).

Culture and society determine guidelines for normal progression of development and behavior patterns. What is normal in one ethnic or racial group may be considered deviant or undesirable in another. Further, deviation from normal may occur in all or only certain areas of function. The child may show abnormally slow development in one area and unusually accelerated or a mature quality in another. Yet despite these differences, the child may be perceived generally by others as a normal person, depending on the degree of deviance.

Throughout life the person strives to reach optimum physical and emotional potential, barring great interferences. An inner drive or motivation propels him or her onward to meet the various developmental tasks. The person tries all types of adaptive behavior when interferences occurs. He or she may regress to work through unsolved problems from the past. Once a need is met or a goal is accomplished, the person is free to move on to new arenas of behavior (42, 85, 129).

General Principles of Development

The following statements apply to the overall development of the person.

Childhood is the foundation period of life. Attitudes, habits, patterns of behavior and thinking, personality traits, and health status established during the early years (the first 5) determine to a large extent how successfully the person will continue to develop and adjust to life as he or she gets older. Early patterns of behavior persist throughout life, within the range of normalcy (33, 42).

Development follows a definable, predictable, and sequential pattern and occurs continually through adulthood. All persons progress through similar stages, but the age for achievement varies because achievement depends on inherent maturational capacity interacting with the physical and social environment. The different areas of growth and development—physical, mental, emotional, social, and spiritual—are interrelated, proceed together, and affect each other; yet these areas mature at their own pace. The stages of development overlap, and the transition from one stage to another is gradual (42, 129).

Growth and development are continuous, but they occur in spurts rather than in a straight upward direction. At times the person will appear to be at a standstill or even regress developmentally.

Growth is usually accompanied by behavior change. As the child matures, he or she retains earlier ways of behaving, but there will be a developmental revision of habits. For example, the high-activity infant becomes a high-activity toddler or adult, but the object of the activity changes from diffuse interests to concentrated play to work. The young child's temperament is a precursor of later behavior, although the person is adaptable and changes throughout life. Behavior changes also occur because of others' reactions and expectations, which change as the person matures physically.

Human behavior has purpose or is goal directed. Therefore, the behavior is commonly preceded by imagining the desired result. The person visualizes the future and tries to bring it about. Behavior is directed to meeting needs and goals.

When one need or goal is met, the person has energy to pursue another need, interest, or goal. Behavior changes direction, but it does not come to an end.

Critical periods in human development *occur when specific organs and other aspects of a person's physical and psychosocial growth undergo marked rapid change and the capacity to adapt to stressors is underdeveloped. During these critical periods when tremendous demands are placed on the person, the individual has an increased susceptibility to adverse environmental factors that may cause various types and degrees of negative effects.* For example, implantation is a critical period, and at certain times during pregnancy certain substances are more likely to damage fetal structures (26, 66, 134). The form of the brain is established by the 12th week of gestation. Critical periods of brain growth are during early formation (organogenesis) from the 3rd to 9th weeks of gestation; during brain growth spurt from 12 to 20 weeks of gestation; and during the time of rapid neuronal additions from 30 to 40 weeks of gestation and during the first 18 to 24 months after birth. Exposure of the nervous system to a teratogen during these time frames may affect specific brain regions that are growing the most rapidly at that time. During adolescence the rapid physical growth may negatively affect social relationships or feelings about self. Middle or old age may be another critical period (53, 134).

If appropriate stimuli and resources are not available at the critical time or when the person is ready to receive and use particular stimuli for the development of a specific psychomotor skill, the skill may be more difficult to learn later in the developmental sequence. Learning of any psychomotor skill, however, is also influenced by sociocultural factors; the extent to which any skill is influenced by genetics, environmental opportunity, cultural and family values and patterns, and emotional status is not fully known.

Mastering developmental tasks of one period is the basis for mastering the next developmental era, physically and emotionally. Certain periods exist when the task can be best accomplished and the task should be mastered then; if the time is delayed, the person will have difficulty in accomplishing the task. Each phase of development has characteristic traits and a period of equilibrium when the person adjusts more easily to environmental demands and a period of disequilibrium when he or she experiences difficulty in adjustment. Developmental hazards exist in every era. Some are environmental and interfere with adjustment; others come from within the person (32, 42, 91, 116, 129, 147).

Progressive differentiation of the self from the environment results from increasing self-knowledge and autonomy. The young child first separates as an object apart from mother. Gradually he or she becomes less dependent emotionally on the parents. As the child matures into adulthood, an increase in cognitive development enables more control over behavior. The person can think and act on his or her own and become more and more autonomous.

The developing person simultaneously acquires competencies in four major areas: physical, cognitive, emotional, and social. **Physical competency** includes *various motor and neurologic capacities* to attain mobility and manipulation and care for self physically. **Cognitive competency** includes *learning how to perceive, think, solve problems, and communicate thoughts and feelings* that, in turn, affect emotional and social skills. **Emotional competency** includes *developing an awareness and acceptance of self as a separate person, responding to other people and factors in the environment because others have been responsive to him or her, coping with inner and outer stresses, and becoming increasingly responsible for personal behavior.* **Social competency** includes *learning how to affiliate securely with the family first and then with various people in various situations.* These four competencies constantly influence one another. Health of one domain or the extent of competency affects the other domains or competencies. Lack

of care or stimulation in any one area inhibits development of the other three areas. Repetition and practice are essential to learning. Rewarded behavior is usually repeated (66). The person optimally uses personal assets, inner resources, competencies, and abilities to keep energy expenditures at a minimum while focusing toward the achievement of a goal (116, 147).

Readiness and motivation are essential for learning to occur. Hunger, fatigue, illness, pain, and the lack of emotional feedback or opportunity to explore inhibit readiness and lower motivation.

Many factors contribute to the formation of permanent characteristics and traits, including the child's genetic inheritance, undetermined prenatal environmental factors, family and society when he or she is an infant and young child, nutrition, physical and emotional environment, and degree of intellectual stimulation in the environment.

Progressive differentiation of the self from other people and the environment, the **Principle of Development Toward Self-knowledge and Autonomy,** is made apparent with the individual's increasing self-awareness and emergent self-concept. The young child achieves increasing ability to perceive himself or herself as an initiator of action on the environment and an increasing ability to regulate his or her own behavior, to think and act in an individual and unique way, and to become more autonomous. The ability to be autonomous and interdependent is reworked throughout life (66).

Principles of Growth

Several principles of growth are emphasized in the following pages, but the primary determinant of normal growth is the development of the central nervous system, which, in turn, governs or influences other body systems.

The **Principle of Readiness** states that the *child's ability to perform a physical task depends not only on maturation of neurologic structures in the brain but also on the maturation of the muscular and skeletal systems.* Until a state of physiologic readiness is reached, the child cannot perform a function, such as toilet training, even with parental training or planned practice.

The **Principle of Differentiation** means that *development proceeds from simple to the complex; homogeneous to heterogeneous; and general to specific* (66). For example, movement from *simple to complex* is seen in mitotic changes in fetal cell structures as they undergo cell division immediately following ovum fertilization by a sperm (53). All human embryos are anatomically female for the first 6 weeks of life; only through the action of testosterone does the male embryo develop between the 6th and 12th weeks of life. Androgens or steroids administered prenatally can masculinize a genetic female brain. Differentiation from simple to complex motor skill is seen after birth as the baby first waves his or her arms and then later learns to control finger movements. The general body configurations of male and female at birth are much more similar than during late adolescence, thus indicating *movement from homogeneity to heterogeneity*. The mass of cells in the embryo is at first homogeneous, but the limbs of the 5-week-old embryo show considerable differentiation as the elbow and wrist regions become identifiable and finger ridge indentations outline the progressive protrusion of future fingers from the former paddle-shaped arm bud (53). *General to specific* development is observed in motor responses, which are diffuse and undifferentiated at birth and become more specific and controlled later. Baby first moves the whole body in response to a stimuli; later he or she reacts with a specific body part (116, 147). The behavior of the child becomes more specific to the person or situation with increasing age.

The **Cephalocaudal, Proximodistal, and Bilateral Principles** all indicate that *major physical and motor changes invariably proceed in three bipolar directions*. **Cephalocaudal** (*head to tail*) means that the *upper end of the organism develops with greater rapidity than and before the lower end of the organism*. Increases in neuromuscular size and maturation of function begin in the head and proceed to hands and feet. For example, a comparison of pictures of a 5-week-old embryo during a period of several days clearly shows the extensive head growth, caused mainly by development of the brain, accompanied by further oblongation of the body structure from head to tail. Further, auditory, visual, and other sensory mechanisms in the head develop sooner than motor systems of the upper body. At the same time, the arm buds, first appearing paddle shaped, continue to change in shape and size more rapidly than do the lower limbs. After birth the infant will be able to hold the head erect before being able to sit or walk (116, 147). **Proximodistal** (*near to far*) means that *growth progresses from the central axis of the body toward the periphery or extremities*. **Bilateral** (*side to side*) means that the *capacity for growth and development of structures is symmetric* (116, 147); growth that occurs on one side of the body occurs simultaneously on the other.

The **Principle of Asynchronous Growth** focuses on *developmental shifts at successive periods in development*. A comparison of pictures of persons of different ages indicates that the young child is *not* a "small adult"; the proportional size of the head to the chest and of the torso to the limbs of younger and older persons is vastly different. Length of limbs in comparison to torso length is smaller in the infant than the schoolchild and greater in the aged than the adolescent because of the biological changes of aging (33).

The **Principle of Discontinuity of Growth Rate** refers to the *different rate of growth changes at different periods during the life span*. The *whole* body does not grow as a total unit simultaneously. Instead, various structures and organs of the body grow and develop at different rates, reaching their maximum at different times throughout the life cycle. For instance, in its rudimentary form the heart and circulatory system begin to function during the third week of embryonic life, continue to mature slowly compared with the rest of the body, and after the age of 25 years remain fairly constant in size (66). Before birth the head is the fastest growing body part. The brain grows and develops according to a different pattern; this vital organ grows very rapidly during fetal life and infancy, reaching 80% of its maximum size at the age of 2 years. Full growth is seen at approximately 6 years of age (53). Body growth is rapid in infancy and adolescence and relatively slow during school years.

All body systems normally continue to work in unity throughout the life span. Some physiologic characteristics such as oxygen concentration in the blood remain fairly stable throughout life. Others such as body temperature undergo minor changes, depending on age, hormonal balance, or time of day. Some characteristics such as pulse rate and fluid intake that are affected by changes in body surface, organ size, or maturity change markedly during the life cycle (116, 147). Age-related changes occur at varying chronologic periods. Structural deterioration usually precedes functional decline. Some organs and systems deteriorate more rapidly than others. In late life the capacity for adaptation changes and finally decreases. Before death, decline or deterioration usually affects most structural and many functional centers in the aged person (116, 147).

The study of growth and development processes must focus on the complete continuum of the life cycle—from conception through death—to acquire a comprehensive understanding of the complexity of these processes and how these principles are activated throughout the life span.

DEVELOPING PERSON: PRENATAL STAGES AND INFLUENCES

The Beginning

The cell, the basis for human life, is a complex unit. Refer to the anatomy or physiology text for review of cell structure and function. This chapter presents a brief overview of the prenatal period as the beginning of life. For in-depth study of the biological differences of the male and female, the reproductive process, including fertilization and development of the unborn child in utero, inheritance patterns, and the process of labor and delivery, refer to an anatomy and physiology or developmental text and to a maternity nursing text (27, 33, 53, 66, 116, 147).

All body cells have 22 pairs of rod-shaped particles, nonsex **chromosomes** (*autosomes*), and a pair of sex chromosomes. The biological female has two X chromosomes; the biological male has one X and one Y chromosome. Each of the chromosomes contains approximately 20,000 *segments strung out like lengthwise beads* called **genes.** The genes, apparently located according to function, are made up of deoxyribonucleic acid (DNA), which processes the information that determines the makeup and specific function of every cell in the body. The genes play a major role in determining hereditary characteristics (26, 53).

The female reproductive cycle is more regular and is easier to observe and measure than is the male reproductive cycle (116, 147). In contrast to the normal menstrual cycle, spermatogenesis normally occurs in cycles that continuously follow one another.

Approximately 14 days after the beginning of the menstrual period fertilization may occur in the outer third of the fallopian tube. The sperm cell from a male penetrates and unites with an **ovum** (*egg*) from a female to form a *single-cell* **zygote.** The sperm and ovum, known as **gametes** (*sex cells in half cells*), are produced in the reproductive system through **meiosis,** a *specialized process of cell division and chromosome reduction* (53, 66).

A newborn girl has approximately 400,000 immature ova in her ovaries; each is in a **follicle,** or *small sac.* **Ovulation,** *the expelling of an ovum from a mature follicle in one of the ovaries,* occurs approximately once every 28 days in a sexually mature female (53, 66).

Spermatozoa, much smaller and more active than the ovum, are produced in the testes of the mature male at the rate of several hundred million a day and are ejaculated in his semen at *sexual climax* (**orgasm**). For fertilization to occur, at least 20 million sperm cells must enter a woman's body at one time. They enter the vagina and try to swim through the **cervix** (*opening to the uterus*) and into the fallopian tube. Only a tiny fraction of those millions of sperm cells makes it that far. More than one may penetrate the ovum, but only one can fertilize it to create a new human. The sex of the baby is determined by the pair of sex chromosomes; the sperm may carry either an X or Y chromosome, resulting in either a girl (XX zygote) or a boy (XY zygote). Thus *the man determines the sex of the baby* (53, 66).

Spermatozoa maintain their ability to fertilize an egg for a span of 24 to 72 to 90 hours; ova can be fertilized for approximately 24 hours. Thus there are approx-imately 72 to 90 hours during each menstrual cycle when conception can take place. If fertilization does not occur, the spermatozoa and ovum die. Sperm cells are devoured by white blood cells in the woman's body; the ovum passes through the uterus and vagina in the menstrual product (53, 66).

Multiple births may occur. Twins occur in approximately 1 of 86 births. Occasionally two ova are released within a short time of each other; if both are fertilized, **fraternal** (*dizygotic, or two-egg*) **twins** will be born. Created by different eggs and different sperm cells, the twins are no more alike in their genetic makeup than other siblings. They may be of the same or different sex. If the ovum divides in two after it has been fertilized, **identical** (*monozygotic, or one-egg*) **twins** will be born. At birth these twins share the same placenta. They are of the same sex and have exactly the same genetic heritage; any differences they will later exhibit are due to the influences of environment, either before or after birth. Other multiple births—triplets, quadruplets, and so forth—result from either one or a combination of these two processes (53, 66).

Multiple births have become more frequent in recent years as a result of the administration of certain fertility drugs that spur ovulation and often cause the release of more than one egg. The tendency to bear twins apparently is inherited and more common in some families and ethnic groups than in others. Twins have a limited intrauterine space and are more likely to be premature and of low birth weight. They are therefore at greater risk for survival at birth (26).

After either single or multiple fertilization the zygote travels to the uterus for implantation or imbedding in the uterine wall. Progesterone secretion has prepared the uterus for the possible reception of the fertilized ovum. The continued secretion of ovarian estrogen and progesterone develops the uterus for the 9-month nurturance of the developing embryo and fetus in pregnancy. Continued secretion of estrogen during this period increases the growth of the uterine muscles and eventually enlarges the vagina for the delivery of a child. Continued secretion of progesterone during pregnancy serves to keep the uterus from prematurely contracting and expelling the developing embryo before the proper time. In addition, progesterone prepares the breast cells in late pregnancy for future milk production (26).

Stages of Prenatal Development

Life in utero is usually divided into three stages of development: germinal, embryonic, and fetal. The **germinal stage** lasts *approximately 10 days to 2 weeks after fertilization.* It is characterized by rapid cell division and subsequent increasing complexity of the organism and its implantation in the wall of the uterus. The **embryonic stage,** *from 2 to 8 weeks,* is the time of rapid growth and differentiation of major body systems and organs. The **fetal stage,** *from 8 weeks until birth,* is characterized by rapid growth and changes in body form caused by different rates of growth of different parts of the body (26, 53).

The fetus is a very small but rapidly developing human being who is influenced by the maternal and external environment and to whom the mother responds, especially when fetal movement begins. Table 6–1 summarizes some major milestones in the sequential development of the **conceptus,** the *new life that has been conceived;* however, *being precise about the exact timing is difficult* (26, 33, 53, 116, 147).

Prenatal Influences on Development

Heredity

Genetic information is transmitted from parents of offspring through a complex series of processes. Twenty-three pairs of chromosomes in the human germ cells divide into two gametes by meiosis, giving to each of these mature germ cells (female ovum and male spermatozoon) one half the genetic material necessary for producing a new individual. The specific hereditary information is carried on the chromosomes by thousands of genes, but the expression of gene characteristic is not a preprogrammed, unchangeable process (26, 33).

Further, hereditary factors do not by themselves fully determine what the person will become. Because the hereditability of a trait generally does not exceed 50%, there is much room for environmental factors. The role of genetics may be overrated (104). Innate characteristics and environmental forces are closely related. Genetic endowment with respect to any trait may be compared to a rubber band. The rubber band may remain unstretched because of environmental influences, causing potential to remain dormant. Or the rubber band may be stretched fully, causing the person to excel beyond what seems his or her potential. The person in later maturity, for example, has had many years of changing environmental influences; what he or she has become is no doubt an expression of innate genetic potential and environmental supports and the wisdom to take advantage of both.

Embryologic development and principles of genetics affecting body structure and function are complex. A number of references provide additional information (26, 33, 53, 91, 116, 147).

Parental Age

Age of mother and father and number of previous pregnancies affect the health of the fetus:

- A baby born to a woman who has had three or more pregnancies before age 20 is less likely to be healthy. Pregnancy during the teen years is more frequently associated with prematurity and infant illness (116, 147).
- Pregnancy after age 35 may increase the risk of delivery complications and problems in the neonate: prematurity, low birth weight, Down syndrome, birth defects, fraternal twinning (26, 116, 147).
- The more pregnancies a woman has had, the greater the risk to the infant. Maternal physiology cannot support many pregnancies in rapid succession, and as age increases, the ability to cope with the stresses of pregnancy decreases (26, 116, 147).
- The risk of producing offspring with anomalies linked to autosomal dominant mutations is higher when the father is age 40 or older (48).

Prenatal Endocrine and Metabolic Functions

Fetal growth and development are dependent on maternal endocrine and metabolic adjustments during pregnancy. The placenta helps to provide necessary estrogens, progesterone, and gonadotropin to sustain pregnancy and trigger other endocrine adjustments that involve primarily the pituitary, adrenal cortex, and thyroid. Fetal endocrine function is regulated independently from the mother, but endocrine drugs given to the mother may produce undesirable effects in the fetus (26, 53, 116, 147).

Animal research indicates that later sexual characteristics and behavior may be affected by administration of or presence or absence of sex hormones during fetal development. *The fetal period is the first critical period for sexual differentiation.* Although the fetus has a chromosomal combination denoting male or female, the fetus must be exposed to corresponding hormones during pregnancy. If the male fetus is insensitive to androgen (a masculinizing hormone) and exposed to large amounts of estrogens (a feminizing hormone), the child may possess many female characteristics (26, 116, 147). Testicular inductor substance causes production of fetal androgens that suppress anatomic precursors of the oviducts and ovaries and, in turn, cause the male genital tract to develop during the 7th to 12th weeks. The male embryo's testosterone offsets the maternal hormone influences. Unless androgens are present, the external

TABLE 6–1. SUMMARY OF THE SEQUENCE OF PRENATAL DEVELOPMENT

Time Period After Fertilization	Developmental Event
Germinal Stage	
30 hours	First division or cleavage occurs.
40 hours	Four-cell stage occurs.
60 hours	**Morula,** *a solid mass of 12 to 16 cells;* total size of mass not changed because cells decrease in size with each cleavage to allow morula to pass through lumen of fallopian tube. Ectopic pregnancy within fallopian tube occurs if morula is wedged in lumen.
3 days	Zygote has divided into 32 cells; travels through fallopian tube to uterus.
4 days	Zygote contains 70 cells. Morula reaches uterus; forms a **blastocyst,** *a fluid-filled sphere.*
4½–6 days	Blastocyst floats in utero. **Embryonic disk,** *thickened cell mass from which baby develops,* clusters on one edge of blastocyst. Mass of cells differentiates into two layers: (1) **ectoderm,** *outer layer of cells* that become the epidermis of skin, nails, hair, tooth enamel, sensory organs, brain and spinal cord, cranial nerves, peripheral nervous system, upper pharynx, nasal passages, urethra, and mammal glands; (2) **endoderm,** *lower layer of cells* that will develop into gastrointestinal system, liver, pancreas, salivary glands, respiratory system, urinary bladder, pharynx, thyroid, tonsils, lining of urethra, and ear.
6–7 days	**Nidation,** *implantation of zygote* into upper portion of uterine wall, occurs.
7–14 days	Remainder of blastocyst develops into the following: (1) **Placenta,** *a multipurpose organ connected to the embryo by the umbilical cord* that delivers oxygen and nourishment from the mother's body and absorbs the embryo's body wastes, combats internal infection, confers immunity to the unborn child, and produces the hormones that (a) support pregnancy, (b) prepare breasts for lactating, and (c) stimulate uterine contractions for delivery of the baby. Placenta circulation evidenced by 11 to 12 days. (2) **Umbilical cord,** *a structure that contains two umbilical arteries and an umbilical vein and connects embryo to placenta.* Approximately 20 inches long and 1½ in diameter. Rapid cell differentiation occurs. (3) **Amniotic sac,** *a fluid-filled membrane that encases the developing baby,* protecting it and giving it room to move.
2–8 weeks	Period during which embryo firmly establishes uterus as home and undergoes rapid cellular differentiation, growth, and development of body systems. This is a *critical period when embryo is most vulnerable to deleterious prenatal influences.* All developmental birth defects occur during *first trimester (3 months)* of pregnancy. If embryo is unable to survive , a **miscarriage** or **spontaneous abortion,** *expulsion of conceptus from the uterus,* occurs.
Embryonic Stage	
15 days	Cranial end of elongated disk has begun to thicken.
16 days	**Mesoderm,** *the middle layer,* appears and develops into skin dermis, tooth dentin, connective tissue, cartilage, bones, muscles, spleen, blood, gonads, uterus, and excretory and circulatory systems. Yolk sac, which arises from ectoderm, assists transfer of nutrients from mother to embryo.
19–20 days	Neural fold and neural grove develop. Thyroid begins to develop.
21 days	Neural tube forms, becomes spinal cord and brain.
22 days	Heart, the first organ to function, initiates action. Eyes, ears, nose, cheeks, and upper jaw begin to form. Cleft palate may occur if defective development.
26–27 days	Cephalic portion (brain) of nervous system formed. Leg and arm buds appear. Stubby tail of spinal cord appears.
28 days	Crown to rump length, 4–5 mm.
30 days	Rudimentary body parts formed. Limb buds appear. Cardiovascular system functioning. Heart beat 65 times per minute; blood flow through tiny arteries and veins. Lens vesicles, optic cups, and nasal pits forming. By end of first month, new life has grown more quickly than it will at any other time in life. Swelling in head where eyes, ears, mouth, and nose will be. Crown to rump length, 7–14 mm ($\frac{1}{4}$ to $\frac{1}{2}$ inches).
31 days	Eye and nasal pit developing. Primitive mouth present.
32 days	Paddle-shaped hands. Lens vesicles and optic cups formed.
34 days	Head is much larger relative to trunk. Digital rays present in hands. Feet are paddle shaped. Crown to rump length, 11–14 mm.
35–38 days	Olfactory pit, eye, maxillary process, oral cavity and mandibular process developing. Brain has divided into three parts. Limbs growing. Beginning of all major external and internal structures. Crown to rump length, 15–16 mm.
40 days	Elbows and knees apparent. Fingers and toes distinct but webbed. Yolk sac continues to (1) provide embryologic blood cells during third through sixth weeks until liver, spleen, and bone marrow assume function; (2) provide lining cells for respiratory and digestive tracts; (3) provide cells that migrate to gonads to become primordial germ cells.
42 days	Crown to rump length, 21–23 mm.

(continued)

TABLE 6–1. SUMMARY OF THE SEQUENCE OF PRENATAL DEVELOPMENT (continued)

Time Period After Fertilization	Developmental Event
50 days	All internal and external structures present. External genitalia present but sex not discernible; yolk sac disappears, incorporated into embryo; limbs, hands, feet formed. Nerve cells in brain connected.
55–56 days	Eye, nostril, globular process, maxilla, and mandible almost completely formed. Ear beginning to develop.
8 weeks	Stubby end of spinal cord disappears. Distinct human characteristics. Head accounts for half of total embryo length. Brain impulses coordinate function of organ systems. Facial parts formed, with tongue and teeth buds. Stomach produces digestive juices. Liver produces blood cells. Kidney removes uric acid from blood. Some movement by limbs. Weight, 1 g. Length, 1–1½ inches (2.5–3.75 cm).
Fetal Stage 9–40 weeks	Remainder of intrauterine period spent in growth and refinement of body tissues and organs.
9–12 weeks	Eyelids fused. Nail beds formed. Teeth and bones begin to appear. Ribs and vertebrae are cartilage. Kidneys function. Urinates occasionally. Some respiratory-like movements exhibited. Begins to swallow amniotic fluid. Grasp, sucking, and withdrawal reflexes present. Sucks fingers and toes in utero. Makes specialized responses to touch. Moves easily but movement not felt by mother. Reproductive organs have primitive egg or sperm cells. Sex distinguishable. Head one-third of body length. Weight, 30 g (1 oz). Length, 3 to 3½ inches at 12 weeks.
13–16 weeks	Much spontaneous movement. Sex determination possible. **Quickening,** *fetal kicking or movement,* may be felt by mother. Moro reflex present. Rapid skeletal development. Meconium present. Uterine development in female fetus. **Lanugo,** *downy hair,* appears on body. Head one-fourth of total length. Weight, 120–150 g (4–6 oz). Length, 8–10 in. Fetus frowns, moves lips, turns head; hands grasp, feet kick. First hair appears. Ova formed in female.
17–20 weeks	New cells exchanged for old, especially in skin. Quickening occurs by 17 weeks. Vernix caseosa appears. Eyebrows, eyelashes, and head hair appear. Sweat and sebaceous glands begin to function. Skeleton begins to harden. Grasp reflex present and strong. Permanent teeth buds appear. Fetal heart sounds can be heard with stethoscope. Weight, 360–450 g (12 oz–1 lb). Length, 12 in.
21–24 weeks	Extrauterine life, life outside uterus, is possible but difficult because of immature respiratory system. Fetus looks like miniature baby. Mother may note jarring but rhythmic movements of infant, indicative of hiccups. Body becomes straight at times. Fingernails present. Skin has wrinkled, red appearance. Alternate periods of sleep and activity. May respond to external sounds. Weight, 720 g (1½ lb). Length, 14 in.
25–28 weeks	Jumps in utero in synchrony with loud noise. Eyes open and close with waking and sleeping cycles. Able to hear. Respiratory-like movements. Respiratory and central nervous systems sufficiently developed; some babies survive with excellent and intensive care. Assumes head-down position in uterus. Weight, 1200 g (2½ lb).
29–32 weeks	Begins to store fat and minerals. Testes descend into scrotal sac in male. Reflexes fully developed. Thumb sucking present. Mother may note irregular, jerky, crying-like movements. Lanugo begins to disappear from face. Head hair continues to grow. Skin begins to lose reddish color. Can be conditioned to environmental sounds. Weight, 1362–2270 g (3–5 lb). Length, 16 in.
33–36 weeks	Adipose tissue continues to be deposited over entire body. Body begins to round out. May become more or less active because of space constriction. Increased iron storage by liver. Increased lung development. Lanugo begins to disappear from body. Head lengthens. Brain cells number same as at birth. Weight, 2800 g (6 lb). Length, 18–20 in.
37–40 weeks	Organ systems operating more efficiently. Heart rate increases. More wastes expelled. Lanugo and vernix caseosa disappear. Skin smooth and plump. High absorption of maternal hormones. Cerebral cortex well-defined; brain wave patterns developed. Skull and other bones becoming more firm and mineralized. Continued storage of fat and minerals. Glands produce hormones that trigger labor. Ready for birth. Weight, 3200–3400 g (7–7½ lb). Length, 20–21 in. Baby stops growing approximately 1 week before birth.

genitalia of the fetus will appear female regardless of the chromosomal pattern. Estrogens are released in the genetically female embryo and are necessary for the fetus to develop female genitalia. Likewise, inspection of the external genitalia of a newborn female may show abnormal fusion of the labia and enlargement of the clitoris caused by an androgen agent taken by the mother early in her pregnancy (26).

The second critical period for sexual differentiation occurs just before or after birth, when sex typing of the brain may occur. Testosterone may influence the hypothalamus so that a noncyclic pattern for release of pituitary hormones, the gonadotropins, will occur in males and a cyclic pattern of gonadotropin release will occur in females (53).

Fetal and placental growth, nourishment, waste excretion, and total function are dependent on the adequacy of the mother's blood system. Inadequate hemoglobin or red blood cells interfere with fetal function (26, 53).

Maternal hyperglycemia helps promote transfer of excessive glucose across the placenta to the fetus, stimulating fetal insulin secretion, a potent growth factor (26, 61, 88, 137). The diabetic mother is at high risk, as is her fetus. These infants have three to four times the incidence of congenital malformations as in the general population (51). The metabolic stress of fetal hyperinsulinism continues to increase anomalies, such as congenital malformations and disorders of fetal growth and pulmonary development. The metabolic stress of fetal hyperinsulinism apparently contributes to increased anomalies (e.g., obesity of the newborn) (26, 88, 137). Many fetal metabolic defects can now be diagnosed (26). Congenital heart defects are the most common (116, 147). Careful regulation of maternal glycemia through aggressive therapy with insulin and diet is often warranted (73). As most of the anomalies occur in the first few weeks of pregnancy, strict glycemic control beginning before conception appears mandated.

Maternal Nutrition

Nutrition is one of the most important variables for fetal health and prevention of prenatal and intrapartal complications. Scientists know that at least 60 nutrients are basic to maintenance of healthy growth and development (26, 144). Lack of these nutrients over a period may depress appetite, encourage disease, and retard growth and development, including causing mental retardation. If the mother's nutritional state is not adequate, the fetus is deprived of nutrients. Intrauterine growth retardation (IUGR) occurs with later effects on the child. For example, anemic mothers have average lower-birth-weight infants than nonanemic mothers (126). During the first 2 months of pregnancy, the developing embryo consists mostly of water; later more solids in the form of fat, nitrogen, and certain minerals are added. Because of the small amount of yolk in the human ovum, growth depends on nutrients obtained from the mother (26). Although nutritional requirements for the embryo/fetus are quantitatively small during the first trimester, nutritional deprivations can negatively impact placental structure and the ultimate birth weight. Lack of vitamin A, folate, and iron is linked to growth retardation, whereas supplements of calcium and magnesium may increase birth weight and length of gestation (81).

Caloric and *protein* intake are of particular importance. Calories are implicated in cell multiplication, and protein is believed primarily related to enlargement of these cells. Therefore, failure of the cells to receive sufficient protein and calories during critical periods of growth can lead to slowing down and ultimate cessation of the ability of these cells to enlarge, divide, and develop specialized functions. Lack of protein also affects later intellectual performance. Further, sufficient calories from fats and carbohydrates are needed so that protein is not used for energy. On the other hand, an excessive intake of protein and calories may produce excessive fat storage cells that do not disappear and may contribute to later obesity (92, 116, 147).

Caloric requirements for the pregnant woman are approximately 300 calories higher than for the nonpregnant woman, contributing to a total weight gain of approximately 25 pounds. If the woman has not gained at least 10 pounds by 5 months' (20 weeks') gestation, she is at risk for delivery of an ill child. Low maternal weight at conception and little weight gain during pregnancy are associated with birth of a child who is underweight for gestational age and prone to developmental hazards (137, 144). The overweight woman jeopardizes the fetus if she tries to lose weight during pregnancy; the effects of ketoacidosis, which results from calorie limitations, have been associated with neuropsychological defects in the infant (92, 116, 137, 144, 147).

Protein requirements are 1.5 g/kg daily for the pregnant woman, compared with the usual 1 g/kg daily (144). More protein is needed for growth and repair of the fetus, placenta, uterus, and breasts and for increased maternal blood volume. High-protein diets have not demonstrated improvement in birth weight and are not recommended prenatally.

Minerals, especially calcium and phosphorus, follows protein as the next most essential requirement. Calcium is mostly deposited in the infant during the last month of gestation; a good supply must be stored from the early months of pregnancy to meet this demand and minimize depletion of maternal reserves (103).

The recommended intake of phosphorus, sodium, zinc, iodine via iodized salt, magnesium, potassium, and fluoride remains essentially unchanged during pregnancy. Substantial decreases in minerals can predispose the offspring to debilitating conditions; for example, profound zinc deficiency can cause dwarfism, and severe iodine deficiency can lead to endemic cretinism characterized by multiple severe neurologic defects. Most diets that supply sufficient calories for appropriate weight gain also supply adequate minerals if iodized salt is used. The only exception is *iron, which should be supplemented during pregnancy because the maternal blood volume may double* as a result of increases in both plasma and erythrocytes. In addition, almost one-fourth of the maternal iron is transferred to the placenta and fetus. These iron requirements are more prominent during the last two trimester periods of gestation (26, 116, 117). Supplementation with 30 to 60 mg of ferrous iron during the last 3 to 4 months of pregnancy is beneficial in building and protecting maternal reserves and preventing iron deficiency anemia, which predisposes to being underweight and to congenital defects in the newborn. Salt should not be restricted unless edema develops.

Folic acid supplementation is used to prevent fetal malformations, especially neural tube defects and maternal anemia (26). Additional iodine prevents inadequate physical and mental growth (92, 144). Further information on diet for the pregnant woman, including the vegetarian, is found in Chapter 12.

An adequate intake of *vitamins* acquired through foods affects normal metabolism. Vitamin and mineral supplements are necessary but should not be substituted for food (26, 41). *Vitamins B_{12} and B_6* contribute to the plasma demands during pregnancy. The requirement for *vitamin C* increases by one third; a reasonable diet can supply this amount. Large doses of vitamin C can interfere with vitamin B_{12} absorption and metabolism (26). As a vitamin C source, orange juice should be taken in moderation because of the emetic effect related to hyperacidity.

Maternal malnutrition, which usually is related to a lifetime of inadequate nutrition in the mother, has an adverse effect on her children. The fetal central nervous system is the structure most damaged; impaired intelligence performance results late in life (144).

Effects of inadequate nutrition are most severe for the pregnant adolescent, who herself has growth requirements, and for the mother with accumulated effects of several pregnancies, especially closely spaced ones. Nutritional deficiencies of the mother during her own fetal and childhood periods contribute to structural and physiologic difficulties in supporting a fetus. Malnutrition at the time of conception has been linked to schizophrenia in adulthood for men and women. Improvement of the pregnant woman's diet when she has previously been poorly nourished does not appreciably benefit the fetus. The fetus apparently draws most of its raw materials for development from maternal body structure and lifetime reserves (116, 144, 147). You have a significant role in teaching proper nutrition to children and adolescents.

In a Canadian study in which dietary needs for calories and protein were individually calculated for each woman based on body weight for height, with adjustments for protein deficiency and being underweight, the quality of maternal diets significantly improved and the incidence of low-birth-weight infants, stillbirths, neonatal mortality, and perinatal mortality was drastically reduced (144). Refer to Appendices I and II at the end of the book for the recommended daily allowances and major sources and functions of nutrients.

The small or growth-retarded fetus has a much greater short illness and death rate compared with its normal counterpart. The long-term cost of some survivors illuminates the importance of prevention and prediction of pregnancies with fetal growth problems. Better education and nutrition to promote healthy pregnancies and use of ultrasound to safely monitor and manage cases at risk can improve pregnancy outcomes (56). Ultrasound assesses gestational age, fetal size, fetal structure, and fetal function (98).

Anemia. The effects of maternal anemia on the fetus are less clear than those on the mother. **Anemia** denotes a *decrease in the oxygen-carrying capability of the blood,* which is directly related to a reduction in hemoglobin concentration. Anemia, regardless of its cause, has been associated with spontaneous abortion, prematurity, low birth weight, and fetal death, even in mild cases (hemoglobin level, 8–11 g). A direct relationship between anemia and fetal distress has not been established unless the anemia of the mother is severe (hemoglobin < 6 g) (26). The common association of anemia and inadequate maternal nutritional intake with lower educational levels and socioeconomic background is prominent in the literature (116, 144, 147).

Iron Deficiency Anemia (IDA) accounts for 75% of all the anemias diagnosed during pregnancy (92). The iron requirements of pregnancy are considerable—close to 800 mg, of which 300 mg go to the fetus and placenta and 500 mg are used to expand the maternal hemoglobin mass (137, 144). IDA (as well as underweight and congenital defects) develops unless adequate replacement of these and other natural maternal iron losses occur. The developing fetus may not suffer severe ill effects of the mother's decreased iron supply if its own hemoglobin production is maintained at a normal level (i.e., if the placental source of iron is of sufficient amounts for the fetus to establish and maintain normal hemoglobin levels) (26).

Sickle cell anemia in the mother, associated with sickle cell disease seen predominantly in the African-American population, may show a number of negative effects on the developing fetus. Changes in the mother's pathophysiologic state may lead to intrauterine growth retardation, premature labor, a reduction of 250 to 500 g in average birth weight, and even stillbirth related to the "sickling" or clumping of malshaped erythrocytes within the placental vascular system (26, 116, 137, 144, 147).

Pica. **Pica** is *eating nonfood substances* such as clay, unprocessed flour, cornstarch, coal, soap, toothpaste, mothballs, petrol, tar, paraffin, wood, plaster, soil, chalk, charcoal, cinders, baking powder, baking soda, powdered bricks, and refrigerator frost scrapes. Pica is common in children and women of all cultures who are hungry, poor, malnourished, and desire something to chew (116, 147). Sometimes secrecy or superstitious beliefs accompany this habit. Some people such as African-Americans in the southern part of the United States and their descendants believe that eating red and white clay overcomes the chances of disfigured offspring. The practice of pica declined between 1950 and 1970, remaining steady at this time and affecting about one fifth of high-risk pregnancies (64). A study conducted among African-Americans in Washington, DC, noted that eating of clay or dirt was not observed in these women; rather they ingested large quantities of ice and freezer frost, from $\frac{1}{2}$ to 2 cups from 1 to 7 days per week (36). Although other newborn measurements were not significantly different, head circumferences of infants delivered to pica-practicing women were smaller than those of non-pica-practicing women. It was also noted that the support system for pica-practicing women was less than that of their counterparts (106). Pica is usually associated with iron deficiency; whether anemia is the cause or the effect is unknown. Certainly pica interferes with normal nutrition by reducing appetite. Some clays interfere with the absorption of iron, zinc, and potassium (116, 137, 144, 147).

Environmental Hazards to the Fetus: Teratogenic Effects

Teratogens. A **teratogen** is an *agent that interrupts normal development and causes malformation.* **Teratogenesis** is *development of abnormal structures.* Teratogenesis is time specific; the stimulus is nonspecific; timing is more important than the nature of the insult or negative stimulus. Development is characterized by a precise order; the timing, intensity, and duration of insult, injury, teratogen, or abnormal stimulus or event is important for the consequence. Teratogenic agents affect genes in several ways: (1) genes cease protein production so that development ceases, (2) genes fail to complete development already begun, or (3) excess growth of part of the organism occurs (134).

Prominent environmental factors that have the potential of damaging the fetus include radiation, chemical wastes, contaminated water, heavy metals such as lead, some food additives, various pollutants, chemical interactions, nicotine from smoking tobacco, pica, drugs, alcohol, maternal and paternal infections, and maternal stress. The timing of fetal contact with a specific teratogen is a crucial factor (Figs. 6–1 and 6–2). Susceptibility to teratogens, in general, decreases as organ formation advances (26). For instance, a teratogen introduced into the system of an embryo between 3 and 8 weeks of gestation when principal body systems are being established is likely to do much more harm than if it came in contact with the same conceptus during the third or eighth month. During the implantation period when the fertilized ovum lies free within the uterus and uses uterine secretions as its nutrition source, teratogens can kill the embryo (26, 53, 104, 116, 147). Even during the third trimester fetal cerebral vascular reaction to certain teratogens can be detrimental (19–21, 26).

There is no evidence that congenital malformations will always be produced when a teratogen is present, for the embryo has the inherent capacity to replace damaged cells with newly formed cells. Once implantation has occurred (7 or 8 days after fertilization), the embryo undergoes very rapid and important transformations for the next 4 weeks. The sequence of embryonic events shows that each organ (brain, heart, eye, limbs, and genitalia) undergoes a critical stage of differentiation at precise times. During these individual critical periods the embryo is highly vulnerable to teratogens, producing specific gross malformations. Each teratogen acts on a selected aspect of cellular metabolism (26).

In many malformations, a genetic predisposition combined with a teratogen is required to produce an abnormality (26). A substance can have adverse effects on the central nervous system but not on normal development of limbs. A teratogen may cause a variety of gross anomalies; a few show a preferential action on specific organs. For example, thalidomide anomalies are characterized by skeletal malformation; no other form of growth retardation is noted (26, 27, 116, 134, 147).

A complicated interplay exists among the father, mother, offspring, and teratogen. In addition to the critical period of developmental stage and genetic susceptibility, the degree to which a teratogen causes abnormalities depends on its dosage, absorption, distribution, metabolism, physical state of the mother, and excretion by the separate body systems of mother and fetus. A teratogen that enters a mother's system also enters the system of her developing child, meaning that the so-called *placental barrier is practically nonexistent* (66, 116, 147).

External Environmental Factors. Prenatally, environmental teratogens may interfere with the development of the embryo or fetus directly or may cause hormonal, circulatory, or nutritional changes in the mother that in turn damage the organism. Examples include the following (26, 33, 66, 126, 134):

- Soaks in hot tubs or sauna baths in early pregnancy, which may cause fetal neural-tube defects
- High levels of noise

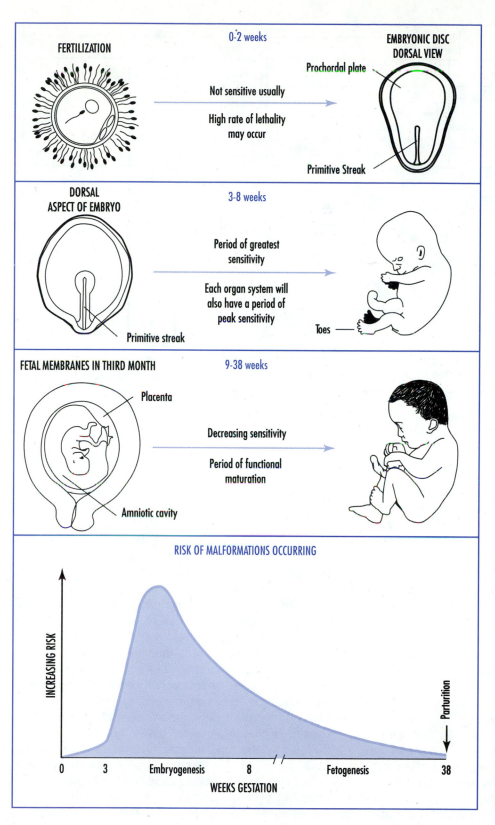

Figure 6–1. Periods of susceptibility to teratogens. *(From Sadler, T.W., Langman's Medical Embryology [5th ed.]. Baltimore: Williams & Wilkins, 1985.)*

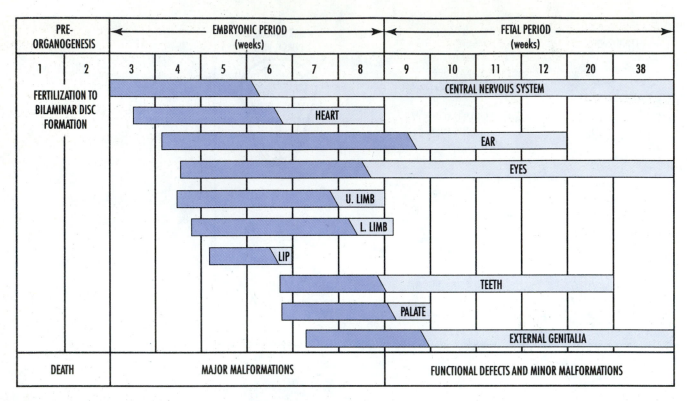

Figure 6–2. Susceptibility of organ systems to teratogens. Solid bars denote highly sensitive periods. *(From Sadler, T.W., Langman's Medical Embryology, 5th ed.. Baltimore: Williams & Wilkins, 1985.)*

- Radiation from multiple sources at work or from diagnostic tests (Most procedures cause low-level fetal x-ray exposure if performed accurately, but the pregnant woman should inform diagnosticians.)
- Ultraviolet light from excessive sun or a sun-lamp
- Air, water, and food pollutants
- Trace minerals linked to the work setting
- Chemicals and drugs in food

Depending on dosage, radiation can be responsible for cell destruction that is linked to embryonic death, gross malformations, growth retardation, and an increased risk of malignancy in later life.

Occupational hazards include transfer of drugs and chemicals from the male to the female during intercourse—an action that later can negatively affect fertilization or implantation or, if the woman is already pregnant, can have teratogenic effects on the developing person. For example, decreased sperm count and infertility are related to paternal exposure to dibromochloropropane (DBCP). Paternal exposure to toxic agents is most likely to result in male infertility or spontaneous abortions. Anesthetic gases, vinyl chloride exposure,

chloroprene, or other hydrocarbons have all been connected to spontaneous abortions. Lead present in the environment directly increases sperm abnormalities, induces male infertility, and facilitates spontaneous abortion through either affected sperm or indirect contamination (22, 126). Persistent environmental contaminants, such as dioxin and polychlorobiphenyls (PCBs), alter the activities of several different hormones. More scientific research is needed in this area with implications for policy change (14).

Occupational hazards may also include the effects of physical effort or activity. In a southern Sweden study comparing pregnant manual workers with nonmanual workers, there were no differences in outcomes of pregnancy; however, the manual workers who were younger than their counterparts did have a higher frequency of diseases of the musculoskeletal system, primarily low back pain (55). No experimental research has been done to document that physical activity via employment promotes preterm birth and low birth weight, although causes could include prolonged standing, long working hours, high speed, bending, and lifting heavy objects. Health care providers should be sensitive to the presence of occupational fatigue associated with workload during pregnancy (45, 60, 110, 117).

Agent Orange, named for the orange strip wrapped around 11 million gallons of a chemical shipped to and sprayed in Vietnam, is composed of 2.4.5-T and other chemicals, including dioxin. Dioxin, a widely publicized, highly toxic substance is believed responsible for the many adverse effects of exposure to Agent Orange experienced by Vietnam veterans such as chloracne, latent extreme fatigue, liver damage, and joint pain in back, hips and fingers, plus increases in spontaneous abortions and congenital malformations (spina bifida, cleft lip, and neoplasms). A major study commissioned by the U.S. government was conducted to explain the linkage of Agent Orange to reproductive problems encountered by veterans and the presence of abnormalities in their offspring (22, 126, 131); however, no conclusive research investigations support a causal role between these chemicals and fetal anomalies. Continued research is warranted as veterans of the Gulf War are also complaining of a variety of symptoms some time after return to the United States (133).

Smoking Tobacco. Since 1989, the U.S. Surgeon General has publicized that tobacco smoking is addictive and that nicotine is the substance responsible for the addictive process. Smoking is associated with numerous detrimental effects:

- Decreased maternal pulmonary function; increased carbon monoxide levels (26)
- Vasoconstriction in mother, reducing blood flow to fetus (26, 70)
- Abnormal bleeding during pregnancy (26, 70)
- Decreased fetal oxygen, lower oxygen tension, and fetal apnea/hypoxia from nicotine and cotinine transfer through placenta (26, 70, 132, 135, 147)
- Reduced fetal hemoglobin from carbon monoxide that crosses placenta (26, 70, 135)
- Higher percentage of spontaneous abortions, stillbirths, and preterm or premature births (decreased gestational age) (26, 70, 135, 143, 147)
- Lower birth weight (less than 2.5 kg or 5.5 pounds), which increases as number of cigarettes smoked daily increases (2, 6, 33, 70, 143)
- Higher perinatal mortality for infant at every level of birth weight (143)
- Increased possibility of sudden infant death syndrome (SIDS) (79)
- Later growth retardation in child related to carbon monoxide effects (70, 116, 143, 147)
- Slight retardation in learning skills (reading, mathematics) in child (70, 116, 135, 147)
- Increased respiratory disease, pneumonia, bronchitis, and allergy in infancy and childhood (116, 147)
- Decreased physical and social development in young children of mothers who smoke 10 or more cigarettes daily (47)
- Childhood cancer linked to prenatal smoking by mother or exposure to smoking by others (passive smoking) (135)
- Poor attention span, hyperactivity, slower perceptual-motor and linguistic development and minimal brain dysfunction in school-age children (26, 33, 70, 77, 116, 135, 147)

Although data on smoking related to pregnancy are usually collected via self-report, a more accurate method is to measure the cotinine level in either maternal or umbilical serum (6). Although the level of antenatal attachment to the fetus is a significant predictor of decrease in alcohol consumption, such a relationship is not found for smoking cessation, suggesting that psychological and physiologic dependence on nicotine may override the effect of an emotional attachment of pregnant woman to developing fetus (23).

Among a sample of almost 300 women who continued to smoke during their pregnancy, most had cut down, and only 40 had quit. Many expressed a desire to quit, feeling guilty about not being able to do so, but reported that smoking offered important benefits related to relaxation and mood control. This type of denial of health risk may well be one of the most adaptive ways of coping with the fact that one engages in a behavior widely promoted as harmful (140).

In a Japanese-based population study, 35% of almost 7000 pregnant women had been exposed passively to tobacco smoking for 2 hours per day at home or work. After adjustment for age, parity, height, alcohol intake, occupation, and fetal gestation, it was found that there was a small reduction in fetal growth associated with passive smoke exposure during pregnancy (95).

Based on the abundance of evidence pointing to the damaging effects of smoking to both mother and fetus, total avoidance of smoking during pregnancy is a primary objective of the National Cancer Institute and is a major medical recommendation. Health education for pregnant smokers increases the rate of quitting; counseling and information are effective and cost beneficial (146). Smoking cessation programs range from self-help to structured interventions. For males, cigarette advertisements continue to link smoking with virility; however a growing body of research links smoking with lowered birth weight as well as reduced sperm count and abnormal sperm shape (33, 150). Large doses of marijuana smoke produce the same effect. This may explain why men who smoke have higher infertility rates (33).

Drug Hazards to the Fetus: Teratogenic Effects

The Food and Drug Administration (FDA) divides drugs into five categories that indicate a safety factor of maternal use during pregnancy. The question raised is: Do fetal risks outweigh benefits gained through use of a drug?

A drug that has a teratogenic effect in animals does not necessarily have the same effect in humans and vice versa. For instance, thalidomide caused very few malformations in animals but causes many in humans (26).

Drugs That Cross the Placenta. Many drugs cross the placenta to the fetus from the mother's blood. The placenta acts like a sieve, not a barrier. Thus no drug, whether obtained by prescription or over the counter, should be taken during pregnancy unless it is medically prescribed as necessary for the mother (26). Cunningham, MacDonald, and Gant (26) stress two basic points: (1) with rare exception, any drug that exerts a systemic effect in the mother will cross the placenta to reach the embryo or fetus, and (2) if an essential drug is administered during pregnancy, the advantages to be gained must clearly outweigh any risks inherent in its use. Physicians prescribe fewer drugs to pregnant women now than in the past; a drug is prescribed only if withholding it would cause a more serious consequence for the mother than its adverse effects on the fetus. Or a drug that is taken daily, such as lithium, may be discontinued during pregnancy and administered again near the delivery date.

Examples of medication to avoid or use carefully during pregnancy follow (26, 102):

- Aspirin (acetylsalicylic acid) and propoxyphene hydrochloride (Darvon) cross the placenta.
- Medications containing salicylates, including those in combinations with caffeine and phenacetin, are associated with an increased incidence of anemia, hemorrhage, prolonged gestation, perinatal mortality, and low birth weight.
- Nonsteroidal anti-inflammatory drugs such as those containing ibuprofen may produce teratogenic effects during the last trimester.
- Some antibiotics are teratogenic and should be given cautiously during pregnancy: Tetracycline therapy causes minor tooth defects, discoloration of the deciduous teeth, and distortion of bone growth. Streptomycin and other aminoglycosides can result in deafness.

- Penicillin has been used extensively during pregnancy and apparently is harmless to the embryo and fetus.
- Sulfonamides are relatively safe but should be avoided during the last few weeks of pregnancy because of the risk of hyperbilirubinemia.
- Antimicrobial agents may cross the placenta; the period of maximum teratogenicity lasts until the ninth week of gestation.
- Antiepileptic agents, particularly phenytoin and carbamazepine, increase the incidence of infant spina bifida, craniofacial defects, fingernail hypoplasia, and developmental delays. In men, sperm with decreased motility and abnormal structural changes have been identified, which may contribute to abnormalities.
- Most cytotoxic drugs used in the treatment of maternal cancer may cause abortion or fetal anomalies if taken during the first trimester; however, no ill effects on the fetus have been reported in cases in which the drugs were administered to the mother during the remainder of the pregnancy. Furthermore, the circulating cancerous cells of the mother appear not to invade or harm the developing embryo and fetus (7, 149).
- Antineoplastic drug exposure via administration to patients by nurses during the first trimester is associated with a significant increase in fetal loss. Cancer chemotherapy agents damage the sperm; sperm banking before therapy or perhaps artificial insemination of mates is an available option.
- Sex hormones or oral contraceptives either just before or during pregnancy may harm the developing fetus, causing spontaneous abortion and cardiovascular defects in the newborn. A delayed consequence has been observed in adolescents or young women who develop vaginal or cervical cancer, which may be fatal. Adolescent and young adult female offspring of women who received diethylstilbestrol (DES) during the first trimester of pregnancy to prevent miscarriage are more likely to develop such cancers. Daughters of women who were administered DES in the 1950s should have regular pelvic examinations. Sons of women who received DES may experience sterility and testicular abnormalities and cancer.
- Corticosteroids (e.g., prednisone) and other hormones may have adverse effects on the fetus.
- Oral antidiabetic drugs are not recommended because of the risk of neonatal jaundice and hypoglycemia; the diabetic mother should take the

hormone insulin. Large-for-gestational-age infants are generally born to women with insulin-dependent diabetes mellitus because of the influence of this growth factor on the fetus (25, 147)

- Sedatives and central nervous system depressants affect circulation in the mother, cause hypoxia in the fetus, and have sedating or depressant effects.
- Accutane, prescribed for severe acne, may cause hydrocephalus or ear anomalies.

Drug Abuse and Addiction. During pregnancy drug abuse and addiction continue to manifest themselves as major psychosocial and physical problems for both mother and child. Before 1968 only a few published reports documented this complication of pregnancy. Now substances commonly abused during pregnancy, taken individually or in combination, are known to have multiple effects on the developing person, on the outcome of pregnancy, and on neonatal neurobehavior (147). Infants exposed to addictive drugs in utero throughout pregnancy are at great risk for a higher rate of congenital malformations, obstetric complications, and perinatal mortality (22, 26, 33, 66, 104, 126).

Effects of drug use on the fetus, neonate, and child depend on the type of drug ingested, dose, duration of drug use before and during pregnancy, and state of maternal nutrition. There are fewer infant symptoms when the pregnant woman stops drug use in the first trimester of pregnancy than if drug use continues. Thus it is imperative to prevent drug use and to support the mother's efforts to stop drug use and to encourage adequate prenatal care and nutrition (147, 151).

These drugs include amphetamines, barbiturates, cocaine (includes "crack" and "ice," potent and purified versions), ethchlorvynol (Placidyl), heroin, meperidine hydrochloride (Demerol), methadone, morphine, pentazocine hydrochloride (Talwin), propoxyphene hydrochloride, phencyclidine, known as "angel dust" (PCP), tetrahydrocannabinol (THC) or marijuana, and methamphetamine (26, 33, 66, 76, 102). Drugs that act on the central nervous system are often lipophilic and of relatively low-molecular-weight characteristics, which facilitate crossing of the so-called placental–fetal blood–brain barrier (26). Some drugs can be metabolized by the fetal liver and placenta; however, these metabolites are water soluble (26). These drugs may interfere with blood flow to the placenta. A high incidence of maternal nutritional deficiency, anemia, and small pregnancy weight gain is also associated with drug use (116, 144, 147).

Clinical assessment for substance abuse should include an evaluation of physical appearance, a nursing history, and a substance abuse interview. The client's demeanor, neatness, cleanliness, and affect may give subtle or overt clues. Urine samples of mothers are effective to screen for ingestion of illicit drugs; alcohol breath tests are appropriate to check maternal alcohol levels at periodic intervals. Interventions should address the habits of pregnant women comprehensively rather than focus on use of any one substance (116).

Low birth weight, short gestation, small size for gestational age, and major malformations occur more often among offspring of **marijuana** users (76). Numerous adverse effects of maternal drug addiction are reported in the literature, including prematurity, low birth weight and accelerated weight loss in the newborn period, depressed Apgar scores at birth, chromosomal abnormalities, and neuromotor abnormalities (19–21, 116, 147, 151).

Addictive drugs such as heroin, cocaine, and morphine in the mother's blood are related to a high incidence of obstetric complications: hypertension, toxemia, abruptio placenta, intrauterine growth retardation, spontaneous abortion, stillbirth, premature and breech delivery, and postpartum hemorrhage (resulting in part from poor prenatal care). Of the three drugs, cocaine in its various forms is the most devastating (19–21, 33, 148, 151). Cocaine's pattern of use is increasing and includes women of childbearing age and pregnant women (38).

Exposure of the fetus to one teratogen often brings out exposure to others. Cocaine-using women actively smoke more cigarettes and may be exposed to more passive tobacco smoke; both lead and tobacco have been associated with later cognitive and behavioral problems, and lead and cocaine have a demonstrated neurotoxicologic interaction in animal studies (94). Prenatal care must include increased surveillance for drug-related complications in coordinated, comprehensive, family-oriented drug treatment programs. Rehabilitation and support efforts should continue after delivery and address issues that lead to and maintain patterns of abuse (142).

Maternal use of cocaine or heroin results in nutritional deficiencies that cause fetal growth retardation, a shorter gestational period, a greater reduction in birth weight and body length, a smaller head circumference, cardiopulmonary abnormalities, and, later, perceptual, motor, and learning impairments (19, 83, 101, 128, 151).

Chasnoff and associates (19–21) explain that cocaine acts peripherally to inhibit nerve conduction and prevent norepinephrine uptake at the nerve terminals, producing increased norepinephrine levels with subsequent vasoconstriction and a concomitant abrupt rise in blood pressure.

Placental vasoconstriction also occurs, decreasing blood flow to the fetus with an increase in uterine contractibility. In the neonate tachycardia and hypertension are clearly associated with cerebrovascular hemorrhage. Computed tomography (CT) scan of the neonate may confirm the presence of acute focal cerebral infarction.

Children exposed to cocaine in the fetal state have an abnormally high incidence of "severe" physical and emotional problems, including the following (8, 21, 33, 54, 66, 116, 128, 147):

- Brain shrinkage or cerebral atrophy
- Learning difficulties; impaired attention span
- Impaired orientation; decreased ability to orient to auditory and visual stimuli
- Growth retardation
- Severe impairments in motor movements, including simple movements like eating and dressing; nonnutritive sucking

- Irritability, impulsivity
- Tremors
- Sensitivity to sounds
- Disrupted rapid eye movement (REM) sleep patterns, affecting personality
- Various personality-social difficulties
- Permanent physical and mental damage as a result of fetal anoxia or fetal or neonatal cerebrovascular hemorrhage

Many of these children have been born to middle-class and wealthy parents, a group increasingly using cocaine (19–21, 128).

The Brazelton Neonatal Behavioral Assessment Scale can be used to evaluate normality of responses to environmental stimuli (116, 147). Finnegan's Neonatal Narcotic Abstinence Syndrome (NSA) is useful for assessing neonatal withdrawal (128). The specific pattern

---

► **NEONATAL NARCOTIC ABSTINENCE SYNDROME: MANIFESTATIONS OF NARCOTIC WITHDRAWAL**

Central Nervous System (signs appear within first 24 hours)

- Hyperirritability
- Hyperactivity—hard to hold; failure to mold to mother's body
- Restlessness
- Incessant shrill cry
- Inability to sleep, disturbed REM sleep
- Hypertonia of muscles
- Hyperactive reflexes
- Stretching
- Tremors
- Poor temperature regulation; fever
- Possible generalized convulsions

Respiratory System

- Rapid irregular breathing
- Yawning
- Sneezing
- Nasal stuffiness, congestion
- Excessive secretions
- Intermittent cyanosis
- Respiratory alkalosis
- Periods of apnea

Cardiovascular System

- Tachycardia

Gastrointestinal System

- Frantic sucking of hands; disorganized sucking behavior
- Difficulty sucking and feeding; poor closure of lips around nipple
- Appearance of being very hungry
- Sensitive gag reflex
- Regurgitation
- Vomiting
- Diarrhea
- Progressive weight loss

Skin

- Pallor
- Sweating
- Excoriation

Musculoskeletal System

- Small head size
- Short length

of symptoms is dependent on (1) the type, amount, and combination of drugs used by the mother, (2) the length of time between drug exposure and delivery, and (3) the fetal ability to metabolize the drug. See Neonatal Narcotic Abstinence Syndrome for a list of the symptoms and signs that are typically observed in the neonate who has been addicted during pregnancy to cocaine, heroin, or another narcotic (19–21, 128, 151). Newborns may require up to 40 days of treatment during the withdrawal phase (21). The limited ability of the newborn to metabolize and eliminate these fat-soluble drugs may be responsible for postponement of withdrawal symptoms for 2 to 4 weeks in some infants (151).

Withdrawing the addicted woman before delivery causes the fetus to experience withdrawal distress caused by visceral vasoconstriction affecting circulation to the uterus. Intrauterine death may occur. The infant is born with drug addiction and experiences withdrawal symptoms in 2 to 4 days.

Fetal, maternal, paternal, and environmental factors all interact to produce neonatal withdrawal syndrome, which is actually a diverse collection of signs and symptoms demonstrated in the newborn (128).

The monograph *Drug Exposed Infant*, presents information on prevalence, medical risks, developmental effects on the child, treatment programs for the mothers, and legal, ethical, and economic issues related to the drug-addicted mother and child (30). See also the monograph *Effects of In Utero Exposure to Street Drugs,* published by the American Public Health Association, Supplement to December 1993 (Vol 83, Issue 12).

Mood-altering or Psychotropic Drugs. With the exception of phenothiazines used for major psychiatric conditions, administration of these drugs before and during pregnancy should be avoided when possible because of their reported untoward effects on the developing person. Such drugs ingested by the mother before conception or between conception and implantation are known to produce chromosomal anomalies in the embryo (26, 116, 147). Minor tranquilizers and antidepressants can produce damaging effects, depending on the critical period of fetal development when the drug is circulated within the mother's system. For instance, thalidomide shows its teratogenic effects when ingested between days 28 and 42 of pregnancy. If psychotropic drugs are taken late in pregnancy, the neonate is likely to suffer drug toxicity, hypothermia, respiratory depression, hypotonia, convulsions, and withdrawal symptoms (26). Newborns of mothers who had taken lithium have been described as hypotonic, listless, and floppy (26). For treatment of stress-related illnesses in males, cimetidine (Tagamet) and sulfasalazine (Azulfidine) may

temporarily suppress sperm production up to nearly 50% (22, 102).

Drug abuse in the father may also act as a teratogen. For example, marijuana abuse may cause chromosomal breaks in the father and contribute to fetal risk. Cocaine use causes sperm abnormality. Animal studies indicate that morphine-dependent and methadone-dependent males father offspring having decreased birth weight, increased stillbirth rates, and increased neonatal mortality rates (22, 116, 147).

Alcohol. Alcohol ingested before or during pregnancy serves as another common cause of abnormal changes in the fetus (33, 69, 77, 78, 84). The combination of alcohol and smoking may reduce birth weight to a substantial degree (65). New research finds that caffeine (coffee, cola, tea, chocolate) has no detrimental effect on birth weight, except in pregnant women who consume large amounts of alcohol (21–43 drinks per week). Cultural habits regarding smoking and the intake of alcohol and caffeinated beverages can explain the differences between levels of consumption reported for different countries. That is, high levels of alcohol consumption are common to low socioeconomic class, lower level of education, and higher number of pregnancies (74). Ethanol acts as a teratogen, causing brain, craniofacial, and limb abnormalities. It acts as inhibitor in the conversion of vitamin A to a molecule (retinoic acid) needed for normal nervous system and limb development (31). It affects production and release of hormones and neurotransmitters, which in turn may affect later sex differentiation, cognitive skills, and sexual expression and behavior.

Alcoholic beverages should be avoided; drinking as little as 3 ounces of liquor daily increases the chances of congenital defects low birth weight, (77), preterm delivery, stillbirth, abruptio placenta, or spontaneous abortion. In a study of 11,698 Danish women, alcohol consumption of 120 g/week or more was associated with a five times greater reduction in average birth weight in babies of smokers versus babies of nonsmokers (147). Alcoholism in the father may inhibit spermatogenesis and also act as a teratogen that contributes to chromosomal breaks or damaged genes, resulting in spontaneous abortion or birth defects (121). Alcoholic men and women often marry, with each contributing to the development of Fetal Alcohol Syndrome (discussed below) to some degree (127). Even abstinence during the gestation period seems to be "too little too late" for infants born to mothers who have had a history of heavy alcoholic intake before conception (77). Drinking before pregnancy is linked to decrements in fetal development because preparation for pregnancy, at least physically, begins prior to conception (79). The affected newborn may suffer many of the signs and symptoms described in Neonatal Narcotic Abstinence Syndrome (see page 276) caused by maternal drug-related consumption. The term in this case is *Fetal Alcohol Syndrome (FAS)*. FAS, which results from excessive regular or episodic maternal ingestion of alcohol, causes the following characteristics (1, 26, 28, 31, 77–80, 120):

- Low birth weight
- Small head
- Flat facial profile or deformity
- Ear and eye abnormalities
- Poor motor coordination
- Disturbed sleep patterns
- Extra digits
- Heart defects

Research conducted by Larroque, et al. (74, 75) indicates that perinatal mortality is abnormally high, impaired fine and gross motor development is continued as the surviving child matures, and the incidence of mental retardation is abnormally high when evaluated up to age 7. The younger the mother is at the onset of alcoholism, the higher is the incidence of speech and language problems in the offspring. These children who suffer the effects of maternal alcoholic intake via FAS are more prone than the average child to acquiring both classifications of bacterial infections—minor and life threatening (116). Lesser defects may occur in the offspring (10% risk of FAS) when the mother engages in moderate social drinking or when the woman drinks an average of 1 to 2 ounces of absolute alcohol daily in the months before pregnancy. Heavy paternal drinking may also be a factor in FAS (22, 27, 82, 134). Physical growth is retarded throughout childhood, and physical, intellectual, speech, communication, and behavioral skills and capabilities appear limited for life.

New research suggests that continued, regular use of alcohol by the mother who breastfeeds can further impede motor development of the infant (1, 28, 78). Alcohol-induced damage to the developing brain encompasses a long developmental time frame, affects more cell populations, occurs at lower levels of exposure, produces greater numbers of permanent effects, and is modulated by more factors than was initially suspected by earlier studies (141). It is clear that there is a need for effective prevention/intervention programs for alcohol-abusing women of childbearing age. Such programs must address the multiple factors that may exacerbate alcohol's teratogenic effects. Community education, treatment for the alcohol-abusing mother, parenting education, and early identification and intervention with the alcohol-affected child are essential (13, 119).

Recommendations to reduce the estimated 12,000 FAS births yearly include the following (13):

- Research into why some women drink alcohol so heavily during pregnancy, and ways to better assess drinking patterns and help women to consume less alcohol
- Improved data collection about the pregnant woman's drinking patterns
- Intervention techniques emphasizing the role of the entire community in encouraging pregnant women not to drink
- Improved assessment to identify children with FAS
- Research to identify effective treatment for FAS
- Comprehensive services for the FAS-affected child and family, including human service agencies, health clinics, home care, and schools
- Reproductive counseling and contraceptive services for women who are substance abusers

Effects of Folklore

Folklore can be defined as *strong beliefs about certain facets of or influences on basic aspects of life.* Most cultures, especially those that adhere less to scientific thinking, define certain desirable or forbidden activities for the pregnant woman. These superstitions, however, are often believed, feared, or unconsciously practiced even by well-educated or professional people, although they might not confess that they believe in them. The commonly experienced fear of giving birth to an abnormal infant causes the pregnant woman, or even the father-to-be, to act in ways that would otherwise be rejected or opposed. The more tightly the woman is bound by her culture, the more she follows the rules or taboos surrounding food, hygiene, activity, and contacts with other people. Many cultures emphasize that the woman should look at pleasant sights, think positive thoughts, eat certain foods, and pursue certain leisure activities to ensure a healthy, happy, talented child. Cultures usually emphasize that unhappy thoughts, aggressive actions, certain foods, unpleasant sights, or unusual or strenuous activity should be avoided to prevent bearing a sick, deformed, or dead baby. Often folklore practices do not interfere with scientific practices; therefore you should not ridicule or try to convince the mother to drop these practices since the resulting conflict she feels internally or from her culture may have adverse health effects. Further, folklore often evolves so that the pregnant woman is protected from hazards or given extra care that, in turn, meets her needs emotionally and physically.

Various references are available to give you further information about specific folklore that affects prenatal care(116, 147).

Maternal Infections: Hazardous Influence on the Fetus

The pregnant woman is more susceptible to infections. The placenta cannot screen out all infectious organisms; therefore infectious diseases in the vaginal region can travel up to the amniotic sac and penetrate its walls and infect the amniotic fluid. Diseases that have a mild effect on the mother may have a profound effect on the fetus, depending on gestational age (26).

Acquired Immune Deficiency Syndrome (AIDS) is transmitted from mother to fetus at some point near the actual birthing process; the exact mode of transmission is not clearly understood. The incidence of AIDS in the pediatric population is increasing; it is now believed to be one of the five leading causes of death in children (29, 52). In 1991 the majority of 2500 cases of pediatric AIDS patients (< age 5) acquired the infection directly from their mothers (89). In 1995, these figures doubled (17).

Breastfeeding has been identified as a mode of transmission of certain pathogens, such as HIV, from mother to infant; however, breastfeeding continues to be encouraged in the HIV-infected woman unless safe and sufficient quantities of infant formula are available (50). Women who are infected with human immunodeficiency virus (HIV) and women who are at risk for infection, such as intravenous (IV) drug users, Haitian-born, partners of IV drug users, and partners of bisexual men, place the unborn fetus and child in serious jeopardy (17). The incubation period can range from 2 months to 5 years. To protect the health care provider, the Centers for Disease Control (CDC) emphasize the consistent use of blood and body fluid precautions for all patients (18). The CDC also recommends that all pregnant women be voluntarily tested for the AIDS virus. If positive, they can be treated with AZT to cut the risk of transmission of the disease to their unborn fetuses. Without this testing and treatment, as many as 2000 (33%) of infants born to HIV-infected mothers will be infected.

The majority of AIDS cases in the pediatric age range (up to 13 years) result from perinatal acquisition of HIV from infected mothers. Modes also include transfusion, either prenatally or postnatally. Records indicate that the earliest year of birth for children with perinatally acquired AIDS was 1977; the earliest transfusion of blood known to have infected a child with HIV was 1978 (109). CDC statistics for 1994 show more than 1200 cases of infected children between ages 5 and 12 (17).

Except for Kaposi's sarcoma, *clinical manifestations of AIDS in newborns* are different than those observed in adults. Newborns of HIV-seropositive mothers show no difference in birth weight, gestational age, head circumference, or Apgar score when compared with those born to seronegative mothers (89). These differences make the task of identifying and managing infected offspring just that more difficult. Conditions such as neurodevelopmental deficiencies, failure to thrive, *Candida* infections, generalized lymphadenopathy, brain involvement, diarrhea, and bacterial infections (bacteremia, pneumonia, otitis media) persist over time in AIDS-infected infants. Diagnosis of AIDS may take several months and includes intensive blood analysis with particular attention to significant changes in T-lymphocyte activity. Prognosis for infants younger than 1 year is bleak (17, 112). Some children have survived longer than expected with gamma globulin therapy, but AIDS-induced brain damage is ever a threat, along with devastation of other body systems (116, 147).

The number of *adolescent AIDS* cases is rising. In 1994, there were 2000 AIDS cases among 13- to 18-year-olds (17). CDC investigators say that prevention efforts must go beyond providing information and must help adolescents develop motivation, attitudes, and skills to avoid behaviors that place them at risk for HIV infection (17). Information about HIV and AIDS is rapidly changing with new research. The journal *AIDS* is one source of current information.

Rubella (German measles) is another example of maternal infection that may occur during the first trimester with harmful effects. Rubella may go unnoticed by the mother, but it can cause spontaneous abortion, prematurity, fetal growth retardation, serious congenital anomalies in the eyes, ears, heart, or brain, and death. Approximately 1 in 600 children is born with congenital rubella (10, 116, 147). *Congenital rubella syndrome* has a wide variety of severe eye and systemic complications. A 20-year follow-up study of the 1963–1965 worldwide rubella epidemic, which affected thousands of infants, revealed that multiple-organ disease was common, usually of the eye and ear. Although the first trimester is believed to be the most vulnerable time for the fetus, results of this study indicate that rubella can be detrimental at any stage of development. New cases of congenital rubella are fewer compared with years past; however, surviving victims of the epidemic continue to deal with its effects (49). Amniocentesis can be used to detect the presence of rubella in utero (118).

To minimize or prevent clinical features of the disease, large doses of gamma globulin are generally administered to nonimmunized pregnant women who have been exposed to rubella. Immunization of all female children before puberty can effectively retard the spread of rubella. The vaccine should never be administered to pregnant women; the rubella vaccine virus will cross the placenta just as the wild (community-acquired) rubella virus (26). The rubella vaccine is actually a live-virus vaccine containing a strain of rubella virus that has been somewhat altered. Therefore women who are at risk, are not aware of being pregnant, and agree to prevent conception for a 3-month period should be vaccinated according to the U.S. Public Health Service Advisory Committee on Immunization Practices (136).

Small-for-date births are a fetal complication of maternal rubella. The fetus suffers an abnormal decrease in the absolute number of cells in most organs because of the viral interference with cell multiplication. The virus also causes adverse changes in the small blood vessels of the developing fetus and does profuse damage to the placental vascular system as well, thus interfering with the fetus' blood flow and oxygenation (26, 116, 147).

Rubeola ("long measles") is also associated with congenital defects. Viruses causing other infections, such as mumps, smallpox, scarlet fever, and viral hepatitis, may be related to formation of anomalies in utero, and during the last month of pregnancy they may cause a life-threatening fetal infection (26).

Maternal syphilis causes severe adverse effects such as congenital syphilis, brain damage, spontaneous abortion (miscarriage) and stillbirth. Adequate treatment before the 18th week of pregnancy prevents syphilis in the fetus as the fetus appears relatively immune to syphilis, compared with other diseases, in early pregnancy.

Statistics show a drastic rise in congenital syphilis. It is important that maternal syphilis be identified before or early in pregnancy to prevent devastating consequences for the neonate (86, 125). Poor prenatal care with lack of maternal treatment for syphilis contributes to these consequences (105). Although necrosis of the umbilical cord (vein) is a clear indication that the newborn is infected, other symptoms may not appear until the 14th week of life (46). Symptoms include lesions of the skin and mucous membranes, coryza, anemia, and localized septicemia; or the child may appear healthy at birth with symptoms appearing in 2 to 6 weeks. Occasionally, symptoms may not appear for 2 years (27, 116, 147). Treatment of the mother also ensures treatment of the ill fetus because penicillin readily crosses the placenta. Other antibiotics, for example, erythromycin, are available for those persons who are allergic to penicillin (44, 116, 147). Tetracycline is contraindicated during pregnancy (26). Newborns of mothers treated prenatally with erythromycin should be re-treated (26).

Chlamydia trachomatis and *gonorrhea* are two lower genital infections that are easily transmitted that can produce pelvic inflammatory conditions. Younger women (15–24 years) are the most predominant group affected. Tubal adhesions is an important factor in the occurrence of ectopic pregnancies (114, 115, 138). Sexual partners should be tested and treated with appropriate antibiotics. New treatments that include a single dose of azithromycin are under investigation.

Herpes simplex of the genital area is increasing in incidence. Thus, the prevention and treatment of perinatal herpes simplex (type II) is of great public concern. Primary and recurrent genital herpes can range from severe, extensive ulceration to asymptomatic virus shedding. Cesarean section is indicated in women with clinically apparent herpes simplex virus (HSV) at delivery to protect the newborn against infection. Vaginal delivery may mean the development of systemic lesions (encephalitis and/or infection limited to skin, eye, mouth) in the newborn within several days to weeks of birth (147). Prenatal treatment of the mother with acyclovir over a prolonged period can dramatically control and reduce its effects. Studies of oral acyclovir taken during the third trimester are now underway. Work is also in progress on the development of a vaccine to prevent the occurrence of HSV. Its primary source is maternal in nature in that genital herpes infections are sexually transmitted: consequently, affected women are mainly in the childbearing age group. The majority of genital infections are asymptomatic and difficult to recognize on clinical examination, thus making the identification of a mother whose fetus is in jeopardy very difficult (33, 116, 147).

Unlike rubella, which readily crosses the placenta, the potential hazards of herpes simplex generally await the unsuspecting fetus in the maternal cervix or lower genital tract. The virus invades the uterus following the rupture of membranes or after contact is made with the fetus during the normal vaginal birth descent. Cesarean section is the delivery of choice if the infection has been diagnosed as a means of protecting the fetus from contamination (26).

Congenital and neonatal herpes simplex viral infections often prove lethal (147). A mortality rate of 60% and serious central nervous system and eye damage have been identified in half the survivors. Neonates may be asymptomatic. Because drug therapeutic measures taken thus far to cure the mother and newborn are ineffective, research in prevention and treatment of the infectious disease continues (26, 147).

Another dangerous infection is *cytomegalovirus* (*CMV*), which is caused by one of the herpes viruses and occurs in 1 to 3% of pregnant women and approximately half their babies. CMV may go undetected in the mother and in the young child because the disease is asymptomatic, but the virus is transmitted via urine, saliva, tears, semen, and breast milk (18). Laboratory analysis of infant cord blood detects the virus. The disease in the newborn is characterized by microcephaly, impaired growth, impaired intellectual ability, impaired hearing, enlarged liver and spleen, hemolytic anemia, and fracture of long bones (18, 26).

Toxoplasmosis is an infection that was first discovered in 1909 in Africa in a rodent. The parasite can be contracted by eating infected meat or eggs that are raw or undercooked, or through contact with the feces of an infected cat. Should the mother become infected during pregnancy, there is a good possibility that the parasite will cross the placental barrier. Although flulike symptoms can be mild in adults, infants may face blindness, mental retardation, neurologic deficits, and deafness (3). Although usually asymptomatic, 1 to 8 of every 1000 women become infected, with transmission to the fetus in about 40% of cases (5). Health education on how to avoid contact with the parasite should be emphasized by the nurse. Transplacental transmission occurs during acute infection of the mother. The infected mother can be treated with medication, for example, sulfadiazine/pyrimethamine, folinic acid, and spiramycin, which probably reduces fetal damage; however, pregnant women who are not immune should be advised not to handle cats, cat feces, or litter boxes (26). Chronic maternal alcohol use acts as a predisposition to infection. Alcoholics are more susceptible to pulmonary infections; alcohol has adverse effects on all components of the immune system (4).

Fetal Infection

Intrauterine fetal infection caused by group B *Streptococcus* probably occurs with greater frequency than is clinically diagnosed. In the most serious of cases the clinical signs—apnea, respiratory distress, and shock—emerge at birth or within 48 hours (26). Immediate treatment is mandatory for survival. The death rate may be particularly high in preterm infants who show early signs and symptoms. Evidence points to the passage of this infectious agent during the birthing process via the maternal genital tract. Only penicillin is indicated for use as an antibiotic as no severe allergic reaction to the fetus or newborn has been reported (26).

Immunologic Factors

The fetus is immunologically foreign to the mother's immune system, yet the fetus is sustained. Selected antibodies of measles, chicken pox, hepatitis, poliomyelitis, whooping cough, and diphtheria are transferred to the fetus. The resulting immunity lasts several months after birth. Antibodies to dust, pollen, and common allergens do not transfer across the placenta (26).

The most commonly encountered interference with fetal development is incompatibility between maternal and infant blood factors, resulting in various degrees of circulatory difficulty for the baby. This problem is more complex than the commonly known Rh incompatibility. When a fetus' blood contains a protein substance, the Rh factor (Rh-positive blood), but the mother's blood does not (Rh-negative blood), antibodies in the mother's blood may attack the fetus and possibly cause jaundice, spontaneous abortion, stillbirth, anemia, heart defects, mental retardation, or death. Usually the first Rh-positive baby is not affected adversely, but with each succeeding pregnancy the risk becomes greater. A vaccine can be given to the Rh-negative mother within 3 days of childbirth or within 3 days of abortion that will prevent her body from making Rh antibodies. Babies affected by the Rh syndrome can be treated by repeated blood transfusions (26). In-depth information can be attained from a physiology or obstetrics text (26, 53).

Maternal Emotions

The physical–psychological interdependence between mother and fetus still is being studied; effects of the mother's elation, fear, and anxiety on the behavior and other developmental aspects of the baby are poorly understood. Anxiety and fear, resulting from physical abuse, worries about the current living situation or finances, or violence in the neighborhood or community, produce a variety of physiologic changes in the person because of activation of the hypothalamus and the sympathetic division response of the autonomic nervous system, which stimulates the adrenal medulla to produce adrenaline. Adrenaline, in turn, stimulates the anterior lobe of the pituitary to produce adrenocorticotropic hormone (ACTH), which activates the adrenal cortex to release cortisone. The results are increased heart rate, constriction of peripheral vessels, dilation of coronary vessels, decrease in gastrointestinal motility, and changed carbohydrate and protein metabolism, which also affects many body functions and changes in the adrenocortical hormonal system (26). These changes occurring in the pregnant woman contribute to hyperactivity of the fetus because increased maternal cortisone is secreted and enters the blood circulation, crossing the placenta to the fetus (15, 26, 116, 147). Further, fetal circulatory and nutritional processes may be affected, interfering with intrauterine development. Because the fetus experiences only the consequences and not the cause of the emotion itself, the experience may mean nothing to the fetus; however, some studies indicate that maternal fear and anxiety induce the same sensations in the fetus (27, 33, 147). Animal studies indicate that stress-producing situations influence the fetus, causing changes in emotional states and also in learning activity after birth (33). Studies indicate that the human fetus responds with increased activity to loud noises in the environment (27, 33). Maternal stress therefore, may be considered a teratogen, resulting in physical and psychological alterations of the developing person before and following birth.

The effects of job stress on pregnant women have not been adequately researched, and results are contradicting. One study of 15,000 women on perinatal outcome of broken marriages (separated, divorced, widowed) found that these women are at higher risk for low-birth-weight infants than married mothers (odds ratio, 5:1) or single mothers. The low birth weight was attributed to reduced growth rather than to prematurity and was associated with substance abuse (87). Other studies that compared the outcomes of pregnancies of female medical residents with those of wives of male medical residents showed no significant difference despite long work hours, lack of sleep, and high occupational stress of the former group of women (60, 68, 97).

Other studies also showed no direct relationship between work-related psychosocial stress during pregnancy and preterm or low-birth-weight delivery (63, 100); however, personal motivation toward work, as well as physical effect of work, should be considered in evaluating the impact of a job's psychological effects on pregnancy outcome. Women who did not want to remain in the work force were more likely to experience work-related stress and preterm, low-birth-weight delivery (63).

A severe but not uncommon stressor for the pregnant woman is physical abuse or battering, which also involves fear, anxiety, and other feelings related to emotional abuse. Some men grow up rejecting their own needs for love and therefore find it difficult and threatening to meet the pregnant woman's emotional needs. Battering a pregnant woman may present a more extreme response of jealousy toward the unborn baby and anger at being displaced from the center of the woman's attention. Men also may fear and envy women's reproductive power ("womb envy," which is the other side of Freud's concept of women's "penis envy"). Such men deal with fear and envy by asserting physical power over the woman, often forcing themselves sexually on women to the extent of manifesting sexual addiction or rape (15, 62).

Maternal anxiety reactions are also related to physiologic responses of pregnancy, such as nausea and vomiting, backaches, and headaches, which, in turn, affect the fetus.

The woman who begins pregnancy with inadequate psychic reserves is especially vulnerable to the stresses and conflicting moods that accompany pregnancy (33). A study of 8823 married pregnant women revealed that women who did not want their pregnancy were two times more likely to deliver infants who died within the first 28 days of life than were women who had accepted their pregnancies. There was no evidence of intentional injury. The study was conducted from 1959 to 1966, when abortions were illegal (16). Do not assume harmony between the partners or happiness about the coming baby. The mother-to-be may have many feelings to resolve during pregnancy, as may the father-to-be; however, maternal emotionality during pregnancy has not been correlated with specific mother–child behavioral interaction.

Birth Defects Transmitted by the Father

Genes of both mother and father and the prenatal maternal environment may cause birth defects. Genetic

---

► CAUSES OF PATERNAL CONTRIBUTIONS TO BIRTH DEFECTS IN THE CHILD

Direct (occur at conception)

- Damage to spermatozoa caused by chemicals such as fumigants, solvents, vinyl chloride, methylmercury, hypothermia, and radiation.
- Alterations in seminal fluid.
- Factor or agent affects chromosomes or cytogenic apparatus in sperm cells or their precursors.
- Drugs and chemicals cross into testes and male accessory reproductive organs for secretion in semen.

Indirect (occur before conception)

- Genetic constitution contributed by father to fetus may make fetus more susceptible to environmental factors to which it is later exposed. (Responses to teratogens may in part depend on genotype of exposed individual.)
- Transmission of chemicals to the pregnant woman through the man's skin, hair, or contaminated clothing.

Examples of Contributions of Paternal Causes of Fetal Defects

- Down syndrome (trisomy 21): paternal nondisjunction and extra chromosome; 20 to 30% of cases occur when father is 55 years and older at time of conception.
- Sex chromosome disorders in child.
- Adverse outcomes such as spontaneous abortion and perinatal death (stillbirth) due to methadone and morphine dependency, chemicals such as fumigants, solvents, and vinyl chloride.
- Infertility in the couple due to drugs or other chemicals.
- Hemophilia: coagulation disorder in child; deficiency factor VIII.
- Marfan syndrome: connective tissue disorder with elongated extremities, hands.
- Progeria: premature aging, growth deficiency.
- Decreased neonatal survival due to methadone and morphine dependency.
- Birth defects if father is epileptic (especially if taking phenytoin) or if father is exposed to lead, waste, anesthetic gases, Agent Orange, or dioxin.

mutations in sperm are being formed in a greater percent of the population. Mutations may be caused by exposure to irradiation, infection, drugs, and chemicals. These mutations occur more frequently as a man ages and may be responsible for various inborn disorders and congenital anomalies (see Causes of Paternal Contributions to Birth Defects in the Child) (26, 48, 96, 150). For males this "cutoff" is 45 years of age; risks for chromosomal abnormalities may double when the male is 55 years or older (48). The male may affect the unborn child in other ways as well. For example, recent research reveals the sperm of the man who uses cocaine may be affected by the substance and in turn adversely affect the ovum and developing child (148). Refer also to Chapter 2 for additional information on birth defects transmitted by the father, with a focus on Table 2–5.

VARIABLES RELATED TO CHILDBIRTH THAT AFFECT THE BABY

Medications

Analgesics and general anesthetics given during childbirth cross the placental barrier, affecting the newborn for days after delivery. Respiration after birth is negatively affected; artificial resuscitation may be needed for severe respiratory depression. Motor skills are also less adept, and more crying irritability is seen after birth. Local anesthetics also indirectly affect the fetus by reducing blood flow to the uterus, thus affecting the fetal heart rate (26, 116, 147). The APGAR score may be low (see Chapter 7).

Childbirth without drugs was first introduced in 1914 by Grantly Dick Read. He was followed by Dr. Fernand Lamaze. In recent times the natural childbirth method has become popular to both mother and father because they can both actively participate in the birth of their child. During natural childbirth classes parents learn about the physiology of pregnancy and childbirth, exercises that strengthen the mother's abdominal and perineal muscles, and techniques of breathing and relaxation during labor and delivery. The father acts as encourager and coach throughout the prenatal classes and during labor and delivery so that the birth experience is shared between the couple. Equally of benefit is the child who comes into the world without any ill effects from medication. Refer to literature from the American Society for Psychoprophylaxis in Obstetrics and obstetric nursing texts for more information on prepared childbirth.

Method of Delivery

Birth can be difficult, even dangerous. Forceps may be needed to withdraw the baby, because of maternal or fetal reasons, and are safe if the cervix is completely dilated and the head is within 2 in. of the mouth of the vagina. Abdominal surgery, cesarean section, is done when the baby, for a number of reasons, cannot be born vaginally. This major surgery should not be done unless absolutely necessary.

Inadequate Oxygenation

Anoxia, *decreased oxygen supply,* and increased carbon dioxide levels may result during delivery. Some degree almost routinely occurs from compression of the umbilical cord, reduced blood flow to the uterus, or placental separation. Fortunately, newborn babies are better able to withstand periods of low oxygen than are adults. Other causes of asphyxia, however, such as drug-induced respiratory depression or apnea, kinks in the umbilical cord, wrapping of the cord around the neck, very long labor, and malpresentation of the fetus during birth, have more serious effects. Longitudinal studies of anoxic newborns revealed lower performance scores on tests of sensorimotor and cognitive-intellectual skills and personality measures than for children with minimal anoxia at birth. Anoxia is also the principal cause of perinatal death and a common cause of mental retardation and cerebral palsy (26, 27, 116, 147).

Premature Birth and Low Birth Weight

Prematurity may have long-term consequences for the child. **Prematurity** is defined as *the birth at a gestational age of 37 weeks or earlier, combined with birth weight of less than 2500 g or 5½ pounds.* Risk of death is greater to premature babies. Causes have been discussed earlier in this chapter.

Later developmental and behavioral problems such as physical and mental retardation and hyperactivity may also be correlated with prematurity (33, 116, 147). Treatment of the premature neonate in sterile, precisely controlled incubators causes the absence of environmental and sensory stimuli which also contributes to retardation. Research shows that gentle rubbing hourly throughout the 24-hour day promotes positive effects immediately and later for infants in isolettes—they are more active and gain weight faster, and later they perform better on tests of motor development while appearing healthier and more active than premature children who suffer tactile and sensory deprivation.

The small-for-gestation age or **low-birth-weight infants** (*less than 5½ pounds or 2500 g*) may not be premature; some are small for gestational age. Low birth weight is the major factor associated with death of the infant during the first 4 weeks of life. Women who are

Research Abstract

Martinez, F., A. Wright, L. Taussig, and Group Health Medical Associates, The Effect of Paternal Smoking on the Birth Weight of Newborns Whose Mothers Did Not Smoke, American Journal of Public Health, *84, no. 9 (1994), 1489–1491.*

Active maternal cigarette smoking during pregnancy is associated with reduced birth weight in the offspring. There are fewer data on possible effects of the mother's passive exposure to cigarette smoke on the child's birth weight, but findings suggest that father's smoking is associated with lower birth weight of infants. The purpose of this study was to determine the possible effects of paternal smoking on the infant's birth weight.

Subjects included a cohort of 1219 newborns whose parents used one of the largest health maintenance organizations in Tucson, Arizona. Each parent was given a questionnaire concerning, among other issues, his or her smoking habits during the woman's pregnancy. Cord blood specimens were collected for 87% of the enrolled infants; cord serum levels of cotinine (a metabolite of nicotine) were measured by competitive radioimmunoassay in a sample of 175 infants. There was no significant difference in any social or demographic parameter between these 175 infants and the rest of the eligible population. The lower limit of detectability for serum cotinine assay was 1 ng/mL.

Findings revealed a relationship between paternal smoking (passive exposure to the mother) and lower birth weight. A mean decrease in birth weight of 88 g was found in newborns of nonsmoking mothers whose fathers smoked more than 20 cigarettes a day. Detectability of cotinine in cord blood was significantly correlated with the number of cigarettes smoked daily by fathers. These findings support studies showing decreased birth weight of 107 and 120 g in newborns when fathers, but not mothers, smoke, and also support similar studies done in Italy and India.

Health care implications of this study point to the need for smoking cessation education and programs for men when their partner is pregnant. The father, as well as the pregnant woman, should stop smoking during the pregnancy, as fetal growth is adversely affected by not only maternal, but also paternal smoking. Pregnant women should also be advised to avoid environments in which cigarettes are smoked by others. Lower-birth-weight infants are at risk for greater mortality during the first year of life as well as for greater neonatal mortality.

physically abused during pregnancy are more likely to deliver low-birth-weight infants, compared with non-abused women. Being physically abused also doubles the chance of having a miscarriage. Abuse, physical and emotional, may be one of the most frequent problems in pregnancy (15, 59, 116, 147).

The following maternal factors contribute to a higher risk of low-birth-weight babies (15, 27, 116, 137, 144, 147):

- Underweight before pregnancy
- Less than 21 pounds gained during pregnancy
- Inadequate prenatal care
- Age of 16 years or younger or 35 years or older
- Low socioeconomic level
- Poor nutrition during pregnancy
- Smoking cigarettes during pregnancy
- Use of addictive drugs or alcohol during pregnancy
- History of prior abortions

- Complications during pregnancy; poor health status
- High stress levels including suffering physical or emotional abuse

Risk of low birth weight is associated with financial problems or living in high-crime areas, irrespective of the variables of race, poor health habits, and complications during pregnancy (66). A study of low-birth-weight children born to disadvantaged families showed that those who had received sensory stimulation in the nursery and additional sensorimotor stimulation from their mothers throughout the first year of life performed better on tests of intellectual and sensorimotor development at the end of the year than the children who had not received extra stimulation.

A study of 1000 infants for 3 years in eight U.S. cities indicated that the outcomes for premature and low-birth-weight infants can be significantly improved by intensive interventions for the first 3 years of the child's life. Children and families received the following services (34):

- Weekly home visits in the first year of the child's life and biweekly thereafter
- Attendance for the child at a special child development center after 12 months of age
- Bimonthly group meetings for parents

Children who received these services showed higher intelligent quotient scores and fewer behavioral problems than did those who received no intervention (34).

Premature children differ from full-term infants in a number of ways, including sleep patterns, which are poorly organized with poorly differentiated sleep states. Shorter and less regular periods of each sleep state are exhibited and may persist beyond infancy. Because more growth hormone is released during sleep, disturbed sleep patterns in the premature may affect physical growth and size generally (26, 33).

EARLY CHILDHOOD VARIABLES THAT AFFECT THE PERSON

Nutrition

Nutrition can exert an important influence on growth and development, especially if nutritional deficiency diseases occur. It is estimated that 1 of every 8 children under the age of 12 in the United States goes to bed hungry every night, despite available nutrition programs (107). Unfortunately, minimum, optimum, and toxic levels of nutrients are not well researched to date; however, inadequate nutrition may slow normal growth and apparently causes permanent effects of low intellectual ability. As much as 30% of the brain's neurons may never be formed if protein intake is inadequate during the second trimester of pregnancy or the first 6 months of life. Children who suffer starvation do not catch up with growth norms for their group, although later in life adequate nutrition and socioemotional support help to offset the differences (33, 144).

Obesity in childhood more likely is related to eating patterns than to genetics, according to a study of weight differences between infants of obese and nonobese foster mothers. The babies weighed $4\frac{1}{2}$ pounds at birth and entered the foster homes at $3\frac{1}{2}$ weeks of age. Children cared for by obese foster parents also became obese. The mean weight of all children of obese mothers was greater at all ages than for children of nonobese mothers. Children with excess cell mass from excessive caloric intake develop adult adipose cells early in life. Adipose stores continue to increase because of the increased number of adipose cells (116, 144, 147).

Even breastfeeding is not completely safe. Many drugs ingested by the mother are excreted in human milk. The newborn is susceptible to foreign substances because the body's principal detoxifying mechanisms are not functional, the enzyme system is immature, and kidney function is incompletely developed (26, 116, 147). Media reports indicate that pesticides in food and other environmental pollutants unknowingly ingested by the mother are excreted in human milk.

Stress

Stress related to emotional and sensory deprivation causes undesirable physical, emotional, and intellectual effects (9, 16, 33, 99, 107, 122–124, 129). Studies show that severe stress, discomfort, or pain causes the infant to perceive fewer external stimuli and to distort perceptions. Less tolerance for stress develops (99).

Effects of Practice on Neuromuscular Development

Effects of exercise or practice on developing early motor skills remain contradictory in reports. Apparently certain motor behavior appears when the body has the neuromuscular maturity for that behavior; practice of the behavior before its natural appearance does little to speed up long-term development, although it may appear that the child can do an activity earlier. Unpracticed children catch up, often doing the same activity in research studies only a few days later (27, 66, 134).

Endocrine Function

Mediation of hormones is crucial to the child and person throughout life. A **hormone** is a *chemical substance produced by an endocrine gland and carried by the bloodstream to another part of the body (the target organ) where it controls some function of the target organ.* The major functions of hormones include integrative action, regulation, morphogenesis. **Integration,** *permitting the body to act as a whole unit in response to stimuli,* results from hormones traveling throughout the body and reaching all cells of the body. For example, the response of the body to epinephrine during fright is generalized. Estrogen, although more specific in its action, affects overall body function. **Regulation,** *maintaining a constant internal environment or homeostasis,* results from all the hormones. The regulation of salt and water balance, metabolism, and growth are examples. In **morphogenesis,** the *rate and type of growth of the organism,* some hormones play an important part (53).

Growth hormone (GH) or *somatotropic hormone (STH)*, secreted by the anterior pituitary gland and regulated by a substance called *growth hormone-releasing-factor (GHF)*, produced in the hypothalamus, affects morphogenesis by promoting the development and enlargement of all body tissues that are capable of growing. Growth hormone has three basic effects on the metabolic processes of the body: (1) protein synthesis is increased; (2) carbohydrate conservation is increased; and (3) use of fat stores for energy is increased (53).

Growth hormone is secreted in spurts instead of at a relatively constant rate. The lowest concentrations of plasma GH are found in the morning after arising; the highest concentrations occur between 60 and 90 minutes after falling asleep at night. The peak of GH is clearly related to sleep; thus, the folk belief that sleep is necessary for growth and healing has been supported (53, 66).

SOCIOCULTURAL FACTORS THAT INFLUENCE THE DEVELOPING PERSON

Cultural and Demographic Variables

Culture, social class, race, and ethnicity of the parents—foods eaten by the pregnant woman, prenatal care and childbirth practices, childrearing methods, expected patterns of behavior, language development and thought processes during childhood and adulthood, and health practices—variously affect the person from the moment of conception. The person, however, will demonstrate some behaviors outside the cultural norm. If the child's parents are from a different ethnic or social background from most citizens of the area, the child may learn to talk, act, and think differently from most people. Conflict results between the person and the representatives (people and institutions) of the main culture, which, in turn, affects the child's ongoing development and care. Refer to Chapter 1 for in-depth discussion.

The health care given to the child by the parents is related to sociocultural status. For example, in urban areas parents of children who are adequately immunized are likely to have the following characteristics: (1) they perceive childhood diseases as serious; (2) they know about the effectiveness of vaccination; (3) they are older; (4) they are better educated; (5) they have smaller family size (number of children); and (6) they read newspapers, listen to radio or television promotions of immunizations, and respond to these community educational efforts. Inadequately immunized children in urban areas are found in families in which the parents are young, poor, and minimally educated, and have a large number of children. The parents do not perceive childhood diseases as serious, do not know about the effectiveness of vaccines, or do not pay attention to health education in the mass media (66, 147).

All the advantages of inheriting a good brain can be lost if the child does not have the right environment in which to develop it. Animal and human studies demonstrate that lack of physical or social stimulation and nutrition have an effect on later behavior and development.

Child–caregiver interaction; lifestyle factors such as adequate rest, smoking, and drug and alcohol use; use of health promotion measures; poor food habits that result in either malnutrition or obesity; along with toxic factors in the environment and infections all together are major determinants of how closely the genetic potential can be reached. All of these factors affect the child's growth and development, learning ability, functional capacity, and health. All of these factors eventually affect the health and longevity of adults, including into old age, as shown by longitudinal studies in England (113).

Socialization Processes

Socialization is the *process by which the infant is transformed into a member of a particular society and learns the roles appropriate to sex, social class, and ethnic group or subculture* (93).

All humans experience socialization, the shaping of the person into a socially acceptable form, especially during the early years of life. Thus heritage and culture are perpetuated. The newborn is a biological organism with physical needs and inherited characteristics, which will be socialized or shaped along a number of dimensions: emotional, social, cognitive, or intellectual, perceptual, behavioral, and expressive. During the period of socialization various skills, knowledge, attitudes, values, motives, habits, beliefs, needs, interests, and ideals are learned, demonstrated, and reinforced. Various people are key agents in the socialization process: parents, siblings, relatives, peers, teachers, and other adults. Certain forces will impinge on the person and interact with all the individual is and learns; these forces include culture, social class, religion, race or ethnicity, the community, the educational system, mass media, and various organizations. Certain factors may limit or enhance the socialization process: age, sex, rate and stage of development, general constitution, and innate intelligence. Integration of all the various individual and socializing forces will form the adult character, personality traits, role preferences, goals, and behavioral mode.

Socialization is a lifelong process of social learning or training through which the person acquires knowledge, skills, attitudes, values, needs, motivations, and cognitive, affective, and conative patterns that relate to the sociocultural setting. The success of the socialization process is measured by the person's ability to perform in the roles he or she attempts and to respond to rapid social change and a succession of life tasks (93).

The life cycle is seen as a succession of roles or transitions and changing role constellations. Certain order and predictability of behavior occur over time as the person moves through the given succession of roles. The person learns to think and behave in ways consonant with the roles to be played; performance in a succession of roles leads to predictable personality configurations (14, 32, 33, 93).

Community Support System

Community relationships influence primarily the parents, but they also influence the child. An emotional support system for the parents, physical and health care resources in the community, and social and learning opportunities that exist outside the home promote the child's development and prepare him or her for later independence and citizenry roles. If the parents are unable to meet the child's needs adequately, other people or organizations in the community may make the difference between bare survival and eventual physical and emotional normalcy and well-being.

Cultures vary in the degree to which the new mother is given help. For example, in India the mother is assisted with child care and is allowed to do nothing except care for her baby for 40 days after delivery. Several decades ago mothers in the United States were hospitalized for 10 or 12 days, and the family helped at home for another couple of weeks or so. Now the mother is sent home after 24 to 72 hours, often to assume total child care.

Physical health of the baby and emotional health of the mother in the months following delivery depend on whether or not she had assistance with infant care during the first month after delivery (116, 147).

Family Factors

The family structure, developmental level and roles of family members, their health and financial status, their perception of baby, and community resources for the family influence the child's development and well-being, before birth and afterwards. Social and environmental factors that produce low birth weight, for instance, are likely to continue to operate on the infant and child as well. The child learns to behave differently and as an adult, will have different values and expectations if he or she is reared in a single-parent, nuclear, extended, matrifocal, or patriarchal family or in a poor or wealthy family. The number of siblings, their sexes, and birth order influence how the child is treated and perceives self. The stresses on and crises within the family determine how well the child is cared for from birth, how and what is taught to the child, discipline measures, and how he or she looks at life. The family's presence or absence of work, leisure, travel, material comforts, habits of daily living, and the facade put on for society will affect the child's self-concept, learning, physical well-being, and eventual lifestyle. Refer to Chapter 4 for more information.

Spitz (122–124), studied four different childrearing situations to determine the effect on the young child. Children from professional, urban homes had the highest developmental quotient initially, and it stayed high. Children living in an isolated fishing village with poor nutrition, housing, hygiene, and medical care had a low developmental quotient in the first 4 months, and it remained low. Children born to delinquent women and reared in a penal institution by their mothers had a lower development quotient initially than children in the fishing village, but they gained slightly. Children from a Latin, urban background who were raised in a foundling home had an initial high development quotient, but the score was lowest of the groups studied at the end of the first year.

The children in the foundling home had been given minimum mothering by overworked nurses. The presence of the mother is sufficient to compensate for lack of material objects. The lack of development was related to lack of human stimulation, as deterioration of the child was arrested if he or she was removed from the foundling home at 1 year of age.

The mother has traditionally been credited with having the most effect on the child, whether the outcome was good or bad; however, researchers now acknowledge the importance of the father and the effect of the father's presence or absence on the developing child (72, 82). The stability and strength of attachment between the child and family will largely determine the degree to which he or she will become a self-confident, productive citizen. The long-term emotional and physical environments are the most crucial variables in the child's measured performance at 10 years. A positive environment overcomes negative perinatal influences; a negative environment may have lasting effects (116, 147).

Vulnerable and Resilient Children

Both vulnerable and resilient children develop within the same family system. Siblings brought up under chaotic situations, with alcoholic or drug-using parents, or in impoverished circumstances do not all develop the same personality traits. One becomes physically or emotionally ill, whereas the sibling thrives. No single set of qualities or circumstances characterizes such resilient children, but they are different from their vulnerable siblings from birth. **Resilient children** appear to be *endowed with innate characteristics that insulate them from the pain of their families and allow them to reach out to some adult who provides crucial emotional support.* Characteristics of these children include the ability to (27):

- Use some talent or personality traits to draw some adult to them as a substitute parent
- Recover quickly from stressors
- Be more alert to their surroundings from birth
- Establish trust with the mother
- Have warm and secure relationships with the mother, regardless of other circumstances
- Be more independent, easy going, enthusiastic for activities, and able to tolerate frustration by age 2
- Be more cheerful, flexible, and persistent in the face of failure and seek help from adults by age $3\frac{1}{2}$

Vulnerable children *are closest emotionally to the distressed parent and are most likely to show signs of distress.* These children are more likely to be self-derogatory, anxious, depressed, and physically ill; however, hardships can leave even the resilient children with psychological scars, although they tend not to become emotionally disabled. Even apparently well-adjusted, successful, resilient children may pay a subtle psychological cost. In adolescence they are more likely to cling to a moralistic outlook. In intimate relationships they are apt to be disagreeable and judgmental. They tend to be constricted and overcontrolled. If the disturbed parent is of the opposite sex, the resilient person is often emotionally distant in intimate relationships, breaking off relationships as they become more intimate. Some seek partners with problems, with the idea of rescuing or curing them (27).

Child Abuse

Child abuse is a negative influence on the developing person. It is currently an epidemic, and children are suf-fering more serious and brutal injuries. Parents who abuse their children are from every race, color, creed, ethnic origin, and economic level (116, 147). As a nurse, you are crucial in preventing child abuse through your assistance to parents. **Child abuse** is a *pattern of abnormal parent–child interactions and attacks over a period that results in nonaccidental injuries to the child physically, emotionally, or sexually or from neglect.* Other terms are *battered child* or *maltreatment syndrome.* Abused children range in age from neonate through adolescence.

You may be the first health worker to encounter such a child in the community. Be alert for signs of child abuse as you assess the injured or ill child. Nonaccidental physical injury includes multiple bruises or fractures from severe beatings; poisonings or overmedication; burns from immersion in hot water or from lighted cigarettes; excessive use of laxatives or enemas; and human bites. The trauma to the child is often great enough to cause permanent blindness, scars on the skin, neurologic damage, subdural hematoma, and permanent brain damage or death. **Sexual molestation,** *exploitation of the child for the adult's sexual gratification,* includes rape, incest, exhibitionism to the child, or fondling of the child's genitals. **Emotional abuse** includes *excessively aggressive or unreasonable parental behavior to the child,* placing unreasonable demands on the child to perform above his or her capacities, verbally attacking or constantly belittling or teasing the child, or withdrawing love, support, or guidance. **Neglect** includes *failure to provide the child with basic necessities of life* (food, shelter, clothing, hygiene, or medical care), *adequate mothering, or emotional, moral, or social care* (27, 33, 39, 40, 58, 66, 116, 134, 147). The parents' lack of concern is usually obvious. Abandonment may occur. In all forms of abuse the child frequently acts fearful of the parents or adults in general. The child is usually too fearful to tell how he or she was injured.

There are a number of characteristics of the potentially or actually abusive parent(s). Typically the abuser:

- Is young
- Is emotionally unstable, unable to cope with the stress of life or even usual personal problems
- Was insufficiently mothered, rejected, or abused as a child
- Is lonely, has few social contacts, and is isolated from people
- Is unable to ask for help; lacks friends or family who can help with child care
- Does not understand the development or care needs of children
- Is living through a very stressful time such as unemployment, spousal abuse, or poverty

- Has personal emotional needs previously unmet; has difficulty in trusting others
- Is angered easily; has negative self-image and low self-esteem
- Has no one from whom to receive emotional support, including partner
- Expects the child to be perfect and to cause no inconvenience
- May perceive the child as different, too active, or too passive, even if the child is normal or only mildly different

Sometimes the child has mild neurologic dysfunction and is irritable, tense, and difficult to hold or cuddle. The child may have been the result of an unwanted pregnancy or premature or have a birth defect. Usually only one child in a family becomes the scapegoat for parental anger, tension, rejection, and hate. The child who does not react in a way to make the parent feel good about his or her parenting behavior will be the abused one (27, 33, 39, 40, 45, 58, 66, 116, 147).

Additional information about child adolescent abuse is found in Chapters 7 through 11.

Prolonged Separation

Separation for more than 3 months from a mothering person leads to serious consequences because from approximately 3 to 15 months of age the presence of a consistently loving caretaker is essential. Physical and intellectual growth is impaired, and the baby will not learn to form and maintain trust or a significant relationship. He or she will either withdraw or seek precociously to adapt by getting attention from as many people as possible. Death may result even with the best possible physical care (33, 66, 116, 122–124, 147).

Maternal Deprivation and Failure to Thrive

Maternal deprivation and **failure to thrive** are the terms used to describe *infants who have insufficient contact with a mothering one and who do not grow as expected in the absence of an organic defect.* These infants may be institutionalized or have a parent who does not exhibit affectionate maternal behavior. Deprivation during the second 6 months occurs when a previously warm relationship with the mother is interrupted. This deprivation is more detrimental to the child than the lack of a consistent relationship during the first 6 months. Another cause for failure to thrive is **perceptual deprivation,** *lack of tactile, vestibular, visual, or auditory stimuli,* resulting from either organic factors or the lack of mothering (116, 147). Touch and cuddling

are essential for the infant; the skin is the primary way in which baby comes to know self and the environment.

Although damage to the child from maternal deprivation may be severe, not every deprived child becomes delinquent or a problem adult. Some infants who have lacked their mother's love appear to suffer little permanent damage. The age of the child when deprived or abused, the length of separation or duration of abuse, the parent–child relationship before separation or in later childhood, care of the child by other adults during separation from the parents, and the stress produced by the separation or abuse all affect the long-range outcome.

Spiritual Factors

Religious, philosophic, and moral insights and practices of the parents (and of the overall society) influence how the child is perceived, cared for, and taught. These early underpinnings—or their lack—will continue to affect the person's self-concept, behavior, and health as an adult, even when he or she purposefully tries to disregard these early teachings. Refer to Chapter 3 for more information.

Macroenvironmental Factors That Influence the Developing Person

The overall environment of the region in which the person lives and in the home affects development and health. The climate the person learns to tolerate, water and food availability, emphasis on cleanliness, demands for physical and motor competency, social relationships, opportunities for leisure, and inherent hazards depend on whether the child lives on a farm or in the city, on the seacoast or in a semiarid region, in the cold North or sunny South, in a mining town or a mountain resort area. Added to these effects are the hazards from environmental pollution that affect all societies, whether it is excrement from freely roaming cattle or particles from industrial smokestacks. No part of the world is any longer uncontaminated by pesticides; all parts have disease related to problems of waste control. On a more immediate level, the size, space, noise, cleanliness, and safety within the home will affect the person's behavior and health and the home environment he or she will eventually build.

Further discussion of effects of the macroenvironment on the person's health can be found in Chapter 2.

► HEALTH CARE AND NURSING APPLICATIONS

Your support, assistance, and teaching with the pregnant woman and her significant support system will contribute to more nurturing parenting. Refer to texts on obstetric and maternal–child nursing for additional information about nursing care of the woman during pregnancy, labor, delivery, and after delivery. Information is also given in Chapters 2 and 7 through 11 that can be shared with the pregnant woman and parents for health promotion.

The following health promotion strategies are useful:

- Consider the principles of growth and development as you assess people in different developmental eras.
- Carefully assess pregnant women to determine whether they are at risk because of any of the negative influencing factors.
- Consider also the sociocultural and religious background and the lifestyle of the person you are caring for so that you do not overlook or misinterpret factors that are significant to the pregnant woman and her family.
- Help those who are at risk to get the care necessary to prevent fetal damage and maternal illness.
- Teach potential parents about the many factors discussed in this and following chapters that can influence the welfare of their offspring.
- Be aware of community services such as genetic screening and counseling, family planning, nutritional programs, prenatal classes, counseling for prevention of child abuse, and medical services.
- Join with other citizens in attempts to reverse environmental and child abuse hazards.

Your role with the child-abusing parent and the abused child is a significant one. To help parents and child, you must first cope with your own feelings as you give necessary physical care to the child or assist parents in getting proper care for the baby. Often parents who feel unable to cope with the stresses of childrearing will repeatedly bring the child to the emergency room for a variety of complaints of minor, vague illnesses or injuries.

Certain health promotion strategies are useful:

- Be alert to the subtle message; talk with the parent(s) about himself or herself, the management of the child, feelings about parenting and the child, and who helps in times of stress.
- Establish rapport; act like a helpful friend; convey a feeling of respect for them as people (which may be difficult if you feel that the child abuser is a monster).
- Avoid asking probing questions too quickly.
- Do not lecture or scold the parent about his or her childrearing methods.
- Help parents to feel confident and competent in any way possible.
- Form a "cool mothering" relationship with the parent(s) (i.e., make yourself consistently available but do not push too close emotionally). Often the mother responds well to having a grandmotherly person (usually a volunteer) spend time with her. This person could go to the home, where she could mother the mother, assist with a variety of household chores, giving the mother time to spend with her baby while unharried by demands of other children or household tasks.
- Be a model on how to approach, cuddle, and discipline the child; the parent may expect the 6-month-old baby to obey commands.
- Convey that consistency of care is important. Realize that the parent will need long-term help in overcoming the abusive pattern.
- Use the principles of therapeutic communication and crisis intervention discussed in Chapters 4 and 5 to avoid driving the parent away from potential help or becoming more abusive to the child.
- Intervene sensibly with the parents and the child to avoid further harm and to avoid disrupting any positive feelings that might exist between parents and child. Foster home care is not necessarily the answer; foster parents are sometimes abusive, too. Rapid court action may antagonize parents to the point of murdering the child or moving to a different geographic location where they cannot receive help.
- Refer the parents to Parents Anonymous, a self-help parent's group that exists in some large cities, or to other local self-help crisis groups.

Further, cooperate with legal, medical, and social agencies to help the parent(s) and to prevent further child abuse—and possible death or permanent impairment of the child. Child abuse is against the law in every state, and every state has at least one statewide agency to receive and investigate suspected cases of child abuse. Any citizen or health worker can anonymously report a case of child abuse to authorities without fear of recrimination from the abuser. An investigation by designated authorities of the danger to the child is carried out shortly after reporting; the child may be placed in a foster home or institution by court order if the child's life is threatened. The goal of legal intervention is to help the parents and child, not to punish.

Unless the problem of child abuse can be curbed, many of today's children will become the next generation of abusing parents.

Mothers and children constitute approximately two-thirds of the population in any society. They are worth caring for physically and emotionally because of their worth to the future of the society.

SUMMARY

1. Childhood is the foundation period of life, and development follows a definable, predictable, sequential pattern.

2. The person is unique, yet similar to other people in patterns of development, characterized by wholism (physical, emotional, cognitive, social and spiritual/moral dimensions).

3. Growth, development, developmental tasks, maturation, and learning are key terms to understanding the developing person.

4. Several principles of growth explain the pattern of development.

5. Prenatal influences on development include heredity, various physiologic processes, and age, health, and nutritional status of the mother.

6. Environmental hazards, drugs, alcohol, infections, and other conditions are teratogens that may adversely affect the developing organism, especially during the critical period of the first trimester.

7. Certain variables, such as medication in the mother, may negatively affect the fetus during labor and delivery.

8. Early childhood variables that affect the developing person include nurturance from the parents, nutrition, stressors, physiologic functions in the infant, and various sociocultural and family characteristics.

REFERENCES

1. Abkarian, G.G., Communication Effects of Prenatal Alcohol Exposure, *Journal of Communication Disorders,* 25, no. 4 (1992), 221–240.

2. Ahlborg, G., and L. Bodin, Tobacco Smoke Exposure and Pregnancy Outcome Among Working Women: A Prospective Study at Prenatal Care Centers in Orebro County, Sweden, *Preventive Journal of Epidemiology,* 133, no. 4 (1991), 338–347.

3. Ausman, L.F., Toxoplasmosis and Pregnancy, *Canadian Nurse,* 89, no. 4 (1993), 31–32.

4. Baker, R.C., and T.R. Jerrells, Recent Developments in Alcoholism: Immunological Aspects, *Recent Developments in Alcoholism,* 11 (1993), 2491.

5. Bakht, F.R., and L.O. Gentry, Toxoplasmosis in Pregnancy: An Emerging Concern for Family Physicians, *American Family Physician,* 45, no. 4 (1992), 1683–1690.

6. Bardy, A.H., P. Lillsunde, J.M. Kataja, P. Koskela, J. Pikkaraineu, and V.K. Hilesmaa, Objectively Measured Tobacco Exposure During Pregnancy: Neonatal Effects and Relation to Maternal Smoking, *British Journal of Obstetrics and Gynaecology,* 11 (1993), 721–726.

7. Barnicle, M.M., Chemotherapy and Pregnancy, *Seminars in Oncology Nursing,* 8, no. 2 (1992), 124–132.

8. Bateman, D., S. Ng, C. Hansen, and M. Heagarty, The Effects of Intrauterine Cocaine Exposure in Newborns, *American Journal of Public Health,* 83 (1993), 190–193.

9. Beck, C., The Effects of Postpartum Depression on Maternal–Infant Interaction: A Meta-analysis, *Nursing Research,* 44 (1995), 298-303.

10. Berhart-Phillips, P., P.D. Frederick, R.O. Baron, and L. Mascola, Measles in Pregnancy: A Descriptive Study of 58 Cases, *Obstetrics and Gynecology,* 82, no. 5 (1993), 797–801.

11. Berrien, K., *General and Social Systems.* New Brunswick, NJ: Rutgers University Press, 1968.

12. Better Detection, Surveillance Needed for Fetal Alcohol Syndrome, *The Nation's Health,* 25, no. 10 (1995), 14.

13. Birnbaum, L.S., Endocrine Effects of Prenatal Exposure to PVBs, Dioxins, and Other Xenobiotics: Implications for Policy and Future Research, *Environmental Health Perspectives,* 102, no. 8 (1994), 678–679.

14. Buhler, C., The Developmental Structure of Goal Setting in Group and Individual Studies, in Buhler, C., and F. Massarik, eds., *The Course of Human Life,* New York: Springer-Verlag, 1968.

15. Bullock, B.L., and J. McFarlane, The Birth-Weight/Battering Connection, *American Journal of Nursing,* 89, no. 9 (1989), 1153–1155.

16. Bustan, M., and A. Coker, Maternal Attitude Toward Pregnancy and the Risk of Neonatal Death, *American Journal of Public Health,* 84 (3), 1994, 411–414.

17. *AIDS Information* (Document 320200), Atlanta: Centers for Disease Control, 1995.

18. *CMV Virus* (Information Document 362301), Atlanta: Centers for Disease Control, 1995.

19. Chasnoff, I.J., Prenatal Cocaine Exposure Is Associated With Respiratory Pattern Abnormalities, *American Journal of Disabled Children,* 144 no. 2 (1990), 583–587.

20. ———, and D. Griffith, Cocaine: Clinical Studies of Pregnancy and the Newborn. *Annals of the New York Academy of Sciences,* 562 (1989), 260–266.

21. ———, et al., Temporal Patterns of Cocaine Use in Pregnancy: Perinatal Outcomes, *Journal of the American Medical Association,* 261, no. 12 (1989), 1741–1749.

22. Cohen, F.L., Paternal Contributions to Birth Defects, *Nursing Clinics of North America,* 21, no. 1 (March 1986), 51–66.

23. Condon, J.T., and C.A. Hilton, A Comparison of Smoking and Drinking Behaviors in Pregnant Women: Who Abstains and Why, *Medical Journal of Australia,* 148 (1988), 381–385.

24. Corcoran, G.D., and G.L. Ridgway, Antibiotic Chemotherapy of Bacterial Sexually Transmitted Diseases in Adults: A Review, *International Journal of SID and AIDS,* 5, no. 3 (1994), 165–171.

25. Cordero, L., and M.B. Landen, Infant of the Diabetic Mother, *Clinics in Perinatology,* 20, no. 3 (1993), 635–648.

26. Cunningham, F., P. MacDonald, and N. Gant, *Williams Obstetrics* (18 th ed.). Norwalk, CT: Appleton & Lange, 1989.

27. Dacey, J., and J. Travers, *Human Development Across the Lifespan* (3rd ed.). Madison, WI: Brown & Benchmark, 1996.

28. Day, N.L., and G.A. Richardsen, Prenatal Alcohol Exposure: A Continuum of Effects, *Seminars in Perinatology,* 15, no. 4 (1991), 271–279.

29. Dowe, D.A., E.R. Heitzman, and J.J. Larking, Human Immuno-deficiency Virus Infection in Children, *Clinical Imaging,* 16, no. 3 (1992), 145–151.

30. Drug Exposed Infant, *The Future of Children,* 1, no. 1 (Spring 1991), 1–200.

31. Duester, G.A., Hypothetical Mechanism for Fetal Alcohol Syndrome Involving Ethanol Inhibition of Retinoic Acid Synthesis at the Alcohol Dehydrogenase Step, *Alcohol: Clinical and Experimental Research,* 15, no. 3 (1991), 568–572.

32. Duvall, E., and B. Miller, *Marriage and Family Development* (6th ed.). New York: Harper & Row, 1984.

33. Dworetzky, J., *Human Development: A Lifespan Approach* (2nd ed.). St. Paul/Minneapolis: West, 1995.

34. Early Intervention Improves the Developmental Outcome of Premature Infants, New Study Says, *Advances: Newsletter of the Robert Wood Johnson Foundation,* 3, no. 2 (1990), 3.

35. Edelman, C., and C. Mandle, *Health Promotion Throughout the Lifespan* (3rd ed.). St. Louis: Mosby, 1994.

36. Edwards, C.H., A.A. Johnson, E.M. Knight, U.J. Oyemade, O.J. Cole, O.E. Westney, S. Jones, H. Laryea, and L.S. Westney, *Journal of Nutrition,* 124, 6 Suppl. (1994), 954s–962s.

37. Elango, S., Aetiology of Deafness in Children From a School for the Deaf in Malaysia, *International Journal of Pediatric Ophthalaryngology,* 27 (1993), 21–27.

38. Ellis, J.E., L.D. Byrd, S.R. Sexson, and C.A. Patterson-Barnett, In Utero Exposure to Cocaine: A Review, *Southern Medical Journal,* 86, no. 7 (1993), 725–731.

39. Elmer, E., *Children in Jeopardy: The Study of Abused Minors and Their Families.* Pittsburgh: University of Pittsburgh Press, 1962.

40. ———, Child Abuse: The Family's Cry for Help, *Journal of Psychiatric Nursing,* 5, no. 4 (1967), 338ff.

41. Enstrom, J.E., L.E. Kanim, and L. Breslow, The Relationship Between Vitamin C Intake, General Health Practices, and Mortality in Alameda County, California, *American Journal of Public Health,* 76, no. 9 (September 1986), 1124-1129.

42. Erikson, E., *Childhood and Society* (2nd ed.). New York: W.W. Norton, 1963.

43. Erkhart, C.B., Clinical Correlations Between Ethanol Intake and Fetal Alcohol Syndrome, *Recent Developments in Alcoholism,* 9 (1991), 127–150.

44. El Tabbakh, G.H., B.R. Elejalde, and F.F. Broekhuizen, Primary Syphilis and Nonimmune Fetal Hydrops in Penicillin-allergic Women: A Case Report, *Journal of Reproductive Medicine,* 39, no. 5 (1994), 412–414.

45. Florack, E.I., G.A. Ziehhuis, J.E. Pellegrino, and R. Rolland, Occupational Physical Activity and the Occurrence of Spontaneous Abortion, *International Journal of Epidemiology,* 22, no. 5 (1993), 878–884.

46. Fojaco, R.M., G.T. Hensley, and L. Moskowitz, Congenital Syphilis and Necrotizing Funisitis, *Journal of American Medical Association,* 261, no. 12 (1989), 1788–1790.

47. Fox, N.L., M. Sexton, and J.R. Hebel, Prenatal Exposure to Tobacco: Effects on Physical Growth at Age Three, *International Journal of Epidemiology,* 19, no. 1 (1990), 66–71.

48. Friedman, J.M., Genetic Diseases in the Offspring of Older Fathers, *Obstetrics and Gynecology,* 57, no. 6 (1981), 745–749.

49. Givens, K.T., D. A. Lee, T. Jones, and D.M. Ilstrup, Congenital Rubella Syndrome: Ophthalmic Manifestations and Associated Systematic Disorders, *British Journal of Ophthalmology,* 77, no. 6 (1993), 358–383.

50. Goldfarb, J., Breastfeeding: AIDS and Other Infectious Diseases, *Clinics in Perinatology,* 20, no. 1 (1993), 225–243.

51. Goto, M.P., and A.S. Goldman, Diabetic-Embryopathy: Current Opinion, *Pediatrics,* 6, no. 4 (1994), 486–491.

52. Griffith, B.P., and J. Booss, Neurologic Infections of Fetus and Newborn, *Neurologic Clinics,* 12, no. 3 (1994), 541–564.

53. Guyton, A. *A Textbook of Medical Physiology* (9th ed.). Philadelphia: W.B. Saunders, 1996.

54. Habitual Cocaine Use May Cause Brain Shrinkage, *Professional Nurses Quarterly,* 5, no. 1 (1990), 8–9.

55. Hakansson, A., Equality in Health and Health Care During Pregnancy: A Prospective Population-Based Study From Southern Sweden, *Acta Obstetricia et Gynecologica Scandinavica,* 73, no. 9 (1994), 674–679.

56. Harrington, K., and S. Campbell, Fetal Size and Growth, *Current Opinion in Obstetrics & Gynecology of North America,* 18, no. 4 (1991), 907–931.

57. Hayman, L., J. Meininger, P. Coales, and P. Gallagher, Nongenetic Influences of Obesity on Risk Factors for Cardiovascular Disease During Two Phases of Development, *Nursing Research,* 44 (1995), 277–282.

58. Helberg, J., Documentation in Child Abuse, *American Journal of Nursing,* 83, no. 2 (1983), 236–239.

59. Helton, A., Battering During Pregnancy, *American Journal of Nursing,* 86, no. 8 (1986), 910–913.

60. Henriksen, T.B., D.A. Savitz, M. Hedegaard, and N.J. Secher, Employment During Pregnancy in Relation to Risk Factors and Pregnancy Outcomes, *British Journal of Obstetrics and Gynaecology,* 101, no. 10 (1994), 858–865.

61. Hill, J.D., and R.D. Milner, Insulin as a Growth Factor, *Pediatric Research,* 19 (1955), 879–886.

62. Hoff, L., *Battered Women as Survivors,* New York: Routledge, 1990.

63. Homer, C., S. James, and E. Siegel, Work-Related Psychosocial Stress and Risk of Preterm, Low Birthweight Delivery, *American Journal of Public Health,* 80 (1990), 173–177

64. Horner, R.D., C.J. Lackey, K. Kolasa, and K. Warren, Pica Practices of Pregnant Women, *Journal of the American Dietetic Association,* 91, no. 1 (1991), 34–38.

65. Isen, J., A. de Costa Pereira, and S.F. Olsen, Does Maternal Tobacco Smoking Modify the Effect of Alcohol on Fetal Growth? *American Journal of Public Health,* 81, no. 1 (1991), 69–73.

66. Jolley, J., and M. Mitchell, *Lifespan Development: A Topical Approach.* Madison, WI: Brown & Benchmark, 1996.

67. King, I., *Theory for Nursing: Systems, Concepts, Process.* New York: Delmar, 1981.

68. Klebnoff, M.A., P.H. Shione, and G.G. Rhoads, Outcomes of Pregnancy in a National Sample of Resident Physicians, *New England Journal of Medicine,* 323, no. 15 (1990), 1040–1045.

69. Klein, J., et al., Drinking During Pregnancy and Spontaneous Abortion, *Lancet,* 2, no. 7 (1980), 1976.

70. Kleinman, J.C., and A. Kopstein, Smoking During Pregnancy, *American Journal of Public Health,* 77, no. 7 (July 1987), 823–825.

71. Kozier, B., G. Erb, K. Blais, and J. Wilkinson, *Fundamentals of Nursing: Concepts, Process, and Practice* (5th ed.). Redwood City, CA: Addison-Wesley, 1995.

72. Lamb, M. *The Father's Role,* New York, John Wiley & Sons, 1986.

73. Landon, M.B., and S.G. Gabbe, Fetal Surveillance in the Pregnancy Complicated by Diabetes Mellitus, *Clinics in Perinatology,* 20, no. 3 (1993), 549–560.

74. Larroque, B., M. Kaminski, N. Lelong, D. Subtil, and P. Dehaene, Effects on Birth Weight of Alcohol and Caffeine Consumption During Pregnancy, *American Journal of Epidemiology,* 137, no. 9 (1993), 941–950.

75. Larroque, B., M. Kaminski, P. Dehaene, D. Subtil, M. Delfosse, and D. Querleu, Moderate Prenatal Alcohol Exposure and Psychomotor Development at Preschool Age, *American Journal of Public Health,* 85 (1995), 1654–1661.

76. Levin, S., et al., The Association of Marijuana Use With Pregnancy, *American Journal of Public Health* 73, no. 10 (1983), 1161–1164.

77. Little, R.E., et al., Decreased Birth Weight in Infants of Alcoholic Women Who Abstained During Pregnancy, *Journal of Pediatrics,* 96, no. 6 (1980), 974.

78. ———, et al., Maternal Alcohol Use During Breastfeeding and Infant Mental and Motor Development at One Year. *New England Journal of Medicine,* 321, no. 7 (1989), 425–430.

79. ———, and D.R. Petersen, Sudden Infant Death Syndrome Epidemiology: A Review and Update, *Epidemiology Review,* 12 (1990), 241–246.

80. ———, and J.K. Wendt, The Effects of Maternal Drinking in the Reproductive Period: An Epidemiologic Review, *Journal of Substance Abuse,* 3, no. 2 (1991), 187–204.

81. Luke, V., Nutritional Influences on Fetal Growth, *Clinical Obstetrics and Gynecology,* 37, no. 3 (1994), 538–549.

82. Lynn, D., *The Father: His Role in Child Development.* Monterey, CA: Brooks Cole, 1974.

83. MacGregor, S.N., et al., Cocaine Abuse During Pregnancy: Correlation Between Prenatal Care and Perinatal Outcome, *Obstetrics and Gynecology,* 74, no. 6 (1989), 882–885.

84. Marbury, M., et al., The Association of Alcohol Consumption with Outcome of Pregnancy, *American Journal of Public Health,* 73, no. 10 (1983), 1165–1168.

85. Maslow, A., *Motivation and Personality* (2nd ed.). New York: Harper & Row, 1970.

86. McFarlin, S., S.F. Bottoms, B.S. Dock, and N.B. Isada, Epidemic Syphilis: Maternal Factors Associated With Congenital Infection, *American Journal of Obstetrics and Gynecology,* 170 (1994), 535–540.

87. McIntosh, L.J., N.E. Roumayah, and S.F. Bottoms, Perinatal Outcome of Broken Marriage in the Inner City, *Obstetrics and Gynecology,* 85 (1995), 233–236.

88. Menton, R.K., et al., Transplacental Passage of Insulin in Pregnant Women With Insulin-Dependent Diabetic Macrosomia, *New England Journal of Medicine,* 323, no. 5 (1990), 309–315.

89. Minoff, H.L., et al., Pregnancy Outcomes Among Mothers With Human Immunodeficiency Virus and Uninfected Control Subjects, *American Journal of Obstetrics and Gynecology,* 163, no. 5 (1990), 1598–1604.

90. Murray, R., and M. Huelskoetter, *Psychiatric/Mental Health Nursing: Giving Emotional Care* (3rd ed.). E. Norwalk, CT: Appleton & Lange, 1991.

91. Mussen, P., et al., *Child Development and Personality* (7th ed.). New York: Harper & Row, 1990.

92. National Academy of Sciences Institute of Medicine, Subcommittee on Nutritional Status Weight Gain During Pregnancy. *Nutrition During Pregnancy.* Washington, DC: National Academy Press, 1990.

93. Neugarten, B., Adaptation and the Life Cycle, *Counseling Psychologist,* 6, no. 1 (1976), 16–20.

94. Neuspiel, D.R., M. Markewitz, and E. Drucker, Intrauterine Cocaine, Lead, and Nicotine Exposure and Fetal Growth, *American Journal of Public Health,* 84, no. 9 (1994), 1492–1495.

95. Ogawa, H., S. Tominaga, K. Hori, K. Noguschi, I. Kanou, and M. Matsubara, Passive Smoking by Pregnant Women and Fetal Growth, *Journal of Epidemiology and Community Health,* 45 (1991), 164–168.

96. Olson, J., A. de Costa Pereira, and S. Olsen, Does Maternal Tobacco Smoking Modify the Effect of Alcohol on Fetal Growth? *American Journal of Public Health,* 81, no. 1 (1991), 69–73.

97. Osborn, L.M., D.C. Harris, M.C. Reading, and M.B. Prather, Outcome of Pregnancies Experienced During Residency, *Journal of Family Practice,* 31, no. 6 (1990), 618–622.

98. Otto, C., and L.D. Platt, Fetal Growth and Development, *Obstetrics and Gynecology Clinics of North America,* 18, no. 4 (1991), 907–931.

99. Overcrowding, Environmental Risks Mark Many Children's Lives, *The Nation's Health,* July, 1993, 7.

100. Peoples-Sheps, M., E. Siegel, C. Suchindran, H. Origisa, A. Ware, and A. Barakat, Characteristics of Maternal Employment During Pregnancy: Effects on Low Birthweight, *American Journal of Public Health,* 81 (1991), 1007–1012.

101. Petitt, D., and C. Coleman, Cocaine and the Risk of Low Birth Weight, *American Journal of Public Health,* 80, no. 1 (1990), 25–28.

102. *Physicians' Desk Reference.* Oradel, NJ: Medical Economics, 1995.

103. Pitkin, R.M.. Calcium Metabolism in Pregnancy and the Perinatal Period, *American Journal of Obstetrics and Gynecology,* 151, no. 1(1985), 99–109.

104. Plomin, R., and R. Rende, Human Behavioral Genetics, in Rosenzsweig, R., and L. Porter, eds., *Annual Review of Psychology,* Vol. 42. Palo Alto, CA: Annual Reviews, 1991.

105. Rawstron, S.A., S. Jenkins, P.W. LiBlanchard, and K. Bromberg, Maternal and Congenital Syphilis in Brooklyn, N.Y.: Epidemiology, Transmission, and Diagnosis, *American Journal of Diseases of Children,* 147 (1993), 7727–7731.

106. Reid, R.M., Cultural and Medical Perspectives on Geophasia, *Medical Anthropology,* 13, no. 4 (1992), 337–351.

107. Reports Indicate U.S. Children Often Undernourished, Stressed Out, *The Nation's Health,* July (1993), 7.

108. Rogers, M., *Theoretical Basis of Nursing.* Philadelphia: F.A. Davis, 1970.

109. Rogers, M.F., et at., Acquired Immunodeficiency Syndrome in Children: Report of the Center for Disease Control National Surveillance, 1982 for 1985, *Pediatrics,* 79, no. 6 (1987), 1008–1012.

110 Saurel-Cubizolles, M.J., D. Subtil, and M. Kaminski, Is Preterm Delivery Still Related to Physical Working Conditions in Pregnancy? *Journal of Epidemiology and Community Health,* 45, no. 1 (1991), 29–34.

111. Schnoor, T.M., et al., Video Display Terminals and the Risk of Spontaneous Abortion, *New England Journal of Medicine,* 324, no. 11 (1991), 727–733.

112. Scott, G.B., et. al., Survival in Children With Perinatally Acquired Human Immunodeficiency Virus Type 1 Infection, *New England Journal of Medicine,* 321, no. 26 (1989), 1791–1796.

113. Scrimshaw, N., The New Paradigm of Public Health Nutrition, *American Journal of Public Health,* 85 (1995), 622–624.

114. Sheffield, P.A., D.E. Moore, L.F. Boigt, D. Scholes, S.P. Wang, J.T. Grayston, and J.R. Darling, The Associations Between *Chlamydia Trachomatis* Serology and Pelvic Damage in Women With Tubal Ectopic Gestations, *Fertility and Sterility,* 60 (1993), 870–876.

115. Sherman, K.J., J.R. Daling, A. Stergachis, N.S. Weiss, H.M. Foy, S.P. Wang, and J.T. Grayston, Sexually Transmitted Diseases and Tubal Pregnancy, *Sexually Transmitted Diseases,* 17, no. 3 (1990), 115–121.

116. Sherwen, L., M. Scoleveno, and C. Weingarten, *Nursing Care of the Childbearing Family,* Norwalk, CT: Appleton & Lange, 1991.

117. Simpson, J.L., Are Physical Activity and Employment Related to Preterm Birth and Low Birth Weight? *American Journal of Obstetrics and Gynecology,* 168, no. 4 (1993), 1231–1238.

118. Skovorc-Ranko, R., H. Lavola, P. St. Denis, M. Gagnou, R. Chicoine, M. Boucher, J. Guimond, and Y. Dontigny, Intrauterine Diagnosis of Cytomegalovirus and Rubella Infections by Amniocentesis, *Canadian Medical Association Journal,* 145 (1991), 649–664.

119. Smith, I.E., and C.D. Coles, Multilevel Intervention for Prevention of Fetal Alcohol Syndrome and Effects of Prenatal Alcohol Exposure, *Recent Developments in Alcoholism,* 9 (1991), 165–180.

120. Smith, K.J., and M.J. Eckardt, The Effects of Prenatal Alcohol on the Central Nervous System, *Recent Developments in Alcoholism,* 9 (1991), 151–164.

121. Spagnolo, A., Teratogenesis of Alcohol, *Annali dell' Instituto Suyperidi Sanitá,* 29, no. 1 (1993), 89–96.

122. Spitz, R., Hospitalism, in *The Psychoanalytic Study of the Child,* Vol. 1, New York: International University Press, 1945.

123. ———, Hospitalism: The Genesis of Psychiatric Conditions in Early Childhood, in Sze, W., ed., *Human Life Cycle,* New York: Jason Aronson, 1975, pp. 29–43.

124. ———, and K.M. Wolf, Anaclitic Depression: An Inquiry into the Genesis of Psychiatric Conditions in Early Childhood, in *The Psychoanalytic Study of the Child,* Vol. 2, New York: International University Press, 1946, pp. 313–342.

125. Starling, S.P., Syphilis in Infants and Young Children, *Pediatric Annals,* 23 (1994), 334–340.

126. Stellman, J.M., The Effects of Toxic Agents on Reproduction, *Occupation Health and Safety* (April 1979), 36–43.

127. Stenchover, M., Fetal Risks from Paternal Medication, *Journal of American Medical Association,* 211 (February 1970), 1382.

128. Strachan-Lindenberg, C., et al., A Review of the Literature on Cocaine Abuse in Pregnancy, *Nursing Research,* 40, no. 2 (1991), 69–75.

129. Sullivan, H.S., *Interpersonal Theory of Psychiatry.* New York: W.W. Norton, 1953.

130. Swain, S., S. Singh, B.D. Bhatia, S. Pandey, and N. Krishna, Maternal Hemoglobin and Serum Albumin and Fetal Growth, *Indian Pediatrics,* 31, no. 7 (1994), 777–782.

131. Theiler, P., A Vietnam Aftermath, *Common Cause Magazine,* (November–December 1984), 29–34.

132. Toubas, P., et al., Effects of Maternal Smoking and Caffeine Habits on Infantile Apnea: A Retrospective Study, *Pediatrics,* 78 (July 1986), 159–163.

133. Tracking the Second Storm, *Newsweek* (March 1994), 56–57.

134. Turner, J., and D. Helms, *Lifespan Development* (5th ed.). Ft. Worth: Harcourt Brace College, 1995.

135. U.S. Department of Health and Human Services, *The Health Consequences of Smoking: Nicotine Addiction. A Report of the Surgeon General.* Bethesda, MD: Centers for Disease Control, 1989.

136. U.S. Public Health Service Advisory Committee on Immunization Practices, Revised Recommendations on Rubella Vaccine, *Pediatrics,* 65, no. 6 (1980), 6.

137. Uphold, C., and M. Graham, *Clinical Guidelines in Family Practice* (2nd ed.), Gainesville, FL: Barmarrae Books, 1994.

138. Ville, Y., M. Lernez, E. Glowaczower, J.N. Robertson, and M.E. Ward, The Role of *Chlamydia Trachomatis* and *Neisseria Gonorrheae* in the Aetiology of Ectopic Pregnancy in Gabon, *British Journal of Obstetrics and Gynaecology,* 98 (1991), 1260–1266.

139. Von Bertalanffy, L., *General Systems Theory.* New York: George Braziller, 1968.

140. Wakefield, M.A., and W.R. Jones, Cognitive and Social Influences on Smoking Behavior During Pregnancy, *New Zealand Journal of Obstetrics and Gynecology,* 31, no. 3 (1991), 235–239.

141. West, J.R., and C.R. Goodlet, Teratogenic Effects of Alcohol on Brain Development, *Annals of Medicine,* 22 (1990), 319–325.

142. Wheeler, S.F., Substance Abuse During Pregnancy, *Primary Care in Office Practice,* 20, no. 1 (1993), 191–207.

143. Wilcos, A.J., Birth Weight and Perinatal Mortality: The Effect of Maternal Smoking, *American Journal of Epidemiology,* 137, no. 20 (1993), 1098–1104.

144. Williams, S., *Nutrition and Diet Therapy* (10th ed.). St. Louis: C.V. Mosby, 1995.

145. Windsor, R., C. Li, J. Lowe, L. Perkins, D. Ershoff, and T. Glynn, The Dissemination of Smoking Cessation Methods for Pregnant Women: Achieving the Year 2000 Objectives, *American Journal of Public Health,* 83 (1993), 173–178.

146. Windsor, R., J. Lowe, L. Perkins, D. Smith-Yoder, L. Artz, M. Crawford, K. Amburgy, and N. Boyd, Health Education for Pregnant Smokers: Its Behavioral Impact and Cost Benefit, *American Journal of Public Health,* 83 (1993), 201–206.

147. Wong, D., *Whaley and Wong's Nursing Care of Infants and Children* (5th ed.). St. Louis: C.V. Mosby, 1995.

148. Yazigi, R., R. Odem, and K. Polakoski, Demonstration of Specific Binding of Cocaine to Human Spermatozoa, *Journal American Medical Association,* 266, no. 14 (1991), 1956–1959.

149. Zemlickis, D., M. Lishner, P. Degendorfer, T. Panzarella, S.B. Sutcliffe, and G. Koren, Fetal Outcome After in Utero Exposure to Cancer Chemotherapy, *Archives of Internal Medicine,* 152, no. 3 (1992), 573–576.

150. Zhang, J., and J. Ratcliffe, Paternal Smoking and Birthweight in Shanghai, *American Journal of Public Health,* 83, no. 2 (1993), 207–210.

151. Zuckerman, B., et al., Effect of Maternal Marijuana and Cocaine Use on Fetal Growth, *New England Journal of Medicine,* 320 (1989), 762–768.

III

The Developing Person and Family: Infancy Through Adolescence

chapter seven

Assessment and Health Promotion for the Infant

A baby is God's opinion that the world should go on.

—Carl Sandberg

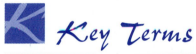

Key Terms

Neonate/newborn

Infant

Mother (parent[s])

Crisis

Attachment

Bonding

Engrossment

Binding-in

   Identification

   Claiming

   Polarization

Shaken baby syndrome

Psychological abuse, battering, or maltreatment

Autistic behavior

Anterior fontanel

Posterior fontanel

Acrocyanosis

Lanugo

Vernix caseosa

Milia

Hemangiomas

Mongolian spots

Jaundice

Physiologic jaundice

Desquamation

Umbilical cord

Circumcision

Phimosis

Caput succedaneum

Cephalohematoma

Brown fat

Surfactant

Meconium

Reflex

   Consummatory

   Avoidant

   Exploratory

   Social

   Attentional

Micrographia

Ptosis

Hydrocele

Hernia

Imperforate anus

Spina bifida

Amblyopia

Colic

Stools

Colostrum

Burping

Weaning

Phenylketonuria (PKU)

Immunizations

Herd immunity

Atopic dermatitis

Diaper dermatitis (rash)

Seborrheic dermatitis

Oral candidiasis (thrush)

Constipation

Iron deficiency anemia

Roseola infantum

Psychosocial development

Intelligence

Cognitive behavior

Speech awareness

Speech

Language

Undifferentiated cry	Basic trust	Adaptive mechanisms	Displacement
Cooing	Mistrust	Symbolization	Sexuality
Babbling	Body image	Condensation	Premature infant
Lalling	Self-concept	Incorporation	Congenital anomalies
Autistic			

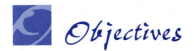

Objectives

Study of this chapter will enable you to:

1. Define terms and give examples of basic developmental principles pertinent to the neonate and infant.

2. Discuss the crisis of birth for the family, factors that influence parental attachment and family response, and your role in assisting the family to adapt to this crisis and perform their developmental tasks.

3. Describe the adaptive physiologic changes that occur at birth.

4. Assess the neonate's physical characteristics and the manner in which psychosocial needs begin to be filled.

5. Contrast and assess the physiologic, motor, cognitive, linguistic, emotional, and social characteristics and adaptive mechanisms of the infant.

6. Discuss and assess the nutritional, sleep, movement, and play needs and patterns and sexuality development of the infant.

7. Interpret the immunization schedule and other safety and health promotion measures for a parent.

8. Discuss your role in assisting parents to foster the development of trust and a positive self-concept and to nurture the infant physically.

9. State the developmental tasks for the infant and behavior that indicates that these tasks are being met.

10. Compare parental behavior toward the infant who thrives with parental behavior toward the infant who fails to thrive.

11. Discuss your role in promoting parental attachment and preventing maternal deprivation and child abuse.

12. Begin to implement appropriate intervention measures with parents and baby after delivery and during the first year of life.

This chapter discusses the normal growth and development of the baby during the first year of life, baby's effect on the family, and the family's influence on baby. Measures to promote his or her welfare that are useful in nursing practice and that can be taught to parents are described throughout the chapter.

In this chapter the term **neonate,** or **newborn,** refers to the *first 4 weeks of life;* **infant** refers to the *first 12 months* **Mother** or **parent(s)** *is* the term used to *denote the person(s) responsible for the child's care and long-term welfare.*

You can refer to an embryology and obstetric nursing book for detailed information on fetal development, prenatal changes, and the process of labor and delivery. This chapter builds on information presented in Chapters 4 and 6 and focuses on the developmental tasks of the infant and family after birth. The authors are aware

that some characteristics and developmental tasks of the infant and family described here may vary in other countries. Certainly the infant will be slower to develop some characteristics if he or she is born where there is famine, economic deprivation, political unrest or war, or devastation due to natural disaster. For example, for the child born in a refugee camp or between bombings, the parents have survival as the main task.

FAMILY DEVELOPMENT AND RELATIONSHIPS

The coming of the child is a **crisis,** a *turning point in the couple's life in which old patterns of living must be changed for new ways of living and new values* (53, 54, 65). The crisis may first be felt by the woman as she recognizes body changes and new emotional responses.

The crisis may relate to losing the slim figure; determining how long she can work if she is in a career or profession and whether or not she can balance working and childrearing; making spatial changes in the home or moving to a new home to accommodate the baby; and balancing the budget to meet additional expenses. The crisis will be less if the baby is wanted than if the couple had planned on having no children. But having a baby is always a crisis—a change.

The crisis is greater when the baby is not planned for or wanted. Do no assume that either the woman or her partner is happy about the pregnancy. The woman may not deliberately seek an abortion, but she may not eat or may exercise vigorously in an effort to maintain a slim figure; not gain too much weight, or deny the pregnancy. Sometimes the man fears becoming a father and the consequent responsibility and loss of freedom. As the woman's pregnancy progresses and as she looks more pregnant and activity must be curtailed, the man may withdraw emotionally, be apathetic about the baby, spend more time with male friends, work associates, or other women, and avoid preparation for the baby's arrival. In turn, the woman spends more time alone and feels increasingly rejected, abandoned, depressed, and angry. The woman may challenge the man's behavior, and more bickering, tension, resentment, and verbal (and sometimes physical) fighting may occur in the marital relationship. The couple may separate unless both the man and woman are helped to admit and work through their feelings and recommit their love for each other. It is important that such assistance be given—for the future of both the baby and the parents.

"Your life will never be the same again." A starry-eyed expectant couple often hears this phrase. Being caught up in the romantic adventure of pregnancy, these words may fall on deaf ears. What do these words really imply?

With the advent of parenthood, a couple is embarking on a journey from which there is no return. To put it simply, parents cannot quit. Most losses in today's world are reversible. If the marriage partner is lost, the individual can remarry; if a job is lost, a new position can be found. But an "I'll-try-it" attitude cannot be assumed toward parenthood. The child's birth brings a finality to many highly valued privileges and a permanence of responsibilities.

The young couple who has enjoyed an intense relationship suddenly finds a not-always-so-welcome onlooker and intruder. Gone for many years are sleeping late on Saturday mornings, last-minute social invitations or plans for a weekend trip, spontaneous sex, quiet meals by candlelight, an orderly house, and naps when desired. Of course, some of these activities can still be accomplished but never as freely as before. What was

previously taken for granted now becomes a luxury. The "childhood" of parents comes to a screeching halt as the infant's needs take precedence.

Going to work, to visit friends, or even to shop is no easy task. Even a few hours away from home means making sure you have everything baby needs—bottle, food, pacifier, a few toys, a clothing change, and more than enough diapers. In addition to this armful, an infant seat or stroller must also be packed, By the time baby is dressed and everything is packed, Mom may want a nap more than anything else. Making sure baby is wearing a dry diaper before the final exit through the door becomes more important than the finishing touches of makeup or putting on the special jewelry for the outfit. If there are several small children to care for in addition to baby, the planning and effort are compounded, and older brothers and sisters can help with various tasks only to a certain point.

The intensity of the newcomer's demands may call for massive changes in lifestyle. Life changes have been correlated with illness susceptibility in the Social Readjustment Scale by Holmes and Rahe (54). When enough life changes occur within a year and add up to more than 300 points, trouble may lie ahead. Changes that may be connected with the addition of a family member total up to an ominous 397, as shown by the following list (53, 54). For some the score may be higher.

Pregnancy	40
Sex difficulties	39
Gain of new family member	39
Change in financial state	38
Change in number of arguments with spouse	35
Trouble with in-laws	29
Wife begins or stops work	26
Change in living conditions	25
Revision of personal habits	24
Change in recreation	19
Change in church activities	19
Change in social activities	18
Change in sleeping habits	16
Change in number of family get-togethers	15
Change in eating habits	15
	397

Whether perceived as positive or negative, change always involves a sense of loss of the familiar, for the way it used to be. The vacuum created by the loss is a painful one and one for which parents are usually ill-prepared. The couple's life will never again be "normal" as they once knew it, but together the family now needs to find a "new normal."

If pregnancy and parenting create a crisis for a couple who want a baby, they are even more upheaving for the adolescent or for the woman who is the single-parent family—either unmarried, or, if married, left by the husband or father to face pregnancy, birth, and child rearing alone. This adolescent/woman needs the support of and help from at least one other person during this period. A parent, relative, or friend can be a resource. Often the support and help of a number of people are needed. As a nurse, you may be the primary source of support. Your empathetic listening, acceptance, practical hints for better self-care and baby care, and general availability can make a real difference in the outcome of the pregnancy and in the mother's ability to parent and to handle future crises. Referral to other resources and self-help groups such as Coping With Overall Parenting Experience (COPE) and Parents Without Partners or to a counselor may also be of great help to the mother.

Growth and Development of Parents

An increasing number of people are not prepared either intellectually or emotionally for family life because of the lack of nurturing or because of the difficult family life they experienced in childhood. Creating and maintaining a family unit are difficult in today's society. Many occupations demand travel, frequent change of residence, and working on Sundays and holidays, the traditional family days. The rapid pace of life and available opportunities interfere with family functions. The close-knit interdependence of the old family unit is being replaced with a group of individuals whose lives seem merely thrown together.

Expectations for self and others have increased. For example, the woman may be striving for success in several areas. No longer is being a wife and mother enough: many women seek a career as well. All these expectations conflict with a strong family life, for children demand parents become other-centered instead of self-centered.

Despite today's difficulties in maintaining a family unit, the norm still exists to have children. Thus, many couples wander rather naively into the developmental crisis of parenthood. In a culture in which adolescence may last until the midtwenties, most young people are just getting used to being called Ma'am or Sir when suddenly they become Mom and Dad. Thus, along with the developmental tasks of finding identity and intimacy may be superimposed the task of being generative as well.

Pregnancy is preparation for the birth event, whereas parenting is a process that continues for many years. Becoming a parent involves grieving the loss of one's own childhood and former lifestyle. The person must be in touch with and be able to express and work through feelings of loss before he or she can adapt and move on to a higher level of maturation. Being aware of the tremendous influence of parents on their children's development, parents may feel challenged to become the best persons they are capable of being. New parents may need to develop a confidence that they do not feel, an integrity that has been easy to let slide, and values that can tolerate being scrutinized. To grow and develop as a parent, the person needs to make peace with his or her past so that unresolved conflicts are not inflicted on the child.

After a baby joins the family, a number of problems must be worked through. The mother must deal with the separation from a symbiotic relationship with the baby. The reality of child care and managing a household may be a disillusionment after exposure to the American ideals inculcated by the mass media and advertising.

One of the potential problem areas that you can explore with parents is that of reestablishing a mutually satisfying sexual relationship, which is not a simple psychological process but has intricate psychological overtones for man and woman. You may also need to address the couple's desire for family planning (see Table 12–3 for information on contraceptive measures). Sexual relationships usually decrease during pregnancy, childbirth, and the postpartum period. By 6 weeks after birth the woman's pelvis is back to normal; lochia has ceased; involution is complete; and physically she is ready for an active sex life. But the mother may be so absorbed in and fatigued by the challenges and responsibilities of motherhood that the father is pushed into the background. Father may feel in competition with baby, resenting both the baby and his wife.

Either one may take initiative in renewing the role of lover, in being sexually attractive to the other. The woman can do this by getting a new hairdo or stylish clothes for the now slimmer outward figure. Inwardly, she can strengthen flabbly perineal muscles through prescribed exercise. Patience on the part of the husband is also necessary, for if an episiotomy was done before delivery, healing continues for some time, and the memory of pain in the area may cause the woman involuntarily to tense the perineal muscles and wish to forego intercourse. Happy couples who have a sound philosophy and communication system soon work out such problems, including the fact that the baby's needs will sometimes interrupt intimacy. For couples whose earlier sex life was unsatisfactory and who do not work together as a team, such problems may be hard to surmount. The woman may prolong nursing, complain of fatigue, ill health, or pain. The man may find other outlets.

Husband and wife must reestablish effective communication so that they can share feelings of pride, joy, anxiety, insecurity, and frustrations of early parenthood, avoid eclipsing their marriage by the new family roles, and understand the involvement of the multiple roles of mate, parents, and persons. Your support, suggestions, and assistance in helping the couple seek and accept help from family and friends foster their ability to manage.

Given the whole realm of stresses and life changes associated with a baby's birth, it is understandable that at least initially parenting is at best a bittersweet experience. Parents feel strong ambivalence and what Angela Barron McBride (72) calls "normal crazy" thoughts and feelings toward this child whom they have together created.

The following stress factors may be used in your assessment to predict the likelihood of postpartum difficulties (122):

- Woman is having her first baby (primipara).
- No relatives are available to help with baby care.
- Complications occurred during pregnancy.
- Woman's mother is dead.
- Woman is ill apart from pregnancy.
- Woman was ill during pregnancy.
- Woman has distant relationship or conflict with own mother.
- Male partner is often away from home or not involved with pregnancy or childrearing.
- Woman has no previous experience with babies.

Postpartum difficulties are also more likely if the parent is an adolescent or has suffered child abuse. The more past and present stresses, the more difficulty the woman has in coping with the postpartum experience.

Parenting is a risky process. It involves facing the unknown with faith because no one can predict the outcome when the intricacies of human relationships are involved. Parents grow and develop by taking themselves and their child one day at a time and by realizing the joy that can be part of those crazy, hectic early weeks and months. The feelings of joy and involvement increase as the parent–child attachment is cemented.

Because establishing this attachment is crucial to the long-term nurturing of the child and parental interest in the child, the process is explored in depth to assist you in assessment and intervention.

Infant–Parent Attachment

Attachment *is an affectional tie between two persons.* Thus, it is *a human phenomenon characterized by certain behaviors.* It is described as a *close, reciprocal relationship between two people that involves contact with and proximity to another that endures over time.* It is only when these behaviors are directed to one or a few persons rather than to many persons that the behaviors indicate attachment (Fig. 7–1). Health care professionals often use the term *attachment* to describe behaviors between caregivers and their infants. Authors and investigators have devoted considerable attention to and interest in the formation of early maternal–infant and, more recently, paternal–infant affectional ties. Authors often use the term *attachment* interchangeably with the term *bonding*. **Bonding** first appeared in behavioral research and referred to the *sensitive period for the establishment of a tie between animal mothers and their offspring.* The term now *refers to the initial maternal feeling and attachment behavior immediately following delivery.* **Engrossment** is the term authors use to describe the *father's initial paternal response to the baby.* Interest in the concept of bonding went beyond the maternal–infant dyad to consider the father–infant dyad. This concept developed in a manner of thinking parallel to the development of the concept of maternal–infant bonding (2, 11, 48, 61, 89).

Rubin describes the beginning of the mother–child relationship as similar to the beginning of any new rela-

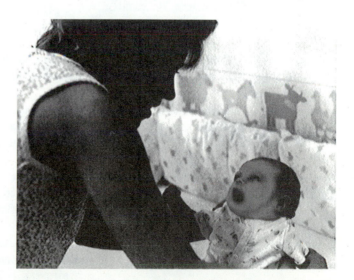

Figure 7–1. Mother–infant attachment develops mutually over the first year of life. *(From Sherwen, L.N., M.A., Scoloveno, and C.T. Weingarten, Nursing Care of the Childbearing Family. Stamford, CT: Appleton & Lange, 1991, p. 44.)*

tionship. She writes that "identification of the partner in the relationship is a universal prerequisite. Even before any interaction occurs, there are certain relevant pieces of information to be obtained about the newcomer—sex, condition and size. Each member must obtain introductory information before any interaction can occur" (92). Table 7–1 outlines some behaviors of the infant, mother, and father in the typical order of progression in establishing this initial relationship (2, 11, 12, 48, 91–97, 111).

Recent investigations and review articles conclude that there is no firm scientific evidence supportive of immediate parent–infant bonding (47, 82). But Palkovitz found that media presentations, anecdotal reports, and survey data indicate that a majority of lay respondents expressed a strong belief not only in the phenomenon of bonding, but also in the existence of scientific evidence to support this concept. In view of the general public's beliefs concerning bonding, health care workers, especially childbirth educators, must present scientific information in an objective manner to decrease the possibility that parents will experience guilt or disappointment concerning their role in the intrapartum or postpartum period. It is important that childbirth educators inform parents that early contact with the infant in the postpartum period can be a fulfilling, but neither necessary nor sufficient, experience (82, 83).

Some research shows that all mothers do not initially follow the sequence of handling that is described in most of the literature and in Table 7–1. Some mothers initially use palms or arms to handle the infant and then their fingers to explore the infant. Often mothers simultaneously use fingers and palms and then arms and trunk to explore and hold the baby. Some mothers may be initially hesitant or awkward in touching or holding the baby, or hold the baby differently than most mothers, and yet feel very maternal. These differences should be considered in assessment of maternal bonding and attachment (113). Realize also that there are cultural differences in expression of attachment. In some cultures, the parents of the woman or the man take care of the newborn and mother for a designated time. Further, out of respect for the elderly, the new parents will do whatever their parents tell them to do, regardless of what professionals tell the young parents.

The state of the infant is a strong predictor of the relative frequency with which fathers display interactional behavior, affection, and comfort toward the infant. Very young crying infants are comforted or shown affectional behavior. One study found that fathers are most likely to stimulate by touch those infants who are awake but not crying. Fathers are as likely to talk in a stimulating manner to crying as noncrying and to sleeping as awake infants. Perhaps fathers perceive talking

TABLE 7–1. INFANT–PARENT ATTACHMENT BEHAVIORS

Infant	Mother	Father
Reflexly looks into mother's face, *establishes eye-to-eye contact* or *"face tie"*; molds body to mother's body when held	*Reaches* for baby; *holds high against breast–chest–shoulder area*; handles baby smoothly	Has great *interest in baby's face and notes eyes*
Vocalizes, cries, and *stretches out arms* in response to mother's voice; responds to mother's voice with *"dance"* or *rhythmic movements*	Talks softly in *high-pitched voice* and with intense interest to baby; puts baby face-to-face with her (*en face position*); eye contact gives baby sense of identity to mother	*Desires to touch, pick up, and hold baby;* cradles baby securely; shows more fingertip touching and smiling to male baby; has more eye contact with infant delivered by forceps or cesarean section
Roots, licks, then *sucks* mother's nipple if in contact with mother's breast; cries, smiles	*Touches* baby's extremities; examines, strokes, massages, and kisses baby shortly after delivery; puts baby to breast if permitted; oxytocin and prolactin released	*Looks for distinct features;* thinks newborn resembles self; perceives baby as beautiful in spite of newborn characteristics
Reflexly embraces, clambers, clings, using hands, feet, head, and mouth to maintain body contact	*Calls baby by name;* notes desirable traits; *expresses pleasure* toward baby; *attentive* to reflex actions of grunts and sneezes	*Feels elated,* bigger, proud after birth; has strong *desire to protect and care for child*
Odor of mother distinguished by breastfeeding baby by fifth day	*Recognizes odor* of own child by third or fourth day	

NOTE: Similar behaviors are seen with a premature baby but the timing will vary.

as less soothing to crying infants than touch and less disturbing than touch to sleeping infants. Infant state behaviors are strongly related to affectional paternal responses, indicating that new fathers begin early to read and respond to infant cues (65).

Studies in bonding and attachment have been done primarily on middle-class, reasonably well-educated Caucasians. Bonding and attachment behaviors, especially for the male, could be different in other racial and cultural groups. Some cultures emphasize the mother as caretaker of the infant; the bond or attachment between father and child is less overt and may be emphasized later in childhood.

One study indicates that the first hour after birth is a critical time for stimulating attachment feelings and bonding in the parents, as then the baby tends to have eyes open, gazes around, has stronger sucking reflexes, cries more, and shows more physical activity than in subsequent hours (48). Other investigators found a positive relationship between the first holding of the infant and the development of attachment feelings, but indicated attachment began when the infant was first held regardless of how long after delivery the holding occurred. (75).

Some authors believe that in addition to causing increased alertness in the baby, effective maternal–infant bonding can promote baby's physical health: (1) transference of maternal nasal and respiratory flora to baby may prevent him from acquiring hospital strains of infectious organisms; (2) maternal body heat is a reliable source of heat for the newborn; and (3) regular breastfeedings can pass on the antibodies IgA and T and B lymphocytes to baby to protect against enteric pathogens (61).

Binding-in is the term Rubin (93, 94, 96, 97) uses to describe the *maternal–child relationship as a process that is active, intermittent, and accumulative over a period of 12 to 15 months.* Maternal identity is essential for the binding-in process, and both maternal identity and binding-in are either enhanced or inhibited by the infant's behavior and society. The process involves:

- Identification of the infant by the mother as part of self and belonging to self
- Claiming the child as her own emotionally and physically
- Polarization or separating the infant from the unity of self and fetus

Maternal binding-in is stimulated and augmented by fetal movement during pregnancy and the physical needs of the newborn. After birth, fantasies about the child are replaced by an object to see, touch, hear, smell, and care for, which organizes material behavior and attitudes. Sex, size, and condition of the infant are critical to the material response. Complete **identification** occurs when the *mother knows by looking, touching, hearing, or smelling that the child is well or unwell, hungry or satisfied, comfortable or in distress.* **Claiming** *occurs with the mother's commitment to the child in labor and delivery and is seen in the pleasure with the birth of the child.* Claiming also occurs by association with significant others in the social environment who claim the infant and her. **Polarization,** *separating from the symbiotic relationship with the fetus, begins with labor and delivery.* Gradually the woman realizes the baby is not inside of her. The infant is held, nurtured, and compared to self and family members but is increasingly seen as a separate, unique individual and less as an extension of self and her own body image. Family life is reorganized; the baby is included in family activities. Over the period of the first year the mother can let go of the child as he or she gains motor, social, and emotional competence. The psychological loosening allows the mother also to give the child more physical space (93, 94, 96, 97).

Development of attachment between parent and baby continues through infancy. It involves emotional, cognitive, and socialization processes: loving through cuddling, touching, stroking, kissing, cooing and talking to, laughing, playing with, and reinforcing and teaching baby. Such contact should be consistent and done while caring physically for baby. The touching, cooing, talking, and laughing can also be focused on baby while mother (or father) is preparing a meal, doing a household task, or waiting in a grocery line. The parent's voice across the room can also soothe and promote attachment. Further, just as the parent may need to learn to respond to the infant, sometimes the child needs prompting to be responsive to the parent and to signal needs and not just wait for every need to be automatically met.

Factors Influencing Maternal Attachment

Motherly feelings do not necessarily accompany biological motherhood. Various factors affect the mother's attachment and caretaking. Variables that are difficult or impossible to change include the woman's level of emotional maturity, how she was reared, what her culture encourages her to do, relationships with her family and partner, experience with previous pregnancies, and planning for and events during the course of this pregnancy (16, 61, 93, 95, 122).

Deterrents to adequate mothering include the mother's own immaturity or lack of mothering, stress situations, fear of rejection from significant people, loss of a loved one, financial worries, lack of a supportive partner, and even the sex and appearance of the child.

Separating mother and infant the first few days of life, depersonalized care by professionals, rigid hospital routines, and the current practice of early discharge from the hospital without adequate help also interfere with establishing attachment and maternal behaviors (2, 6, 12, 44, 71, 122). Assess for these deterrents. Your nurturing of the mother and helping her seek additional help may offset the negative impact of these factors.

Nurturing will be essential for the mother who returns home within the 24-hour period after delivery. She will be exhausted, sore, and possibly overwhelmed with emotion and responsibility. The home health nurse is one support system; relatives or friends will also be needed for help. The nurse's assessment is critical related to the mother's physical and emotional status and need for information about child care. The nurse's assessment is also essential to determine status of the newborn. The first 72 hours of baby's life is a significant period of transition and stabilization, and also a time when malformations or cardiorespiratory or feeding problems are evidenced. Infection in both mother and baby may occur in this initial period.

Parenting skills can be manifested in various ways. Although eye contact, touch, and cuddling are important, love can be shown by a tender, soft voice and loving gazes. Observe other indications of warm parenting feelings:

- Calls the baby by name
- Expresses enjoyment of the baby and indicates that the baby is attractive or has other positive characteristics
- Looks at the baby and into baby's eyes
- Talks to the baby in a loving voice
- Takes safety precautions for the baby
- Responds to the baby's cues for attention or physical care

Factors Influencing Paternal Attachment

Fatherly feelings do not necessarily accompany fatherhood. Bonding and attachment feelings in the father appear related to various factors: general level of education, participation in prenatal classes, sex of infant, role concept, attendance at delivery, type of delivery, early contact, and feeding method for baby (48, 111).

Support from the mother is most effective in reducing stress levels in expectant fathers; support from others is critical only if the expectant woman cannot be supportive. This may be because intimacy and self-disclosure for men are maintained primarily in the partner relationship. For the expectant woman, support from both the partner and others is critical in coping with stress, perhaps because women are socialized to value and depend on social relations to a greater extent than men (19).

Father is increasingly recognized as an important person to the infant and young child, not only as a breadwinner but also as a nurturer. Lack of a father figure can cause developmental difficulties for the child. Just as the mother is not necessarily endowed with nurturing feelings, the father is not necessarily lacking nurturing feelings. Some fathers seem to respond better to this role than their spouses (39, 65, 66, 75, 98).

The man who nurtures his children may meet some resistance in a society in which this role is sometimes considered unmanly, although social attitudes are changing. One father who was taking the basic child-raising responsibilities while his wife pursued the major family career was ostracized when he appeared at a meeting calling for "scout mothers." No women sat with him until he initiated conversation explaining why he was there. Occasionally the mother herself cannot understand when the father seems to cherish the nurturing role. She feels that her position is threatened, her husband is not acting "as a man," or he loves the children more than he loves her. Actually, the man who is allowed to express these feelings often simultaneously develops an even closer feeling for his wife.

Behavior Characteristic of Parental Difficulty in Establishing Attachment

Realize that parents tend to project their own feelings onto their child, turning the child into a figure from their own past. Negative feelings in the parent can create a dysfunctional relationship with the child.

Note the methods of relating to and holding the infant that would indicate the parent's *difficulty in establishing attachment* (61, 93, 95, 105, 122).

- Maintains little or no eye contact with baby
- Does not touch baby, or picks up baby at times to meet own needs
- Does not support baby's head
- Holds baby at a distance, at arm's length after initial visits, loosely, or not at all
- Appears disinterested in baby, is preoccupied with something else when baby is present, and has a flat, fixed facial expression or unconvincing smile in response to your enthusiasm about baby
- Perceives baby as unattractive or looking like someone who is disliked
- Talks or coos to baby little or not at all
- Has passive response to baby; allows baby to be placed in arms rather than reaching out to baby

- Calls baby "it" rather than saying "my baby" or calling baby by name
- Notes defects or undesirable traits in baby, even if baby is normal, or is convinced baby is abnormal
- Avoids talking about baby, even when someone else initiates the topic
- Expresses dissatisfaction with or revulsion about care of baby
- Ignores baby's communications of cries, grunts, sneezes, and yawns
- Gets upset when baby's secretions, feces, or urine touch body or clothes; perceives care of baby as revolting
- Readily gives baby to someone else
- Does not take adequate safety precautions with baby (e.g., in relation to diapering, feeding, covering baby, or baby's movements)
- Handles the baby roughly, even after the baby has eaten or vomited
- Gives inappropriate responses to baby's needs such as over- or underfeeding, over- or underhandling
- Thinks baby does not love him or her
- Expresses dislike of self, finds attribute in baby that is disliked in self
- Complains of being too tired to take care of baby
- Expresses fears that baby might die of a minor illness

You may not observe all these behaviors in the mother, initially or in the mother or father later, but a combination of several should alert you to actual or potential difficulty with being a parent.

Three components must be present before child abuse occurs: (1) the parents must have the potential for abuse; (2) there must be a special child; and (3) there must be a crisis or series of crises. The cycle of abuse can be prevented or treated by intervening with one of these components (122).

Parents Anonymous, a nationwide organization of and for adults with child abuse problems, recognizes six forms of child abuse: (1) physical abuse, (2) physical neglect, (3) emotional abuse, (4) emotional neglect, (5) verbal abuse, and (6) sexual abuse (122).

Be aware of the parent who has such *difficulty with attachment that maltreatment or abuse of the child results*. Types of abuse, signs and symptoms of the abused child, and characteristics of the child who suffers abuse, neglect, or material deprivation and characteristics of the abusing parent are presented in Chapter 6. Chapter 4 also describes characteristics and behaviors of the parent who has difficulty with parenting.

More than 2 million children are the victims of abuse and neglect each year; death rates from abuse continue to escalate. In 1995, an estimated 142,000 children were seriously injured and almost 20,000 permanently disabled because of abuse. Many of these children were infants. A common form of physical abuse in

▶ SHAKEN BABY SYNDROME

At Risk

Infants and small children because of physical characteristics: heavy head, weak neck muscles, soft and rapidly growing brain, thin skull wall, lack of control over head and neck, lack of mobility

Clinical Presentation

- Unexplained seizures
- Vomiting, associated with drowsiness or lethargy
- Irritability
- Listlessness
- Bradycardia
- Hypothermia
- Unexplained bulging or full fontanels, or large head circumference
- Apnea
- Coma
- Retinal hemorrhage
- Subdural hematoma
- Mild form may be mistaken for viral illness.

Risk Factors

- Behavioral difficulties of parent; unconscious desire for role reversal when parent expects child to provide love and nurture.
- Immaturity or illness in parent, inability to manage normal crying and colic other than with anger and abuse
- Addiction in mother, resulting in drug-addicted baby who is more irritable and difficult to manage
- Lack of knowledge about child behavior, how to handle baby, and danger of shaking
- Male sex, caregiver at time of incident (Male may or may not be related to baby.)

Prevention

- Education about parenting, infant, and child care.
- Education about dangers of shaking child
- Stress management education and counseling
- Prenatal classes, support groups after baby is born

infancy is the **Shaken Baby Syndrome**, *a complex of symptoms that results from vigorous shaking of the child that produces acceleration and deceleration forces in the head and consequent damage.* Butler describes specific pathophysiologic changes. Shaken Baby Syndrome on the previous page summarizes risk factors, manifestations, and prevention strategies (21).

Garbarino, Guttmann, and Seeley (43) describe types of psychological abuse, battering, or maltreatment. **Psychological abuse, battering or maltreatment** is a *deliberate pattern of attack by a parent or an adult on a child's developmental status, sense of self, or so-cial competence.* As the infant fears loss of support, sudden or unexpected motion, and looming objects, especially with loud noise or bright lights, shaking the baby can constitute psychological as well as physical abuse.

Parental Behaviors Characteristic of Psychological Maltreatment of the Infant presents parental behaviors that are characteristic of psychological abuse or maltreatment. As a result of maltreatment, the child becomes vulnerable to negative forces in the broader social environment, does not develop a sense of trust, and becomes emotionally, socially, and sometimes physically ill (43).

Garbarino, Guttmann, and Seeley (43) discuss strategies and tools for identification and intervention with the family, individual child, and institutional network of social services.

Helberg (51) gives specific criteria for documentation of child abuse. The article by Mittelman, Mittelman, and Wetu (76) shows pictures of both subtle and obvious abuse and gives detailed and specific description for clues that will assist you in assessing the child. Reporting child abuse is required of the professional. Each state has a central agency to follow up reported cases.

► **PARENTAL BEHAVIORS CHARACTERISTIC OF PSYCHOLOGICAL MALTREATMENT OF THE INFANT**

Rejecting

- Refuses to accept the child's attachment behavior or spontaneous overtures
- Refuses to return smiles and vocalizations

Isolating

- Denies child the experience of enduring patterns of interaction
- Leaves the child in its room unattended for long periods
- Denies access to the child by interested others

Terrorizing

- Exposes the child consistently and deliberately to intense stimuli or frequent change of routine
- Teases, scares, or gives extreme or unpredictable response to child's behavior

Ignoring

- Fails to respond to infant's spontaneous behavior that forms basis for attachment
- Does not respond to infant's smiles; vocalizations, or developing competence and changing skill

Corrupting

- Reinforces bizarre habits
- Creates alcohol or drug addictions
- Reinforces the child for oral sexual contact

From Garbarino, J., E. Guttmann, and J. Seeley, The Psychologically Battered Child: Strategies for Identification, Assessment, and Intervention. San Francisco: Jossey-Bass, 1987. Copyright 1986 by Jossey-Bass, Inc., Publishers.

Personalizing Nursing Care to Promote Attachment

Certain interventions directed to the parents will assist them to develop attachment with the infant:

- Call the child, mother, and father by their names during your care.
- Inquire about the mother's well-being; too often all the focus is on the baby. She is in a receptive state and must be emotionally and physically cared for.
- Father also needs nurturance before he can show caring and be helpful to mother and baby.
- Make favorable comments about the infant's progress.
- Compliment the mother on her intentions or ability to comfort, feed, or identify her baby's needs. Speak of the pleasure baby shows in response to the parent's ministrations.
- Reassure parents that positive changes in baby are a result of their care, and avoid judgmental attitudes or guilt statements.

Interventions *that support, teach, and counsel parents about how to* **promote attachment** *and optimum infant stimulation follow*:

- Encourage both parents to cuddle, look at, and talk to the baby; if necessary, demonstrate how to stroke, caress, and rock baby.
- Encourage parents to be prompt and consistent in answering the infant's cry.
- Assist parents in gaining confidence in responding effectively to baby's cry through recognizing the meaning of the cry and using soothing measures such as rocking, redundant sounds, and swaddling.
- Explain the infant's interactive abilities and help the mother develop awareness of her own initial effective responses to the newborn's behavior.
- Explain the basis of early infant learning as the discovery of associations, connections, and relationships between self and repeated occurrences. Explore how to provide variety; a gradually increasing level of stimulus complexity, sights, sounds, smells, movements, positions, temperatures, and pressure all provide learning opportunities and opportunities for emotional, perceptual, social, and physical development.
- Call attention to baby and those behaviors that indicate developmental responsiveness such as reflex movements, visual following, smiling, raising chin off bed, rolling over, and sitting alone. Pupil dilation in the presence of the parent begins at approximately 4 weeks of age. During the first few weeks of life baby prefers the human face to other visual images.
- Differentiate between contact stimulation and representative behaviors present in fetal life. Pressure and touch sensation is present a few months before birth; thus the newborn responds well to touch and gentle pressure. Rooting and hand–mouth activity occur in fetal life and is a major adaptive activity after birth.
- Emphasize the importance of visual and auditory skills for developing social behaviors during the first 2 months of life.
- Encourage mutual eye contact between parent and baby; all infant's efforts to vocalize should be reinforced. Eye contact between the parent and baby increases during the first 3 months of life and is soon accompanied by other social responses—smiling and vocalization.
- Encourage regular periods of affectionate play when the infant is alert and responsive. Mother and father may pick up and hold the baby close, encourage visual following and smiling, and talk to the infant, repeating sounds. Rhythm and repetition are enjoyed. Often baby is most alert after a daytime feeding.
- Promote awareness in other family members of baby's competencies so that they can also respond to and reinforce the infant.

Several tools are designed to help you assess baby, mother and mother's attitude toward baby as you continue their care (15, 122). The *Neonatal Behavioral Assessment Scale* points out unique characteristics and strengths of the neonate (15). For example, you can demonstrate to the parents how the newborn can follow the direction of the mother's soft high-pitched voice as she moves from the line of baby's vision.

The *Blank Infant Tenderness Scale* can be used to measure mother's perceptions of infant tenderness needs and ability to give physical and emotional nurturance (9). The *Dyadic Interaction Code* is a tool for studying over time the interaction process between mother and newborn. There is rhythmicity in the mother–infant interaction, associated with synchronous interactions, heightened levels of positive affect, and extended periods of attention. The baby who is preterm, not healthy, or suffering from congenital anomalies may not be as responsive to the mother, thus interrupting rhythmicity and attachment (24). The tool can be used for several visits, combining repeated observations and interviews, to obtain an accurate and comprehensive assessment. As you pinpoint problems, you should be able to intervene or direct the parents to a helpful resource.

Incorporate the parents' cultural beliefs, values, and attitudes into your nursing care and modern health care practices whenever possible (105, 122). Maintaining important cultural traditions is one way to individualize care. Satz (100) gives specific examples of how she incorporated the values of the Navajo in promoting attachment. Specific traditions may extend to naming or bathing the baby, prenatal and postnatal care of mother, how to hold or dress baby, inclusion or exclusion of father from the delivery, and roles of various family members. Be sensitive to the preferences of clients who represent a culture different from your own. Listen to and observe carefully their requests. Listen to what is not said but is implied. Suggest rather than advise or direct when you teach.

Listen attentively for information and signs that give you clues to the parents' feelings about themselves, where they are in their own developmental growth, who they rely on for strength, their ideas about child discipline, and their expectations of the new child. As you see weaknesses or gaps in necessary information, you can instruct. If your approach is right, the parents will recognize you as a helpful friend. Mothers are receptive to your information and to your reinforcement of the mother's mothering skills.

Help parents realize that soon the complete focus on mother–father–new baby will be gone. Other roles will be reestablished: husband, wife, employer or employee, student, daughter, son, friend. The new parents will have to allow for all aspects of their personalities to function again. Baby will have to fit in.

While you are caring for baby, you will no doubt feel great satisfaction. Remember, however, that the child belongs to the parents; this is not *your* baby. Do not become so involved that through your actions you push aside the parents and cause them to feel ineffective.

Baby's Influence on Parents

Some babies have a high activity level and warm up easily to the parent; some are quiet, withdrawn, with a low activity level; and various other mixtures of activity level and temperament exist. The infant's dominant reaction pattern to new situations manifests an innate temperament, and the temperament affects the reactions of others, especially the parents. They in turn will mold baby's reaction pattern (28, 58, 114).

It is easy to love a lovable baby, but parents have to work harder with babies who are not highly responsive. Assess the reactions between baby and parents, as the style of child care that will develop has its basis here. A highly active mother who expects an intense reaction may have a hard time mothering a low-activity, quiet baby because she may misinterpret the baby's behavior, feel rejected, and in turn reject the child. Baby will be denied the stimulation necessary for development. If the mother is withdrawn, quiet, and unexpressive and has a high-activity baby, she may punish the baby for normal energetic or assertive behavior and ignore the bids for affection and stimulation. The child needs to feel his or her behavior will produce an effect or he or she will stop contacting the parents. Extreme parental rejection or lack of reaction causes the syndrome of neglect and deprivation, emotional illness, and **autistic behavior,** characterized by *self-absorption, isolation from the world, obsession with sameness, repetitive behavior, and lack of language communication with others* (8, 78). An assertive child may become controlling with an indecisive mother and not learn that others also have needs and rights. If baby is controlled by mother, he or she cannot develop trust, independence or ability to cope with persons on equal terms. If the mother overanticipates the child's needs, the child becomes passive and dependent.

Help parents understand the *mutual response* between baby and themselves, and help them learn to read the baby's signals and to give consistent signals to the baby. All parents feel incompetent and despairing at times when they are unable to understand the child's cues and meet needs, but if self-confidence is consistently lacking, the parent's despair may turn to anger, rejection, and abuse.

Expansion of Intrafamily Relationships

Grandparents-to-be and other relatives frequently become more involved with the parents-to-be, bringing gifts and advice, neither of which is necessarily desired. Yet their gifts and supportive presence can be a real help if the grandparents respect the independence of the couple, if the couple has resolved their earlier adolescent rebellion and dependency conflicts, and if the grandparents' advice does not conflict with the couple's philosophy or the doctor's advice. The couple and grandparents should collaborate rather than compete. Grandparents should be reminded not to take over the situation, and the couple's autonomy should be encouraged in that they can listen to the various pieces of advice, evaluate the statements, and then as a unit make their own decision. In addition, parents should refrain from expecting the grandparents to be built-in babysitters and to rescue them from every problem. Grandparents usually enjoy brief rather than prolonged contact with baby care. For the single parent, the grandparents or other relatives can be a major source of emotional and financial help and can provide help with child care.

You may assist the parent(s) in working with grandparents, resolving feelings of either being controlled or not adequately helped, understanding grandparents' feelings, accepting help, and avoiding excessive demands.

In some cultures the maternal grandmother has a major role in care of the pregnant and postpartum daughter and in care of the infant. The grandmother may give advice about nutrition, self-care, or baby care to the daughter; however, the advice may be contrary to scientific and medical knowledge and practices. Establish rapport with both the grandmother and the pregnant woman or the mother. Respect the role of the grandmother. Often the advice she gives is culturally based—the practices have maintained the group for centuries. The practices may be carried out along with modern-day health and medical practices. If the advice is truly harmful to the mother or baby, your rapport, nonjudgmental approach, and well-timed, low-key teaching to the grandmother may help her to accept the teaching you direct to the pregnant woman/mother. Indeed, if either or both grandparents are considered the head of the household, direct your attention initially to them and direct your teaching to them. Initial or exclusive focus on their daughter is likely to alienate them so that they discontinue coming for care or become resistive and not allow their daughter to carry out your teaching.

PHYSIOLOGIC CONCEPTS

Neonate — Physical Characteristics

The neonatal period of infancy includes the critical transition from parasitic fetal existence to physiologic independence. The normal newborn is described in the following pages (28, 34, 58, 105, 114, 122). Transition begins at birth with the first cry. Air is sucked in to inflate the lungs. Complex chemical changes are initiated in the cardiorespiratory system so that the baby's heart and lungs can assume the burden of oxygenating the body. The foramen ovale closes during the first 24 hours; the ductus arteriosus closes after several days. For the first time, baby experiences light, gravity, cold, and firm touch.

The newborn is relatively resistant to stress of anoxia and can survive longer in an oxygen-free atmosphere than an adult. The reason is unknown, as are the long-term effects of *mild* oxygen deprivation.

General Appearance

The newborn does not match the baby ads and may be a shock to new parents. The misshapen head, flat nose, puffy eyelids and often undistinguished eye color, discolored skin, large tongue and undersized lower jaw, short neck and small sloping shoulders, short limbs and large rounded abdomen with protruding umbilical stump that remains to 3 weeks, and bowed skinny legs may prove very disappointing if the parents are unprepared for the sight of a newborn. The head, which accounts for one-fourth of the total body size, appears large in relation to the body.

The **anterior fontanel,** a *diamond-shaped area at the top of the front of the head,* and the **posterior fontanel,** a *triangular-shaped area at the center back of the head,* are often called **soft spots.** These unossified areas of the skull bones, along with the suture lines of the bones, allow the bones to overlap during delivery and also allow for expansion of the brain as they gradually fill in with bone cells. The posterior fontanel closes by 2 or 3 months; the anterior fontanel closes between 8 and 18 months. These soft spots may add to the parents' impression that the newborn is too fragile to handle.

Reassure the parents that the newborn, although in need of tender, gentle care, is also resilient and adaptable. The head and fontanels can be gently touched without harm, although strong pressure or direct injury should be avoided. Reassure them also that the baby will soon take on the features of the family members and look more as they expected.

Apgar Scoring System

The physical status of the newborn is determined with the Apgar tool 1 minute after birth and then 5 minutes later. The newborn's respirations, heart rate, muscle tone, reflex activities, and color are observed. A maximum score of 2 is given to each sign, so that the score could range from 0 to 10, as indicated by Table 7–2. A score less than 7 means that the newborn is having difficulty adapting, needs even closer observation than usual, and may need life-saving intervention.

Gestational Age Assessment

In addition to using the Apgar score, assessment includes estimating gestational age to use parameters other than weight to assess an infant's level of maturity. By considering *both birth weight* and *gestational age,* you can categorize infants into one of several groupings. Problems can then be anticipated and, if present, be identified and treated early. Assessment can be done

TABLE 7–2. ASSESSMENT OF THE NEWBORN: APGAR SCORING SYSTEM

Sign	0	1	2
Heart rate	Absent	Less than 100 beats/min	More than 100 beats/min
Respirations	Absent	Slow, irregular	Cry; regular rate
Muscle tone	Flaccid	Some flexion of extremities	Active movements
Reflex irritability	None	Grimace	Cry
Color	Body cyanotic or pale	Body pink; extremities cyanotic	Body completely pink

Modified from refs. 105 and 122.

as early as the first day of life and should be done no later than the fifth day of life, as external criteria such as hip abduction, square window, dorsiflexion of foot, and size of breast nodules change after 5 to 6 days of life. If the neonate is examined on the first day of life, he or she should be examined again before the fifth day to detect neurologic changes. The score can be affected by asphyxia or maternal anesthesia.

To assess gestational age, several scales can be used. The *Classification of Newborns by Intrauterine Growth and Gestational Age* scale uses weight, length, and head circumference to determine gestational age (Fig. 7–2) (5). The *Dubowitz Guide to Gestational Age Assessment* examines 10 neurologic and 11 external signs (31). Ballard et al. modified the Dubowitz scale. The *Ballard Gestational Age Assessment* determines neuromuscular and physical maturity in relation to gestational age (Fig. 7–3) (4). This will place the infant in one of nine categories based on *age* and *weight*.

Skin

The skin is thin, delicate, and usually mottled, varies from pink to reddish, and becomes very ruddy when the baby cries. **Acrocyanosis,** *bluish color of the hands and feet,* is the result of the sluggish peripheral circulation that occurs normally only a few days after birth. **Lanugo,** *downy hair of fetal life,* most evident on shoulders, back extremities, forehead, and temples, is lost after a few months and is replaced by other hair growth. The *cheesy skin covering,* **vernix caseosa,** is left on for protective reasons; it rubs off in a few days. **Milia,** *tiny white spots that are small collections of sebaceous secretions,* are sprinkled on the nose and forehead and should not be squeezed or picked; they will disappear. **Hemangiomas,** *pink spots* on the upper eyelids, between eyebrows, on the nose, upper lip, or back may or may not be permanent. **Mongolian spots,** *slate-colored areas* on buttocks or lower back in Black, Asian, or Mediterranean babies, fade without treatment. If a birthmark is present, parents should be assured it is not their fault. **Jaundice,** *yellowish discoloration of skin,* should be noted. If it occurs during the first 24 hours of life, it is usually caused by blood incompatibility between mother's and baby's blood and requires medical investigation and possibly treatment. **Physiologic jaundice** normally appears on the third or fourth day of life because the excess number of red blood cells present in fetal life that are no longer needed are undergoing hemolysis, which in turn causes high levels of bilirubin (a bile pigment) in the bloodstream. The jaundice usually disappears in approximately 1 week when the baby's liver has developed the ability to metabolize the bilirubin. If bilirubin levels are excessively high, the neonate is placed under full-spectrum lights (phototherapy) to promote bilirubin breakdown. The baby's eyes must be covered during phototherapy.

Parents should be reassured about these and other conditions of the skin that normally occur. Foot or hand prints are made for identification, as these lines remain permanently. **Desquamation,** *peeling of skin,* occurs in 2 to 4 weeks.

Umbilical Cord

The *bluish-white, gelatinous structure that transports maternal blood from placenta to fetus* is the **umbilical cord.** It is cut 1½ to 3 in. from baby's abdominal wall. Because of the high water content, the stump of the cord dries and shrinks rapidly, losing its flexibility by 24 hours after birth. By the second day, it is a very hard yellow or black (blood) tab on the skin. Slight oozing where the cord joins the abdominal wall is common and offers an excellent medium for bacterial growth.

The area should be cleaned with cotton balls and alcohol several times daily until the cord has dropped off (6–14 days) and for 2 or 3 days after the cord falls off when the area is completely healed. Parents should be taught this procedure.

Circumcision

The *surgical removal of the foreskin,* **circumcision,** is done almost automatically on newborn males. In contrast to past belief, this is a painful procedure for the baby, as shown by the cry (81). The same reasons are given by people in different cultures either to do or not to do circumcision. These reasons include:

- Sign of manhood
- Cultural norms
- Sexuality concerns
- Hygienic, cosmetic, or comfort concerns
- Biblical or religious mandate
- Prevention of later genitourinary problems
- Medical advice

The main difference among various cultural groups related to circumcision is the issue of pain. Some people believe the procedure is not harmful or even very painful to infants; others believe it is traumatic and dangerous (49). Although it is part of religious ritual for the Jewish male, most families have the boy circumcised to facilitate hygiene of the penis and to decrease the risk of penile cancer.

Although there are risks to circumcision, these complications occur infrequently. Irritation and infec-

CLASSIFICATION OF NEWBORNS (BOTH SEXES)
BY INTRAUTERINE GROWTH AND GESTATIONAL AGE[1,2]

NAME _____   DATE OF BIRTH _____   BIRTH WEIGHT _____

HOSPITAL NO. _____   DATE OF EXAM _____   LENGTH _____

RACE _____   SEX _____   HEAD CIRC. _____

GESTATIONAL AGE _____

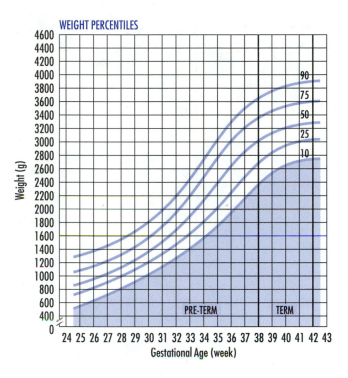

WEIGHT PERCENTILES

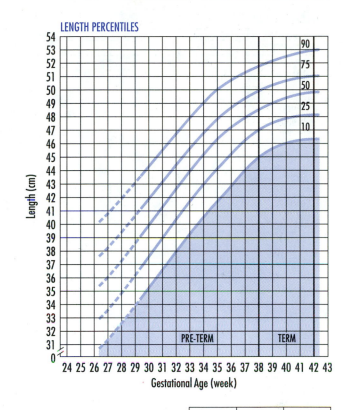

LENGTH PERCENTILES

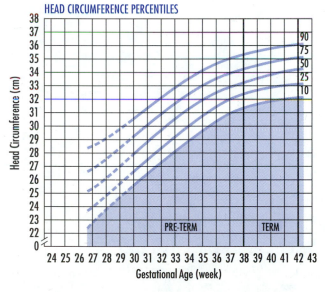

HEAD CIRCUMFERENCE PERCENTILES

CLASSIFICATION OF INFANT*	Weight	Length	Head Circ.
Large for Gestational Age (LGA) (>90th Percentile)			
Appropriate for Gestational Age (AGA) (10th to 90th percentile)			
Small for Gestational Age (SGA) (<10th percentile)			

*Place an "X" in the appropriate box (LGA, AGA, SGA) for weight, for
length and for head circumference.

Figure 7–2. Classification of newborns (both sexes) by intrauterine growth and gestational age. *(Courtesy of Ross Laboratories, Columbus, OH, A Division of Abbott Laboratories, USA.)*

GESTATIONAL AGE ASSESSMENT (Ballard)

NAME _____   DATE/TIME OF BIRTH _____   BIRTH WEIGHT _____

HOSPITAL NO. _____   DATE/TIME OF EXAM _____   LENGTH _____

_____   AGE WHEN EXAMINED _____   HEAD CIRC. _____

RACE _____   SEX _____   EXAMINER _____

APGAR SCORE: 1 MINUTE _____   5 MINUTES _____

NEUROMUSCULAR MATURITY

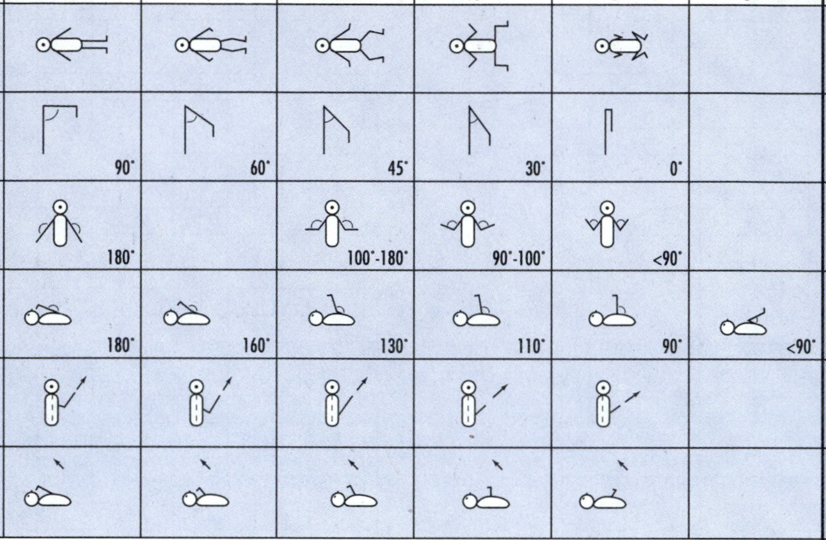

NEUROMUSCULAR MATURITY SIGN	SCORE						RECORD SCORE HERE
	0	1	2	3	4	5	
POSTURE							
SQUARE WINDOW (WRIST)	90°	60°	45°	30°	0°		
ARM RECOIL	180°	100°-180°	90°-100°	<90°			
POPLITEAL ANGLE	180°	160°	130°	110°	90°	<90°	
SCARF SIGN							
HEEL TO EAR							

TOTAL NEUROMUSCULAR MATURITY SCORE

PHYSICAL MATURITY

PHYSICAL MATURITY SIGN	SCORE						RECORD SCORE HERE
	0	1	2	3	4	5	
SKIN	gelantinous red, transparent	smooth pink, visible veins	superficial peeling, &/or rash few veins	cracking pale area rare veins	parchment deep cracking no vessels	leathery cracked wrinkled	
LANUGO	none	abundant	thinning	bald areas	mostly bald		
PLANTAR CREASES	no crease	faint red marks	anterior transverse crease only	creases ant. 2/3	creases cover entire sole		
BREAST	barely percept.	flat areola no bud	stippled areola 1-2mm bud	raised areola 3-4mm bud	full areola 5-10mm bud		
EAR	pinna flat, stays folded	sl. curved pinna; soft with slow recoil	well-curv. pinna; soft but ready recoil	formed & firm with instant recoil	thick cartilage ear stiff		
GENITALS (Male)	scrotum empty no rugae		testes descending, few rugae	testes down good rugae	testes pendulous deep rugae		
GENITALS (Female)	prominent clitoris & labia minora		majora & minora equally prominent	majora large, minora small	clitoris & minora completely covered		

TOTAL PHYSICAL MATURITY SCORE

SCORE

Neuromuscular _____

Physical _____

Total _____

MATURITY RATING

TOTAL MATURITY SCORE	GESTATIONAL AGE (WEEKS)
5	26
10	28
15	30
20	32
25	34
30	36
35	38
40	40
45	42
50	44

GESTATIONAL AGE (weeks)

By dates _____

By ultrasound _____

By score _____

Figure 7–3. Gestational age assessment. *(From Ballard, J., et al., A. Simplified Score for Assessment of Fetal Maturation in Newly Born Infants,* Journal of Pediatrics, 95 *(1979), 769–774.)*

tion can occur. Hemorrhage is the most common complication, requiring sutures or pressure dressings that can cause scarring, deformity, or **phimosis** (*tightening of the foreskin*). If the physician is not skilled, various surgical mishaps may occur. Although rare, septicemia with osteomyelitis, pulmonary abscess, and death may occur. Physicians are now questioning the necessity of circumcision. Good hygiene provides the same medical benefits without the risk of surgery and the pain (81, 105). Parents may feel they have no choice about circumcision. Discuss the procedure with them so that their action is based on information. Further, you may share that the American Academy of Pediatrics states there are no medical indications for circumcision; however, urologists report that a small percentage of uncircumcized males develop genitourinary infections, inflammation of the glans, or phimosis (tightening of the foreskin) (105).

Weight, Length, and Head Circumference

In newborns these circumferences provide an index to the normality of development, and measurements should be accurate. The **average birth weight** of Caucasian male infants in America is $7\frac{1}{2}$ pounds (3400 g) and for girls is 7 pounds (3180 g). Newborn infants of African-American, Indian, and Asian-American population groups are smaller, on the average, at birth (80). There is a difference in risk for low birth weight among ethnic groups in general and among major Asian-American groups in particular. The risk of low birth weight was greatest for African-Americans and Filipinos (106). In a comparison of Mexican-Americans and Mexicans in Mexico City, the lower birth weight of babies born in Mexico City appeared to be due to the effects of altitude and greater prevalence of pathologic conditions and high-risk delivery (79). Maternal age, parity, lifestyle, and the woman's previous state of nutrition and prenatal care also influence birth weight. In all instances female babies are somewhat smaller than males. Shortly after birth the newborn loses weight, up to 10% of birth weight, because of water loss, and parents should be told that this is normal before a steady weight gain, which begins in 1 or 2 weeks. Tissue turgor shows a sense of fullness because of hydrated subcutaneous tissue (105, 122).

In developing countries a large percentage of babies are born at home. Babies are not weighed at birth because scales are not available; however, measurements within 24 hours of birth of chest circumference (at nipple line) and midarm circumference (midway between acromium process and bend of elbow), when combined, were predictors of birth weight in one study.

Based on accurate (92–97%) studies of 402 newborns in Thailand, the *Chulalongkorn University Birthweight Estimation Device,* a circular nomographic chart, has been developed. Estimation, if not precise measurement, of birth weight is important because low birth weight is the major factor associated with death of infants within the first 4 weeks of life (32).

Length is measured by having the child supine on a hard surface, extending the knees, placing the soles upright, and measuring from the soles of the feet to the vertex (tip) of the head. The **average length** of American infants at birth is just under 20 in. (50.8 cm). Boys range from 19 to 21 in. (48.2–53.3 cm); girls average slightly less. The bones are soft, consisting chiefly of cartilage. The back is straight and curves with sitting. The muscles feel hard and are slightly resistant to pressure (105, 122).

Measurement of **head circumference** is important in assessing the speed of head growth to determine if any abnormalities such as too rapid or too slow growth are present. The measurement is taken over the brow just above the eyes and across the posterior occipital protuberance. This standard measure of head size averages approximately 12.4 to 14.8 in. (31–37 cm) at birth, but variations of $\frac{1}{2}$ in. are common. Chest circumference is usually approximately an inch less than head size (105, 122). Parents should be prepared for molding of the skull during vaginal delivery; **caput succedaneum,** *irregular edema of the scalp,* which disappears approximately the third day; or for **cephalohematoma,** *a collection of blood beneath the fibrous covering of the skull bones,* usually the parietal bones.

The baby's characteristic *position* during this period is one of flexion, closely imitating the fetal position, with fists tightly closed and arms and legs drawn up against the body. The baby is aware of disturbances in equilibrium and will change position, reacting with the Moro reflex.

Ethnic differences for weight, length, head circumference, and other measurements have been noted in Anglo and Mexican-American children ages 48 to 56 weeks. The Mexican-American child has shorter stature and greater weight for length than the Anglo child, with greater chest circumference, subscapular skinfolds, and estimated body fat, with no difference by sex. Head circumference is greater for males than females in both ethnic groups but is greater in Anglo than Mexican-American children. Thigh circumference is greater in Mexican-Americans than Anglos and in females than in males (64).

Despite widespread poverty and lack of access to medial care, Latinos in the United States, especially Mexican-Americans, have less risk of low-birth-weight babies and less infant mortality than do Caucasians or

African-Americans. In Latin cultures the prevalence of traditional family values, better prenatal diets, fewer single mothers, strong extended families, and lower smoking rates may account for the difference. Health practices of Mexican-Americans deteriorate the longer they live in the United States as they become more likely to eat fast foods, smoke, and drink alcohol, activities that have serious health effects (79).

Neonate — Other Characteristics

Several other characteristics are also normal and resolve themselves shortly after birth: swollen breasts that contain liquid in boys and girls; swollen genitalia with undescended testicles in the boy; and vaginal secretions in the girl, caused by maternal hormones. Genital size varies for boys and girls. Urine is present in the bladder, and the baby voids at birth. Obstruction of the nasolacrimal duct is also common, and the excessive tearing and pus accumulation usually clear up when the duct opens spontaneously in a few months.

Vital Signs

In the newborn vital signs are not stable.

Respiratory Efforts. Respiratory efforts at birth are critical, and immediate adaptations must occur to counter the decreasing oxygen level and increasing carbon dioxide level in the blood. Causes of respiratory initiations include cutting of the umbilical cord, which causes hypoxia, resulting in carbon dioxide accumulation; physical stimulation of the birth process; the sudden change in baby's environment at birth; the exposure to firm touch; and the cool air. If the mother were medicated during labor or if the baby is premature, the respiratory center of the brain is less operative, and baby will have more difficulty with breathing. *Respirations* range from 50 to 80 per minute during the first hour after birth and then decrease to 30 to 60 per minute. Respirations are irregular, quiet, and shallow and may be followed by an intermittent 5- to 10-second pause in breathing (105, 122).

Body Temperature. Body temperature ranges from 97 to 100°F (36.1–37.7°C) because:

- The heat-regulating mechanism in the hypothalamus is not fully developed.
- Shivering to produce heat does not occur.
- There is less subcutaneous fat.
- Heat is lost to the environment by evaporation, conduction, convection, and radiation.

At birth amniotic fluid increases temperature loss by evaporation from the skin; thus, diligent efforts to dry the skin are necessary. The wet newborn can lose up to 200 calories of heat per kilogram per minute (90 calories/min is the maximum the adult can lose). If the room is cool and the baby is placed in contact with cold objects, heat loss occurs by convection, radiation, and conduction. Excessive heat loss or cold stress may lead to apnea, respiratory depression, and hypoglycemia (105, 122).

Thus, baby should be placed next to mother's abdominal skin or breast initially and then wrapped well in blankets before being placed in a warm crib. Several mechanisms occur to help the newborn conserve heat:

- Vasoconstriction, by which constricted blood vessels maintain heat in the inner body
- Flexion of the body to reduce total amount of exposed skin (the premature baby does not assume a flexion of the extremities onto the body)
- Increased metabolic rate, which causes increased heat production
- Metabolism of adipose tissue that has been stored during the eighth month of gestation

This *adipose tissue* is called **brown fat** because it is *brown in color from a rich supply of blood vessels and nerves,* and it is unique in that it *aids adaptation to the stress of cooling.* Brown fat, located between the scapulae around the neck, behind the sternum, and around the kidneys and adrenal glands, accounts for 2 to 6% of the neonate's body weight and is metabolized quickly (105, 122).

Body temperature of the baby normally drops 1 to 2°F immediately after birth, but in a warm environment begins to rise slowly after 8 hours. Thus, prevention of heat loss, especially during the first 15 minutes, is crucial to adaptation to extrauterine life (105, 122). Also, babies who have lost excessive amounts of heat cannot produce surfactant. **Surfactant** is a *thin lipoprotein film produced by the alveoli that reduces surface tension of the alveoli, allows them to expand, and allows some air to remain in alveoli at end of expiration.* Thus it takes less effort to reexpand the lungs (105, 122).

The temperature should be taken at the axillary site for 5 minutes. Rectal temperatures may cause infection, raise blood pressure, lower arterial blood oxygen, and unnecessarily stimulate defecation, causing loss of fluid and calories (109).

Heart Rate. Heart rate ranges at birth from 100 to 160 beats per minute because of the immature cardiac regulatory mechanism in the medulla. The heart rate may increase to 170 to 180 beats per minute when the newborn cries and drop to 90 during sleep. The pulse rate gradually decreases during the first and subsequent years (105, 122).

Blood Pressure.
Blood Pressure. Blood pressure may range from 40 to 50 mm Hg systolic, depending on cuff size or the instrument used for measurement. By the end of the first month, blood pressure averages 80/40, increases slowly the first year, and remains under 90/60 (105, 122).

Meconium

The *first fecal material* is sticky, odorless, and tarry. This **meconium** is passed from 8 to 24 hours after birth. Transitional stools for a week are loose, contain mucus, are greenish-yellow and pasty, and have a sour odor. There will be two to four stools daily. If the neonate takes cow's milk, the stools will become yellow and harder and average one to two daily.

Reflex Activity

Reflex activity is innate or built in through the process of evolution and develops while the baby is in utero. **Reflex** is an *involuntary; unlearned response elicited by certain stimuli,* and it indicates neurologic status or function (28, 34, 105, 122). Individual differences in the newborn's responses to stimulation are apparent at birth. Some respond vigorously to the slightest stimulation; others respond slowly, and some are in between. Several types of reflexes exist in the neonate and young infant; consummatory, avoidant, exploratory, social, and attentional. **Consummatory reflexes** *such as rooting and sucking promote survival through feeding.* **Avoidant reflexes** are *elicited by potentially harmful stimuli* and include the Moro, withdrawing, knee jerk, sneezing, blinking, and coughing reflexes. **Exploratory reflexes** *occur when infants are wide awake and are held upright so that their arms move without restraint.* The visual object at eye level elicits both reaching and grasping reflexes. **Social reflexes** such *as smiling promote affectionate interactions between parents and infants* and thus have a survival value. Crying in response to painful stimuli, loud noise, food deprivation, or loss of support; quieting in response to touch, low soft tones, or food; and smiling in response to changes in brightness, comforting stimuli, or escape from uncomfortable stimuli are examples of innate reflexes that can be modified by experience and that persist throughout life. **Attentional reflexes,** including orienting and attending, *determine the nature of the baby's response to stimuli* and have con-

tinuing importance through development (28, 34, 105, 122).

The nervous system of the newborn is both anatomically and physiologically immature, and reflexes should be observed for their presence and symmetry. These reflexes are described in Table 7–3.

Sensory Abilities

The newborn has more highly developed sensory abilities than was once supposed. Apparently a moderately enriched environment, one without stimulus bombardment or deprivation, is best suited for sensory motor development. Even premature babies placed in a stimulus-rich environment until discharged from the hospital learn more quickly and are healthier at 4 months than premature babies who lived in the traditional environment (63, 105, 122).

The infant's use of the senses, innate abilities, and environment lay the ground work for intellectual development. Studies show that 20 minutes of extra handling a day will result in earlier exploring and grasping behavior by the infant. He or she is very sensitive to touch and vestibular (rocking, holding upright) stimulation; cutaneous and postural stimulation is necessary for development of the nervous system, skin sensitivity, and emotional health (16, 63). Moderate, gentle kinesthetic stimulation daily results in a baby who is quieter, gains weight faster, and shows improved socioemotional function.

The first impressions of life, security, warmth, love, pleasure, or lack of them come to the infant through touch. Knowledge of the people around him or her, initially of mother, is gradually built from the manner in which baby is handled. He or she soon learns to sense mother's self-confidence and pleasure as well as her anxiety, lack of confidence, anger, or rejection. These early touch experiences and the infant's feelings through them apparently lay the foundation for feelings about people throughout life.

Sensitivity to Pain, Pressure, and Temperature.
Sensitivity to Pain, Pressure, and Temperature. Sensitivity to pain, pressure, and temperature extremes is present at birth; pain is shown by a distinct cry (42, 105, 122). The baby is especially sensitive to touch around the mouth and on the palms and soles. Females are more responsive to touch and pain than males (68). The newborn reacts diffusely to pain, as he or she has little ability to localize the discomfort because of incomplete myelinization of the spinal tracts and cerebral cortex (105, 122); however, the baby's response to pain increases each day in the neonate period. Visceral sensations of discomfort such as hunger, overdistention of

TABLE 7–3. ASSESSMENT OF INFANT REFLEXES

Reflex	Description	Appearance/Disappearance
Rooting	Touching baby's cheek causes head to turn toward the side touched.	Present in utero at 24 weeks; disappears 3–4 months; may persist in sleep 9–12 months
Sucking	Touching lips or placing something in baby's mouth causes baby to draw liquid into mouth by creating vacuum with lips, cheeks, and tongue.	Present in utero at 28 weeks persists through early childhood, especially during sleep
Bite	Touching gums, teeth, or tongue causes baby to open and close mouth.	Disappears at 3–5 months when biting is voluntary, but seen throughout adult years in comatose person
Babkin	Pressure applied to palm causes baby to open mouth, close eyes.	Present at birth; disappears in 2 or 4 months
Pupillary response	Flashing light across baby's eyes or face causes constriction of pupils.	Present at 32 weeks of gestation; persists throughout life
Blink	Baby closes both eyes.	Remains throughout life
Moro or startle	Making a loud noise or changing baby's position causes baby to extend both arms outward with fingers spread, then bring them together in a tense, quivery embrace	Present at 28 weeks of gestation; disappears at 4–7 months
Withdrawing	Baby removes hand or foot from painful stimuli.	Present at birth; persists throughout life
Colliding	Baby moves arms up and face to side when object is in collision course with face.	Present at birth or shortly after; persists in modified form throughout life
Palmer grasp	Placing object or finger in baby's palm causes his or her fingers to close tightly around object.	Present at 32 weeks of gestation; disappears at 3–4 months, replaced by voluntary grasp at 4–5 months
Plantar grasp	Placing object or finger beneath toes causes curling of toes around object.	Present at 32 weeks of gestation; disappears at 9–12 months
Tonic neck or fencing (TNR)	Postural reflex is seen when infant lies on back with head turned to one side; arm and leg on the side toward which he or she is looking are extended while opposite limbs are flexed.	Present at birth; disappears at approximately 4 months
Stepping, walking, dancing	Holding baby upright with feet touching flat surface causes legs to prance up and down as if baby were walking or dancing.	Present at birth; disappears at approximately 2–4 months; with daily practice of reflex, infant may walk alone at 10 months
Reaching	Hand closes as it reaches toward and grasps at object at eye level.	Present shortly after birth if baby is upright; comes under voluntary control in several months
Orienting	Head and eyes turn toward stimulus of noise, accompanied by cessation of other activity, heartbeat change, and vascular constriction.	Present at birth; comes under voluntary control later; persists throughout life
Attending	Eyes fix on a stimulus that changes brightness, movement, or shape.	Present shortly after birth; comes under voluntary control later; persists throughout life
Swimming	Placing baby horizontally, supporting him under abdomen, causes baby to make crawling motions with his or her arms and legs while lifting head from surface as if he or she were swimming.	Present after 3 or 4 days; disappears at approximately 4 months; may persist with practice
Trunk incurvation	Stroking one side of spinal column while baby is on his or her abdomen causes crawling motions with legs, lifting head from surface, and incurvature of trunk on the side stroked.	Present in utero; then seen at approximately third or fourth day; persists 2–3 months
Babinski	Stroking bottom of foot causes big toe to raise while other toes fan out and curl downward.	Present at birth; disappears at approximately 9 or 10 months; presence of reflex later may indicate disease
Landau	Suspending infant in horizontal, prone position and flexing head against trunk cause legs to flex against trunk.	Appears at approximately 3 months; disappears at approximately 12–24 months
Parachute	Sudden thrusting of infant downward from horizontal position causes hands and fingers to extend forward and spread as if to protect self from a fall.	Appears at approximately 7–9 months; persists indefinitely
Biceps	Tap on tendon of biceps causes biceps to contract quickly.	Brisk in first few days, then slightly diminished; permanent
Knee jerk	Tap on tendon below patella or on patella causes leg to extend quickly.	More pronounced first 2 days; permanent

Data from References (105, 114, 122).

the stomach, passage of gas and stool, and extremes of temperature apparently account for much of the newborn's crying. At first the cry is simply a primitive discharge mechanism that calls for help. He or she wails with equal force regardless of stimulus. In a few weeks baby acquires subtle modifications in the sound of the cry that provide clues to the attentive parent about the nature of the discomfort so response can be adjusted to the baby's need (45, 122).

Vision. The following are characteristics of newborn vision (71):

- *Initial state:* Vision is blurred.
- *Acuity:* Clarity of vision at a specific distance begins within the first day; 8 to 20 in. is necessary for focus.
- *Fixation:* The newborn is able to direct his or her eyes at the same point in space for a specific time (4–10 seconds).
- *Tracking:* The newborn visually follows large moving objects beginning a day after birth.
- *Discrimination:* The newborn demonstrates a preference for particular sizes, shapes, colors, or patterns; discriminates large from small and intensity of color; and prefers less complex stimuli and large pictures or objects.
- *Conjugation:* The newborn is able to move the eyes together; frequency of refixation is more frequent.
- *Sensitivity to light:* The newborn's sensitivity to light is equal to that of adults.
- *Scanning:* The newborn is able to move her or his eyes over the visual field and focus on a satisfying image.
- *Accommodation:* The newborn is able to adjust the eyes for distance. The preferred distance is 8 in. up to 1 month; at 2 months, the lenses become more flexible; and at 4 months, the ability to adjust is on an adult level.

The infant maintains contact with the environment through visual fixation, scanning, and tracking and pays more attention to stimuli from the face than to other stimuli (Fig. 7–4). The newborn looks at mother's face while feeding and while sitting upright, follows the path of an object, crying or pulling backward if it comes too close to his or her face.

He or she apparently has innate depth perception, can define stripe and edge, and correlates touch with sight. He or she apparently sees colors and prefers black and white to red, orange, or yellow. The newborn looks longer at colors of medium intensity (yellow, green, pink) than at bright (red, orange, blue) or dim (gray, beige) colors. The newborn focuses attention on patterned objects such as geometric shapes, large circles, dots, and squares in preference to solid colors. Babies also prefer real faces to mobiles: by 1 month, baby distinguishes the mother's face from a stranger's, by 6 or 7 months, infants distinguish people by their faces. Pupils respond sluggishly to light; bright lights cause discomfort, and the newborn will blink and withdraw (28, 34, 71, 105, 114, 122).

Teach parents that baby needs eye contact and the opportunity to see the human face and a variety of changing scenes and colors. Providing a mirror or chrome plate that reflects light and objects and rotating the bed help the baby use both eyes, avoiding one-sided vision. Hang cardboard black and white mobiles, especially those that make sound, and have them within the reach of baby's kicking feet. Later the infant enjoys other colors and designs that are within grasp. By age 2 months, baby can see the ceiling and decorations on it. As baby grows older the crib should be low enough that he or she can see beyond the crib (71).

Parents should be reassured that the antibiotic ointment correctly placed in baby's eyes at birth will not damage vision but prevents blindness if the mother should have an undetected gonorrheal infection (122).

Hearing. Hearing is developed in utero when the fetus is exposed to internal sounds of mother's body, such as the heartbeat and abdominal rumbles (heard at 5 months), and external sounds, such as voices, music, and a cymbal clap (heard at 7 months). Hearing is blurred the first few days of life because fluid is retained in the middle ear, but hearing loss can be tested as early as the first day (122). The neonate cannot hear whispers but can respond to voice pitch changes. A low pitch quiets and a high pitch increases alertness. Baby responds to sound direction—left or right—but responds best to mother's voice, to sounds directly in front of his or her face, and to sounds experienced during gestation (28, 34, 58, 105, 114, 122). Baby often sleeps better with background songs or a tape recording of mother's heartbeat. By 3 days of age, the newborn discriminates between the voice of mother and another female (34, 122). Differentiation of sounds and perception of their source take time to develop, but there are startle reactions. The baby withdraws from loud noise (105).

The presence of congenital (born deaf) hearing loss is more common than ordinarily understood. It is believed that approximately 1.5 to 3% of infants born in the United States each year have a hearing loss severe enough to require special education or help. The Checklist to Detect Presence of Hearing in Infancy (see p. 319) is

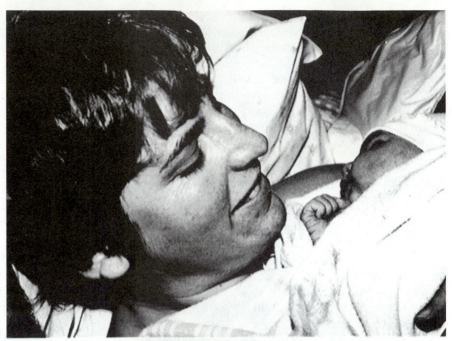

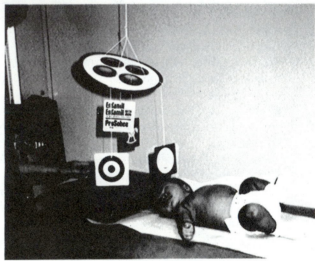

Figure 7–4. Infant has the ability to fix on the mother's face beginning 1 day after birth and finds geometric objects interesting. *(From Sherwen, L.N., M.A. Scoloveno, and C.T. Weingarten,* Nursing Care of the Childbearing Family. *Stamford, CT: Appleton & Lange, 1991, pp. 635, 847.)*

a guide for parents and health care professionals to check for hearing ability in the neonate and infant (34, 114).

Taste and Smell. Taste is not highly developed at birth, but acid, bitter, salt, and sweet substances evoke a response. Taste buds for sweet are more abundant in early than late life. Breathing rhythm is altered in response to fragrance, showing some ability to smell. The sense of smell is well developed in the newborn; infants can sense the odors that adults sense (34).

Neonates differ in their appearance, size, function, and response. Girls are more developmentally advanced than boys and African-Americans more than Cauca-

sians. The most accurate assessment is made by comparing the neonate against norms for the same sex and race (105, 122).

Special Considerations in Physical Assessment of the Neonate

When a newborn is examined, the primary concerns are neurologic status, congenital deformities, and metabolic disturbances. Any history of hereditary diseases and pregnancy and delivery information is essential. See Table 7–3 because reflex status indicates neurologic and some congenital deformities. The following are particular aspects to check when physically assessing the neonate (55, 105, 122).

► CHECKLIST TO DETECT PRESENCE OF HEARING IN INFANCY

From Birth to 2 Weeks Does Baby:

- Jump or blink when there is a sudden loud sound
- Stop crying when you start to talk
- Seem aware of your voice
- Stir in sleep when there is continuous noise close by
- Jump or blink when there is a sudden soft click such as a light switch or a camera click when the room is otherwise quiet
- Stop sucking momentarily when there is a noise or when you start to talk
- Look up from sucking or try to open eyes when there is a sudden noise

From 2 to 10 Weeks Does Baby:

- Stop crying when you talk to him or her
- Stop movements when you enter the room
- Seem aware of your voice
- Sleep regardless of noises
- Waken when the crib or bassinet is touched
- Respond to comforting only when held against mother or familiar caretaker
- Cry at sudden loud noises
- Blink or jerk at sudden loud noises

From 2½ to 6 Months Does Baby:

- Always coo with pleasure when you start to talk
- Turn eyes to the speaker
- Know when father comes home and wriggle in welcome (if awake)
- Startle when you bend over the crib after awakening
- Seem to enjoy a soft musical toy (e.g., a crib musical toy)
- Cry when exposed to sudden, loud unexpected noise
- Stop movements when a new sound is introduced
- Try to turn in the direction of a new sound or a person who starts to talk
- Make many different babbling sounds when alone
- Try to "talk back" when you talk
- Start wriggling in anticipation of a bottle when you start preparing it (if the baby is awake and the preparation is out of sight, as the refrigerator door opening, and so on)
- Know own name (smiles, turns, or otherwise gives an indication)

NOTE: If the child is hearing impaired or deaf, a source of information about treatment facilities and/or other educational materials for parents can be obtained from Galludet College, Washington, DC.

A *small chin,* called **micrograthia,** may mean that the neonate will experience breathing difficulties, as the tongue can fall back and obstruct the nasopharynx.

Ear position is important because there is a strong association between low-set ears and renal malformation or a chromosomal aberration such as Down syndrome. The top of the ear should be in alignment with the inner and outer canthi of the eyes. The eustachian tube is shorter and wider than in the adult. To examine the neonate with an otoscope, the head should be stabilized and the pinna of the ear pulled back and up.

Discharges from the eye may be due to chemical irritation or to ophthalmic neonatorum from gonorrhea in the mother. A mongoloid slant in a Caucasian infant may suggest a chromosome abnormality.

Ptosis (*drooping*) of the eyelids should be a cause for concern. Drooping eyelids reduce the amount of light entering the retina and can decrease development of sight.

Conjunctival hemorrhage is usually of no significance. An infant lid retractor may be used to view the fundus if the muscles of the newborn keep the eyelids closed.

The **nose** should be patent. Flaring of the nostrils usually represents respiratory distress. A thick bloody discharge from the nose suggests congenital syphilis.

The **mouth** should be inspected for cleft lip and cleft palate. Although spitting up is common in the newborn, projectile vomiting is not. The newborn should have very little saliva, and tonsillar tissue should not be present at birth.

The **chest** and **abdomen** are considered a unit in the newborn. The anteroposterior diameter is usually equal to the transverse diameter. Wide-set nipples may indicate Turner syndrome, a genetic disorder. Smaller breasts that contain liquid are not uncommon in both male and female. The breath sounds in the infant are bronchovesicular. If heart murmurs exist, they are usually best heard over the base of the heart rather than at the apex.

The **umbilical cord** should have two arteries and one vein. Auscultation of bowel sounds should precede palpation for masses, an extremely important procedure in the newborn.

The **genitalia** are examined for deformities. Only the external genitalia are examined in children. In uncircumcised males up to 3 months of age, the foreskin should not be retracted to avoid tearing the membrane. The testes should be palpated in the scrotum, although sometimes they are still undescended. A **hydrocele,** *a collection of watery fluid in the scrotum or along the spermatic cord,* and **hernia,** *a protrusion of part of the intestine through the abdominal muscles,* are common findings in males.

A bloody or mucous vaginal discharge may be present in girls. Fused labia are a serious anomaly, but simple adhesion may be due to inflammation.

Rectal temperatures will rule out **imperforate anus** (*lacking normal anal opening*).

The spine should be palpated for **spina bifida,** *a congenital neural tube defect characterized by anomaly in posterior vertebral arch.* Observation for symmetric bilateral muscle movements of the hips and knees is essential. The **hips** should be examined for dislocation by rotating the thighs with the knees flexed.

Extremities should be noted for the right number of fingers and toes and bilateral movements, and position of hands and feet should be checked.

Signs of prematurity include low birth weight and small size, thick lanugo, excess vernix, slow or absent reflexes, undescended testicles in the male, and nipples not visible (55, 122).

Infant — Physical Characteristics

General Appearance

The growing infant changes in appearance as he or she changes size and proportion (28, 34, 58, 105, 114, 122). The face grows rapidly; trunk and limbs lengthen; back and limb muscles develop; and coordination improves. By 1 month the baby can lift the head slightly when prone and hold the head up briefly when the back is supported. By 2 months the head is held erect, but it bobs when he or she is sitting unsupported.

Skull enlargement occurs almost as rapidly as total body growth during the first year and is determined mainly by the rate of brain expansion. From birth to 4 weeks, the head size increases to 14.75 in. (37.5 cm); at 3 months to 15.75 in. (39.5 cm); at 20 weeks to 16.5 in. (41 cm); and at 30 weeks to 17 in. (43 cm). By the end of the first year the head will be two-thirds of adult size.

Physical Growth and Emotional, Social, and Neuromuscular Learning

Physical growth and these areas of learning are concurrent, interrelated, and rapid in the first year. The first year of life is one of the two periods of rapid physical growth after birth. (The other period is prepuberty/postpuberty.) Baby gains $\frac{2}{3}$ oz per day in the first 5 months and $\frac{1}{2}$ oz per day for the next 7 months. Birth weight doubles by 5 to 6 months and triples by 12 months. Baby grows approximately 1 ft in the first year.

Physical and motor abilities are heavily influenced by genetic, biological, and cultural factors, nutrition, maturation of the central nervous system, skeletal formation, overall physical health status, environmental conditions, stimulation, and consistent loving care. African-American infants mature ahead of Caucasian infants in motor skills, bone ossification, and walking. This is apparently due to genetic factors and has evolutionary adaptive value. The skeletal system should be assessed for any orthopedic problems (69).

Table 7–4 divides further developmental sequence into 3-month periods for specific assessment (28, 34, 45, 58, 68, 105, 114). *It is only a guide,* not an absolute standard. Great individual differences occur among infants, depending on their physical growth and emotional, social, and neuromuscular responses. Girls usually develop more rapidly than boys, although the activity level is generally higher for boys. Even with these cautions, the table can be a useful tool if you observe overall behavior patterns rather than isolated characteristics.

Neurologic System

The neurologic system is immature, but it continues the fetal pattern of developing a functional capacity at a rapid rate. Consistent stimulation of the nervous system is necessary to maintain growth and development, or function is lost and cannot be regained (28, 34, 58, 105, 114, 122).

Vision. Under 4 months of age baby does not look for an object hidden after seeing it, and when the same object reappears, it is as if the object were a new object. The infant has no knowledge that objects have a continuous existence: the object ceases to exist when it is not seen (86, 87). The baby coordinates both eyes, and attends to and prefers novel stimuli. At 4 months he or she can focus for any distance and perceive shape constancy when the object is rotated at different angles. Infants look longer at patterned stimuli of less complexity than at stimuli that have more complex designs or no lines or contours and can detect change of pattern. The infant prefers faces but is attracted by checkerboard designs, geometric shapes, and large pictures (circles, dots, and squares at least 3 in. high and with angles rather than contours). Full depth perception develops at approximately 9 months when the images received in the central nervous system from the macula of each eye are integrated. Visual stimulation of both eyes simultaneously is necessary for the baby to develop binocular vision. Otherwise **amblyopia** (*lazy eye*), *which is a gradual loss of the ability to see in one eye because of lack of stimulation of visual nerve pathways,* develops without damage to

TABLE 7–4. ASSESSMENT OF PHYSICAL CHARACTERISTICS OF THE INFANT

1–3 Months	3–6 Months	6–9 Months	9–12 Months
Many characteristics of newborn, but more stable physiologically	Most neonatal reflexes gone		Temperature averages 99.7°F (37.7°C)
Heartbeat steadies at about 120–130 beats/min	Temperature stabilizes at 99.4°F (37.5°C)	Pulse about 115/min	Pulse about 100–110/min
Blood pressure about 80/40; gradually increases		Blood pressure about 90/60	Blood pressure 96/66
Respirations more regular at 30–40/min; gradually decrease		Respirations about 32/min	Respirations 20–30/min
Appearance of salivation and tears			
Weight gain of 5–7 oz (141.75–198.45 g) per week	Weight gain of 3–5 oz (85.05–141.75 g) per week		Weight gain of 3–5 oz (85.05–141.75 g) per week
Weight at 8–13 lb (3629–5897 g)	Weight at 15–16 lb (6.8–7.3 kg) by 6 months	Birth weight doubled by 6 months	Birth weight tripled; average 22 lb (10 kg)
Head circumference increases 1 in. up to 16 in. (40 cm)	Head size increases 1 in. (2.54 cm)	Head size 17.8 in. (43.21 cm)	Head size increases slightly more, about ½ in. (18.3 in. or 45–46 cm)
Chest circumference 16 in. (40 cm)	Chest size increases more than 1 in. (17.3 in. or 43–44 cm)	Chest circumference increases ½ in. (17.8 in. or 44–45 cm)	Chest circumference increases about ½ in. (18.3 in. or 45–46 cm)
Growth of 1 in. (2.54 cm) monthly	Growth of ½ in. (1.27 cm) monthly	Growth of ½ in. (1.27 cm) monthly	Growth of ½ in. monthly; height 29–30 in. (72.5–75 cm), increased by 50% since birth
Tonic neck and Moro reflexes rapidly diminishing	Most neonatal reflexes gone		
Arms and legs found in bilaterally symmetric position	Palmar reflex diminishing		
Limbs used simultaneously, but not separately	Movements more symmetric		
Hands and fingers played with			
Clenched fists giving way to open hands that bat at objects			
Reaches for objects	Reaches for objects with accurate aim and flexed fingers	Palmar grasp developed	Throws objects
Plays with hands		Picks up objects with both hands; bangs toys	
	Objects transferred from one hand to another by 6 months	Holds bottle with hands; holds own cookie	Puts toys in and out of container
	Bangs with objects held in one hand	Preference for use of one hand	
	Scoops objects with hands		
	Begins to use fingers separately	Probes with index finger	Points with finger
		Thumb opposition to finger (prehension) by 7 months	Brings hands and thumb and index finger together at will to pick up small objects
			Releases objects at will
Can follow moving objects with eyes when supine; begins to use both eyes together at about age 2 months	Binocular depth perception by about 5 months	Explores, feels, pulls, inspects, tastes, and tests objects	Makes mark on paper
	Looks for objects when they are dropped		
	Improving eye–hand coordination	Hand–mouth coordination	
		Feeds self cracker and other finger foods	Eats with fingers; holds cup, spoon
	Eruption of one or two lower incisors	Begins weaning process	Has six teeth, central and lateral incisors; eruption of first molars at about 12 months

(continued)

TABLE 7–4. ASSESSMENT OF PHYSICAL CHARACTERISTICS OF THE INFANT (continued)

1–3 Months	3–6 Months	6–9 Months	9–12 Months
Attends to voices	Binaural hearing present		
Raises chin while lying on stomach at 1 month	Turns head to sound	Turns to sounds behind self	
Raises chest while lying on stomach at 2 months; raises head and chest 45° to 50° off bed, supporting weight on arms			
Holds head in alignment when prone at 2 months; holds head erect in prone position at 3 months			
Supports self on forearms when on stomach at 3 months	Rolls over completely by 6 months		Rolls easily from back to stomach
Sits if supported	Sits with support at 4 months		
	Holds head steady while sitting		
	Pulls self to sitting position		
	Begins to sit alone for short periods	Sits erect unsupported by 7 months	Sits alone steadily
	Plays with feet		Pivots when seated
	Kicks vigorously		Puts feet in mouth
	Begins to hitch (scoot) backward while sitting	Creeps or crawls by 8 or 9 months	Hitches with backward locomotion while sitting
	Bears portion of own weight when held in standing position	Pulls self to stand by holding onto support	Sits from standing position without help
	Pushes feet against hard surface to move by 3 or 4 months	Cruises (walking sideways while holding onto object with both hands) by 10 months	Stands alone for a minute
			Walks when led by 11 months
		Begins to walk with help	Walks with help by 12–14 months
			Lumbar and dorsal curves developed while learning to walk
			Turning of feet and bowing of legs normal
			Beginning to show regular bladder and bowel patterns; has one or two stools per day; interval of dry diaper does not exceed 1 to 2 hours
			Not ready for toilet training
Smiles at comforting person reflexly	Smiles at person deliberately during interaction	Experiences separation anxiety about 7–9 months	
			Begins to cooperate in dressing; puts arm through sleeve; takes off socks
Coos, chuckles, laughs	Babbles; plays with sounds		Improves previously acquired skills throughout this period

the retina or other eye structures. If visual stimulation is not lacking for too many weeks, the condition reverses itself. If one eye continues to do all the work for several months, blindness results in the other eye.

Vital Signs. During infancy vital signs (temperature, pulse, respirations, and blood pressure) stabilize, as shown in Table 7–4.

Intersensory integration. To infancy, information from two sense modalities is interrelated. Four-month-old infants respond to relationships between visual and auditory stimuli that carry information about an object. Six-month-old infants look longer at television when both picture and sound are on than when only the picture is on. They look longer at patterns on television than other types of stimuli.

Touch. The haptic system is that body system pertaining to tactile stimulation. There are different neural receptors for heat, warmth, cold, dull pain, sharp pain, deep pressure, vibration, and light touch. At birth all humans possess central nervous system ability to register and associate sensory impressions received through receptor organs in the skin and from kinesthetic stimuli that originate with neuromuscular stimulation from their contact with other humans. Sensory pathways subserving kinesthetic and tactile activities are the first to complete myelinization in infancy, followed by auditory and visual pathways (34, 105, 122).

Touching the infant from birth on provides the basis for higher-order operations in the neurologic, perceptual, muscular, skeletal, and cognitive systems. Each tactile act carries a physiologic impact with psychological and sociocultural meaning. Much information is gained through discriminating one physical stimulus from another, with the form or quality of touch changing the perception of the tactile experience. Tactile stimulation is essential for both beginning body image development and other learning (77). Encourage parents to stroke, massage, and cuddle baby; to talk and sing to baby; and to provide toys that have primary colors, different textures, and movement.

Endocrine System

The endocrine system begins to develop primarily in infancy and childhood; it is limited in fetal life. Thus the child is very susceptible to stress, including fluid and electrolyte imbalance, during the first 18 months because the pituitary gland and adrenal cortex do not function well together and the adrenal gland is immature. The pituitary gland continues to secrete growth hormone and thyroid-stimulating hormone (begun in fetal life), which influence growth and metabolism (105).

Respiratory System

The structures of the upper respiratory tract remain small and relatively delicate and provide inadequate protection against infectious agents. Close proximity of the middle ear, wide horizontal eustachian tube, throat, short and narrow trachea, and bronchi result in rapid spread of infection from one structure to the other. Mucous membranes are less able to produce mucus, causing less air humidification and warming, which also increases susceptibility to infection. The rounded thorax, limited alveolar surface for gas exchange, and amount of anatomic dead air space in the lungs or portion of the tracheobronchial tree where inspired air does not participate in gas exchange means that more air must be moved in and out per minute than later in childhood, causing increased respiratory rate. By age 1 year the lining of the airway resembles that of the adult. Respiratory rate at rest decreases gradually during the first year (105).

Gastrointestinal System

The gastrointestinal system matures somewhat after 2 to 3 months when the baby can voluntarily chew, hold, or spit out food. Saliva secretion increases and composition becomes more adultlike. Stomach Capacity of the Infant (below) depicts capacity by age. The stomach's emptying time changes from $2\frac{1}{2}$ to 3 hours to 3 to 6 hours. Gastric hydrochloric acid is low; pepsinogen secretion nears adult levels at 3 months. Tooth eruption begins at approximately 6 months and stimulates saliva flow and chewing (122).

The small intestine is proportionally longer than it is in an adult; the large intestine is proportionally

► **STOMACH CAPACITY OF INFANT**

Newborn	10–20 mL
1-week-old	30–90 mL
2- to 3-week-old	75–100 mL
1-month-old	90–150 mL
3-month-old	150–200 mL
1-year-old	210–360 mL

shorter. Peristaltic waves mature by slowing down and reversing less after approximately 8 months; then stools are more formed and baby spits up or vomits less. **Colic,** a term that indicates *daily periods of distress,* usually occurs between 2 to 3 weeks and 2 to 3 months and seems to have no remedy. X-ray films taken of such infants show unusually rapid and violent peristaltic waves throughout the intestinal tract. These movements are normally set off by a few sucking movements. Gas pressure in the rectum is also three times greater than in the average infant (105, 122). Some physicians believe colic is caused by a deficiency of vitamin K, A, or E. Some mothers find that changing formula and giving plain, low-fat yogurt helps reduce the pains. When small yogurt feedings do not help, vitamin A and E supplements have been found effective. Apparently colic disappears as digestive enzymes become more complex, and normal bacterial flora accumulate as baby ingests a larger variety of food. By 2 months baby usually has two **stools** (*bowel movements*) daily. By 4 months there is a predictable interval of time between feeding and bowel movements. Breastfed babies usually have soft, semiliquid stools that are light yellow. Breastfed babies may vary more in the bowel movement pattern: the baby may have three or four watery stools a day or may go several days without a bowel movement. The stools of the formula-fed baby are more brown and formed.

The liver occupies a larger part of the abdominal cavity than an adult's liver does and remains functionally immature until age 1 year. Glycogen and vitamin storage is less effective than it is later in life.

As the autonomic nervous system and gastrointestinal tract mature, interconnections from between higher mental functions and the autonomic nervous system; the infant's gastrointestinal tract responds to emotional states in self or someone close to him or her (105, 122).

Muscular Tissue

At birth muscular tissue is almost completely formed; growth results from increasing size of the already existing fibers under the influence of growth hormone, thyroxine, and insulin. As muscle size increases, strength increases in childhood. Muscle fibers need continual stimulation to develop to full function and strength (105, 122).

Skin

Structures typical of adult skin are present, but they are functionally immature; thus baby is more prone to skin disorders. The epidermal layers are very permeable, causing greater loss of fluid from the body. Dry, intact skin is the greatest deterrent to bacterial invasion. Sebaceous glands, which produce sebum, are very active in late fetal life and early infancy, causing milia and cradle cap, which go away at approximately 6 weeks. Production of sebum decreases during infancy and remains minimal during childhood until puberty, which accounts for the dry skin.

Eccrine (sweat) glands are not functional in response to heat and emotional stimuli until a few months after birth, and function remains minimal through childhood. The inability of the skin to contract and shiver in response to cold or perspire in response to heat causes ineffective thermal regulation (105, 122).

Urinary System

Renal structural components are present at birth; by 5 months tubules have adultlike proportions in size and shape. The ureters are relatively short, and the bladder lies close to the abdominal wall. Renal function, however, is not mature until approximately 1 year; therefore, the child is unable to handle increased intake of proteins, which are ingested if cow's milk is given too early (105, 122).

Immune System

Components of the immune system are present or show beginning development. The phagocytosis process is mature, but the inflammatory response is inefficient and unable to localize infections. The ability to produce antibodies is limited; much of the antibody protection is acquired from the mother during fetal life. Development of immunologic function depends on the infant's gradual exposure to foreign bodies and infectious agents (105, 122).

Red Blood Cell and Hemoglobin Levels

High at birth, red blood cell and hemoglobin levels drop after 2 or 3 months and then gradually increase when erythropoiesis begins. Iron deficiency anemia becomes apparent around 6 months of age if the physiologic system does not function adequately to sustain red blood cell and hemoglobin levels. By the end of infancy white blood cells, high at birth, decline to reach adult levels. Red blood cell and hemoglobin levels reach adult norms in late childhood (105, 122).

Increasingly, studies show that the health of the adult is influenced considerably by the person's health status in early life. Obesity, discussed in Chapters 10, 11, and 12, is an example. Blood pressure in adult years is apparently set by age 1; the mix of genetic and environmental influences such as diet, stress, and infections is unknown. One measure of childhood onset of a tendency toward hypertension (high blood pressure) and a possible screening method are being sought in the enzyme kallikrein, released by the kidney and found in the urine. Kallikrein causes the release of materials that dilate blood vessels and is lowest in people with hypertension; kallikrein is also lower in African-American children than in Caucasian children, even before a difference in their blood pressure is seen (80, 105, 122).

Nutritional Needs

The feeding time is a crucial time for baby and mother: a time to strengthen attachment, for baby to feel love and security, a time for mother and baby to learn about self and each other, and a time for baby to learn about the environment. See Table 7–5 for a summary of the changing schedule and amount of food during the first year of life.

Breastfeeding

Breastfeeding of infants has come in and out of fashion. The American Academy of Pediatrics recommends breastfeeding for the first 6 to 12 months of life; however, a large percent of infants are bottle-fed. Human milk is considered ideal because it is sterile, digestible, available, inexpensive, and contains the necessary nutrients except vitamins C and D and iron. Further, even in undernourished women, the composition of breast milk is adequate, although vitamin content depends on the mother's diet (50). Breast milk is all that baby needs the first 6 months of life. It contains higher levels of lactose, vitamin E, and cholesterol and less protein than cow's milk. The additional cholesterol may induce production of hormones required for cholesterol breakdown in adulthood. Breast milk has a more efficient nutritional balance of iron, zinc, vitamin E, and unsaturated fatty acids (119).

Because of the host-resistant factors in human milk, breast milk offers many advantages to the infant, including the premature infant. Immunoglobulins and antibodies to many types of microorganisms, especially those found in the intestinal tract, and enzymes that destroy bacteria are obtained from human milk. Living milk leukocytes, which further promote disease resistance, are also present in breast milk. Respiratory and gastrointestinal diseases, infantile obesity, and meningitis occur two to three times less frequently in breastfed than in bottle-fed babies. Breastfed babies are also less

TABLE 7–5. FEEDING SCHEDULES AND AMOUNTS DURING THE FIRST YEAR OF LIFE

Age of Infant	Schedule for Milk and Food	Amount of Milk Each Feeding
1 week	Every 2–4 hours (six to eight feedings)	60–90 mL (2–3 oz)
2–4 weeks	Every 4 hours (six feedings)	90–120 mL (3–4 oz)
1 month	Every 4–5 hours (five or six feedings)	90–120 mL (3–4 oz)
2–3 months	Five feedings. Sleeps through night. May add rice cereal (fewest allergic reactions)	120–180 mL (4–6 oz)
4–5 months	Five to six feedings. May add iron-fortified cereals; cooked, strained, pureed vegetables; and meat	150–210 mL (5–7 oz). Average serving size for food, 1–2 tablespoons
6–7 months	Four to five feedings. Enjoys finger foods. May add foods with eggs, fruits, oven-dried toast, and soy or wheat flour. Ready to eat solid foods, not just thickened feedings	210–240 mL (6–8 oz). Serving size, 2 tablespoons
8–9 months	Three to four feedings. Eats regular food, mashed or chopped; follows eating pattern of family. Will accept variety of foods	240 mL (8 oz). Needs additional fluids during days
9–12 months	Three feedings. May add juice by cup	Whole milk added at 12 months

Data from References (38, 119).

prone to allergies. Breast milk has growth-promoting substances not found in formula or cow's milk. Human milk kept refrigerated in a sterile container (not pasteurized and not frozen) can be given to premature infants to prevent necrotizing enterocolitis, a frequently fatal bacterial invasion of the colon wall. *Even a brief period of breastfeeding gives immunologic and other benefits* (38, 119).

The mother's decision either to breastfeed or to bottle-feed can be influenced by the obstetrician, pediatrician, hospital staff, husband, friends, and how her own mother fed her children, or there may be no decision making at all. It may be assumed from the start that the mother will feed either one way or the other. Recently in the United States more Anglo women, both of lower and higher economic status, are returning to breastfeeding.

In the study by Scrimshaw et al. (104) 82% of Mexican-American women planned to breastfeed for at least 1 month; 30% planned to breastfeed for more than 6 months. Mexican-American women who were more acculturated were less likely to breastfeed. Women who are married or planning to marry, rather than unmarried women, were more likely to breastfeed. Women who were less anxious prenatally and in postpartum were more likely to breastfeed. Bottle feeding, on the other hand, seemed more often a decision made by the woman herself. Reasons for not breastfeeding included no milk, pain, husband against breastfeeding, and dislike for the procedure. Fewer women planned to breastfeed if they planned to return to work soon—a mandatory choice if the woman did not have economic support from the father or was not married.

The woman who works can be encouraged to breastfeed when at home, although in some work sites women can bring their babies so breastfeeding could be continued. The mother can be told of the benefits of breastfeeding to the baby and informed about community resources such as La Leche League.

Any woman is physiologically able to nurse her baby, with very rare exceptions (119). But childbirth, breastfeeding, and childrearing are sexual experiences for the woman. The woman's success in breastfeeding is related to other aspects of her psychosexual identity (18). She may choose not to breastfeed or to limit the lactation period because of personal preference, illness, or employment in a place where she cannot take baby with her. Further, in the United States feelings of embarrassment, shame, guilt, and disgust about breastfeeding are still apparent, despite today's openness about the subject; often medical personnel convey these feelings to women who wish to breastfeed. In cultures in which breastfeeding is accepted, women breastfeed without difficulty. Mother keeps baby nearby day and night and feeds baby whenever he or she is hungry or needs comfort. Babies fed in this way seldom cry and are satisfied. In societies with a leisure class in which women are objects of amusement and pleasure and technology is king, women are less likely to breastfeed or to have success if they try. Breastfeeding is a learned social behavior. A positive social support system is essential for the woman who breastfeeds as fear of failure, embarrassment, anxiety, exhaustion, frustration, humiliation, anger, fear, or any stress-producing situation can prevent the effect of oxytocin and can block the flow of milk (18). The woman who really wants to breastfeed will develop the courage to do so as comfortably as possible when in public places. Rentscler (90) found that the pregnant woman's level of information and motivation for achievement were positively related to successful breastfeeding.

Preparation for breastfeeding begins during pregnancy. An adequate diet during pregnancy is an initial step toward successful lactation and breastfeeding. Teach the woman the importance and method of preparation. The woman may consult La Leche League literature for help.

During pregnancy the progesterone level is high, like just before menstruation. If a mother nurses after delivery, the pituitary gland secretes prolactin. The high levels of estrogen from the placenta that inhibited milk secretion during pregnancy are gone. As the baby sucks, the nipple is in the back of the mouth, and the jaws and tongue compress the milk sinuses. These tactile sensations trigger the release of the hormone oxytocin from the pituitary gland, which, in turn, causes the "let-down" response. The sinuses refill immediately, and milk flows with very little effort to the baby. This is the crucial time to learn breastfeeding. Oxytocin also causes a powerful contraction of the uterus, lessening the danger of hemorrhage (105, 122).

Every effort should be directed toward making breastfeeding a comfortable, uninterrupted time. Effective techniques for mother getting into a comfortable position, holding the baby, and putting the baby to nipple are described in La Leche League literature, obstetric nursing and other child care books, and some booklets prepared by formula companies. Mother needs an encouraging partner or family member, knowledgeable and supportive nursing and medical personnel to assist, acquaintance with other successful nursing mothers, and hospital routines that allow the baby to be with her for feeding when the baby is hungry and her breasts are full. The mother should not automatically receive medication to stop lactation, and the baby should not be fed in the nursery between breastfeedings. The mother whose milk does not let-down may need oxytocin, a period of relaxation, or perhaps a soothing liquid before feeding. She should, in any case, be encouraged to increase her fluid intake and meet the increased recommended dietary allowances for lactating women (60, 105, 119, 122).

The baby may be put to breast immediately after delivery and fed within 8 hours of birth to reduce hypoglycemia and hyperbilirubinemia (105). That is also a key time to promote bonding (122).

The first nourishment the baby receives after delivery from breastfeeding is **colostrum,** a *thin yellow secretion.* Colostrum is rich in carbohydrates, which the newborn needs, and serves as a laxative in cleaning out the gastrointestinal tract. Colostrum fed immediately after birth prevents against infection because it triggers antibody production. Depending on how soon and how often the mother nurses, true milk comes in the first few days (105, 119).

The baby may nurse every hour or two at first or on demand, perhaps 15 to 30 minutes each time, but graduate to 3- to 4-hour intervals, by 4 months, obtaining more milk in shorter feeding sessions. If anxieties, excessive stimuli, and fatigue are dealt with appropriately, the mother's milk supply will increase or decrease to meet the demand. Alternating breasts with each feeding and emptying the breasts will prevent caking. The infant should grasp the areola completely to avoid excess pressure on the nipples. Generally breastfeeding babies get enough to eat; the child whose growth and weight are within the norm is being breastfed adequately. The large or active infant may need supplemental feeding in addition to breast milk, even when mother's supply is not compromised; however, usually extra formula or baby food is not necessary before the fourth month. Food in addition to breast milk (or formula) should be introduced by the end of the sixth month. If mother received ample amounts of iron during pregnancy, her baby's iron stores should last 4 to 12 months, even on an iron-poor diet (38, 119).

Premature infants can breastfeed earlier and with less effort than they can bottle-feed, but they need time to learn to suck. Physiologically, breastfeeding is an advantage; premature infants suck for approximately 25 minutes at one time, but the longer feeding fills the stomach more slowly. The infant controls the pace of breastfeeding and also avoids gastric distention, in contrast to bottle feeding and the caregiver's controlling feeding pace, amount, and time (17).

Breastfeeding the premature infant is possible and desirable and can be a rewarding option for the mother and nutritionally and emotionally beneficial to the baby. Breast milk is more digestible, and milk from mothers with preterm babies has adequate protein, sodium, potassium, and chloride. It is not at that point adequate in calcium, phosphorus, iron, zinc, and copper. These substances can be provided in supplementary feedings designed for premature infants (38). Boggs and Rau (10) describe (1) the specific procedure for pumping the breasts; (2) how the mother can maintain a milk supply; (3) ways to enhance the experience for the mother, baby, and intensive care nursery staff; and (4) continuation of breastfeeding after discharge.

Alcohol, nicotine, many medications, including laxatives and barbiturates, and drugs and foreign substances such as chemical pollutants and pesticides pass into the milk and to the infant. The mother should be informed of these hazards to her baby if she breastfeeds so that she can avoid harmful substances if possible. Foods without preservatives or dyes can be purchased; some food can be homegrown by families if they wish to exert the effort and use the space. All medications except essential ones should be avoided by the lactating woman; even prescribed medications should be taken with caution.

Weaning gradually, whether to a bottle or a cup, will lessen the discomfort of temporarily having a greater supply than demand. There are normal growth spurts during the first few months when the baby may demand more milk, or the mother may notice a lag as the infant's interests are directed more to the surroundings. She can assume that the infant is receiving enough milk if weight gain is normal, if he or she has six or more wet diapers a day, and if the urine is pale (105, 119).

Commercial Formulas

Commercial formulas are similar to each other and to human milk, but they are not exactly the same. Most have a slightly higher renal solute load than does breast milk. Special formulas have been developed to meet the needs of infants with phenylketonuria, fat malabsorption, and protein hypersensitivity. Modular formula, made by Ross Laboratories, consists of a core of proteins and vitamins and minerals to which different carbohydrates and fats can be added in increasing amounts. Normal growth and development are possible without breastfeeding; however, formula feeding causes greater deposits of subcutaneous fat (105).

Higher protein intake from formula produces a higher blood urea nitrogen level and serum or urine level of amino acids (except taurine). If soy protein isolate is used as a substitute for milk protein, it is supplemented with the amino acid methionine in the formula. Soy protein isolate formula supports growth similar to that of breastfed babies except the preterm baby. Soy-based formulas are used for infants with lactose deficiency or galactosemia, for the baby in a vegetarian family, or for the baby who is allergic to cow's milk and regular formulas. Protein hydrolysate or meat-based formulas can be used for infants allergic to cow's milk or who have malabsorption problems. If the osmolality is too high, water is drawn from the tissue, causing dehydration. Necrotizing enterocolitis may also be more likely to result (119). Wink (120) compares human milk and formulas. This comparison is shown in Table 7–6.

Infants should receive supplemental iron by 4 months of age and preterm babies by 2 months. Iron-fortified formulas are the best source for formula-fed babies. Too high a sodium level in the formula may cause transient elevation of blood pressure in neonates (119, 120).

Teach parents that care must be taken if the bottle is heated; it is not essential to heat it. Instruct the par-

TABLE 7–6. COMPARISON OF HUMAN MILK AND FORMULA

Nutrient or Component	Human Milk	Formula (by National Standards)
Protein	1.6 g/100 kcal; whey:casein ratio of 60:40	1.8–4.5 g/100 kcal; average, 2.3 g/100 kcal; whey: casein ratio of 60:40
Carbohydrates	Lactose, 70 g/L (39% of calories)	Lactose, sucrose, corn syrup, corn syrup solids, maltodextrins, or tapioca starch (40–50% of calories)
Fats	50% of calories	3.3–6 g/100 kcal; at least 300 mg/100 kcal must be linoleic acid, polyunsaturated fat (30–54% of calories)
		Butterfat of cow's milk excreted; soy, coconut, corn, oleo, safflower, or medium-chain triglyceride oils added
Osmolality	300 mOsm/kg	400 mOsm/kg
Iron	1 mg/L	0.15 mg/100 kcal
Sodium		Higher than human milk
Potassium		Higher than human milk
Chloride		Same as human milk

Modified from Wink, D., *Getting Through the Maze of Infant Formulas*, American Journal of Nursing, 85, no. 4 (1985), 388–392.

ents why baby bottles should preferably not be heated in the microwave. The bottle, nipple, and milk all become too hot and will cause oropharyngeal and esophageal burns. Further, the formula-filled disposable plastic liner of a commercial nurser may explode after removal of the heated bottle from the microwave, causing body burns.

Water intoxication is a growing concern with babies who are bottle-fed, especially in poor families when the mother receives Special Supplemental Food Program for Women, Infants, and Children (WIC) formula supplements. The formula allotment of one can per day is often consumed before the end of the month so that the baby is given either very diluted formula or only water to drink. The baby, receiving excess water and inadequate protein and other nutrients, retains water and suffers cerebral edema and electrolyte imbalance, and convulsions ensue. The condition can be life-threatening. Thus, mothers in the lower socioeconomic levels are being encouraged to breastfeed.

Cow's Milk

Cow's milk is designed for another animal; thus, it is not surprising that it varies considerably in composition from human milk. Cow's milk is unsuitable for the infant less than 6 months of age. Cow's milk contains from two to three times as much protein as does human milk, and a much greater percentage of the protein is casein, which produces a large, difficult-to-digest curd. It is higher in saturated fats and lower in cholesterol than is human milk, but the total fat content is comparable; however, the butterfat is poorly absorbed. Cow's milk contains half as much total sugar as human milk and also has galactose and glucose. Although it contains more sodium, potassium, magnesium, sulfur, and phosphorus than human milk, like human milk it is a relatively poor source of vitamins C and D and iron. One striking difference between cow's milk and human milk is the calcium content: cow's milk contains more than four times as much calcium, and babies fed cow's milk have larger and heavier skeletons. Whether or not this is normal or better is debatable. Two percent or skim milk should not be fed to infants because they will not gain weight and they need the fat content (119, 120).

Water

The baby needs approximately 100 to 150 mL of water per kilogram of body weight daily to offset normal fluid losses. Some of this is obtained through the milk, but hot weather, fever, diarrhea, or vomiting quickly leads to dehydration. Infants become dehydrated more quickly than adults because they have a smaller total fluid volume in the body compared with body size (119). Water should be offered at least twice daily. Parents should know the *signs of dehydration:* dry, loose, warm skin; dry mucous membranes; sunken eyeballs and fontanels; slowed pulse; lower blood pressure and increased body temperature; concentrated, scanty urine; constipation or mucoid diarrhea; lethargy; a weak cry. Any combination of these symptoms implies the need for medical treatment.

Nutrient Requirements

After the initial period of adjustment (7–10 days after birth), the baby needs a daily average of 2.2 g of protein and 117 calories per kilogram (or 36 per pound) of body weight to grow and gain weight satisfactorily. Moderate protein intake is apparently well used and increases growth. No specific fat requirement is set, but some fats are necessary because they contain essential fat-soluble vitamins, furnish more energy per unit than carbohydrates and protein, promote development of the nervous system, and contribute to diet palatability. Adequate intake of vitamins and minerals, especially iron and fluoride, is essential. If the water supply is not fluorinated, supplementation should be given until 12 years of age to prevent dental caries. Recommendations for various ages can be found in Appendix I and in a nutrition text (119).

Feeding Comfort

Mothers frequently need instruction about times and methods of **burping** (*bubbling, or gently patting baby's back*) the baby to reduce gaseous content of the stomach during feeding because the cardiac sphincter is not well developed (60). Young babies must be bubbled after every ounce and at the end of a feeding. Later they can be bubbled halfway through and again at the end. The infant should be moved from a semireclining to an upright position while the feeder gently pats the back. Because a new infant's gastrointestinal tract is unstable, milk may be eructated with gas bubbles. Adequate bubbling should occur before the infant is placed into the crib to prevent milk regurgitation and aspiration. The infant should be positioned on back or on side.

Solid Foods

There is no rigid sequence in adding solid foods to the infant's diet. (See Table 7–5 for guidelines.) Whatever solid food is offered first or at what time is largely a matter of individual preference of the mother or of the pediatrician. Ideally the infant's needs and developmental achievements such as eye–hand–mouth coordination and fine pincer grasp should be considered when introducing solids. A large, active baby may need cereal added to the diet at 2 months to satisfy hunger. A smaller, more lethargic baby may find it awkward to accept such supplements before 3 or 4 months.

The mother or nurse introducing the baby to solid foods should make it a pleasant experience. The foods offered should be smooth and well diluted with milk or formula. The infant should not be hurried, coaxed, or allowed to linger more than 30 minutes. New foods should be offered one at a time and early in the feeding while he or she is still hungry. Emphasize *not to add* salt or sugar to feedings to please the feeder's taste buds. Honey should *not* be added to feedings the first year because of the possibility of honey botulism (38, 119).

Because fetal iron stores may last up to 6 to 12 months and because of an increasing incidence of allergies in infants introduced to a variety of solids before 3 months, many physicians now recommend later introduction of solids. Many pediatricians are also concerned about early feedings because of the possible relationship between overfeeding and infant and adult obesity (14% of overweight 6-month-old babies become overweight adults (38). Some even encourage a total milk diet as a nutritionally adequate diet during the first 6 months.

Help the parents realize that when the baby is first fed puréed foods with a spoon, he or she expects and wants to suck. The protrusion of the tongue, which is needed in sucking, makes it appear as if baby is pushing food out of the mouth. Parents misinterpret this as a dislike for the food, but it really is the result of immature muscle coordination and possibly surprise at the taste and feel of the new items in the diet. This reflex gradually disappears by 7 to 8 months. The baby should not be punished for spitting out food. Further, baby begins to exercise some control over the environment by pacing the feeding.

When you or the physician suggests that the mother offer "table food" to the infant, ask what table food is in their home. Depending on the level of the household hygiene or the family food pattern, table food may or may not constitute an adequate or healthy diet. Family diet counseling may be necessary to ensure continued health of the family unit. Food supplies not only physical sustenance but also many personal and cultural needs. The introduction of foods characteristic of a culture provides the foundation for lifelong food habits and the basis for teaching a cultural pattern of eating.

Infant nutritional status can be assessed by measuring head circumference, height, and weight. The fat baby, with a differential of two or more percentiles between weight and length, more likely will become an overweight adult (122); however, weight at birth or weight gain in infancy is not an accurate predictor of obesity in children. Small stature may indicate undernutrition unless there is a genetic influence from small-sized parents. Signs of nutritional deprivation include smaller-than-normal head size, pale skin color, poor skin turgor, and low hemoglobin and hematocrit levels (119, 122).

Teach parents to avoid overfeeding—either milk or foods. Theories hold that babies who are fed more calories than they use daily develop additional fat cells to store unused energy sources. These fat cells proliferate in infancy and continue to replace themselves during childhood. Adults who were fat infants will have excess fat cells to fill through life and may have difficulty with weight control or may be obese. Another theory about the effect of infant feeding on adult weight is that eating patterns are difficult to change, especially if food symbolizes love, attention, or approval.

In addition to discussing the food quantities, quality, and nutrients needed by the baby, help parents to realize that food and mealtime are learning experiences. The baby gains motor control and coordination in self-feeding; he or she learns to recognize color, shape, and texture. Use of mouth muscles stimulates the ability to make movements necessary for speech development. He or she continues to develop trust with the consistent, loving atmosphere of mealtime. Food should not be used as reward or punishment (by withholding food). The child should learn moderation in feeding quantity, and between-feeding snacks should be avoided or, if used, should be healthful, small in quantity, and given because the child is hungry despite eating at mealtime (119).

Unless you are an experienced mother, you may feel uncomfortable in teaching about feeding or other child care. Yet, you can share information gleaned from the literature, experiences of other mothers you have helped, and your own experiences if you have worked in the newborn nursery or helped a family member with a new baby. Do not tell the mother what method is best; give her the available information and then support her in *her* decision. Because feeding is one of the first tasks as a mother, she will need your guidance, assistance, and emotional support. You can offer suggestions such as the posture that will assure a comfortable position for her as she cradles the baby in her arms close to her body. Whether breast- or bottle-fed, the baby needs the emotional warmth and body contact. The bottle should never be propped because choking may result. Further, nursing-bottle mouth may develop: tooth decay is much higher in children when mothers use the bottle of milk, juice, or sugar water as a pacifier. The upper front teeth are most affected because liquids pool around these teeth when baby is drowsy or asleep (38).

Mother–child contacts after birth are a continuation of the symbiotic prenatal relationship. The dependence of the baby on the mother and the reciprocal need of the mother for satisfaction from the child, proving her dependability and giving her confidence, are necessary to develop and continue the relationship. A successful feeding situation sets the foundation for the infant's personality and social development. It is the main means of establishing a relationship with another person and consequently the most basic opportunity to establish trust. Thus, feeding is much more than a mechanical task. Your teaching attitude can convey its importance. If a father will be a primary nurturer, teach him the same way you would teach the mother.

Mercer (74) explored early psychophysiologic mother–infant interaction using the tenderness and anxiety theorems of Harry Stack Sullivan. Maternal anxiety and perception were assessed and related to changes in healthy infant satiety, anxiety, and bottle-feeding behavior. Blood samples were obtained from the infants just before and 60 minutes after feeding for determination of glucose and cortisol. Formula consumption was also noted. An empathetic linkage exists in healthy postpartum mother–infant couples. The interaction of both a mother's transitory anxiety around feeding time and overall anxiety is associated with changes in her infant's satiety and anxiety levels and feeding behavior. Relatively low maternal anxiety at feeding time is associated with both increased formula intake and decreased postfeed cortisol, the latter being indicative of a feeling of security. Extremely low maternal anxiety or apathy (which can result from anxiety) around feeding time is associated with both decreased formula intake and increased postfeed cortisol, the latter reflecting a feeling of insecurity. Thus maternal anxiety levels are a threat physically and emotionally to the infant. A mother's perception of the infant tenderness needs is related to her prefeed and feed anxiety level. Increased maternal tenderness is associated with low maternal anxiety before and during infant feeding.

Weaning

The *gradual elimination of breastfeeding or bottle feeding in favor of cup and table feeding* (**weaning**) is usually completed by the end of the first year. Baby shows signs of making this transition: muscle coordination increases, teeth erupt, and he or she resists being held close while feeding. The two methods should overlap and allow baby to take some initiative and allow mother to guide the new method. Mother's consistency in meeting the new feeding schedule is important to development of a sense of trust.

The most difficult feeding to give up is usually the bedtime feeding because baby is tired and is more likely to want the "old method." After the maxillary central incisory teeth erupt, a night bottle should contain no carbohydrate to reduce decay in the deciduous teeth. During periods of stress the baby will often regress. Baby is also learning to wait longer for food and may object vigorously to this new condition.

The need to suck varies with different children. Some children, even after weaning, will suck a thumb or use a pacifier (if provided). The baby should not be shamed for either of these habits because they are not likely to cause problems with the teeth or mouth during the first 2 years.

Weaning coincides with a slower growth rate and will be accompanied by a decrease in appetite. Baby should not be forced to eat at the old rate during this period. Teach parents the meaning of the baby's behavior and how to adapt to this new period of development.

Asian infant feeding patterns differ from those of many other countries, including the dominant culture in the United States, United Kingdom, and Europe. Some Asian-born immigrants have traditionally breastfed the baby for 1 to 3 years, after which the child is fed a plain diet of rice, lentils, some vegetables, occasionally eggs, fish or fruit, and rarely meat. The Moslem parent, a vegetarian, cannot use, for religious purposes, commercially prepared baby food that has any meat product in it. They may occasionally eat animals slaughtered according to Moslem religious laws and rituals (meat is then classed as *halal*), but such meat is difficult to find in non-Moslem countries. Thus, eggs and milk are the primary sources of protein. If the diet for the weaned child is well planned, it can be adequate. Assess for steady weight gain; normal developmental behavior; healthy-appearing hair, skin, teeth, and eyes; energy; ability to play and sleep; and infrequent colds or other infections. The main difference between Western and Asian infant feeding practices is lack of variety in diet and prolonged use of milk and certain baby foods (67).

A study was conducted by Thomas and DeSantis to compare Cuban and Haitian immigrant mothers' beliefs and practices related to feeding, weaning, and introduction of supplemental foods, and how living in the U.S. affected these. Both groups of women believed that breastfeeding was better, but some did not breastfeed for fear of transferring sickness to the baby through the mother's milk, need for employment outside the home, and inadequate supply of breast milk. Some had been told by family or friends not to breastfeed. In contrast to the norm in the United States of weaning from the bottle at about 1 year of age, Cuban and Haitian mothers weaned their children from the bottle at ages 4 and 2 years, respectively, although supplemental foods, often of high carbohydrate content, had been introduced by 6 months of age. Both populations believe that a fat child is a healthy child. Implications for transcultural nursing care were discussed in the study (110).

Sleep Patterns

One of the most frequent concerns of a new mother is when, where, and how much baby sleeps. Awake, alert periods are altered by different types of feeding schedules. Sleep patterns are unique to each infant, but some generalizations can be made.

The infant exhibits at least six states or levels of arousal (105, 122):

- Regular or quiet sleep: Eyes are closed, breathing is regular, and the only movements are sudden, generalized startle motions. Baby makes little sound. This is the low point of arousal; infant cannot be awakened with mild stimuli.
- Irregular, active rapid eye movement (REM) sleep: Baby's eyes are closed, breathing is irregular, muscles twitch slightly from time to time, and there are facial responses of smiles or pouts in response to sounds or lights. Baby may groan, make faces, or cry briefly.
- Quiet wakefulness: Eyes are open, the body is more active, breathing is irregular, and there is varying spontaneous response to external stimuli.
- Active wakefulness: Eyes are open; there is visual following of interesting sights and sounds, body movements, and vocalizations that elicit attention.
- Crying.
- Indeterminate state: transition from one state of alertness to another.

The newborn and young infant spend more time in REM sleep than adults. In this state baby shows continual slow rolling eye movements on which are superimposed rapid eye movements. Additionally, respirations increase and are irregular, and small muscle twitchings are seen (105, 122).

As the infant's nervous system develops, baby will have longer periods of sleep and wakefulness that gradually become more regular. By 6 weeks, baby's biological rhythms usually coincide with daytime and nighttime hours, and he or she will be sleeping through the night. Babies sleep an average of 16 to 20 hours a day for the first week. By 12 to 16 weeks these hours will be reduced to 14 or 15 a day. Usually this pattern will continue through the first year, with nap times getting shorter until the morning nap is eliminated. By 7 or 8 months, baby may sleep through the night without awakening. By the end of the first year, the baby may sleep 12 to 14 hours at night and nap 1 to 4 hours during the day (105).

Help parents understand that when a baby goes through the stage of separation anxiety about 8 months of age, bedtime becomes more difficult because he or she does not want to leave mother. Because the baby needs sleep, the parent should be firm about getting the child ready for bed. Prolonging bedtime adds to fatigue and separation fears. Caressing or singing softly while holding baby in a sleeping position in bed is calming; restraint is perceived as helpful rather than punitive. If the mother is available when the baby first awakes, he or she anticipates this pleasure, and sleep is associated with return of mother. If the baby awakes and cries during the night, the parent should wait briefly. Many times the crying will subside with the baby's growing ability to control personal anxiety feelings. Persistent crying indicates unmet needs and should be attended.

Frequently a mother becomes concerned if baby sleeps too long during the day, perhaps 6 or 7 hours without a feeding. If this happens frequently, it may help to awaken the baby during the day for regular feedings and attempt to establish a better routine with longer sleeping periods at night. Occasional oversleeping is little cause for concern. The physical preparations for sleep ideally include a room and a bed for the baby, especially after the first few weeks. Sharing the parents' bed or room may lead to later sleep problems for the infant and can be detrimental to the husband–wife relationship. The infant should at least have a consistent place for sleeping (be it box, drawer, or crib) and a clean area for supplies. Sometimes baby does not seem to sleep enough. Some babies sleep less and remain healthy. Other babies have chronic sleeplessness, which may be due to allergy to cow's milk; if so, a suitable milk substitute should be used (59).

A baby can sleep comfortably in an infant crib or bassinet during the first few weeks, but as soon as active arms and legs begin to hit the sides he or she should be moved to a full-sized crib. The crib slats should be no more than 2½ inches apart. No pillows should be used. The crib should have a crib border placed at the bottom of the slats to prevent catching the head between the bars. It should be fitted with a firm, water-proofed, easy-to-clean mattress and with warm light covers loosely tucked in. The sides of the crib should fit closely to the mattress so that the infant will not get caught and crushed if he or she should roll to the edge. Thin plastic sheeting can cause suffocation and should never be used on or around the baby's crib. Teach these safety measures to the parents.

Play Activity

The infant engages in play with self: with the hands or feet, by rolling, getting into various positions, and with the sounds he or she produces. Baby needs playful activity from both mother and father to stimulate development in all spheres. Share the following information with parents. You may need to teach the parents how to touch, cuddle, talk to, and play with the baby.

Certain toys are usually enjoyed at certain ages because of changing needs and developing skills. Guide to Play Activities lists age, characteristics that influence play interest and activities, and suggested activities, toys, and equipment (45, 114, 116, 117).

The baby can remain satisfied playing with self for increasing amounts of time but prefers to have people around. Baby enjoys being held briefly in various positions, being rocked, swinging for short periods, being taken for walks.

Because much of baby's play involves putting objects into the mouth, a clean environment with lead-free paint is important. A small object that baby swallows such as a coin is passed through the digestive tract; however, small batteries used in cameras, calculators, and other electronic equipment may be hazardous if swallowed because they can rupture and release poisonous chemicals. Surgical removal may be necessary. Children gradually build an immunity to the germs encountered daily on various objects; however, health may be threatened by that which goes unnoticed. Sitting and playing in dirt or sand contaminated by dioxin, other pesticides or herbicides, or radiation is dangerous to the developing physiologic systems. Children's or parents' reading material, which can become play objects, may also be hazardous. The high lead content of the glossy color pages of magazines and newspaper inserts may account for some cases of lead poisoning in young children, who are eaters of the inedible. A study conducted by researchers at the Connecticut Agricultural Experiment Station revealed that the lead content of glossy paper printed in color—especially pages containing the color yellow—is so high that a child devouring a 4-in. square of it every day for 6 weeks could be at a critical stage of lead poisoning. Although black-and-white newsprint, the comics, and the black-and-white magazine stock are scarcely recommended for snacking, their lead content is dramatically lower than that of the shiny, colored pages, the research showed. Ideally, the child does not eat paper; yet most children have been observed sucking or chewing on corners of magazines or pieces of paper.

Toys need not be expensive, but they should be colorful (and without leaded paint), safe, sturdy, and easily handled and cleaned. They should be large enough to prevent aspiration or ingestion; they should be without rough or sharp edges or points, detachable parts, or loops to get around the neck, and some should make sounds and have moving parts.

Baby needs an unrestricted play area that is safe, although use of a playpen is necessary for short peri-

► GUIDE TO PLAY ACTIVITIES

AGE	CHARACTERISTIC DEVELOPMENT	SUGGESTED ACTIVITIES & EQUIPMENT
4 weeks	Tonic neck reflex attitude Rolls partway to side Disregards ring in midplane Eyes follow ring toward midplane Hand clutches on contact Drops rattle immediately Attends bell Activity diminishes Marked head lag when pulled to sitting position Head sags forward; back evenly rounded Head rotation; in prone position Startles easily to sudden sounds or movements	Much tender loving care Mobiles and other hanging objects which can be followed by eyes but which can't be grasped — bright in color Musical mobiles
16 weeks	Head position in midplane Plays with hands at midplane Regards ring immediately, arms activate Holds rattle in fist Head fairly steady in sitting position On verge of rolling Laughs aloud; coos; carries on "conversation" Spontaneous social smile Knows mother; stares at strangers Smiles at strangers who are friendly	Enjoys cuddling and motion Cradle gym for brief periods (20–30 minutes) Rattles Soft, stuffed, small toys to touch and squeeze Soothing music (humming, singing, phonograph records) Rattles, bells, musical toys Crinkling paper, clap or snap of fingers Large wooden or nonsplintering plastic toys, beads, spools
28 weeks	Transfers small toys (blocks, bells, etc.) from one hand to the other Mouths objects Lifts head in supine position Reaches with one hand Sits momentarily by self-leaning on hands Feet to mouth Regards image in mirror Polysyllabic vowel sounds Bounces actively Prompt grasp Pivots in prone position Plays contentedly alone	Small toys Soothing music Cradle gym (30–40 minutes) Peek-a-boo Pat-a-cake Noise makers (bells, squeak toys) Moderately active bouncing on lap Use of mirror to see self and others Outdoor excursions — walks Reading to child, letting child touch and pat books Splashing in water, water toys
40 weeks	Knocks blocks together in hands Approaches objects with index finger Prehends pellet, inferior pincer grasp Grasps bell by handle and waves it Sits with good control Goes from sitting to prone position Creeps Pulls to standing position Waves bye-bye Increasing imitation Adjusts to simple commands	Small one-square-inch blocks Soft, small toys Assorted objects of varying color having interesting texture Peek-a-boo Pat-a-cake Rides in buggy or stroller Parallel play Is fascinated with words and other sounds Nesting, stack, or climbing boxes and blocks Kitchen utensils Bath toys Cups and boxes to pour (water, sand) and fill
12 months	Walks with help Throws and rolls ball Offers objects, but frequently does not release them Vocabulary of 3–10 words Vigorous imitative scribble	Open and close simple boxes Empty and fill toys Push-pull toys Strongly strung large beads Small, brightly-colored blocks Rag and oil cloth books Balls, bells, floating bath toys Cuddle toys Nursery rhymes Music and singing to child

ods. Excess restriction or lack of stimulation inhibits curiosity, learning about self and the environment, and development of trust. Therefore baby should not wear clothing that is restraining, he or she should not be kept constantly in a playpen or crib, and he or she needs play objects and a loving parent who provides stimulating surroundings.

Verzemnieks discusses ways to stimulate sensory development of the hospitalized child during routine care measures and common items in the hospital that can be used as toys, such as medicine cups, souffle cups, empty tape cylinders, and various boxes (116). She also lists common household items that can be used in the home for toys that can provide fun and stimulate creativity, more so than some of the expensive toys on the market.

Parents should know the dangers of overstimulation and rough handling. Fatigue, inattention, and injury may result. The playful, vigorous activities that well-intentioned parents engage in such as tossing the baby forcefully into the air or jerking the baby in a whiplash manner may cause bone injuries or subdural hematomas and cerebrovascular lesions that later could cause mental retardation. Premature infants and male babies are twice as vulnerable as full-term girls, because of the relative immaturity of their brains.

Health Promotion and Health Protection

In addition to measures already discussed, including the safety measures in the previous section on play activity, the following measures also promote health.

At birth the neonate should have silver nitrate drops or ointment instilled in the eyes. Although less than 3% of mothers have gonorrhea, the possibility of blindness in the infant, along with the low cost and effectiveness of the treatment, makes this procedure mandatory (105).

Injecting 1 mg of vitamin K is effective in preventing hemorrhagic disease, which is caused in 1 of 2000 to 1 of 3000 live births by a transient deficiency of factor VIII production. Sickle cell screening can be obtained from in-cord blood (105).

During the first week of life the infant should be screened for **phenylketonuria (PKU)**, *an inborn metabolic disorder characterized by abnormal presence of phenylketone and other metabolites of phenylalanine in the urine.* Hypothyroid screening is also recommended for all newborns. Refer to Chart 1 in Appendix IV for a schedule of health screening measures for the infant.

Immunizations

Immunizations, *promoting disease resistance through injection of attenuated, weakened organisms or products produced by organisms,* are essential to every infant as a preventive measure. Before birth baby is protected from certain organisms by the placental barrier and mother's physical defense mechanisms. Birth propels baby into an environment filled with many microorganisms. Baby has protection against common pathogens for a time, but as he or she is gradually exposed to the outside world and the people in it, further protection is needed through routine immunizations, available from private physicians or public health clinics. Annually, millions of children in the developing world either are permanently disabled or die from childhood diseases that are preventable. The World Health Organization (WHO) has as its goal to immunize every child against diphtheria, polio, measles, tetanus, and whooping cough and to protect against tuberculosis (105).

The immunization schedule presented in Chart 4 in Appendix IV should be followed. Vaccination is essential to provide **herd immunity,** *immunity to all susceptible persons,* especially for pregnant women in the first trimester.

OPV should not be administered in households with immunodeficient individuals because OPV is excreted in the stool and could infect an immunodeficient person. Poliovirus vaccine inactivated (IPOL) is safe to give in these households. A primary series of IPOL for children and adults consists of three 0.5-mL doses administered subcutaneously at least 4 weeks, preferably 8 weeks, apart. (The first two doses can be given with the DTP immunizations at 2 and 4 months of age.) The third dose should follow at least 6 months, preferably 12 months, after the second dose. Use of IPOL is contraindicated in persons with a history of hypersensitivity to any component of the vaccine, including neomycin, streptomycin, and polymyxin B. If allergic reaction occurs within 24 hours of the first dose, no further doses should be given (57).

Parents should be told the importance of immunizations and should be helped to get them, for example, through flexible clinic hours or low-cost mass immunizations in a community. Parents should also keep a continuing record of the child's immunizations. Your teaching, encouragement, community efforts, and follow-up are vital.

One study showed that a mailed reminder about the date for immunization of the 6-month-old infant increased the chances that baby would receive the scheduled immunization, especially in families that had a record of not keeping clinic appointments. A telephone reminder may help in getting mothers to return for well-baby immunizations.

As a result of worldwide efforts, worldwide immunization of children is now increasing, according to WHO. The biggest recent improvements in administration rates has been in Africa. WHO estimates that 3 million child deaths were prevented because of immunization programs; yet about 2 million children died in 1994 in the world from three vaccine-preventable deaths: measles (1 million), neonatal tetanus (500,000), pertussis or whooping cough (almost 500,000) (46).

Safety Promotion and Injury Control

Safety promotion and injury control are based on the understanding of infant behavior. Accidents are a major cause of death to individuals less than 26 years of age. Risk factors that influence the occurrence of fatal childhood accidents include (1) host factors such as age and sex; (2) environmental factors such as hazardous play equipment, flammable clothing, and accessible poisons; and (3) parental characteristics such as socioeconomic status (122). Although infant mortality rates in the United States have decreased in the past four decades, in 1988 the United States ranked 23rd in infant mortality, higher than most industrialized countries. Differences in infant mortality are noted in terms of socioeconomic and educational variables. Substantial differences in infant mortality between the various ethnic/racial groups have been documented (107).

Epidemiologic studies report that the main causes of death for the infant are drowning; suffocation by inhalation and/or ingestion of food or by mechanical means (in bed or cradle, by plastic bag, or by polystyrene-filled pillows); transport accidents; and falls (27, 88, 122). Contrary to common belief, the baby is not immobile: he or she will not necessarily stay where placed. Baby rolls, crawls, creeps, walks, reaches, and explores. As he or she is helpless in water, the baby should never be left alone or with an unresponsible person while in water. The home and car have many often unnoticed hazards; thus, the baby should never be left alone in either and should never roam freely in the car while it is in motion. Parents should use an approved car infant seat or harness (Fig. 7–5).

Falls can be avoided if the parents or nurse is responsible for doing the following:

- Keep crib rails up.
- Maintain a firm grasp of the baby while carrying or caring for him or her and support the head during the first few months.
- Use a sturdy high chair and car infant seat or harness with fasteners in place (this is law in many states).

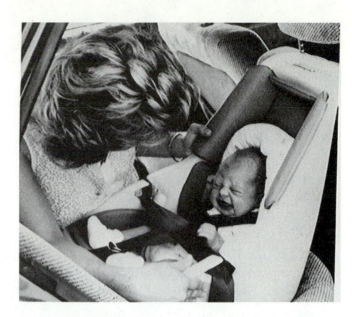

Figure 7–5. Infants should be transported in an approved automobile infant seat or harness. *(From Sherwen, L.N., M.A. Scoloveno, and C.T. Weingarten, Nursing Care of the Childbearing Family. Stamford, CT: Appleton & Lange, 1991, p. 926.)*

- Have a gate at the top of the stairs or in front of windows or doors that are above the first story.
- Keep room free of loose rugs or trailing cables or cords to avoid child falling over them as he or she becomes mobile.
- Keep furniture secure so child does not pull it on self when becoming mobile.

Suffocation at home and in the health care setting can be avoided:

- Remove any small objects that could be inhaled or ingested (safety pins, small beads, coins, toys, nuts, raisins, popcorn, balloons).
- Keep plastic bags, Venetian blind cords, or other cords out of reach.
- Avoid the use of pillows in the crib or excessively tight clothing or bedcovers.

Burns can also be avoided:

- Place the crib away from radiators or fireplaces.
- Use warm-air vaporizers with caution.
- Cover electric outlets.
- Avoid tablecloths that hang over the table's edge.
- Turn pot handles inward on the stove.
- Avoid excessive sun exposure.
- Avoid smoking around the baby.

Encourage parents to take a first-aid course (one directed to cardiopulmonary resuscitation, preventing airway obstruction, and other home and family concerns) that enables them to recognize hazards and take appropriate measures to avoid injury to loved ones. Teaching parents about the child's normal developmental patterns will also enable them to foresee potential accidents and take precautions.

Parents must also consider another threat to the safety of the child and to the integrity of their family unit: stealing, kidnapping, or abduction of their infant.

Burgess et al. describe characteristics of the abductor and legal ramifications of the crime (20).

Common Health Problems: Prevention and Treatment

Various conditions are common in the infant. Table 7–7 summarizes the problems, their signs or symptoms, and methods to prevent or treat them (55).

TABLE 7–7. COMMON HEALTH PROBLEMS IN INFANCY

Problem	Definition	Symptoms/Signs	Prevention/Treatment
Atopic dermatitis	Chronic inflammatory disease of skin, characterized by itching	Family history of allergic disease, especially asthma Onset: usually after 2 months Rough, red, papular scaling areas, mainly on scalp, behind ears, on forearms and legs	Use warm water for baths. Apply lotions. Use soft cotton clothing. Keep fingernails short.
Diaper dermatitis	Inflammation of skin covered by diaper	Itching, irritability Redness on buttocks, genitalia papules, vesicles, and pustules	Keep area clean and dry. Allow air to circulate. Apply bland ointment or Burrow's solution.
Seborrheic dermatitis ("cradle cap")	Oily, scaly condition occurring in areas with large numbers of sebaceous glands	Scaly eruption spreading to eyebrows, eyelids, nasolabial folds	Shampoo and massage scalp. More severe cases may require a selenium sulfide (e.g., Selsun) shampoo.
Oral candidiasis ("thrush")	Fungal infection found in mouth of infants	White, irregular plaques found in mouth	Administer oral medication (e.g., nystatin [Mycostatin]).
Constipation	Difficulty in passing stool; excessive firmness of stool; decreased frequency of defecation	Straining on defecation, lack of stool passage Sometimes anal tissue or perianal abscess	Give warm sitz bath. Apply petroleum jelly to anus. Give additional water to drink.
Iron deficiency anemia	Anemia associated with inadequate supply of iron for synthesis of hemoglobin	Hematocrit value less than 30 Pallor, lethargy Anorexia Poor weight gain Splenomegaly	Discontinue whole cow's milk and substitute commercial formula. Increase intake of foods high in iron content. Give ferrous sulfate.
Roseola infantum	Acute benign febrile illness; fever stops as rash appears	High sudden fever lasting 3–4 days with few other symptoms Rash lasts 24–48 hours	Use antipyretic therapy.
Colic	Periods of unexplained irritability, usually in first 3 months; apparently associated with abdominal pain	Intense crying, legs drawn up to abdomen, hands clenched, pass flatus	Reassure parents. Consider formula change. If breastfeeding, review mother's intake. Review feeding and feeding technique. Apply warmth to abdomen. Let sleep in prone position. Apply rhythmic movement. Feed warm water during attack. Try Mylicon drops.
Umbilical cord granuloma	Small pink lesion that forms at the base, believed to be result of mild infection	Pink granulation tissue on umbilicus, seropurulent discharge	Keep area cleaned. Cauterize with silver nitrate stick. Wash 3–5 minutes after cauterizing. Clean with alcohol at least three times daily.

Data from References (5, 13, 105, 122).

The incidence of *acute respiratory disease, bronchitis,* and *pneumonia* increases with the increasing number of cigarettes smoked by the mother or other family members, particularly in infants aged 6 to 9 months. Infants of smoking mothers have significantly more admissions for bronchitis or pneumonia and more injuries. In households in which the mother smokes, the infant's urine cotinine levels are higher, especially in breastfed babies during nonsummer months; however, infants in a family in which any member smokes will suffer the effects of passive smoking from absorption of environmental tobacco smoke (26, 28).

A study in Sweden that included screening of more than 10,000 newborn infants for cytomegalovirus infection and hearing loss concluded that cytomegalovirus infection accounted for 40% of the hearing loss (40). Ophthalmologists now recommend eye examinations for neonates and at 6 months, $3\frac{1}{2}$ years, and 5 years.

The common health problems presented throughout these chapters reflect what are considered common today. Even in the last 25 years, striking changes have occurred in patterns of disease caused by transmissible agents: thus, what was common in 1945 is not even seen in the 1990s. On the other hand, we have some diseases today that were not even named in 1945.

PSYCHOSOCIAL CONCEPTS

The *intellectual, emotional, social, and moral components can be combined into what is often referred to as* **psychosocial development.** The separation of these facets of growth is artificial for they are closely interrelated. Similarly, psychosocial, physical, and motor development greatly influence each other. Babies are born cognitively flexible rather than with preset instinctual behavior. A level of physiologic maturation of the nervous system must be present before environmental stimulation and learning opportunities can be effective in promoting emotional and cognitive development. In turn, without love and tactile, kinesthetic, verbal, and other environmental stimuli, some nervous system structures do not develop. Babies adapt and react to the environment with which they are confronted. Low-birth-weight and premature infants have neurologic deficits that predispose to an increased risk for developmental delays, and they are apt to have behavioral styles that are more difficult to handle, which reduces maternal involvement and the stimulation needed for development (105, 122).

Cognitive Development

Intelligence is the *ability to learn or understand from experience, to acquire and retain knowledge, to respond to a new situation, and to solve problems.* It is a system of living and acting developed in a sequential pattern through relating to the environment. Each stage of operations serves as a foundation for the next (87). **Cognitive behavior** includes *thinking, perceiving, remembering, forming concepts, making judgments, generalizing,* and *abstracting.* Cognitive development is learning and depends on innate capacity, maturation, nutrition, gross and fine motor stimulation, touch, stimulation of all senses through various activities, language, and social interaction (68).

Case Situation: Infant Development

Michael, 8 months old, is sitting on the lap of his babysitter, Aunt Jennifer, who is reading a story to him. Aunt Jennifer smiles and chuckles as she reads. Michael responds by mimicking her mouth movements. She says "Ooooohh" with a widened O-shaped mouth, and Michael imitates the O-shape of her mouth while she speaks. Michael makes a long, loud "Ooooohh" sound. Aunt Jennifer responds with smiles and exclamations of enthusiasm, recognizing his achievement. Michael smiles and continues to repeat "Ooooohh."

Michael then attempts to imitate Aunt Jennifer's actions in reading the book. He reaches toward the book and makes babbling sounds as he swats at the book. Michael's coordination of vision, hearing, and tactile senses as he repeatedly imitates his aunt's facial expressions, reaches for the book, and engages in prespeech babbling demonstrates a common behavior of children in this age group. These behaviors demonstrate Piaget's stage 3, Secondary Circular Reactions of the Sensorimotor Stage of cognitive development.

Sequence in Intellectual Development

The sequence described by Piaget corresponds rather roughly in time span to those described for emotional development. The infant is in the *Sensorimotor Period of cognitive development* (86, 87, 117).

The infant arrives in the world with great potential for intellectual development, but at birth intellectual capacities are completely undifferentiated.

Stage 1: The Reflex Stage. This stage covers the neonatal period when behavior is entirely reflexive. Yet all stimuli are being assimilated into beginning mental images through reflexive behavior and from human contact.

Stage 2: Primary Circular Reactions. Primary circular reactions are response patterns where a stimulus creates a response and gratifying behavior is repeated. At 1 to 4 months, life is still a series of random events, but hand–mouth and ear–eye coordination is developing. The infant's eyes follow moving objects; eyes and ears follow sounds and novel stimuli. Responses to different objects vary. Baby does not look for objects removed from sight. He or she spends much time looking at objects in the environment and begins to separate self from them. Beginning intention of behavior is seen; he or she reproduces behavior previously done. For example, the 8-week-old infant can purposefully apply pressure to a pillow to make a mobile rotate, smile at familiar faces, and anticipate a routine such as diapering.

Stage 3: Secondary Circular Reactions. Stage 3 covers 4 to 8 months. Baby learns to initiate and recognize new experiences and repeat pleasurable ones. Intentional behavior is seen. Increasing mobility and hand control help him or her become more oriented to the environment. Reaching, grasping, listening, and laughing become better coordinated. Memory traces are apparently being established: baby anticipates familiar events or a moving object's position. The child repeats or prolongs interesting events. Activities that accidentally brought a new experience are repeated. Behavior becomes increasingly intentional. Habits developed in previous stages are incorporated with new actions. Baby will imitate another's behavior if it is familiar and not too complex.

Stage 4: Coordination of Secondary Schemata. In this stage, from 8 to 12 months, baby's behavior is showing clear acts of intelligence and experimentation. Baby uses certain activities to attain basic goals. He or she realizes for the first time that someone other than self can cause activity, and activity of self is separate from movement of objects. He or she searches for and retrieves a toy that has disappeared from view. Shapes and sizes of familiar objects are recognized, regardless of the perspective from which they are viewed. Because of the baby's ability to differentiate objects and people from self and the increased sense of separateness, he or she experiences separation (eighth month) anxiety when the mothering figure leaves. Baby is more mobile; sitting, creeping, standing, or walking gives a new perception of the environment. Baby understands words that are said. Thus coordination of schema involves using one idea or mental image to attain a goal and a second idea or image to deal with the end result (45, 86, 87, 117). Baby systematically imitates another while observing another's behavior.

Reaffirm with parents that they can greatly influence the child's later intellectual abilities by the stimulation they provide for baby, the loving attention they give, and the freedom they allow for baby to explore and use his or her body in the environment (8). Many educational toys are on the market, but common household items can be made into educational toys. For example, a mobile of ribbons and colorful cutouts will attract as much attention as an expensive mobile from the store. Unbreakable salt and pepper shakers or small cardboard boxes partly filled with rice, sand, or pebbles make good rattles.

Communication, Speech, and Language Development

Communication between people involves facial expressions, body movements, other nonverbal behavior, vocalizations, speech, and use of language. A newborn is ready to communicate if parents and caretakers know how to read the messages. The first communications are through eye contact, crying, and body movements.

Speech awareness *begins before birth. In utero the fetus hears a melody of language,* equivalent to overhearing two people talk through the walls of a motel room. *This creates a sensitivity that after birth provides the child with clues about sounds that accompany each other.* If babies have been read to in utero, after birth they appear to prefer the sound of the stories they had heard in utero (28, 34).

Speech is the *ability to utter sounds;* **language** refers to *the mother tongue of a group of people,* the *combination of sounds into a meaningful whole to communicate thoughts and feelings.* Speech development begins with the cry at birth, and the cry remains the basic form of communication for the infant. Baby's **cry** is **undifferentiated** for the first month; the *adult listener cannot distinguish between cries of hunger, pain, fear, and general unhappiness.* Parents learn to distinguish the meanings of different cries and grunts the baby makes in the first 2 or 3 months. At first baby responds to both soothing and distressing stimuli with similar sounds. Then other prespeech sounds heard are as follows:

- **Cooing,** *the soft murmur or hum of contentment,* beginning at 2 to 3 months
- **Babbling,** *incoherent sounds made by playing with sounds,* beginning at 2 to 3 months (The number of sounds produced by babbling gradually increases, reaches a peak at 8 months, and gives way for true speech and language development.)
- *Squealing* and *grunting*
- **Lalling,** *the movement of the tongue with crying and vocalization,* such as "m-m-m"
- *Sucking sounds*
- *Gestures*

Smiles, frowns, and other facial expressions often accompany the baby's vocalizations as do gestures of reaching or withdrawing to convey feelings (28, 34).

There is a biological basis for speech; the brain has amazing ability to process and interpret verbal expressions over an infinite range; however, parent–child interaction is essential for the child to learn language and conversation. Further, there is a critical period during which young children need environmental stimuli, or they will not learn to speak even when the sensory stimulation is exchanged for sensory deprivation (105, 122).

At first vocalizations are reflexive: no difference exists between the vocalizations of hearing babies and deaf babies before 6 months of age. Later, vocalizations are self-reinforcing, that is, the baby finds pleasure in making and hearing his or her own sounds, and responses from others provide further reinforcement. Reinforcement when desired sounds are made and when certain sounds are omitted is necessary for the infant to progress to language development. The child must also hear others speak to reinforce further the use of the sounds and language of the culture. Effective mothers speak to their children frequently, even while they are doing their housework (8, 68).

By 9 months baby will have made every sound basic to any human language. The sounds made in infancy are universal, but when he or she learns the native language, the potential to say all universal sounds is lost (68).

At every age the child comprehends the meaning of what others say more readily than he or she can put thoughts and feelings into words. In speech comprehension, the child first associates certain words with visual, tactile, and other sensations aroused by objects in the environment. Between 9 and 12 months, baby learns to recognize his or her name and the names of several familiar objects, responds to "no," echoes and imitates sounds, repeats syllables, and may occasionally obey the parent (8, 68).

Baby tries to articulate words from the sounds heard. Words are invented such as "didi" to mean a toy or food. Language is **autistic;** *he or she associates meanings with sounds made by the self, but the sounds are not meaningful to others,* often even to the parents. By trial and error and by imitation and as a result of reinforcement from others, the baby makes the first recognizable words, such as "mama," "dada," "no," and "bye-bye" between 10 and 18 months of age. (If the correct sound is directed to the appropriate parent, the sound is reinforced, and the baby continues speech.) Words such as "mama" and "nana" are universal to babies in every culture because they result from the sounds the infant normally makes in babbling. By age 1 year baby has a vocabulary of approximately six words. Nouns typically are learned first. He or she learns to associate meaning with an object such as its name, size, shape, texture, use, and sound; then a word becomes a symbol or label for the object. Learning to speak involves pronouncing words, building a vocabulary, distinguishing between sounds such as "p*e*t" and "p*a*t" or "*h*ear" and "*n*ear" and then making a sentence. The baby's first sentence usually consists of one word and a gesture (8, 34, 68).

Teach parents that many factors influence speech and language development: innate intelligence, ability to hear, modification of the anatomic structures of the mouth and throat, sense of curiosity, parental verbal stimulation and interest, and encouragement to imitate others (34, 68).

Emotional Development

Eight psychological stages in the human life cycle are described by Erikson (35). He elaborates on the core problems or crisis with which each person struggles at each of these levels of development. In addition to these problems, the child has other tasks to accomplish that relate to the psychosocial crisis such as learning to walk. Emotional or personality development is a continuous process. No person succeeds or fails completely in attainment of the goal to reach at a particular point in personality development.

Developmental Crisis

According to Erikson (35), the psychosexual crisis for infancy is trust versus mistrust. **Basic trust** involves *confidence, optimism, acceptance of and reliance on self*

► CONSEQUENCES OF MISTRUST

Infant

- Is lethargic
- Fails to gain weight
- Eats poorly
- Sleeps poorly
- Experiences excessive, persistent colic
- Fails to thrive

Child and Adult

- Is pessimistic, hopeless
- Lacks self-confidence
- Is gullible, easily hurt
- Is suspicious, unsure of self or others
- Is dependent on others, clings to others
- Is antagonistic toward others
- Is bitter to others
- Is withdrawn, asocial
- Avoids new relationships or new experiences, or
- Bullies others; is aggressive, sarcastic, controlling
- Is pathologically optimistic (takes risks, gambles on everything, sure nothing can go wrong)
- Is unable to delay gratification

and others, faith that the world can satisfy needs, and a sense of hope or a belief in the attainability of wishes in spite of problems and without overestimation of results. A sense of trust forms the basis for a sense of hope and for later identity formation, social responsiveness to others, and ability to care about and love others. The person accepts self, develops reachable goals, assumes life will be manageable, and expects people and situations to be positive. A sense of trust may be demonstrated in the newborn and infant by the ease of feeding, the depth of sleep, the relaxation of the bowels, and the overall appearance of contentment. **Mistrust** is a *sense of not feeling satisfied emotionally or physically, an inability to believe in or rely on others or self.* See Consequences of Mistrust for further insight.

Security and trust are fostered by the prompt, loving and consistent response to the infant's distress and needs and by the positive response to happy, contented behavior. You can teach parents that they do not "spoil" a baby by promptly answering the distress signal—his

or her cry. Rather, they are teaching trust by relieving tension. Parents should understand the meaning they convey through such care as changing diapers. Even if the techniques are not the best, baby will sense the positive attitude if it exists. If the parents repeatedly fail to meet primary needs, fear, anger, insecurity, and eventual mistrust result. If the most important people fail him or her, there is little foundation on which to build faith in others or self and little desire to be socialized into the culture. The world cannot be trusted. If the baby is abused, neglected, or deprived, he or she may suffer irreversible effects, as discussed in Chapter 6, pp. 287 and 289.

The infant who is in a nurturing, loving environment and who has developed trust is a happy baby most of the time. He or she is sociable and responsive to others. Attachment to the parent has been formed so that separation or stranger anxiety is experienced at approximately 7 to 9 months of age and may extend to 10 to 12 months. After a time the infant will again respond to strangers. Sociable babies have sociable mothers, and sociable, friendly babies score higher on cognitive tests than less sociable or mistrusting infants (8, 34).

The working mother may discuss her situation with you. Emotional development of the infant is not compromised by the working mother if she has time and energy to maintain consistent, loving, and stimulating responses when she is with baby. Quality of care rather than quantity of time is the essence of parenting and promoting emotional development. When work is not stressful and is a source of personal satisfaction for the mother, she is a more contented mother and gives the baby better care. The father's nurturance is also important, and often he is more involved in caring for the child when the mother works, which contributes to quality care. The lowest scores of adequate mothering are found in dissatisfied homemakers. Further, the effective mother does not devote the bulk of her day in the home to childrearing but instead designs an environment that is loving, adequately stimulating, and helpful to the child in gaining competency (68).

Because so many mothers work today, an important subject to discuss is child-care arrangements or babysitting services. Even if the parent does not work, some time away from the baby is rejuvenating and enhances the quality of parenting. Each parent has different ideas about how often, if at all, to leave the baby with a sitter. Discuss characteristics to consider in a sitter. Point out that parents will probably be most satisfied with a sitter whose childrearing philosophy and guidance techniques coincide with theirs and who has had some child-care training or experience.

The *sitter* or nanny should be physically and emotionally healthy, be acquainted with the baby and the home, and like the baby. If possible, parents should keep the baby with the same person consistently, especially around 7 or 8 months when baby is experiencing separation anxiety. The sitter or nanny should have exact instructions about where the parents can be reached; special aspects of care; telephone numbers of doctor, police, and fire department; name and telephone number of another family member; and telephone number of a poison control center, if nearby. As more mothers return to work shortly after childbirth, there has been an increasing trend toward infant day-care centers. Factors to consider in choosing day-care services are discussed in Chapter 9.

Development of Body Image

Body image, the *mental picture of one's body,* includes the external, internal, and postural picture of the body, although the mental image is not necessarily consistent with the actual body structure. Included also are attitudes, emotions, and personality reactions of the individual in relation to his or her body as an object in space, with a distinct boundary and apart from all others and the environment. The body image, gradually formulated over a period of years, is included in the **self-concept** (*awareness of self or me*) and *derives from reactions of others to his or her body, perceptions of how others react, experiences with his or her own and other bodies, constitutional factors, and physiologic and sensory stimuli* (101).

At birth the infant has diffuse feelings of hunger, pain, rage, and comfort but no body image. Pleasurable sensations come mainly from the lower face, the mouth–nose area, which has considerable nerve innervation. At first all the baby knows is self. Baby has the same attitude toward his or her body as toward other objects in the environment; the external world is an extension of self. Gradually, baby disinguishes his or her body from other animate and inanimate objects in the environment as he or she bites a hand, bangs the head, grasps and mouths a toy, and experiences visceral, visual, auditory, kinesthetic, and motor sensations (101).

A primitive ego or self-development begins at approximately 3 months. Weaning, contact from others, and more exploration of the environment also heighten self-awareness. As the child approaches the first birthday, there is some coordination of these sensory experiences that are being internalized into the motor body image. He or she is aware that some body parts give greater pleasure than other parts and that there are differences in sensation when his or her body or another object is touched (101).

Without adequate somatosensory stimulation, body image and ego development are impaired as shown by studies of premature incubator infants who lacked rocking, stroking, and cuddling (63). The infant's initial experiences with his or her body, determined largely by maternal care and attitudes, are the basis for a developing body image and how he or she later likes and handles the body and reacts to others.

Adaptive Mechanisms

Adaptive mechanisms are *learned behavioral responses that aid adjustment and emotional development.* At first the baby cries spontaneously. Soon baby learns that crying brings attention; therefore, he or she cries when uncomfortable, hungry, or bored. Other tools besides crying used in adaptation are experimentation, exploration, and manipulation. Baby uses the body in various ways to gain stimulation. He or she grabs and plays with whatever is within reach, whether it is father's nose or a toy. By the end of infancy, emotions of anger, fear, delight, and affection are expressed through vocalization, facial expression, and gestures.

The young infant does not understand waiting. But a baby meets with security and feels a sense of tenderness from caretakers, he or she begins to wait a short time between feeling hunger pains and demanding food. Instead of immediately screaming when a toy cannot be reached, baby will persist in repeating the action that will get him or her to the object. The baby is beginning to respond to the expectations of others and adapt to the family's cultural patterns.

If, however, care does not foster trust, the infant constantly feels threatened. At first he or she cries and shows increased motor activity, perhaps expressing rage, but may eventually feel powerless and become apathetic.

Adaptive mechanisms in infancy are called *primary process.* Some of these rudimentary methods of handling anxiety are symbolization, condensation, incorporation, and displacement. **Symbolization** *occurs when an object or idea comes to stand for something else because of associated characteristics.* For example, taking milk from mother's breast satisfies hunger. Soon the act also means pleasurable body contact, emotional response, and security. **Condensation** is the *reverse process. Several objects are fused into a single symbol.* The word *toy,* for example, comes to represent a variety of objects. **Incorporation** occurs when the *representation of mother or other objects is taken into the self and becomes a part of the understanding* and is the basis for the child's separation anxiety or attachment to parents. **Displacement** occurs when *emotions are transferred from an original object to* *another* such as from the mother to other family members or the babysitter (8, 68).

Adaptive behavior is developed through structuring of the baby's potential. He or she needs both freedom to explore and exercise and consistent, pleasant restraints for personal safety, which together enable learning of self-restraint. Constantly saying "No" or confining the child to a walker or playpen does not help the learning of adaptive behavior.

One study compared the temperament of very-low-birth-weight (VLBW) infants with that of full-term infants at 6 and 12 months of age, assessed patterns of change in temperament from 6 to 12 months, and investigated effects of the neonatal experience on manifestations of temperament. The infants were free of congenital anomalies and appropriate for gestational age. At 6 months the VLBW infants were significantly less adaptable and more intense than full-term infants. There were significantly more "difficult" and fewer "easy" infants in the study group. However, although at 12 months the VLBW infants were less persistent than a full-term infant, the behavioral style clusters of the VLBW children did not differ significantly from those of full-term infants. The social environment of the VLBW infant plays an important role in the manifestation of childhood temperament as early as 6 months of age, but behavioral styles are modified during the first year of life with corrective nurturing (73).

Findings of another study confirm other researchers' findings that environmental factors can assist or sabotage developmental progress in a child who was originally at biological risk. Developmental progress in VLBW infants may be more sensitive to subsequent environmental influences than it is to past perinatal insults. The impact of the environment appears to become more powerful as the child matures (103).

There are two possible explanations for this finding. One explanation concerns the infant's natural self-righting tendencies. The infant may be temporarily deflected off course by premature birth, prolonged hospitalization, and illness around the time of birth, but once he or she is exposed to an even minimally appropriate environment, natural self-righting mechanisms have the potential to bring him or her back into the maturational trajectory characteristic of their species. A second explanation lies in the view of human development; the infant is changing and growing within the context of a transactional, organismic milieu. Negative past events become less important as the child, the parents, and the environment influence one another. The child elicits and reinforces parental responses, and parental behaviors and characteristics support developmental gains. The quality of the home environment and the passage of time significantly affect the outcome (7, 103).

Sexuality Development

Sexuality may be defined as a *deep, pervasive aspect of the total person and the sum total of one's feelings and behavior as a male or female, the expression of which goes beyond genital response.* Sexuality includes the attitudes that are necessary to maintain a stable and intimate relationship with another person. Sexuality culminates in adulthood, but it begins to develop in infancy (68, 114).

Sex is determined at the moment of fertilization. Chromosome combination and hormonal influences affect sexual development prenatally, as discussed in Chapter 6. Sometimes mothers respond to the fetus in a sex-differentiated way: an active fetus is interpreted as a boy, a quiet one as a girl. Prenatal position, according to folklore, relates to sex: boys are supposedly carried high, and girls are carried low.

Gender or sex assignment occurs at birth. The parents' first question is usually "Is it a boy or a girl?" The answer to this question often stimulates a set of adjectives to describe the newborn: soft, fine-featured, little, passive, weak girl; robust, big, strong, active boy, regardless of size or weight. The name given to baby also reflects the parents' attitudes toward the baby's sex and may reflect their ideas about the child's eventual role in life. Mothers, however, engage in less sex-typing stereotypes than fathers (68, 114).

Occasionally external genitalia are ambiguous in appearance, neither distinctly male nor distinctly female. When this occurs, parents should be given as much support and information as possible to cope with the crisis; sex assignment based on chromosomal studies or appearance should be made as soon as possible (122).

The stereotypes about sex do have some basis in fact because at birth males usually are larger and have more muscle mass, are more active, and are more irritable than girls. Females are more sensitive to auditory, touch, and pain stimuli. At 3 weeks of age males are still more irritable and are sleeping less than females (114).

Initially, mothers seem to respond more to male infants than to female infants (perhaps because male infants have traditionally been more highly valued). But by 3 months this reverses, and mothers are thought to have more touch and conversational contact with female infants, even when they are irritable. This reverse may occur because mothers are generally more successful in calming irritable daughters than irritable sons (68, 114).

By 5 months baby responds differently to male and female voices, and by 6 months he or she distinguishes mother from father and as distinct people. At 6 months the female infant has a longer attention span for visual stimuli and better fixation to a human face, is more responsive to social stimuli, and prefers complex stimuli. The male infant has a better fixation response to a helix of light and is more attentive to an intermittent tone (34, 114).

Also, when the babies are 6 months old, mothers imitate the verbal sounds of their daughters more than their sons, and mothers continue to touch, talk to, and handle their daughters more than their sons. Throughout infancy and childhood, female children talk to and touch their mothers more, whereas boys are encouraged to be more independent, exploratory, and vigorous in gross motor activity (68).

Fathers tend to treat the baby girl more softly and the baby boy more roughly during the last 6 months of infancy. At 9 months, a baby girl behaves differently with her mother than with her father. She will be rougher and more attention seeking with her father (8).

By 9 to 12 months, baby responds to his or her name, an important link to sex and role. Research indicates that girl babies are more dependent and less exploratory by 1 year than boys because of different parental behaviors to each sex. Parents appear to reinforce sex-coded behavior in infancy so that sex role behavior is learned on the basis of parental cues (68).

Infants receive stimulation of their erogenous zones during maternal care. The mouth and lower face are the main erogenous zones initially, providing pleasure, warmth, and satisfaction through sucking. Both sexes explore their genitalia during infancy. Erection in the male and lubrication in the female occur.

Explore sexuality development with parents. Help them be aware of the importance for sexuality development of their tone of voice, touch, behavior, and feelings toward the boy or girl. Help them develop ways to relate optimally to and promote trust and well-being in the child.

Developmental Tasks

Infancy is far from what some have assumed—a time for rigidly and mechanically handling the baby because he or she seems to have so little capability as an adapting human being. The following developmental tasks are to be accomplished in infancy (33):

- Achieve equilibrium of physiologic organ systems after birth
- Establish self as a dependent person but separate from others
- Become aware of the alive versus inanimate and familiar versus unfamiliar and develop rudimentary social interaction

- Develop a feeling of and desire for affection and response from others
- Adjust somewhat to the expectations of others
- Begin to manage the changing body and learn new motor skills, develop equilibrium, begin eye–hand coordination, and establish rest–activity rhythm
- Begin to understand and master the immediate environment through exploration
- Develop a beginning symbol or language system, conceptual abilities, and preverbal communication
- Direct emotional expression to indicate needs and wishes

Explore these tasks with parents. Help them realize specific ways they enable their baby to achieve these tasks.

► HEALTH CARE AND NURSING APPLICATIONS

Your role with the infant and family has been discussed with each section throughout this chapter. You can also be instrumental in establishing or working with community agencies that assist parents and infants. You may be called on to work with families who have adopted a child or with the single parent or with the reconstituted family who then has their own child (see also Chapter 4). You may work with a family whose child is not healthy or perfect or is born prematurely (see also Chapter 4), or you may work with a family who experiences sudden death of the infant. For more information, see Selected Nursing Diagnoses Related to the Infant.

Establishment and Use of Community Resources for Continuity of Care

Some sources of help that may be found in your community are summarized in Community Resources for Parents.

In one large city two maternity nurses identified a need for a local organization that would offer courses in parenting. In addition to course offerings, the organization now hosts discussion groups for expectant and new mothers and for parents of toddlers. Recently a "postpartum hot line" was started. The despair of couples who experience postpartum problems is pointed out repeatedly. For example, "This is Julie. . . . We had our baby on the fourteenth. But (*tears*) you must have to be a pediatrician to be a mother. The baby is crying all the

► **SELECTED NURSING DIAGNOSES RELATED TO THE INFANT***

Pattern 1: Exchanging

Altered Nutrition: More Than Body Requirements
Altered Nutrition: Less Than Body Requirements
Altered Nutrition: Potential for More Than Body Requirements
Constipation
Diarrhea
Impaired Gas Exchange
Risk for Infection
Risk for Injury
Risk for Suffocation
Risk for Poisoning
Risk for Trauma
Risk for Aspiration
Altered Protection
Risk for Impaired Skin Integrity

Pattern 6: Moving

Impaired Physical Mobility
Sleep Pattern Disturbance
Ineffective Breastfeeding
Altered Growth and Development

Pattern 7: Perceiving

Sensory/Perceptual Alterations
Unilateral Neglect

Pattern 9: Feeling

Pain
Anxiety

*Other of the NANDA diagnoses are applicable to the ill infant.
From North American Nursing Diagnosis Association, NANDA Nursing Diagnoses Definitions & Classification 1995–1996. Philadelphia: North American Nursing Diagnosis Association, 1994.

tion time and more directly involving father in care. Every woman or family, however, is not a candidate for early discharge, even though many insurance plans cover only 2 days or less. Prenatal preparation is necessary. Mother and baby must show no potential complications. Medical backup care must be quickly available. Further, at times mother may get more rest and emotional support in the hospital than at home, depending on home and family conditions. In fact, visits by a nurse 1 hour daily for 2 or 3 days may *not* provide sufficient care.

► **COMMUNITY RESOURCES FOR PARENTS**

Classes on Parenting, Prenatal or Postnatal Care, Lamaze or Psychoprophylaxis Method of Childbirth

- Junior or senior college presenting nonacademic courses
- Hospital clinics
- Individual childbirth educators who are members of local and international Childbirth Education Association
- Crisis agencies such as Parent and Child, St. Louis
- Local Red Cross chapter
- Community health nursing services

Breastfeeding Information

- La Leche League

Parent Support

- Voluntary self-help agencies such as Cesarean Support Group
- Mother's Center
- A Mother Experiencing Neo-Natal Death (AMEND)
- Association for Retarded Citizens
- Mothers of Twins Club
- Association of Family Women
- Coping With Overall Parenting Experience (COPE), Boston, Massachusetts
- Compassionate Friends, Box 1347, Oakbrook, IL 60521
- National Foundation for SIDS (Sudden Infant Death Syndrome), 1501 Broadway, New York, NY 10036
- National Sudden Infant Death Syndrome Foundation, 310 South Michigan Avenue, Chicago, IL 60604

Crisis Attendance or Counseling

- Crisis hotlines such as Life Crisis Center or Parent and Child, St. Louis
- Family and Children's Services
- Clergy or other counselors

time; I don't know if I can continue to nurse her.... Everything is horrible!" (A home visit and a series of follow-up phone calls played a part in this mother's nursing her baby happily for 8 months.)

Instead of using referral to a community agency, a hospital may provide its own postpartum home care services, especially for mothers and babies who are discharged from the hospital 12 to 24 hours after delivery. Early discharge can have the advantages of treating mother and baby as well, not ill, reducing family separa-

Research Abstract

Saarinen, U., and M. Kajosoari, Breastfeeding as Prophylaxis Against Atopic Disease: Prospective Follow-up Study Until 17 Years Old, Lancet, 346 (October 21, 1995), 1065–1069.

Although heredity has been thought to be a great influence on the development of allergy, the purpose of this prospective study, conducted over 17 years, was to determine the extent to which breastfeeding helps to prevent allergies.

The sample consisted of healthy infants born in 1975 at Helsinki University Central Hospital. Of the initial 236 infants selected, 150 completed follow-up at 2 weeks and 1, 2, 4, 6, 9, and 12 months, and were divided into three groups. The groups were infants breastfed less than 1 month, 1 to 6 months, or 6 to 12 months. All babies started solid foods at 3 to 5 months. The 150 children were then monitored at ages 3, 5, 10, and 17 years through history, physical examination, and laboratory tests.

The results indicated that breastfed babies had a better chance than formula-fed babies of reaching adulthood free of allergies. Even children breastfed for less than 1 month had a lower prevalence of atopic eczema, food allergy, and respiratory allergy in childhood than did children who were not breastfed at all. At age 17, 65% of children breastfed less than 1 month had some atopic allergy, compared with 36% of those who had breastfed 1 to 6 months and 42% of those who had breastfed more than 6 months. There was even less multiorgan allergy in adolescents who were breastfed longer: 8% among those who had nursed longer than 6 months, 23% among those who had nursed 1 to 6 months, and 54% among those who had nursed under 1 month.

Prevalence of different allergies peaked at different times—eczema at about 1 year, food allergies at about 3 years, and respiratory allergies at about 17 years—and the peaks were lowest among the breastfed children. The data indicated that 6 months or more of breastfeeding was needed to prevent eczema; only a month of breastfeeding was enough to reduce the chances of food or respiratory allergy. Breastfeeding may help prevent allergies by promoting maturation of intestinal mucus and humoral immunity in the infant or by reducing absorption of food allergens. Health care providers can assist the woman during pregnancy and after delivery in the decision about breastfeeding, and to prepare for and continue breastfeeding. Information about the benefits of breastfeeding should include long-term health of the child.

Whenever visits are made in the home, assessment tools that can be used, if administered by a qualified person, are the *Denver II—Revision and Restandardization of the Denver Developmental Screening Test (DDST)* (see Fig. 9–2), a general scale that measures personal and social skills, language, and gross and fine motor abilities (41); the *Infant Temperament Questionnaire (ITQ),* which addresses various areas of temperament and behavior (28); and the *Home Observation for Measurement of the Environment (HOME)* in which the home-rearing situation is assessed (22).

Care of the Premature Baby and the Baby With Congenital Anomalies

The principal threats to infant health are low birth weight and birth defects. The infant mortality rate is higher than the national average in areas where there is higher unemployment and, consequently, a lack of health insurance and lack of prenatal and obstetric care. Minority groups and adolescents are especially affected. Preterm and low-birth-weight infants have higher rates of morbidity and mortality than normal-weight infants. Preterm delivery accounts for approximately 7% of all births and 65% of prenatal deaths. Of those who survive, 50% have neurologic defects requiring lifelong social and financial commitment. A preterm infant usually develops complications that necessitate neonatal intensive care at considerable cost (34).

Birth defects are a leading cause of infant death in the United States. The most common defects are heart problems, central nervous system disorders, and defects of the respiratory system. Another leading cause of death is a combination of low birth weight, prematurity, and respiratory distress syndrome. These children also receive neonatal intensive care unit (NICU) treatment. The average total lifetime cost per survivor for NICU graduates was estimated in 1989 to range from $40,647 to $362,992, depending on infant birth weight and morbidity. Costs have escalated since then. Another major cause is sudden infant death syndrome (SIDS).

The United States is experiencing an epidemic of children born to mothers addicted to alcohol, cocaine, crack, and other such drugs. A generation of babies have already been affected and will present major problems to our society because of their developmental disabilities, uncontrollable behavior and rage, learning deficits, and lack of superego and remorse. There is an inadequate number of treatment centers and foster homes. Mothers or grandmothers are likely to bear the brunt of this crisis. For many parents and their families, birth of a baby will not bring joy but fear, grief, and depression—for a long time (30).

There are times, however, when the baby is preterm or premature or has a lasting problem for no known reason. Further, there are families who reach out to these babies with love and caring; as a result, the baby develops to the maximum potential. Supportive nursing care is a key factor for these families (7).

Cultures vary in the care of the premature. Premature babies in some countries are placed with their mothers 2 to 3 hours after birth and are sent home soon after birth because of economic status of the parents, problems with cross and nosocomial infections, and deep respect for natural processes. In some countries the premature child has no chance of survival.

Parents of the baby with **congenital anomalies** (*defects in physical structure or function*) will need the same considerations as parents of the premature infant. They should be encouraged to see their infant as soon as possible to avoid fantasies that are often worse than the anomaly. Show them the normal parts and emphasize the baby's positive features. Above all, show your acceptance of the infant: hold, cuddle, and look at the infant as you talk to him or her. Give information about the anomaly and the possible prognosis. This is a difficult time for parents, and they will need ample time to express their grief, guilt, and worries. Your patience and support will be most helpful. Various references provide more in-depth information to share with parents pertinent to the specific disability (105, 122). Refer to Chapter 4 for additional information on nursing practice with the family.

There are *ethical dilemmas* with care of the premature infant, especially if he or she is greatly preterm and very low birth weight, and with care of the infant that has a severe congenital anomaly. Infants who in 1975 would have had no chance for survival are today receiving care from health professionals armed with extensive knowledge and state-of-the-art technologies. Many infants with multiple and serious handicaps can now survive anywhere from weeks to years, which raises questions about the cost of their care and the quality of their lives.

Parents and members of the health care and judicial systems continue to debate hotly the anticipated length and quality of many of those infants' lives. Some infants who are saved will continue as a financial and care burden for their parents the rest of the parents' and the child's lives.

The ethical, personal, and economic dilemmas posted by the use of life-sustaining technologies are considerable and have caused policymakers to consider withholding treatment from selected infants. Using high-technology treatment methods may be experimentation and research, shrouded in the guise of treatment. The pivotal case of Baby Doe has come to exemplify just such an event. The case is discussed at length by Wakefield-Fisher (118).

The advanced technology to maintain life has posed a major ethical dilemma for parents and professionals: Should life be continued with machines, *or* when and how the critically ill infant or child should be allowed to die. Schloman and Fister describe the perspectives of parents in their study (102).

Nurses increasingly have understanding of both the questions and legal and ethical responses related to withholding life-sustaining treatment from infants. Nurses must participate in the decision making, based on adequate knowledge of the issue.

Care of the Family Experiencing Adoption and Infant Death

Mothers Who Adopt Out Their Newborns

These mothers are confronted with a crisis that involves bereavement. Ambivalence prevails during the prenatal period: love for baby, guilt about abandonment, and concern for his or her future. Therapeutic intervention begins prenatally by exploring with the mother the anticipatory grief, anger, depression, decisions about seeing the baby, and choice of postdelivery care. To promote bonding would be cruel, but the mother should have the opportunity—the reality—of holding and inspecting. Not to recognize the infant is to deny the pregnancy; seeing the infant gives concrete focus to the mother's grief. A maternity nurse-specialist should consult the relinquishing mother on a scheduled basis to promote the woman's personal growth, self-respect, and dignity. Refer also to Chapter 4 for more information on the adoptive process and family.

Parents Whose Infants Die

If the newborn dies, there are no magic words. Certain actions are helpful: (1) give parents momentos, such as a footprint sheet, identification band, or photograph; (2)

be patient and compassionate; and (3) help the family say goodbye. Parents must work through the affectional-symbiotic bond developed in anticipation of the baby as perfect. Full expression of the grief, guilt, and anger is necessary. Many hospital practices tend to discourage these reactions by removing all evidence of the baby's existence. Nothing is left to confirm the reality of the baby's death. Parents should, if they desire, be permitted to view, touch, and hold their dead infant. Within the beliefs of the parents, some traditional bereavement service should be arranged to promote grieving and making the death real. Meeting with the parents after the death of the infant or attending the funeral can assist them through mourning. Contact or meet with the parents within the next 2 to 3 weeks and in 3 to 6 months. During these visits you can effectively listen, encourage expression of feelings, and assist the parents in working through their feelings and reactions (29, 61, 122).

Although SIDS is at least as old as Biblical times, it did not become acceptable as a term for use on death certificates until the early 1970s. Formerly it was called *crib death*. This disease is a primary cause of death in infants after the first week of life (105). A typical case might be an apparently healthy infant, possibly with a slight cold, usually between the ages of 3 weeks and 7 months, who is put to bed and then found dead when the caretaker goes to check him or her. Usually the baby has not made a sound, and there is no evidence of struggle. Autopsy is the only means of making a diagnosis and may reveal widely diffuse petechiae across the pleura, minor inflammation of the upper respiratory tract, minor lung congestion and common viruses, or no unusual findings (122).

No one knows what causes SIDS but there are many theories: (1) the mild viral infection may affect nerves that affect lung activity; (2) inherent nerve deficit may affect the larynx, causing laryngospasm; (3) there may be decreased carbon dioxide sensitivity or sleep apnea, and (4) suffocation may result from rebreathing face down in polystyrene-filled cushions. SIDS may be increased eightfold in offspring of heroin or cocaine addicts because the respiratory center and feedback mechanisms are poorly developed in utero in addicted pregnant women. Some believe baby should not be placed on the abdomen to sleep. Close monitoring may aid prevention. Special monitoring devices for use in the home can be purchased (105, 122).

The thrust for the nurse is in helping the parents or caretakers deal with their guilt, grief, and future psychological balance. You should be able to direct these people to national or local help. National organizations are listed in Community Resources for Parents, found earlier in this chapter. In some health departments

► CONSIDERATIONS FOR THE INFANT AND FAMILY IN HEALTH CARE

- Cultural background and experiences of the family of the infant
- Reaction of the mother and father to the crisis resulting from the baby's birth
- Attachment behaviors and the binding-in process of the mother; attachment of father and other family members
- Parental behaviors that indicate difficulty in establishing attachment or potential/actual abuse of the infant
- Physical characteristics and patterns, such as eating, sleeping, elimination, and activity in the neonate/infant, that indicate health and are within the age norms for growth
- Cognitive characteristics and behavioral patterns in the neonate/infant that indicate age-appropriate norms for intellectual development
- Communication characteristics and behavioral patterns in the neonate/infant that indicate intact neurologic and sensory status, speech awareness, and ability to respond with age-appropriate sounds (prespeech)
- Overall appearance and behavioral and play patterns in the neonate/infant that indicate development of trust, rather than mistrust, and continuing age-appropriate emotional development
- Behavioral patterns and characteristics that indicate the infant has achieved developmental tasks
- Parental behaviors that indicate knowledge about how to care physically and emotionally for the neonate/infant
- Parental behaviors that indicate they are promoting positive self-concept and sexuality development in the infant
- Evidence that the parents provide a safe and healthful environment and the necessary resources for the neonate/infant
- Parental behaviors that indicate they are achieving their developmental tasks for this era

there are nurses who are designated to make visits for as long as needed. Self-help groups have been formed to assist parents with mourning and feelings of guilt, failure, and isolation after their infant's death.

No matter what birth takes place—normal or abnormal—the family is going through a type of *rebirth* in that their lives are forever changed by the event. Your guidance in this process may be felt for years.

SUMMARY

The neonatal period, the first 30 days of life, and infancy, the first year of life, constitute an era that is a critical period for the child. Physiologic adaptations are necessary to survive after birth, and this first year is a period of rapid growth physically. This year is also critical emotionally, in that the child must be consistently loved and cared for as a whole person to thrive, learn to trust, and achieve developmental tasks.

Considerations for the Infant and Family in Health Care and Chart 1 in Appendix IV summarize what you should consider in assessment and health promotion with the infant; the family of the infant is included in Considerations. Chart 1 in Appendix IV presents the American Academy of Family Physicians Periodic Health Examination Birth to 18 Months to assist in screening the infant, promoting health, preventing injury, counseling parents, and determining immunization schedules and risk categories.

► REFERENCES

1. Abernathy, J., The Long and Short of It: Brief Maternity Stays May Not Fill the Bill, *Citizen Journal,* 7, no. 5 (July 16, 1995), 1.
2. Ainsworth, M.D., The Development of Infant–Mother Attachment. In Caldwell, B., and Ricciuti, H. eds., *Child Development Research.* Chicago: University of Chicago Press, 1973, pp. 1–94.
3. American Academy of Family Physicians, *Age Charts for Periodic Health Examination.* Washington, DC: Author, 1995.
4. Ballard, J., et al., A Simplified Score for Assessment of Fetal Maturation in Newly Born Infants, *Journal of Pediatrics,* 95 (1979), 769–774.
5. Battaglia, F.C., and L.O. Lubchenco, A Practical Classification of Newborn Infants by Weight and Gestational Age, *Journal of Pediatrics,* 71 (1967), 159–163.
6. Beck, C., The Effects of Postpartum Depression on Maternal–Infant Interaction: A Meta Analysis, *Nursing Research,* 44 (1995), 298–302.
7. Becker, P., et al., Outcomes of Developmentally Supportive Nursing Care for Very Low Birth Weight Infants, *Nursing Research,* 40, no. 3 (1991), 150–155.
8. Bettelheim, B., and A. Freedgood, *A Good Enough Parent: A Book on Child-rearing.* New York: Random, 1988.
9. Blank, D., Development of the Infant Tenderness Scale, *Nursing Research,* 34, no. 4 (1985), 211–215.
10. Boggs, K., and P. Rau, Breastfeeding the Premature Infant, *American Journal of Nursing,* 83, no. 10 (1983), 1437–1439.
11. Bowlby, J., *Attachment and Loss, Vol. 1.* New York: Basic Books, 1969.
12. ———, Disruption of Affectional Bonds and Its Effect on Behavior, *Canada's Mental Health Supplement,* no. 59 (January–February, 1969), 2–12.
13. Boynton, R.W., E.S. Dunn, and G.R. Stephens, *Manual of Ambulatory Pediatrics* (3rd ed.). Philadelphia: J. B. Lippincott, 1994.
14. Bozett, F., and S. Hanson, eds., *Fatherhood and Families in Cultural Context.* New York: Springer, 1991.
15. Brazelton, P.T., *The Neonatal Behavioral Assessment Scale* (2nd ed.). Philadelphia: J.B. Lippincott, 1984.
16. Brazelton, T., and B. Cramer, *The Earliest Relationship.* Reading, MA: Addison-Wesley, 1990.
17. Breast Is Best—For Premies Too, *American Journal of Nursing,* 87, no. 11 (1987), 1403–1404.
18. Brock, D., Social Forces, Feminism, and Breast-feeding, *Nursing Outlook,* 23, no. 8 (September 1975), 556–561.
19. Brown, M., Social Support, Stress, and Health: A Comparison of Expectant Mothers and Fathers, *Nursing Research,* 36, no. 2 (1986), 74–76.
20. Burgess, A., E. Dowdell, C. Hartman, C. Nakemy, and J. Rabun, Infant Abductors, *Journal of Psychosocial Nursing,* 33, no. 9 (1995), 30–37.
21. Butler, G., Shaken Baby Syndrome, *Journal of Psychosocial Nursing,* 33, no. 9 (1995), 47–50.
22. Caldwell, B., *Home Inventory for Infants.* Fayetteville, AK: Fayetteville Center for Development and Education, University of Arkansas, 1978.
23. Carey, W.B., and S.C. McDevitt, A Review of the Infant Temperament Questionnaire, *Pediatrics,* 61 (1978), 735–738.
24. Censullo, M., B. Lester, and J. Hoffman, Rythmic Patterning in Mother–Newborn Interactions. *Nursing Research,* 34, no. 6 (1985), 342–348.
25. Centers for Disease Control and Prevention General Recommendations on Immunization: Recommendations of the Advisory Committee on Immunization Practices (ACIP), *Morbidity and Mortality Weekly Report,* 43 (January 28, 1994), 23.
26. Chilmonczyk, B., et al., Environmental Tobacco Smoke Exposure During Infancy, *American Journal of Public Health,* 80, no. 10 (1990), 1205–1208.
27. Cushions May Cause Infant Death, *Washington University School of Medicine Outlook,* Fall (1991), 2–3.
28. Dacey, J., and J. Travers, *Human Development Across the Lifespan* (3rd ed.), Madison, WI: Brown & Benchmark, 1996.
29. Diaz, M., When a Baby Dies, *American Journal of Nursing,* 95, no. 11 (1995), 54–56.
30. Dorris, M., *The Broken Cord.* New York: Harper Collins, 1991.
31. Dubowitz, L., and V. Dubowitz, *A Clinical Manual: Gestational Age of the Newborn.* New York: Addison-Wesley, 1977.
32. Dusitin, N., et al, Development and Validation of a Simple Device to Estimate Birthweight and Screen for Low Birthweight in Developing Countries, *American Journal of Public Health,* 81, no. 9 (1991), 1201–1205.
33. Duvall, E., and B. Miller, *Marriage and Family Development* (6th ed). New York: Harper & Row, 1984.
34. Dworetzky, J., *Human Development: A Life Span Approach* (2nd ed.). St. Paul/Minneapolis: West, 1995.
35. Erikson, E., *Childhood and Society* (2nd ed.). New York: W.W. Norton, 1963.
36. ———, *Toys and Reasons.* New York: W.W. Norton, 1977.
37. Eyer, D.E. *Mother–Infant Bonding: A Scientific Fiction.* New Haven, CT: Yale University Press, 1992.
38. Feeding Your Child, *Parenting: Glennon Hospital for Children,* St. Louis (1990), 10–11.
39. Ferketich, S., and R. Mercer, Predictors of Role Competence for Experienced and Inexperienced Fathers, *Nursing Research,* 44 (1995), 89–95.
40. Fowler, K., and R. Pars, Cytomegalovirus Infection as a Cause of Hearing Loss Among Children, *American Journal of Public Health,* 85, no. 5 (1995), 734.
41. Frankenburg, W.K., and J.B. Dodd, The Denver Developmental Screening Test, *Journal of Pediatrics,* 71 (1967), 181–191.
42. Fuller, B., Acoustic Discrimination of Three Types of Infant Cries, *Nursing Research,* 40, no. 3 (1991), 156–160.
43. Garbarino, J., E. Guttmann, and J. Seeley, *The Psychologically Battered Child: Strategies for Identification, Assessment, and Intervention.* San Francisco: Jossey-Bass, 1987.

44. Gelfand, D., and D. Teti, How Does Maternal Depression Affect Children? *The Harvard Mental Health Letter,* 12, no. 5 (1995), 8.
45. Gesell, A., et al., *The First Five Years of Life.* New York: Harper Brothers, 1940.
46. Global Immunization of Children, Showing Increase, Saving Lives, Reports WHO, *The Nation's Health,* 25, no. 10 (1995), 7.
47. Goldberg, S., *Parent–Infant Bonding: Another Look.* Child Development, 54 (1983), 1355–1382.
48. Greenburg, M., and N. Morris, Engrossment: The Newborn's Impact Upon the Father, *American Journal of Orthopsychiatry,* 44 (1974), 520–531.
49. Harris, C., Cultural Values and the Decision to Circumcise, *Image,* 18, no. 3 (1986), 98–103.
50. Hartwick, N., Infant Formula: A Threat to Third-World Babies, *Graduate Woman,* 75, no. 6 (1981), 26–31.
51. Helberg, J., Documentation of Child Abuse, *American Journal of Nursing,* 83, no. 2 (1983), 234–239.
52. Hill, S., The Child With Ambiguous Genitalia, *American Journal of Nursing,* 77, no. 5. (May 1977), 810–814.
53. Holmes, T.H., and M. Masuda, Life Change and Illness Susceptibility, *Separation and Depression AAAS* (1973), 161–186.
54. ———, and R.H. Rahe, The Social Readjustment Rating Scale, *Journal of Psychosomatic Research,* 2 (1967), 213–218.
55. Hoole, A., C. Pickard, Jr., R. Ouimette, J. Fohr, and R. Greenberg, *Patient Care Guidelines for Nurse Practitioners* (4th ed.). Philadelphia: J. B. Lippincott, 1994.
56. Horn, B., Cultural Concepts and Postpartal Care, *Journal of Transcultural Nursing,* 2, no. 1 (1990), 48–51.
57. IPOL (Poliovirus Vaccine Inactivated), *Nation's Health,* September (1991), 6.
58. Jolley, J., and M. Mitchell, *Lifespan Development: A Topical Approach.* Madison, WI: Brown & Benchmark, 1996.
59. Kahn, A., et al., Insomnia and Cow's Milk Allergy in Infants. *Pediatrics,* 76 (December 1985), 880–884.
60. Kelly, P., ed., *First Year Baby Care: An Illustrated Step-by-Step Guide for New Parents.* Deephaven, MN: Meadowbrook Press, 1983.
61. Klaus, M., and J. Kennell, *Parent–Infant Bonding* (2nd ed.). St. Louis: C.V. Mosby, 1982.
62. Kleimhuizen, J., Traditions Guard Hispanic Babies' Health. *USA Today,* February 4 (1991), Sect. D, p. 4.
63. Kramer, M., et al., Extra Tactile Stimulation of the Premature Infant, *Nursing Research,* 24, no. 5 (September–October 1975), 324–334.
64. Krantz, L., Comparison of Body Proportions of One-year Old Mexican American and Anglo Children, *American Journal of Public Health,* 71, no. 3 (1981), 280–282.
65. Lamb, M., The Emergent American Father, in Lamb M., ed., *The Father's Role: Cross Cultural Perspectives.* Hillsdale, NJ: Erlbaum, 1987.
66. LaRossa, R., Fatherhood and Social Change, *Family Relations,* 37 (1988) 451–457.
67. Lee, E., Asian Infant Feeding, *Nursing Mirror,* 160, no. 21 (May 22, 1985), 14–15.
68. Lidz, T., *The Person: His and Her Development Throughout the Life Cycle* (2nd ed.). New York: Basic Books, 1983.
69. Linley, J., Screening Children for Common Orthopoedic Problems, *American Journal of Nursing,* 87, no. 10 (1987), 1312–1316.
70. Lubchenco, L.O., C. Hansman, and E. Boyd, Intrauterine Growth in Length and Head Circumference as Estimated From Live Births at Gestational Ages From 26 to 42 Weeks, *Pediatrics,* 37 (1966), 403–408.
71. Lundington-Hoe, S., What Can Newborns Really See? *American Journal of Nursing,* 83, no. 9 (1983), 1286–1289.
72. McBride, A.B., *The Growth and Development of Mothers.* New York: Harper & Row, 1973.
73. Medoff-Cooper, B., Temperament in Very Low-Birth-Weight Infants, *Nursing Research,* 35, no. 3 (1986), 139–142.
74. Mercer, D., Relating Mother's Anxiety and Perception to Infant Satiety, Anxiety, and Feeding Behaviors, *Nursing Research,* 35, no. 6 (1986), 347–361.
75. Mercer, R.T., and Ferketich, S.L., Predictors of Parental Attachment During Early Parenthood, *Journal of Advanced Nursing,* 15 (1990) 268–280.
76. Mittelman, R., H. Mittelman, and C. Wetu, What Child Abuse Really Looks Like, *American Journal of Nursing,* 87, no. 9 (1987), 1185–1188.
77. Montagu, A., *Touching: The Human Significance of the Skin* (3rd ed.). New York: Columbia University Press, 1986.
78. Murray, R., and M. Huelskoetter, *Psychiatric Mental Health Nursing: Giving Emotional Care* (3rd ed.). Norwalk, CT: Appleton & Lange, 1991.
79. Notzon, F., J. Bobadilla, and I. Coria, Birthweight Distributions in Mexico City and Among U.S. Southwest Mexican Americans: The Effect of Altitude, *American Journal of Public Health,* 82 (1992), 1014–1017.
80. Owen, G., and A. Lubin, Anthropometric Differences Between Black and White Preschool Children, *American Journal of Diseases of Children,* 126 (1973), 168–169.
81. Owens, M., A Crying Need, *American Journal of Nursing,* 86, no. 1 (1986), 73.
82. Palkovitz, R., Fathers: Birth Attendance, Early Contact and Extended Contact With Their Newborns: A Critical Review, *Child Development,* 56, no. 2 (1985), 392–406.
83. ———, R., Laypersons: Beliefs About the "Critical" Nature of Father–Infant Bonding: Implications for Childbirth Educators, *Maternal–Child Nursing Journal,* 15, no. 1 (Spring 1986), 39–46.
84. ———, Sources of Father–Infant Bonding Beliefs: Implication for Childbirth Educators, *Maternal–Child Nursing Journal,* 17, no. 2 (Summer 1988), 101–113.
85. Paltiel, F.L., Child-rearing, a Task for Fathers as Well as Mothers. *World Health Forum,* 10 (1989), 249–257.
86. Piaget, J., *The Construction of Reality in the Child* (M. Cook, transl.). New York: Basic Books, 1954.
87. ———, *The Origins of Intelligence in Children.* New York: International University Press, 1952.
88. Pitch the Polystyrene-Filled Pillows, *Washington University Magazine,* Fall (1991), 3.
89. Pressler, J., Promoting Attachment, in Craft, M., and J. Denehy, eds., *Nursing Interventions for Infants & Children.* Philadelphia: W.B. Saunders, 1990, pp. 4–17.
90. Rentscler, D., Correlates of Successful Breast Feeding, *Image,* 23, no. 3 (1991), 151–154.
91. Robson, K., The Role of Eye-to-Eye Contact in Maternal–Infant Attachment, *Journal of Child Psychology and Psychiatry,* 8 (1976), 13–25.
92. Rubin, R., The Family–Child Relationship and Nursing Care, *Nursing Outlook,* 8(1964), 36–39.
93. Rubin, R., Attainment of the Maternal Role—Part I, *Nursing Research,* 16, no. 3 (1967), 237–245.
94. ———, Attainment of the Maternal Role—Part II, *Nursing Research,* 16, no. 4 (1967), 342–346.
95. ———, Cognitive Style in Pregnancy, *American Journal of Nursing,* 70, no. 3 (1970), 502–508.
96. ———, Binding-in in the Postpartum Period, *Maternal–Child Nursing Journal,* 6 (1977), 67–75.

97. ———, *Maternal Identity and the Maternal Experience.* New York: Springer, 1984.

98. Rustia, J.G., and D.A. Abbott, Father Involvement in Infant Care: Two Longitudinal Studies, *International Journal of Nursing Studies,* 30, no. 6 (1993), 467–476.

99. Salk, L., The Role of the Heartbeat in the Relations Between Mother and Infant, *Scientific American,* 228 (May 1973), 24–29.

100. Satz, K., Integrating Navajo Tradition Into Maternal–Child Nursing, *IMAGE, Journal of Nursing Scholarship,* 14, no. 3 (1982), 89–91.

101. Schilder, P., *The Image and Appearance of the Human Body.* New York: International University Press, 1951.

102. Schloman, P., and S. Fister, Parental Perspectives Related to Decision-making and Neonatal Death, *Pediatric Nursing,* 21 (1995), 243–248.

103. Schraeder, B., Developmental Progress in Very Low-Birth-Weight Infants During the First Year of Life, *Nursing Research,* 35, no. 4 (1986), 237–242.

104. Scrimshaw, S., et al., Factors Affecting Breast-feeding Among Women of Mexican Origin or Descent in Los Angeles, *American Journal of Public Health,* 77, no. 4 (1987), 467–470.

105. Sherwen, L., M. Scoloveno, and C. Weingarten, *Nursing Care of the Childbearing Family.* Norwalk, CT: Appleton & Lange, 1991.

106. Singh, G., and S. Yu, Birthweight Differentials Among Asian Americans, *American Journal of Public Health,* 84 (1994), 1444–1449.

107. ———, Infant Mortality in the United States: Trends, Differentials, and Projections, 1950 Through 2010, *American Journal of Public Health,* 85 (1995), 957–964.

108. Stearns, P.N., Fatherhood in Historical Perspective: The Role of Social Change, in Bozett, F.W., and Hanson, S.M.H., eds., *Fatherhood and Families in Cultural Context.* New York: Springer, 1991, pp. 28–52.

109. Temperature Recording in Infants and Children, *Pediatric Nursing,* 19 (1992), n.p.

110. Thomas, J., and L. DeSantis, Feeding and Weaning Practices of Cuban and Haitian Immigrant Mothers, *Journal of Transcultural Nursing,* 6, no. 2 (1995), 34–42.

111. Toney, L., The Effects of Holding the Newborn at Delivery on Paternal Bonding, *Nursing Research,* 32, no. 1 (1983), 16–19.

112. Troy, N., Early Contact and Maternal Attachment Among Women Using Public Health Care Facilities, *Applied Nursing Research,* 6, no. 4 (1993), 161–166.

113. Tulman, L., Mothers and Unrelated Persons' Handling of Newborn Infants, *Nursing Research,* 34, no. 4 (1985), 205–210.

114. Turner, J., and D. Helms, *Lifespan Development* (5th ed.). Ft. Worth: Harcourt Brace College, 1995.

115. Uphold, C., and M. Graham, *Clinical Guidelines in Family Practice* (2nd ed.), Gainesville, FL: Barmarrae Books, 1994.

116. Verzemnieks, I., Developmental Stimulation for Infants and Toddlers. *American Journal of Nursing,* 84, no. 6 (1984), 749–752.

117. Wadsworth, B., *Piaget's Theory of Cognitive and Affective Development* (4th ed.). New York: Longman, 1989.

118. Wakefield-Fisher, M., Balancing Wishes with Wisdom: Sustaining Infant Life, *Nursing and Health Care,* no. 11 (1987), 517–520.

119. Williams, S.R., *Nutrition and Diet Therapy* (6th ed.). St. Louis: Times Mirror/Mosby, 1989.

120. Wink, D., Getting Through the Maze of Infant Formulas, *American Journal of Nursing,* 85, no. 4 (1985), 388–392.

121. ———, Better Breast Milk for Preemies, *American Journal of Nursing,* 89, no. 1 (1989), 48–49.

122. Wong, D., *Whaley and Wong's Nursing Care of Infants and Children* (5th ed.). St. Louis: Mosby, 1995.

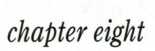
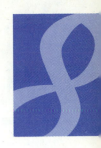
Assessment and Health Promotion for the Toddler

Train up a child in the way he should go, and when he is old, he will not depart from it.

—Proverbs 22: 6

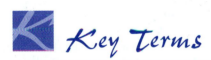

Key Terms

Toddler stage

Separation anxiety

Protest

Despair

Denial

Myelinization

Accommodate

Hyperopic

Juvenile hypertension

Spider nevi

Mongolian spots

Café au lait spots

Bruises

Parallel play

Myopia

Astigmatism

Strabismus

Hearing impairment

Otitis media

Dental caries

Malabsorption syndrome

Impetigo

Pharyngitis

Acute nonspecific gastroenteritis
  (diarrhea)

Varicella (chickenpox)

Rubella

Pinworms (*Enterobius
  vermicularis*)

Miliaria rubra

Viral croup

Parataxic mode

Egocentric

Syncretic speech

Telegraphic speech

Contraction

Expansion

Autistic

Autonomy

Shame

Doubt

Anal stage

Self-concept

Self-system

  Good-me

  Bad-me

  Not-me

Primary identification

Repression

Suppression

Denial

Reaction formation

Projection

Sublimation

Discipline

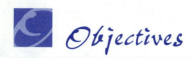

Objectives

Study of this chapter will enable you to:

1. Discuss the effects of family and toddler on each other, the significance of attachment behavior and separation anxiety, and the family developmental tasks to be achieved.

2. Explore with parents ways to adapt to the toddler while they simultaneously socialize the child and meet their developmental tasks.

3. Assess a toddler's physical and motor characteristics and related needs, including nutrition, rest, exercise, play, safety, and health protection measures.

4. Assess a toddler's general cognitive, language, emotional, and sexuality development.

5. Describe specific guidance and discipline methods for the toddler and the significance of the family's philosophy about guidance and discipline.

6. Discuss with parents their role in contributing to the toddler's cognitive, language, emotional, self-concept, and moral development.

7. Discuss the commonly used adaptive mechanisms that promote autonomy and your role in assisting parents to foster the development of autonomy.

8. State the toddler's developmental tasks and ways to help him or her achieve them.

9. Work effectively with a toddler and the family in the healthcare and nursing situation.

In this chapter development of the toddler and the family relationships are discussed. *Nursing responsibilities for health promotion of the child and family are discussed throughout the chapter.* The information in this chapter is the basis for care of the toddler and family in any setting.

Within the first year of life children make remarkable adaptation internally and externally to their environment. They sit, walk, remember, recognize others, begin to socialize, communicate more purposely with speech, and show more specific emotional responses.

The **toddler stage** *begins when the child takes the first steps alone at 12 to 15 months and continues until approximately 3 years of age.* The family is very important during this short span of the child's life as he or she acquires language skills, increases cognitive achievement, improves physical coordination, and achieves control over bladder and bowel sphincters. These factors lead to new and different perceptions of self and the environment, new incentives, and new ways of dealing with problems.

FAMILY DEVELOPMENT AND RELATIONSHIPS

Behaviorally, the toddler changes considerably between 12 months and 3 years, a change that in turn affects family relationships. Because of new skills, the child begins to develop a sense of independence, establishes physical boundaries between self and mother, and gains the sense of a separate, self-controlled being who can do things on his or her own. From the age of 2

years the child moves toward independence—from the protracted dependency of childhood toward adulthood independence, self-reliance, and object relations. The child attempts self-education through mastery and engaging parents and others in help when necessary. Without the myriad attempts to do things for himself or herself, the child would obtain no degree of autonomy in skills. The periods of practice that ensure reliable performance and skills are often periods of independent action; however, dependence on others and gratification of dependency needs are essential for optimum ego development. Dependency does not mean passivity, for the child is quite active in obtaining help by crying, screaming, taking an adult by the hand and pulling him or her to another area, or asking how to solve a problem. The toddler should neither be kept too dependent nor forced too quickly into independence (25).

The family of a toddler can be quiet and serene one minute and in total upheaval the next, resulting from the imbalance between the child's motor skills, lack of experience, and mental capacities. One quick look away from the toddler can result in a broken object, a spilled glass of milk, or an overturned dish. The toddler's quickly changing moods from tears to laughter or anger to calm, combined with energy, sense of independence, and curiosity, also account for parents' labeling their toddler a *terrible two*.

Help parents realize this behavior is normal and necessary for maturation. Expecting, planning for, and trying to handle patiently each situation will reduce parent frustration.

The toddler is frequently jealous of younger siblings because of having to vie for the center of attention that was once his or her own: older siblings are resented because they are permitted to do things he or she cannot. Power struggles focusing on feeding and toilet training occur between parent and child. Family problems may also arise when the toddler's activities are limited because of parental anxieties concerning physical harm or because of their intolerance of the child's energetic behavior and unknowing infractions of societal rules.

You can inform parents that their social teaching likely will center on cleanliness and establishing reasonable controls over anger, impulsiveness, and unsafe exploration.

Influence of the Family

The chief molder of personality is the family unit, and home is the center of the toddler's world. Family life nurtures in the child a strong affectional bond, a social and biological identity, intellectual development, attitudes, goals, and ways of coping and responding to situations of daily life. The family life process also imparts tools such as language and an ethical system in which the child learns to respect the needs and rights of others and provides a testing ground before he or she emerges from home. A loving, attentive, healthy, responsible family is essential for maximum physical, mental, emotional, social, and spiritual development in childhood (1). The importance of the father's role with the child and the mother is being affirmed (1, 5, 23–25).

Parents with high self-esteem provide the necessary conditions for the toddler to achieve trust, self-esteem, and autonomy (self-control) through allowing age-appropriate behavior. Parents with low self-esteem provoke feelings of shame, guilt, defensiveness, decreased self-worth, and "being bad" in the child by overestimating the child's ability to conform, inappropriately or forcefully punishing or restraining the child, denying him necessities, and withdrawing love (37).

Help parents work out their feelings about self in relation to the child. Changing parental attitudes are often evident. If the parent is delighted with a dependent baby and is a competent parent to an infant, the parent may be threatened by the independence of the toddler and become less competent. Some parents have difficulty caring for the dependent infant but are creative and loving with the older child. But if the parent's development was smooth and successful, if the inner child of the past is under control, and if he or she understands self, parental behavior can change to fit the maturing child.

Attachment Behavior

Attachment behavior is very evident during the toddler years. The symbiotic mother–child relationship is slowly being replaced by the larger family unit, but the toddler still needs mother close. Children need to be touched, cuddled, hugged, rocked. All young mammals need physical contact for normal brain tissue development and for the brain to develop receptors that inhibit secretion of adrenal hormones (glucocorticoids)—the stress hormones. Thus, both the immune and neurologic systems are affected positively by touch and by emotional attachment (35).

In a classic study in the 1950s two groups of young Ugandan children were compared: those reared in the traditional African way with much attention focused on the child and those reared in the emerging European or Western way with the child left with other caretakers. In the African model the mother never left the child, carried the child on her back, and played with and stimulated the child. The European model was to bottle-feed the child and leave it alone a great deal. The children raised in the African way were, at 2 years of age, more advanced in motor development, language, adaptivity, and personal–social relationships. Good health and the ability to relate are the result of loving relationships (1, 18). Other authors validate these results (5–7, 14, 25, 30, 35).

The toddler shows attachment behavior by maintaining proximity to the parent. Even when out walking, the child frequently returns part or all the way to the parent for reassurance of the parent's presence, to receive a smile, to establish visual, and sometimes touch, contact, and to speak before again moving away (7).

Although attachment is directed to several close people such as father, siblings, babysitter, and grandparents, it is usually greatest toward one person, mother. Attachment patterns do not differ significantly between children who stay home all day versus those who go to day-care centers, as attachment is related to the intensity of emotional and social experience between child and adult rather than to physical care and more superficial contact. Attachment is as great or greater if the mother shows warm affection less frequently than if she is present all day but not affectionate. In comparing children raised in Israeli kibbutzim to American children, both groups are equally attached to their parents, although young children in the kibbutzim had greater attachment to peers than did young American children because they depended more on peers for approval (5).

Separation anxiety, the *response to separation, from mother,* intensifies at approximately 18 and 24 months. Anxiety can be as intense for the toddler as for the infant if the child has had a continuous warm attachment to a mother figure because he or she thinks an object ceases to exist when it is out of sight. The child who is more accustomed to strangers will suffer less from a brief separation. When separated, the child experiences feelings of anger, fear, grief, and revenge. An apathetic, resigned reaction at this age is a sign of abnormal development. The child who is separated from the parent for a period, as with hospitalization, goes through three phases of *grief and mourning*—protest, despair, and denial, which may merge somewhat—as a result of separation anxiety (7).

During **protest,** *lasting a few hours or days and seen for short or long separations, the need for mother is conscious, persistent, and grief laden. The child cries continually, tries to find her, is terrified, fears he or she has been deserted, feels helpless and angry that mother left him or her, and clings to her on her return.* If he or she is also ill, additional uncomfortable body sensations assault the toddler (7). The child needs mother at this time.

Despair *is a quiet stage, characterized by hopelessness, moaning, sadness, and less activity. The child does not cry continuously but is in deep mourning. He or she does not understand why mother has deserted him or her. The child makes no demands on the environment nor responds to overtures from others, including at times the mother. Yet the child clings to her if permitted.* Mother may feel guilty and want to leave to relieve her distress, as she may feel her visits are disturbing to the child, especially when the child does not respond to her.

Mother needs help in understanding that the child's and her reactions are normal and that the child desperately needs her presence (7). If she can be present, you can promote family-centered care through your explanations to the mother and child, by not being rigid about visiting hours, by attending to mother's (or father's) comfort and needs, and by letting the parent help care for the child. Protests, in the form of toddler's screams and crying, will thus be less intense. Be accepting if a parent cannot stay with the child. Parents may live great distances from the hospital or have occupational or family responsibilities that indeed prevent them from visiting the child as often as they desire. The parent may also be ill or injured. Be as nurturing to the toddler as possible while the parent is away. Tell the toddler how much Mommy and Daddy love him or her and want to be present but cannot. If possible, have the parent leave an article with the child that is a familiar representation of the parent.

Denial, *which occurs after prolonged separation, defends against anxiety by repressing the image of and feelings for mother and may be misinterpreted for recovery.* The child now begins to take more interest in the environment, eats, plays, and accepts other adults. Anger and disappointment at mother are so deep that the child acts as if he or she does not need her and shows revenge by rejecting her, sometimes even rejecting gifts she brings. To prevent further estrangement, mother should understand that the child's need for her is more intense than ever (7).

Continue the above interventions that promote family-centered care. Give mother (father) and child time together undisturbed by nursing or medical care procedures. Provide toys that help the child to act out the fears, anxiety, anger, and mistrust experienced during the hospitalization and separation. Encourage the parent to talk about and work through feelings related to the child's illness and absence from the family.

With prolonged hospitalization, the child may fail to discover a person to whom he or she can attach for any length of time. If the child finds a mother figure and then loses her, the pain of the original separation is re-experienced. If this happens repeatedly, the child will eventually avoid involvement with anyone but invest love in self and later value material possessions more highly than any exchange of affection with people.

Teach parents that immediate aftereffects of separation include changes in the child's behavior—regression, clinging, and seeking out extra attention and reassurance. If extra affection is given to the child, trust is gradually restored. If the separation has been prolonged, the child's behavior can be very changed and disturbed for months after return to the parents. The parent needs support in accepting the child's expressions of hostility and in meeting his or her demands. Counteraggression or withdrawal from the child will cause further loss in trust and regression.

Child abuse or maltreatment may begin or continue at this age. Even when parents seem concerned and loving, a child is not immune from abuse. Further, children today are exposed to a variety of potential abusers—babysitters, day-care workers, the parent's live-in lover or occasional friend, stepparents, extended family members, and neighbors. Be alert to signs and symptoms of child abuse, discussed in Chapters 4, 6, and 7.

You often must be very patient and observant to detect child abuse because the child does not have the language skills to tell you what has happened. The child's nonverbal behavior, play, and artwork may provide clues. Observation of the latter takes time and patience as well as the parent's presence (25, 31). Parental Behavior Characteristics of Psychological Maltreatment of the Toddler, Physical Signs of Abuse of a Child, and Interaction Signs of Parental Abuse of a Child present information to aid you in recognizing signs of abuse.

Family Developmental Tasks

The family with a toddler faces many new developmental tasks:

- Meeting the spiraling costs of family living
- Providing a home that is safe and comfortable and has adequate space

▶ PARENTAL BEHAVIOR CHARACTERISTIC OF PSYCHOLOGICAL MALTREATMENT OF THE TODDLER

Rejecting
- Excludes actively from family activities
- Refuses to take child on family outings
- Refuses to hug or come close to child
- Places the child away from the family

Isolating
- Teaches the child to avoid social contact beyond the parent–child relationship
- Punishes social overtures to children and adults
- Rewards child for withdrawing from opportunities for social contact

Terrorizing
- Uses extreme gestures and verbal statements to threaten, intimidate, or punish the child
- Threatens extreme or mysterious harm (from monsters or ghosts or bad people)
- Gives alternately superficial warmth with ranting and raging at the child

Ignoring
- Is cool and apathetic with child
- Fails to engage child in daily activities or play
- Refuses to talk to child at mealtimes or other times
- Leaves child unsupervised for extended periods

Corrupting
- Gives inappropriate reinforcement for aggressive or sexually precocious behavior
- Rewards child for assaulting other children
- Involves the child sexually with adolescents or adults

From Garbarino, J., E. Guttman, and J. Seeley, The Psychologically Battered Child: Strategies for Identification, Assessment, and Intervention. San Francisco: Jossey-Bass, 1987. Copyright 1986 by Jossey-Bass, Inc., Publishers.

▶ PHYSICAL SIGNS OF ABUSE OF A CHILD

- An injury for which there is no explanation or an implausible explanation is present.
- Injury is not consistent with the type of accident described. (e.g., child would not suffer both feet burned by stepping into hot tub of water; he or she would step in with one foot at a time. Or a child who tips a pot of hot coffee on his or her hand has a splash-effect burn, not a mitten appearance.
- Inconsistencies exist in the parents' stories about the reason for child's injuries.
- Parents quickly blame a babysitter or neighbor for an accidental injury.
- Child does not have total appearance of an accident—dirty clothes, face smudged, hair tousled.
- Large number of healed or partially healed injuries are observed.
- Large bone fracture, multiple fractures, or tearing of periosteum caused by having limb forcibly twisted are evident.
- Child flinches when your fingers move over an area not obviously injured, but it is tender due to abusive handling.
- Human bite marks are evident.
- Fingernail indentations or scratches are noted.
- Old or new cigarette burns are evident.
- Loop marks from belt beating are present.
- Soft tissue swelling and hematomas are noted.
- Clustered or multiple bruises are observed on trunk or buttocks, in body hollows, on back of neck, or resembling hand prints or pinch marks.
- Bald spots are observed.
- Retinal hemorrhage from being shaken or cuffed about the head is assessed.
- History of unusual number of accidents exists.

Data from references 25, 37.

- Maintaining a sexual involvement that meets both partners' needs
- Developing a satisfactory division of labor
- Promoting understanding between the toddler and the family
- Determining whether or not they will have any more children.
- Rededicating themselves, among many dilemmas, to their decision to be a childbearing family (12)

Help parents to be cognizant of these tasks. Encourage them to talk through concerns, feelings, and practical aspects related to fulfilling these tasks. Refer them to a counselor or community agency if help is desired.

► INTERACTION SIGNS OF PARENTAL ABUSE OF A CHILD

- Child flinches or glances about nervously when you touch him or her.
- Child seems afraid of parents or caregivers and is reluctant to return home.
- Parent issues threat to crying child such as "Just wait 'til I get you home."
- Parent remains indifferent to child's distress.
- Parent(s) blames child for his or her own injuries (e.g., "He's always getting hurt" or "He's always causing trouble").
- Parental behavior suggests role reversal; parent solicits help or protection from child by acting helpless (when child cannot meet parent's needs, abuse results).
- Parent repeatedly brings healthy child to emergency room and insists child is ill (parent feeling overwhelmed by parental responsibilities and may become abusive).
- Child has had numerous admissions to an emergency room, often at hospitals some distance from the child's home.

Data from references 25, 37.

PHYSIOLOGIC CONCEPTS

Physical Characteristics

General Appearance

The appearance of the toddler has matured from infancy. He or she has lost the roly-poly look of infancy by 12 to 15 months, with abdomen protruding, torso tilting forward, legs at stiff angles, and flat feet spaced apart. Limbs are growing faster than torso, giving a different proportion to the body. By 12 to 15 months, chest circumference is larger than head circumference. The child increasingly looks like a family member as face contours fill out with the set of deciduous teeth. By age 2, he or she has 16 teeth. Gradually the chubby appearance typical of the infant is lost; muscle tone becomes firmer as the fat-storing mechanisms change. Less weight is gained as fat; more weight is gained from muscle and bone (10, 25, 37).

Rate of Growth

During toddlerhood, _growth is slower than in infancy; but it is even, and development follows the cephalocaudal, proximodistal, and general-to-specific principles discussed in Chapter 6._ Although the rate of growth slows, bone growth continues rapidly with the development of approximately 25 new ossification centers during the second year (37).

Between the first and second years the average height increase is 4 to 5 in. (10–12 cm). Average height increase the next year is $2\frac{1}{2}$ to $3\frac{1}{2}$ in. (6–8 cm). Weight gain averages 5 to 6 pounds (2.27–2.72 kg) between the first and second years. _Birth weight is quadrupled by age 2._ The 2-year-old child stands 32 to 33 in. (81–84 cm) and weighs 26 to 28 pounds (11–13 kg). At 30 months average height is 36 in. (91.5 cm), and weight is approximately 30 pounds (13.6 kg). _By age 2, the girl has grown to 50% of final adult height; by age $2\frac{1}{2}$, the boy to 50% of adult height_ (10, 13, 19, 22, 32).

Neuromuscular Maturation

Neuromuscular maturation and repetition of movements help the child further develop skills. **Myelinization,** _covering of the neurons with the fatty sheath called myelin,_ is almost complete by 2 years. This enables the child to support most movement and increasing physical activity and to begin toilet training. Additional growth also occurs as a greater number of connections form among neurons, and the complexity of these connections increases. Lateralization or specialization of the two hemispheres of the brain has been occurring; evidence of signs of dominance of one hemisphere over the other can be seen. The left hemisphere matures more rapidly in girls than in boys; the right hemisphere develops more rapidly in boys. These differences may account for language ability in girls and spatial ability in boys. Handedness is demonstrated, and spatial perception is improving (10, 13, 22, 32). (Spatial ability will be complete at approximately age 10.) The limbic system is mature; sleep, wakefulness, and emotional responses become better regulated. The toddler responds to a wider range of stimuli and has greater control over behavior. The brain reaches 80% of adult size by age 2 (37). The growth of the glial cells accounts for most of the change (27, 37).

Motor Coordination

Increasing gross motor coordination is shown by leg movement patterns and by hand–arm movements. Table 8–1 summarizes the increasing motor coordination skills manifested during the toddler years (10, 13, 22, 32).

TABLE 8–1. MOTOR COORDINATION DURING THE TODDLER YEARS

Age (months)	Characteristics
12–15	Walks alone; legs appear bowed
	Climbs steps with help; slides down stairs backward
	Stacks two blocks; scribbles spontaneously
	Grasps but rotates spoon; holds cup with both hands
	Takes off shoes and socks
15–18	Runs but still falls
	Walks backward and sideways (17 months)
	Climbs to get to objects
	Falls from riding toys or in bathtub
	Hammers on pegboard
	Grasps with both hands
	Picks up small items off floor; investigates electric outlets; grabs cords and table cloths (15 months)
	Clumsily throws ball
	Unzips large zipper
	Takes off easily removed garments
	Stacks three to four blocks (18 months)
18–24	Falls from outdoor play equipment
	Walks stairs with help (20 months)
	Walks up and down stairsteps alone, holding rail, both feet on step before ascending to next step
	Can reach farther than expected, including for hazardous objects
	Fingers food
	Brushes paint; fingerpaints
	Takes apart toys; puts together large puzzle pieces
24–30	Runs quickly; falls less
	Walks downstairs holding to rail; does not alternate feet
	Jumps off floor with both feet (28 months)
	Throws ball overhand
	Puts on simple garments
	Stacks six blocks
	Turns door handles
	Plays with utensils and dishes at mealtimes; pours and stacks
	Turns book pages
	Uses spoon with little spilling; feeds self
	Brushes teeth with help
30–36	Walks with balance; runs well
	Balances on one foot; walks on tiptoes (30 months)
	Jumps from chair (32 months)
	Pedals tricycle (32 months)
	Jumps 10–12 in. off floor (36 months)
	Climbs and descends stairs, alternating feet (36 months)
	Rides tricycle
	Sits in booster seat rather than high chair
	Stacks 8–10 blocks; builds with blocks
	Pours from pitcher
	Dresses self completely except tying shoes; does not know back from front
	Turns on faucet
	Assembles puzzles
	Draws; paints

Data from References 10, 13, 19, 22, 32, and 37.

Vision

Visual acuity and the ability to **accommodate**, *to make adjustments to objects at varying distances from the eyes,* are slowly developing. Vision is **hyperopic,** *farsighted,* testing approximately 20/10 at 2 years. Visual perceptions are frequently similar to an adult's, even though the child is too young to have acquired the richness of symbolic associations. The child's eye–hand coordination also improves. At 15 months he or she reaches for attractive objects without superfluous movements (10, 37).

Endocrine System

Endocrine function is not fully known. Production of glucagon and insulin is labile and limited, causing variations in blood sugar. Adrenocortical secretions are limited, but they are greater than in infancy. Growth hormone, thyroxine, and insulin remain important secretions for regulating growth (37).

Respiratory System

Respirations average 20 to 30 per minute. Lung volume is increased, and susceptibility to respiratory infections decreases as respiratory tract structures increase in size (37).

Cardiovascular System

The pulse decreases, averaging 105 beats per minute. Blood pressure increases, averaging 80 to 100 systolic and 64 diastolic. The size of the vascular bed increases, thus reducing resistance to flow. The capillary bed has increased ability to respond to hot and cold environmental temperatures, thus aiding thermoregulation. The body temperature averages 99°F (37.2°C) (37).

Juvenile hypertension has been defined as *sustained blood pressure levels above the 95th percentile on at least three measurements at different visits in circumstances where anxiety is minimized.* Another definition for children 3 to 12 years is a *diastolic pressure greater than 90 mm Hg* (21, 37).

If hypertension is suspected, a complete investigation is warranted by a specialist interested in hypertension in children. Tell parents that many children will respond to an overall cardiovascular health program. If at all possible, drug therapy will be avoided (21, 37).

Gastrointestinal System

Foods move through the gastrointestinal tract less rapidly, and digestive glands approach adult maturity. Acidity of gastric secretion increases gradually. Liver and pancreatic secretions are functionally mature. Stomach capacity is 500 mL (37).

Skin

The skin becomes more protective against outer invasion from microorganisms, and it becomes tougher with more resilient epithelium and less water content. Less fluid is lost through the skin as a result. The skin remains dry because sebum secretion is limited. Eccrine sweat gland function remains limited. At this age eczema improves and the frequency of rashes declines (37).

Urinary System

By age 3, the bladder has descended into the pelvis, assuming adult position. Renal function is mature; except under stress, water is conserved, and urine is concentrated on an adult level (37).

Immune System

Specific antibodies have been established to most commonly encountered organisms, although the toddler is prone to gastrointestinal and respiratory infections when he or she encounters new microorganisms. Despite environmental exposure, antibody IgC increases, IgM reaches an adult level, and IgA gradually increases. Lymphatic tissues of adenoids, tonsils, and peripheral lymph nodes undergo enlargement, partly because of infections and partly from growth. By age 3 years, the adenoid tissue reaches maximum size and then declines, whereas tonsils reach peak size around 7 years (37).

Blood Cell Components

Blood cell counts are approaching adult levels, although the hemoglobin and erythrocyte (red blood cell) count are lower. Sufficient iron intake is necessary to maintain an adequate erythrocyte level. Erythrocytes are formed in the bone marrow of the ribs, sternum, and vertebrae as in adulthood. During stress, the liver and spleen also form erythrocytes and granulocytes (37).

Overall Development

Development does not proceed equally or simultaneously in body parts and maturational skills. Sometimes a child concentrates so intently on one aspect of development (e.g., motor skills) that other abilities (e.g., toilet training) falter or regress. Illness or malnutrition may slow growth, but a catch-up growth period occurs later so that the person reaches the developmental norms. The brain is more vulnerable to permanent injury because destroyed cells are not replaced, although some brain cells may take over some functions of missing cells. Most children also show seasonal spurts in growth. Caucasians, for example, show more height increase in spring and more weight increase in fall. There are also cultural differences in growth and development. The African-American child develops motor skills at a greater pace than the Caucasian until age 3. The African-American child may be walking alone at 7 or 9 months, in contrast to 12 or 15 months. If all variables are controlled, the African-American child probably will be heavier and have more advanced skeletal development (10, 13, 22, 32, 37).

Discuss physical characteristics of the toddler with the parents to help them adjust to his or her changing competencies.

Physical Assessment of the Young Child

The approach to the physical examination depends on the age of the individual. Adequate time should be spent in becoming acquainted with the child and the accompanying parent. A friendly manner, quiet voice, and relaxed approach help make the examination more fruitful. Hands should always be warmed before giving an examination, but especially so in the case of the child.

No assessment is complete without knowing the antenatal, natal, and neonatal history. When the child is old enough, let him or her tell what conditions surround the visit even if the message is only "stomach hurt."

Many times you will be learning about the young child from the mother and will be learning about the mother's attitude. If other siblings are present, observe the interaction among the family members.

What are the mother's facial expressions? In what tone of voice does she talk? Does she look away or comfort the child if the child seems disturbed with a procedure?

What are the other siblings' reactions toward the toddler, the mother, and the health care worker? What are the siblings' reactions in general?

Although the child may not talk much, general appearance can reveal much information. Does the child look ill or well? What is the activity level? Coordination? Gait, if walking? Reactions to parents, siblings, and examiner? Nature of cry, if present? Facial expressions (28, 29)?

Before 6 months of age the infant usually tolerates the examining table. Between 6 months and 3 to 5 years, most of the examination can be done from the mother's or caretaker's lap. After age 4, much depends on the relationship established with the child.

The sequence of the examination with the young should be from least discomfort to most discomfort. Undressing can be a gradual procedure as children are often shy about this process. Some examiners prefer to go from toe to head or at least to start with auscultation, which is painless and sometimes fascinating to the child. It is best to leave the ears, nose, and mouth to the end because examination of these areas often initiates a negative response.

Generally the temperature should be taken rectally during the first years of life. Through the age of 2, the head circumference is measured at its greatest width and plotted on a growth curve scale that is compared with the norm (28, 29).

Blood pressure should be taken with the cuff that will snugly fit the arm. The first reading is recommended at age 3. The inflatable bladder should completely encircle the arm but not overlap. Artificially high blood pressure results if the cuff is too narrow or too short (28, 29). Because this procedure causes some discomfort and it is important to get readings in a low-anxiety state, sensitive timing is needed to get desired results. It sometimes helps to make a game out of the procedure by allowing the toddler to help pump up the bulb or read the numbers on the gauge.

The skin can be examined for turgor by feeling the calf of the leg, which should be firm. **Spider nevi,** *pinhead-sized red dots from which blood vessels radiate,* are commonly found, as are **Mongolian spots,** *large, flat black or blue-and-black spots.* One or two *patches of light brown, nonelevated stains,* called **café au lait spots,** are within normal findings, but more may be indicative of fibromas or neurofibromas. **Bruises** (*ecchymoses*) are not abnormal in healthy active children, but their location is important. Bruises not on the extremities or on areas easily hit when falling may indicate child abuse, or excessive bruising may indicate blood dyscrasias (21, 28, 29).

Lymph nodes are palpable in almost all healthy young children. Small, mobile, nontender nodes often point to previous infection (28, 29).

When examining the head region, consider the following:

- The auricles of the ears should be pulled back and down in young children and back and up in older children.
- A complete hearing test with an audiometer should be done before a child enters school. Before that, the whisper technique or the use of a tuning fork is adequate.
- A Snellen E chart can be used for testing visual acuity before the child knows the alphabet. Visual acuity at 3 years is 20/40, and at 4 to 5 years is 20/30.
- Other aspects of the visual examination depend on the child's age and the suspected problem (e.g., after surgery for congenital cataracts).
- Teeth should be examined for their sequence of eruption, number, character, and position (21, 29).

When examining the thorax and lungs, remember that breath sounds of young children are usually more intense and more bronchial and expiration is more pronounced than in adults. The heart should be examined with the child erect, recumbent, and turned to the left. Sinus arrhythmia and extrasystoles can be benign and are not uncommon (21, 29).

When standing, a child's abdomen may be protuberant; when lying down, it should disappear. The skilled examiner should be able to palpate both the liver and the spleen (29).

When examining the male genitalia, the testicles should be examined while the male is warm and in a sitting position, holding his knees with heels on the seat of the chair or examining table. Without warmth and abdominal pressure, the testes may not be in the scrotum (21).

Examination of the female genitalia is basically visual unless a specific problem in the area has developed.

When examining the extremities, the examiner may note bowlegs, which are common until 18 months. Knock-knees are common until approximately age 12. The toddler may appear flat-footed when first walking. All these characteristics are usually short term (21, 28, 29).

The neurologic examination is conducted throughout and is not much different from the sequence in the adult examination; however, the appropriate maturation level must be kept in mind.

► RECOMMENDED NUTRITIONAL INTAKE
FOR TODDLERS (AGES 12–24 MONTHS)

• Meat or fish, an egg or cheese	Two (1-oz) servings
• Milk (whole)	Maximum of 4 cups (1 qt), preferably 3 cups
• Green and yellow vegetables	Two or more ($\frac{1}{4}$-cup) servings
• Fruit	At least two servings
• Cereal, bread	At least two servings
• Fats and carbohydrates	To meet caloric needs

Nutritional Needs

See Recommended Nutritional Intake for Toddlers (Ages 12–24 Months) for a listing of dietary requirements by food group. Children less than age 2 should not receive low-fat (2%) milk because they need the extra calories from fat for energy, for growth, and for brain development. Liver or another high-iron food should be served at least once a week. Toddlers like breads, sweets, mashed potatoes, milk, and snack foods; such a diet, if served exclusively, would impair health. Too much milk without adequate amounts of other foods is also undesirable because omission of meats and vegetables could lead to iron deficiency anemia (16, 36).

The average serving sizes for the child of 2 to 3 years are as follows (16, 36):

- Milk, 6 oz ($\frac{3}{4}$ glass); cheese, $\frac{1}{2}$ oz or $\frac{1}{4}$ cup; yogurt, $\frac{1}{2}$ cup
- Juice, 3 to 4 oz ($\frac{1}{3}$ to $\frac{1}{2}$ cup)
- Meat, $\frac{1}{6}$ pound
- Egg, one medium size
- Cereal, 3 tablespoons cooked; $\frac{1}{2}$ cup ready-to-eat
- Bread, one half slice; cookies, 2; rice, $\frac{1}{2}$ cup; pasta, $\frac{1}{4}$ cup
- Fruits and vegetables, one half of raw fruit, 2 to 4 tablespoons (up to $\frac{1}{4}$ cup) cooked

Each day offer the toddler three regular meals and three snacks; snacks may be fruits, vegetables, crackers, yogurt, small sandwich, or juice. Avoid high-sugar, fat, and high-salt snacks; they may be permitted for special occasions. Caloric needs are not high and increase slowly throughout the toddler period. The toddler's appetite typically declines at approximately 18 months. The child has finished a major growth spurt and needs fewer calories. Approximately 1000 calories per day are needed at age 1, and only 1300 to 1500 calories are required by age 3 (100 cal/kg/d) because the child is growing less rapidly than during infancy. Body tissues are developing slowly; thus, protein needs are not high, between 1 g of protein per pound or 1.8 g per kilogram of body weight daily. Vitamin supplements are rarely needed if food intake is balanced in nutrients. (Refer to Appendix I.) Fluoride supplements are helpful in areas without fluorinated water. Fluid requirements are approximately 115 to 125 mL/kg/d (16, 36).

Food intake, or its refusal, is one way for the toddler to show increasing independence. Decreased food intake may result from a (1) slower growth rate; (2) short attention span and distractibility by other stimuli; and (3) increased interest in the surroundings. How well the child eats, however, is determined to a great extent by how parents manage mealtime, parental behavior toward food, and the atmosphere surrounding the meal.

Some suggestions to teach parents to avoid having mealtime be a battleground are (16, 36):

1. Serve food in small portions.
2. Serve finger foods or cut food so that it can be eaten with the fingers.
3. Let the child choose (it is not necessary for the toddler to sample every food served).
4. Avoid high-fat, high-salt, or carbohydrate foods such as soda, candy, and cake or empty nutrition snack foods in the choice.
5. Offer a food again if it has been rejected one time, without fussing about it.
6. Avoid insisting that the child eat everything on the plate.

The toddler is a great imitator; he or she eats the kind of foods eaten by the parents. Parental pressure or reprimands when the child does not eat a particular food convey anxiety or anger and reinforce not eating, because of either the negative attention received or the stress response felt by the child. Toddlers can be fussy eaters or go on "food jags," preferring only a certain food. Advise parents to give the requested food for a few days until the child gets bored with it, while continuing to offer alternative foods. Or the toddler may overeat if parents overeat. If there is a high caloric intake, obesity may result. Excessive weight gain interferes with the physical mobility that is a part of being a normal toddler.

Teach parents about the nutritional needs and eating patterns of the toddler. Avoid serving too large a portion, which can be the beginning of overeating or cause refusal to eat all the food, with resultant conflict between parent and toddler.

Malnutrition may lead to slower growth, tooth decay, lowered resistance to disease, and even death. Signs of malnutrition include abdominal swelling, lethargy, lack of attention to stimuli, lack of energy, diminished muscle strength and coordination, changes in skin color, and hair loss. Females apparently are buffered better against effects of malnutrition or illness than males. Malnutrition delays growth, but children have great recuperative powers if malnutrition does not continue too long. When nutrition improves, growth takes place unusually fast until norms for weight, height, and skeletal development are reached. For example, children who suffered early malnutrition but were provided good nutrition later performed as well on intellectual tests as their peers (16, 36, 37).

A hospitalized toddler frequently regresses; refusing to feed self is one manifestation. The child needs a lot of emotional support and to feel some kind of control over his or her destiny and that he or she is not totally helpless and powerless. A way of assuring some area of control is by permitting the child to choose foods and encouraging him or her to feed self (37).

Play, Exercise, and Rest

Play and Exercise

Play is the business of the toddler. During play he or she exercises, learns to manage the body, improves muscular coordination and manual dexterity, increases awareness and organizes the surrounding world by scrutinizing objects, and develops beginning spatial and sensory perception. The child learns language and to pay attention and releases emotional tensions as he or she channels unacceptable urges such as aggression into acceptable activities; translates feelings, drives, and fantasies into action; and learns about self as a person. Through play the toddler becomes socialized and begins to learn right from wrong. The child learns to have fun and to master.

The child has little interest in other children except as a curious explorer. **Play** is solitary and **parallel;** *he or she plays next to but not with other children.* There is little overt exchange, but there is satisfaction in being close to other children. Toddler is unable to share toys

Case Situation: Toddler Development

The setting is an urban day-care center. The outdoor fenced, grassy play area, with a sandbox, a variety of climbing and swing play equipment, and wheeled toys, looks inviting. Indoors the wide hallways, a cubicle for each child's clothing and personal items, and a large room where the children play indicate that this is a busy center. The large room has several distinct play areas: a house corner, a large block corner, a music area with piano and other children's instruments, a reading corner with books, and an art area with large sheets of paper and crayons, pencils, chalk, and finger paints. Tables in the middle of the room are piled with toys. Large windows face the playground; potted plants and an aquarium add life to the bustling room.

Luis, 18 months of age, is a typical toddler: 24 pounds, 28 in. tall. He occasionally falls as he walks around the room but rises to his feet without help. He pulls a toy truck, then sits on a tractor and pushes himself with his feet. In a few minutes a pink ball on a shelf catches his attention, and he runs to it, grasping it with hands and forearms. He repeatedly sets the ball on the shelf to play with a nearby toy but returns again for the ball.

While Luis is holding the ball, another toddler approaches him to get the ball. Luis yanks away, displaying the typical toddler's egocentricism and inability to share. The other child hits Luis, who cries to get the teacher's attention and support. The teacher talks to each child, encourages both to hug and be friendly, and plays with the two children briefly as they share the ball. In a few minutes each child has been distracted to engage in another activity in the room.

Before lunch the teacher calls the group together for story time, which is limited to 10 minutes because of the toddler's short attention span. During this time the toddlers repeat a nursery rhyme that was part of the story and then sing the rhyme, demonstrating rote memory. Luis and the other toddlers enjoy music and rhyming play.

and is distressed by demands of sharing as he or she has a poorly defined sense of ownership. Toddler will play cooperatively with guidance, however. By the end of 2 years, most children imitate adults in dramatic play by doing such things as setting the table and cooking. When selecting play materials for the toddler, remember likes and dislikes and choose a variety of activities because the attention span is short. (Safety and durability aspects of toys, as discussed in Chapter 7, must be considered.)

Table 8–2 presents suggested play activities and equipment for the child 18 months or 2 years of age.

TABLE 8–2. SUGGESTED PLAY ACTIVITIES AND EQUIPMENT FOR TODDLERS

Age (months)	Toy, Equipment, or Activity
18	Push–pull toys (cars, trucks, farm tools)
	Boxes and toys for climbing
	Empty and fill toys (plastic food containers, kitchen utensils, small boxes, and open–close toys)
	Big picture books—thick-paged, colorful, sturdy (child will turn two or three pages at a time, tear at thin pages, can identify one picture at a time)
	Stuffed animals with no detachable parts
	Baby dolls, large enough to hug, carry, cuddle, dress, feed
	Big pieces of plain paper or newspaper layers and crayons for scribbling
	Small blocks—builds a tower of two or three at a time
	Shape-sorting blocks or cube
	Small chair; small furniture to play "house"
	Toy farm animals or equipment
	Rubber or soft ball; throws overhand
	Phonograph record, preferably sturdy plastic that child can manipulate by self; musical and sound toys; musical instruments simple to use
	Rocking horse; rocking chair
24	All of the above are enjoyed; child now turns book or magazine pages singly—still tears; builds tower of seven blocks and aligns cubes
	Makes circular strokes with crayon, enjoys fingerpaints
	Puppets
	Pedal toys; dumping toys (dump trucks)
	Sandbox toys
	Playdough and clay; mud
	Jungle gym for climbing; sand box; small water pool for waterplay
	Pounding toys—hammer and pegs, drums, small boards
	Picture puzzles—two to four pieces (wooden or thick cardboard)
	Large, colored wooden beads to string
	Simple trains, cars, boats, planes to push–pull or sit on and pedal
	Kick ball
	Likes to run

Help parents understand the importance of play and safety. A relation exists between the quality of attachment between mother and baby and the quality of play and problem-solving behavior at 2 years of age. Toddlers who are securely attached at 18 months of age are more enthusiastic, persistent, cooperative, and able to share than if secure attachment has not developed. There is also more frequent and sophisticated interaction with peers at 3 years when secure attachment has formed in infancy (25). Discuss play patterns and toys with the parents.

Help parents realize the importance of offering playthings that can transform into any number of toys, depending on his or her mood and imagination at the time. The adult can be available or initially start a play activity with the child; however, the child should be encouraged to play independently, developing mastery, autonomy, and self-esteem in the process.

Verzemnieks (33) describes developmental stimulation, play activities, and toys for the hospitalized child. See Techniques for Using Play While Caring for the Child for a summary of how play can be used effectively with the ill child.

Rest

Rest is as essential as exercise and play, and although a child may be tired after a day full of exploration and exerting boundless energy, bedtime is often a difficult experience. Bedtime means loneliness and separation from fun, family, and, most important, the mother figure. The toddler needs an average of 10 to 12 hours of sleep nightly plus a daytime nap.

Teach the following guidelines to parents for establishing a bedtime routine for the toddler.

- Set a definite bedtime routine and adhere to it. If the child is overly tired, he or she becomes agitated and difficult to put to sleep.
- Establish a bedtime ritual, including bath, a story, and a tucking-in routine. Begin approximately 30 minutes before bedtime. The tucking-in should be caring and brief.
- If the child cries, which most children do briefly, go back in a few minutes to provide reassurance. Do not pick up the child or stay more than 30 seconds. If the crying continues, return in 5 minutes and repeat the procedure. Thus the parent can determine whether there is any real problem, and the child feels secure.
- If extended crying continues, lengthen the time to return to the child to 10 minutes. Eventually fatigue will occur, the cry will turn to whimpers, and the child will fall asleep.

► TECHNIQUES FOR USING PLAY WHILE CARING FOR THE CHILD

Physical Assessment

- Talk soothingly and calmly. Explain what you are doing as you do it.
- Blow on the stethoscope. Ask child to imitate.
- Have child listen to own heartbeat with stethoscope.
- Name body parts and touch them. "Foot. Here is my foot." "Where are your eyes?" "There are your eyes!" "Where is your nose?" Guide the child's hands to touch.
- Use diversions—another toy, tickles (especially abdomen).
- Play peek-a-boo: cover your eyes, then child's. Hide your head with blanket, then child's head. When child covers own head, say, "Where's (name?)" Then delight in discovery.
- Use body movement, exercising child's arms and legs rhythmically while doing assessment.
- Sing a nonsense tune or talk animatedly.
- Talk about sensations: warm or cold, soft or rough as sensations are presented.
- Name body position: up or down, over.
- Encourage child to do examination of doll, teddy bear, toy animal.

Bathing

- Experiment with the properties of water in a small tub. Use items that float and sink—washcloth, plastic soap dish, paper cup, plastic lid, empty plastic cylinders, or toys at child's cribside. Talk about what happens.
- Identify body parts as you wash them. Give simple directions: "Close your eyes." "Raise your arms." "Wash your hair.") Be sure to praise all help.
- Encourage child to "bathe" a doll, teddy bear, or toy animal.

Feeding

- Place the child in high chair or walker when he or she can sit unsupported. Tie toy or utensil to high chair to facilitate retrieval.
- Discuss the food: hot or cold, colors, textures, which utensils to use.
- Use an extra spoon and cup: one for you, one for baby.
- Experiment with food: fingerpaint with food on tray, make lines.

Diagnostic Procedures

- Explain to the child what you plan to do and are doing. Be honest but gentle.
- Tell the child it is all right to cry; comfort if child cries.
- Set up situation so child can do procedure on doll or toy animal. While child is imitating, talk about how much it hurts. Cuddle and comfort the child, cooing, singing softly, rocking after the procedure.
- Distract the child with empty dressing packages, encouraging crushing and listening to sounds.
- Make the sounds and touch different parts of child's body.
- Vocalize sounds related to procedure. Have child imitate you.

- The child should remain in his or her bed rather than sleep for all or part of the night with parents. Bedtime routine becomes a precedent for other separations; however, if the parents make an occasional exception such as during a family crisis of major loss, trauma, or transition or if the child is ill, neither the marriage relationship nor the child's development will be hindered. It is important that the exception not become the routine.
- As the child grows older, limit the number of times the child can get up, for any reason, after going to bed.

Sleep problems during hospitalization may show up through restlessness, insomnia, and nightmares. Increasingly, hospitals are permitting parents to spend the night in the child's room to lessen fears and separation anxiety. Cuddling is still important to a toddler, especially if hospitalized. If a parent cannot remain with a frightened child, you can hold and rock him or her while he or she holds a favorite object.

Health Promotion and Health Protection

Routine Immunizations

These immunizations remain a vital part of health care. Refer to Chart 2 in Appendix IV for an immunization schedule. The tine test is repeated at 3 years of age. If the parent refuses to have the child immunized for religious reasons, emphasize the need to prevent exposure to these diseases, if possible, and the importance of continued good hygiene and nutrition. As a way to reduce the number of children in the Latino community who were susceptible to measles (15) the age for MMR immunization was lowered to 12 months by the Los Angeles County Health Department.

Common health threats at this age are respiratory infections and home accidents. The causes for accidents are motor vehicles, burns, suffocation, drowning, poisoning, and falls. Accidents are the leading cause of death, and deaths from poisonings continue to increase. Areas outside the home—the yard, the street, the grocery cart—have greater hazard because today there is more contact with them. Communicable diseases are less a health threat than parasitic diseases.

Safety Promotion and Injury Control

Accidents are a major cause of death. Thus it is necessary to childproof the home. Teach parents they can prevent injury from furniture by:

- Selecting furniture with rounded corners and a sturdy base
- Packing away breakable objects.
- Putting safety catches on doors to prevent the child opening furniture doors or pulling furniture on self

They can prevent falls by:

- Avoiding hazardous waxing
- Discarding throw rugs
- Keeping traffic lanes clear
- Placing gates at tops of stairways (Fig. 8–1) and screens on the windows
- Placing toys and favorite objects on a low shelf

Burns are prevented by blocking access to electric outlets, heating equipment, matches, lighters, hot water or hot food, and stoves, fireplaces, and appliances that heat. Handles of pans should be turned to the back of the stove. Electric cords attached to appliances that heat should not drape over the top edge of a work or counter surface. Fireworks should never be used when a young child is nearby. Placing tools and knives high on the wall or in a locked cabinet can prevent lacerations or more serious injury. Any surface that is sharp may cut the child and should be covered, if possible, or kept out of the way of the child.

Parents may call you to help when their child has been injured or is ill. Know emergency care. A poison treatment chart is available from the National Poison Center Network, Children's Hospital, 125 DeSoto Street, Pittsburgh, PA 15213. Many cities also have poison control centers to treat and give information to parents and professionals. The Red Cross is also a source of first-aid information. Refer to Parent Teaching to Prevent Poisoning for more tips to share with parents.

Thoroughly explore safety promotion with the parents, as the following normal developmental characteristics make the toddler prone to accidents. He or she:

- Moves quickly and is impulsive
- Is inquisitive and assertive
- Enjoys learning by touch, taste, and sight
- Enjoys playing with small objects
- Likes to attract attention
- Has a short attention span and unreliable memory
- Lacks judgment
- Has incomplete self-awareness
- Imitates the actions of others

Tell parents to teach the toddler to swim and always stay with the child when he or she is near water; not to allow boisterous play or sharp objects near a swimming pool, jungle gym, or sandbox; and to provide safety equipment and supervision.

Common Health Problems: Prevention and Treatment

The child must be carefully assessed for infections and other disease conditions because he or she lacks the cognitive, language, and self-awareness capacities to de-

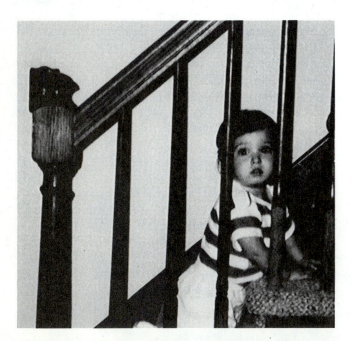

Figure 8–1. Toddlers should be prevented from climbing stairs, for example, by a portable gate. *(From Sherwen, L.N., M.A. Scoloveno, and C.T. Weingarten, Nursing Care of the Childbearing Family. Stamford, CT: Appleton & Lange, 1991, p. 926.)*

► PARENT TEACHING TO PREVENT POISONING

- Teach the child that medication and vitamins are not candy; keep them locked. Discard old medicine.
- Keep medicines, polishes, insecticides, drain cleaners, bleaches, household chemicals, garage products, and other potentially toxic substances in a locked cabinet out of the child's reach. Do not store them in containers previously used for food.
- Store nonfood substances in original containers with labels attached, not in food or beverage containers.
- If you are interrupted while pouring or using a product that is potentially harmful, take it with you. The toddler is curious and impulsive and moves quickly.
- Keep telephone numbers of the physician, poison control center, local hospital, and police and fire departments by the telephone.
- Teach the child not to eat berries, flowers, or plants; some are poisonous.

scribe discomforts. Table 8–3 summarizes common conditions.

Consult pediatric nursing texts for additional information on childhood illnesses and their assessment, care, and prevention (37).

PSYCHOSOCIAL CONCEPTS

Cognitive Development

The intellectual capacity of the toddler is limited. The child has all the body equipment that allows for an assimilation of the environment, but he or she is just beginning intellectual maturity.

Learning occurs through several general modes (5, 19, 25):

- Natural unfolding of the innate physiologic capacity
- Imitation of others
- Reinforcement from others as the child engages in acceptable behavior
- Insight, gaining understanding in increasing depth as he or she plays, experiments, or explores
- Identification, taking into self values and attitudes like those he or she is closely associated with through use of the other modes

The toddler experiences the world in a **parataxic mode,** in that *wholeness of experience and cause–effect relationships do not exist.* He or she experiences parts of things in the present; they are not necessarily events connected with past and future (30). Repeating simple and honest explanations, for example, why a certain tool works or why he or she should not play in the street, will eventually lead to understanding of cause and effect (30).

The toddler's attention span lengthens. He or she likes songs, nursery rhymes, and stories, even though he or she does not fully understand simple explanations of them. He or she can name pictures on repeated exposure. The toddler plays alone sometimes but prefers being near people. He or she is aware of self and others in a new way.

Part of the toddler's learning is through imitation of the parents, helping them with simple tasks such as bringing an object, trying new activities on his or her own, ritualistic repetition of activity, experimenting with language, and expressing self emotionally. According to Piaget, the toddler finishes the fifth and sixth stages of the Sensorimotor Period and begins the Preoperational Period at approximately age 2 (34).

In the **fifth stage of the Sensorimotor Period** (12–18 months) the child consolidates previous activities involving body actions into *experiments* to discover new properties of objects and events and achieve new goals instead of applying habitual behavior. He or she no longer keeps repeating the same behavior to achieve a goal and performs familiar acts without random maneuvers. The child differentiates self from objects in the environment. Understanding of *object permanence, space perception,* and *time perception* can be observed in new ways. The child is aware that objects continue to exist even though they cannot be seen; he or she accounts for sequential displacements and searches for objects where they were *last* seen. Toddler manipulates objects in new and various ways to learn what they will do. For the first time, objects outside the self are understood as causes of action. Activities are now linked to internal representations or symbolic meaning of events or objects (memories, ideas, feelings about past events) (34).

The **sixth stage of the Sensorimotor Period** (18–24 months) seems primarily a transitional phase to the preoperative period. Now the child does less trial-and-error thinking but uses memory of past experience and imitation to act as if he or she arrived at an answer. He or she imitates another who is out of sight. Toddler begins to solve problems, to foresee maneuvers that will succeed or fail, and to remember an object that is absent and search for it until it is found (10, 13, 22, 32, 34).

In the **Preoperational Period** (2–7 years) thought is more symbolic; memory continues to form; and the child internalizes mental pictures of people, the environment, and ideas about rules and relationships. The child begins to arrive at answers mentally instead of through physical activity, exploration, and manipulation. Symbolic representation is seen in (1) the use of language to describe (symbolize) objects, events, and feelings, (2) the beginning of symbolic play (crossing two sticks to represent a plane), and (3) delayed imitation (repeating a parent's behavior hours later) (19, 34). The toddler can understand simple abstractions, but thinking is basically concrete (related to tangible events) and literal. He or she is **egocentric** (*unable to take the viewpoint of another*); the ability to differentiate between subject and object, the real object and the word symbol, is not developed. He or she knows only one word for any object and cannot understand how the one word *chair* can refer to many different styles of chairs. If the flower is called *flower* and *plant,* the child will not understand that more than one word can refer to the same object. Concept of time is *now* and concept of distance is whatever can be seen. The child imitates the thinking and behavior observed in another but lacks

TABLE 8–3. COMMON HEALTH PROBLEMS OF TODDLERS

Problem	Definition	Signs/Symptoms	Prevention/Treatment
Myopia	Nearsightedness	Squinting, not seeing far away	Prescribed glasses, use Allen cards to check vision; 30 ft represents the maximum distance at which child should identify object; if identified at 15 ft, vision is 15/30
Astigmatism	Unequal curvature in the refractive surfaces of the eyes	Cannot clearly focus	Prescribed glasses, use Allen cards to check vision; 30 ft represents the maximum distance at which child should identify object; if identified at 15 ft, vision is 15/30
Strabismus	Eyes are not straight or properly aligned	One or both eyes may turn in, turn out, turn up or down; may be consistent or come and go	Prescribed treatment to bring the deviating eye back into binocular vision before age 6 by wearing a patch over the better aligned eye
Hearing impairment	Hearing less than normal for age group	Inability to speak by age 2; failure to respond to out-of-sight noise; tilting the head while listening	Observe child carefully for appropriate hearing; check with practitioner to see if ear or upper respiratory problem is to blame; teach lip reading and sign language if appropriate
Otitis media	Infection of middle ear with accumulation of seropurulent fluid in middle ear cavity	Earache; fever; upper respiratory infection; decreased hearing; bulging tympanic membrane; disappearance of landmarks	Medication (antibiotic), sometimes decongestant; follow-up examination
Dental caries	Tooth decay often related to excess concentrated sweets or bottle mouth syndrome	Obvious dark places or breakdown of teeth; pain	Supplemental fluoride; avoidance of sweets; directions to parents for cleaning teeth (hydrogen peroxide on gauze before 18 months; then a soft toothbrush); Prepare for first dental visit with explanation, role play, positive image If problem with discolored teeth, infection, chipping, see dentist immediately
Malabsorption syndrome	Lactose intolerance	Chronic vomiting; diarrhea; abdominal discomfort; flatulence, irritability; poor sleep pattern	Try other products besides milk (e.g., soybean formula)
Impetigo	Lesions caused by microorganism (usually *Streptococcus*), often a complication of insect bites, abrasions, or dermatitis.	Upper layers of skin have honey-colored, fluid-filled vesicles that eventually crust, surrounded by a red base	Identification of lesions significant because acute glomerulonephritis can follow if not properly treated; trim fingernails to avoid scratching; wash and scrub lesions gently three times daily; wash towels used or infected areas separately; oral or topical antibiotics
Pharyngitis	Inflammation of pharynx or tonsils, or both, caused by virus or group A *Streptococcus* and rarely *Mycoplasma pneumoniae* and *Corynebacterium diphtheriae*	Red throat, exudate, enlarged lymph nodes; fever; other upper respiratory infectious symptoms	Get specific diagnosis with throat culture; treat with antibiotic if bacterial cause to avoid further disease complications; antipyretic medicine if fever present (Do not give salicylates to children because of possible Reye's syndrome, a rare but sometimes fatal disease. Warm saline gargle if able; increased fluid intake
Acute nonspecific gastroenteritis (simple *diarrhea*)	Inflammation of the gastrointestinal tract during which stools are more liquid and frequent than usual	May cause dehydration with signs of sunken eyes, dry mucous membranes, decreased skin turgor, and weight loss	Discontinue milk; give small amounts of clear liquids such as flat cola (at room temperature) alternating with an electrolyte solution; add simple foods slowly

(continued)

TABLE 8–3. COMMON HEALTH PROBLEMS OF TODDLERS (continued)

Problem	Definition	Signs/Symptoms	Prevention/Treatment
Varicella (*chickenpox*)	Acute, highly contagious disease caused by varicella–zoster virus	Rash consisting of lesions that appear in crops and that go from flat macules to fluid-filled vesicles that crust in 6–8 hours; spread is from trunk to periphery and sometimes into the mouth; itching; fever; headache; general malaise; loss of appetite	Give vaccine when available; keep fingernails short; use lotions such as Calamine or prescription drug if itching intense; antipyretic drug if fever; isolate until lesions are all crusted
Rubella (*3-day measles*)	Viral disease characterized by rash and lymph node enlargement	Rash on face or neck, spreading to trunk and extremities; rash usually gone in 3 days	Prevention: immunization — a very serious disease for the pregnant female, associated with high degree of congenital malformation; mild disease treated symptomatically for the toddler, but to be avoided by all
Pinworms (*Enterobius vermicularis*)	Most common parasite infestation in the United States; cycle begins with oral infection of pinworm eggs which pass through intestinal tract in 15–28 days, hatch into larva and then into adult worms	Possibly asymptomatic; itching around anus; 1-in. white thready worms visible on perineum, especially when child at rest	Medication (treat all family members); personal hygiene; washing all laundry and bedclothes in hot water; clean favorite stuffed animals, chairs, and rugs, which may harbor eggs
Miliaria rubra (*"heat rash"* or *"prickly heat"*)	Erythematous papular rash distributed in area of sweat glands	Fine red, raised rash; itching, pustules in neck and axillary region	Keep environment cool and dry; use air conditioner/fan; tepid baths; light clothing; use Caldesene powder; use sparingly 1% hydrocortisone cream
Viral croup (*laryngotracheobronchitis;* usually caused by parainfluenza virus in late fall or early winter)	Inflammation of the respiratory mucosa of all airways; edema of the larynx and subglottic area	Gradual onset of upper respiratory infection; inspiratory stridor; low-grade fever; barking cough; wheezing; hoarseness; high-pitched sound on inspiration	Keep child well hydrated; use cool mist vaporizer; force liquids; take child in bathroom and turn on hot water; take child outside; if airway obstruction present, seek help immediately

the past experience and broader knowledge that is essential for logical thought. This level of learning will continue through the preschool era (10, 13, 22, 32, 34).

Pushing children to read and write at an early age has not been shown to produce long-lasting positive effects. It may cause the child to lose initiative, curiosity, desire to use ingenuity, and ability to cope with ordinary life stresses. The child knows inside what he or she can do. If the parents whom the child looks to for support and guidance are manipulating him or her to meet their needs, the child may come to mistrust parents and self. Before parents put the child in a preschool that emphasizes formal academics, they should consider what the child is not learning from missed playtime. Play that is parallel to and cooperative with peers helps the child develop language, motor, cognitive, nonverbal, and social skills; positive self-esteem; a sense of worth as an individual; and unique problem-solving skills in the face of stress (1, 25, 27).

Teach parents about this aspect of development. This period can be trying and should be tempered by supportive guidance and discipline: parents' saying what is meant, providing environmental stimulation, showing interest in the child's activities and talking and working with the child, reinforcing intellectual attempts, and showing a willingness to teach with simple explanations. Much of the intellectual development now depends on the achievements of infancy, how parents used the baby's potential, and the *quality* of parent–child interaction rather than the *amount* of time, per se, that is spent with the child (25). The child learns to enjoy learning, which forms the basis for later school achievement.

Language Development

Learning to communicate in an understandable manner begins during this era. Through speech the toddler will gradually learn to control unacceptable behavior, exchange physical activity for words, and share the view of reality held by society.

The ability to speak words and sentences is not governed by the same higher center that controls understanding. The child understands words before they are used with meaning, and some children develop adequate comprehension but cannot speak (25).

Various theories explain language acquisition. Although behavioral or learning theory explains some language learning through receiving reinforcement for imitation of language sounds, the number of specific stimulus–response connections that would be necessary to speak even one language could not be acquired in a lifetime. Nor do behaviorists explain the sequence of language development, regardless of culture; however, learning principles can be used to modify acquired language deficits (5, 25).

Interactionist Theory is used by most theorists to explain language development. Language develops through interaction between heredity, maturation, encounters with people and environmental stimuli, and life experiences. Humans are biologically prepared for language learning, but experience with the spoken word and with loving people who facilitate language acquisition is equally essential. Further, the child has an active role in learning language rather than a passive one. Adults modify their speech when talking to a child, and the child is more attentive to simplified speech. Mothers and fathers use different conversational techniques to talk with the child, who, in turn, teaches language in a broader way (5, 25).

Speech and language are major adaptive behaviors being developed during the second year. Speech enables the child to become more independent and to better make needs known. Speech is the mediation for thought processes. The greater the comprehension and vocabulary a child has, the further a child can go in cognitive processes. As the child and parents respond verbally and nonverbally to each other, the child learns attitudes and values and behaviors and ideas. The child first responds to patterns of sounds rather than to specific word sounds; if others speak indistinctly to the child, he or she will also speak indistinctly. The normal child will begin to speak by 14 months, although some children may make little effort to speak until after 2 years. By age 3, he or she may still mispronounce more than half the sounds (5).

The toddler speaks in the present tense initially, using **syncretic speech,** in which *one word stands for a certain object, and has a limited range of sounds.* Single words represent entire sentences; for example, "go" means "I want to go." By 18 to 20 months he or she uses **telegraphic speech**, *two- to four-word expressions that contain a noun and verb and maintain word order,* such as "go play" and "go night-night." Variety on intonation also increases. A 2-year-old will introduce additional words and say "I go play" or "I go night-night." Conversation with parents involves contraction and expansion. The *child shortens into fewer words what the parent says but states the main message* (**contraction**); the *parent elaborates on, uses a full sentence, and interprets what the child says* (**expansion**). Expansion helps the child's language development (32). The toddler frequently says "no," perhaps in imitation of the parents and their discipline techniques, but may often do what is asked even while saying "no." Stuttering is common because ideas come faster than the ability to use vocabulary.

Recognizable language develops sequentially. See Table 8–4 for a summary of language and speech development.

The toddler's speech is **autistic** because *vocalizations have specific meaning only to the child.* He or she plays with sounds and incorrectly produces the majority of consonant sounds.

Apparently the child learns to speak in a highly methodical way, breaking down language into its simplest parts and developing rules to put the parts together. Children proceed from babbling to one-word and two-word sentences, use of word order and plurals, use of negative sentences, and the importance of phonetics or a sound system. To communicate effectively, the child must learn not only the language and its rules, but also the use of social speech, which takes into account the knowledge and perspective of another person (19, 32). This begins in toddlerhood and continues to develop through childhood as the child gains interpersonal and social experiences.

Teach parents that this is facilitated when they teach social language strategies to the child as they introduce him or her to life experiences. Through conversation with the family at mealtime and in other activities, vocabulary is enlarged, and the child learns family expressions that aid socialization. Mealtime provides a miniature society in which the toddler can feel secure in attempting to imitate speech. He or she gets positive reinforcement for speech efforts, especially for words that are selected, repeated frequently, and reinforced by eager parents. In addition, *being talked with, using adult words rather than baby talk frequently throughout the day, being read to, and having an opportunity to explore the environment increases the child's comprehension of words and rules of grammar as well as organization and size of vocabulary and use of word inflections* (6).

Language development *requires a sense of security and verbal and nonverbal stimulation.* For a child to speak, he or she must have a loving, consistent relationship with a parent or caretaker. Unless the toddler feels that this person will respond to his or her words, toddler will not be motivated to speak. The toddler may not

Research Abstract

Russell, K., and V. Champion, Health Beliefs and Social Influence in Home Safety Practices of Mothers with Preschool Children, IMAGE: Journal of Nursing Scholarship, 28 (1996), 59–64.

One of every five children experiences an injury requiring treatment. Each year about 600,000 children are hospitalized for injuries; 16 million are treated in the emergency room, and more than 30,000 are permanently disabled from injuries. Young children are especially vulnerable to unintentional injuries in the home. Injury risks are higher in children when the child has suffered previous injury, and when parents are of low income status, are African American, and have little knowledge about injury prevention.

The purpose of this study was to determine relationships among health beliefs, social influence, and behavior that prevent injury in the home. It was hypothesized that a combination of injury experience, knowledge, demographic characteristics, health beliefs, and social influence variables could predict home hazard accessibility and frequency of occurrence.

The sample was composed of 140 women residing in two inner-city public housing complexes in a Midwestern metropolitan city. The children were between 1 and 3 years of age (55% were boys and 45% were girls) and free of physical and mental handicapping conditions. Except for number of bathrooms and bedrooms per dwelling, the public housing units were identical in structure, scheduling of maintenance, and smoke detector devices. Most of the women (97.2%) were African American, aged 15 to 41 years, never married, with an educational range of 8 to 14 years, and unemployed. The majority (88.3%) reported household incomes at or below the poverty level.

The research instruments consisted of a questionnaire measuring health beliefs, social influence, and injury prevention knowledge variables; an observational tool for measuring presence of hazards in the home; and an interview form. After the interview, observations for safety hazards were made in the home. As hazardous items were identified, they were pointed out to the subjects and information was given on how to eliminate the hazard. General childhood injury prevention materials and injury-related packets, including soaps, band-aids, and socket covers, were discussed and distributed.

Bivariate and regression analysis was performed to analyze data. The top seven accessible hazards, in order of frequency out of a possible 20, were uncovered electric outlet sockets, missing nonskid surface in the bathtub, personal hygiene/beauty products, medications, unguarded stairs, missing electric plates, and clutter on the floor. Neither frequency nor accessibility of hazards varied when the number of rooms for a resident was controlled. Hazard accessibility decreased when the mother had previous injury experience, had more education, had a perception of self-efficacy, or was older. Self-efficacy was the strongest predictor of the mother's safetyproofing the home.

Mothers who perceived barriers to preventing injuries in their children were less likely to safetyproof their homes against injury hazards. Barriers included limited access to information, maternal fatigue, and inefficient household management.

Health care implications are to increase self-efficacy in mothers through four approaches:

1. Give mothers the opportunity to perform injury prevention tasks until they can successfully sustain each activity over time.

2. Health care workers demonstrate or model the desired action or provide vicarious experience.

3. Use health education materials to teach mothers injury-prevention behaviors. The content should be culturally relevant and use similar language, be socially acceptable, and depict homes and parents with similar characteristics. Prevention actions should provide strategies within the resource capacity of the family.

4. Explore the mother's feelings about her ability to perform injury prevention.

TABLE 8–4. ASSESSMENT OF LANGUAGE AND SPEECH DEVELOPMENT

Characteristic	1 Year	1½ Years	2 Years	2½ Years
Language understanding and basic communication	Understands "no-no" inhibition; knows "bye-bye" and pat-a-cake; says "mama," "dada," or some similar term for caretakers	Understands very simple verbal instructions accompanied by gesture and intonation; identifies 3 body parts; points to 5 simple pictures; points for wants	Identifies 5 body parts; finds 10 pictures; obeys simple commands	Points to 15 pictures; obeys 2 or 3 simple commands
Appearance of individual sounds	10 vowels, 9 consonants in babbling and echoing	p, b, m, h, w in babbling		t, d, n, k, g, ng in words
Auditory memory imitation and repetition	Lalls; imitates sound; echoes or repeats syllables or some words (may not have meaning)		Meanings increasingly becoming associated with words	Repeats 2 digits; remembers 1 or 2 objects
Numerical size of vocabulary	1 or 2 words	Adds 10–20 words a week	50–250–300 words if consistently spoken to	400–500 words
Word type	Nouns	Nouns, action verbs, some adjectives	Nouns, verbs, adjectives, adverbs	Pronouns, "I"
Sentence length	Single word	Single words expanding to 3 or 4 words, noun and verb	2–5 words; elemental sentence	
Description of vocalization and communication	Babbling, lalling, echolalia (repeating sounds)	Leading, pointing, jargon, some words, intonations, gestures	Words, phrases, simple sentences	Developmental language problems first seen
Purpose of vocalization and communication	Pleasure	Attention getting	Meaningful social control; wish requesting	
Speech content and style			Possessive "mine"; pronouns last grammar form learned; grammar depends on what is heard	
Percent intelligibility		20–25% for person unfamiliar with child	60–75%; poor articulation of some words	Vowel production—90%

Data from References 10, 13, 19, 22, 32, and 37.

talk when separated from mother, such as during hospitalization or the first day at day-care. When being prepared for hospital procedures, the toddler needs simple and succinct explanations, with gestures pointing to the areas of the body being cared for, and verbal and physical displays of affection.

If a child is *delayed in speech,* carefully assess the child and family. Causes may include deafness or the inability to listen, mental retardation, emotional disturbance, maternal deprivation or separation from the parents, lack of verbal communication within the family and to the child, inconsistent or tangential responses to the child's speech, presence of twins, or parents' anticipating the needs of the child before he or she has a chance to communicate them.

Verbal interaction, an environment with a variety of objects and stimuli, and freedom to explore are crucial to help the young child use his or her senses and emerging motor skills and thereby are necessary to learn during the Sensorimotor and Preoperational Stages.

Emotional Development

The toddler is a self-loving, uninhibited, dominating, energetic little person absorbed in self-importance, always seeking attention, approval, and personal goals. Sometimes the toddler is cuddly and loving. At other times, he or she bites or pinches and looks almost happy, feeling no sense of guilt or shame. There is little self-control over exploratory or sadistic impulses. The toddler only slowly realizes that he or she cannot have everything desired and that some behavior annoys others.

He or she experiments with abandon in the quest for independence yet becomes easily frightened and runs to the parent for protection, security, reassurance, and approval.

Because the toddler still relies so much on the parents and wants their approval, he or she learns to curb the negativism without losing independent drives, to cooperate increasingly, and to develop socially approved behavior. Need for attention and approval is one of the main motivating forces in ego development and socialization.

The toddler often repeats performances and behavior that are given attention and laughed at; he or she likes to perform for adults and pleases self as much as the audience. He or she has a primitive sense of humor, laughs frequently, especially at surprise sounds and startling incongruities, and laughs with others who are laughing and at his or her own antics. Parents should give sufficient attention but not make the child show off for an audience, verbally or physically, and they should not overstimulate with laughter or games. Further, adults must realize the child fears separation, strangers, the dark, sudden or loud noises, large objects and machines, and hurtful events such as traumatic procedures.

Developmental Crisis

The psychosexual crisis for the toddler is autonomy versus shame and doubt (14). **Autonomy** is *shown in the ability to gain self-control* over motor abilities and sphincters; to make and carry out decisions; to feel able to cope adequately with problems or get the necessary help; to wait with patience; to give generously or to hold on, as indicated; to distinguish between possessions or wishes of self and of others; and to have a feeling of good will and pride. Autonomy is characterized by the oft-heard statement, "Me do it." Mastery accomplished in infancy sets the basis for autonomy.

Using negativism, even displaying temper, dawdling, and rituals; exploring even when parents object; developing language skills; saying "no" although he or she may do as asked; and increasing control over his or her body or situations are some apparent ways the toddler is demonstrating developing autonomy and maintaining a sense of security and control. Ritualistic behavior is normal and peaks at 2½ years, especially at bedtime and during illness. Although autonomy is developing, emotions are still contagious. The toddler reflects others' behavior and feelings. For example, if someone laughs or cries, he or she will imitate for no apparent reason.

Shame and doubt are felt if autonomy and a positive self-concept are not achieved (14). **Shame** is *the feeling of being fooled, embarrassed, exposed, small, impotent, dirty, of wanting to hide, and rage against self.* **Doubt** is *fear, uncertainty, mistrust, lack of self-confidence, and feeling that nothing done is any good and that one is controlled by others rather than being in control of self* (14).

There is a limit to how exposed, dirty, mean, and vulnerable one can feel. If the child is pushed past the limit or disciplined or toilet trained too harshly, or abused, he or she can no longer discriminate about self, what he or she should be and can do. If everything is planned and done *for* and *to* the child, he or she cannot develop autonomy. The toddler's self-concept and behavior will try to measure up to the expectations of parents and others, but there is no close attachment to an adult. Consequences of Shame and Doubt outlines traits and behaviors of a child who develops stronger feelings of shame and doubt than of autonomy. Too much shaming does not develop a sense of propriety but rather a secret determination to get away with things.

Discourage parents from creating an emotional climate of excessive expectations, criticism, blame, punishment, and overrestriction for the toddler because within the child's consciousness a sense of shame and doubt may develop that will be extremely harmful to further development. The child should not be given too much autonomy, or he or she will feel all-powerful. When a toddler fails to accomplish what he or she has been falsely led to believe could be achieved, the self-doubt and shame that result can be devastating. Aggressive behavior results if the child is severely punished or if parents are aggressive. With the proper balance of guidance and discipline, the toddler gains a sense of personal abilities and thus has the potential to deal with the next set of social adjustments (5, 25).

Toilet Training

Toilet training is a major developmental accomplishment and relates directly to the crisis of autonomy versus shame and doubt or to what Freudian theory calls the **anal stage** (25). Independence and autonomy (self-control), not cleanliness, are the critical issues in teaching the child to use the toilet. For the process to work, the parents must do little more than arrange for the child to use the toilet easily. The parent supports rather than acts as a trainer and is interested in the child, not just the act (1). The toddler is interested in the products he excretes. The toddler gradually learns to control

► CONSEQUENCES OF SHAME AND DOUBT

- Has difficulty with eating, digestion, elimination, sleep
- Has low self-esteem
- Has low frustration tolerance, gives up easily
- Is apathetic, withdrawn
- Is passive, too compliant, easily controlled or manipulated
- Is excessively negativistic, defiant
- Is impulsive
- Is physically overactive, aggressive
- Is angry about being controlled or manipulated by others
- Is stubbornly assertive, obstinate
- Has little sense of responsibility
- Is sneaky, wanting to get away with things
- Is compulsive
- Hoards
- Is overmeticulous or excessively messy

bowel and bladder. *Neuromuscular maturity,* which occurs from 1 to 3 years, with bowel before bladder control, *is necessary for regular, self-controlled evacuation* (37).

Many factors are involved besides biological readiness, as the toddler's fears, goals, and conflicting wishes also influence this learning experience. Psychologically, toilet training is complex. Mother gives approval not only for defecating properly but also for withholding feces. The sensations of giving and withholding feces, imitation of parents and siblings, approval from family, and pride in the accomplishments hasten toilet training. Being forced to do the parents' will may cause problems of negativism.

Bowel training is a less complex task than bladder training and should be attempted first. You can assist parents by alerting them to signs of readiness. The toddler shows physical readiness for bowel training when he or she defecates regularly and shows some signs of being aware of defecation such as grunting, straining, and tugging at the diaper. It also helps if the child can speak, understand directions, and manipulate the clothing somewhat. *Mental readiness* includes the child's wanting to watch people use the toilet (which should be allowed), wanting to flush the toilet, and asking questions about it. *Emotional readiness* includes feeling secure about using the toilet, pretending to use it, and asking to use it.

Some toddlers, after defecation, cry and indicate distress until they are changed. Others do not indicate discomfort and will play with and smear feces. They are curious, explore, and see nothing shameful about such behavior. They have not learned the aesthetic and cultural connotations of feces being "dirty" and "smelly" and not an object for play. But because play with feces must be restricted because it is unsanitary and nonaesthetic, changing diapers immediately after defecation, using safety pins to keep the diaper on snugly, having well-fitted training pants, and showing parental disapproval are ways to prevent such play. In addition, encourage parents to provide opportunities for play and smearing with clay, sand, mud, paste, and finger paints to help the child develop natural potentials and divert instinctual urges into socially accepted behavior.

Parents may demonstrate inordinate interest in this aspect of development, producing anxiety over bowel training with possible harmful physical effects such as constipation or psychological effects, which result from trying to meet excessive demands. Be aware of the development problems associated with toilet training, but remember that elimination is a natural process. In fact, some authors say toilet training can be learned in less than a day if parents follow behavioral learning principles (4, 13). Teach parents to approach toilet training in a matter-of-fact and relaxed way, to expect some resistance, and not to push the child or reflect anxiety. Every child by age 3 can carry on this task with some help as to where and how. Culturally, American society seems to demand that mothers begin toilet training somewhere around 2 years of age, but $2\frac{1}{2}$ years would be soon enough (25); however, when younger parents follow the directions given in this chapter, grandma may defy them and secretly sit 1-year-old Suzie on the potty. Toilet training should not be started in turbulent periods such as hospitalization of the toddler, homecoming of a new baby, absence of the main caretaker from home, or a family crisis. Even when started in a calm period, some regression is natural.

Encourage the parents to have the child use a potty chair as it is mechanically easier than the family toilet, and the chair is his or her own. The potty chair should be in a place convenient for the child. Recommend that the child wear training pants and that training take place when disruptions in regular routine are at a minimum. The toddler should be praised for success. Parents should remain calm, reassuring, and supportive, if the child has an accident.

Bladder training is more complex because the reflexes appropriate for bladder training are less explicit, neurologic maturation comes later, and urination is a reflex response to bladder tensions and must be inhibited. Bladder control demands more self-awareness and self-discipline from the toddler and is usually achieved between the ages of $2\frac{1}{2}$ and $3\frac{1}{2}$ years when physiologic development has progressed enough that the bladder can retain urine for approximately 2 hours. Waking hours and sleeping hours present two phases of control and differences in awareness of bladder function.

The series of events necessary for bladder training is that the toddler must first realize he or she is wet, then know he or she is wetting, next recognize impulses that tell that he or she is going to urinate, and finally control urinating until he or she is at the toilet. A physically ready child is able to stay dry for 2 or more hours during the day, and wake up dry from naps and may wake up dry in the morning.

You may help the parents by explaining the process of urination. Make it clear to the parents that both boys and girls can sit down while urinating and that both may try to stand like daddy. Sleeping control will be effective when the child responds to bladder reflexes and not before. Cutting down on fluids and other devices to reduce enuresis, or bed wetting, are not effective in gaining reflex control.

After waking control has been well established, sleeping control usually follows. Past 5 years of age, however, if nighttime control has not been achieved, there might be a physiologic or psychological problem. Encourage medical attention if this problem persists, and consider possible emotional causes. Enuresis is discussed further in Chapter 9.

Body Image and Self-Concept Development

Body Image

Body image development gradually evolves as a component of self-concept. The toddler has a dim self-awareness, but with a developing sense of autonomy, he or she becomes more correctly aware of the body as a physical entity and one with emotional capabilities. Toddler is increasingly aware of pleasurable sensations in the genital area and on the skin and mouth and is learning control of the body through locomotion, toilet training, speech, and socialization.

The toddler is not always aware of the whole body or the distal parts and might even consider distal parts such as the feet as something apart from self. By age 3, the child can depict self in simple drawings or stick figures; however, assessment of body image must include the child's total behavior, language, and play, not just art work (11). Toddler does not always know when he or she is sick, tired, or too hot or when the pants are wet. The child also has difficulty realizing that body productions such as feces are separate from self; therefore he or she may resist flushing the toilet. Toddler is not aware of the influences on his or her body but is aware of general feelings and thoughts and increasingly of others' reactions to his or her body and behavior. For example, when the toddler is in control of the environment, the body feels good, wonderful, and strong. When things are not going well, if he or she cannot succeed or is punished excessively, the child feels bad and shameful.

Self-Concept

Self-concept is also made up of the *feelings about self, adaptive and defensive mechanisms, reactions from others, and one's perceptions of these reactions, attitudes, values, and many of life's experiences.*

As the child incorporates approval and disapproval, praise and punishment, gestures that are kind and forbidding, he or she forms an opinion about self as a person. How the person feels about self is determined to a great degree by the reactions of others and, in turn, later determines how he or she views others. The young child is very aware of the gradient of anxiety: mild, moderate, or severe. He or she watches for signs of approval and disapproval from others in relation to self. Increasingly there is recall about what caused discomfort or anxiety. Experiences of discomfort are first with mother and then are generalized to other people, and much behavior becomes organized to avoid or minimize discomfort around others. Thus, he or she gradually evolves adaptive and defensive behaviors and learns what to do to get along with others. The **self-system** gradually develops as an *organization of experiences that exists to defend against anxiety and to secure satisfaction* (30).

The various appraisals of others cause the child to form feelings of good-me, bad-me, or not-me, as the self-concept. The child is fully aware of reactions that convey approval, love, security, and because these make him or her feel good, a concept of **good-me** forms. *He or she likes self because others do, the basis of a positive self-concept.* Reactions of disapproval or punishment from significant adults increase the child's anxiety, and if this cycle continues, **bad-me,** a *negative self-concept,* results. If negative reaction is neverending, the child may evolve defensive behaviors such as denial that prevent noticing the negative evaluations. Some appraisals from others evoke severe discomfort or panic; these *feelings and awareness of the situation are repressed and dissociated from the rest of the personality,* forming the **not-me** part of the self. These are the *ideas, feelings, or body parts that later seem foreign to the person.* For example, severe toilet training or punishing the child for masturbating or touching the genitals may be so traumatic and panic producing that he or she becomes almost unaware of the genital area. Later the person does not include the lower half of the body or the genital area in self-drawings or does not speak of sexual matters; he or she may be very inhibited about toileting, and a disturbed sex identity may be evident through behavior. The more feelings or life experiences that are dissociated, the more rigid the personality and the less aware of self he or she is in later life. Each person attempts to find ways to keep feelings of *good-me* and reduce the uncomfortable feelings elicited by the *bad-me* (30).

The direction of the self-concept and personality often follows the impetus given it in early childhood; the person remains fairly consistent in behavior and attitudes, although there are some changes throughout life as the person encounters new experiences and people. For example, if the young child internalizes feelings of being bad, unworthy, inadequate, perhaps because of race, color, or neighborhood, he or she will later have difficulty believing that he or she is good or competent, even when that is realistic. If the person has good, happy, adequate feelings about self because of childhood experiences, occasional failures will not dampen self-esteem or feelings of competence.

The child's major caretaker should have a positive self-concept and feel good about being a mother (father). If others in the family or if society debase the mothering one, there is injury to the child's self-esteem. Thus, the issue of equality of women becomes critical. Equality as a person, the importance of the mother and homemaker role, and the importance of women to society and to the work world are all critical to successful childrearing. If the female caretaker doubts her own worth, is resentful of societal oppression, and has doubts about her own power and status, these negative feelings will be conveyed nonverbally to the child and will have a direct bearing on his or her sense of security and self-worth. This critical phase of development lies between 18 and 36 months (1, 2, 25).

Be mindful of body image and self-concept formation as you care for toddlers, for it determines their reaction. Only through repetitious positive input can you change a negative self-concept to one that is positive. By stimulating a positive self-image, you are promoting emotional health. Teach parents to provide an environment in which the child can successfully exercise skills such as running, walking, and playing and feel acceptance of his or her body and behavior. Help them realize that as the child's autonomy develops, so too will a more appropriate mental picture of his or her body and emotions.

Adaptive Mechanisms

Before the child is 2 years old, he or she is learning the basic response patterns appropriate for the family and culture; a degree of trust and confidence, or lack of it, in the parents; how to express annoyance and impatience and love and joy; and how to communicate needs.

The toddler begins to adapt to the culture because of **primary identification.** He or she *imitates the parents* and responds to their encouragement and discouragement. With successful adaptation, the child moves toward independence. Other major adaptive mechanisms of this era include repression, suppression, denial, reaction formation, projection, and sublimation (25).

Repression *unconsciously removes from awareness the thoughts, impulses, fantasies, and memories of behavior that are unacceptable to the self.* The *not-me* discussed earlier is an example and may result from child abuse. **Suppression** *differs from repression in that it is a conscious act.* For example, the child forgets that he or she has been told not to handle certain articles. **Denial** is *not admitting, even when warned, that certain factors exist,* for example, that the stove is hot and will cause a burn. **Reaction formation** is *replacing the original idea and behavior with the opposite behavior characteristics.* For example, the child flushes the toilet and describes feces as dirty instead of playing in them, thus becoming appropriately tidy. **Projection** occurs when *he or she attributes personal feelings or behaviors to someone else.* For example, if the babysitter disciplines toddler, he or she projects dislike for her by saying, "You don't like me." **Sublimation** is *channeling impulses into socially acceptable behavior rather than expressing the original impulse.* For example, he or she plays with mud, finger paints, or shaving cream instead of feces, which is socially unacceptable.

Teach parents that the child's adaptive behavior is strengthened when he or she is taught to do something for self and permitted to make a decision *if that decision is truly his or hers to make.* If the decision is one that must be carried out regardless of the toddler's wish, it can best be accomplished by giving direction rather than by asking the child if he or she wants to do something.

Sexuality Development

Traditionally parents have handled sons and daughters differently during infancy, and the results became evident in toddlerhood.

Because parents encourage independent behavior in boys and more dependency in girls, by 13 months the boy ventures farther from mother, stays away longer, and looks at or talks to his mother less than does the girl. The girl at this age is encouraged to spend more time touching and staying near mother than is the boy; however, the separation process later seems less severe for girls. Perhaps boys should be touched and cuddled longer (5, 25).

Boys play more vigorously with toys than do girls, and they play more with nontoys such as doorknobs and light switches. Yet basically there is no sexual preference for toys, although parents may enforce a preference. A boy responds with more overt aggression to a barrier placed between him and his mother at 13 months of age than do girls. Boys show more exploratory and aggressive behavior than girls, and this behavior is encouraged by the father. The female remains attentive to a wide variety of stimuli and complex visual and auditory stimuli. The female demonstrates earlier language development and seems more aware of contextual relationships, perhaps because of the more constant stimulation from the mother (5, 25).

Society has traditionally been easy on girls in terms of achievement. If they excel, this is an added plus; if they do not, no one cares. Boys, however, are expected to achieve. As early as the toddler years this influence can be seen: girls are allowed to be more dependent, but boys are pushed to achieve. Attitudes, however, are changing about women's roles and abilities.

Primary identification, *imitation, and observation of the same-sexed parent,* contributes to sex identity. The child by 15 months is interested in his or her own and others' body parts. Both boys and girls achieve sexual pleasure through self-stimulation, although girls masturbate less than boys (possibly because of anatomic differences).

By 21 months the child can refer to self by name, an important factor in the development of identity. By 2 years of age, the child can categorize people into boy and girl and has some awareness of anatomic differences if he or she has had an opportunity to view them (13).

By the end of toddlerhood, the child is more aware of his or her body, the body's excretions, and his or her actions, and he and she can be more independent in the first steps of self-care. Ability to communicate verbally expands to the point that he or she can ask questions and talk about sexual topics with parents and peers.

Help parents to understand the developing sexuality of their child and to be comfortable with their own sex identification and sexuality so that they can cuddle the child and answer questions. Help them understand that a wide variety of play experiences will prepare the child for adult behavior and competence. They may talk through their concerns about a son's becoming a sissy if he plays with dolls or wears mother's high heels in dramatic play. Help parents realize that a daughter's playing with trucks does not mean she will become a truck driver.

Guidance and Discipline

Discipline is *guidance that helps the child learn to understand and care for self and to get along with others.* It is not just punishing, correcting, or controlling behavior, as is commonly assumed.

Everything in the toddler's world is new and exciting and meant to be explored, touched, eaten, or sat on, including porcelain figurines from Spain or boiling water. In moving away from complete dependency, the toddler demonstrates energy and drive and requires sufficient restrictions to ensure physical and psychological protection and at the same time enough freedom to permit exploration and autonomy. Because mother must now set limits, a new dimension is added to the relationship established between mother and toddler. Before, mother met his or her basic needs immediately. With the toddler's increasing ability, freedom, and demands, the parent sometimes makes him or her wait or denies a wish if it will cause harm. The transition should be made in a loving, consistent, yet flexible manner so that the child maintains trust and moves in the quest for independence. Excessive limitations, overwhelming steady pressure, or hostile bullying behavior might cause an overly rebellious, negativistic, or passive child. Complete lack of limitations can cause accidents, poor health, and insecurity.

Mother is usually the main disciplinarian at this age, and her approach is important. When the mother is under high acute or chronic stress, support and help from others are the most significant factors in reducing a negative discipline approach to the child(ren), regardless of the mother's age, education, or marital status (1, 5).

Through guidance and the parent's reaction, the child is being socialized, learning what is right and wrong. Because the child cannot adequately reason, he or she must depend on and trust the parents as a guide for all activities. He or she can obey simple commands. Later, the child will be capable of internalizing rules and mores and will become self-disciplined as a result of having been patiently disciplined. Setting limits is not easy. Parents should not thwart the toddler's curiosity and enthusiasm, but they must protect him or her from harm. Parents who oppose the toddler's desire of the moment are likely to meet with anything from a simple "no" to a temper tantrum.

Teach parents the importance of constructive guidance and discipline. Temper tantrums result because the toddler hates being thwarted and feeling helpless. Once the feelings are discharged, the child regains composure quickly and without revenge. If temper tantrums, a form of negativism, occur, the best advice is to ignore the outburst; it will soon disappear. The child needs the parent's reaction for the behavior to continue. Belittling or beating the child does not help temper tantrums. If he or she is given more frustration than can be handled, fear, hostility, and anger mount, and the lack of verbal ability inhibits adequate outlet. Hence he or she strikes out, bites, or hits physically. Now toddler desperately needs mother's support, firm control, and mediation. The parent's calm voice, expressing understanding of feelings, and introduction of an activity to restore self-esteem are important to teaching self-control.

Because parents are sometimes confused about handling the toddler's behavior, you can assist them by teaching some simple rules for guiding the toddler (1, 5, 25):

- Provide an environment in which the child feels respected.
- Decide what is important and what is not worth a battle of will. For example, the child may not be wearing matched clothing but resists parental attempts to change. Avoid negativism and an angry scene by deciding that today it is all right for the child to wear an unmatched outfit.
- Changing the mind, pursuing an alternate activity, or letting the child have his or her way is not giving in, losing face, being a poor parent, or letting the child be manipulative. When limits are consistent, changing a direction of behavior can be a positive learning experience for the child. The child is becoming aware of being a separate person, able to assert self and influence others.
- Remove or avoid temptations such as breakable objects within reach or candy that should not be eaten to avoid having to repeatedly say "no."
- Try not to ask open-ended questions for the child to decide about an activity when the decision is not really one the child can make.
- Consider limits as more than restrictions but also as a distraction *from* one prohibited activity

to another in which the child can freely participate. Distraction with alternatives or a substitute is effective with the toddler because attention span is short.
- Reinforce appropriate behavior through approval and attention. The child will continue behavior that gains attention, even if the attention is punitive, because negative attention is better than none to the child.
- Set limits consistently so that the child can rely on the parent's judgment rather than testing the adult's endurance in each situation.
- State limits clearly, concisely, simply, positively, and in a calm voice. For example, if the child cannot play with a treasured object, he or she should not be allowed to handle it. Say "Look with your hands behind your back" or "Look with your eyes, not your hands" rather than "Don't touch."
- Set limits only when necessary. Some rules promote a sense of security, but too many confuse the child.
- Provide a safe area where the child is free to do whatever he or she wants to do.
- Do not overprotect the child; he or she should learn that some things have a price such as a bruise or a scratch.
- Do not terminate the child's activity too quickly; tell him or her that the activity is ending.

Each situation will determine the extent of firmness or leniency needed. The toddler needs grades of independence.

Moral–Spiritual Development

Birth through the toddler era might be termed the *prereligious stage*. This label does not deny religious influences but simply points out that the toddler is absorbing basic intellectual and emotional patterns regardless of the religious conviction of the caretakers. The toddler may repeat some phrases from prayers while imitating a certain voice tone or body posture that accompanies those prayers. The child only knows that when he or she imitates or conforms to certain rituals, affection and approval come that add to the sense of identification and security. The "good" and "bad" are defined in terms of physical consequences to self.

Teach parents that the toddler can benefit from a nursery-school type of church program in which emphasis is on positive self-image and appropriate play and rest rather than on a lesson to learn. Toddler also needs to have others to imitate who follow the rules of society, and he or she needs rewards and reinforcement for good or desirable behavior.

According to Kohlberg's Theory of Moral Development, the toddler is in the Preconventional Stage. Refer to Chapter 5, pp. 228, 231, and 232, and Table 5–12.

Developmental Tasks

Developmental tasks for the toddler may be summarized as follows (12):

- Settling into healthy daily routines
- Mastering good eating habits
- Mastering the basics of toilet training
- Developing the physical skills appropriate to the stage of motor development
- Becoming a family member
- Learning to communicate efficiently with an increasing number of others

The constantly sensitive situation of the toddler, gaining autonomy and independence—at times overreaching and needing mother's help, at times needing the freedom from mother's protection—is one you can help parents understand. The child's future personality and health will depend partially on how these many opportunities are handled now. Your role in teaching and support is critical.

► HEALTH CARE AND NURSING APPLICATIONS

Your role with the toddler and family has been discussed with each section throughout this chapter. Selected Nursing Diagnoses Related to the Toddler lists some *nursing diagnoses* based on assessments that would be accomplished from knowledge presented in this chapter. Interventions include your role modeling of caring behavior to the toddler and family; parent and family education, support, and counseling; or direct care to meet the toddler's physical, emotional, cognitive, and social needs.

SUMMARY

The toddler grows at a slower pace physically than the infant, but physical growth is steady and there is considerable gain in neuromuscular skills. Emotionally, socially, and behaviorally, the toddler makes great strides

► SELECTED NURSING DIAGNOSES RELATED TO THE TODDLER*

Pattern 1: Exchanging

Altered Nutrition: More than Body Requirements
Altered Nutrition: Less than Body Requirements
Altered Nutrition: Potential for More Than Body Requirements
Risk for Infection
Risk for Injury
Risk for Suffocation
Risk for Poisoning
Risk for Trauma
Risk for Aspiration

Pattern 2: Communicating

Impaired Verbal Communication

Pattern 3: Relating

Impaired Social Interaction

Pattern 6: Moving

Impaired Physical Mobility
Altered Growth and Development

Pattern 7: Perceiving

Self-Esteem Disturbance
Sensory/Perceptual Alterations
Unilateral Neglect

Pattern 9: Feeling

Pain
Anxiety
Fear

*Other of the NANDA diagnoses are applicable to the ill toddler. *From North American Nursing Diagnosis Association, NANDA Nursing Dignoses Definitions & Classification 1995–1996. Philadelphia: North American Nursing Diagnosis Association, 1994.*

in development during these 2 years. The child gains control over basic physiologic processes, for example, toileting, and a competency in behavior patterns. Developmental or autonomy tasks are achieved in his or her own unique way as parents and family members pro-

► CONSIDERATIONS FOR THE TODDLER AND FAMILY IN HEALTH CARE

- Family cultural background and support systems for the family of the toddler
- Attachment behaviors of the parents; separation reactions of the toddler
- Parental behaviors that indicate difficulty with attachment or potential/actual abuse of the toddler
- Physical characteristics and patterns, such as eating, toilet training, sleep/rest, and play, that indicate health and are within age norms for growth
- Cognitive characteristics and behavioral or play patterns in the toddler that indicate age-appropriate norms for intellectual development
- Communication patterns and language development that indicate age-appropriate norms for the toddler
- Overall appearance and behavioral or play patterns in the toddler that indicate development of autonomy rather than shame and doubt, positive self-concept, sense of sexuality, and continuing age-appropriate emotional development
- Behavioral patterns that indicate the toddler is beginning moral–spiritual development
- Behavioral patterns and characteristics that indicate the toddler has achieved developmental tasks
- Parental behaviors that indicate knowledge about how to physically and emotionally care for the toddler
- Parental behaviors and communication approaches that indicate effective guidance of the toddler
- Evidence that the parents provide a safe and healthful environment and the necessary resources for the toddler
- Parental behaviors that indicate they are achieving their developmental tasks for this era

vide consistent love and guidance and adequate resources to foster physical, cognitive, emotional, social, and moral development.

Considerations for the Toddler and Family in Health Care and Charts 1 and 2 in Appendix IV summarize what you should consider in assessment and health promotion with the toddler. The family is included in Considerations. Chart 1 presents the American Academy of Family Physicians Periodic Health Examination Birth to 18 Months, and this chart includes information pertinent to screening the toddler aged 12 to 18 months, counseling parents, and determining immunization schedules and risk categories for that age group. Chart 2 presents the American Academy of Family Physicians Periodic Health Examination 19 Months to 6 Years and thus presents information pertinent to screening the toddler aged 19 to 36 months, health care, and parent counseling.

► REFERENCES

1. Adams, D., *The Child Influencers.* Cuyahoga Falls, OH: Home Team Press, 1990.
2. Adams, P., What Women's Inequality Means to Children and Adolescents, *American Journal of Social Psychiatry,* 1, no. 1 (April 1981), 6–8.
3. *Age Charts for Periodic Health Examination.* Washington, DC: American Academy of Family Physicians, 1995.
4. Azrin, N., and R. Foxx, *Toilet Training—In Less Than a Day.* New York: Simon & Schuster, 1974.
5. Bettelheim, B., *A Good Enough Parent: A Book on Child-Rearing.* New York: Random, 1988.
6. Bossard, J.H.S., and E.S. Boll, *The Sociology of Child Development* (4th ed.). New York: Harper & Row, 1966.
7. Bowlby, J., *Attachment and Loss,* Vol. I: *Attachment.* New York: Basic Books, 1969.
8. Boynton, R., E. Dunn, and G. Stephens, *Manual of Ambulatory Pediatrics* (3rd ed.). Philadelphia: J.B. Lippincott, 1994.
9. Centers for Disease Control and Prevention, General Recommendations on Immunization: Recommendations of the Advisory Committee on Immunization Practices (ACIP), *Morbidity and Mortality Weekly Report,* 4 (January 28, 1994), 23.
10. Dacey, J., and J. Travers, *Human Development Across the Lifespan* (3rd ed.), Madison, WI: Brown & Benchmark, 1996.
11. DiLeo, J., *Children's Drawings as Diagnostic Aids.* New York: Brunner/Mazel, 1973.
12. Duvall, E., and B. Miller, *Marriage and Family Development* (6th ed.). New York: Harper & Row, 1986.
13. Dworetzky, J., *Human Development: A Life Span Approach* (2nd ed.). St. Paul/Minneapolis: West, 1995.
14. Erikson, E.H., *Childhood and Society* (2nd ed.). New York: W.W. Norton, 1963.
15. Ewert, D., et al., Measles Vaccination Coverage Among Latino Children Aged 12 to 59 Months in Los Angeles County: A Household Survey, *American Journal of Public Health,* 81, no. 8 (1991), 1057–1059.
16. Feeding Your Child, *Parenting: Glennon Hospital for Children* (1990), 10–11.
17. Feigenberg, M., and J. Sotman. A Toddler with a Malabsorption Syndrome, *American Journal of Nursing,* 75, no. 6 (1975), 978–979.
18. Geber, M., The Psycho-motor Development of African Children in the First Year and the Influence of Maternal Behavior, *The Journal of Social Psychology,* 47 (1958), 185–195.
19. Gesell, A., et al., *The First Five Years of Life.* New York: Harper & Brothers, 1940.
20. Gottlieb, L., and J. Bailles, Firstborn's Behaviors During a Mother's Second Pregnancy, *Nursing Research,* 44 (1995), 356–362.
21. Hoole, A., C. Pickard, R. Ouimette, J. Lohr, and R. Greenberg, *Patient Care Guidelines for Nurse Practitioners* (4th ed.). Philadelphia: J.B. Lippincott, 1995.
22. Jolley, J., and M. Mitchell, *Lifespan Development: A Topical Approach.* Madison, WI: Brown & Benchmark, 1996.
23. Lamb, M., The emergent father, in Lamb, M.E., ed., *The Father's Role: Cross-cultural Perspectives.* Hillsdale, NJ: Lawrence Erlbaum, 1987, pp. 1–26.
24. LaRossa, R., Fatherhood and Social Change, *Family Relations,* 37 (1988), 451–457.
25. Lidz, T., *The Person: His and Her Development Throughout the Life Cycle* (2nd ed.). New York: Basic Books, 1983.

26. Linley, J., Screening Children for Common Orthopedic Problems, *American Journal of Nursing,* 87, no. 10 (1987), 1312–1316.

27. Murphy, B., Pushing Up Baby, *Washington University School of Medicine Outlook,* 24, no. 3 (1987), 16.

28. Sherman, J.L., Jr., and S. Fields, *Guide to Patient Evaluation* (5th ed.). Garden City, NY: Medical Examination Publishing, 1987.

29. Silver, H., II, C.H. Kempe, and H. Bruyn, *Handbook of Pediatrics* (15th ed.). Los Altos, CA: Lange, 1987.

30. Sullivan, H.S., *Interpersonal Theory of Psychiatry.* New York: W.W. Norton, 1953.

31. Taking Care of Toddlers' Teeth, *Health Scene,* Fall (1987), 11.

32. Turner, J., and D. Helms, *Lifespan Development* (5th ed.). Ft. Worth: Harcourt Brace College, 1995.

33. Verzemnieks, I., Developmental Stimulation for Infants and Toddlers, *American Journal of Nursing,* 84, no. 6 (1984), 749–752.

34. Wadsworth, B., *Piaget's Theory of Cognitive and Affective Development* (5th ed.). New York: Longman, 1996.

35. Why Children Need Their Parents' Time, *AFA Journal,* April (1991), 17–18.

36. Williams, S., *Nutrition and Diet Therapy* (10th ed.). St. Louis: C.V. Mosby, 1995.

37. Wong, D., *Whaley and Wong's Nursing Care of Infants and Children* (5th ed.). St. Louis: C.V. Mosby, 1995.

chapter nine

Assessment and Health Promotion for the Preschooler

> *If the child is safe, the people are safe.*
>
> —*Marian Wright Edelman*

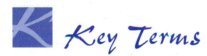

Key Terms

Preschool years	Minor lacerations	Juvenile hypertension	Concepts of causality
Peers	Burns	Hypochromic anemia	Animistic
Oedipal or Electra stage	First degree	Child abuse and neglect	Egocentric
Identification	Second degree	Physical abusive acts	Preconceptual Phase
Day-care	Third degree	Psychological abuse	Intuitive Phase
Family day-care	Encephalopathy	Child sexual abuse	Transductive logic
Nursery school	Strabismus	Pressured sexuality	Absolute thought
Early school experiences	Conjunctivitis	Ritualistic abuse	Centering
Montessori programs	Hearing loss	Neglect	Reversibility
Compensatory programs	Otitis media	Concepts	Peer
Kindergarten	Acute cervical adenitis	Concept formation	Peer group
Siblings	Urinary tract infection	Action space	Physical activity
Dyads	Enuresis	Body space	Dramatic play
Growth hormone deficiency	Nonspecific vulvovaginitis	Object space	Creative playthings
Active immunity	Measles	Map space	Quiet play
Passive immunity	Diarrhea	Abstract space	Permissive discipline
Minor head injury	Postural problems	Quantitative concepts	Overpermissive discipline

Initiative	Articulate	Secondary identification	Superego
Guilt	Integration	Fantasy	Sexual abuse
Differentiation	Introjection	Anthropomorphism	Sexual intrusion

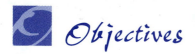

Objectives

Study of this chapter will enable you to:

1. Compare the family relationships between the preschool and previous developmental eras and the influence of parents, siblings, and nonfamily members on the preschooler.

2. Explore with the family the expected developmental tasks and ways to meet them.

3. Visit several day-care centers and nursery schools, compare their values and services to parents and child, and discuss necessary adaptation by the preschooler in each setting.

4. Assess physical, motor, mental, language, play, and emotional characteristics of a 3-, 4-, and 5-year-old.

5. Describe the health needs of the preschooler, including nutrition, exercise, rest, safety, and immunization, and measures to meet these needs.

6. Explore with parents their role in contributing to the preschooler's cognitive, language, self-concept, sexuality, moral–spiritual, and emotional development and physical health.

7. Discuss measures to diminish the trauma of hospitalization for this age group.

8. Explore with parents effective ways for communication with and guidance and discipline of the preschooler to enhance his or her development.

9. Describe the developmental crisis of initiative versus guilt, the adaptive mechanisms commonly used that promote a sense of initiative, and the implications of this crisis for later maturity.

10. Discuss the developmental tasks and your role in promoting achievement of them.

11. Work effectively with a preschooler in the nursing situation.

In this chapter development of the preschool child and the family relationships are discussed. *Nursing responsibilities for health promotion for the child and family are discussed throughout the chapter. The information regarding normal development and needs serves as a basis for assessment.* Your role is to use information on assessment and health promotion in health education and counseling of families and in your care of the preschooler. You will find opportunity in many settings—the neighborhood, day-care center, church group, clinic, doctor's office, school, industrial setting, or hospital—to correct parents' misconceptions and validate their sound thinking about their child's development and the importance of the family's behavior for the child's emotional, physical, and social health. Principles of communication, health teaching, and crisis work also apply. Become active as a citizen to educate the public about needs of hospitalized children, promote needed legislation, or directly offset problems that affect children's health such as child abuse and lead poisoning. Promote quality day-care or preschool programs. The range of possible effective intervention is wide and will depend on your work setting and interest.

The **preschool years,** *ages 3 through 5,* along with infancy and the toddler years, form a crucial part of the person's life. The preschool child is emerging as a social being. He or she participates more fully as a family member but begins to grow slowly out of the family, spending more time in association with **peers,** *children of the same age.* Physical growth is slowing, but the body is well proportioned and control and coordination are increasing. Many body activities are becoming routine. Emotional and intellectual growth is progressively apparent in the ability to form mental images; express self in anger; become acquainted with the environment; have some perception of social relationships and the status of self as an individual compared with others; identify with the play group and follow rules; control primitive (*id*) impulses; and begin to be self-critical with references to a standard set by others (*superego formation*).

The parents, too, must learn to separate themselves from their growing child and revise decisions about how much free expression and initiative to permit the child while at the same time setting certain limits. The child's long step into the outside world is not always accomplished with ease for either the child or the parent. Thus gradually promoting more independence during the preschool years allows both the child and parents to be more comfortable about the separation that occurs when he or she goes to school.

FAMILY DEVELOPMENT AND RELATIONSHIPS

The family unit, regardless of the specific form, is important to the preschooler, and in turn the preschooler affects relationships within the family by his or her behavior. The close relationship of the baby to the mother and father gradually expands to include other significant adults living in the home, siblings, and other relatives, and they will have some effect on the child's personality.

There are several dominant parenting styles:

- **Authoritarian:** *Parents are demanding and expect instant obedience.* Reasons for rules or punishment are not given; no consideration is given to the child's view.
- **Authoritative:** *Parents exert control but give reasons for behavior and expect mature behavior.* They encourage independence and the child's meeting his or her potential. They try to maintain a balance between socialization and individualization.
- **Permissive:** *Parents are accepting of a wide range of behavior; they rarely make demands.* The child is encouraged to make almost all his or her own decisions. These parents may seem indulgent.
- **Secure:** *Parents are confident in their techniques.* If they make mistakes, they can change. They assume they and the child will cope successfully.
- **Insecure:** *Parents feel overwhelmed by the parenting role.* Any aspect of child care is a major issue.

- **Intimidated:** *Parents lack the ability to be firm with the child.*

The important thing is the match between parenting behaviors and the child's temperament. Parenting behaviors also vary with the culture. In addition, the child's temperament also affects the parent's behavior (22).

Effect of parenting styles on preschoolers and their parents can be divided into several categories of behavior as depicted in Effect of Parenting Style on Child's Behavior.

Another study showed that the child's behavior affects parental reactions and is different toward each parent. When the child is more dependent in behavior, both parents interact more physically and verbally with the child and display more controlling behavior. In one study the girl child appeared to engage in specific tasks with father and in more personal interaction with mother. The father was more likely to help the child physically or become detached, whereas mother was more likely to encourage independence and to explain or question the child. More study must be done on the reciprocity of parent–child relationships and the effect of each on the other. For example, perhaps the parent who has been authoritarian and controlling over the child from birth on fosters dependent behavior in the child, which in turn stimulates more controlling behavior (7, 47).

► EFFECT OF PARENTING STYLE ON CHILD'S BEHAVIOR

Parent's Behavior	Child's Behavior
More controlling, demanding, loving overtly than most parents	Friendly, self-controlled, self-reliant
Controlling, detached, rather than loving and warm	Discontented, withdrawn
Highly permissive, warm and friendly	Low self-reliance, low self-control
Relatively demanding, loving	Self-reliant, more independent, better adjusted
Warm, loving, expect a great deal of child at early age, demanding of child, show interest in child's activities	Highly creative, high achievement need, independent, highly competent, work toward set goals

Relationships With Parents

The preschooler's early emotional and physical closeness to the parents now leads to a different kind of relationship with them. This is the stage of the *family triangle, family romance,* or what Freud called the *Oedipal** or *Electra†* *Complex* (47).

Various authors say that knowledge of the Oedipal or Electra conflict as it exists in general Western culture, the manner in which it is resolved, and the significance of it in the preschool era are essential for understanding the development of the adolescent and adult in American culture. Others feel that this theory has been overpublicized. The intensity of this situation appears related to family attitudes and culture (47).

During this **Oedipal** or **Electra stage** or *phase of pregenital sexuality, positive, possessive, or love feelings are directed mainly toward the parent of the opposite sex, and the parent of the same sex may receive competitive, aggressive, or hostile feelings.* The daughter becomes "Daddy's girl" and tries to imitate the mother's role; the father responds to her femininity. The son is "Mommy's boy" and imitates the father's role; the mother responds to his masculinity. The parent of the same sex may be told, "I hate you. Go away." The child may declare to the opposite-sex parent that he or she will marry the parent someday. Help parents recognize these feelings as developmentally normal. During this phase the child is establishing a basis for his or her own eventual mate relationship; the parents' positive handling of the Oedipal conflict is crucial.

Help the parents feel comfortable with the sexuality of the child and with their own sexuality so that they are neither threatened by nor ignore or punish the child's remarks and behavior.

As the parent of the opposite sex continues to show love to his or her mate and the child, and as the parents desexualize the relationship with the child, the erotic aspects gradually disappear. The child can then get on with one of the major preschool tasks—identification. **Identification** *occurs first through imitation of the same-sex parent's overt behavior. In the preschool years, secondary identification occurs through introjection of atti-*tudes, feelings, and values about sexual, moral, social, and occupational roles and behavior* (43, 45, 47).

In the *one-parent or stepparent family* (or in the abusive home), achieving identification may be more difficult. The little girl raised by a male may not fit in with other girls at school or be able to feel comfortable and relate to women later in life. The boy raised by a woman may relate to women but not to men.

Explore with parents the importance of identification with the same-sex parent or adult and ways to achieve this if the parent of the same sex as the child is not in the home. *Divorced parents* must understand that to the child divorce signifies rejection and that the missing parent no longer loves the child. The child feels at blame, and there may be guilt about the separation or about the relief felt after the separation if much discord preceded the divorce. Family discord may cause more distress than the absence of a parent; but the separation is still difficult. There are often practical problems such as financial or lifestyle changes and emotional trauma. After the divorce the child may manifest insomnia, grief and depression, digestive and elimination problems, irritability, anger, aggression, regressive behavior, fear, anxiety, and withdrawal. The child needs help in expressing feelings (through art, play, music, and talking) and in adapting to the change. The child needs loving interactions with an adult relative or friend who is of the same sex, and the mother or father should foster such a relationship. After divorce the child may have difficulty relating to or identifying with a stepparent. If possible, the child needs an ongoing involvement with the divorced parent who is no longer in the home. The child loves and needs both parents in most cases and needs to learn to live with and feel affection for and from the stepparent as well. The child needs help to develop a sense of history with the family of origin and the stepparent family, to maintain allegiance to the absent parent, and to develop new traditions. The effects of divorce on the child are considerable and long-term (43, 45, 58, 73).

The monograph Children and Divorce presents not only the epidemiology of divorce, but also the emotional effects on the child, the financial strains on the mother, the role of the father after divorce, the life span adjustment of the child, and legal issues (19).

These families benefit from (1) your empathy; (2) your listening ear; (3) your exploration of their own and the child's feelings; (4) your suggestions of practical ways of helping the child spend time with both biological parents; (5) your discussion of ways to help the child mourn the loss he or she feels and adjust to the changed life situation; and (6) your counseling efforts and skills as the family works to resolve the crisis of separation, divorce, or remarriage.

---

*Oedipus, a hero of Greek mythology, was the son of King Laius and Queen Jocasta. At the time of Oedipus' birth, the oracle prophesied that Oedipus would kill his father and marry his mother. To avoid the prophecy, Laius ordered the infant abandoned so that he would die. Through a series of uncontrollable events, the infant survived, and the prophecy came true.

†Electra was a legendary Greek woman who was obsessed by an intense love for her murdered father and plotted with her brother to kill her mother and mother's lover, whom she blamed for the father's death.

Sex or Sexual Identity

Help parents realize that sex is reinforced through name, clothing, color of clothing and room, behavior toward, and expectations of the child. The innumerable contacts between the child and significant adults contribute to sex or sexual identification and should occur in this developmental period (7, 26, 47, 70). The sex of the child is a great determinant in personality development because each sex has different tasks and roles in every culture. Achieving a firm identity as a man or woman is basic to emotional stability and ego development.

In the United States most parents are less rigid about what clothing or colors are appropriate for boys and girls and are making an effort to teach both daughters and sons to talk about feelings, to do the same household tasks, and to engage in the same play activities. In some homes, however, the daughter is reinforced for being cuddly, domestic, and emotional, and the son is reinforced for being physically aggressive or "tough." The 5-year-old son is not expected to set the table or help with dusting. Parents who have fixed ideas about sex role behavior may not be responsive to your suggestions about the importance of both daughters and sons having the same play, learning, or social experiences or the appropriateness of pants and skirts for the daughters. Parental ideas frequently reflect their subcultural values and norms.

Explain parental reactions to and expectations of the child. Help them clarify their feelings and behavior and convey their respect to the child, regardless of sex. The sex assigned to the child by significant adults may be physically realistic or unrealistic. The feelings and needs of the parents strongly influence their reactions to the child so that sex assignment within the family can override biological factors. The parent can "make" little boys out of infant girls or vice versa by the way they name, handle, dress, play with, touch, or talk to the child. Attitudes about activity and passivity and feelings of mastery or being mastered go into development of male and female traits in most cultures.

The Oepidal or Electra phase brings the development of sexuality to the foreground. The child is interested in the appearance and function of his or her own body, in variations of clothing and hairstyles (the child at first assigns sex on this basis) and in the bodies of others, especially in their sex organs (47). Children at this age feel a sense of excitement in seeing and feeling their own and others' nude bodies and of exposing themselves to other children or adults.

Although some body exposure goes on in the average American home, help parents realize that the child needs to learn clothing norms for the culture. Unless the parents live in a nudist camp, there are limits to undressing in public. Help the parents realize that their nudity may stimulate considerable fantasy in the child during this stage and that sexual feelings aroused in the child may be difficult for child or parents to handle.

The girl learns that she is equal to or surpasses boys in size, intelligence, and physical capacities and that there are obvious differences in their genital organs. The so-called *penis envy* of Freudian theory is not so much envy as fascination with the difference. It becomes envy if the parents convey the attitude that masculinity is superior to femininity. Questions about the boy's penis can be answered along with the information that she will later have breasts and be able to bear children.

The child has many questions about conception and childbirth and usually develops or expands a personal theory: babies come from a seed placed in the mother's mouth, from eating foods with seeds, from kissing, or from animals; babies are manufactured like household items; prenatally the baby sits on the mother's stomach, ingesting food as she eats; and babies come out of the anus or the navel.

Teaching Sexuality

Teaching sexuality to the child is enmeshed in the acquisition of sex identity and positive feelings about the self. The basis for sex education begins prenatally with the parents' attitudes about the coming child. Parents and other child educators or caretakers, including nurses, continue daily thereafter to form attitudes in the child and impart factual knowledge in response to questions. You can assist parents in acquiring information to answer the child's questions.

Because of the child's consuming curiosity, he or she asks many questions: Will the man in the television come out? How do I tie my shoes? Why is that lady's tummy so big? What is lightning? These questions are originally asked with equal curiosity. The adult's response will determine into what special category the child places questions about sex.

If parent-child communication has been open—if the child feels free to ask questions about sex and other topics, and if the parent gives satisfactory and correct answers without embarrassment—the basis for a healthy sexual attitude exists.

Although sex education must be tailored to the individual child's needs and interests and to the cultural, religious, and family values, the following suggestions are applicable to all children and can be shared with parents:

- Recognize that education about the self as a sexual person is best given by example in family life through parents' showing respect and love for the self, mate, and the child.
- Understand that the child who learns to trust others and to give and receive love has begun preparation for satisfactory adulthood, marriage, and parenthood.
- Observe the child at play; listen carefully to statements of ideas, feelings, and questions and ask questions to understand better his or her needs.
- Respond to the child's questions by giving information honestly, in a relaxed, accepting manner, and on the child's level of understanding. Avoid isolated facts, myths, or animal analogies. The question, "Where does baby come from?" could be answered, "Mommy carried you inside her body in a special place" rather than saying "The stork brought baby," "Baby was picked up at the hospital after a special order," or "God makes babies." Religious beliefs can be worked into the explanation while acknowledging human realities.
- Teach the child anatomic names rather than other words for body parts and processes. Parents may hesitate to do this because they do not want the child to blurt out *penis* or *vagina* in public. Parents can teach the child that certain topics such as sexual and financial matters are discussed in the home, just as certain activities such as urinating are done in private.
- Grabbing the genitals and some masturbation are normal. Children explore their bodies, especially body parts not easily seen and that give pleasurable sensations when touched. Masturbation should be accepted if it occurs in the home. The child should be taught that this is not normal behavior in public.
- Playing doctor or examining each other's body parts is normal for preschool children. Parents should not overreact and should calmly affirm that they want the children to keep their clothes on while they play. Diversion from "playing doctor" is useful. If children seem to be using each other in a sexual way, they should be instructed that this is not acceptable.
- Realize that sex education continues throughout the early years. The child's changing self motivates the same or different questions again and again. Remain open to his or her ongoing questions. Explanation about reproduction may begin with a simple statement, for example: "A man and a woman are required to be baby's father and mother. Baby is made from the sperm in the daddy's body and an egg in the mother's body." A simple explanation of sperm and egg would be needed. Later the child can be given more detail.

Influence of Nonfamily Members

Help parents realize that other people may be significant to the child, depending on frequency and duration of contact, warmth of the relationship and how well the parents meet the child's needs (25, 47).

Other significant adults may include relatives, especially grandparents, aunts, uncles, and cousins who are peers; the teacher at the day-care center or nursery school; the babysitter; or neighbors. Servants, live-in help, the in-home caretaker, the babysitter, or the child's nurse–caretaker may provide positive or negative identification figures and should be chosen with care, especially those who live in the home. Relatives and friends also contribute to development of identity if contact is frequent.

Guests introduce the child to new facets of family life and parents' behavior, to different people with unfamiliar behavior, and to different ideas, religions, or occupations. Visits to others' homes aid socialization through comparison of the households, ability to separate from home, and interaction with people in new places.

Even domestic pets can be useful in meeting certain needs: loving and being loved; companionship; learning a sense of responsibility; and learning about sex in a natural way.

If the family uses day-care, nursery school, or other early schooling for the child, the adults in the agency may exert a strong influence on the child.

Parents may ask you about each agency: the differences between them, their significance for the child, and the criteria for selection. Share the following information.

Day-care is a *program to provide daily care away from home for any part of a 24-hour day, for compensation, or otherwise.* This program can be an important resource to many families: for example, when the single parent works and is the sole support of the family; when both parents work; when one parent is ill or a full-time student and the other parent works; or when the mother needs relief from child care for health or other urgent personal reasons. Some day-care programs are intergenerational, so that both preschoolers and elders come to the same site. A positive relationship is fostered between preschoolers and grandparents, or surrogate grandparents (44).

Family day-care is the *arrangement by a woman to care for mixed-aged children in the home.* Many home-care providers are former working women who want to remain in the home with their own children while continuing to contribute to the family budget by caring for several other children in the home. In most cases the number of children in the home is limited by law to six. The mixed ages of the children provide stimulation for each other, and the small number of children usually ensures that each child gets the attention he or she needs.

Nursery school is usually a *half-day program that emphasizes an educational, socialization experience for the children to supplement home experiences.*

Early school experiences may include a *Montessori program, a compensatory program,* or *kindergarten,* which has now become the first step before school entry for most children in the United States. **Montessori programs** evolved from the Italian educator, Maria Montessori, who developed preschool education in Europe. They *emphasize: (1) self-discipline of the child; (2) intellectual development through training of the senses; (3) freedom for the child within a structure and schedule; and (4) meaningful individual cognitive experiences that are provided in a quiet, pleasant, educational environment.* **Compensatory programs,** which first began as Head Start and Follow Through Projects in the 1960s, *focus on making up for deprived conditions in the child's life, and include (1) giving physical care (good nutrition, dental care, immunizations); (2) fostering curiosity, exploring creativity, and learning about the self and environment; (3) promoting emotional health through nurturing, positive self-concept, self-confidence, and self-discipline; and (4) teaching social skills and behaviors, how to interact with peers, teachers, and parents* (70). **Kindergarten** is a *half- or whole-day educational program* for the 5-year-old child that may be an extension of either a nursery school or a part of the elementary school system. In some parts of the country, kindergarten attendance is mandatory for entry into first grade because the cognitive learning that is begun is a foundation for the cognitive program of the first grade. The social behaviors that are learned also prepare the child to be better disciplined in the school setting and to interact appropriately with teacher and peers. The half-day program also helps the child and parents to separate from each other for a period if that has not been done through nursery school or day-care.

Criteria for selection of the day-care center or nursery school may be discussed with parents as they seek assistance with child care and education. Some of the same criteria are useful in selecting a family day-care, Montessori, or compensatory program (Table 9–1).

The criteria in Table 9–1 also are applicable to **family day-care,** although they would be applied to one

TABLE 9–1. CRITERIA FOR SELECTION OF DAY-CARE FACILITY

1. Operated by reputable person, agency, or industry. Either profit or non-profit programs can offer quality care.
2. Licensed or certified by local and state regulatory bodies. However, this only ensures meeting minimum standards.
3. Located convenient to home or workplace, open at the hours needed by the parent(s).
4. Committed to a philosophy of and beliefs about childrearing and discipline that are similar to those of the parents.
5. Staffed with certified teachers and other workers in appropriate staff/child ratio. Teacher and staff have a low turnover rate in employment.
6. Provision of an environment in which children and staff are happy and interacting. Children are having fun and learning.
7. Provision for grouping children according to age and developmental level so that children are safe and can learn from each other.
8. Provision of adequate space that is safe with well-controlled temperature; attractive; clean (but not sterile in appearance) and appropriate for age of child; psychomotor and sensory stimulation (height of windows, level floor); colorful but simple decor.
9. Provision of safe space and a variety of equipment, materials, and supplies for different types of play, such as:
   - Creative: art, music, reading, water play
   - Quiet: games, puzzles
   - Active: pedal toys, blocks
   - Outdoor: jungle gym, balls
   - Dramatic: Playhouse, farm, fire station
10. Provision of place for child to keep personal belongings.
11. Provision for snacks and mealtime. Kitchen facilities meet health department standards. Tables and chairs are available for children and staff to sit and eat together.
12. Provision for child to be alone for short period, if desired, and for midday rest (floor mats provided).
13. Provision of age-appropriate toilet facilities and sinks.
14. Provision of separate room supplied to give emergency health services to an impaired or ill child until parents, or their designate, or emergency medical services can arrive.
15. Provision for occasional extra events, or short trip, such as a visit by a fireman or trip to the local fire station.
16. Operated at a cost comparable to other similar facilities or programs or on a sliding scale basis.
17. Willingness by staff for anyone to visit unannounced.
18. Daily interaction of teachers with parents and talk with parents about child's behavior, progress, or health, as indicated.
19. Discussion between teachers and administrator(s) and parents about policies and procedures and their rationale, and explanation of planned changes well in advance.
20. Satisfaction of parents, child, teachers, administrator(s), and staff with decision to have child attend program.

adult in a home setting. The following questions should additionally be asked:

- Is there backup help available to the adult if it is needed (e.g., in case she is ill or if her child or another child was injured or became ill)?
- Does the adult take the children for trips in a vehicle? If so, are there child safety seats or belts appropriate to the child's age?
- Is care provided on weekends, holidays, or in the evening.

The *nursery school* operated by a reputable person or organization provides the aforementioned except for a full noon meal. Usually only a midsession snack is served. In either center the parent should observe the program to learn about the philosophy of the staff regarding childrearing, care, and discipline; administrative policies; the use of professional consultants for educational, social, or medical concerns; and the educational qualifications of the staff. They should note the warmth, emotional characteristics, and competence of the staff as they and children work and play together. Cost of the program, when services are available, and the parents' obligations to the agency are other aspects to consider.

In *either type of program,* the child, under guidance of qualified staff, will have many experiences and develop a variety of skills:

- Socializing with others
- Investigating the environment
- Doing imaginative experimentation
- Developing creative abilities
- Doing basic problem solving
- Becoming more independent, secure, and self-confident in a variety of situations
- Handling emotions, broadening self-expression
- Learning basic hygiene patterns
- Learning about the surrounding community

You can help parents be aware of these resources, answer their questions, and give suggestions regarding criteria for selection. As a nurse, you may also assist with primary prevention and health consulting to teachers, children, and parents in such an agency. For example, public health workers in Hennepin County, Minnesota, designed a program to promote optimum health and safety of children in day-care settings through health education to staff, technical assistance support, nurse–child assessment, and evaluation of policies and procedures (37). The articles by Wenger et al. (75) and Johansen et al. (39) describe conditions of day care usually associated with disease. Bartlett et al. (5) describe

control strategies. Other sources are also helpful (6, 9, 38, 71, 77).

There are no accurate predictors of later academic success for preschool children. Some studies show that when infants and young children in a ghetto were given a planned educational experience aimed at preventing retardation and promoting parental interaction, environmental stimulation, and experiential opportunity, the experimental group showed superior cognitive abilities at 5.5 years compared with children in a control group raised in the usual way. Other studies showed that 3-year-old children who were given special educational opportunities showed better intellectual performance at the end of second grade than did children in a control group (70). Other authors say that pushing the child to develop reading and mathematics skills too early will create problems: fatigue, stress-related illnesses, disciplinary problems, and parental burnout (29).

If parents use a day-care center, family day-care, nursery school, or early school program, help them understand that they remain the most important people to the child and that their love and involvement with the child are crucial for later learning and adjustment to life. The care or enrichment of a preschool center or program where children attend a few hours daily cannot undo deprivation or abuse that is present in a family. Help the working mother realize that her working does not necessarily deprive the child. Many career women tend to do better than full-time homemakers. They do not see the child as an end in itself; they allow the child to develop autonomy and initiative in creative ways because they have a sense of self-fulfillment in their own lives.

You can help the parents and child prepare for the separation if the child will be enrolled in a nursery school or day-care center. Help the parents realize, too, that the child's emotional and social adjustment and overall learning depend on many factors. Because each child interprets entrance into the agency on the basis of his or her own past experience, each differs in adjustment. Being with a number of children can be an upsetting experience. The child needs adequate preparation to avoid feeling abandoned or rejected. The mother must have confidence in the agency so that she can convey a feeling of pleasurable expectation to the child. The child should accompany the mother to see the building, observe the program, and meet the teachers and other children before enrollment. Ideally the child should begin attending when both mother and child feel secure about the ensuing separation, and the mother should be encouraged to stay with the child the whole first day or for a shorter period for several days until he or she feels secure without mother. If possible, the parent, rather than a neighbor or stranger, should take the child each day, assuring the child of the parent's return at the end of the day.

Relationships with Siblings

The discussion in Chapter 4 on the effect of the child's sex and ordinal position on family interaction is significant for understanding the preschooler.

Often the preschool child has **siblings,** *brothers or sisters,* either younger or older, so that family interaction is complex with many **dyads,** *groups of two people.* Siblings become increasingly important in directing and crystallizing the child's early development, partly because of their proximity but also because the parents change in their role with each additional child. Parents often are emotionally warmer after the firstborn, possible because they feel more experienced and relaxed. In the following discussion you should realize that the relationships described could occur at other developmental eras in childhood, but in the preschool years siblings begin to make a very definite impact (25, 26, 47).

The sibling may be part of a multiple birth: twins, triplets, or more. Identical twins share traits, emotional bonds, and pain and communicate with each other in their own language in uncanny or mysterious ways, often when they are miles apart. Studies of identical twins who are reared separately in different environments can help to sort out the relative influence of heredity and environment. Twins seem to think about each other more than other siblings, so some of the ESP-like communication or experiences may be coincidence. Yet the extreme intimacy can be pathologic; there may be jealousy of each other or a symbiotic interdependence that interferes with identity formation of each individual. For the parents, raising twins creates a delicate balance.

You may give the following suggestions: (1) by the way parents talk to, dress, and handle twins (or other multiple births), help the children realize they are individuals first and twins second; (2) encourage each to develop separate interests, pursue different hobbies and subjects, or go to different schools to reduce competition and rivalry; (3) talk to the twins about different kinds of relationships, their own special closeness, the rewards of developing separate friendships, and the importance of separate intimate relationships, and (4) get help from the magazine *Twins* (Overland Park, Kansas), The National Organization of Mothers of Twins Clubs (Albuquerque, New Mexico), and the chapters of TWINLINE (Berkeley, California), which can provide information to parents (2). Refer also to Chapter 4 for more information on multiple births.

Preschooler and New Baby

The arrival of a new baby changes life: the preschooler is no longer the center of attention but is expected by the parents to delight in the baby. It is important for parents to prepare the young child (toddler or preschooler) for a new arrival (Fig. 9–1). Although a space of 3 to 4 years is ideal, such ideal spacing does not always occur.

When pregnancy is apparent, there are some ways for parents to prepare the older child:

- Share the anticipation in discussions and planning. Let the child feel fetal movements. Show the child a picture of when he or she was a newborn. Talk about what he or she needed as a baby and the necessary responsibilities. Read books that explain reproduction and birth on his or her level.
- Include the child as much as possible in activities such as shopping for furniture for the baby or decorating baby's room. The preschool child likes to feel important, and being a helper enhances this feeling.
- Accept that the child may act out, regress, or express dependency or separation anxiety during the pregnancy as well as after the new baby arrives.

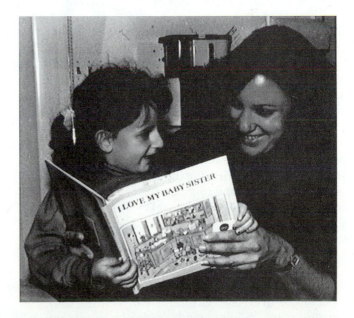

Figure 9–1. As birth approaches, parents can help prepare the preschooler for the arrival of the new sibling. *(From Sherwen, L.N., M.A. Scoloveno, and C.T. Weingarten,* Nursing Care of the Childbearing Family. *Stamford, CT: Appleton & Lange, 1991, p. 537.)*

- Have child attend sibling preparation classes, if available. Encourage relatives and friends to bring a small surprise gift for the older child when they visit and bring a gift for baby. Have them spend time with the older child also rather than concentrating only on baby.
- Prepare child to be with mother during birth, if family considers this appropriate and if permitted by birthing center. Have the child visit mother and baby at the hospital, if rules permit, after delivery, or the older child can talk to mother by phone (69).

Accepting the family's affection toward the baby is difficult for the firstborn, and jealousy is likely to occur if more attention is focused on the baby than on him or her. As a result, the preschooler may regress, overtly displaying a need to be babied. He or she may ask for the bottle, soil self, have enuresis, lie in the baby's crib, or demand extra attention. The child may harm the baby, directly or indirectly, through play or handling baby roughly. He or she may appear to love the baby excessively, more than is normal. The child may show hostility toward the mother in different ways: direct physical or verbal attacks, ignoring or rejecting her, or displacing anger onto the day-care, nursery, or Sunday school teacher.

Teach parents that these outward behaviors and the underlying feelings should be accepted, for they are better handled with overt loving behavior than repressed through punishment. Jealousy can be handled by the parents in a variety of ways: tell the child about the pregnancy but not too far in advance because a young child has a poor concept of time. Convey that the child is loved as much as before, provide a time for him or her only, and give as much attention as possible. In addition, avoid ridicule; emphasize pleasure in having the child share in loving the new arrival and give increasing responsibility and status without overburdening him or her. Encourage the child to talk about the new situation or express hostility in play and involve him or her in preparing for the new baby. Although the preschooler may have to give up a crib, getting him or her a new big bed can seem like a promotion rather than a loss. Reading stories about feelings of children with new siblings can help the child express personal feelings. There is other effective advice you can give about ways to handle jealous behavior: (1) do not leave the preschooler alone with the baby; (2) give him or her a pet or doll to care for as mother cares for the baby; (3) encourage the child to identify with the parents in helping to protect the baby because he or she is more grown up; and (4) avoid overemphasis of affection for the baby.

Older Child and Preschooler

The older sibling in the family who is given much attention for accomplishments may cause feelings of envy and frustration as the preschooler tries to engage in activity beyond his or her ability to get attention also. If the younger child can identify with the older sibling and take pride in the accomplishments while simultaneously getting recognition for his or her own self and abilities, the child will feel positive about self. If the younger child feels defeated and is not given realistic recognition, he or she may stop emulating the older sibling and regress instead. In turn, the older sibling can be helpful to the younger child if he or she does not feel deprived or is not reprimanded too much because of the preschooler.

Explore sibling relationships with parents and present suggestions for preventing conflicts. Often positive feelings exist between siblings. Quarrels are quickly forgotten if parents do not get overly involved. Because siblings have had a similar upbringing, they have considerable empathy for each other, similar values, similar superego development, and related perceptions about situations. Sibling values may be as important as the parents' values in the development of the child. Often recognition and other feelings of the sibling are of such importance to the child that he or she may conceal ability rather than move into an area in which the sibling has gained recognition, or he or she may engage in activity to keep the sibling from being unhappy. The children will learn to develop roles and regulate space among themselves to avoid conflicts unless conflictual behavior is given undue attention or the children are manipulated against each other by the significant adults.

Developmental Tasks of the Family

While the preschool child and siblings are achieving their developmental tasks, the parents are struggling with childrearing and their own personal developmental tasks. A discussion of parental developmental tasks while raising a preschooler follows (25):

- Encourage and accept the child's evolving skills rather than elevating the parent's self-esteem by pushing the child beyond his or her capacity. Satisfaction is found through reducing assistance with physical care and giving more guidance in other respects.
- Supply adequate housing, facilities, space, equipment, and other materials needed for life, comfort, health, and recreation.

- Plan for predicted and unexpected costs of family life such as medical care, insurance, education, babysitter fees, food, clothing, and recreation.
- Maintain some personal privacy and an outlet for tension of family members while including the child as a participant in the family.
- Share household and child-care responsibility with other family members, including the child.
- Strengthen the partnership with the mate and express affection in ways that keep the relationship from becoming humdrum.
- Learn to accept failures, mistakes, and blunders without piling up feelings of guilt, blame, and recrimination.
- Nourish common interests and friendships to strengthen self-respect and self-confidence and to remain interesting to the spouse.
- Maintain a mutually satisfactory sexual relationship and plan whether or not to have more children.
- Create and maintain effective communication within the family.
- Cultivate relationships with the extended family.
- Tap resources and serve others outside the family to prevent preoccupation with self and family.
- Face life's dilemmas and rework moral codes, spiritual values, and a philosophy of life.

Explore with parents the challenges and practical ways of meeting these tasks within the specific family unit.

PHYSIOLOGIC CONCEPTS

Physical Characteristics

Growth

Growth during the preschool years is *relatively slow,* but changes occur that transform the chubby toddler into a sturdy child who appears taller and thinner. Limb growth is greater in proportion to trunk growth. Although development does not proceed at a uniform rate in all areas or for all children, *development follows a logical, precise pattern or sequence* (32, 33, 70, 78). The preschool child grows approximately $2\frac{1}{2}$ to 3 inches (6–7.5 cm) and gains less than 5 pounds (2.2 kg) *per year.* The child appears tall and thin because he or she grows proportionately more in height than in weight. The average height of the 3-year-old is 37 in. (94 cm); of the 4-year-old, 41 in. (104 cm) (*or double the birth length*); and of the 5-year-old, 43 to 52 in. (110–130 cm). At 3 the child weighs approximately 33 pounds (15 kg);

at 4 years, 38 pounds (17 kg); and at 5 years, approximately 40 to 50 pounds (18–23 kg).

Vital Signs

The *temperature* is 98° to 99°F (36.7°–37.2°C). The *pulse rate* is normally 80 to 110 and the *respiratory rate* approximately 30 per minute. Blood pressure is approximately 90/60 mm Hg, systolic and diastolic.

Other Characteristics

Vision in the preschooler is farsighted; the 5-year-old has 20/40 to 20/30 vision and is visually discriminative. Eye-hand coordination improves. By age $4\frac{1}{2}$, the motor nerves are fully myelinated and the cerebral cortex is fully connected to the cerebellum, permitting better coordination and control of bowel and bladder and fine muscle movements, such as tying shoelaces, cutting with scissors, or holding a pencil or crayon. Internal organs are larger; at 5 years the brain is at 90% of the weight of the adult brain. The child has 20 teeth, and by the end of the preschool period the child begins to lose deciduous teeth (70, 77). *Physical characteristics to assess in this child are listed in Table 9–2. Because each child is unique, the normative listings indicate only where most children of a given age are in the development of various characteristics.* Characteristics are listed by age in all following tables for reasons of understanding sequence and giving comparison. Consideration of only the chronologic age is misleading as a basis for assessment and care. The development of the whole and unique child and interrelationships among various aspects must be considered. For example, opportunity for muscle movement and exercise and nutritional status, rather than gender, influences strength. Still, by using the norms for the child at a given age, you can assess how far the child deviates from the norm. W*ith more parental guidance, the child may reach norms ahead of age.* Certain situations, such as prenatal alcohol or drug exposure, are likely to cause the child to be below the norms (77).

Developmental Assessment

The Denver II—Revision and Restandardization of the Denver Developmental Screening Test (DDST) evaluates four major categories of development: gross motor, fine motor-adaptive, language, and personal-social (Fig. 9–2). It is used to determine whether a child is within normal range for various behaviors or is developmentally delayed. Like the original DDST, the Denver II is applicable to children from birth through 6 years of age.

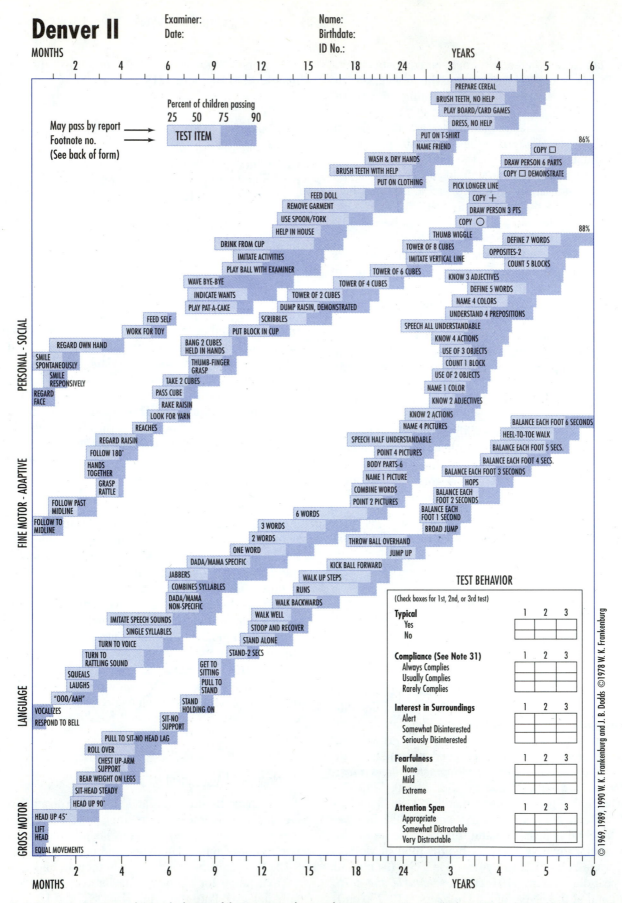

Figure 9–2. Denver II — Revision and Restandardization of the Denver Developmental Screening Test *(From Frankenberg, W.K., and J.B. Dobbs,* Denver II — Revision and Standardization of the Denver Developmental Screening Test. Denver Developmental Materials, 1990.)*

DIRECTIONS FOR ADMINISTRATION

1. Try to get child to smile by smiling, talking or waving. Do not touch him/her.
2. Child must stare at hand several seconds.
3. Parent may help guide toothbrush and put toothpaste on brush.
4. Child does not have to be able to tie shoes or button/zip in the back.
5. Move yarn slowly in an arc from one side to the other, about 8" above child's face.
6. Pass if child grasps rattle when it is touched to the backs or tips of fingers.
7. Pass if child tries to see where yarn went. Yarn should be dropped quickly from sight from tester's hand without arm movement.
8. Child must transfer cube from hand to hand without help of body, mouth, or table.
9. Pass if child picks up raisin with any part of thumb and finger.
10. Line can vary only 30 degrees or less from tester's line. ⅴ
11. Make a fist with thumb pointing upward and wiggle only the thumb. Pass if child imitates and does not move any fingers other than the thumb.

   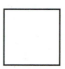

12. Pass any enclosed form. Fail continuous round motions.
13. Which line is longer? (Not bigger.) Turn paper upside down and repeat. (pass 3 of 3 or 5 of 6)
14. Pass any lines crossing near midpoint.
15. Have child copy first. If failed, demonstrate.

When giving items 12, 14, and 15, do not name the forms. Do not demonstrate 12 and 14.

16. When scoring, each pair (2 arms, 2 legs, etc.) counts as one part.
17. Place one cube in cup and shake gently near child's ear, but out of sight. Repeat for other ear.
18. Point to picture and have child name it. (No credit is given for sounds only.)
    If less than 4 pictures are named correctly, have child point to picture as each is named by tester.

 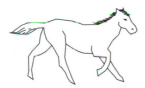 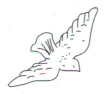 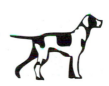 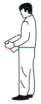

19. Using doll, tell child: Show me the nose, eyes, ears, mouth, hands, feet, tummy, hair. Pass 6 of 8.
20. Using pictures, ask child: Which one flies?...says meow?...talks?...barks?...gallops? Pass 2 of 5, 4 of 5.
21. Ask child: What do you do when you are cold?...tired?...hungry? Pass 2 of 3, 3 of 3.
22. Ask child: What do you do with a cup? What is a chair used for? What is a pencil used for?
    Action words must be included in answers.
23. Pass if child correctly places *and* says how many blocks are on paper. (1, 5).
24. Tell child: Put block **on** table; **under** table; **in front of** me, **behind** me. Pass 4 of 4.
    (Do not help child by pointing, moving head or eyes.)
25. Ask child: What is a ball?...lake?...desk?...house?...banana?...curtain?...fence?...ceiling? Pass if defined in terms of use, shape, what it is made of, or general category (such as banana is fruit, not just yellow). Pass 5 of 8, 7 of 8.
26. Ask child: If a horse is big, a mouse is _____ ? If fire is hot, ice is _____? If the sun shines during the day, the moon shines during the _____ ? Pass 2 of 3.
27. Child may use wall or rail only, not person. May not crawl.
28. Child must throw ball overhand 3 feet to within arm's reach of tester.
29. Child must perform standing broad jump over width of test sheet (8 1/2 inches).
30. Tell child to walk forward ⬭⬭⬭ ➞ heel within 1 inch of toe. Tester may demonstrate.
    Child must walk 4 consecutive steps.
31. In the second year, half of normal children are non–compliant.

OBSERVATIONS:

Figure 9–2. **Denver II — Revision and Restandardization of the Denver Developmental Screening Test** (*From Frankenberg, W.K., and J.B. Dobbs,* Denver II — Revision and Standardization of the Denver Developmental Screening Test. *Denver Developmental Materials, 1990.*)

TABLE 9–2. ASSESSMENT OF PHYSICAL CHARACTERISTICS: MOTOR CONTROL

3 Years	4 Years	5 Years
Occasional accident in toileting when busy at play; responds to routine times; tells when going to bathroom	Independent toilet habits; manages clothes without difficulty	Takes complete charge of self; does not tell when going to bathroom
Verbalizes difference between how male and female urinate	Insists on having door shut for self but wants to be in bathroom with others	Self-conscious about exposing self
Needs help with back buttons and drying self	Asks many questions about defecation function	Boys and girls to separate bathrooms
Nighttime control of bowel and bladder most of time		Voids four to six times during waking hours; occasional nighttime accident
Runs more smoothly, turns sharp corners, suddenly stops; trunk rotates with run	Runs easily with coordination	Runs with skill, speed, agility, and plays games simultaneously
	Skips clumsily	Starts and stops abruptly when running
	Hops on one leg	Increases strength and coordination in limbs
	Legs, trunk, shoulder, arms move in unison	
	Aggressive physical activity	
Walks backward	Heel–toe walk	May still be knock-kneed
Climbs stairs with alternate feet	Walks a plank	Jumps from three to four steps
Jumps from low step	Climbs stairs without holding onto rail	
	Climbs and jumps without difficulty	
Tries to dance but has inadequate balance, although sense of balance improving	Enjoys motor stunts and gross gesturing	Balances self on toes and on one leg; dances with some rhythm
		Balances on one foot approximately 10 sec
Pedals tricycle	Enjoys new activities rather than repeating same ones	Jumps rope
Swings		Roller skates
		Hops and skips on alternate feet
		Enjoys jungle gym
Sitting equilibrium maintained but combined awkwardly with reaching activity	Sitting balance well maintained; leans forward with greater mobility and ease	Maintains balance easily
	Exaggerated use of arm extension and trunk twisting; touches end of nose with forefinger on direction	Combines reaching and placing object in one continuous movement
		Arm extension and trunk twisting coordinated
		Tummy protrudes, but some adult curve to spine
Undresses self; helps dress self	Dresses and undresses self except tying bows, closing zipper, putting on boots and snow suit	Dresses self without assistance; ties shoelaces
Undoes buttons on side or front of clothing	Does buttons	Requires less supervision of personal duties
Goes to toilet alone if clothes simple	Distinguishes front	Washes self without wetting clothes
Washes hands, feeds self	Brushes teeth alone	
May brush own teeth		
Catches ball with arms fully extended one out of two to three times	Greater flexion of elbow	Uses hands more than arms in catching ball
More refined hand movement	Catches ball thrown at 5 ft two to three times	Pours fluid from one container to another with few spills; bilateral coordination
Increasing coordination in vertical direction	Throws ball overhand	Uses hammer to hit nail on head
Pours fluid from pitcher, occasional spills	Judges where a ball will land	Interest and competence in dusting
Hits large pegs on board with hammer	Helps dust objects	Likes water play
Builds tower of 9 to 10 blocks; builds three-block gate from model	Likes water play	Builds things out of large boxes
Imitates a bridge	Builds complicated structure extending vertically and laterally; builds five-block gate from model	Builds complicated three-dimensional structure and may build several separate units
	Notices missing parts or broken objects; requests parents to fix	Able to disassemble and reassemble small object
Copies circle or cross; begins to use scissors; strings large beads	Copies a square	Copies triangle or diamond from model
Shows hand preference	Uses scissors without difficulty	Folds paper diagonally
Trial-and-error method with puzzle	Enjoys finer manipulation of play materials	Definite hand preference
	Surveys puzzle before placing pieces	Does simple puzzles quickly and smoothly
	Matches simple geometric forms	Prints some letters correctly; prints first name
	Prefers symmetry	
	Poor space perception	
Scribbles	Less scribbling	Draws clearly recognized lifelike representatives; differentiates parts of drawing
Tries to draw a picture and name it	Form and meaning in drawing apparent to adults	

Data from References 30, 32, 33, 37, 70, and 77.

The age divisions are monthly until 24 months and then every 6 months until 6 years of age (18, 30).

Although it is not the purpose of this discussion to describe the administration and interpretation of the Denver II, the following points should be noted. First, to avoid errors in administration and interpretation, and hence invalid screening results, the examiner should carefully follow the protocol outlined by the test's authors. A manual–workbook, videotape, and proficiency test have been developed to ensure accurate administration and interpretation by examiners. Second, before administering the test, explanations should be given to both the child and parent(s). Parents should be advised that the Denver II is not an intelligence test but rather a means of assessing what the child can do at a particular age (18, 30).

Because the Denver II is nonthreatening, requires no painful or unfamiliar procedures, and relies on the child's natural activity of play, it is an excellent way to begin the health assessment. It provides a general assessment tool that can help guide treatment and teaching. The Denver II form and instruction manual can be obtained from Denver Developmental Materials, Inc., P.O. Box 6919, Denver, CO 80206–0919; (303) 355–4729.

It is important to consider genetics, family factors, nutrition, and social environment when you assess and care for children who are developmentally delayed (22, 26, 40, 70). Occasionally a child does not attain height within the norms for his or her age, although torso–leg proportions are normal, because the pituitary gland does not produce enough growth hormone (70, 77). **Growth hormone deficiency,** *which causes dwarfism in a preschool child,* can now be treated with a synthetic growth hormone. The person still remains short in stature but is within a normal height range. The treatment is important because children who lag behind peers in growth are often teased, are kept from participating in certain play activities, and may have difficulty finding clothes or play equipment such as a bicycle that is of correct size. The child may be regarded by others as retarded intellectually. He or she may feel inferior, suffer a negative self-concept, lack initiative, and become withdrawn, depressed, or antisocial in later childhood or adult years (71, 77).

Nutritional Needs

The child needs the same food groups as the adult each day, but in smaller quantities. The child needs a gradual increase in caloric intake (1250–1600 cal/day or 90–100 kcal/kg/day). Slower growth rate and heightened interest in exploring the environment may lessen interest in eating. Stomach size is larger and mouth muscles are stronger; thus, a greater amount and variety of foods are eaten. The box outlines the daily nutritional needs of the preschool child. A rule of thumb for the size of servings is 1 tablespoon for each year of age: 3 tablespoons of fruit or vegetables for a 3-year-old; 5 tablespoons for a 5-year-old. Protein requirements remain high—30 to 36 g daily (or 3 g/kg/day). Without adequate fruits and vegetables, vitamins A and C usually are lacking. Calcium (800 mg to age 10) and iron (10 mg/day) are needed for storage and are ensured through eating the foods described in Recommended Nutritional Intake for Preschoolers (71, 76). (Refer to Appendices I and II). Desserts should furnish protein, minerals, vitamins, and calories and should be a natural part of the meal, not used as a reward for finishing the meal or omitted as punishment.

Children who are reared in vegetarian families may be shorter and weigh less, but by the end of the preschool era, the child's growth velocity approaches the norm. In contrast, children reared in migrant families may be both inadequately nourished and below the norms for physical growth (71, 77).

Midmorning, midafternoon, and evening snacks are necessary because of the child's high level of activity but should be wisely chosen: milk; juice; fruit wedges; vegetable strips; cereals without added sugar that are unrefined and with fiber; cheese cubes; peanut butter with crackers or bread; or plain cookies. Sweets (candy, raisins, sodas, sugar-coated cereals) should be offered only occasionally, not as a reward for behavior and not before a meal. This pattern will help prevent now and later the health problems associated with overeating sweet foods, such as dental caries, malnutrition, and obesity, and associating only pleasure with food. Lifetime food habits are being formed (48, 68, 76).

► RECOMMENDED DAILY NUTRITIONAL INTAKE FOR PRESCHOOLERS

Meat or meat substitutes	2 to 3 (1½ to 2 oz) servings
Milk or equivalent milk servings	1–1½ pints
Vegetables and fruits	5 or more servings
Bread and cereals	4 or more servings
Fats, oils, sweets	Use sparingly
Adequate water	12–16 small glasses

Weight gains between 2 and 3 years for girls and 4 and 6 years for boys are the earliest times that are highly related to later obesity (65).

Teach parents about eating patterns, for they differ in each developmental era. Eating assumes increasing social significance for the preschooler and is still an emotional and physiologic experience. The child needs the right foods physically and a warm, happy atmosphere in which he or she is included in mealtime conversation. The family mealtime promotes socialization and sexual identification in relation to meal preparation, behavior during mealtimes, language skills, and understanding of family rituals and situation. The training is positive or negative, depending on the parents' example. Such learning is missed if there are no family mealtimes. Table manners need not be rigidly emphasized; accidents will happen, and parental example is the best teacher.

The preschooler's eating habits are simple. There may be periods of overeating or not wanting to eat certain foods, but they do not persist. The overall eating pattern from month to month is more pertinent to assess. Parental feeding practices, values related to food, preference for chubby children, and parental obesity were related to the preschooler's being obese in a study of Mexican-American children (1). In another study of Mexican children in a rural village, the benefits of a nutritious supplement added to an inadequate diet were apparent for the 15 years that a follow-up study was conducted (63). Preschoolers who follow their own appetite patterns are likely to maintain normal weight (1, 76).

The sense of taste is keen; color, flavor, form, and texture are important. Foods should be attractively served; mildly flavored; whole; plain; separated and distinctly identifiable in flavor and appearance rather than mixed as in creamed foods, casseroles, and stews, except for spaghetti and pizza; and preferably lukewarm rather than too hot or too cold, including drinks. The preschooler likes to eat one thing at a time. Of all food groups, vegetables are least liked, whereas fruits are a favorite. He or she prefers vegetables and fruits crisp, raw, and cut into finger-sized pieces. Strong-tasting vegetables such as cabbage, onions, cauliflower, and broccoli and those with tough strings such as celery and green beans are usually disliked. Meats should be easily chewed and cut into bite-sized pieces. New foods can be gradually introduced; if a food is refused once, offer it again after several days.

A child may be eating insufficiently, for the following reasons:

- Eating too much between meals
- Unhappy mealtime atmosphere
- Attention seeking
- Example of parental eating habit
- Excessive parental expectations
- Unavailability of adequate variety and quantity
- Tooth decay, which may cause nausea or toothache with chewing
- Sibling rivalry
- Overfatigue
- Physical illness
- Emotional disturbance

Parents should consider, too, the difference in eating pattern of the 3-, 4-, and 5-year-old, which can influence food intake. The 3-year-old either talks or eats, gets up from the table during meals but will return to eat more food, and rarely needs assistance to complete a meal. The 4-year-old normally combines talking and eating, rarely gets up from the table, and likes to serve self. The 5-year-old eats rapidly and is sociable during mealtime, so that family atmosphere is crucial (25, 47).

Measures to increase food intake include letting the child help plan the menu, set the table, wash dishes, or prepare foods such as stirring instant puddings or gelatin desserts, beating cake or cookie mix, or kneading dough. Other aids are serving meals in courses in a quiet environment in which there are few distractions; avoiding coaxing, bribing, or threatening; providing a premeal rest period; giving small, attractive servings; providing comfortable chair and table; allowing sufficient time for eating; and avoiding between-meal nibbling. Making food an issue and forcing the child to eat create eating problems, and the child is likely to win the battle. The child's appetite will improve as his or her growth rate increases nearer school age.

Although vitamin-mineral supplements should not be a food substitute, many pediatricians recommend them, especially during these years when appetite fluctuates. Fluoride supplements should be continued if there is insufficient fluoride in the water.

Share information about nutritional needs and eating patterns and the psychological aspects of food and mealtime with parents.

Exercise, Rest, and Sleep

This is the period when the child has a seeming surplus of energy and is on the move. The child needs time and space for physical exercise through play. Clothing and shoes should be comfortable and allow for movement. Shoes should provide flexibility, yet be stable, and conform to the plantar arch contours (62). The child may play to the point of fatigue. Thus the adult must initiate rest periods alternated with activity. Share the following information with parents.

The 3-year-old child does not always sleep at naptime but will rest or play quietly for 1 or 2 hours if undisturbed. The 4-year-old child resists naps but needs a quiet period. The 5-year-old child is unlikely to nap if he or she gets adequate sleep at night.

The preschooler may still take a favorite toy to bed; he or she likes to postpone bedtime and is ritualistic about bedtime routines such as prayers, a story, or music. Sleeping time decreases from 10 to 12 hours for the younger preschooler to 9 to 11 hours for the older preschooler. Dreams and nightmares may awaken the 3- or 4-year-old, causing fear and a move into bed with parents or older siblings. The 5-year-old sleeps quietly through the night without having to get up to urinate and has fewer nightmares.

If the parent responds with special attention to the child who awakens during the night, the sleep disturbance becomes worse. Parents should not become a sleep adjunct to the child (e.g., holding child in lap until he or she falls asleep again, picking up child as soon as he or she cries) because the child will not learn to fall asleep alone. The parent reinforces the waking behavior. Instead help the restless child develop sleep strategies such as cuddling a teddy bear or blanket or babbling to an imaginary friend. Parents should provide reassurance and set and stick to limits (29).

Dreams and nightmares occur during the light stages of sleep as a way to resolve emotional conflicts. During deep stages of sleep the child may sleepwalk or have night terrors. Often children do not awaken after they sleepwalk. In night terrors the child screams or cries, may thrash and squirm, is confused, does not respond to parents, behaves abnormally, and has tachycardia and tachypnea, dilated pupils, and sometimes facial contortions and diaphoresis.

Help the parents understand that calm reassurance is needed with night terrors. Wait out the attack without trying either to comfort or to arouse the child. Further stimulation intensifies agitation. After 15 minutes or so, the child collapses back into sleep without memory of what happened. Sleep problems usually subside spontaneously, but the child and parents may need therapy if the problem persists several times weekly or over a period.

Health Promotion and Health Protection

Immunization Schedules

These schedules will be adjusted to the individual child; however, before school entry the child should receive a DTP booster, an MMR booster, and a refeeding of oral polio virus vaccine (20). Frequency of tuberculin testing depends on geographic region and personal environ-ment. Inoculation for hepatitis B and influenza are also recommended if they have not been done before (20).

Help parents realize that the state law of requiring immunizations before school entry is indeed a beneficial one as the organisms that cause childhood communicable diseases cannot be eliminated from the environment. The decrease in these diseases and their harmful effects has resulted only because of mass *inoculations of a disease antigen* (**active immunity**) or an *antibody* (**passive immunity**). The minimum reaction is far better than acquiring the disease.

In Manitoba, Canada, a centralized, computerized childhood immunization system provides an age-at-immunization profile for individuals and groups. Such a system would be useful to health maintenance organizations in the United States. (57).

Before giving an immunization, ask yourself the following questions (77).

- Has the parent given consent? Members of some religious groups such as Church of Christ, Scientist (Christian Scientist), do not believe in immunizations. (The school district may allow these children to attend without immunization, based on parents' rights regarding their children.)
- Is the vaccination (immunization) indicated based on the child's age and previous immunization record?
- Are there any contraindications such as allergy to any of the constituents of the vaccine; presence of another infectious disease (febrile condition, dermatitis) or immunodeficiency disease; presence of malignancy or immunosuppressive therapy; or administration of gamma globulin, plasma, or blood transfusion in the previous 6 to 8 weeks that would have given passive antibodies?
- Has the parent been informed of the method (route of administration) and benefits and risks involved in inoculation?
- Has the parent informed you of any reactions or difficulties that occurred with or after previous immunizations? If the child has a minor reaction, remaining doses may be cut in half or thirds to decrease the possibility of a systemic reaction. The child then returns an additional number of times to receive the full immunization series.
- Has the parent been told that the antigens to the various diseases may be given separately but are usually combined for convenience of administration?

- Has the vaccine been stored according to manufacturer's recommendations (usually refrigerated) and is there a date of expiration?

Dental Care

Because caries frequently begin at this age and spread rapidly, dental care is equally important. Deciduous teeth guide in the permanent ones; they should be kept in good repair. Fluoride is important for preventing caries. If the child has teeth with deep grooves, a plastic coating can be applied to the teeth to prevent tooth decay and loss. If deciduous teeth are lost too early, permanent teeth grow in abnormally. Teeth should be brushed after eating, using a method recommended by the dentist, and intake of refined sugars limited to help prevent tooth decay.

Before entering school the child is usually required to have a physical examination (including urinalysis) and a dental examination. Refer to Appendices III and IV for a schedule of health screening measures for the preschool child.

Safety Promotion and Injury Control

The preschooler has more freedom, independence, initiative, and desire to imitate adults than the toddler but still has an immature understanding of danger and illness. This combination is likely to get him or her into hazardous situations.

A major responsibility of caretaking adults is safety promotion and injury control: the child needs watchfulness and a safe play area. The adult serves as a bodyguard while slowly teaching caution and keeping the environment as safe as possible. Other siblings can also take some, but not total, responsibility for the preschooler. Protecting the firstborn is simple as you can put dangerous objects away and there is likely to be more time and energy for supervision. When there are a number of children in a family, the activities of the older children may provide objects or situations that are dangerous to the younger ones.

Preschoolers need clear-cut safety rules, explained simply, repeatedly, and consistently; and you can help parents establish them. As the child learns to protect self, he or she should be allowed to take added responsibility for personal safety and should be given appropriate verbal recognition and praise that reinforce safe behavior. Constant threats, frequent physical punishment, and incessant "don'ts" should be avoided, for the child will learn to ignore them, feel angry or resentful, and purposefully rebel or defy adults, thus failing to learn about real danger. Also if the parent voices fear constantly, natural curiosity and the will to learn will be dulled; the child may fear every new situation.

Explore information in this section with parents so that they and you can use these safety suggestions:

- Begin safety teaching early. Teaching done in the toddler years, for example, pays off later.
- When you must forbid, use simple command words in a firm voice without anger to convey the impression that you expect the child to obey, for example, "stop," "no."
- Phrase safety rules and their reasons in positive rather than negative terms when possible. For example, say: "Play in the yard, not the street, or you'll get hurt by cars"; "Sit quietly in the car to avoid hurt"; "Put tiny things (coins, beads) that you find in here (jar, bowl, box)."
- Teach the child his or her full name, address, and telephone number (including zip code), and teach the child how to use the police or adults in service roles for help (e.g., 991—Emergency Services, Fire Department).
- Teach the child not to give information over the phone about himself or herself or the family.
- Encourage the child to share any "secrets"; emphasize that he or she does not have to be afraid to say anything.
- Tell the child not to leave home alone or with a stranger. He or she should use a "buddy" system when going somewhere.
- Never leave the child alone in public or unattended in a car.
- Teach the child escape techniques, for example, how to unlock home doors or car doors.
- Never leave the child home alone. Make sure that the babysitter is reliable.
- Never allow play in or near a busy driveway or garage. Forbid street play if other play areas are available. Teach children to look carefully for and get away from cars. Drivers must take all possible precautions. A fenced yard or playground is ideal, although not always available.
- Teach the child how to cross the street safely.
- Teach the child to refuse gifts or rides from strangers, to avoid walking or playing alone on a deserted street, road, or similar area, and about the possibility of child molesters or abductors.
- Keep matches in containers and out of reach.
- Dispose of or store out of reach and in a locked cabinet as many poisons as possible: rat and roach killer, insecticides, weed killer, kerosene, cleaning agents, furniture polish, medicines. Suntan lotion, shampoo, deodorants, nail polish, and cosmetics remain potential hazards; the

child should be taught their *correct* use. The child is less likely to pull them out of cabinets or swallow them than when he or she was a toddler, but brightly colored containers or pills, powders, or liquids raise curiosity and experimentation. Keep medications out of the child's reach. Bright-colored pills can be mistaken for candy. Keep the Poison Control Center telephone number readily seen.

- Observe your child closely while he or she plays near water. Cover wells and cisterns. Fence ponds or swimming pools.
- Keep stairways and nighttime play areas well lit.
- Equip upstairs windows with sturdy screens and guards. Have hand rails for stairways.
- Store knives, saws, and other sharp objects or lawn or power tools out of reach.
- Remove doors from abandoned appliances or cars and campaign for legislation for appropriate disposal of them and for mandatory door removal.
- Discourage playing with or in the area of appliances or power tools while they are in operation: a washing machine with a wringer, a lawn mower, a saw, or a clothes dryer.
- Use safety glass in glass doors or shower stalls; place decals on sliding doors at child's eye level (and adult's eye level, too) to prevent walking or running through them.
- Use adhesive strips in the bathtub.
- Avoid scatter rugs, debris, or toys cluttered on the floor in areas of traffic.
- Use seatbelts in the car that are appropriate for the weight of the child.
- Teach the child sun safety rules: cover up, find shade, and use sun-safe products/sunscreens.

If the child continually fails to listen and obey, ask the following questions: Is the child able to hear? Is he or she intellectually able to understand? Are demands too many and expectations too great? Are statements too lengthy or abstract? Is anger expressed with teaching and discipline to the point that it interferes emotionally with the child's perception and judgment? Perhaps most important, do the parents demonstrate safety-conscious behavior with equipment, movements, or use of sun safety rules? Imitation is a major way to learn.

Accidents

Accidents are the most common cause of death. Approximately one-third of the accidental deaths are caused by motor vehicles; the next most common

causes are drowning, burns from fire or hot water, and poisonings. Running through sliding glass doors in homes, locking self in an abandoned refrigerator or freezer, and electric shocks from electric equipment also frequently cause severe injury or death. Falls can cause minor bumps, bruises, and lacerations. Animal bites are common (77).

Minor head injury is *any trauma to the head that does not alter normal cerebral functioning*. What appears a very minor head injury can result in a subdural or epidural hematoma—the preschooler bears very close monitoring. Parents or caretakers should be taught to check the preschooler every 2 hours in the first 24 hours after injury. If the preschooler cannot be awakened, is mentally confused, is unusually restless, disturbed, or agitated, starts vomiting, has a severe headache, has different sized pupils (unless previously that way), has weakness of arms or legs, has drainage from ears or nose, or has some sort of fit or convulsion, medical help must be sought (38, 66, 71, 77).

Minor lacerations, *cuts,* should be examined for dirt and foreign objects even after they have been cleaned with warm water and soap. The laceration should be covered with a loose bandage that will keep out dirt and protect the wound from additional trauma. The parent or caretaker should watch for signs of infection: redness, heat, swelling, and drainage. The child should have updated tetanus prophylaxis (71, 77).

Burns are *thermal injuries to the skin*. A **first-degree burn** usually *shows redness only;* a **second-degree burn** causes *blister formation,* sometimes with peeling and weeping. Scalds often produce this type of burn. A **third-degree burn** *chars the skin, causing a whitish appearance, and involves tissue under the skin*. It may cause anesthesia. Flame and hot metal often cause third-degree burns (38, 71, 77).

For a first-degree burn the affected area should be plunged into cold water for a few minutes. Gentle washing with soap and water should be sufficient. A second-degree burn should have the same initial treatment. Blisters that form should be left intact, and the burned area should be covered with a nonadherent gauze and a bulky, dry, sterile dressing. Tetanus immunization should be up to date. A third-degree burn, any second-degree burn that covers an area greater than an adult's hand size, any facial burns, and any burn in which child abuse or neglect is suspected should be seen by the health care provider and physician (38, 71, 77).

Accidental ingestions and poisonings occur under the age of 5, sometimes even when preventive measures as discussed in Chapter 8 are used. These ingestions can cause a great variety of symptoms and signs. The following guidelines should be taught to parents:

1. Look for an empty container nearby if sudden unusual symptoms or abnormal odor to breath or clothes is observed.
2. Try to determine what and how much was ingested and when.
3. Call the poison control center for help.
4. If there are no contraindications to vomiting (either from reading the side of the container or from getting directions at the poison control center), induce vomiting with syrup of ipecac. Mechanical stimulation of the posterior pharynx can be used to induce vomiting *except* with ingestion of corrosive agents such as lye, gasoline, and kerosene.
5. Take the child to the nearest clinic that is set up to deal with these problems (38, 71, 77).

The *bite of any animal* will probably have few symptoms other than pain at the site of puncture wounds or small lacerations. Dog bites are most common, although the child may have contact with other animals that bite or scratch. Bites from other children can also occur. The chief concern is the possibility of rabies. It is essential to establish the vaccination status of the biting animal, if possible, for if the animal is properly vaccinated, there is little chance of acquiring and transmitting the disease to humans. Rabies prophylaxis will be determined by the physician. The wound should be washed with copious amounts of soap and water. After the soap is well removed, zephiran chloride or 40 to 70% alcohol or povidone–iodine solution should be applied. Tetanus prophylaxis should be up to date (77).

Lead poisoning, especially in preschoolers, will produce **encephalopathy,** or *brain dysfunction.* The onset is insidious, with weakness, irritability, weight loss, and vomiting followed by personality changes and developmental regression. Convulsions and coma are late signs. Often history will reveal pica involving cracking paint in old homes, lead toys, old yellow and orange crayons, artist's paints, leaded gasoline, or fruit tree sprays (3, 77).

A study investigated the average daily dietary lead intake of a cross-sectional sample of American children from birth to 5 years. Daily lead intake should not exceed 100 mg, and the study showed a daily average of 62 mg but a range from 15 to 234 mg. The higher levels may represent mouthing of objects and hands and the ingestion of some nonfood substances in addition to the lead content in food (3, 77).

Prevention lies in keeping the preschooler in a lead-free environment as much as possible. You may call the housing inspector, with the family's permission, to test paint for lead. In many cities landlords are required to repaint the house interior when lead paint is found. Treatment for severe cases of lead poisoning involves hospitalization. General measures are to prevent reexposure to lead and to give the preschooler a high-calcium, high-phosphorus diet (milk) and large doses of vitamin D to help in removing lead from the blood by depositing it in the bones (3, 77).

Common Health Problems: Prevention and Treatment

Teach parents that scheduled health maintenance visits to the doctor or nurse practitioner are important for early detection of problems. Table 9–3 summarizes some common health problems (10, 38, 66, 71, 77).

Chart 2 in Appendix IV presents the American Academy of Family Physicians' Periodic Health Examination for Children ages 19 months to 6 years. It includes guidelines for screening and parent and child counseling, summarizes an immunization schedule, and categorizes risks for which to assess.

Abuse

An all-too-common health problem for the young child is *abuse, neglect,* or *maltreatment.* Garbarino, Guttmann, and Seeley (31) describe behaviors of the psychologically abusing parents (see Chapters 7 and 8) toward the young child.

Be aware that when you encounter children with some of the previous accidental occurrences or health problems, the origin of the problems may be the beatings, burns, shakings, handling, sexual abuse or incest, or neglect received at the hands of the parents, stepparents, day-care teacher, or other adult caretaker (49).

Role relationship of the child to the offender may be intrafamilial or extrafamilial (day-care worker, teacher, babysitter, family acquaintance). When the abuser is older, the age difference conveys that others will not believe the accusations of the child but the denial of the offender. Further, the role of the offender often also involves one of caretaker so that trust would be the normal feeling for the child (13–17, 55).

The Federal Child Abuse Prevention and Treatment Act defines **child abuse and neglect** as the *"physical or mental injury, sexual abuse, negligent treatment, or maltreatment of a child under the age of 18 by a person who is responsible for the child's welfare under circumstances which indicate that the child's health or welfare is harmed"* (78).

The three types of abuse (physical, psychological, and sexual) may be present simultaneously, but frequently the child's symptoms and perceptions convey that one abuse experience is dominant (14).

TABLE 9–3. COMMON HEALTH PROBLEMS OF PRESCHOOLER

Problem	Definition	Signs/Symptoms	Prevention/Treatment
Strabismus	Eyes not straight or properly aligned	Double vision (diplopia), followed by irreversible loss of vision in suppressed eye (amblyopia)	Appropriate vision testing E chart or Allen cards Use toy to go through visual field testing Test for color blindness Functional amblyopia remedied through corrective lens, contact lens, and prisms
Conjunctivitis	Inflammation of the eyelids or conjunctivae or both; caused by bacteria or virus	Redness of conjunctivae; mild irritation; excessive lacrimation; normal vision	Cool compresses Appropriate eye drops
Hearing loss	Hearing less than normal for age group	Inability to speak by age 2; failure to respond to out-of-sight noise; tilting the head while listening	Use play technique to evaluate hearing Use earphones to transmit sounds and have child put peg in board when hearing sound
Otitis media	Infection of middle ear with accumulation of seropurulent fluid in middle ear cavity	Earache, fever, upper respiratory infection; decreased hearing; bulging tympanic membrane; disappearance of landmarks	Lymphatic tissue, tonsils, and adenoids more abundant now than later and, therefore, are often involved in the infectious process
Acute cervical adenitis	Inflammation of one or more cervical nodes in response to an infection in the ear, nose or throat; group A Strep often etiology	Painful swelling of neck; possibly high fever; usually unilateral cervical nodes enlarged and tender	Appropriate antibiotic Antipyretic Warm compresses
Urinary tract infection	Bacterial infection of part or all of urinary tract, collecting system of kidneys, and bladder	May be asymptomatic; urgency and frequency of urination; dysuria; flank and suprapubic pain; foul-smelling urine; fever	Appropriate antibiotic Increased water intake Personal hygiene
Enuresis	Involuntary passage of urine; occurs at night in 10–15% of 5-year-olds	Bedwetting	Reduction of liquid intake in the evening Maintaining appropriate attitude Signal device sometimes helpful Getting child up at specified times to urinate
Nonspecific vulvovaginitis	Inflammation of vulva and vagina; usually nonspecific organism responsible	Discharge; pruritus; erythema	Personal hygiene Wearing cotton underwear Avoidance of bubble baths and perfumed soaps Cold compresses to vulva
Measles	Highly contagious viral disease with severe complications	Rash (beginning at face and descending down body); 3C's—coryza, cough, conjunctivitis; Koplik's spots (red) on buccal mucosa; fever	Prevention: immunization *If disease: isolation* No specific therapy Symptomatic treatment
Diarrhea	Inflammation of gastrointestinal tract caused at this age by *Giardia lambdia* and *Salmonella*	Stools more frequent and liquid than usual	Sometimes antibiotics Personal hygiene Staying out of wading pools
Postural problems	Deviation of normal posture and normal spinal curves	Deviation seen as child bends anteriorly, laterally, posteriorly	Exercises prescribed by knowledgeable health care practitioner
Juvenile hypertension	Child more than age 3 who has diastolic pressure greater than 90 mm Hg	Probably none other than blood pressure elevation	Referral for overall cardiovascular investigation
Hypochromic anemia	Prevalent nutritional problem in childhood, caused by inadequate intake of absorbable iron	Associated with poor hygiene, chronic disease; major part of diet is milk or milk products	Encourage parents to feed child eggs, meat, fish, fruits, cereals, and dark green leafy vegetables Normal, not excessive, milk

Data from References 10, 37, 66, 71, and 77.

Physical abusive acts *include being bit, punched, cut, burned, physically restrained, and tied up.* It is also considered abuse if the child witnesses this behavior between an adult and a child or between adults (14).

Psychological abuse *is characterized by behaviors, activities, and words that intimidate, threaten, humiliate, shame, or degrade the child; blaming the child for the abuse; and threatening the child with harm* such as

being locked in a box, removal of body parts, and death to self or family members if he or she tells about the abuse (14, 31).

Child sexual abuse is defined to *include immature children and adolescents engaged in sexual activities who do not fully comprehend the sexual act, who are unable to give informed consent, or who are forced to engage in activities that violate social taboos of family roles.* The

Research Abstract

Gottlieb, L., and J. Baillies, Firstborns' Behaviors During a Mother's Second Pregnancy, Nursing Research, 44 (1995), 356–362.

Preparation for a new sibling can be stressful for the young child, as the child must adjust to shifts in quality and quantity of time with the parents, changes in living arrangements, and increased maturity demands from the mother. The mother's pregnancy may be used as a time to teach about reproduction and birth, the older sibling role, and what it means to be a family. The child may resort to distress behaviors, such as temper tantrums, to elicit mother's attention during pregnancy or after birth.

The purposes of this study were to (1) examine firstborn's behaviors at different weeks in the mother's pregnancy and how these behaviors related to firstborns' sex and age, and (2) study the stress of the mother's pregnancy for the sibling by comparing firstborns' behaviors with behaviors of only children of nonpregnant women.

The sample consisted of 80 women who had a young child between 18 and 60 months of age. There were three groups of pregnant women, 20 in each group, who were in either early (12–20 weeks), middle (21–28 weeks), or late (28–38 weeks) pregnancy. One group consisted of 20 women who were not pregnant. All families were Caucasian, middle class, well-educated, and intact. The women were employed less than 21 hours weekly. To examine how behaviors differed as a function of the child's age and/or sex, each group was balanced for age (toddlers, 18–36 months; and preschoolers, 37–60 months) and sex. Within each group of mothers there were 5 young boys, 5 older boys, 5 young girls, and 5 older girls. The groups were comparable in demographic characteristics.

The Preschool Behavioral Rating Scale, a 48-item maternal rating questionnaire, was used to assess the firstborn child's reaction to the sibling's birth. The questionnaire sought the mother's information about the child's distress, separation anxiety, anger, dependence, and autonomy (independence) behaviors. The items were age-appropriate for the child. Each group was followed for 3 months: ratings were done monthly.

Results indicated that some firstborn children from each phase of pregnancy were rated more distressed by their mothers at the first rating time (weeks 12, 20, and 28) than at the other two rating times. There were variations in the children's distress as a function of time, age, and sex. At 12 weeks of pregnancy, toddler girls were more dependent than preschool girls or the toddler and preschool boys. During first trimesters mothers may be more tired or nauseated and thereby less responsive to their toddler daughter's needs. Preschool children may have more outside interests; fathers may be more involved with toddler sons than daughters. All children in the middle phase of pregnancy group were more dependent at 20 than at 24 or 28 weeks. This may be related to having learned about the baby; mother's usually tell their children about the fifth month of pregnancy. During the late phase of pregnancy, boys were more distressed than girls; they reacted more to separation and were angrier. It may be during this period that the child begins the complex psychological work of becoming a sibling. Boys tend to react to stress with more externalizing behavior, and parents tend to respond more negatively to boy's acting out behaviors. Further, girls, in contrast to boys, continue to identify with their mothers and engage in dramatic play throughout the preschool period, and mothers may remain more sensitive to their needs. Finally, differences in sex reactions may be related to the possibility that boys are biologically more vulnerable to change and appraise situations as more stressful than girls.

More research is needed to understand how the child's temperament and situational factors, such as family changes and maturity demands, influence children's coping during pregnancy. Parents may need education or assistance related to the effects of changes during pregnancy on the child and consequent effects on intrapersonal, relationship, and systems levels.

child is victimized by the lack of choice involved. Sexual abuse is defined as pressured or ritualistic (15, 42, 49, 64).

Pressured sexuality is an *adult's dominance used to ensure sexual control over the child so that there is loss of choice of consent and right to say no to the perpetrator; it often is accompanied by threats of violence to the child or family members (13, 41).*

Sexual activity that is child sexual abuse includes enforcing nudity or disrobing, genital exposure, observation of the child, photographing, kissing, fondling, masturbation, fellatio, cunnilingus, digital penetration of the anus or vagina, penile penetration of the vagina, and dry intercourse or forcing the child to perform sexual acts on other children or to watch sexual behavior between children and adults (13–17, 42).

Ritualistic abuse refers to the *systematic and repetitive sexual, physical, and psychological abuse of children by adults engaged in cult worship. The purpose of ritualistic abuse is to induce religious or mystical experiences for the adult participants.* Ritualistic behavior is linked with symbols of overriding power, authority, and purpose, often pseudoreligious or satanic in nature ("It is God's will that you be punished in this way for your sins"). There is the determined intent by the offender to convert the abused person to a victim role (14, 41).

Indications of satanic ritual abuse include the following (41):

- Use of special table or altar
- Sex involving unusual practices
- Imitations and reversals of the Catholic Mass
- Ritual use of body fluids and excrement
- Ritual use of a circle
- Ritualized use of chants and songs, especially using names of demons
- Use of animals and insects in ceremonies
- Wearing of special masks and robes in ceremonies
- Use of torches, candles, darkness, and body parts in ceremonies
- Administration of drugs and potions
- Dismemberment of infants and young children
- Cannibalism of animals or humans; drinking of human or animal blood in ceremonies

The autonomic response to abuse is of two types: numbing and hyperarousal. Affective states may include passivity, anxiety, depression, anger, hostility, defiance, and rebellion. With *hyperarousal,* night terrors, stomach-ache, startle reflexes, avoidance of people and places, crying, and enuresis may be noted. Alcohol and drug use may be a way to avoid the emotional pain. With *numbing,* there may be acting out of aggressive and sexualized behaviors and a lack of empathy for oth-

ers (14, 17, 41, 59). Federation (28) and Polk-Walker (55) also discuss feelings of the abused child and causes of abuse and treatment. More information about nursing assessment and intervention for the abused child is discussed in the section, Health Care and Nursing Applications later in this chapter. See Signs and Symptoms of Sexual Abuse of a Child (13–17, 41, 42, 64).

A study of two groups of children attending daycare who were sexually abused revealed differences using the TRIAD tool. One group (N = 32) was subjected to patterned sexual abuse. In this group the children's relationship with adult caretakers was sexual. Physical abuse and control of these children usually was opportunistic and aimed at immediate conquest of the child. The second group (N = 35) was subjected to sexual abuse within the context of ritual activities. Each form of abuse was scripted and aimed at performance of aggressive, erotic, and sadistic impulses of the abuser. Ritualistic abuse was more severe, and the child's fears continued longer after ritualistic abuse than after nonritualistic abuse. With ritualistic abuse there were significantly more physical abuse, more sexual acts, greater variation of sexual acts, and more offenders. The ritualistically abused children scored higher than the other abused children, although that group also had more symptoms than normal children. Of particular harmful impact were acts demanding sexual activity with other children, pornographic photography, and forced participation in rituals. Both groups had been highly stressed so that the children vacillated between great anxiety and numbness, for when the children reached a panic state, they went into dissociation (14, 41).

The monograph Sexual Abuse of Children presents the incidence of sexual abuse, consequences for the child and family, prevention, treatment of the child and offender, and legal issues. For further information, see Resources for Information and Prevention of Child Abuse (64).

Neglect

Not all abused children are battered. Some suffer just as cruelly from another type of abuse—parental neglect, either willful or unintentional. **Neglect** is a *lack of adequate food, clothing, shelter, love, concern, and attention.* Neglect can take many forms. A parent may neglect a child by simply "forgetting" about him or her (e.g., leaving him or her behind at a bus terminal after rounding up the other children), or a parent may sedate a rejected child to keep him or her quiet; belittle the child until he or she is convinced he or she is worthless; or

► SIGNS AND SYMPTOMS OF SEXUAL ABUSE OF A CHILD

Disclosures

- States that someone removed child's clothes or handled or had contact with the genital area in some way
- Complains that an adult or older child touched or penetrated child's bottom, vagina, rectum, or mouth or that child touched an older child or adult's bottom, vagina, penis, or rectum
- Refers to blood or "white stuff" in genital area
- Describes detailed and age-inappropriate understanding of sexual behavior
- Hints about engaging in sexual activity

Physical Symptoms

- Somatic complaints: stomachaches, nausea, vomiting, headaches, leg aches
- Underwear excessively soiled due to reluctance to clean self or to a relaxed anal sphincter
- Semen or blood stains on child's underwear, skin, or hair or in mouth
- Bruises or abrasions in the genital or rectal area
- Vaginal or anal pain, burning when washed, pain when urinating or defecating
- Chronic constipation or urinary infections
- Constant fatigue, illness, flare-ups of allergies, vomiting
- On examination, relaxed anal sphincter, anal or rectal lacerations or scarring; child relaxes rather than tenses rectum when touched
- On examination, enlargement of vaginal opening and vaginal lacerations in girls, sore penis in boys; blood or trauma around genital area
- Presence of venereal disease, including infections such as trichimonas, herpes, and monilia

Behavior of Child

- Uncontrolled, hyperactive, wild
- Accident-prone or deliberately hurts self

- Negativistic; resistant to authority; mistrusts adults
- Overcompliant with authority; overly pleasing with adults
- Withdrawn; does not play; plays in lethargic, unfocused way
- Exhibits short attention span; has difficulty staying on task
- Does not learn readily
- Regressive, babyish, delayed, or disordered speech; significantly decreased speech production
- Sleep disorders: nightmares or night terrors, bed wetting, fear of going to bed
- Does not clean himself or herself after going to the bathroom
- Masturbates excessively; attempts to insert finger or other object in rectum or vagina
- Pulls down pants, lifts dress, or takes off clothes inappropriately
- Touches others sexually or asks for sexual activity
- Is sexually provocative or seductive in behavior
- Excessive bathing; preoccupation with cleanliness of self and surroundings
- Unusual reluctance to remove clothes (e.g., during visit to pediatrician, insistence on wearing underwear to bed)

Emotional Responses

- Low self-esteem, feeling of being "bad"; feels deserving of punishment
- Perceives self as dumb, ugly, unloved
- Is fearful and clingy; regresses to "baby" behavior
- Shows an unusual fear of people of a particular age group, sex, of policemen, doctors
- Is angry, aggressive, acts out
- Shows rapid mood changes inappropriate to the circumstances
- Sudden onset of anxiety or anxiety-related behavior (e.g., nail biting, grinding teeth, rocking)
- Is fearful of being touched; fears having genital area washed

---

hurt the child by physically abusing his or her pet or favorite toy.

Signs of a neglected child include the following (14, 77):

- Signs of malnutrition, including wasting of subcutaneous tissue, abdominal distention, thinness, pallor, dull eyes, sore gums
- Inadequate clothing in cold weather
- Apathy or hyperexcitability in the child
- Behavior problems or emotional or developmental immaturity in the child
- Parasitic infections

- Depression or psychosomatic illness
- Parental role-playing among siblings (when all the children in a family are neglected, older children will sometimes "mother" the younger ones)

Reactions to Illness and Hospitalization

During this stage, when the child has heightened feelings of sexuality, fears of dependency and separation, fantasies, feelings of narcissism, and rivalry with parents, he or she is particularly vulnerable to fears about body damage. The child perceives and fears dental, medical,

► ## RESOURCES FOR INFORMATION AND PREVENTION OF CHILD ABUSE

American Humane Association, Children's Division

- 63 Inverness Drive East, Englewood, CO 80122-5117 (303) 792-9900 or (800) 227-5242

  Health care and other professionals share goal of ensuring effective services for families at risk for abuse and neglect. Information, policy and legislation, and advocacy are the focus.

American Professional Society on the Abuse of Children

- 332 South Michigan Ave., Suite 1600, Chicago, IL, 60604 (312) 554-0166

  Interdisciplinary professional society for those who work in the field of child maltreatment.

C. Henry Kempe Center for Prevention and Treatment of Child Abuse and Neglect

- 1205 Oneida Street, Denver, CO 80220 (303) 321-3963

  Provides a clinically based resource for training, consultation, program development and evaluation, and research, with a commitment to multidisciplinary approaches. Staff conduct a number of prevention, treatment, and research programs.

Clearinghouse of Child Abuse and Neglect Information

- 3998 Fair Ridge Drive, Suite 350, Fairfax, VA 22033-2907, General Address: P.O. Box 1182, Washington, DC 20013-1182 (703) 385-7565 or (800) 394-3366 (outside DC metropolitan area)

  Collects, processes, and disseminates information in the areas of research and practice, prevention and treatment programs, and public awareness. Maintains data bases and develops publications.

National Center on Child Abuse and Neglect (NCCAN)

- Administration on Children, Youth, and Families, U.S. Department of Health and Human Services, P.O. Box 1182, Washington, DC 20013 (202) 205-8586

  The primary federal agency for assisting states and communities in prevention, identification, and treatment of child abuse. Allocates child abuse and neglect funds appropriated by Congress, coordinates federal child abuse and neglect prevention activities.

National Committee for Prevention of Child Abuse

- 332 South Michigan Avenue, Suite 1600, Chicago, IL 60604 (312) 663-3520

  A volunteer-based organization of concerned citizens working with community, state, and national groups to disseminate knowledge about child abuse prevention.

National Resource Center on Child Sexual Abuse

- 107 Lincoln Street, Huntsville, AL 35801 (205) 534-6868 or (800) 543-7006

Provides technical support information and referrals for treatment and expert consultation to all professionals working with sexually abused children and their families.

The U.S. Advisory Board on Child Abuse and Neglect

- 200 Independence Avenue, S.W., Washington, DC 20201 (202) 690-8137

  Prepares annual reports for the Secretary of Health and Human Services and appropriate committees of Congress. Evaluates the nation's efforts to accomplish the proposed goals of the Child Abuse Prevention and Treatment Act. Provides recommendations for federal child abuse and neglect prevention activities, research, and program initiatives.

Family Resources Coalition

- 200 South Michigan Avenue, Suite 1520, Chicago, IL 60604 (312) 341-0900

Provides information.

Harvard Family Research Project

- 38 Concord Avenue, Cambridge, MA, Mail c/o Harvard Graduate School of Education, Longfellow Hall, Appian Way, Cambridge, MA 02138 (617) 495-9108

  Provides information.

Hawaii's Healthy Start Program

- Family Health Services Department Maternal and Child Health Branch, State of Hawaii, Department of Health, 741-A Sunset Avenue, Honolulu, HI 96816 (808) 733-9022

  Provides information.

Maternal and Child Health Bureau

- U.S. Department of Health and Human Services, 5600 Fisher's Lane, The Parklawn Building, Room 18A-39, Rockville, MD 20857 (301) 443-2250

  Provides information.

MotherNet

- International Medical Services for Health, 45449 Severn Way, Suite 161, Sterling, VA 22170 (703) 444-4477

  Provides information.

Parents as Teachers National Center

- 9374 Olive Boulevard, St. Louis, MO 63132 Contact: Mildred Winter, Executive Director (314) 432-4330

  Provides information.

and surgical procedures as mutilating, intrusive, punishing, or abandonment. The resulting conflicts, fears, guilt, anger, or excessive concern about the body can persist and influence personality development into adulthood.

Teach parents that many of these negative reactions can be averted by introducing the child to medical facilities and health workers when he or she is well. The best teaching is positive example. If the parent takes the child with him or her to the physician and dentist and if the child observes courteous professionals, a procedure that does not hurt (or an explanation of why it will hurt), and a positive response from the parent, a great deal of teaching is accomplished. These visits can be reinforced with honest answers to the many questions the preschooler will have.

Hospitalization should be avoided if possible. Preparation for hospitalization is important to reduce the separation anxiety and grief and mourning response described in Chapter 8. Most families have had some experience with a hospital and can give some explanation to the child.

Although children are forbidden in certain areas of a hospital, parents may arrange for a tour of the pediatric ward. The child should be told that special caring people work there and that if he or she is ever hospitalized, the parents will stay close by. The child can be further prepared through play, books, and appropriate films. Emphasize the importance of continued, ample contact with the child whenever either parent or child is hospitalized. Advise parents to (1) trust their intuition (they know the child best); (2) shop for a doctor and hospital; (3) prepare themselves so that they can prepare the child; (4) prepare the child a few days before hospitalization; and (5) be present at important times.

As a nurse, you will be in a position to offset the negative effects of hospitalization through planning individualized care, use of play or art therapy, and involvement in decision and policy making. The hospital personnel must make the ward as homelike as possible through gay decor and furnishings and provision for toys, a playroom, and central dining area. The staff can wear pastel uniforms or smocks and provide for the child to remain in his or her own clothes, keep a favorite toy, eat uninterrupted by procedures, and follow normal living routines when possible. Flexible visiting hours are essential, as the presence of the mother can dramatically revive a child's interest in getting well and improve eating, sleeping, and general behavior. Because a mother feels concern, partial helplessness, and perhaps guilt when her child is hospitalized, she may have an impaired relationship with her child and consequently the entire family. Family affection, concern, and questions should never be considered an interference. Instead, the family should be seen as collaborators in care. Answer questions and ask questions related to parents' questions to clarify further and inform or reinforce their ideas. Ideally, if the parent wishes, he or she should be allowed to stay with the child during care, procedures, tests, or treatments. If not feasible, one nurse should consistently care for the child while involving the parent as much as possible.

The parent needs to see the child receiving competent care and to feel that he or she is important to the child and capable as a parent, even if staying with the child is not possible. Encourage the parent to talk about feelings of fear, anxiety, guilt, shame, or sadness that may be present and related to the child's illness or hospitalization or children left at home. Avoid a critical attitude, voice tone, or disapproving nonverbal behavior that conveys to the parent that he or she is not managing well as a parent. Help parents to talk about the unique aspects of their child's or family life so that care can be truly individualized. For example, the child may prefer to wear his shorts instead of pajamas in bed. If an African-American child with an intricate hairstyle that was just arranged before admission is admitted, do not automatically do a routine admission shampoo. Realize that the Asian or American Indian child may not talk as freely, at least initially, as the average Caucasian child, but this response reflects family and cultural childrearing practices and does not mean that the child is retarded or does not understand you.

Obtain a developmental history from the mother on admission and use it to plan care to follow the child's usual living routine. Of great importance is the attitude of the staff caring for the child. The staff should be like the ideal parent: loving, honest, respectful, accepting, consistent. Cajoling, threatening, or rejection cannot help the child cope with problems. Acknowledge that children suffer great physical and emotional pain. Help the child get in touch with feelings and the pain. Do not tell him or her not to cry or that a procedure will not hurt when it will. Help the child displace aggression onto toys or staff rather than onto parents. Allow the child to be angry. Objective involvement is also important to avoid showing favoritism to only certain children. Several authors describe practical ways to help the child prepare for and cope with painful procedures (35, 77).

PSYCHOSOCIAL CONCEPTS

Cognitive Development

The child in the Preoperational Stage is perceptually bound, unable to reason logically about concepts that are discrepant from visual cues. The child learns by being confronted with others' opinions and being actively involved with objects and processes (74). More important than the facts learned are the attitudes the child forms toward knowledge, learning, people, and the environment. Cognition and learning, at least partly a result of language learning and perceptual ability, can be studied through the child's handling of the physical environment and in connection with the concepts of number, casualty, and time, abstractions highly developed in Western civilization (67).

By helping parents understand the cognitive development of their child, including concept formation, you will help them stimulate intellectual growth realistically, without expecting too much. **Concepts** *come about by giving precepts (events, things, and experiences) a meaningful label; the name or label implies similarity to some other things having the same name and difference from things having a different name.* **Concept formation** *develops with perception progressing from diffuse to roughly differentiated and finally to sharply differentiated awareness of stable and coordinated objects.* The first concept is formed when a word comes to designate a crudely defined area of experience. As the late toddler and early preschooler acquire a number of words, each presenting a loosely defined notion or thing, the global meaning becomes a simple concrete concept. As perceived characteristics of things and events become distinguished from each other, the child becomes aware of differences among words, objects, and experiences such as dog and cat, baby and doll, men and daddy, approval and disapproval; however, the preschooler cannot yet define attributes and cannot make explicit comparisons of the objects. The attributes are an absolute part of the object such as bark and dog; hence the child is said to *think concretely*. What he or she sees or hears can be named, which is different from conceptual or abstract thinking about the object (54, 67, 72).

Concrete concepts become true concepts when the late preschooler can compare, combine, and describe them and think and talk about their attributes. At this point the child can deal with differences between concepts such as "dogs bark, people talk," but not until after age 6 or 7 will he or she be able to deal with opposites and similarities together (22, 40, 54, 67, 72). See Categories of Concepts that Develop in the Preschool Years for more information.

Some of the influences on concept development include the following:

- The child's inability to distinguish between his or her own feelings and outside events
- The ability to be impressed by the external, obvious features of a situation or thing rather than its essential features
- Awareness of gaps in a situation
- Emotional or contextual significance of words.

▶ CATEGORIES OF CONCEPTS THAT DEVELOP IN THE PRESCHOOL YEARS

- **Life:** ascribes living qualities to inanimate objects
- **Death:** associates death with separation, lack of movement; thinks dead people capable of doing what living people do
- **Body functions:** has inaccurate ideas about body functions and birth process
- **Space:** judges short distances accurately; aware of direction and distance in relation to body
- **Weight:** estimates weight in terms of size; by age 5 can determine which of two objects feels heavier; notion of quantity—more than one, big, small
- **Numbers:** understands up to 5
- **Time:** has gradually increasing sense of time; present oriented; knows day of week, month, and year
- **Self:** knows sex, full name, names of outer body parts by age 3; when begins to play with other children, self-concept begins to include facts about his or her abilities and race but not socioeconomic class
- **Sex roles:** has general concept of sex, identity, and appropriate sex roles developed at age 5 or 6
- **Social awareness:** is egocentric but forms definite opinions about others' behavior as "nice" or "mean"; intuitive; concept of causality is magical, illogical
- **Beauty:** names major colors; prefers music with definite tune and rhythm
- **Comic:** considers as comic funny faces made by self or others, socially inappropriate behavior, and antics of pets

---

The concreteness typical of a preschooler's concepts is found in the rambling, loosely jointed circumstantial descriptions. Everything is equally important and must be included. One must listen closely to get the central theme as young children learn things in bunches and not in a systematic, organized way. They can memorize and recite many things, but they cannot paraphrase or summarize their learning (22, 40, 47, 67).

Concepts of Relationships

These concepts involve time, space, number, and causation, are more abstract than those based on the immediately observable properties of things, and are greatly determined by culture (22, 67).

Time Concept

For the preschooler, time is beginning to move; the past is measured in hours, and the future is a myth. At first formal time concepts have nothing to do with personal time. Adults are seen as changeless, and the child believes that he or she can mature in a hurry; thus the preschooler thinks he or she can grow up fast and marry his or her parent. Time concepts are further described in Table 9–4 (22, 33, 40, 54, 67, 72, 74).

Spatial Concepts

These concepts differ markedly in children and adults. There are five major stages in the development of spatial concepts. First, there is **action space,** *consisting of the location or regions to which the child moves.* Second, **body space** *refers to the child's own awareness of directions and distances in relation to his or her own body.* Third, there is **object space,** *in which objects are located relative to each other and without reference to the child's body.* The fourth and fifth stages, **map space** and **abstract space,** are *interrelated and depend on knowing directions of east, west, south, and north; allocating space in visual images to nations, regions, towns, rooms; and the ability to deal with maps, geographic or astronomic ideas, and three-dimensional space* that use symbolic (verbal or mathematical) relationships (67).

The preschool child has action space and moves along familiar locations and explores new terrain. He or she is beginning to orient self to body space and object space through play and exploration of his or her own body, up and down, front and back, sideways, next to, near and far, and later left and right. The child is not able until approximately age 6 to understand object space as a unified whole; he or she will first see a number of unrelated routes or spaces. He or she is generally aware of specific objects and habitual routes. The child does not see self and objects as part of a larger integrated space with multiple possibilities for movement. *Map space and abstract space are not understood until later.*

Quantitative Concepts

Notions of quantity such as one and more than one, bigger, and smaller are developed in the early preschool years. Understanding of the quantity or amount represented by a number is not related to the child's ability to count to 10, 20, or higher, nor can he or she transfer numbers to notions of value of money, although he or she may imitate adults and play store, passing money back and forth. Ordinal numbers, indicating successions rather than totals, develop crudely in "me first" or "me last"; the concept of second or third develops later. The preschooler cannot simultaneously take account of different dimensions such as 1 quart equals 2 pints and equal volume in different-shaped containers (33, 40, 67, 70, 72). (See also Table 9–4.)

Concepts of Causality

The way of perceiving cause and effect is marginal. Things simply are. The child may be pleased or displeased with events but does not understand what brought them about. He or she does precausal thinking, confusing physical and mechanical causation or natural phenomena with psychological, moral, or sequential causes. He or she frequently says "n' then," indicating causal sequence. When the child asks "why?" he or she is probably looking for justification rather than causation. Most things are taken for granted; the child assumes that people, including self, or some motivated inanimate being is the cause of events. Perception of the environment is **animistic,** *endowing all things with the qualities of life Westerners reserve for human beings.* There is little notion of accident or coincidence. It takes some time to learn that there are impersonal forces at work in the world. Thinking is also **egocentric:** *things and events are seen from a personal and narrow perspective and are happening because of self* (7, 47, 67).

The late preschooler fluctuates between reality and fantasy and a materialistic and animistic view of the world; most adults never completely leave behind the magical thinking typical of the preschooler. The child plays with the idea of a tree growing out of the head, what holes feel like to the ground, and growing up starting as an adult. The adult finds no meaning in music, art, literature, love, and possibly even science and mathematics without fantasy or magic.

Preoperational Stage

The Preoperational Stage is divided into the Preconceptual and Intuitive Phases (22, 26, 70, 72). During the **Preconceptual Phase,** *from 2 to 4 years of age, the child gathers facts as they are encountered but can neither separate reality from fantasy nor classify or define events in a systematic manner.* Ability to define properties of an object or denote hierarchies or relationships among elements in a class is lacking. He or she is beginning to develop mental strategies from concept formation; concepts are constructed in a global way. He or she is capable of perceiving gross outward appearances but sees only one aspect of an object or situation at a time. For example, if you say, "Take the yellow pill," he or she will focus on either yellow or pill but cannot focus on both aspects at once. The child is unable to use time, space, equivalence, and class inclusion in concept formation. During the **Intuitive phase,** *lasting from approximately 4 to 7 years, the child gains increasing, but still limited, ability to develop concepts.* He or she defines one property at a time, has difficulty stating the defini-

TABLE 9–4. ASSESSMENT OF MENTAL DEVELOPMENT

3 Years	4 Years	5 Years
Knows he or she is a person separate from another Knows own sex and some sex differences	Senses self one among many	Aware of cultural and other differences between people and the two sexes Mature enough to fit into simple type of culture Can tell full name and address Remains calm if lost away from home
Resists commands but distractible and responsive to suggestions Can ask for help Desire to please Friendly Sense of humor	States alibis because more aware of attitude and opinions of others Self-critical; appraises good and bad of self Does not like to admit inabilities; excuses own behavior Praises self; bosses or criticizes others Likes recognition for achievement Heeds others' thoughts and feelings; expresses own	Dependable Increasing independence Can direct own behavior; but fatigue, excessive demands, fantasy, and guilt interfere with assuming self-responsibility Admits when needs help Moves from direct to internalized action, from counting what he or she can touch to counting in thought; uses more clues
Uses language rather than physical activity to communicate	Active use of language Active learning Likes to make rhymes, to hear stories with exaggeration and humor, dramatic songs Knows nursery rhymes Tells action implied in picture books	Improves use of symbol system, concept formation Repeats long sentences accurately Can carry plot in story Defines objects in terms of use States relationship between two events
Imaginative Better able to organize thoughts Can bargain with him or her Sacrifices immediate pleasure for promise of future gain	Highly imaginative yet literal, concrete thinking Can organize his or her experience Increasing reasoning power and critical thinking capacity Makes crude comparisons	Less imaginative Asks details Can be reasoned with logically More accurate, relevant, practical, sensible than 4-year-old Asks to have words defined Seeks reality
Understands simple directions; follows normal routines of family life and does minor errands	Concept of 1, 2, 3; counts to 5; does some home chores Generalizes	Begins to understand money Does more home chores with increasing competence Can determine which of two weights heavier Idea in head precedes drawing on paper or physical activity Interested in meaning of relatives
Knows age Meager comprehension of past and future Knows mostly today	Realizes birthday is one in a series and that birthday is measure of growth Knows when next birthday is Knows age Birthday and holidays significant because aware of units of time Loves parties related to holiday Conception of time Knows day of week	Understands week as a unit of time Knows day of week Sense of time and duration increasing Knows how old will be on next birthday Knows month and year Adults seen as changeless Memory surprisingly accurate
Has attention span of 10–15 minutes	Has attention span of 20 min	Has attention span of 30 minutes

tion, but knows how to use the object. The child uses **transductive logic,** *going from general to specific in explanation,* rather than deductive or inductive logic. He or she begins to label, classify in ascending or descending order, do seriation, and note cause–effect relationships, even though true cause–effect understanding does not occur (26, 56, 70, 72).

The Preoperational Stage is characterized by the following (47, 54, 56, 72):

- Egocentric thought
- Literal thinking with absence of reference system
- Intermingling of fantasy, intuition, and reality
- **Absolute thought,** *seeing all or nothing without shades of gray or any relativity*
- **Centering,** *focusing on a single aspect of an object,* causing distorted reasoning
- Lack of concept of **reversibility,** *for every action, there is one that cancels it*
- Static thinking
- Difficulty remembering what he or she started talking about so that when the sentence is finished he or she is talking about something else
- Inability to state cause–effect relationships, categories, or abstractions, believing that events that occur together belong together

In general, the preschooler has a consuming curiosity. Learning is vigorous, aggressive, and intrusive. The imagination creates many situations he or she wishes to explore. Judgment is overshadowed by curiosity and excitement. The preschooler has begun to develop such concepts as friend, aunt, uncle; accepting responsibility; independence; passage of time, spatial relationships; use of abstract words, numbers, colors; and the meaning of cold, tired, and hungry. Attention span is lengthening.

The child's ability to grasp reality varies with individual intelligence and potential intelligence, the social milieu, and opportunities to explore the world, solve problems independently, ask questions, and get answers. Table 9–4 summarizes major characteristics of mental development to help you in assessment (32, 33, 54, 56, 67, 70, 72).

An educational trend is underway to teach the preschooler more factual content and to provide some schooling from infancy on as seen in the large number of preschoolers in the United States who are enrolled in pre-primary-school programs. Impetus for this trend stems from the following:

- Head Start program in the 1960s
- Women's liberation campaigns for day-care centers

- Growing realization by the middle class that competition for school achievement and college entrance will remain intense
- Awareness that most of the brain is developed by age 4
- Theory that at least half of all human intelligence is developed by age 4, possibly even earlier (Another theory states that by age 5 the intelligence quotient [IQ] is basically established, that attitudes toward learning and patterns of thinking will guide the child for the rest of his or her life [67, 70]; however, he or she needs informal learning opportunities, not facts.)

Parents can enhance the child's growth by realizing the importance of the following approaches. Share this information with them. Refer to the article by Pontious (56) for ways to explain nursing procedures to a child.

The single most critical factor in the child's learning is a loving caretaker, as that is whom the child imitates. How the mothering person speaks to, touches, and plays with the child governs the potential for socialization and cognitive development. This is true even for the child who had a low birth weight and was at risk for developmental lag or disability (67). A child's problem-solving abilities are shaped by the parents' method for handling problems and by opportunities for problem solving. In families in which everyone gets a chance to speak out and jointly explore a problem, the child learns to express him or herself logically. Automatic obedience or acceptance of parental commands or decisions will interfere with reasoning (7). Important also are the opportunities provided for the child to learn, encouraging him or her to handle objects, explore, ask questions, and play a variety of games. In the home the child learns how to learn or how not to learn. Teaching the child is more than telling him or her what to do. It involves demonstration, listening, and talking about the situation in direct and understandable terms and giving reasons. Cognitive development includes more than fluency with words, a good verbal memory, and information. It includes ability to use imagination, form mental pictures, and engage in fantasy appropriately, along with art, music, and other creative activities. It includes expanding skills in logical thinking. Most important, it involves increasing integration of many kinds of brain functions. Much integrated learning comes from the child's engaging in motor activity, play, and language games; talking with adults and peers; and paying attention to both trivial and important aspects of the environment (7, 47).

Creative methods of teaching for preschoolers are seen in educational programs such as *Sesame Street and Mister Rogers' Neighborhood. Sesame Street,* presented as a lively, fast-moving, colorful program, emphasizes the alphabet, number concepts, similarities and differences, and positive body image. *Mister Rogers' Neighborhood* emphasizes positive body image, learning how things are done, and a personal one-to-one relationship between Mister Rogers and each child. It is difficult to assess the effect of these programs on the overall cognitive development of the child. Such programs appear to improve rote learning, although there is not much evidence that long-range concept formation is much different from what develops in children not exposed to these programs.

Because television is essentially a passive and solitary activity, more than occasional viewing may interfere with the purposes that more traditional play activities offer (see section on Play Patterns). Thus, television viewing can negatively affect self-concept and social skills, as well as motor, cognitive, and emotional learning (22, 70).

Explore the use of television with parents. You can teach parents to see themselves as a parent educator rather than as "only a housewife" or "his pal, Dad." Parents can stimulate the intellectual development of their child by providing various practices: creating many and varied opportunities to learn about people and their environment; avoiding doing too much for the child; sharing activities with him or her; talking to him or her about situations the adult and child are in (shopping, cooking a meal, laundering); providing an interesting home; giving the child freedom to roam and follow natural curiosity within safe limits; giving daily individual attention to the child; obtaining information about child development and rearing from books, films, and other parents; experimenting with games and childrearing practices and observing feedback from the child to determine which meet his or her needs; and avoiding the push to learn academic subjects too early, causing undue frustration and a negative attitude about learning and school later. The child will sense which activities provide interest and challenges without excess difficulty. Let him or her develop his or her own learning style and see you and other adults as sources of information and ideas.

Communication Patterns

People have three types of communication at their disposal: (1) somatic or physical symptoms such as flushed skin color and increased respirations; (2) action such as play or movement; and (3) verbal expression. The preschool child uses all of them.

Learning to use verbal expression—language—to communicate is an ongoing developmental process that is affected directly by the child's interaction with others. Language skills are enhanced, expanded, and refined as the child explores ideas with others and experiences a variety of social and educational environments. Language, cognition, and socialization are complex and interwoven. Verbal reasoning ability is dependent on the audible monologue of early toddler thinking, which then develops into inner speech and verbal thought (22, 26, 40, 70).

The child uses *language* for many reasons:

- To maintain social rapport
- To gain attention
- To get information
- To seek meaning about his or her experience
- To note how others' answers fit personal thoughts
- To play with words
- To gain relief from anxiety

He or she asks why, what, when, where, how, repeatedly.

A child learns language from hearing it and using it. Words are at first empty shells until he or she has experiences to match. Parents should provide age-appropriate experiences so the child learns that words and actions go together. Equally important, parents should avoid saying one thing and doing another. Attaining trust in the utility and validity of verbal communication, learning that talking helps rather than hinders life, is crucial to transition from infancy to school years. If talking does not gain response from others or help the child solve problems and relate to those he or she needs or if the world is too troublesome, the child is likely to find refuge in fantasy and neglect social, communicative meanings of language.

Directing his or her own life depends on language and an understanding of the meaning of words and logic with which they are used. When the child acquires language, he or she gradually becomes freed from tangible, concrete experiences and can internalize visual symbols, develop memory and recall, fragment the past, project the future, and differentiate fantasy from reality.

Language is also learned from being read to and having printed material available. Share the following suggestions with parents for choosing books for the preschooler. The book should be durable, have large print that does not fill the entire page, and be colorfully illustrated. The concepts should be expressed concretely in simple sentences and should tell a tale that fits the child's fantasy conception of the world, such as a story with animals and objects who can talk and think like people. Or the story should tell about the situations he or she ordinarily faces such as problems with playmates, discovery of the preschooler's world, night-mares, and the arrival of a new baby.

Follow and share with the significant adults in the child's life these *effective ways of talking with the preschooler* listed in Table 9–5.

Table 9–6 is a guide for assessing language skills of the preschooler. During assessment keep in mind that how the child's parents and other family members

TABLE 9–5. GUIDELINES FOR COMMUNICATION WITH A PRESCHOOLER

1. Be respectful as you talk with the child.

2. Do not discourage talking, questions, or the make-believe in the child's language; verbal explorations are essential to learn language. Answers to questions should meet needs and give him or her an awareness of adult attitudes and feelings about the topics discussed.

3. Tell the truth to the best of your ability and on the child's level of understanding. Do not say an injection "won't hurt." Say, "It's like a pin prick that will hurt a short time." Admit if the answer is unknown, and seek the answer with the child. A lie is eventually found out and causes a loss of trust in that adult and in others.

4. Do not make a promise unless you can keep it.

5. The child takes every word literally. Do not say, "She nearly died laughing," or "I laughed my head off." Do not describe surgery as "putting you to sleep."

6. Respond to the relationship or feelings in the child's experience rather than the actual object or event. Talk about the child's feelings instead of agreeing or disagreeing with what he or she says. Help the child understand what he or she feels rather than why he or she feels it.

7. Precede statements of advice and instruction with a statement of understanding of the child's feelings. When the child is feeling upset emotionally, he or she cannot listen to instructions, advice, consolation, or constructive criticism.

8. Do not give undue attention to slang or curse words, and do not punish the child for using them. The child is demonstrating initiative and uses these words for shock value, and attention or punishment emphasizes the importance of the words. Remain relaxed and give the child a more difficult or different word to say. If he or she persists in using the unacceptable word, the adult may say, "I'm tired of hearing that word, say_____"; ask him or her not to say the word again since it may hurt others, or use distraction. Children learn unacceptable words as they learn all others, and parents would be wise to listen to their own vocabulary.

9. Sit down if possible when participating or talking with children. You are more approachable when at their physical and eye level.

10. Seek to have a warm, friendly relationship without thrusting yourself on the child. How you feel about the child is more important than what you say or do.

11. Through attentive listening and interested facial expression, convey a tell-me-more-about-it attitude to encourage the child to communicate.

12. Regard some speech difficulties as normal. Ignore stuttering or broken fluency that does not persist. Do not correct each speech error and do not punish. Often the child thinks faster than he or she can articulate speech. Give the child time when he or she speaks.

13. Talk in a relaxed manner. Do not bombard the child with verbal information.

speak and the language opportunities the child has influence considerably his or her language skills.

Play Patterns

Play is the work of the child. Play occupies most of the child's waking hours and serves to consolidate and enlarge his or her previous learning and promote adaptation. Play has elements of reality, and there is an earnestness about it. Piaget described play as assimilation; play behavior involves taking in, molding, and using objects for pleasure and learning (54).

The preschooler is intrusive in play, bombarding others by purposeful or accidental physical attack. He or she is into people's ears and minds by loud, assertive talking; into space by vigorous gross motor activities; into objects through exploration; and into the unknown by consuming curiosity (27).

The preschool years are the pregang stage in which the child progresses from solitary and parallel play to cooperating for a longer time in a larger group. He or she identifies somewhat with a play group; follows rules; is aware of the status of self compared with others; develops perception of social relationships; begins the capacity for self-criticism; and states traits and characteristics of others that he or she likes or dislikes. At first the child spends brief, incidental periods of separation from the parents. The time away from them increases in length and frequency, and eventually the orientation shifts from family to peer group (25, 47, 51, 53, 67, 70).

A **peer** is a *person with approximately equal status, a companion, often of the same sex and age,* with whom one can share mutual concerns. The **peer group** is a *relatively informal association of equals who share common play experiences with emphasis on common rules and understanding the limits that the group places on the individual.* The preschool play group differs from later ones in that it is loosely organized. The activity of the group may be continuous; but membership changes as the child joins or leaves the group at will, and the choice of playmates is relatively restricted in kind and number. This is the first introduction to a group that assesses him or her as a child from a child's point of view. The preschooler is learning about entering a new, different, very powerful world when he or she joins the group. Although social play is enjoyed, the child feels a need for solitary play at times (26, 70).

The number and sex of siblings and the parent's handling of the child's play seem to influence behavior with the play group. If the family rejects the child, he or she may feel rejected by peers, even when the child

TABLE 9–6. ASSESSMENT OF LANGUAGE DEVELOPMENT

3 Years	4 Years	5 Years
Appearance of individual sounds *y, f, v* in words	Appearance of individual sounds *sh, zh, th* in words	Appearance of individual sounds *s, z, th, r, ch, j* in words
Vocabulary of at least 900, up to 2000, words	Vocabulary of at least 1500, up to 3000, words	Vocabulary of at least 2100, up to 5000, words
Uses language understandably; uses some sounds experimentally	Uses language confidently	Uses language efficiently, correctly
Understands simple reasons	Concrete speech	No difficulty understanding others' spoken words
Uses some adjectives and adverbs	Increasing attention span	Meaningful sentences; uses future tense
	Uses "I" and other pronouns	Increasing skill with grammar
	Imitates and plays with words	Knows common opposites
	Defines a few simple words	
	Talks in sentences; uses past tense	
	Uses plurals frequently	
	Comprehends prepositions	
Talks in simple sentences about things	Talks incessantly while doing other activities	Talks constantly
Repeats sentence of six syllables	Asks many questions	No infantile articulation
Uses plurals in speech	Demands detailed explanations with "why"	Repeats sentences of 12 or more syllables
Collective monologue; does not appear to care whether another is listening	Carries on long involved conversation	Asks searching questions, meaning of words, how things work
Some random, inappropriate answers	Exaggerates; boasts; tattles; may use profanity for attention	Can tell a long story accurately, but may keep adding to reality to make story more fantastic
Intelligibility is 70–90%	Frequently uses "everything"	Intelligibility good; some distortion in articulation of *t, s*
Sings simple songs	Tells family faults outside of home without restraint	Sings relatively well
	Tells story combining reality and fantasy; appears to be lying	
	Intelligibility is 90%; articulation errors with *l, r, s, z, sh, ch, j, th*	
	Variation in volume from a yell to a whisper	
	Likes to sing	
Knows first and family name	Calls people names	Counts to 10 or further without help
Names figures in a picture	Names three objects he or she knows in succession	Repeats five digits
Repeats three digits	Counts to 5 without help	Names four colors, usually red, green, blue, yellow
Likes to name things	Repeats four digits	
	Knows which line is longer	
	Names one or more colors	
Talks to self or imaginary playmate	Talks with imaginary playmate of same sex and age	Sense of social standards and limits seen in language use
Expresses own desires and limits frequently	Seeks reassurance	
	Interested in things being funny	
	Likes puns	

is not rejected, causing self-isolation, inability to form close friendships, and ultimately real rejection.

Purposes of Play

The natural mode of expression for the child is play. Purposes of play include the following:

- Develop and improve muscular strength, coordination, and balance; define body boundaries
- Work off excess physical energy; provide exercise
- Communicate with others, establish friendships, learn about interpersonal relations, and develop concern for others
- Learn cooperation, sharing, and healthy competition
- Express imagination, creativity, and initiative
- Imitate and learn about social activity, adult roles, and cultural norms
- Test and deal with reality, gain mastery over unpleasant experiences
- Explore, investigate, and manipulate features of the adult world; sharpen the senses and concentration

Case Situation: Preschooler Development

Kalisha is an active, 38-month-old girl, who weighs 34 pounds (15.45 kg) and is 38 in. (95 cm) tall. She is playing on the sidewalk in front of her parents' home with her brother Marvin, 4 years old, and her next-door neighbor Lori, aged 5 years.

Kalisha is riding her small, two-wheeled bicycle, which has training wheels. Marvin and Lori are riding their small bicycles or scooters. Kalisha rides for a while, then stops to watch the others. Although involved in the same activity, she plays next to rather than with the older children. Several times Kalisha rides her bicycle into the path of her brother's approaching bicycle. The preschooler is typically intrusive in play, bombarding others by purposeful or accidental attack. Kalisha continues to ride and stop, always staying within her mother's view as she moves farther away and then nearer on her bicycle. She demonstrates the attachment behavior typical of this age by maintaining proximity to her mother.

When Marvin and Lori ride down the street, leaving Kalisha, she asks her mother to go with her to join them. She pulls her mother's hand insis-tently several times, and they walk together down the street. When she approaches the other children, Kalisha runs to them, laughing, and then gives Lori a hug. Lori chases Kalisha up the street, and Kalisha laughs and runs to her mother, seeking protection, security, assurance, and approval. Through this behavior she affirms that her mother is still the most important person in her life.

As the older children ride their bicycles on the sidewalk toward Kalisha, she laughs and shouts, then waves her arms, telling them, "I am the stop sign." She tells Lori to stop, but Lori rides by, laughing and saying, "You'll have to give me a ticket." On the return trip, Lori stops at Kalisha's command. Kalisha and Lori repeat this pattern several times, and each time Kalisha becomes more animated. She demonstrates autonomy and beginning initiative in these interactions, displaying the egocentrism typical of the preschooler as she commands events for her own needs and purposes and gains a sense of power through symbolic play.

- Learn about rules of chance and probability and rules of conduct and that at times one loses, but it is all right
- Build self-esteem
- Feel a sense of power, make things happen, explore and experiment
- Provide for intellectual, sensory, and language development and dealing with concrete experiences in symbolic terms
- Assemble novel aspects of the environment
- Organize life's discrepancies privately and with others
- Learn about self and how others see him or her
- Practice leader and follower roles
- Have fun, express joy, and feel the pleasure of mastery
- Act out and symbolically work through a painful physical or emotional state by repetition in play so that it is more bearable and assimilated into the child's self-concept; master overwhelming stimuli
- Develop the capacity to gratify self and to delay gratification
- Formulate a bridge between concrete experiences and abstract thought

Types of Play Related to Social Characteristics and Common Themes in Children's Play give more insight into children's play (46, 67, 70, 77).

Play Materials

These materials should be simple, sturdy, durable, and free from unnecessary hazards. They need not be expensive. The child should have adequate space and equipment that is unstructured enough to allow for creativity and imagination to work unfettered. He or she will enjoy trips to parks and playgrounds. (The parents should be sure the child is not playing at dumps or at contaminated landfills.) Often creative, stimulating toys can be made from ordinary household articles: plastic pot cleaners, empty thread spools, a bell, yarn, or empty boxes covered with washable adhesive paper. The child may like the box more than the toy.

Increasing emphasis is being placed on high-technology, interactive, and weaponry toys. These toys actually stifle imagination and discovery, and weaponry toys may cause fears, heighten aggressive fantasies, and cause injury and sometimes death. Weaponry toys should be avoided as much as possible. Young children

► **TYPES OF PLAY RELATED TO SOCIAL CHARACTERISTICS**

- **Onlooker play:** Child watches others with no interactions or movement toward participation (e.g., use of television).
- **Parallel play:** Child plays independently but next to other children; displays no group association.
- **Associative play:** Children play together in similar or identical play without organization, division of labor, leadership, or mutual goals.
- **Cooperative play:** Play is organized in group with others. There are planning and cooperation before play starts to form goals, division of labor, and leadership.
- **Solitary play:** Child, either by choice or because of lack of peers, entertains self in play. Play is often imaginative or studylike in nature.
- **Supplementary play:** Play shifts from large group activities or games to focus on smaller group or board games.

Data from references 67 and 77.

► **COMMON THEMES IN CHILDREN'S PLAY**

- Various issues in the child's life will be repeated four to five times in each play session. These issues are shown in different styles of play, but the theme is the thread that ties all the different styles together, as the pieces of a quilt unite to form the pattern of the whole.
- Power/control
- Anger/sadness
- Trust/relationships/abandonment
- Nurturing/rejection/security
- Boundaries/intrusion
- Violation/protection
- Self-esteem
- Fears/anxiety (separation, monsters, ghosts, animals, the dark, noises, bad people, injury, death)
- Confusion
- Identity
- Loyalty/betrayal
- Loss/death
- Loneliness
- Adjustment/change

need to direct their games to be in control of their play and their fantasies. They use play to work out problems, to practice skills, and to act out roles in preparation for later real life experiences. If the toy is too limiting, it will be cast aside by the child, regardless of how much the parent enjoys it. Some toys from infancy and toddlerhood are still enjoyed.

The play materials that are available will determine the play activities. Play materials are enjoyed for different reasons. For example, **physical activity,** *which facilitates development of motor skills,* is provided through play with musical instruments and records for marching and rhythm, balls, shovel, broom, ladder, swing, trapeze, slide, boxes, climbing apparatus, boards, sled, wagon, tricycle, bicycle with training wheels, wheelbarrow, and blocks. Swimming, ice skating, roller skating, and skiing are being learned. **Dramatic play,** *which is related to the ability to classify objects correctly, take another's perspective, and do problem solving,* is afforded through large building blocks, sandbox and sand toys, dolls, housekeeping toys, nurse and doctor kits, farm or other occupational toys, cars and other vehicles, and worn out adult clothes for dress-up. This is a predominant form of play in childhood and also can include aspects of physical play. **Creative playthings,** *which promote constructive, nonsocial, cognitive, and emotional development,* include blank sheets of paper, crayons, finger or water paints, chalk, various art supplies, clay, plasticine, or other manipulative material, blunt scissors, paste, cartons, scraps of cloth, water-play equip-

ment, and musical toys. **Quiet play,** *which promotes cognitive development and rest from physical exertion,* is achieved through books, puzzles, records, and table games. Children's songs, nursery rhymes, and fairy tales can absorb anxiety, entertain, soothe, reassure that life's problems can be solved, and support the child's superego (7, 23, 24, 47, 51, 53, 70).

The role of the adult in child's play is to provide opportunity, equipment, and safety and to avoid interference or structuring of play. (However, parents may need to restrict television watching, and children often want the structure of bedtime stories.) Allow the child to try things and enjoy personal activities. Assist only if he or she is in need of help. The child is not natural in play when he or she thinks adults are watching; avoid showing amusement or ridicule of play behavior or conversation. Allow playmates to work out their own differences. Distract, redirect, or substitute a different activity if the children cannot share and work out their problems. There are times to play with the child, but avoid overstimulation, teasing, hurry, talking about him or her as if he or she were not present, or doing the activity for the child. Let him or her take the lead. Try to enter the child's world. If he or she wants you to attend the teddy bear's 100th birthday party, go. A book that is creatively illustrated and gives many ideas for play activity for and with the preschooler is *Learning Through Play* by Jean Marzolla and Janice Lloyd (51).

Table 9–7 summarizes play characteristics as a further aid in assessment and teaching (7, 23, 24, 32, 33, 47, 51, 53, 70).

Share the above information with parents and explore their feelings about child's play and their role with the child.

Guidance and Discipline

The child learns how to behave by imitating adults and by using the opportunities to develop self-control. If the adult tells the child, "Tell him I'm not home" when the child answers the door, the child may at first be astonished, then accept the lie, and eventually use this behavior too.

The child needs consistent, fair, and kind limits to feel secure, to know that the parents care for and love him or her enough to provide protection—a security he or she does not have when allowed to do anything, regardless of ability. Limits should be set in a way that preserves the self-respect of the child and parent and should not be applied angrily, violently, arbitrarily, or capriciously, but rather with the intent to educate and build character. Only when the child can predict the behavior of others can he or she accept the need to inhibit or change some of his or her behavior and work toward predictable and rational behavior. The parent should be an ally to the child as he or she struggles for control over inner impulses and convey to the child that he or she need not fear impulses.

The preschooler needs discipline that is permissive with limits; however, *permissive discipline* must be distinguished from *overpermissive* discipline. **Permissive discipline** *accepts the childish behavior of the child as normal and recognizes that the child is a person with a right to have all kinds of feelings and wishes that may be expressed directly or symbolically.* It sets realistic limits but is not harsh or demanding of perfection. The adult should distinguish between the wish and act and set limits on the act, not on the wish. Feelings and wishes must be identified and expressed verbally or through other outlets; it may be necessary to limit or redirect actions as destructive behavior cannot be tolerated.

Overpermissive discipline *permits undesirable behavior that can become harmful or destructive.* It causes the child to feel insecure and anxious; he or she perceives others' disapproval and believes that the parents do not care. Further, the child is unable to accomplish what he or she is ready to do because of lack of external or self-control; and he or she does not learn to

like self. In turn, fantasies will increase, and the child will demand more privileges than should be granted. The vicious circle is uncomfortable for adult and child alike.

Share the above information, and explore with parents the importance of their guidance to the child. *Techniques for guidance and limit setting* that would be helpful to you personally in working with children and should be shared with parents when indicated are as follows (7, 47, 52):

- Convey authority without anger or threat to avoid feelings of resentment, fear, or guilt.
- Be positive, clear, and consistent; let the child know what is acceptable behavior.
- Place specific limits on special actions when the occasion arises, maintaining some flexibility in rules.
- Recognize the child's wish, and put it into words, "You *wish* you could have that but ...." Point out ways the wish can be partially fulfilled when possible.
- Help the child express some resentment likely to arise when restrictions are imposed. "I realize you don't like the rules but ...."
- Enforce discipline by adhering to the stated rules kindly but firmly. Do not argue about them nor initiate a battle of wills. Spanking is one way to discipline, but it may show the child an undesirable way of handling frustration. Spanking may interfere with superego development by relieving guilt too easily; the child feels he or she has paid for the misbehavior and is free to return to mischievous activity.
- Positive suggestions rather than commands and "don'ts" help the child to learn how to get what he or she wants at the time and how to form happy relationships with others.
- If the child has no choice about a situation, give direction that conveys what he or she has to do, for example, "It is time now to ...."
- Convey that adults are present to help the child solve problems that cannot be solved alone.
- Control the situation if the child has temporarily lost self-control; remove him or her from the stimulating event; stay with the child; talk quietly; use distraction or diversion if necessary; encourage thinking through the problem and finding a fair solution after he or she has become calm. Convey that you feel the child can regain self-control and handle the situation and can rejoin the group or continue the former activity when he or she feels ready.

TABLE 9–7. ASSESSMENT OF PLAY CHARACTERISTICS

3 Years	4 Years	5 Years
Enjoys active and sedentary play	Increasing physical and social play	More varied activity More graceful in play
Likes toys in orderly form Puts away toys with supervision	Puts away toys when reminded	Puts away toys by self
Fantasy not yielding too much to reality Likes fairy tales, books	Much imaginative and dramatic play Has complex ideas but unable to carry out because of lack of skill and time	More realistic in play Less interested in fairy tales More serious and ready to know reality Restrained but creative
Likes solitary and parallel play with increasing social play in shifting groups of two or three	Plays in groups of two or three, often companions of own sex Imaginary playmates Projects feelings and deeds onto peers or imaginary playmates May run away from home	Plays in groups of five or six Friendships stronger and continue over longer time Chooses friends of like interests Spurred on in activity by rivalry
Cooperates briefly Willing to wait turn and share with suggestion	Suggests and accepts turns but often bossy in directing others Acts out feelings spontaneously, especially with music and arts	Generous with toys Sympathetic, cooperative, but quarrels and threatens by word or gesture Acts out feelings Wants rules to do things right; but beginning to realize peers cheat, so develops mild deceptions and fabrications
Some dramatic play-house or family games Frequently changes activity Likes to arrange, combine, transfer, sort, and spread objects and toys	Dramatic and creative play at a peak Likes to dress up and help with household tasks; plays with dolls, trucks Does not sustain role in dramatic play; moves from one role to another incongruous role No carry over in play from day to day Silly in play	Dramatic play about most life events, but more realistic Play continues from day to day Interested in finishing what started, even if it takes several days More awareness of yesterday and tomorrow
Able to listen longer to nursery rhymes Dramatizes nursery rhymes and stories Can match simple forms Enjoys cutting, pasting, block building Enjoys simple puzzles, hand puppets, large ball Enjoys sand and water play Enjoys dumping and hauling toys Rides tricycle	Concentration span longer Sometimes so busy at play forgets to go to toilet Reenacts stories and trips Enjoys simple puzzles and models with trial-and-error method Poor space perception Uses constructive and manipulative play material increasingly Enjoys sand and water play; cups, containers, and buckets for carrying and pouring Enjoys crayons and paints, books Enjoys swing, jungle gym, toy hammer or other tools, pegboards	Perceptive to order, form, and detail Better eye–hand coordination Rhythmic motion to music; enjoys musical instruments Likes excursions Interested in world outside immediate environment; enjoys books Enjoys cutting out pictures, pasting, working on special projects, puzzles Likes to run and jump, play with bicycle, wagon, and sled Enjoys sand and water play; dramatic and elaborative in play Enjoys using tools and equipment of adults

Data from References 32, 33, and 51.

A behavior modification technique that can be used to discipline an aggressively acting out child is *time-out*. Time-out involves immediately placing the child after a mean act in a quiet, uninteresting place (hall, small room, or corner of a room) for 5 to 15 minutes to remove the child from positive reinforcement. Time-out stops the misbehavior and is unpleasant enough to increase the possibility that the child will not repeat the undesirable act. The child learns accountability for behavior when time-out is linked to rules, limits, and extreme behavior. The child as part of the family unit should have input into formulating the rules and limits and the discipline method of time-out. This method should not be viewed by the child as a way to get out of cleanup or other tasks. During time-out the child may be requested to write sentences—positive and no longer than five words ("I will be polite"). Time-out is a method to help parents avoid nagging, spanking, screaming, lecturing, or being abusive and yet help parents feel in control and handle misbehavior so the child's behavior can improve. *The child should be helped to realize time-out means his or her behavior, not him or her, is rejected; thus, use of rewards to reinforce desired behavior is necessary* in conjunction with this time-out method.

Emotional Development

If the child has developed reasonably well and if he or she has mastered earlier developmental tasks, the preschooler is a source of pleasure to adults. He or she is more a companion than someone to care for. The various behaviors discussed under development of physical, mental, language, play, body image, and moral–spiritual aspects contribute to his or her emotional status and development. The beginning motor self-control, high-energy level, use of language, ability to delay somewhat immediate gratification, ability to tolerate separation from mother, curiosity, strong imagination, and desire to move, all propel him or her to plan; attack problems; start tasks; consider alternatives; learn aggressively; direct behavior with some thought, logic and judgment; and appear more self-confident and relaxed. Tolerance of frustration is still limited, but flares of temper and frustrations over failure pass quickly. As the child is learning to master things and handle independence and dependence, so is he or she increasing mastery of self and others and learning to get along with more people, both children and adults. The preschooler attempts to behave like an adult in realistic activity and play and is beginning to learn social roles, moral responsibility, and cooperation, although he or she still grabs, hits, and quarrels for short bursts of time. Table 9–8 summarizes common causes and emotional manifestations of various emotional states in preschoolers (32, 33, 47).

If the child has the opportunity to resolve the Oedipal triangle, to establish a sense of gender, and to identify with mature adults, if the attitude about self is sound and positive, and if he or she has learned to trust and have some self-control, he or she is ready to take on the culture. The preschooler begins to decide what kind of person he or she is, and self-concept, ego strength, and superego will continue to mature. Self is still very important, but he or she does not feel omnipotent.

TABLE 9–8. COMMON EMOTIONAL PATTERNS OF PRESCHOOLER

Emotion	Cause	Manifestation
Anger	Conflicts over playthings, thwarting of needs or wishes, attacks from another child	Temper tantrums; cries, screams, stomps, kicks, jumps, hits
Fear	Conditioning, imitation, and memories of unpleasant experiences; stories; pictures; TV; movies; dark; being locked in closed-in space or room	Panic reaction; runs away and hides, cries, avoids situation; withdraws from source of punishment
Jealousy	Attention from parent shifted to someone else in family, especially younger sibling	Open expression; regresses to infantile behavior; pretends to be ill; is naughty; seeks attention
Curiosity	Anything new; their own and others' bodies; replaces normal fears	Sensorimotor exploration, questions
Envy	Abilities or material possessions of another, e.g., older sibling	Complains about what he or she has, states wish for something else, steals object wanted
Joy	Physical well-being; uncongruous situation; sudden or unexpected noises; slight calamities; playing pranks on others; accomplishment of difficult task; music; drama; art	Smiles, laughs, claps hands, jumps up and down, hugs object or person
Grief	Loss, separation from loved person, pet, or object	Cries, is apathetic about daily activities, appears sad
Affection	Pleasure-giving persons, objects, or situations	Expresses verbally or nonverbally through smile, laugh, shout, hug, or words

Developmental Crisis

The psychosexual crisis for this era is initiative versus guilt, and all the aforementioned behaviors are part of achieving initiative (27). **Initiative** is *enjoyment of energy displayed in action, assertiveness, learning, increasing dependability, and ability to plan.* Natural initiative is desirable; however, it is important for parents not to expect too much or to push the child excessively. Studies indicate that teachers can identify type A behaviors in young children (competitiveness, impatience, hostility, pseudoleadership) and that these children have a cardiovascular responsivity similar to that of adults with type A behavior. Some of the type A behavior may be the result of innate temperament, but parental practices or behavior may also have an influence (11, 12).

If the child does not achieve the developmental task of initiative, there is an overriding sense of guilt from the tension between the demands of the superego, or expectations, and actual performance. One study indicated that children whose mothers were depressed for some duration (e.g., 1 year) scored lower in social competence and had more behavior problems (34).

Guilt is a *sense of defeatism, anger, feeling responsible for things that he or she is not really responsible for, feeling easily frightened from what he or she wants to do, feeling bad, shameful, and deserving of punishment.* A sense of guilt can develop from sibling rivalry, lack of opportunity to try things, or restriction on or lack of guidance in response to fantasy or when parents interfere with the child's activity. They stifle initiative by doing things for the child or by frequently asking, "Why didn't you do it better?" If the guilt feelings are too strong, the child is affected in a negative way. Excessive guilt does not enhance moral or superego development, although the child must experience realistic guilt for wrong behavior (7, 27, 47, 61). See Consequences of Guilt for a summary of this topic (27).

You can help parents understand that if the child is to develop a sense of initiative and a healthy personality, they and other significant adults must encourage use of imagination, creativity, activity, and plans. Punishment must be limited to those acts that are truly dangerous, morally wrong, socially unacceptable, or with a harmful or unfortunate consequence for self or others. Parents should encourage the child's efforts to cooperate and share in the decisions and responsibilities of family life. The child develops best when he or she is commended and recognized for accomplishments. Appropriate behavior should be reinforced so that it will continue. Affirming a child's emotional experience is as important as affirming his or her physical development. Parents

► **CONSEQUENCES OF GUILT**

- Guilt is an expression of a rigid superego. The child exercises strong self-control but displays evidence of resentment or bitterness to the restrictive adult.
- Stammering speech
- Poor motor coordination
- Eating and elimination problems
- Regressed or immature behavior
- Inability to separate from mother without extreme anxiety
- Fear of strangers
- Temper tantrums
- Lack of interest in childhood activities or peers
- Anxiety, easily frightened, irritability
- Nightmares
- Disorganized in behavior, not demonstrating age-appropriate neuromuscular, mental, or social skills

should set aside a time each day, perhaps near bedtime, for the child to review emotional experiences. If there has been joy, pride, or anger, it can be recounted to the parents. In talking, the child conjures up the feelings once again and integrates these feelings with the event. This promotes emotional growth. The preschooler needs to learn what feelings of love, hate, joy, and antagonism are and how to cope with and express them in ways other than physically. He or she needs guidance toward mature behavior.

Self-Concept: Body Image and Sexuality Development

Self-concept, including body image and sex role behavior, are gradually developing in these years (26, 32, 33, 40, 47, 70, 77). Positive self-concept develops from parental love, effective relations with peers and others, success in play and other activities, and gaining skills and self-control in activities of daily living. Body boundaries and sense of self become more definite to the preschooler because of developing sexual curiosity and awareness of how he or she differs from others, increased motor skills with precision of movement and maturing sense of balance, improved spatial orientation, maturing cognitive and language abilities, ongoing play activities, and relationship identification with his or her parents.

The pleasurable feelings associated with touching the body and genitals and with masturbation and play involving rocking or riding toys heighten self-awareness but also anxiety and anticipation of punishment. If the child is threatened or punished because of sexual curiosity, he or she may repress feelings about and awareness of the genitals or other body parts and develop a distorted body image. Of course, he or she must be taught that society does not condone handling of genitals in public. The preschooler must be able to stroke the body with affection; he or she needs adult caresses as well.

Learning about the body—where it begins and ends, what it looks like, and what it can do—is basic to the child's identity formation. Included in the growing self-awareness is discovery of feelings and learning names for them. The child is beginning to learn how he or she affects others and others' responses, and he or she is learning the rudiments of control over feelings and behavior. The concept of body is reflected in the way the child talks, draws pictures, and plays. The child with no frame of reference in relation to self has increased anxiety and misperception of self and others. Fantasies about self affect later behavior.

Parental and cultural attitudes about sex-appropriate behavior for boys and girls may heighten anxiety and body image confusion, especially if the child's behavior and appearance do not match the expectations of others.

The artistic productions of the preschooler tell us about self-perceptions. The 3-year-old draws a man consisting of one circle, sometimes with an appendage, a crude representation of the face, and no differentiation of parts. The 4-year-old draws a man consisting of a circle for a face and head, facial features of two eyes and perhaps a mouth, two appendages, and occasionally wisps of hair or feet. Often the 4-year-old has not really formulated a mental representation of the lower part of the body. The 5-year-old draws an unmistakable person. There is a circle face with nose, mouth, eyes, and hair; there is a body with arms and legs. Articles of clothing, fingers, and feet may be added. The width of the person is usually approximately one-half the length (24, 32, 33). The child may think of the body as a house (47). For example, while eating, he or she may name the various bites as fantasy characters who will go down and play in his or her house. The child may create an elaborate play area for them. (You can take advantage of this fantasy if eating problems arise.)

When the 3-year-old is asked his or her sex, the child is likely to give his or her name; the 4-year-old can state sex, thus showing a differentiation of self (26, 70).

Discuss with the parents the concept of body image and how they can help the child's formulation of self. The child needs opportunities to learn the correct names and basic functions of body parts and to discover his or her body with joy and pride. Mirrors, photographs of the child, drawings of self and others such as parents and siblings, weighing, and measuring height enhance the formation of his or her mental picture. The child needs physical and mental activity to learn body mastery and self-protection and to express feelings of helplessness, doubt, or pain when the body does not accomplish what he or she would like or during illness. The preschooler needs to manipulate the tools of his or her culture to learn the difference between self and machines, equipment, or tools. The child needs to be encouraged to "listen" to the body—the aches of stretched muscles, tummy rumblings, stubbed toes—and to understand what he or she feels. To deny, misinterpret, misname, or push aside physical or emotional activities and feelings promotes an unrealistic self-understanding and eventually a negative self-concept and unwhole body image. Specific nursing measures after illness or injury help the child reintegrate body image (7, 24, 77).

Adaptive Mechanisms

Development proceeds toward increasing differentiation, articulation, and integration. **Differentiation** involves a *progressive separation of feeling, thinking, and acting and an increased polarity between self and others.* Differentiation is seen in the child's ability to **articulate** or *talk about the perceived experience of the world and the experience of self as a being.* **Integration** is seen in the *development of structured controls and adaptive or defensive mechanisms* (47, 70).

With increasing differentiation, articulation of language, perceptions, and experience, and integration of experience and adaptive mechanisms into self, the child is better able to talk about fears and other feelings. The infant demonstrates behaviorally and through crying that he or she fears sudden movements, loud noises, loss of support, flashing lights, pain, strange people, objects, or situations, and separation from familiar people. The toddler's fears of being alone, the draining bathtub, the vacuum cleaner, the dark, dogs or other animals, high places, insecure footing, and separation from familiar people are expressed behaviorally and vocally, although the adult may have difficulty determining which fear is being expressed because of imprecise language skills. The preschooler has gained both language and conceptual ability, greater experience, and a greater imagination. Now he or she can talk about and play out the fears of being alone, ghosts, masks, the dark, strange noises, strangers, dogs, tigers, spiders, bears, and snakes, closed places, thunderstorms, and separation from loved ones. These fears decline by age 5 but may persist until age 7 or 8.

What the preschool child sees through the media or hears in stories (including traditional fairy tales) may produce great fear. The child has no way of knowing, unless explanations are given, that the big bad wolf will not eat him or her, or that the Indians attacking wagon trains will not attack his or her home next. Fears of ghosts, monsters, robbers, kidnappers, and other fantasized characters last through the preschool years until age 7 or 8, especially if parents do not talk about them and help the child differentiate between reality and imagination. Help parents realize that to instill realistic fear is adaptive: viewing and reading experiences that do not emphasize violence, bad people, or fearsome objects or animals, but rather gentle and calm experiences, are helpful for the child to gain a sense of self-control over fears.

The child encounters a variety of frustrations as he or she engages in new activities, expects more of self, and others expect more of the child. Disappointments arise. The child must learn to cope with frustrations just as he or she learns to handle and overcome fears. Teach parents that they can help by (1) showing concern and acceptance of the child's feelings; (2) helping the child talk about the feelings; (3) exploring with the child possible causes for the feelings; (4) helping the child realize that emotions have reasons and that they can discover causes for personal feelings; (5) emphasizing that the child is neither expected to be perfect nor should expect that everything will always go as desired; and (6) helping the child make a decision about handling the frustrating situation, thus learning problem-solving strategies. How the parent handles frustrations and problems sets an example for the child.

During the preschool years certain adaptive mechanisms are at a peak. They include introjection, primary and secondary identification, fantasy, and repression. These mechanisms may be used in other developmental eras to aid or hinder adjustment. Mechanisms previously discussed are also used in response to situations.

Introjection, *taking attitudes, information, and actions into the self through empathy and learning,* along with primary identification (imitation) is essential for secondary identification to occur. Through **secondary identification** the *child internalizes standards, moral codes, attitudes, and role behavior, including sex, as his or her own, and in his or her own unique way.*

Through **fantasy,** or *imagination,* the child handles tension and anxiety related to the problems of becoming socialized into the culture, family, and peer group. As the child mentally restructures reality to meet personal needs, he or she is gradually learning how to master the environment realistically. Because the child has difficulty distinguishing between wish and reality, parents must be gently realistic when necessary without shattering fantasies when they are needed or cause no problem. Parents must realize that an active imagination is normal at this age and provides tension release.

The child has fantasies about many things, shown in fondness for fairy tales and in the fears expressed. Some cultures allow magic, symbols, and fantasy to play a significant part in life; all cultures retain some. If the child is forced to distinguish reality too early or too quickly, if imaginings are not accepted, and if creativity is not encouraged, he or she is likely to lose the attributes that contribute to the creative adult—a personal and social loss to be avoided.

Repression occurs as the culture and parents continue to insist firmly on reality and following the rules. Excessive repression is related to guilt feelings, harsh punishment, or perceived strong disapproval and will later interfere with memories of this period and result in constricted creativity and restricted behavior. Some repression such as that related to the Oedipal conflict is necessary to free the child's energies for new tasks to be learned.

You can help parents understand the processes of differentiation, articulation, and integration as related to emotional development, ways to help the child learn coping skills, and the normality and importance of these adaptive mechanisms.

Moral-Spiritual Development

A great influence on the child during these early years is the parents' attitude toward moral codes (the human as creative being, spirituality, religion, nature, love of country, the economic system, and education), and their behavior in the presence of the child. They convey to the child what is considered good and bad, worthy of respect or unworthy. With the developing superego and imitation of and identification with adults, the child is absorbing a great deal of others' attitudes and will retain many of them throughout life. He or she is also beginning to consider how his or her actions affect others.

There are some general considerations you may find helpful pertaining to moral and religious education. The child cannot be kept spiritually neutral. He or she hears about morals and religion from other people and will raise detailed questions about the basic issues of life: Where did I come from? Why am I here? Why did the bird (or Grandpa) die? Why is it wrong to do . . . ? Why can't I play with Joey? How come Billy goes to church on Saturday and we go to church on Sunday? What is God? What is heaven? Mommy, who do you like best: Santa Claus, the Easter Bunny, the tooth fairy, or Jesus? These questions, often considered inappropriate from the adult viewpoint, should not be lightly brushed aside, for how they are answered is more important than the information given.

Example is the chief teacher for the child; if adult actions do not match the words, he or she quickly notices and learns the action. For the child, the parent is like God, omnipotent. Parents would be wise to remember this and try to live up to the high ideals of the child while at the same time introducing him or her to the reality of the world, for example, that parents do make mistakes. Talking with the child about such a mistake and asking forgiveness (if the child was wronged) will help him or her understand the redeeming power of a moral code, religion, or an ideal philosophy.

There are two major methods of religious education: indoctrination or letting the child follow the religion of his choice. Help parents realize that neither meets the real issues. The preschooler does not follow any religion because he or she understands it but because it encompasses daily life, offers concomitant pleasure, and is expected of him or her. The preschooler accepts the religion of the parents because to the child they are all-powerful. He or she is trusting and literal in the interpretation of religion. The first religious responses are social in nature; bowing the head and saying a simple prayer is imitated but is like brushing teeth to the young preschooler. The child likes prayers before meals and bedtime, and the 3-year-old may repeat them like nursery rhymes. The 4-year-old elaborates on prayer forms, and the 5-year-old makes up prayers.

Interpretation of religious forms and practices, influenced by the child's mental capacity and experiential contact, is marked by mental processes normal for the age: (1) egocentricism; (2) **anthropomorphism,** *in which the child relates God to human beings he or she knows;* (3) fantasy rather than causal or logical thinking; and (4) animism. The child thinks either God or human beings are responsible for all events. God pushes clouds when they move; wind is God blowing; thunder is God hammering; the sun is God lighting a match in the sky.

Thus the child needs consistent, simple explanations matched with the daily practices and religious ceremonies, rituals, or pictures. Encourage parents to discuss religion and related practices with the child. The preschool child is old enough to go to Sunday school, vacation Bible school, or classes in religious education that are on an appropriate level for the child. Religious holidays raise questions, and the spirit of the holiday and ceremonies surrounding it should be explained. In America where Christmas and Easter have become secularized and surrounded with the myths of Santa Claus and Easter Bunny, the child's fantasy and love of parties are likely to minimize the religious significance of the days. There is no harm to moral–spiritual development in telling the child about these myths so long as they are used to convey the religious spirit of the days rather than used as an end in themselves. The child thinks concretely, and embodiments of ideas such as the material objects used in any religion convey abstract meanings that words alone do not. When he or she expresses doubt about the myths, a more sophisticated explanation may be presented.

Conscience, or Superego, Development

This development is related to moral–spiritual training, discipline, conditioning of behavior (smiles, loving words), modeling of parents and others for correct behavior, being given reasons for behavior, and other areas of learning. The **superego,** *that part of the psyche that is critical to the self and enforces moral standards,* forms as a result of identification with parents and an introjection of their standards and values, which at first are questioned (47). At this point the child is in the Preconventional Period, Stage 2, of moral development (see Chapter 5, Table 5–12). The preschooler usually behaves even if there is no external authority standing around, to avoid disapproval, although he or she will slip at times. The superego can be cruel, primitive, and uncompromising. The child can be overobedient or resentful because parents do not live up to what the child's superego demands. The child is likely to overreact to punishment. This all-or-nothing quality of the superego is normally tempered later; a strict superego does not necessarily mean that the child has strict parents, but rather that he or she perceives them as strict. It is the result of the child's interpretation of events, teaching, admonitions, demands of the environment, discipline, punishment, fears, and guilt and anxiety about fantasized and real deeds.

Superego development will continue through contact with teachers and other significant adults through the years. If the superego remains too strict, self-righteous, or intolerant of others, the person in adulthood will develop a reaction formation of moralistic behavior so that prohibition rather than initiative will be a dominant pattern of behavior.

If the superego does not develop and if no or few social values are internalized, the child will be increasingly regarded as mischievous or bad in his or her behavior. Eventually he or she may have no guilt feelings and no qualms about not following the rules. The child is then on the way to truancy, delinquency, or becoming mentally ill, emotionally inadequate and unable to form mature relationships or follow social or ethical standards.

The child continues the moral development previously begun, learning a greater sense of responsibility, empathy, mercy, compassion, and fairness. The parents are the major teachers as they relate to the child fairly with compassion and gentleness. They teach also by being reliable and responsive. Further, they teach when they point out to the child the consequences of his or her behavior to others. If the child hurts another child physically or emotionally, the child needs to know that. Then the child learns an appropriate sense of guilt. That does *not* mean that the parent abuses the child or uses brute force to teach pain. Rather, discussion and reasoning, along with asserting authority (restraining and calming an angry, aggressive child) when necessary, are ways to influence positively the child's moral outlook. Withdrawal of love and physical punishment are not effective ways to teach moral behavior. In response to physical punishment, the child acts out even more physically or verbally from the consequent anger. Withdrawal of love results in a terrified, withdrawn, passive child who cannot respond to messages to be caring to others (61). If the child feels valued and values self, he or she will in turn treat other people, animals, the environment, and things as if they are valuable.

Discuss with parents the importance of superego development and beginning moral development during this period. Share the preceding information.

Developmental Tasks

In summary, the developmental tasks for the preschooler are the following (25):

- Settle into a healthful daily routine of adequately eating, exercising, and resting.
- Master physical skills of large- and small-muscle coordination and movement.
- Become a participating member in the family.
- Conform to other's expectations.
- Express emotions healthfully and for a wide variety of experiences.
- Learn to communicate effectively with an increasing number of others.
- Learn to use initiative tempered by a conscience.
- Develop ability to handle potentially dangerous situations.
- Lay foundations for understanding the meaning of life, self, the world, and ethical, religious, and philosophical ideas.

Discuss with parents how these tasks may be achieved and encourage them to talk about their con-

cerns or problems as they help the child mature in these skills.

When the preschool child becomes more realistic, relinquishes some fantasies, substitutes identity for rivalry with the parent of the same sex while seeking admiration of the parent of the opposite sex, and feels a sense of initiative rather than excessive guilt, he or she is ready to enter the period of latency.

If maladaptive behavior such as failure in language development, destructiveness, or excessive bedwetting persists, the parents and child need special guidance. You can obtain information on causes, associated behavior, and care for these and other special problems from a pediatric nursing book.

▶ HEALTH CARE AND NURSING APPLICATIONS

Your role with the preschooler and family has been discussed in each section throughout this chapter. Selected Nursing Diagnoses Related to the Preschooler lists some *nursing diagnoses* that may apply to the preschooler based on assessments that would result from knowledge presented in this chapter. Interventions include your role modeling of caring behavior to the preschooler and family; child, parent, and family education, support, and counseling; and direct care to meet the preschooler's physical, emotional, cognitive, social, or spiritual and moral needs.

Because child abuse, especially sexual abuse, is epidemic in this country, some detail about the nurse's role is described. It is critical that the nurse and other health team members intervene to protect the child and work with the family to improve parenting. Neither the child who is being abused nor the abusive family can develop and mature normally. The same is true for the family in which the child has been abused by someone from outside the family.

Assessment

Assessment must be done carefully. The TRIADS checklist assesses the dimensions of child abuse (14). This acronym represents the following assessment areas:

Type of abuse (physical, psychological, sexual)
Role relationship of victim to offender (intrafamilial or extrafamilial)
Intensity of abuse (way abuse began and ended, number of times abuse occurred, and number of offenders involved)
Autonomic response of the child

► SELECTED NURSING DIAGNOSES RELATED TO THE PRESCHOOLER*

Pattern 1: Exchanging

Altered Nutrition: More than Body Requirements
Altered Nutrition: Less than Body Requirements
Altered Nutrition: Potential for More Than Body Requirements
Risk for Infection
Risk for Injury
Risk for Poisoning
Risk for Impaired Skin Integrity

Pattern 2: Communicating

Impaired Verbal Communication

Pattern 3: Relating

Impaired Social Interaction

Pattern 5: Choosing

Impaired Adjustment

Pattern 6: Moving

Sleep Pattern Disturbance
Feeding Self-Care Deficit
Toileting Self-Care Deficit
Altered Growth and Development

Pattern 7: Perceiving

Body Image Disturbance
Self-Esteem Disturbance
Sensory/Perceptual Alterations
Unilateral Neglect
Hopelessness

Pattern 8: Knowing

Knowledge Deficit

Pattern 9: Feeling

Pain
Anxiety
Fear

*Other NANDA diagnoses are applicable to the ill preschooler.
From North American Nursing Diagnosis Association, NANDA Nursing Diagnoses Definitions & Classification 1995–1996. Philadelphia: North American Nursing Diagnosis Association, 1994.

Duration of abuse (length of time over which abuse occurred, ranging from days to years)
Style of offender or abuse

Style of abuse relates to the offender's techniques and access to the child (14): (1) whether it occurs spontaneously and explosively and without anticipation on the part of the child; (2) if there are antecedent cues that alert the child to a series of acts; or (3) if acts are repetitively patterned, ritualistic, or ceremonial to control how the child can act.

If you suspect abuse, establish rapport and talk with the child alone; however, do not pry. If the child finds it difficult to talk, gently offer to draw some pictures or play with the child to gain information as follows:

- What has happened to you? The child may not answer because he or she (a) thinks abuse is normal, (b) is terrified that parents will be more abusive if they knew he or she told, (c) feels loyalty to the parents and fears desertion, or (d) believes abuse is deserved.
- Tell me everything that happened just before that.
- Has anyone ever told you to take off your panties?
- Has anyone ever put his or her finger (or another object) between your legs?
- Does anyone ever get in bed with you at night?

Obtain information related to the points on the TRIADS checklist. Such information must also be obtained if incest is the issue.

When you talk with the parents about the subject of child abuse, do not give the impression that you are criticizing them, trying to impart your own values, or acting as their judge. Putting them on the defensive will not make them cooperate, and it may keep them from accepting help from other health care professionals. Do your best to be tolerant and understanding. Try to determine how realistically they perceive the child, how they cope with the stresses of parenting, and to whom they turn for support. As you talk, attempt to get the parents' answers to the following questions (14, 28, 56, 78):

- What do you do when he or she cries too much? If that does not work, what do you do?
- Does the child sleep well? What do you do when he or she does not sleep?
- How do you discipline him or her?
- How do you feel after you have disciplined the child?
- Are you ever angry because the child takes up so much of your time?

- Does he or she take up more time than your other children or require more disciplining? If yes, why?
- Do you think he or she misbehaves on purpose?
- Whom do you usually talk to when your child upsets you? Is that person available now?
- Does the child remind you of a relative or former spouse that is disliked? (Explore this possibility with gentle questions: "It must be really upsetting for you when he acts like his father. What goes through your mind then?" "In what ways is she like your mother? Do those characteristics irritate you?").

As you discuss things, try to determine what the situation is at home. Does one or both of the parents seem unduly distressed? Perhaps they are facing other stresses with which they cannot cope such as a job loss, loneliness, illness, or alcoholism.

Explain your suspicions to the parents, obtain necessary information, and indicate you want to help. The parents may be relieved that someone recognized the problem; however, they may also object strenuously and try to take the child home. The doctor may have to get an order from the police or other legal authorities to retain the child.

If you suspect **sexual abuse** (*intercourse* or *intrusion physically into the body*) or **sexual intrusion** (*touching the genital area*), find out the following from the parents:

- What words or names does the child use to describe various body parts?
- What are the names of family members and frequent visitors?
- Who babysits for the child?
- What are the family's sleeping arrangements?
- Does the child have behavioral problems such as excessive masturbation?
- Does the child have any phobias or excessive fears of any person or place? Any nightmares?

Parents may not be involved in the sexual abuse and may be unaware of its occurrence. Work up gradually to the subject of their child's being abused. Inform them of your suspicions in private and without judgment. Do not bombard the parents with questions they will interpret as accusatory. Offer your support, telling them of your concern for the child. Suggest counselors who would be helpful for the child and parents. Give them ideas on how to help the child work through feelings about the trauma. Advise parents not to punish or scold the child when he or she works through emotions through masturbation or by playing with dolls (14, 78).

A pelvic examination is necessary if the child has been sexually abused; however, this procedure should be done carefully after explanation is given to the child, questions are answered, rapport is established, and the child feels some sense of security. A visual examination of the whole body, including the genital and rectal regions, should be done before a pelvic examination. Allow plenty of time for every step of the examination. The prepubescent vagina is extremely sensitive, and the doctor may want to sedate or anesthetize the child before the examination. A sterile plastic medicine dropper lubricated with sterile water should be used to obtain specimens. A nasal speculum or infant-sized vaginoscope, lubricated with water and warmed, can be used with the young child. Test the child for venereal disease (girls who are past menarche should be tested for pregnancy) (14, 78).

Selected Nursing Diagnoses Related to the Preschooler lists some *nursing diagnoses* based on your assessment, to be used in planning care.

Intervention

You are a key factor in *intervention;* however, do not engage in rescue fantasies. You are limited in what you can do, although reporting to the appropriate professionals is necessary action for intervention.

Interventions for the abused child include the following (13, 14, 21, 28, 31, 49, 55, 77):

1. Relaxation techniques and psychopharmacology to reduce hyperactivity, nightmares, enuresis, and startle responses—sensory disruption
2. Thought stopping, clarification, and reframing of beliefs and linking distress directly to the trauma experience to reduce perceptual–cognitive disruptions
3. Desensitizing the child to fearful involvement with others, focused role-playing to discriminate threatening exploitative behavior from safe behavior, and empathy training to reduce interpersonal disruption

Treatment objectives for the sexually abused child, using play therapy include the following:

1. Child will express feelings about being sexually abused.
2. Child will reenact incidents of sexual trauma; anatomic dolls will be used for the child to show where she or he has been touched by the adult and to allow the child to vent anger felt for the adult.

3. In an appropriate but satisfying way, child will diffuse anger, shame, humiliation, tension from secrecy, fear, and guilt and work through feelings of being damaged.
4. Child will learn to respect her or his body and the right to have physical and psychological boundaries.
5. Child will learn to improve judgment process with adults and strangers and to handle sexual confrontations.
6. Child will demonstrate less acting out at school or home.
7. Child will discuss bad dreams and nightmares to be reassured of safety.

Crayons, paints, chalkboards, punching bags, bean bags, and dolls are media to use in treatment. Simple teaching tools, basic vocabulary, and keen observation are essential. Repetition of stories, recreation of telephone conversations with the perpetrator, and drawing and painting are essential for beginning resolution (28, 77).

If you are in a health care facility and suspect child abuse, report it to the doctor and appropriate health team members. Also report your suspicions to the proper agency—the police, the district attorney's office, a child-protective service, or a social service group. *Carefully document all evidence of abuse,* your interview of and actions with parents and child, any agencies or persons contacted about the abuse, and any agencies to which the parents were referred. All 50 states and the District of Columbia provide immunity to professionals who report suspected or actual abuse. In some states failure to report abuse is a crime (78).

List the names of children who are repeatedly brought to the hospital with injuries. Make sure the notes on the chart include what the parents said, how they reacted, and how they explained the accident. Provide other hospitals in the area with the names on file. Urge them to do the same with their files. Take the time to check with other hospitals when you have a case you question (78).

A **neglected child** needs help as much as one who has been abused. Careful assessment and interviewing of child and parents are essential. Notify your community's child protection service and document thoroughly your findings and interventions. Many of the guidelines described above are applicable.

SUMMARY

The preschooler grows at a steady pace and gains considerable neuromuscular, cognitive, emotional, and so-cial competencies. The child develops the ability to carry out basic hygiene, to participate within the family, and to relate more effectively with adults who are either extended family, friends, or authority figures in the community. The child slowly grows out of the family, establishing beginning peer relationships. As parents provide consistent love and guidance and new experiences, the preschooler demonstrates physical, cognitive, emotional, social, and moral–spiritual development.

► CONSIDERATIONS FOR THE PRESCHOOL CHILD AND FAMILY IN HEALTH CARE

- Family, cultural background and values, support systems, and community resources for the family
- Parents as identification figures for the child; secondary identification of the preschool child with the parents
- Behaviors that indicate gender identity and sense of sexuality in the preschool child
- Behaviors that indicate ability of the preschool child to relate to siblings, adults in the extended family, and other adults and authority figures in the environment
- Parental behaviors that indicate difficulty with parenting or potential/actual abuse of the preschool child
- Physical characteristics and patterns, such as neuromuscular development, nutrition, exercise, and rest/sleep, that indicate health and are within age norms for growth for the preschool child
- Cognitive characteristics and behavioral patterns in the preschool child that demonstrate curiosity, increasingly realistic thought, expanding concept formation, and continuing mental development
- Communication patterns—verbal, nonverbal, and action—and language development that demonstrate continuing learning and age-appropriate norms for the preschool child
- Behaviors that indicate that the child can participate in and enjoys early childhood education experiences
- Overall appearance and behavior and play patterns in the preschool child that indicate development of initiative rather than excessive guilt, positive self-concept, body image formation, and sense of sexuality
- Use of adaptive mechanisms by the preschool child that promote a sense of security, control of anxiety, and age-appropriate emotional responses
- Behavioral patterns that indicate the preschool child is forming a superego or conscience and continuing moral–spiritual development
- Behavioral patterns and characteristics that the preschool child has achieved developmental tasks
- Parental behaviors that indicate knowledge about and how to guide and discipline the child and assist the child in becoming more independent
- Parental behaviors that indicate they are achieving their developmental tasks for this era

Considerations for the Preschool Child and Family in Health Care and Chart 2 in Appendix IV summarize what you should consider in assessment and health promotion with the preschooler. The family is included in Considerations. Chart 2 presents the American Academy of Family Physicians Periodic Health Examination 18 months to 6 years, and thus presents information pertinent to screening the preschooler, counseling parents, and determining immunization schedules and risk categories.

▶ REFERENCES

1. Alexander, M., and J. Blank, Factors Related to Obesity in Mexican-American Preschool Children, *IMAGE: Journal of Nursing Scholarship* 20, no. 2 (1988), 79–81.

2. Anderson, M., The Mental Health Advantages of Twinship, *Perspectives in Psychiatric Care,* 23, no. 3 (1985), 114–116.

3. Bander, L.K., et al., Dietary Lead Intake of Preschool Children, *American Journal of Public Health,* 73, no. 7 (1983), 789.

4. Barnett, W., Benefit–Cost Analysis of Preschool Education: Findings From a 25-Year Follow-up, *Journal of Orthopsychiatry,* 63 (1993), 500–508.

5. Bartlett, A., et al., Controlled Trial of *Giardia lamblia:* Control Strategies in Day Care Centers, *American Journal of Public Health,* 81, no. 6 (1991), 1001–1006.

6. Bell, D., et al., Illness Associated with Child Day Care: A Study of Incidence and Cost, *American Journal of Public Health,* 78, no. 4 (1988), 479–484.

7. Bettelheim, B., *A Good Enough Parent: A Book on Child-Rearing.* New York: Alfred A. Knopf, 1987.

8. Bobak, M., B. Kriz, D. Leon, J. Danova, and M. Marmot, Socioeconomic Factors and Height of Preschool Children in the Czech Republic, *American Journal of Public Health,* 84 (1994), 1167–1170.

9. Bonner, A., and R. Dale, *Giardia lamblia:* Day Care Diarrhea. *American Journal of Nursing,* 86, no. 9 (1986), 918–920.

10. Boynton, R., E. Dunn, and G. Stephens, *Manual of Ambulatory Pediatrics* (3rd ed.). Philadelphia: J.B. Lippincott, 1994.

11. Brown, M., and C. Tanner, Type A Behavior and Cardiovascular Responsivity in Preschoolers, *Nursing Research,* 37, no. 3 (1988), 152–155.

12. ———, and C. Tanner, Measurement of Type A Behavior in Preschoolers, *Nursing Research,* 39, no. 4 (1990), 207–211.

13. Burgess, A., Intra-familial Sexual Abuse, in Campbell, J., and Humphreys, I. eds., *Nursing Care of Victims of Family Violence.* Reston, VA: Reston, 1984.

14. ———, C. Hartman, and S. Kelley, Assessing Child Abuse: The TRIADS Checklist, *Journal of Psychosocial Nursing and Mental Health Services,* 28, no. 4 (1990), 6–14.

15. ———, C. Hartman, and T. Baker, Memory Presentations of Childhood Sexual Abuse, *Journal of Psychosocial Nursing,* 33, no. 9 (1995), 9–16.

16. ———, M. McCausland, and W. Wolbert, Children's Drawings as Indicators of Sexual Trauma, *Perspectives in Psychiatric Care,* 19, no. 2 (1981), 50–58.

17. ———, et al., Child Molestation: Assessing Impact in Multiple Victims (Part I), *Archives of Psychiatric Nursing,* 1, no. 1 (1987), 33–39.

18. Cadman, D., et al., The Usefulness of the Denver Developmental Screening Test to Predict Kindergarten Problems in a General Community Population, *American Journal of Public Health,* 74, no. 110 (1984), 1093–1097.

19. Center for the Future of Children, *The Future of Children, Children and Divorce,* 4, no. 1 (1994), 1–247.

20. Centers for Disease Control and Prevention General Recommendations on Immunization: Recommendations of the Advisory Committee on Immunization Practices (ACIP), *Morbidity and Mortality Weekly Report,* 43 (January 28, 1994), 23.

21. Critchley, D., Therapeutic Group Work With Abused Preschool Children, *Perspectives in Psychiatric Care,* 20, no. 2 (1982), 79–85.

22. Dacey, J., and J. Travers, *Human Development Across the Lifespan* (3rd ed.), Madison, WI: Brown & Benchmark, 1996.

23. De Santis, V., Nursery Rhymes: A Developmental Perspective, in Solnit, A., and Neubauer, P. eds. *The Psychoanalytic Study of the Child,* Vol. 41, New Haven, CT: Yale University Press, 1986, pp. 601–626.

24. DiLeo, J.H., *Young Children and Their Drawings.* Springfield, IL: Springer, 1971.

25. Duvall, E., and B. Miller. *Marriage and Family Development* (6th ed.). New York: Harper & Row, 1984.

26. Dworetzky, J., *Human Development: A Life Span Approach* (2nd ed.). St. Paul/Minneapolis: West, 1995.

27. Erikson, E.H., *Childhood and Society* (2nd ed.). New York: W.W. Norton, 1963.

28. Federation, S., Sexual Abuse: Treatment Modalities for the Younger Child, *Journal of Psychosocial Nursing,* 24, no. 7 (1986), 21–24.

29. Foster, R., M. Hunsberger, and J. Anderson, *Family-Centered Nursing Care of Children.* Philadelphia: W.B. Saunders, 1989.

30. Frankenburg, W., and J.B. Dobbs, *Denver II—Revision and Restandardization of the Denver Developmental Screening Test.* Denver: Denver Developmental Materials, 1990.

31. Garbarino, J., E. Guttmann, and J. Seeley, *The Psychologically Battered Child: Strategies for Identification, Assessment, and Intervention.* San Francisco: Jossey-Bass, 1987.

32. Gesell, A., and F. Ilg, *The Child From Five to Ten* (rev. ed.) New York: Harper & Collins, 1977.

33. ———, et al., *The First Five Years of Life,* New York: Harper & Brothers, 1940.

34. Gross, P., B. Conrad, L. Fogg, L. Willis, and C. Garvey, A Longitudinal Study of Maternal Depression and Preschool Children's Mental Health, *Nursing Research,* 44 (1995), 96–101.

35. Heiney, S., Helping Children Through Painful Procedures, *American Journal of Nursing,* 91, no. 11 (1991), 20–24.

36. The Hennepin County Child Care Consultation Program, *American Journal of Public Health,* 76, no. 11 (1986), 1357–1358.

37. Hoole, A., C. Pickard, R. Ouimette, J. Lohr, and R. Greenberg, *Patient Care Guidelines for Nurse Practitioners* (4th ed.). Philadelphia: J.B. Lippincott, 1995.

38. Injury-Proofing the School-Age Child, *Patient Care,* 23, no. 15 (1989), 178.

39. Johansen, A., A. Leibowitz, and L. Waite, Child Care and Children's Illness, *American Journal of Public Health,* 78, no. 9 (1988), 1175–1177.

40. Jolley, J., and M. Mitchell, *Lifespan Development: A Topical Approach.* Madison, WI: Brown & Benchmark, 1996.

41. Kelley, S., Parental Stress Response to Sexual Abuse and Ritualistic Abuse of Children in Day Care Centers, *Nursing Research,* 39, no. 1 (1990), 25–29.

42. Kempe, C., Sexual Abuse: Another Hidden Pediatric Problem, *Pediatrics,* 62 (1978), 582.

43. Lamb, M., The Emergent Father, in Lamb, M.E., ed., *The Father's Role: Cross-cultural Perspectives.* Hillsdale, NJ: Lawrence Erlbaum, 1987, pp. 1–26.

44. Latimer, D., Involving Grandparents and Other Older Adults in the Preschool Classroom, *Dimensions of Early Childhood,* 22, no. 2 (1994), 26–30.

45. LaRossa, R., Fatherhood and Social Change, *Family Relations,* 37, (1988), 451–457.

46. LeVieux-Anglin, L., & E. Sawyer. Incorporating Play Interventions into Nursing Care, *Pediatric Nursing,* 19 (1993), 459–462.

47. Lidz, T., *The Person: His and Her Development Throughout the Life Cycle* (2nd ed.). New York: Basic Books, 1983.

48. Liebman, B., and J. Hurley, How to Pick a Cereal, *Nutrition Action Health Letter,* 22, no. 5 (1995), 11.

49. Lieske, A., Incest: An Overview, *Perspectives in Psychiatric Care,* 19, no. 2 (1981), 59–62.

50. Loescher, L., J. Emerson, A. Taylor, D. Christensen, and M. McKinney, Educating Preschoolers About Sun Safety, *American Journal of Public Health,* 85 (1995), 939–943.

51. Marzolla, J., and J. Lloyd, *Learning Through Play.* New York: Harper & Row, 1972.

52. Messer, A., *The Individual in His Family, An Adaptational Study,* Springfield, IL: Charles C Thomas, 1970.

53. Millar, S., *The Psychology of Play.* Harmonds-Worth, England: Penguin Books, 1974.

54. Piaget, J., *Origins of Intelligence in Childhood* (2nd ed.). New York: International Universities Press, 1953.

55. Polk-Walker, G., What Really Happened? Incidence and Factor Assessment of Abused Children and Adolescents, *Journal of Psychosocial Nursing,* 28, no. 11 (1990), 17–22.

56. Pontious, S., Practical Piaget: Helping Children Understand, *American Journal of Nursing,* 82, no. 1 (1982), 114–117.

57. Roberts, J., L. Poffenroth, L. Roos, J. Bebchuk, and A. Carter, Monitoring Childhood Immunizations: A Canadian Approach, *American Journal of Public Health,* 84 (1994), 1666–1668.

58. Runyon, N., and P. Jackson, Divorce: The Impact on Children, *Perspectives in Psychiatric Care,* 24, nos. 3 and 4 (1987/1988), 101–105.

59. Salzinger, S., R. Feldman, M. Hammon, and M. Rosario, The Effects of Physical Abuse on Children's Social Relationships, *Child Development,* 64 (1993), 169–187.

60. Schilder, P., *The Image and Appearance of the Human Body.* New York: International Universities Press, 1951.

61. Schulman, M., *Moral Development Training: Strategies for Parents, Teachers, and Clinicians.* Menlo Park, CA: Addison-Wesley, 1985.

62. Schuster, R., Footgear Modifications for Children in the Preschool to Pre-Teen Ages, *Proceedings National Academies of Practice Fourth National Health Policy Forum,* April 24–25 (1992), 81–85.

63. Scrimshaw, N., The New Paradigm of Public Health Nutrition, *American Journal of Public Health,* 85 (1995), 622–624.

64. Sexual Abuse of Children, *The Future of Children,* 4, no. 2 (1994), 1–247.

65. Shapiro, L., et al., Obesity Prognosis: A Longitudinal Study of Children From Age 6 Months to 9 Years, *American Journal of Public Health,* 74, no. 9 (1984), 968–972.

66. Sherman, J., Jr., and S. Fields, *Guide to Patient Evaluation* (5th ed.). Garden City, NY: Medical Examination Publishing, 1989.

67. Stone, J., and J. Church, *Childhood and Adolescence: Psychology of the Growing Person* (5th ed.). New York: Random House, 1984.

68. Sugar-Coated Cereal Talk, *Tufts University Diet & Nutrition Letter,* 13, no. 7 (1995), 1.

69. Troy, P., et al., Sibling Visiting in the NICU, *American Journal of Nursing,* 88, no. 1 (1988), 68–69.

70. Turner, J., and D. Helms, *Lifespan Development* (5th ed.). New York: Harcourt & Brace, 1995.

71. Uphold, C., and M. Graham, *Clinical Guidelines in Family Practice* (2nd ed.), Gainesville, FL: Barmarrae Books, 1994.

72. Wadsworth, B., *Piaget's Theory of Cognitive and Affective Development* (5th ed.). New York: Longman, 1996.

73. Wallerstein, J., Children After Divorce: Wounds That Don't Heal, *Perspectives in Psychiatric Care,* 24, nos. 3 and 4 (1987/1988), 107–113.

74. Webb, P., Piaget: Implications for Teaching, *Theory Into Practice,* 19, no. 2 (1980), 93–97.

75. Wenger, J., et al., Day Care Characteristics Associated With *Haemophilus Influenza Disease, American Journal of Public Health,* 80, no. 12 (1990), 1455–1458.

76. Williams, S. *Nutrition and Diet Therapy* (10th ed.). St. Louis: C.V. Mosby, 1995.

77. Wong, D., *Whaley and Wong's Nursing Care of Infants and Children* (5th ed.). St. Louis: C.V. Mosby, 1995.

78. Yorker, B., The Prosecution of Child Sexual Abuse Cases, *Journal of Child Psychiatric Nursing,* 1, no. 2 (1988), 50–57.

chapter ten

Assessment and Health Promotion for the Schoolchild

If you are concerned about yourself, plant rice. If you are concerned about your family, plant trees. If you are concerned about your nation, educate your children.

—Chinese Proverb

Key Terms

School-age years

Middle childhood

Late childhood

Juvenile period

Preadolescence/prepubescence

Power-assertive discipline

Love-withdrawal discipline

Inductive discipline

Latch key child

Fluoride mottling

Scoliosis

Obesity

Accommodative esophoria

Otitis externa

Serous otitis media

Allergic rhinitis

Asthma

Herpes type I

Contact dermatitis

Tinea corporis

Tinea capitis

Warts

Pediculosis humanus capitis

Mumps

Diabetes mellitus type I

Fifth disease (erythema infectiosum)

Hand-foot-and-mouth disease

Pityriasis rosea

Rabies

Cognitive style

Conceptual tempo

Impulsive

Reflective

Sociocentric

Concrete operations

   Classification

   Seriation

   Nesting

   Multiplication

   Reversibility

   Transformation

   Conservation

   Decentering

Cognitive conflict

School phobia

Perfectionistic child

Gifted child

Syntaxic, consensual communication

Gang

Chum

Altruism

Competition

Morality of constraint

Compromise

Cooperation

Morality of cooperation

Collaboration

Industry

Inferiority

Stress

Vulnerable

Resilient

Sexuality education	Reaction formation	Fantasy	Rationalization
Sex education	Undoing	Regression	Sublimation
Ritualistic behavior	Isolation	Malingering	

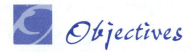

Objectives

Study of this chapter will enable you to:

1. Discuss the family relationships of the schoolchild and the influence of peers and other adults on him or her.

2. Explore with the family members their developmental tasks and ways to achieve them.

3. Compare and assess the physical changes and needs, including nutrition, rest, exercise, safety, and health protection, for the juvenile and preadolescent.

4. Assess intellectual, communication, play, emotional, self-concept, sexuality, and moral–spiritual development in the juvenile and preadolescent and influences on these areas of development.

5. Discuss the crisis of school entry and ways to help the child adapt to the experience of formal education, including latch key care.

6. Discuss the physical and emotional adaptive mechanisms of the schoolchild and how they contribute to his or her total development, including meeting the developmental crisis of industry versus inferiority.

7. Discuss the significance of peers and the chum relationship to the psychosocial development of the child.

8. Explore with parents their role in communication with and guidance of the child to foster healthy development in all spheres of personality.

9. Discuss influence of media on behavior.

10. State the developmental tasks of the schoolchild and discuss your role in helping him or her to achieve them.

11. Work effectively with the schoolchild in the nursing setting.

As growth and development continue and the child leaves the confines of the home, he or she emerges into a world of new experiences and responsibilities. If previous developmental tasks have been met and the child has developed a healthy personality, he or she will continue to acquire new knowledge and skills steadily. If previous developmental tasks have not been met and the child's personality development is immature or warped, the child may experience difficulties mastering the developmental tasks of the school-age child. Peers, parents, and other adults can have a positive, maturing influence if the child is adequately prepared for leaving home, if individual needs are considered, and if he or she has some successful experiences.

The **school-age years** can be divided into **middle childhood** (*6–8 years of age*) and **late childhood** (*8–12 years of age*) (58). The school-age years can also be divided into the juvenile and preadolescent periods. *At approximately age 6, the* **juvenile period** *begins, marked by a need for peer associations.* **Preadolescence** *usually begins at 9 or 10 years of age and is marked by a new ca-*

pacity to love, when the satisfaction and security of another person of the same sex is as important to the child as personal satisfaction and security (205). *Preadolescence ends at approximately 12 years with the onset of puberty. Preadolescence is also called* **prepubescence** *and is characterized by an increase in hormone production in both sexes,* *which is preparatory to eventual physiologic maturity. Psychological and social changes also occur as the child slowly moves away from the family. This chapter discusses characteristics to assess and intervention measures for you to use in relation to health care for the child and family.*

Some of the characteristics described in this chapter will not be applicable to every child in the United States or children in war-torn or famine-stricken countries. Children in rural Appalachia and the Horn of Africa may grow up stunted in physical and intellectual potential from the malnutrition they now suffer. The children of Beirut and Sarajevo may grow up with the haunted eyes of battle fatigue. Children in city slums worldwide may die early from communicable diseases and violence. Both the diary of Zlato Filipovic, age 10, a Bosnian girl of mixed heritage (69), and the diary of Anne Frank, a Dutch Jewish girl in World War II, more than 50 years ago (72), reveal the horrors of war and represent the uncertainty that many school-age children face. Millions of children in the world are homeless—street children—living on garbage, outcasts, sold for prostitution, dying young unless some humanitarian or religious agency takes them in for care and education.

Combating poverty and violence and their effects on children means that money, effort, and time are necessary to:

- Help children who are at risk of dropping out of school with special tutoring so that academic performance and self-esteem can be strengthened.
- Counsel parents and children in homes where abuse and violence are present.
- Assist parents with child care; support efforts of parents who are trying to improve their incomes and life.
- Provide day-care or after-school care for children when parents cannot be in the home because of job demands.
- Advocate at federal, state, and local governmental levels for policies and programs that will assist children, such as healthy school lunches, as well as eliminate causes of poverty, such as employment conditions.
- Work at the community level to reduce violence in the neighborhoods, community, and school.

FAMILY DEVELOPMENT AND RELATIONSHIPS

Relationships With Parents

Although parents remain a vital part of the schoolchild's life, the child's position within the family is altered with his or her entry into school. Parents play a major role in socializing the child to the adult world. They contribute to the socialization process in at least five ways: (1) by assuming the role of love providers and caretakers; (2) by serving as identification figures; (3) by acting as active socialization agents; (4) by determining the sort of experiences the child will have; and (5) by participating in the development of the child's self-concept (58, 129).

The schoolchild now channels energy into intellectual pursuits, widens social horizons, and becomes familiar with the adult world. He or she has identified with the parent of the same sex and, through imitation and education, continues to learn a social role. The fam-

ily atmosphere has much impact on the child's emotional development and future response within the family when he or she becomes an adolescent. Research indicates that children can become positive in their behavior whether they are reared in either authoritarian or permissive homes if parents are consistent in their approach. The permissive childrearing style does not necessarily produce a child with undisciplined behavior, and the authoritarian style does not necessarily produce aggressive or inhibited children (16, 129). Nevertheless the disciplinary style and parenting practices used in the home are important influences on the child, and several different disciplinary styles are used by parents. In **power-assertive discipline,** the *parent uses threats, commands, spankings, and withdrawal of privileges.* The parent controls the behavior of the child because the parent is in a position of power. With **love-withdrawal discipline,** the *parent relies on the child's fear that he or she will lose the emotional support, affection, and/or approval of the parent. The parent may also appeal to the child's reason, pride, or desire to be grown up;* this is **inductive discipline,** the form of discipline that apparently is the most effective in establishing self-regulation (58).

Although parental support is needed, the schoolchild pulls away from overt signs of parental affection. Yet during illness or when threatened by his or her new status, he or she turns to parents for affection and protection. Parents get frustrated with behavioral changes, antics, and infractions of household rules.

The romantic notion of the "typical American two-parent family with a male wage earner and a mother who stays home to care for two children" has been prevalent in the United States. This stereotype represents few American families (only 7% of school-age children) (142). The stereotype ignores the following (197):

- Families of the millions of children whose mothers work outside the home (73% of mothers with school-age children)
- Millions of single-parent families who are more likely to be poor (25% of all children less than 18 years of age live with a single parent)
- Millions of families who have at least one child with a physical, mental, or emotional handicap
- Hundreds of thousands of children who do not have homes of their own—who live with relatives or doubled up or in shelters, which may serve as home and school
- Millions of teenage parents, themselves merely children, struggling to raise another generation

In the United States, only 58% of children live with two biological parents, although 79% live in two-parent households. About 26% of all children under 18 years live with a divorced, separated, or stepparent. About 10% of all children live with a divorced, single parent; almost 8% were living with a single, never-married parent, most of whom are mothers. As of 1991, 39% of divorced women with children lived in poverty. Employment of divorced mothers does not provide an adequate buffer against economic deprivation. It is projected that nearly one-half of the babies born today will experience divorce.

Marital conflict, separation, and divorce are all stressful events for the whole family, especially the child. Considerable stress is economic, in that there may be inadequate or no support for the mother and children from the father, whether or not custodial. The change in lifestyle is often dramatic (36). Children growing up in homes without fathers more often have lowered academic performances, more cognitive and intellectual deficits, increased adjustment problems, and higher risks for psychosexual development problems (173).

Children who experience parental divorce, compared with children in continuously intact two-parent families, exhibit more conduct disorders, symptoms of psychological maladjustment, and social problems; lower academic achievement; and lower self-concept. Considerable variations in reactions exist, however, depending on the (1) amount and quality of contact with the noncustodial parent, (2) custodial parent's psychological adjustment and parenting skills, (3) level of interparental conflict preceding and following divorce, (4) degree of economic hardship, and (5) number of stressful life experiences that accompany and follow divorce (3).

Table 10–1 summarizes the tasks that must be resolved by children after divorce (219). Many schools have counselors to conduct group sessions 12 to 14 times a semester for students who are experiencing separation or divorce of parents. These sessions are designed to help students toward resolution of the tasks listed in Table 10–1, which in turn should enhance their scholastic ability.

The monograph *Children and Divorce* gives considerable information about the scope and effects of divorce, as well as legal issues (36).

The media report that children constitute the poorest age group in the United States, for at least 20% of all children are below the poverty line. One-half of African-American children and more than one-third of Latino children live in poverty. Being poor affects all dimensions of development (16, 33, 186).

Not only poor, minority, or single-parent families need help, however. Many middle-class or upper-class families do not feel confident about raising their children. They may have all the help that professionals,

TABLE 10–1. PSYCHOLOGICAL TASKS FOR CHILDREN AFTER DIVORCE

Task I: Understanding the Divorce
Schoolchildren
1. Understand the immediate changes.
2. Differentiate fantasy from reality.
3. Manage concerns regarding abandonment, placement in foster care, not seeing departed parent again.

Adolescents/Young Adults
1. Understand what led to marital failure.
2. Evaluate parents' actions.
3. Draw useful conclusions for their own lives.

Task II: Strategic Withdrawal
1. Acknowledge concern and provide appropriate help to parents and siblings.
2. Avoid divorce as the total focus and get back to their own interests, pleasures, activities, peer relationships.
3. Children allowed to remain children.

Task III: Dealing With Loss
1. Deal with loss of intact family and loss of presence of one parent, usually the father.
2. Deal with feelings of rejection and blame for making one parent leave.
3. Task is easier if child has good relationship with both parents; this may be most difficult task.

Task IV: Dealing With Anger
1. Manage anger at parents for deciding to divorce.
2. Be aware of parents' needs, anxiety, and loneliness.
3. Diminish anger and forgive.

Task V: Working Out Guilt
1. Deal with sense of guilt for causing marital difficulties and driving wedge between parents.
2. Separate guilty ties and get on with their lives.

Task VI: Accepting Permanence of Divorce
1. Overcome early denial and fantasies of parents getting back together.
2. Task may not be completed until parent remarries or child mourns loss.

Task VII: Taking a Chance on Love
1. Remain open to love, commitment, marriage, fidelity.
2. Able to turn away from parents' model.
3. Most important task for growing children, adolescents, and young adults.

housekeepers, and nursemaids can give and may not be able to exercise effective control over what their children see on television or eat (129).

Although the poor child frequently shares the helplessness of an unemployed parent, the higher-income child often feels the relentless pressure on the parent who is a high-powered corporate executive, lawyer, professor, or government official preoccupied with his or her own survival. Too often the demands of the workplace encroach on the needs and happiness of the family (129).

In some families abuse, neglect, or maltreatment occurs. Refer to Chapters 4, 6, 7, and 9 for background information about precipitating factors, characteristics of abusing parents, and signs, symptoms, and treatment of abuse. Table 10–2 summarizes risk factors for sexual abuse. The research of Garbarino, Guttmann, and Seeley shows that psychological abuse or maltreatment of the schoolchild is demonstrated by the behavior described in Parental Behavior Characteristic of Psychological Maltreatment of the Schoolchild. Refer also to references 22, 23, 25, 68, 89, 97, 102, 113, 131, 171, 182, 207, 236, 238, and 239.

The **latch key child,** the *child who has the door key because no one is home when the child returns from school,* is seen increasingly as more than 70% of women with children under 18 work. Children voice different feelings about the working mother and having no one home to meet them after school. Some like it. They enjoy the solitude, privacy, responsibility, and closeness of each other at day's end. Some hate it for the same reasons. Some tolerate it out of necessity, disliking the separation and lack of time together. Some are afraid for themselves and their mothers. Some are proud of mother and how they are managing together. Some become discipline problems. All understand the financial reasons and sometimes the career and emotional reasons that are usually the basis for mother working. Some girls say they want to work as a result, and some want to be homemakers when they grow up. More programs such as YWCA Latch Key Programs and daycare centers that provide longer hours of care are being

TABLE 10–2. SEXUAL ABUSE OF THE SCHOOLCHILD*

Risk Factors
- Having a stepfather
- Poor relationship between child and parent
- Mothers who work outside the home or are emotionally distant
- Having a parent who does not live with the child
- Sex: 25% of all females; 10% of all males by age 18 years

Family Characteristics
- An emotionally dependent adult male in the home
- Sexual estrangement between the parents or parental figures
- Mother deserted the family (literally or figuratively)
- Sexual offender suffers a crisis, i.e., loss of job
- Daughter begins to mature sexually
- Parent has poor impulse control
- Problems such as substance abuse, personality disorders, psychoses, and mental retardation in parent(s)

*The legal definition differs from state to state.

► PARENTAL BEHAVIOR CHARACTERISTIC OF PSYCHOLOGICAL MALTREATMENT OF THE SCHOOLCHILD

Rejecting
- Communicates negative definitions of self to the child
- Creates a sense of "bad-me" or negative self-concept by consistently calling child negative names such as stupid, dummy, monster
- Belittles child's accomplishments regularly
- Scapegoats child in the family system

Isolating
- Removes child from normal social relations with peers
- Prohibits child from playing with or inviting children into the home
- Withdraws child from school

Terrorizing
- Places child in double bind
- Demands opposite or conflicting behavior or emotions simultaneously from the child
- Forces child to choose one of the two parents
- Changes rules of the house or of relationship with parents frequently
- Criticizes constantly so that child has no prospect of meeting expectations

Ignoring
- Fails to protect child from threats or intervene on behalf of the child
- Does not protect child from assault from siblings or other family members
- Does not respond to child's request for help or feedback

Corrupting
- Rewards child for stealing, substance abuse, assaulting other children, and sexual precocity
- Goads child into attacking other children
- Exposes child to pornography
- Encourages drug use
- Reinforces sexually aggressive behavior
- Involves child sexually with adolescents or adults

From Garbarino J., E. Guttman, and J. Seeley, The Psychologically Battered Child: Strategies for Identification, Assessment and Intervention. San Francisco: Jossey-Bass, 1987. Copyright 1986 by Jossey-Bass, Inc., Publishers.

established to accommodate the child after school. Safety measures are critical. If the child is to return home before the parent arrives, the child should be taught the following measures:

- Teach children not to display keys and always to lock doors. Keep a spare key at a neighbor's house.

- Tell children not to go into the house after school if the door is ajar, a window is open, or anything looks unusual. Teach children not to open the door to anyone unless the person has been approved by the parent.
- Teach children not to get in cars with strangers.
- Teach children first-aid procedures and prepare a safety kit.
- Teach safety rules to children who are expected to cook. Microwave ovens are the safest. Parents should not expect too much from the child.
- Emphasize such fire safety rules as leaving the house and not returning to it if a fire starts and practicing fire drills and evacuation at home, including determining a safe place to meet outside the home.
- Teach children about weather-related safety: (a) stay in the house in an electric storm; (b) stay in the storm cellar or in the safest part of the house during a tornado warning (practice tornado drills with children); and (c) keep a flashlight handy in case of power failures.
- Prevent drowning by (a) instructing children that they should never swim without adult supervision and (b) teaching older children caring for infants and toddlers about safe bathing methods.
- Use locked storage for firearms. Instruct children that only adults may handle the firearms.
- Teach children to tell callers that their parents are busy rather than saying "They're not here."
- Keep police, fire department, and other important telephone numbers by the phone. Be sure children know how to report emergencies.
- Investigate the neighborhood for families who will be at home and available for help with emergencies.
- Establish clear rules about what may or may not be done until parent gets home.
- Offer children a choice of activities.
- Discuss with children what to do after school. Recommend specific activities other than television.

The child must be given time—physically, emotionally, mentally, and socially—to be a child and to learn about the world around him or her at an individual pace. Too often parents want to hurry the child into adulthood. The result will be a chronologic adult who still acts and feels like a child. Television, firms, advertisements, peers, and neighbors all exert pressure to wear adult clothes, to be sexually precocious, to manipulate parents into fewer limits and less guidance, to take technology, materialism, and money for granted, and often to participate in a multitude of after- (or before-)

school activities. Parents believe their child must be the "early maturer." The pressures and hurry, especially in the middle-class and lower-upper-class urban family, are contributing to a growing number of troubled children who are emotionally distressed or ill or who are antisocial. The child abuses self and others with alcohol, drugs, and sexual activity. He or she also may search for peace among various cults or even through suicide. If the child must be *hurried* through childhood and if the child cannot be accepted for who he or she is, feelings of being unloved, rejected, and inferior grow ever deeper and bigger.

If we are committed to the family remaining the basic childrearing institution—and we have not invented anything better for children than parents—our attitudes and policies must catch up with the fact that millions of American families need help at different times for various reasons to raise their children well. As a nurse, you care for the family and the individual. Help parents clarify and act on their values. As a school nurse, your assessment may be the key to a child's receiving necessary care, as many children do not have a family doctor. You can conduct many health promotion activities described throughout this chapter. You can counsel and teach both parents and children. Be aware of cultural beliefs and practices as you work with children and families. A family who has lived in this country for several generations may follow the same cultural patterns as the family who is a new immigrant. Finally, as a citizen, your vote on action to pass health-related legislation is important and may be as crucial to health promotion as immunizations.

Relationships With Siblings

Although parental influence is of primary importance, the child's relationship with siblings affects personality formation. The influence of siblings on the development of the school-age child depends on a number of factors, including age and sex of the siblings, number of children in the family, proximity of their ages, and type of parent–child interaction (58).

Relationships between the school-age child and siblings vary from jealousy, rivalry, and competition to protectiveness and deep affection. Siblings tend to get along more harmoniously when they are the same sex, but boys usually are more physically aggressive at all ages. School-age children need privacy and personal space. Quarrels and conflicts erupt when this need is violated (58, 151, 211). Although sibling jealousy is less acute in school-age children than in preschool children, it still exists. An older child may be jealous of the attention given to younger siblings and may resent having to help with their care. The younger school-age child may feel jealous of the freedom given to older siblings. School-age children may feel the need to compete for parental attention and academic excellence. Parental comparisons of siblings' scholastic and artistic abilities or behavior should be avoided as they add to jealousy and resentment.

Adjustment outside the home is generally regarded as easier for the child with siblings than for the only child, who may develop a very close, intense relationship with the parents. The only child may cling to the notion of being the center of the family and may expect to be the center of attention in other groups as well. As a result, he or she may find the give and take of social living difficult (58). The differences in socialization between small and large families and for the only child are discussed in Chapter 4.

Sibling relationships are likely to influence social interactions in later life. Siblings teach each other how to negotiate, cooperate, compete, support, and reward one another and how to work and play with others. One child's illness or disability will have an effect on a healthy sibling, either positive or negative. Siblings of chronically ill children may work hard at being helpful to parents and the ill child, or even be overprotective, to receive attention and approval as well as to convey love, depending on how the family approaches care of the ill child. The siblings may also become depressed, withdraw, or act out in various ways to receive attention. They may have more school problems, or they may excel at school if that is the reinforcer. In part, how the siblings react depends on the psychological health of parents and their marital adjustment, and on the parents' ability to allow siblings to express anger, guilt, exclusion, deprivation, jealousy, fears of family breakup, or other feelings related to how their life differed from the life patterns of their friends (e.g., fewer outings, increased chores, less money for desired items). Siblings should have an opportunity to talk with health care professionals about the illness and their feelings.

Family Development Tasks

Family activities with the school-age child revolve around expanding the child's world. Family development tasks include the following (57):

- Take on parenting roles.
- Adjust the marital system and the lifestyle to allow physical, emotional, and social space for the child(ren).
- Keep lines of communication open among family members.

- Work together to achieve common goals.
- Plan a lifestyle within economic means.
- Find creative ways to continue a mutually satisfactory married life or satisfactory single parenthood.
- Maintain close ties with relatives.
- Realign relationships with the extended family to include parenting and grandparenting roles.
- Expand family life into the community through various activities.
- Validate the family philosophy of life. The philosophy is tested when the child brings home new ideas and talks about different lifestyles he or she encountered, forcing the family to reexamine patterns of living.

These tasks are manifested differently by families from various cultural backgrounds; those who are homeless, live in poverty, or are migrants; or those who live in war-torn or Third World countries. As you care for families and assist them to meet these tasks, consider the uniqueness of the family situation.

Adoptive families have the same developmental tasks as other families. An issue for adoptive parents, however, is how to help their adopted child(ren) feel a part of the family, especially if adoption occurs at an age when the child remembers the process.

Table 10–3 describes the adopted child's perception of adoption during the school years and how adoptive parents may respond. Prepare parents for when the adopted child may initiate search for the birth parent. Jenkins describes the reasons for the search and how the adoptive parents can help (109).

The adopted child especially struggles with identity issues because of uncertainties about the past, especially when the child is of different racial or ethnic origin than parents. The adolescent may become especially rebellious, saying, for example, "I don't have to obey you—you're not my real mom." Parents must remain open to the youth's questions, sustain an accepting and open atmosphere, expect turbulence, and help him or her find other supportive adults. Parents should not smother with concern, give in to unreasonable demands, or hold a grudge against the child who is acting ungratefully. (Most adolescents do.) Adoption is not a constant issue, but parents cannot ever completely retreat from it (141, 183).

Relationships Outside the Family

As the child's social environment widens, other individuals begin to function as role models and to influence the child. The child strives for independence and estab-

TABLE 10–3. ADOPTED CHILD'S PERCEPTIONS AND SUGGESTED PARENTAL RESPONSES

Age	Child's Perception	Suggested Parental Response
5–7	Begins to grasp full notion of adoption, that parents are not blood relatives, and that most children live with biological parent(s) Feels sense of loss	Emphasize that child is important to them and was chosen. Answer questions comfortably and naturally. Explain it is normal for child to have mixed emotions about adoption.
8–11	Fantasizes and wonders about birth parents Realizes he or she is different from nonadopted children Wants to question parents about adoption but fears appearing disloyal or ungrateful Feels grief and goes through mourning process Frequently asks questions about why birth parents relinquished him or her, parents' appearance, and whether there are siblings	Discuss the adoption openly, when appropriate, to help the child vent curiosity and feelings. Help child accept fact he or she is different and emphasize other differences as well. Answer questions truthfully. Do not criticize or overpraise birth parents. Adjust depth of answer to age of child. Realize children who are not adopted also fantasize they are.

lishes meaningful relationships with peers, teachers, and other significant adults. These relationships provide the child with new ideas, attitudes, perspectives, and modes of behavior. Although the parents remain role models, the influence of the family and the time spent with family diminish. Parents may feel a loss of control and may actually experience ambivalent feelings toward the child's peers and new adult role models. Influences outside the family may cause the child to verbalize less love and respect for parents, to resent limits imposed by the family, and to question ideas, attitudes, and beliefs held by the family. Through contacts with the peer group, the child acquires a basis for judging the parents as individuals and learns that parents can make mistakes (58, 74, 211).

The schoolchild has a growing sense of community that changes with increased mobility and independence and added responsibility. His or her understanding broadens to include a sense of boundaries, distance, location, and spatial relationships of resources and organizations, demographic characteristics, and group identity.

As a nurse or health care worker, you are in a key position to listen to and explore with families their con-

cerns about being parents, achieving the expected developmental tasks, and adjusting to the growing and changing child as he or she interacts with parents, siblings, other relatives, peers, and other adults outside the home. At times you may validate their approach to a given situation. At other times you may help them clarify their values so they can, in turn, better guide the child. Such practical suggestions as how to plan more economically a nutritious meal or handle sibling rivalry can help a distraught parent feel and become more effective.

Most parents try to do right by their children, but they may lack access, confidence, information, and power to deal alone with the people and institutions who could give help. Your ability to see beyond the obvious and to help the family use community resources effectively to meet basic needs is often the first step in promotion of both physical and emotional health. Your help may involve much effort over a period as you deal with a bureaucratic system and gain increasing empathy for the struggling family.

PHYSIOLOGIC CONCEPTS

Physical Characteristics

The child between 6 and 12 years old exhibits considerable change in physical appearance. Growth during this stage of development is hypertrophic (cells increase in size) instead of hyperplastic (cells increase in number). The growth rate is usually slow and steady, characterized by periods of accelerations in the spring and fall and by rapid growth during preadolescence (47, 58, 79, 80, 111, 211, 233).

Weight, Height, and Girth

These measurements vary considerably among children and depend on genetic, environmental, and cultural influences. African-American children and Caucasian children from lower socioeconomic groups usually are smaller in weight and height (233). Growth retardation is more reflective of socioeconomic than ethnic and genetic factors (212).

The average schoolchild grows 2 to 2½ inches (5–6 cm) per year to gain 1 to 2 ft (30–60 cm) in height by age 12. A weight gain of 4 to 7 pounds (2–3.5 kg) occurs per year. The average weight for a 6-year-old boy is 48 pounds (21.5 kg), and the average height is 46 in. (117 cm). By age 12 the average child weighs approximately 88 to 90 pounds (40 kg) and is more than 59 in. tall (150 cm). By age 12, the child has usually attained 90% of adult height. During the *juvenile* or *middle childhood period* girls and boys may differ little in size; their bodies are usually lean, with narrow hips and shoulders. There is a gradual decrease in the amount of baby fat with an increase in muscle mass and strength. Although the amount of muscle mass and adipose tissue is influenced by muscle use, diet, and activity, males usually have more muscle cells, and females have more adipose tissue. Muscle growth is occurring at a rapid rate. The muscles are changing in composition and are becoming more firmly attached to the bones. Muscles may be immature in regard to function, resulting in children's vulnerability to injury stemming from overuse, awkwardness, and inefficient movement. Muscle aches may accompany skeletal growth spurts as developing muscles attempt to keep pace with the enlarging skeletal structure. As the skeletal bones lengthen, they become harder. Ossification, the formation of bone, continues at a steady pace. The schoolchild loses the pot-bellied, swayback appearance of early childhood. Abdominal muscles become stronger; the pelvis tips backward and posture becomes straighter (212, 233).

Vital Signs

Vital signs of the schoolchild are affected by size, sex, and activity. Temperature, pulse, and respiration gradually approach adult norms with an average *temperature* of 98° to 98.6°F (36.7°–37°C), *pulse rate* of 70 to 80 per minute, resting pulse rate of 60 to 76 per minute, and *respiratory rate* of 18 to 21 per minute. The average *systolic blood pressure* is 94 to 112, and average *diastolic blood pressure* is 56 to 60 mm Hg. As respiratory tissues achieve adult maturity, *lung capacity* becomes proportional to body size. Between the ages of 5 and 10, the respiratory rate slows as the amount of air exchanged with each breath doubles. Breathing becomes deeper and slower. By the end of middle childhood, the lung weight will have increased almost 10 times. The ribs shift from a horizontal position to a more oblique one; the chest broadens and flattens to allow for this increased lung size and capacity (85, 233).

Cardiovascular System

The *heart* grows slowly during this age period; the left ventricle of the heart enlarges. After 7 years of age, the apex of the heart lies at the interspace of the fifth rib at the midclavicle line. Before this age, the apex is palpated at the fourth interspace just to the left of the midclavicle line. By age 9, the heart weighs 6 times its birth weight. By puberty, it weighs 10 times its birth weight. Even though cardiac growth does occur, the heart remains small in relation to the rest of the body. Because the heart is smaller proportionately to body size, the child may tire easily. Sustained physical activity is not desirable. The schoolchild should not be pushed to run, jog, or engage in excessively competitive sports such as football, hockey, and racquetball (212).

Hemoglobin levels are higher for Caucasian than African-American 10- to 15-year-olds. In all likelihood racial differences in hemoglobin levels during childhood exist independent of nutritional values. Racial differences are consistent with those for infants, preschool children, teenagers, pregnant women, and athletes, unrelated to nutritional variables (154).

Head

The growth of the *head* is nearly complete; head circumference measures approximately 21 in. (53 cm) and attains 95% of its adult size by the age of 8 or 9. The sinuses strengthen the structured formation of the face, reduce the weight of the head, and add resonance to the voice. The child loses the childish look as the face takes on features that will characterize him or her as an adult. Jaw bones grow longer and more prominent as the mandible extends forward, providing more chin and a place into which *permanent teeth* can erupt. Girls lose teeth earlier than boys; deciduous or baby teeth are lost and replaced at a rate of four teeth per year until approximately age 11 or 12. The "toothless" appearance may produce embarrassment for the child. The first permanent teeth are 6-year molars that erupt by age 7 and are the keystone for the permanent dental arch. Evaluation for braces should not be completed until all four 6-year molars have appeared. The second permanent molars erupt by age 14, and the third molars (wisdom teeth) come in as late as age 30. Some persons' wisdom teeth never erupt (Fig. 10–1). When the first permanent central incisors emerge, they appear too large for the mouth and face. Generally the teeth of boys are larger than those of girls (212, 233). Children who live in areas with high fluoride content in the drinking water may demonstrate **fluoride mottling** (*brownish permanent discoloration*) of the teeth in late childhood and adolescence (28).

Gastrointestinal System

Secretion, digestion, absorption, and excretion become more efficient. The stomach shape changes and its capacity increases; capacity at age 10 is 750 to 900 mL. Maturity of the gastrointestinal system is reflected in fewer stomach upsets, better maintenance of blood

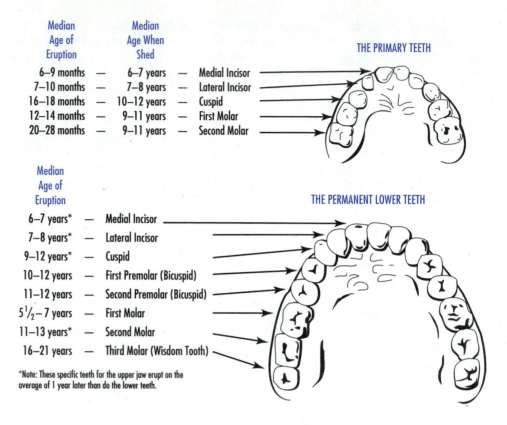

Median Age of Eruption		Median Age When Shed			THE PRIMARY TEETH
6–9 months	—	6–7 years	—	Medial Incisor	
7–10 months	—	7–8 years	—	Lateral Incisor	
16–18 months	—	10–12 years	—	Cuspid	
12–14 months	—	9–11 years	—	First Molar	
20–28 months	—	9–11 years	—	Second Molar	

Median Age of Eruption			THE PERMANENT LOWER TEETH
6–7 years*	—	Medial Incisor	
7–8 years*	—	Lateral Incisor	
9–12 years*	—	Cuspid	
10–12 years	—	First Premolar (Bicuspid)	
11–12 years	—	Second Premolar (Bicuspid)	
5½–7 years	—	First Molar	
11–13 years*	—	Second Molar	
16–21 years	—	Third Molar (Wisdom Tooth)	

*Note: These specific teeth for the upper jaw erupt on the average of 1 year later than do the lower teeth.

Figure 10–1. Normal tooth formation in the child.

sugar levels, and an increased stomach capacity (212, 233).

Urinary System

The urinary system becomes functionally mature during the school years. Between the ages of 5 and 10, the kidneys double in size to accommodate increased metabolic functions. Fluid and electrolyte balance becomes stabilized, and bladder capacity is increased, especially in girls. Urinary constituents and specific gravity become similar to those of an adult; however, 5 to 20% of school-age children have small amounts of albuminuria (233).

Vision

The shape of the eye changes during growth, and the normal farsightedness of the preschool child is gradually converted to 20/20 vision by age 8. By age 10 the eyes have acquired adult size and shape. Binocular vision is well developed in most children at 6 years of age; peripheral vision is fully developed. Girls tend to have poorer visual acuity than boys, but their color discrimination is superior. Large print is recommended for

reading matter and regular vision testing should be part of the school health program (233).

Immune System

Lymphoid tissues reach the height of development by age 7, exceeding the amount found in adults. The body's ability to localize infection improves. Enlargement of adenoidal and tonsillar lymphoid tissue is normal, as are sore throats, upper respiratory infections, and ear infections, which are caused by the excessive tissue growth and increased vulnerability of the mucous membranes to congestion and inflammation. The frontal sinuses are developed near age 6. Thereafter, all sinuses are potential sites for infection. Immunoglobulins G and A reach adult levels by age 9, and the child's immunologic system becomes functionally mature by preadolescence (233).

Neuromuscular Development

By age 7 the brain has reached 90% of adult size. The growth rate of the brain is greatly slowed after age 7, but by age 12 the brain has virtually reached adult size. Myelinization is complete; memory has improved. The child can listen better and make associations with incoming stimuli. Neuromuscular changes are occurring along with skeletal development. Neuromuscular coordination is sufficient to permit the schoolchild to learn most skills he or she wishes (233).

The transformation of the "clumsy" 6-year-old into the coordinated 12-year-old is due in part to maturation of the *central nervous system* and improved transmission of nerve impulses. The 6-year-old moves constantly—hopping, running, roller skating. The child walks a chalk mark with balance. Hands are used as tools in manipulative skills of hammering, cutting, pasting, tying shoes, and fastening clothes. Large letters or figures are made as he or she awkwardly grasps a pencil or crayon (47, 79, 80, 111, 212, 233).

Children of 7 have a lower *activity level* and enjoy active and quiet games. The child sees small print without difficulty, reverses letters less frequently while printing, and prints sentences. The 8-year-old moves energetically but with grace and balance, even in more active sports. Increased myelinization improves the child's reaction time and coordination. Longer arms permit more skillful throwing. He or she grasps objects better and writes rather than prints because the hands are larger and he or she has better small muscle coordination. The 9-year-old moves with less restlessness, is skillful in manual activities because of refined hand–eye coordination, and uses both hands independently. This child strives to improve coordination and to perfect physical skills, strength, and endurance. The preadolescent, aged 10 to 12, has energetic, active, restless movements with tension releases through finger drumming or foot tapping. Skillful manipulative movements nearly equal those of the adult, and physical changes preceding pubescence begin to appear (79, 80, 212, 233).

Prepubertal Sexual Development

During the *preadolescent* or *prepuberty period,* both males and females develop preliminary characteristics of sexual maturity. This period is characterized by the growth of body hair, a spurt of physical growth, changes in body proportion, and the beginning of primary and secondary sex characteristics. They demonstrate some of the same physical changes such as increased weight and height, vasomotor instability, increased perspiration, and active sebaceous glands. There is an increase in fat deposition approximately 1 year before the height spurt. These fat deposits last approximately 2 years or until skeletal growth and muscle mass increase. Females have more subcutaneous fat deposits, and the fat is lost at a slower rate, accounting for

the fuller appearance of the female figure (47, 58, 111, 212, 233).

The girl's growth spurt begins as early as 8 years; the average is 10, and maximum height velocity is reached around 12 years. The boy's growth spurt begins near 12 years; maximum height velocity is reached by approximately 14 years. The male grows approximately 4 in. (10 cm) per year for $2\frac{1}{2}$ years and then begins a slower rate of growth. The female grows an average of 3 in. (7.5 cm) per year until menarche begins. For both males and females, the growth spurt begins in the hands and feet and progresses to the calves, forearms, hips, chest, and shoulders; the trunk is the last to grow appreciably (47, 58, 111, 212, 233).

As sebaceous glands of the face, back, and chest become active, acne (pimples) may develop. These skin blemishes are caused by the trapping of collected sebaceous material under the skin in small pores. The preadolescent and later the adolescent are concerned with their appearance; these blemishes cause considerable embarrassment. The young person and the family may resort to use of numerous techniques such as skin specialists, sun lamps, diets, makeup, lotions, and creams to alleviate this problem. Basically, the skin should be kept clean. If the problem persists, a dermatologist should be seen. To prevent the youth's withdrawal from social contact, the parents and youth should be encouraged to seek medical attention as early as possible after acne occurs. Acne is further discussed in Chapter 11.

► ## PHYSICAL CHANGES IN GIRLS DURING PREADOLESCENCE

- Increase in transverse diameter of the pelvis
- Broadening of hips
- Tenderness in developing breast tissue and enlargement of areolar diameter
- Axillary sweating
- Change in vaginal secretions from alkaline to acid pH
- Change in vaginal layer to thick, gray, mucoid lining
- Change in vaginal flora from mixed to Döderlein's lactic acid–producing bacilli
- Appearance of pubic hair from 8 to 14 years (hair first appears on labia and then spreads to mons; adult triangular distribution does not occur for approximately 2 years after initial appearance of pubic hair)

These physical changes for females are listed in the approximate sequence of their occurrence (47, 58, 111, 212, 233).

► PHYSICAL CHANGES IN BOYS DURING PREADOLESCENCE

- Axillary sweating
- Increased testicular sensitivity to pressure
- Increase in size of testes
- Changes in color of scrotum
- Temporary enlargement of breasts
- Increase in height and shoulder breadth
- Appearance of lightly pigmented hair at base of penis
- Increase in length and width of penis

These physical changes for males are listed in the approximate sequence of their occurrence (47, 58, 111, 212, 233).

Vasomotor instability with rapid vasodilation causes excessive and uncontrollable blushing. This condition usually disappears when physical growth is completed.

For a summary of physical changes, refer to Physical Changes in Girls During Preadolescence and Physical Changes in Boys During Preadolescence.

Teach parents about the physical and growth characteristics of the school-age child and the importance of nutrition, rest, immunizations, healthful activity, and regular medical and dental care. The rest of the chapter refers to variables that influence physical health.

Physical Assessment of the School-Age Child

Information will be gained from the child, the parents or caretakers, or both when assessing the child.

A child may be better at drawing than at explaining what is wrong. For example, when asked to draw a big circle where it hurts, the child can normally identify the part if given a simple outline drawing of a child.

The child over age 10 may wish to talk to the health care provider without the parent present. Being alert to the child's chronologic and developmental stage and his or her relationship with parents or caretakers will guide you in interviewing. Remember that the child is not there in isolation. Where the child lives (house or apartment, rural or urban area), how much personal space he or she has (own room, own bed), parents' marital situation, presence or absence of siblings, what is usually eaten, how much exercise and rest in 24 hours, who cares for the child after school if parents are working, and how he or she spends free time are all important in assessing the health status.

When doing a review of systems, remember to use words the child understands. For example, instead of asking if the child has ever experienced any otitis problems, simply ask as follows: Do your ears ever ache? Can you always hear when people talk to you?

In assessing skin, remember that the school-age child is subject to allergic contact dermatitis, warts, herpes type 1, ringworm, and lice. When seeing any rash, a thorough history is in order to determine the diagnosis and necessary treatment.

Understanding that visual function is more than reading the 20/20 line on a Snellen chart will help you suggest a more comprehensive visual examination when a child is experiencing difficulty with school work.

Children and their parents do not always react predictably when there is a need for corrective lenses. Some children may feel self-conscious with their peers when wearing glasses. Parents may react as if the child's visual problem were a flaw and will deny it, stating that they are sure the child will outgrow the problem, ignore the information, or even go from doctor to doctor in search of reassurance.

If you are able to provide accurate information, using the principles of therapeutic communication, it will be exceedingly valuable to a child and family who are having difficulty adjusting to the need for therapy for a visual impairment. (This also holds true when therapy or a corrective device is needed on another body area.)

When assessing a child's hearing and ears, remember that hearing should be fully developed by age 5. By age 7, most children should speak clearly enough to be understood by adults. If either of these factors seems deficient, a thorough investigation into congenital or inherited disorders and how this deficiency affects daily activities and communication is in order (212).

In the young child, because the ear canal slants up, pull the auricle down, but not back as you would in an adult, when using the otoscope. Also, the ear canal is short in the young child, so take care not to insert the ear tip too far. The otoscope should be controlled so that if the young child moves suddenly, you can protect against the otoscope's hitting the ear drum. The cone of light is more indistinct in a child than in an adult (212).

Keep in mind the following as you continue assessment of the child's body systems: (1) if you think you hear fluid in the lungs, check the child's nose because sounds caused by nose fluid can be transmitted to the lungs; (2) an S_3 sound and sinus arrhythmia are fairly common in children's heart sounds; (3) a child's liver and spleen usually will enlarge more quickly than an adult's in response to disease; (4) the bladder is normally found much higher in a child than in an adult, and the kidneys can more often be palpated; (5) the genitalia should be inspected for congenital abnormalities that may have been overlooked and for irritation, inflammation, or swelling; and (6) developmental guidelines must be used to assess the nervous system, specifically language development, motor and sensory functions, and cerebral function (15, 233).

In the last 10 years musculoskeletal and posture problems, especially scoliosis detection, have gained wide attention. **Scoliosis,** *lateral curvature of the spine,* is more common in girls than in boys and is of two types, functional and structural. Ask the child to bend over and touch the toes without bending the knees and keeping the palms of the hands together. If the child has functional scoliosis, the external curve will disappear with this exercise; if it is structural, the curve will remain and sometimes become more pronounced. Early diagnosis is extremely important to arrest this problem (212, 233). Refer the child and family to an orthopedic specialist. If scoliosis is not corrected early in life, it can result in mobility problems, obstructive pulmonary disease, and problems with body image later in life.

Nutritional Needs

Although caloric requirements per unit of body weight continue to decrease for the schoolchild, nutritional requirements remain relatively greater than for the adult. (See Appendix I) The young schoolchild requires approximately 80 calories per kilogram daily or 35 calories per pound. By age 10 there is a decrease in the calories per kilogram for both boys (45 calories/kg) and girls (38 calories/kg). An individual child may require more or fewer calories than the Recommended Dietary Allowances (RDAs), depending on size, activity, and growth rate. Therefore the total caloric range is approximately 1600 to 2200 daily. Daily caloric needs can be approximated for the child by the following formula: 1000 calories the first year plus 100 calories for each additional year (227).

Protein requirement for growth is 1 g per pound or 36 to 40 g of protein daily. Vitamin and mineral requirements are similar to those for the preschool child. Because of enlargement of ossification centers in the bone, vitamin D (400 units) and a large intake of calcium (800 mg to age 10; 1200–1500 mg ages 11 until 24) are needed daily. Vitamin C needs are not met as easily as other nutritional requirements (227). Many of the fruit-flavored juices supply significant amounts of ascorbic acid. Vitamin A, iodine, and iron, major micronutrients, are often deficient, and these deficiencies can threaten school and work output and health, and can threaten life (234).

Water intake may be overlooked; the schoolchild needs 1½ to 3 quarts daily, depending on her or his size.

Nutritional needs for the schoolchild include one or more servings daily of the foods listed in Recommended Nutritional Intake for Schoolchildren. (213, 227).

Lunch for schoolchildren is often a cola, bag of potato chips, brownies, and ice cream. They do not eat the food provided by the school lunch program because they "do not like it." Because junk food and fast foods have also permeated the home, the child may get little else to eat. Further, schools have vending machines with junk food readily available. Thus American children eat too much salt, sugar, fat, and cholesterol, and 25% have a cholesterol level greater than 170, which is extremely high for children. By adolescence these same children will show signs of clogged arteries (199).

The school lunch program offers the child the best chance for a nutritious meal. Since 1946 a federally subsidized lunch has included meat or another protein, two servings of fruit and/or vegetables, a grain, and milk for low cost or at no charge if the student is from a low-income family; however, the lunch can be high in fat (40% of total calories for the meal). Thus foods in this program should be baked, not fried (199).

Anyone over the age of 2 should daily consume no more than 30% of their total calories in fat; however, the average person aged 6 to 19 years consumes 37% of his or her calories in fat (227).

Children eat what their parents eat. More fruits and vegetables must be eaten in the home so that chil-

► RECOMMENDED NUTRITIONAL INTAKE FOR SCHOOLCHILDREN

Meat and eggs (alternates: dry beans, dry peas, lentils)	2 or more 2- or 3-oz servings
Milk (whole, skim, or powdered)	2–4 cups
Fruits and vegetables (including dark green or deep yellow vegetable for vitamin A and fruit or vegetable containing vitamin C)	5 or more servings
Breads and cereals	4 or more servings to meet caloric needs
Fats and carbohydrates	Use sparingly

dren develop a taste for them, and school lunch programs must persist in serving them.

To determine whether Latino children were following the recommended 5-A-Day of fruits and vegetables, a study of 214 mother–child pairs was conducted over a 3-year period. The child's intake averaged fewer than two fruits or vegetables a day; only 6.8% of the children ate five or more servings of fruit and vegetables daily. Those children who ate five servings also had higher intake of vitamins A and C, potassium, iron, cholesterol, protein, and fiber. It is recommended that the campaign to eat 5-A-Day take into consideration the existing patterns of the target population (27).

Discuss with parents the importance of a balanced diet and foods that supply specific nutrients.

Nutritional assessment is determined by obtaining a history of the child's food intake; looking at the general appearance and skin color and turgor; correlating height and weight; measuring subcutaneous tissue; checking for dental caries, allergies, and chronic illness; testing hemoglobin and hematocrit levels; and determining physical, cognitive, emotional, and social well-being (228).

Eating Patterns

It is important to discuss the child's eating needs and patterns with parents so that they can provide a diet with adequate caloric intake and nutrients. By age 8, children have increased appetites; by age 10, their appetites are similar to those of adults. Despite increasing appetites, children seldom voluntarily interrupt activities for meals. Television, sports, and other activities compete with mealtimes. Parents should be encouraged to establish a consistent schedule for meals and to allow their school-age child to participate in the meal planning. The schoolchild of 6 or 7 is capable of learning about healthful eating and of helping plan and prepare meals. Such activities develop a healthy sense of industry and independence in the child if they are not overdone.

Mealtime continues to cause dissension within most families. Parents are often upset by their child's terrible table manners. The young child stuffs food in his or her hands, spills it, and incessantly chatters throughout the meal. The time the family spends together eating can be much more pleasant if manners are not overemphasized. If discipline during meals is necessary, it should be kept to a minimum. When mealtime becomes a time of stress, digestive problems, poor eating habits, or a temporary aversion to food may occur. Making a fuss over eating certain foods may cause the child to reject them more strongly. Experience and time will improve eating patterns, as shown in Table 10–4 (79, 80, 212).

Food preferences and dislikes become strongly established during the school years; however, by age 8 the child will try new or previously disliked foods. Food likes and dislikes are often carried over from the eating experiences of the toddler and preschooler. In addition,

TABLE 10–4. SUMMARY OF EATING PATTERNS OF SCHOOLCHILDREN

6 Years	7 Years	8 Years	9 Years	10 Years	11 Years	12 Years
Has large appetite	Has extremes of appetite	Has large appetite	Has controlled appetite	Goes on eating sprees	Has controlled appetite	Has large appetite
Likes between-meal and bedtime snacks	Improves table manners	Enjoys trying new foods	Enjoys trying new foods	Likes sweet foods	Improves table manners when eating in a restaurant	Enjoys most foods
Is awkward at table	Is quieter at table	Handles eating utensils skillfully	Eats approximately an adult meal	Criticizes parents' table manners	Enjoys cooking	Has adultlike table manners
Likes to eat with fingers	Is interested in table conversation	Has better table manners away from home	Acts more adultlike	Has lapses in control of table manners at times		Participates in table discussions in adultlike manner
Swings legs under table, often kicking people and things	Leaves table with distraction		Becomes absorbed in listening or talking	Enjoys cooking		
Dawdles						
Criticizes family members						
Eats with better manners away from family						

it is easy for the schoolchild, influenced by peers, television commercials and other forms of advertisement, and the availability of junk food, to avoid nutritious foods and to fill up on empty calories.

The child mimics family attitudes toward food and eating. In many families food is equated with love and affection, an attitude that may result in the child's becoming overweight. Companionship and conversation at the child's level are essential during mealtime, for the child wants to talk and participate in a group. Mealtime conversation should be enjoyable, provide for learning conversational skills, and allow for participation by all. The give-and-take of good family discussion stimulates learning, confidence, and digestion. The child especially likes picnics and eating with peers. Because food and eating are such vital social and cultural concerns, the source of a nutritional problem may be as much a psychosocial problem as a physiologic one.

Diet is also influenced by a child's activities. If the child has been active all day, he or she will be hungry and ready to eat. On the other hand, if the child has had limited activity or emotional frustrations during the day, he or she may have no appetite. The schoolchild has more freedom to move without parental supervision and often has small amounts of money to spend on candy, soft drinks, and other treats. In addition, the schoolchild is eating on his or her own for the first time. Peer influence will frequently determine the child's lunch. Schools have attempted to satisfy current eating preferences of this age group by offering a la carte selections such as french fries, hot dogs, pizza, and salads as well as balanced meals. Total and saturated fat and sodium content should be reduced in both school lunches and home meals.

Share the following suggestions with parents to improve nutrition and mealtime (228):

1. Create an environment of respect, love, acceptance, and calm.
2. Make food attractive and manageable.
3. Establish basic rules regarding table etiquette and table language, topics of conversation, and behavior. Provide a rest period before meals.
4. Have a firm understanding with the child that play and television do not take precedence over eating properly; keep television and the telephone at a minimum.
5. Between-meal snacks are necessary and enjoyed and do not interfere with food intake at meals if eaten an hour or longer before mealtime. Milk, cheese, fresh fruits and vegetables, peanut butter, and fruit juices are desirable snacks for both general nutritional needs and dental health.

6. Breakfast is crucial for providing the child with sufficient calories to start the day. The child who attends school without breakfast frequently exhibits fatigue and poor attention (228, 233).
7. With a comfortable environment and adults eating the food on the table, the intake is likely to be adequate for the child, as the parents are role models.

Undernutrition in children can be manifested in retarded growth, underweight, fatigue, lassitude, restlessness, irritability, and poor school performance and work output. Anorexia and digestive disturbances such as diarrhea and constipation signal improper utilization of nutrients. Poor muscular development may be evidenced by a child's posture—rounded shoulders, flat chest, and protuberant abdomen. Prolonged undernutrition may cause irregularities in dentition and may delay epiphyseal development and puberty (227).

Undernutrition and overnutrition may have the same causative factors: the child may be reflecting food habits of other family members; the parents and child may displace unrelated anxieties on food and mealtime; or eating may serve as a reward or punishment by both parents and child. *Overnutrition* and overweight are rarely caused by metabolic disturbances. **Obesity** is sometimes defined as an *individual who is 20% or more above ideal weight*. Obesity is the most frequent nutritional disorder of children in developed countries (227). In addition, childhood obesity can have serious social and emotional effects that may carry into adulthood (129). Prevention of childhood obesity through early nutrition education and established exercise habits is important. Forty percent of overweight 7-year-olds and 70% of overweight 10-year-olds become overweight adults (233). In another study, diet and lifestyle factors were major determinants of obesity in childhood and adolescence and of risk for cardiovascular disease (90).

Parents should be encouraged to promote food to their children as nourishment for their bodies, not as a reward or punishment. They should promote food as necessary and enjoyable. A healthy child's appetite corresponds to physiologic needs and should be a valuable index in determining intake. Too often parents expect young children to eat as much as the parents do. The child should be neither forced to eat everything on his or her plate nor made to feel guilty if second portions of mother's special dish are not eaten.

You can help parents learn about adequate nutrition for their child as well as what behavior to expect at each age. You can also aid teachers as they plan lessons on nutrition. For example, learning activities for the schoolchild could include visiting grocery stores, dairies, or farms as well as taking part in tasting parties and playing store. They could plan menus, cook various foods, and taste them. Such activities are unlimited.

Increasingly, dietary intake of excess sugar, food coloring, and other additives is being related to the child's behavior, especially hyperactivity. The whole family can benefit from natural foods, foods that have a minimum of preservatives or additives, and foods that are cooked properly (58, 227).

Rest and Exercise

There is no rule of thumb for the amount of rest a child should have. Hours of sleep needed depend on such variables as age, health status, and the day's activities. Schoolchildren usually do not need a nap. They are not using up as much energy in growth as they were earlier. A 6-year-old usually requires approximately 11 hours of sleep nightly, but an 11-year-old may need only 9 hours (233). The schoolchild does not consciously fight sleep but may need firm discipline to go to bed at the prescribed hour. Sleep may be disturbed with dreams and nightmares, especially if he or she has considerable emotional stimulation before bedtime.

Exercise is essential for muscular development, refinement of coordination and balance, gaining strength, and enhancing other body functions such as circulation, aeration, and waste elimination. The schoolchild should have a safe place to play and simple pieces of equipment. Because there are times when bad weather will keep a child from going outside, supplies should be available that will facilitate exercise indoors.

Parents should play actively with their children sometimes. Children benefit from their parents' knowledge of various activities and are encouraged by the attention. Exercise then becomes fun, not work. In the United States, where the child can be constantly entertained by television, parents must sometimes encourage exercise.

A study of 552 girls of Asian and Hispanic origin who were in the 5th through 12th grades revealed that only 36% of the children met the year 2000 goal for strenuous physical activity. Less physical activity was associated with less muscle mass and excess body weight. Girls may become less active in strenuous physical activity as they enter adolescence for cultural and social reasons (233). In a study of 262 children, boys and girls who were physically fit had lower cholesterol, low-density lipoprotein cholesterol, and triglyceride levels and higher high-density lipoprotein cholesterol levels than unfit children (87).

Review the child's rest and exercise needs with parents. At the same time, you may have an opportunity to discuss with parents how they are meeting their own needs for rest and exercise and how the parents and child can engage in activities that are mutually interesting and healthful.

Health Promotion and Health Protection

Immunizations

Immunizations against measles, mumps, rubella, and polio should be given to the schoolchild if they have not previously been given. Diphtheria and tetanus toxoids combined with pertussis vaccine (DTP) and oral poliovirus vaccine (OPV) must be given as indicated in previous chapters. Booster doses of DTP and OPV should be given by 6 years of age; pertussis vaccine is not necessary for children over this age. Live measles/mumps/rubella vaccine (MMR) should be given between the ages of 11 and 12. Girls should receive rubella vaccine before they enter puberty to prevent congenital defects in a baby should they be exposed to rubella during pregnancy. Boys should be immunized against mumps before the age of 12; mumps contracted during or after puberty can cause sterility. The need for tuberculin tests depends on the prevalence of tuberculosis and the risk of exposure. Influenza virus vaccine, pneumococcal vaccine, and hepatitis B vaccine are recommended for children in certain high-risk groups (32, 214, 233).

In the United States an estimated 88% of Caucasian and 64% of nonwhite children are immunized against one or more preventable major childhood diseases. (In the developing world, the majority of children are not immunized against common contagious diseases [214, 233].)

Emphasize to parents the importance of immunization and record keeping. Supply parents with information about free immunization programs and school requirements for immunization. Inform them of an appropriate immunization schedule. They should know, for example, that if 7-year-old Tommy steps on a rusty nail, he is protected from tetanus because of DTP immunization at age 5. Before a child receives an immunization, he or she should be told why and where it will be given. Such explanations will elicit cooperation and help the child to understand that neither the illness nor the treatment is being imposed because he or she is bad.

Safety Promotion and Injury Control

Accidents are of major concern for this age group and for younger children. Violent deaths, such as from drive-by shootings, and accidents constitute the largest cause of deaths among schoolchildren; they are fatal nearly four times more often than cancer, the next leading cause of death. Motor vehicle accidents account for half of the accidental deaths in this age group. Other accidents that threaten children are fires, falls, drownings, and poisonings (11, 107, 153, 208, 214, 231, 233). Even though school-age children have developed more refined muscular coordination and control, their use of bicycles, skateboards, roller skates, and sports increases their risk for injury. They are susceptible to cuts, abrasions, fractures, strains, sprains, and bruises. The incidence of injury is significantly higher in school-age boys than girls, and the death rate of boys is twice that of girls (192, 233). Some of the injuries sustained during sporting activities may cause permanent disability because of damage to the epiphyseal cartilage or the neuromuscular system.

A study of farm-related deaths in California in children under age 15 from 1980 to 1989 indicated deaths were likely to be from machinery (81%), animals (10%), electricity (5%), and nontraffic motor vehicles (3%). Rates for farm-related fatalities were higher for Hispanic than non-Hispanics, possibly because of their role in agriculture. Rates of death for farm children were lower in California than in the Midwest, possibly because of a larger number of corporate farms, milder climate, and differences in agricultural practices (192).

There are a group of children who apparently are *accident-prone*. They suffer more accidental injuries than the overall childhood population. Although the causative factors have not been completely determined, children who are overreactive, restless, impulsive, hostile, and immature are frequently found in this group (233).

Parents should be encouraged to provide more supervision and attention to these children and to repeat, even to children who are not accident-prone, cautions as necessary. The child forgets when involved in play; conceptual thinking and judgment are not well developed so that the child does not foresee dangers.

Accident prevention should be taught and enforced in school and at home. You must promote safety by helping parents and children identify and avoid hazards. The school-age child has increasing cognitive maturity, including improved ability to remember past experiences and anticipate probable outcomes of his or her actions. This makes the child a good candidate for safety instructions (233).

Safety education should include information about the hazards of risk taking and improper use of equipment (50, 233). Injury prevention should address motor vehicle injuries, drownings, burns, poisonings, falls, and sports-related injuries. The child should be taught the proper use of seatbelts in motor vehicles. Safe pedestrian behavior should be emphasized by teaching the child the proper way to cross streets, how to read traffic signals, and the dangers of street play. You should stress the safety and maintenance of two-wheeled vehicles (such as bicycles) and encourage the use of safety apparel where applicable (112). Water safety and survival skills should be taught with basic swimming skills at an early age. Families who go boating must teach related safety measures to their children.

Farm children are at risk for accidental injury or death when they accompany or assist parents with farm work. Teach farm parents the following rules to reduce hazards (11, 221):

- Do not allow children as extra riders on equipment.
- Do not allow children to play with idle machinery.
- Leave any equipment that might fall, such as front-end loaders, in the down position.
- When self-propelled machinery is parked, brakes should be locked and keys removed from the ignition.
- Always leave a tractor power-takeoff unit in neutral.
- When starting machinery—and especially when reversing it—know where the children are.
- Maintain machinery in good repair, particularly protective shields and seat belts.
- Do not permit children to operate machinery until they have completed safety training.
- Fence farm ponds and manure pits.
- Place fixed ladders out of reach, or fit with a special barrier; store portable ladders away from danger areas.
- Shield dangerous machinery components and electric boxes and wiring and place out of easy reach or fit with locking devices.
- Place warning decals on all grain bins, wagons, and trucks.
- Maintain lights and reflectors for all equipment used on roads.
- Do not expect children to work with farm animals or with machinery that is beyond their maturity physically or mentally.

Death by homicide has increased markedly in the United States and perhaps throughout the world. Child homicides are more common if the mother is unmarried, teenage, or a high-school dropout, and homicide rates are higher for African-Americans (191, 192, 193, 230).

Meal preparation can be fun for the school-age child, but the hazards of sharp knives, hot stoves, microwave ovens (the health effect of microwave radiation leakage is still unknown (237), and hot liquids must be kept in mind. Supervise the use of matches or flammable chemicals, and teach the child the proper behavior if clothing becomes ignited. A family-designed fire escape plan should be initiated and practiced monthly.

Most boys and girls love to climb trees; adults should teach them how to climb in the safest possible way. Explain the dangers involved in climbing electric poles, water towers, and other dangerous structures. Instruct the child in the proper use of playground equipment and in the need to pick up toys from the floor to prevent falls.

Instruct parents to keep potentially dangerous products in properly labeled receptacles. Educate the child about the dangers of taking nonprescription drugs and chemicals. Gun accidents are common during the school-age period. Parents who have a gun should keep it under lock and place the key in a childproof location. Children of this age should be taught safety rules concerning guns.

You can advise parents of the hazards associated with organized contact sports; stress the use of protective head, elbow, and knee gear. Instruct the child in the proper use of sporting equipment, especially the more hazardous devices—skis, trampolines, skateboards, mopeds, and all-terrain vehicles.

You can reinforce any teaching that takes place in the home. Books, films, and creation of a mock situation can all supplement your verbal instruction. You and the parents will repeat the same cautions endlessly. Yet, caution and concern can be overdone. When a child is overly anxious about his or her welfare, tension can lead not only to accident proneness but to being hurt worse when he or she does encounter danger. In the face of danger, panic prevents clear thinking and skillful action. In addition, overcaution stifles independence, initiative, and maturing. It is important to realize the necessity of shifting responsibility to the child with increasing age.

Responsibility for the child's health rests with the parents, but you can emphasize to parents the importance of regular examinations at a clinic or from a family physician and dentist. Every child should have a thorough preschool examination, including visual and auditory screening and posture and general health examination. Correction of health problems is essential, as they may be a cause for injuries, illness, or difficulties with school work or peers. Realize that in the United States millions of children receive basically no health care.

As a nurse you have a responsibility to strengthen the school health program in your community through direct services; teaching the board of education, teachers, parents, and students about the value and use of such a program despite costs; and working for legisla-

tion to finance and implement programs that do more than first-aid care. A school health program should supervise not only the child's physical health, but also emotional, mental, and social health. Instruction in personal hygiene, disease prevention, nutrition, safety, family life, and group living is of interest to the schoolchild and should be under the direction of the school nurse.

If there are chronically ill or disabled students in school, special preparation should be given to the teachers, the students, and the parents. You can promote understanding of the child and his or her condition, of the child's need to use individual potential, and of a total rehabilitation program. Several references will be helpful (200, 202, 234).

Common Health Problems: Prevention and Treatment

Although the child should now remain basically healthy, health problems do exist.

Inform parents of the need to treat both acute and chronic conditions. *Respiratory conditions* (colds, sore throats, and earaches) account for more than 50% of the reported acute illnesses among children in this age group. *Infective and parasitic diseases* (scabies, impetigo, ringworm, and head lice) are of concern because of their health threat to the child and to others. *Diseases of the digestive tract* (stomachaches, peptic ulcers, colitis, diarrhea, and vomiting) may have a psychosocial and a physiologic cause. Visual and hearing impairment, sickle cell anemia, asthma, hyperactivity, epilepsy, migraine headaches, hypertension, diabetes mellitus, and obesity are *chronic health problems* that may affect the school-age child (179, 235). The child may have been born with a congenital anomaly that can be only partially corrected or a disease such as hemophilia that needs continuing treatment. A considerable number of schoolchildren have risk factors that in adults are predictive of coronary heart disease: hypertension, increased serum cholesterol and triglycerides, and obesity. The elementary school population may also be the main reservoir of infectious hepatitis type A, for schoolchildren often have a mild undiagnosed disease that is spread person to person (101).

Because of the short urethra, girls are prone to *urinary infection;* this may be diagnosed by reddened genitals, a feeling of burning on urination, and abnormal appearance and chemical analysis of the urine. Normal urinary output from 6 to 12 years ranges from 500 mL to the adult output of 1500 mL daily. Pinworms accompany urinary tract infections in approximately 50% of the cases (101).

The 7-year-old has fewer illnesses but may complain of *fatigue* or *muscular pain.* It is common to call these "growing pains"; however, this is not accurate, as growing is not painful. Tension, overactivity or exertion, bruising, or injury may cause the leg pains. Pains in the knees with no exertional signs are also common in school-age children. Such pains usually occur late in the day or night and disappear in the morning.

Children with persistent leg pains should be referred to a physician. The 8- and 9-year-olds are generally healthy but may complain of minor aches to get out of disagreeable tasks. Such behavior should not be reinforced by undue attention.

Visual impairments that occur in the younger child may be undetected and untreated until the child attends school. Visual acuity may not develop normally. For more information, see Signs and Symptoms Indicating Defective Vision in Schoolchildren (101, 233). It is essential that visual problems be corrected.

Table 10–5 summarizes other common health problems, their definitions, symptoms and signs, and prevention or treatment measures (20, 60, 101, 212).

There is increasing concern about the school-child's risks for cardiovascular disease. Study of 71 monozygotic and 34 same-sex dizygotic twin pairs ages 6 to 11 in the Philadelphia area revealed that children with characteristics of type A behavior and its subcomponents—high triglyceride levels, systolic blood pressure, and obesity—have a genetic predisposition to cardiovascular disease, but that some people have a greater response to environmental factors, which also influence these characteristics (145).

Type A behavior apparently is an outcome of an interaction between physiologic factors based on (1) sympathetic reactivity, which may be due to genetics or early conditioning; (2) cognitive reactions to certain situations; and (3) psychological traits. Because weight, lipid profiles, and blood pressure have both substantial environmental and genetic origins, nurses should encourage reduction of fat in the diet, increased physical exercise, and smoking cessation (145).

Rabies, an *acute infectious disease characterized by involvement of the central nervous system, resulting in paralysis and finally death,* is fortunately not a common disease but comes from a common problem: the biting of a human by a mammal. Refer to Chapter 9 for treatment. If a diagnosis of rabies is considered, it must be reported to the local health department and Centers for Disease Control (CDC) in Atlanta. The CDC staff will act as consultants for the use of antirabies vaccine and all other factors surrounding the case. Refer to Uphold and Graham (212) for treatment recommendations. Prevention is in keeping the child away from unfamiliar animals, particularly ones that act agitated, in seeing that

all pets are properly vaccinated, and in taking steps to get preexposure immunization for high-risk children—those living or visiting in countries where rabies is a constant threat.

Increasingly, the ill effects of *smoking and drug and alcohol abuse* are emerging as a regular health problem

► SIGNS AND SYMPTOMS INDICATING DEFECTIVE VISION IN SCHOOLCHILDREN

Behavior

- Attempts to brush away blur; rubs eyes frequently; frowns, squints
- Stumbles frequently or trips over small objects
- Blinks more than usual; cries often or is irritable when doing close work
- Holds books or small playthings close to eyes
- Shuts or covers one eye, tilting or thrusting head forward when looking at objects
- Has difficulty in reading or in other schoolwork requiring close use of the eyes; omits words or confuses similar words
- Exhibits poor performance in activities requiring visual concentration within arm's length (e.g., reading, coloring, drawing); unusually short attention span; persistent word reversals after second grade
- Disinterested in distant objects or fails to participate in games such as playing ball
- Engages in outdoor activity mostly (e.g., running, bicycling), avoiding activities requiring visual concentration within arm's length
- Sensitive to light
- Unable to distinguish colors
- Steps carefully over sidewalk cracks or around light or dark sections of block linoleum floors
- Trips at curbs or stairs
- Poor eye–hand coordination for age, excessively hard-to-read handwriting, difficulty with tying shoelaces or buttoning and unbuttoning

Appearance

- Crossed eyes (iris of one eye turned in or out and not symmetric with other eye)
- Red-rimmed, encrusted, or swollen eyelids
- Repeated styes
- Watery or red eyes

Complaints

- Cannot see blackboard from back of room
- Blurred or double vision after close eye work
- Dizziness, headaches, or nausea after close eye work
- Itching or burning eyes

Data from References 101 and 233.

TABLE 10–5. COMMON HEALTH PROBLEMS OF SCHOOLCHILDREN

Problem	Definition	Symptoms/Signs	Prevention/Treatment
Accommodative esophoria	Eyes converge excessively in response to accommodation	Close work becomes exhausting and overwhelming	Eyeglasses and taking "eye breaks" recommended.
Otitis externa	Inflammation of the external auditory canal and auricle	Pain in ear aggravated by moving the auricle; exudate in ear canal	Prevention: Keep instruments out of ears. Keep dirty water out of ear. Use acetic acid (2%) solution in ear after swimming. After the fact, use antibiotic and/or steroid drops.
Serous otitis media	Accumulation of nonpurulent fluid in middle ear	Fullness and crackling in ear; decreased hearing	Administer decongestants (questionable help).
Allergic rhinitis	Allergic reaction affecting nasal mucosa (and sometimes conjunctiva)	Clear, thin nasal discharge; breathes through mouth; often does "allergic salute" (rubs nose upward)	Find offending irritant or antigen and try to eliminate. Take antihistamines. Obtain workup by allergist if problem persists.
Asthma	Disease of lungs characterized by partially reversible airway obstruction, airway inflammation, and airway hyperresponsiveness; caused by hyperreactivity of the tracheobronchial tree to chemical mediators	Wheezing, cough, dyspnea, anxiety, restlessness	Try to stay away from allergens, if known. Avoid being around those with upper respiratory infections; avoid overexertion, rapid temperature or humidity changes, air pollutants, emotional upsets. Follow NAEP (National Asthma Education Program) step-care approach described by Boynton et al. (20) for appropriate timing of essential medications.
Herpes type I	Vesicular eruption of skin and mucous membranes above the umbilicus (usually mouth)	Soreness of mouth from eruption of mucosa; inflammation and swelling; sometimes fever and enlarged lymph glands (submandibular)	Apply Zovirax ointment to slow down severity. Drink adequate fluids. Use saline solution mouthwash. Administer antipyretic. Isolate from susceptible persons.
Contact dermatitis	Vesicular formation on skin, usually from poison ivy or poison oak	Itching and formation of vesicles, sometimes on most body parts	Apply cold compresses and drying lotion. Sometimes administer cortisone-based oral medicine or injections. Learn how to avoid plants.
Tinea corporis (ringworm of nonhairy skin)	Superficial fungal infection involving face, trunk, or limbs	Red, patch areas that scale and are oval in shape; usually asymptomatic or mildly itchy; no systemic signs	Apply a topical antifungal daily for 2 or 3 weeks.
Tinea capitis (ringworm of the head)	Fungal infection involving scalp	Same as tinea corporis	Apply fungal cream persistently. Sometimes it is necessary to shave hair.
Warts	Intradermal papillomas	Usually appear as common on hands or fingers or plantar (on feet)	Dichloroacetic acid will often dissolve them. Other removal methods are available from dermatologist.
Pediculus humanus capitis (head lice)	Infestation of head, hair, scalp with stated organism	Itching scalp; see nits or ova as little dots attached to base hairs	Shampoo with approved medication. Apply antihistamine for itching. Comb out any remaining ova-nits. Boil all head care items.

(continued)

TABLE 10–5. COMMON HEALTH PROBLEMS OF SCHOOLCHILDREN (continued)

Problem	Definition	Symptoms/Signs	Prevention/Treatment
Mumps	Viral disease characterized by acute swelling of salivary gland, especially the parotid	Anterior ear pain; headache; lethargy; anorexia; vomiting; complication orchitis (*inflammation of one or both testes*)	Prevention: obtain vaccine. Use only supportive treatment such as antipyretics (not aspirin products) and encourage fluid intake.
Diabetes mellitus type I (formally called juvenile diabetes)	Inherited disease with metabolic component that causes elevated blood sugar and vascular component that causes effects on eyes and kidneys	Increased urination; increased thirst and hunger; weight loss and fatigue	Obtain workup by appropriate health care practitioner. Follow diabetic diet and exercise recommendations. Administer insulin.
Fifth disease (erythema infectiosum)	Mild viral illness caused by Human parvovirus B19; no ongoing harm to child but maternal infection can cause spontaneous abortions and stillbirths	Three-stage exanthems: (1) slapped cheek appearance; (2) maculopapulary rash on trunk and extremities, looks lacey; (3) rash has evanescence and recrudenesence	If it is a school-related breakout, expect a 25% attack rate. Stay away from pregnant women. There is no specific treatment, only symptomatic, i.e., acetaminophen for aches. Stay away from sun, which can exacerbate rash.
Hand-foot-and-mouth disease	Contagious viral disease caused by Coxsackie virus A.	Abrupt fever; vesicular lesions of the mouth, palms of the hands, and soles of feet; anorexia	As it is highly contagious, keep isolated until temperature is normal for 24 hours. Treat symptomatically: saline mouth rinse; acetaminophen for temperature elevation; fluids; tepid baths.
Pityriasis rosea	An acute, self-limited, presumably viral-caused disease which produces a characteristic rash	Classic lesion on trunk, looks like a Christmas tree; starts with "mother spot"—scaly, salmon colored, spreading peripherally	There is no need to isolate. Expect rash to last as long as 4 months. Use symptomatic treatment such as cool compress, calamine lotion, Benadryl (if pruritis). Exposure to sunlight will relieve itching and shorten duration of rash.

among adolescents. These habits are influenced by the habits of parents, siblings, and peers. The child may not enjoy smoking but will do it to show off; knowledge of the effects of cigarette smoking is not necessarily a deterrent.

In addition to the ill effects caused by actual smoking, children in families with cigarette smokers have an increased rate of respiratory conditions and cancer. These small children have an increased number of days per year when their activities are restricted because of illness (70, 233). Teach parents that smoking may be interfering with the normal growth and development of schoolchildren and that parental and other adult example is important.

Determinants of positive health behavior in a study of 260 9- and 10-year-old boys and girls indicated that age and sex of the child, parental education, and family size influenced self-esteem and personal perception of health. Boys and girls in the fourth grade differed in their reported health habits; girls scored higher than

boys in health behaviors, willingness to report symptoms, and self-concept. These results may reflect socialization patterns and expected role behaviors of men and women in our culture. Intrinsic motivation for health increases during the school years and increases with age. Children from larger families demonstrated higher self-esteem but were more extrinsically motivated. Children from families with higher maternal education had higher motivation for healthful practices. This study indicates that interventions to teach health promotion to children must consider family assessment and the child's self-esteem and motivational levels, and must foster a positive personal responsibility in the child for healthful practices, such as healthy snacks (66). Further, it is essential to consider cultural differences in definitions of health preventive and health promotion practices (53).

The school nurse and teacher can do considerable health teaching, introducing students to positive health habits. Some programs emphasize that the body is a beautiful system, that no one should abuse the system by doing or using anything damaging, and to "just say no." The program should emphasize that people can be happy and active when they avoid the use of alcohol, drugs, or cigarettes to offset the preponderance of advertising that links youth, beauty, and excitement with these activities. Emphasize to adults that more effective than organized educational attempts is the influence of significant adults, those who take a personal interest in the child and who set an example: parents who neither smoke, drink, or use drugs nor give cigarettes, alcohol, or drugs to their children; the teacher who not only teaches content but also lives the teaching; parents and health care providers who have quit smoking; the athletic coach who is committed to no smoking; nurses and obstetricians who can help young women change habits; and the nurse or pediatrician who counsels children and adolescents. Equally important, or more so, is the peer group; leaders of the peer group who have positive health habits should be used as models (16). Peer communication is also effective for initiating hygienic habits. You may have a role in working with the peer group.

Butz and Alexander describe use of health diaries with children for assessment of problems and disease, monitoring of medication compliance, teaching of health behaviors, evaluation of effectiveness of the teaching, and research purposes (30).

The monograph *Health Promotion for Older Children and Adolescents,* by the National Institute of Nursing Research, presents research findings on influences on development and health, critical points for promoting healthy behavior, and approaches for designing and implementing health promotion interventions. Traditional sites (schools, clinics) and nontraditional sites (shelters, social service programs, correctional institutions, shopping malls, religious institutions, and work and recreational settings) in rural and urban areas are described as places to implement health promotion programs and teaching. Baker and Henry (13) also describe school health policy issues, based on data from The Center for the Study of Social Policy.

PSYCHOSOCIAL CONCEPTS

Cognitive Development

The schoolchild has a strong curiosity to learn, especially when motivation is strengthened by interested parents and opportunities for varied experiences in the home and school.

Learning, behavior, and personality are complex and are not easily explained by one theory. This section uses information from a number of theorists. Refer to Chapter 5 for a review of how the major schools of theorists explain the development of learning, behavior, and personality.

Pattern of Intellectual Development

Children manifest a **cognitive style,** *the characteristic way in which information is organized and problems are solved.* The style varies from child to child, but there are four major cognitive styles (211):

1. *Analytic:* Examine minute details of objects or events.
2. *Superordinate:* Observe for shared attributes of objects or similarities of events.
3. *Functional–relational:* Objects or events are linked because they have interactional value.
4. *Functional–locational:* Objects or events have a shared location.

Older children are more likely to use analytic and superordinate cognitive styles.

In addition to cognitive style, children differ in their **conceptual tempo,** *the manner in which they evaluate and act on a problem.* Tempo may be either **impulsive,** *where the first idea is accepted and hurriedly reported without consideration for accuracy or thoughtfulness,* or **reflective,** *where a longer period is used to consider various aspects of a situation.* Reflective children are more likely to be analytic than are impulsive children (211).

Certain kinds of questions or statements help the child learn to think more analytically and reflectively (211):

- Why? Give an explanation.
- If that is so, what follows? What is the cause of _____?
- Aren't you assuming that _____?
- How do you know that?
- Is the point you were making that _____?
- Can I summarize your point as _____?
- Is this what you mean to say?
- What is your reason for saying that?
- What does that word mean?
- Is there another way of looking at _____?
- Is it possible that _____?
- How else can we view this? How else can we approach this situation?

The pattern of intellectual development can be traced through the school years (47, 58, 79, 80, 111, 163,

166, 170, 211). In American culture the 6-year-old is supposed to be ready for formal education. The child in first grade is frequently still in the Preoperational Stage. See Table 10–6 for a summary of cognitive abilities of the child from ages 6 to 12 (79, 80, 167, 218, 222).

At approximately age 7 the child enters the stage of **Concrete Operations,** *which involves systematic reasoning about tangible or familiar situations and the ability to use logical thought to analyze relationships and structure the environment into meaningful categories.* The child must have interactions with concrete materials to build understanding that is basic for the next stage (167, 218, 222).

The following operations are characteristic of this stage (163–170, 172, 222).

- **Classification:** *Sorting objects in groups according to specific and multiple attributes* such as length, size, shape, color, class of animals, and trademark. Schoolchildren can identify which kind of Ford is approaching on the highway.
- **Seriation:** *Ordering objects according to decreasing or increasing measure* such as height, weight, and strength. The child knows A is longer than B, B longer than C, and A longer than C.
- **Nesting:** *Understanding how a subconcept fits into a larger concept.* For example, a German shepherd is one kind of dog; a reclining chair and a dining room chair are both chairs.
- **Multiplication:** *Simultaneously classifying and seriating,* using two numbers together to come out with a greater amount.
- **Reversibility:** *Returning to the starting point or performing opposite operations or actions with the same problem or situation.* The child can add and subtract and multiply and divide the same problems. A longer row of clips can be squeezed together to form a shorter row and vice versa; the child realizes the number of clips has not changed.
- **Transformation:** *Ability to see the shift from a dynamic to static or constant state, to understand the process of change, and to focus on the continuity and sequence, on the original and final states.* For example, the child realizes or anticipates how a shorter row of pennies was shifted to become a longer row or the gradual shift in level of fluid in a container as it is poured into another container and the increasing level of fluid in the second container.
- **Conservation:** *Understanding transformation conceptually and that a situation has not changed, to see the sameness of a situation or object despite*

TABLE 10–6. COGNITIVE CHARACTERISTICS OF THE SCHOOL-AGE CHILD

Age	Cognitive Ability
6	Thinking is concrete and animistic
	Beginning to understand semiabstract concepts; beginning to understand semiabstract symbols
	Defines objects in relation to their use and effect on self
	May not be able to consider parts and wholes in words at the same time
	Likes to hear about his past
	Knows numbers
	Can read
	Learning occurs frequently through imitation and incidental suggestion and also depends on opportunities
	May not be able to sound out words; may confuse words such as *was* and *saw*
	High correlation between ability to converse and beginning reading achievement; may have vocabulary of 8000 to 14,000 words if assisted with language
7	Learns best from interaction with actual materials or visible props
	Learning broad concepts and subconcepts, e.g., car identified as Ford or Chevrolet, based on memory, instruction, or experience
	A number of mental strategies or operations are learned
	Becoming less egocentric, less animistic
	Better able to do cause–effect and logical thinking
	More reflective; has deeper understanding of meanings and feelings
	Interested in conclusions and logical endings
	Attention span lengthened; may work several hours on activity of interest
	More aware of environment and people in it; also interested in magic and fantasy
	Understands length, area, or mass
	Sense of time practical, detailed, present focus, plans the day
	Knows months, seasons, years
	Serious in inventing, enjoys chemistry sets
8	Less animistic
	More aware of people and impersonal forces of nature
	Improvises simple activities
	Likes to learn about history, own and other cultures, geography, science, and social science
	Intellectually expansive; inquires about past and future
	Tolerant and accepting of others
	Understands logical reasoning and implications
	Learns from own experience
	Extremely punctual
	Improvises simple rules
	Can read a compass
9	Realistic in self-appraisal and tasks
	Reasonable, self-motivated, curious
	Needs minimal direction
	Competes with self
	Likes to be involved with activities and complex tasks
	May concentrate on project 2 or 3 hours
	Plans in advance; wants successive steps explained and wants to perfect skills

(continued)

TABLE 10–6. COGNITIVE CHARACTERISTICS OF THE SCHOOL-AGE CHILD (continued)

Age	Cognitive Ability
	Focuses on details and believes in rules and laws (they can be flexible), as much as luck or chance
	Enjoys history
	Tells time without difficulty
	Likes to know length of time for task
	Likes to classify, identify, list, make collections
	Understands weight
10	Is matter-of-fact
	Likes to participate in discussions about social problems and cause and effect
	Likes a challenge
	Likes to memorize and identify facts
	Locates sites on a map
	Makes lists
	Easily distracted; many interests and concentrates on each for a short time
	Greater interest in present than past
11	Curious but not reflective
	Concrete, specific thinking
	Likes action or experimentation in learning
	Likes to move around in the classroom
	Concentrates well when competing with one group against another
	Prefers routine
	Better at rote memorization than generalization
	Defines time as distance from one event to another
	Understands relationship of weight and size
12	Likes to consider all sides of a situation
	Enters self-chosen task with initiative
	Likes group work but more inner motivated than competitive
	Able to classify, arrange, and generalize
	Likes to discuss and debate
	Beginning Formal Operations Stage, or abstract thinking
	Verbal formal reasoning possible
	Understands moral of a story
	Defines time as duration, a measurement
	Plans ahead, so feels life is under own control
	Interested in present and future
	Understands abstractness of space
	Understands conservation of volume

a change in some aspect, and that mass or quantity is the same even if it changes shape or position. For example, six paper clips moved from a 6-in. line to an 8-in. line remain six paper clips. Water in boiled form is vapor, which can return to water and freeze. It is still the same amount of water; nothing is lost in the process.

• **Decentering:** *Coordination of two or more dimensions,* or *the ability to focus on several charac-*

teristics simultaneously. For example, space and length dimensions can be considered; the younger child would consider only one or the other. When 12 paper clips are spread from 6 to 12 in., the child realizes the clips are spread and there are not more clips.

These operations increase in complexity as the child matures from an empirical to logical orientation. The child can look at a situation, analyze it, and come up with an answer without purposefully going through each step. For example, if two rows of coins have been spread out, the child does not have to count the coins. He or she realizes that nothing was added or subtracted to the rows, so each row still has the same number.

The child learns and can recall associations between sequences and groupings of events. At first he or she makes associations within a certain context or environment; later memory is used to transfer these associations to different contexts or environments. The child also rehearses; in the time between a learning experience and a memory test or application of learning he or she goes over mentally what has been learned (218).

Discuss the child's changing cognitive abilities with parents and ways they can contribute to the cognitive achievement. If parents do not understand that certain cognitive behavior is age-appropriate, their interactions with and guidance of the child may be less effective.

Cognitive development and an increasing understanding of implications and consequences and of cause–effect relations may be a factor in the changing *fearfulness* of the child. By age 7 or 8 most fears that are typical of preschoolers (darkness, spooks) have been resolved. The young schoolchild is fearful of natural hazards, unsafe conditions, loss of parents, war (when the country is involved in war), school problems, disease, body injury, separation, excess punishment, death, breaking the moral code, and hell. Ten- and 11-year-olds report fears of dangerous animals, people, machines, weapons, vehicles, natural hazards, war, the bomb, disease, separation from or death of loved ones, personal death, breaking the moral code, and hell. Some of these fears (e.g., fear of vehicles or dangerous people) are realistic as the child increasingly moves out into the community alone. Adults also express some of these same fears (58, 79, 80, 146, 211).

As a nurse, remember that the school-age child has great fear of body injury, disease, separation from loved ones, death, excess punishment (some diagnostic and treatment procedures seem like punishment), and doing wrong actions. In your practice you can help offset the child's fears.

Case Situation: Schoolchild Development

Sarah, age 10, and Joshua, her 6-year-old brother, are visiting their grandmother, aunt, uncle, and cousins for the day. Sarah is thin, with narrow shoulders and hips and little adipose tissue, although she has considerable muscle mass.

A luncheon is being held for her grandmother's birthday, and Sarah is eager to help her aunt and cousins prepare the food, set the table, and make party favors. Sarah and Megan, her 9-year-old cousin, divide the nuts and candies into party cups to set at each person's plate. They do this systematically and logically, using the concepts of seriation and classification, so that each person receives an identical number of candies and nuts. This is typical of the Concrete Operations Stage of cognitive development.

Sarah and Megan go to play school in Megan's room where there are a toy chest, dolls, bookshelves, and chalkboard. Sarah plays the teacher, writing multiplication tables on the board and talking to Megan and to pretend students. She demonstrates concrete transformations as she solves multiplication problems. Sarah pretends the class is being bad and reprimands them as a teacher would. In this behavior she demonstrates understanding of relationships between various steps in a situation. It is apparent that Sarah's teacher is a role model for her; this is common among school-age children.

Sarah asks Megan for advice on solving the problems and on reprimanding the pretend class. This exchange of information is typical of the syntaxic mode of communication and consensual validation that is observed in the schoolchild. By incorporating Megan's ideas and answers, she shows that she cares about Megan's thoughts.

Concept of Time

The concept of time evolves during the early school period. See Table 10–7 for a summary of how the schoolchild develops a concept of time (79, 80, 211).

You can help parents understand that their school-age children do not have adult concepts of time. The mother who is distraught because her 6- or 7-year-old constantly dawdles in getting ready for school can be helped by understanding the child's concept of time. The mother must still be firm in direction but not expect the impossible. She can look forward to improvement in the 8-year-old.

Understanding maturing time concepts will also aid you as you explain the sequence of a procedure to the schoolchild in the doctor's office, school, clinic, or hospital.

Spatial Concepts

Spatial concepts also change with more experience. The 6-year-old is interested in specific places and in relationships between home, neighborhood, and an expanding community. He or she knows some streets and major points of interest. By age 7 the sense of space is becoming more realistic. The child wants some space of his or her own such as a room or portion of it. The heav-

TABLE 10–7. SCHOOL-AGE CHILD'S CONCEPT OF TIME

Age	Conceptualization of Time
6	Time counted by hours; minutes disregarded
	Enjoys past as much as present; likes to hear about his or her babyhood
	Future important in relation to holidays
	Duration of episode has little meaning
7	Interested in present; enjoys a watch
	Sense of time practical, sequential, detailed
	Knows sequence of months, seasons, years
	Plans days; understands passage of time
8	Extremely aware of punctuality, especially in relation to others
	More responsible about time
9	Tells time without difficulty
	Plans days with excess activities; driven by time
	Wants to know how long a task will take to complete
	Interested in ancient times
10	Less driven by time than the 9-year-old
	Interested primarily in present
	Able to get to places in time on own initiative
11	Feels time is relentlessly passing by or dragging
	More adept at handling time
	Defines time as distance from one event to another
12	Defines time as duration, a measurement
	Plans ahead to feel in control
	Interested in future as well as present

ens and various objects in space and in the earth are of keen interest (79, 200, 218).

For the 8-year-old personal space is expanding as the child goes more places alone. He or she knows the neighborhood well and likes maps, geography, and trips. He or she understands the compass points and can distinguish right and left on others as well as self (79, 80, 218).

Space for the 9-year-old includes the whole earth. He or she enjoys pen pals from different lands, geography, and history. For the 10-year-old space is rather specific, the place where things such as buildings are. The 11-year-old perceives space as nothingness that goes on forever, a distance between things. He or she is in good control of getting around in the personal space (79, 80, 218).

The 12-year-old understands that space is abstract and has difficulty defining it. Space is nothing, air. He or she can travel alone to more distant areas and understands how specific points relate to each other (80, 218).

Encourage the parents to discuss spatial concepts with the child to facilitate abstract reasoning. Pontious (172) and Webb (222) give practical suggestions for using Piaget's concepts in care and teaching of children.

Categories of Concepts Developed During the School Years summarizes other concepts formulated at this time.

► CATEGORIES OF CONCEPTS DEVELOPED DURING THE SCHOOL YEARS

- **Life:** Is aware that movement is not sole criterion of life.
- **Death:** Accepts death as final and not like life. Thinks of death as an angel or bogeyman. Thinks personal death can be avoided if one hides, runs fast, or is good. Traumatic situations arouse fear of death. By age 10 or 11, realizes death is final, inevitable, and results from internal processes. Belief in life after death depends on religious teachings.
- **Body functions:** Has many inaccurate ideas about body functions until taught health class. Needs repetitive sex education. Becomes more modest for self but interested in seeing bodies of adults. Performs complete self-care by 9 years.
- **Money:** Begins to understand value of coins and bills.
- **Self:** Clarifies ideas of self when sees self through eyes of teachers and peers and compares self with peers. By 11 or 12 years, considers self to be in brain, head, face, heart, and then total body.
- **Sex roles:** Has clear concept of culturally defined sex role and that male role is considered more prestigious.
- **Social roles:** Is aware of peers' social, religious, and socioeconomic status. Accepts cultural stereotypes and adult attitudes toward status. Group conscious.
- **Beauty:** Judges beauty according to group standards rather than own aesthetic sensibilities.
- **Comedy:** Has concept of comedy or what is funny influenced by perception of what others think is funny.

Entering School

School entry is a crisis for the child and family, for behavior must be adapted to meet new situations. The school experience has considerable influence on the child because he or she is in formative years and spends much time in school. School, society's institution to help the child develop the fullest intellectual potential and a sense of industry, should help the child learn to think critically; make judgments based on reason; accept criticism; develop social skills; cooperate with others; accept other adult authority; and be a leader and follower. The child who attends a school with children from various ethnic or racial backgrounds or with children who have immigrated will also learn about cultures, and possibly several languages, first-hand (Fig. 10–2). The course of instruction should be such that every child has a sense of successful accomplishment in some area. Not only school promotes these cognitive and social skills, however. The home and other groups (e.g., peer or organized clubs) are important in their own way for intellectual and social development and for promoting a sense of achievement and industry.

Regular attendance at school starts early for some children, perhaps at 2½ to 3 years in nursery school. But not all children are emotionally ready for school, even at age 6 or 7. If the child is unprepared for school, separation anxiety may be intense. The demands of a strange adult and the peer group may be overwhelming.

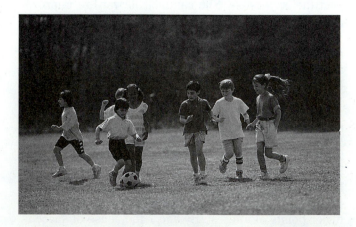

Figure 10–2. Exposure to a variety of peers and learning to work and play cooperatively are important for the school-age child (*Superstock, Inc.*).

Various actions such as teaching the child his or her address and full name, independence in self-care, and basic safety rules help prepare the child for school. The preschool physical and dental examination and an orientation to the school and teacher promote a sense of anticipation and readiness. Parents should examine their attitudes about the child's entering school. Some parents seem eager to rid themselves of a portion of responsibility. Others are worried about the new influences and fear loss of control. Because the parents' attitudes so strongly affect the child, they should verbalize the positive aspects.

The parent or classroom teacher (and the nurse in the health care setting) can *stimulate the child's learning* in the following ways:

- Let each child's success be measured in terms of improved performance.
- Structure for individuation, not for convergence. Avoid having all learning activities structured so that there is only one right answer.
- Provide activities that are challenging, not overwhelming.
- Arrange for the child to accomplish individual activities in the company of peers, when appropriate, as peer interaction provides encouragement and assistance.
- Demonstrate problem-solving and thinking behavior to serve as a model for the child (222).
- Use a multisensory teaching approach (216).
- Include content and experiences that promote understanding of various cultures (6, 56, 188, 226).

There is increasing societal pressure to accelerate the child in the educational process. Piaget contends that optimum comprehension results from numerous experiences over time. Studies of schoolchildren show that a child can quickly learn a specific and advanced task but often with limited retention and transfer. Further, apparent shifts from Concrete to Formal Operations may result from experiences unrelated to education. Direct verbal instruction and use of **cognitive conflict** (*getting the child to question perceptions*) can result in acquisition of conservation abilities, but transfer apparently is limited. Success at learning tasks of increasing complexity depends on levels and interactions of subskills already possessed by the learner. Rather than concentrating on learning of specific tasks, the home or classroom setting should encourage thinking in the child. A variety of experiences and teaching methods increase comprehension, learning, and transfer, which promote acceleration to the next cognitive level. Piecemeal acceleration often results in distorted or incomplete conceptual development that may hamper future thinking (47, 58, 211, 222).

The *teacher–pupil relationship* is important, for it is somewhat similar to the parent–child relationship. Often, however, the classes are so large that the teacher is unable to give much individualized time and attention to each child or to become acquainted with his or her uniqueness. Although the teacher sometimes represents a greater authority figure than the parents, the emotional bond between parent and child is ordinarily stronger than that between teacher and child, and the wise teacher does not act like a substitute parent. The child needs from the teacher a wholesome friendliness, consideration, fairness, sense of humor, and a philosophy that encourages his or her maturity. The teacher should be emotionally and physically healthy and have a thorough understanding of child development.

Most schools today have a culturally *diverse student body;* however, Anglo perspectives usually prevail, and the cultural orientations of American Indians, African-Americans, Asian-Americans, and Hispanic-Americans are frequently misunderstood. Students benefit when educators understand their unique culture; however, *there are many intracultural, socioeconomic, geographic, generational, religious, and individual differences among families and children.* Table 10–8 is meant to be a guide about differences between children and to stimulate you to continue to learn about children through study of their culture and direct contact (137). Further, children of interracial marriages may demonstrate a mix of characteristics.

Teachers may foster personal understanding of cultural differences through the following measures (137):

- Listening to the behavior as well as the words of the child
- Emphasizing that each person is unique and worthy of respectful behavior, regardless of perceived differences
- Reading stories, books, and articles about the history, life patterns, and achievements of people from various cultures and religions
- Having bulletin board displays that commemorate the special days or historical leaders for each cultural group represented in the classroom
- Encouraging parents from various culture groups to come to the classroom, bring artifacts that are important or representative, and discuss commonly held beliefs or practices for the specific cultural group
- Encouraging children to find similarities as well as differences among the cultural and religious groups represented in the classroom

TABLE 10–8. CULTURAL DIFFERENCES THAT CHILDREN BRING TO THE CLASSROOM

American-Indian Children	African-American Children	Asian-American and Pacific Islander Children	Hispanic-American Children	Anglo-American Children
Uniqueness of individual respected and emphasized; person to be treated uniquely and respectfully	Individual recognized; behavior reflects on family and culture	Identity from specific national group; each is unique in outlook	Identity from Latin background as well as national group, geographic area; differences between generations and with acculturation	Individual recognized; emphasize treating everyone fairly and conforming to overall standards and group
Immediate and extended family important for identity; grandparents in leadership and childrearing role	Grandmother or mother may be head; extended family interdependent, close in function; child belongs to and relies on blood relatives and friends, not just parents; kinship felt with all members of community	Father head of household; sex, age, generational status respected by child; eldest son has greater responsibilities and privileges; difference between males' and females' social status slowly decreasing	Father supreme authority, makes all decisions; some redefinition of status of women has occurred; extended family engages in childrearing	Equality among family members; immediate family most important for identity; parents, or parent surrogates, have authoritative and childrearing role in family
Parents and grandparents more lenient, give gentle discipline; child feels isolated and low self-esteem when openly punished	Grandparents, extended family, close friends have responsibility for discipline of child; discipline or punishment openly given	Family expects unquestioning obedience; child's behavior reflects an entire family; guilt and shame instilled to control behavior	Extended family and grandparents as well as parents responsible for child's discipline	Parents emphasize consequences for disobedience; problem solving emphasized; discipline techniques vary
Emphasis on wisdom of elderly and others rather than self; elders esteemed; cooperation rather than competition with others	Emphasis on wisdom of elderly; elders esteemed; children learn to help self and each other; competition to achieve in areas of interest supported by family	Emphasis on wisdom and age of elderly; elders assist in childrearing and are esteemed; cooperation rather than competition with others	Emphasis on cooperation among family members; family comes before personal needs; elders esteemed	Emphasis on youth and self; elders often not considered to have knowledge applicable for today; competition for achievement in family and with others
Emphasis on self-sufficiency, but not at expense of family, tribe, or nature; respect for environment	Emphasis on extended family and community as well as developing own strengths	Loyalty to family and not bringing shame to family emphasized; respect for nature	Emphasis on extended family and loyalty to group	Emphasis on independence from family; mastery over environment emphasized
Seek practical skills useful in life now and later; less emphasis on concepts or abstractions in education	Seek achievement and success; emphasize practical education and skills	Pursue excellence; child pressured to meet high expectations; emphasis on practical knowledge; rote memory; teacher the authority; and future achievements, success, social betterment	Education to promote economic advancement and further goals of family, not just self	Education to be broad, encompass more than learning practical skills; emphasis on concepts abstractions, problem solving
Reserved; restrain strong feelings; formal with authority figures, strangers, elders; polite, indirect responses; silence and time given to answers so spoken word has significance	Expressive of feelings verbally and nonverbally; responses vary with closeness to person; may appear loud or aggressive to others	Restrained and formal; restrained expression of strong feelings expected; polite, reserved, indirect responses; prefer harmony, humility, and compromise instead of self-assertion and emphasis on individual uniqueness, eccentricity; express gratitude for good deed	Expressive of feelings verbally and nonverbally; interpersonal relationships most important; polite, deferential, indirect responses	Expressive of feelings verbally; friendships important; outspoken, friendly, frank, direct responses; rapid answers expected

(continued)

TABLE 10–8.   CULTURAL DIFFERENCES THAT CHILDREN BRING TO THE CLASSROOM (continued)

American-Indian Children	African-American Children	Asian-American and Pacific Islander Children	Hispanic-American Children	Anglo-American Children
Deemphasize materialistic and personal possessions	Emphasis on materialism depends on generation and value system	Body, mind, and spirit related and strength in each is important; hard work, patience, endurance more important than material goods; to have enough is good	Deemphasize materialistic possessions, competition; material goods to be useful, not for status	Some emphasize materialistic and personal possessions, depending on generation and value system
Share possessions; emphasize group welfare				Private ownership, labeling, and care of possessions emphasized; individuality shown in possessions

Problems of the family and child are brought into sharp focus when the child enters school. The teacher sees many difficulties: the loneliness of an only child; the pain of the child with divorce or death in the family; the negative self-image of the child who is not as physically coordinated or intellectually sharp as his or her peers; the child with dyslexia or learning difficulties; the child with separation anxiety or **school phobia,** *fear of or refusal to attend school.* Several theories have developed about the anxious or school-phobic child, one of which describes an overprotective mother, a sense of insecurity and uncertainty, and a sense that mother does not want the child to leave home and gain independence. Very little has been written about the father's role, but he has been viewed by some as passive and by some as firm and controlling. School phobia or separation anxiety can be an indicator of a larger medical problem or it can be nothing more than a normal child with a temporary conflict (155, 211, 233).

School experiences are vivid in the child's memory. The child needs someone to listen to and talk about these experiences when he or she arrives home. This strengthens language skills, self-concept, and self-respect. If the child is put off or no one is there to listen, he or she will increasingly turn inward and may refuse to talk when the adult is ready. The parents' taking a few minutes from supper preparation can be very important to the child.

Help parents realize that the child's ability to learn and achieve in school is affected by factors other than intellectual ability. The educational level of the parents is one of the strongest predictors of a child's academic performance and measured intelligence. Failure to achieve may be the child's reaction to a hostile home environment, poor nutrition, physical illness, a troubled classroom, or a teacher's personal problem. Even the design of the school or physical attributes and appearance of the classroom may contribute to poor achievement. If the child cannot see or hear well, is uncomfortable or bothered by distractions and noise, feels unsafe, or has insufficient space, attention, interest, and learning are reduced. Further, some classrooms are built to foster rigid teacher behavior; some children need more flexibility in the program (197). Parents may project their inferiority feelings onto the child, and he or she believes that it is useless to try. The child may be punishing self out of guilt about past misdeeds, real or imagined, or may be asking for attention; or he or she may have been placed in the wrong learning group, either above or below personal abilities. Occasionally these negative factors cause a child to try harder, to sublimate and overcompensate, and to achieve well if ability is present.

Too much pushing by parents for the child to be a success, perfect in physical skills, the most intellectual, or a hard worker can backfire. The pressure that is generated may be so intense that the child eventually does not succeed at anything. Perfectionistic, highly successful, career- or professionally focused parents are apt to push the child too much. If a parent cannot admit mistakes, he or she is unlikely to tolerate mistakes made by the child, and all of us—parents and children—*do* make mistakes. The child may become a perfectionist from parental example and behavior. Certain signs and symptoms are clues. The **perfectionistic child** manifests (16, 45, 129):

- Extreme concern about appearance.
- Avoidance of tasks, play, or school because of fear of failure.

- Dawdling or procrastinating on easy tasks to avoid harder ones or working so slowly on projects that creativity is lost.
- Jealousy and envy of the apparent success and perfection of others.
- Wanting to do something for which the child has no ability or talent.
- Low tolerance for mistakes (e.g., the boy who wins the race may feel he was not successful because he did not set any records).

If these behaviors are present teach the parents to work on relaxing themselves and the child and developing a sense of tolerance and humor. They can join the child in new activities—done for fun and without competition. They and the child can set realistic goals. They can praise the child's efforts, not focus on the outcome. You may be their counselor, or you may refer them to counseling.

School difficulty may arise from the misuse of intelligence quotient (IQ) testing. IQ scores are not the same as intelligence; IQ scores tell what the child has learned at school. An IQ score can go up or down many points in 1 year. The child with a low IQ score may be placed in the class for slow learners; 1 year in such a group may damage the child for the rest of the school years, even if he or she is later placed with a brighter group. Teachers are likely to respond to this child differently, expecting little and offering little. Attention is usually directed to the child who scored high, which further improves the score. IQ scores can predict academic success generally, but they say nothing about a child's curiosity, motivation, inner thoughts, creativity, ability to get along with people, or ability to be a productive citizen (47, 111, 211). Group standardized aptitude, achievement, and vocational tests used in schools (and the business world) cost more than they are worth. Certainly children should not be separated into gifted or retarded classes only on the basis of IQ scores. Standardized achievement tests should not be the sole determinant of educational decisions as a number of factors, such as hunger and poor nutrition, homelessness, health problems, sensory impairments, lack of concentration, and family stress, may all negatively affect the IQ score (47, 195, 211).

IQ test scores are also affected by very low birth weight, ethnic, racial, cultural, and language biases, the testing environment, and sex (47, 49, 58, 211). Very-low-birth-weight children, when compared with normal-weight children at the end of the first grade, were more likely to have difficulty with information processing and to require special services and less likely to be promoted to second grade. Age of the mother at the time of the child's birth was a more important variable than

birth weight: early childbearing is associated with lower socioeconomic level, lower maternal education, single-parent status, negative attitudes toward children, and larger numbers of offspring (195). For example, many African-Americans score lower than Caucasians on IQ tests; but when the test is given by an African-American person, they score higher than if it is given by a Caucasian, possibly because they turn hostile feelings inward when under the direction of Caucasians. Stress and low self-expectations also adversely affect scores. African-American children score lower than Caucasian children on tests involving abstraction but higher on rote memory tests (58). Male–female differences are also striking. In the early school years boys and girls have equal scholastic standing, although girls may be superior. Later, males surpass females on tests of speed and coordination of gross motor acts, spatial-quantitative problems, mechanical tasks, types of quantitative reasoning, and in the subjects of mathematics, science, social studies, and citizenship. Females surpass males in fine-motor skills, perceptual skills, memory, numerical computations, verbal skills, and in the subjects of writing, music, reading, and literature. The test scores are the result of stereotyped social training and value systems. Girls are rewarded for acting "feminine"; they may drop behind to gain approval. Yet females are as capable as males in all avenues of educational attainment if society allows, expects, or demands it.

The study by the American Association of University Women has revealed the sexism in elementary school education in the United States and how teachers and the educational system favor males over females. As a result, girls experience decreasing self-esteem and academic achievement from the time they begin elementary school to the time they enter high school (143, 147, 148, 158).

The child from a minority group sometimes fares considerably worse in school than does the average child because of being handicapped with fewer verbal skills, the middle-class orientation of school programs and examinations, inadequately trained teachers and inferior school facilities in deprived areas, low motivation to achieve or compete, and the effect of the parents' and teacher's expectations on the child. Research shows that children tend to achieve what adults expect of them (49). Research also indicates that early childhood enrichment programs for disadvantaged children improve performance in the school years, but those enrichment programs should continue into the school years (91, 129).

Research results show a low correlation between IQ scores, cognitive ability, and personality in the preschool years; however, teachers perceive students who show initiative or plunge into a new activity as the brightest and those who participate little or not at all as the least intelligent. Apparently the self-fulfilling prophecy occurs because of differential teacher expectations and differences in teacher interactions with various students; by the seventh grade a high correlation exists between personality characteristics and IQ scores (78, 129, 147, 148, 158, 222).

A classroom with diversity in the children's intellectual ability, skills, and personality is helpful to the child; he or she learns about the real world. A small percentage of disabled, retarded, or maladjusted children in a classroom will not adversely affect the educational process of the normal child. Putting the exceptional child in a normal classroom, however, may not make him or her feel normal; he or she still is perceived and perceives self as different. The exceptional child may need special classes to get the help needed; teachers cannot be expected to specialize in all areas of education, and large classrooms prevent teachers from spending the necessary time with the child who has learning disabilities.

Most students benefit from inclusion (18, 106, 175), but facilities should be available for students who need smaller class size, specially educated teachers, and facilities especially designed for someone who has a disability. The Individuals with Disabilities Education Act (IDEA, 1990) requires states to provide education to all eligible children for preschool and thereafter. Since 1990, the Americans with Disabilities Act (ADA) has broadened educational integration opportunities for all Americans with disabilities, in both private and public schools (18, 106, 175). In October 1995, the Elementary and Secondary Education Act (ESEA) was enacted; it is designed to eliminate sex bias in schools and promote equity for girls and women in schools.

The **gifted child** is *characterized by superior educability and consumption of information and by ability to produce information, concepts, and new forms.* The gifted child demonstrates to a greater extent than other children the seven types of intelligence: logical-mathematical, linguistic, musical, spatial, body-kinesthetic, interpersonal, and intrapersonal. The child is adept at problem solving and problem finding. The gifted child is considered educationally exceptional, and the child's full intellectual, creative, and leadership potential may be neglected if (1) parents are not attuned to the child's abilities and needs; (2) parents or teachers are threatened by the gifted child who grasps concepts more quickly than they; (3) parents do not value cognitive, creative, or leadership abilities; (4) the child is not given freedom to explore and be different; or (5) the school system does not have a program suited for his or her abilities (37, 67, 135, 170). Often the gifted child is misunderstood. Research indicates, however, that

gifted students have higher self-esteem than others and are more popular with their peers than other children (135, 170).

You can encourage parents to respect the individual interests and talents of their child. If parents are not intimidated by the child's unusual interests and behavior, they will not fear deviations from neighborhood patterns and thereby not crush budding interests or creativity. That is perhaps the essence of raising a gifted child—to facilitate, provide opportunity, let alone, not hold back or insist that something be done a certain way. Likewise, the wise parent will be able to await the sprouting of interests that do not come quickly to the surface, even if the child is behind other children or group norms. It takes courage and patience to let a child develop at his or her pace. You can be supportive to parents as they let their child assert his or her own initiative in a situation, even if the child is not at first successful. The impulse toward growth and development must first come from the individual's budding inclinations, not from a desire to conform to another's expectations.

Some parents believe the present public school system is inadequate to teach their children the needed skills. They are usually well-educated professionals and wish to teach their own children at home. References by several authors (44, 177, 180) explore various facets of this movement.

The *ill child* poses unique problems for the school and parents. An issue of mounting emotional intensity in many communities is whether children who have HIV or AIDS, regardless of cause, can attend school with other children. Although not a common health problem, the child with AIDS has a unique problem in school, at home, or when hospitalized. Although no spread by casual contact has been reported, the dilemma of how to handle these children is overwhelming.

Currently, these children are being treated. School systems are handling the child in a variety of ways. In some systems no one except a small panel knows which child, if any, has AIDS, which prevents the child from stigma but does not protect him or her from asserting self too much or getting into situations in which an already low resistance might be compromised even further. Other school districts mandate that the child be taught at home. The lack of financial aid is a problem at all levels of living and treatment. Most children with AIDS do not have a family financial or insurance support system (2, 95, 115).

Klug (115), Uphold and Graham (212), and Wong (233) have detailed information on AIDS in the child from birth on and its effects and complications. They state that children with AIDS can remain in school except when viral infections in others threaten the infected child's immune system and health. The school nurse is in a key role to work with parents, teachers, school administrators, members of the school board, and schoolchildren to help them understand the disease; to reduce fear, myths, and irrationality; and to ensure health and welfare of all the people in the school building. Your communication and negotiation skills and knowledge place you in a special role to be listened to by others, to be an advocate for the child and family, and to facilitate sensible decisions.

In working with parents, you may describe parenting as analogous to growing a garden. The gardener is successful because he or she does not thrust impossible patterns on the plants, respects and even nurtures their peculiarities, tries to provide suitable conditions, protects them from serious threats to life, does not continually poke or probe to make plants sprout more quickly, does not seize the new sprouts to pull open the leaves, and does not trim them all to look alike. As with plants, so it is with children. *They* must do the growing and developing and only through their own motivation (Fig. 10–3).

You, the teachers, and administrators must work together for the health and safety of the child. Guns and other weapons do not belong in school, and the school must be kept safe from gunmen and snipers. All adults must know how to protect the children and themselves (173). The teacher can pass his or her observations about the child and environment on to you. You can work with the child, parents, teachers, and administrators as a consultant or counselor. Treating difficulties early is likely to prevent major and long-term problems. Help the parents understand that they are ultimately responsible for their child's behavior and learning. Suggestions for Parents About Children's Homework summarizes how parents can assist the child. Their understanding of growth and development through your teaching and their knowledge of the school and its functions gained by attending parent–teacher association meetings will help them in this demanding job. Parents with little education may need to learn the same subjects their children are learning to be able to help their children. Special classes could be arranged.

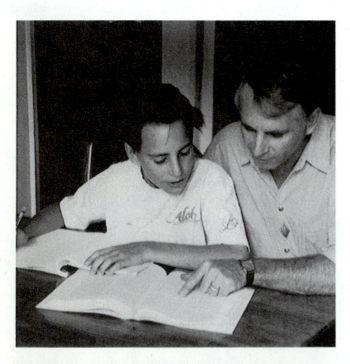

Figure 10–3. Parents nurture their children by providing support and encouraging their efforts and activities. (*From Berger, K.J., and M.B. Williams, Fundamentals of Nursing: Collaborating for Optimal Health. Stamford, CT: Appleton & Lange, 1992, p. 313.*)

► SUGGESTIONS FOR PARENTS ABOUT CHILDREN'S HOMEWORK

Do's

- Let your children know you believe they can do well. Encourage self-evaluation.
- Minimize time spent watching television.
- Help your children organize. Encourage them to do the most difficult task first.
- Talk and read to your children.
- Go to your children's school and volunteer.
- Encourage outside activities and having friends at home.
- Work with your children's teachers and let the teachers know you understand and are supportive.
- Insist on good eating habits.
- Plan activities with your children.
- Be a good example.

Don'ts

- Dwell on the negative by criticizing.
- Allow the television to be your babysitter.
- Do it for the children.
- Leave them to their own devices.
- Forget to encourage verbal exchange.
- Push them to have every minute scheduled or send them off to play.
- Criticize and interfere with everything you do not understand.
- Allow constant eating.
- Send them off without you to family functions (e.g., school plays, pot-luck dinners).
- Say, "Do as I say and not as I do."

Intellectual Needs of the Hospitalized Child

You can help meet the hospitalized child's needs. A hospital tour, if it can be prearranged, helps the child feel acclimated during illness when his or her energy reserve is low. Because the child is beginning logical thought, he or she needs simple information about the illness to decrease the fear of the unknown and promote cooperation in the treatment plan. He or she needs to handle and become familiar with the equipment used. Heiney (93) describes practical ways to help the child deal with painful procedures. Wong (233) is also a thorough reference.

The child who must spend long periods in the hospital needs to learn about the outside world. Some hospitals take chronically ill children to the circus, athletic events, and restaurants. Teachers are also employed so that the child can continue with formal education.

Use of Nonschool Time

Help parents realize the importance of the use of time by the child when he or she is not in school. One study of more than 200 children in grades 3, 6, 7, 9, and 11 gave interesting results, although results may have been influenced by the fact that these children lived in an affluent community in the East (203). These results may help you talk with parents about their awareness of the child's activity and the importance of how the child uses time. In this study children preferred activities with parents, such as going to museums or theaters and working on hobbies or projects, to watching television. These children spent little time on "learning-related" activities, such as model building, stamp collecting, and visits to museums and art exhibits. In fact, they expressed a strong desire for "more interesting after school activities." Homework and reading received little time, from a daily weekday average of 45 minutes for third graders to 75 minutes for ninth graders. One-half as much time was spent on homework on weekends. Almost one-half of the students enjoyed reading "often," but most stated that they opposed more homework. Students at all grade levels were not involved in attending church and community events or in volunteering in community service activities. Yet they expressed a strong desire to participate in such programs at all ages.

If parents cannot initiate attendance at learning-related activities with their children, for whatever reasons, perhaps school and other education-related agencies should offer learning-related activities held at convenient, accessible locations throughout the community. A number of school districts have developed school–business partnerships, internship programs, and other work-related projects designed to help students better understand the realities of the world of work. In a Midwest school district one seventh-grade science teacher has held, for more than a decade, well-attended weekend family field trips to interesting places, related to classwork, for parents and seventh graders. The teacher believes the extra time and effort are well spent; the school system is supportive. Parents endeavor to get their children into his class, partly for the field trip experiences.

Parents, teachers, and school administrators may wish to examine "the seventh-grade slump." Seventh graders watch more television than do all other groups, participate less in learning-related activities, and dislike school more than do other groups. A reexamination of seventh-grade academic programs, extracurricular activities, and out-of-school opportunities for growth would be useful (203).

At all grade levels studied, parents seem to spend little time with children. Children want more time with parents. *Talk with parents to help them examine the role they now play in their children's lives, their various commitments, their priorities, and their importance to the child.* This is difficult when children come from homes with working mothers or from one-parent homes. Nevertheless, this issue is worth raising. Perhaps other caring adults are available also to spend time with the children. Human interaction is an important need for children—in fact, for people of all ages (142, 204).

Communication Patterns

Many factors influence the child's communication pattern, vocabulary, and diction. Some of these factors have been referred to in previous chapters. Influences include (1) speech and verbal and nonverbal communication pattern of parent(s), siblings, other adults such as teachers and peers; (2) attitudes of others toward the child's efforts to speak and communicate; (3) general environmental stimulation; (4) opportunity to communicate with a variety of people in a variety of situations; (5) intellectual development; (6) ability to hear and articulate; (7) vocabulary skills; and (8) contact with television or other technology (47, 130).

The 6-year-old has command of nearly every form of sentence structure. The child experiments less with language, using it more as a tool and less for the mere pleasure of talking than during the preschool period. Now language is used to share in others' experiences. He or she also swears and uses slang to test others' reactions. The child enjoys printing words in large letters (47, 58, 79, 80, 129).

At 7, the child can print several sentences, and at 8 he or she is writing instead of printing. By 9, the child participates in family discussions, showing interest in family activities and indicating an individuality. Verbal fluency has improved, and common objects are described in detail. Writing skill has improved; he or she usually writes with small, even letters. By 10, he or she can write for a relatively long time with speed. The preadolescent may seem less talkative, withdrawing when frustrated instead of voicing anger. Sharing feelings with a best friend is a healthy outlet (47, 58, 79, 80, 129).

As the child shares ideas and feelings, he or she learns how someone else thinks and feels about similar matters. The child expresses self in a way that has meaning to others, at first to a chum and then to others. Thus he or she is validating vocabulary, ideas, and feelings. The child learns that a friend's family has similar life patterns, demands of the child, and frustrations. He or she learns about self in the process of learning more about another. The child recalls what has happened in the past, realizes how this has affected the present, and considers what effect present acts will have on future events. The child uses **syntaxic, or consensual, communication** *when he or she sees these cause-and-effect relationships in an objective, logical way and can validate them with others* (205). By sixth grade, the child who has had opportunity to learn may have a vocabulary 10 to 20 times that of the 6-year-old (211).

Convey love and caring, not rejection, when you talk with children. Love is communicated through nonverbal behavior such as getting down to the child's eye level and through words that value feelings and indicate respect. Children understand language directed at their feelings better than at their intellect and the overt action. Do not overreact to normal behavior. Avoid talking about touchy areas, if possible, or the child's babyhood. He or she is struggling to be grownup; any reminder of younger behavior creates anxiety about potential regression (129). The principles of communicating with the preschooler discussed in Chapter 9 are also applicable to the schoolchild.

Effects of Television on the Child

Television and movies, video and computer games, and the Internet exert a powerful influence on a child's communication and behavior patterns. Children watch an average of 4 to 6 hours of television daily—more time than is spent on school homework or any activity except sleeping (47, 58, 130, 211, 220). The average child will have viewed from 15,000 to 22,000 hours or more of television by high school graduation; he or she will have spent fewer hours in formal classroom study (47, 58, 124, 130, 201, 211, 220).

If watching television is controlled by responsible parents, cognitive and social learning can be enhanced. Educational programs can (1) present information about specific topics as well as the whole universe; (2) model prosocial behaviors; and (3) present and reinforce techniques associated with various sports (47, 58, 130, 211). For the person unable to attend church, the religious programs can be a substitute. Scenic programs have an aesthetic value. Geographic, scientific, historical, and dramatic presentations are educational and relaxing and broaden horizons. Television has the potential to educate, socialize, and teach content and communication skills. Television can be used for health teaching (52, 58, 70). Even viewing ordinary programs, however, has serious limitations (Table 10–9) (7, 47, 52, 58, 61, 65, 67, 81, 86, 124, 148, 160, 176, 184, 201, 211, 217, 220).

Heavy television viewing is associated with lower school achievement. Schoolteachers report that more children are entering school with decreased imaginative play and creativity and increased aimless movement, low frustration level, poor persistence and concentration span, and confusion about reality and fantasy. Rapid speech and constantly changing visuals on television prevent reflection. The child does not learn correct sentence structure, use of tenses, or the ability to express thought or feeling effectively. The result may be a child who is unable to enunciate or use correct grammar and who is vague in the sense of time and history and cause-and-effect relationships (47, 52, 58, 138, 176, 211).

Understanding television can involve active mental work for the young child, but often the child does not understand content, motives, or feelings; integrate events shown; or infer conditions not shown (52, 58, 176, 211). Those are the mental processes that are stimulated by adult and peer interactions and reading literature. Often television is used in the home to the extent that it stifles family interaction and bombards with noise, excitement, speed, and misdirected humor. The stereotypic, simplistic, and often romanticized view of family life shown by most programs is unrealistic and probably not attainable. False expectations about things and people are raised; most advertising is sexist, ageist, and racist, showing women as uninterested in or incapable of anything except putting on diapers and using detergents. Most advertisements are directed to middle-class young Caucasians.

Science fiction conveys that life in the future may be scary and difficult at best. The child may have nightmares. A steady diet of science fiction may influence the child's present and future value systems (52, 170).

Some television programming is frankly pornographic; the values depicted are lack of loyalty or com-

TABLE 10–9.   NEGATIVE EFFECTS OF TELEVISION

1. Promotes passive rather than active learning
2. Increases passivity from continual overstimulation
3. Encourages low-level, nonconceptual thinking
4. Takes time away or distracts from more creative and stimulating activity; reduces creativity and fantasy of the child
5. Encourages short attention span and hyperactivity through its use of snappy attention-getting techniques
6. Causes lack of understanding or comprehension of what is seen or inability to grasp consequences of behavior because of fast pace of programming
7. Causes loss of interest in less exciting but necessary classroom or home activities
8. Creates a desire for the superficial rather than depth of information; teaches superficial judgments
9. Creates uncertainty about what is real and unreal in life and family
10. Creates a confusion of values
11. Promotes a desire for unhealthy products such as high-sugar and high-salt snacks, other products not normally used by the family, or toys or other products that may be unhealthy or dangerous
12. Interferes with correct pronunciation of words, vocabulary use, reading comprehension, and spelling achievement
13. Promotes sedentary lifestyle rather than participation in play, sports, physical exercise, community events, or activities with parents
14. Increases aggressive behavior because of program content, loud music, fast pace, and camera tricks
15. Increases passive acceptance of aggressive behavior toward people as a way to solve problems
16. Becomes a way to keep the child occupied—a passive babysitter
17. Increases suspicion of others, fears, and anxiety
18. Competes with parents, school, and peers as a socializing agent
19. Promotes passivity and withdrawal from direct involvement in real life
20. Deemphasizes complexity of life with simplistic plots, fast action, no lasting consequences, no visual or cognitive depth
21. Conveys unrealistic and stereotyped view of men and women and sex roles; women usually portrayed as sex objects, ornamental, young, with limited speaking and/or problem-solving behaviors
22. Emphasizes overt sexual behavior; portrays nudity, perversions, homosexuality, and sometimes pornographic content
23. Fosters increased incidence of aggressive and violent behavior
24. Promotes excessive fears about war and the bomb, about walking in one's own neighborhood, about the "violent" world, and about the police who use only force
25. Increases emotional problems, including conduct disorders and posttraumatic stress disorder (nightmares, flashbacks, paranoia, poor concentration, impaired attachment to people)

mitment to relationships, the beautiful and young body, immediate gratification, and narcissism. Movies and daytime dramas depict "jumping into bed and from bed to bed." Consequences of such behavior and relationships are not shown. Often such programming is at prime viewing time. The child who has unsupervised television watching cannot miss programs about family life that teach unhealthy values (47, 52, 130, 170, 211).

The violence in television programming is graphic, explicit, realistic, and intensely involving and affects both children and adults but children more so because they have less ego control. Children act out more directly what they see and hear. Many programs directly or indirectly teach violent behavior, showing specifically how to carry out violent acts. It is not unusual when arson, rape, hostage taking, suicide, or homicide is described on the evening news on television to have, either locally or nationally, a number of such incidents repeated within a few days (130). The live and explicit portrayals of violence suggest that violence is normal and justified. Realistic or punitive consequences of violent behavior are not shown. The viewer gets the idea and forms an attitude over time that aggressive or violent behavior should be used to solve problems, that it is normal or courageous to be violent, that violence is rewarded or socially acceptable, and that the violent person is the hero with whom to identify. Further, continual viewing of violence desensitizes the person to violence in general; it is no longer a noteworthy act in the home or society. Even worse, television violence shows inequality and domination; the most frequent victims are women, the old, and children.

Teach parents that, increasingly, research indicates that seeing **violent, sexually seductive programs or pornographic material** on television or on films has **long-term negative effects on children** (130, 138, 144, 185, 201).

Research over the past 25 years indicates that our increasing national violence is linked to increased portrayal of violence in the media. One study estimated that there would be 10,000 fewer homicides per year if our youth saw less media violence (124). There are an average of 32 violent acts per hour on television. The average 15-year-old who watches 28 hours of television per week will have seen 13,000 televised killings (211). Although television programming has appeared to reduce smoking behavior in the youth (70), it has contributed to increased alcohol intake (86). Most studies emphasize that children are more likely to be violent after watching violence on television if they see violence in their own home, receive harsh discipline, or have no nurturing father in the home, and if there is excessive television viewing without parental supervision or discussion (7, 211, 220) (also see Table 10–9).

Teach parents about these effects and the importance of controlling media viewing. Children who have grown up in stable families, who feel secure and loved, and who have a variety of interests and relationships will not be adversely affected by the aggression, violence, and sex of television. They can separate fantasy from fact and all of their fantasy is not based on television. Children growing up without positive identification models, who are already shaky in their self-concept and identity formation, are affected very negatively. Likewise, children from troubled or dysfunctional homes lack the supervision or guidance to help them handle and sort through what they see and hear (47, 58, 81, 144, 160, 211).

Discuss with parents the need to limit the amount of television viewing (2 hours a day); do alternative activities with their children; screen what their children are viewing; and work to reduce the trend to more violent and pornographic programming. Parents can be more vigilant about programs their children watch. Television programming can be improved. Networks and advertisers, of course, hope that parents will disregard research findings that make-believe violence makes for real violence in many settings. As long as violence on television is profitable, programming will contain violence. Parents can rebel: writing letters to stations, writing letters to advertisers, and refusing to buy the products advertised. This is a significant area of life that affects the child's and the family's physical, emotional, cognitive, social, and spiritual health.

Organizations such as the American Medical Association, National Education Association, and Parent–Teacher Association have united in opposition against programming containing violent and sexual excesses. Many parent, school, community, health care, and religious leaders are joining efforts to gain more educational and less destructive programming, including the National Coalition on Television Violence, which is directed by a psychiatrist. Opposition against video games is mounting in the belief that they foster some of the same problems as excess television (130, 160).

In essence, interaction with parents and others and real experiences, not passive observations, help the child learn to work through conflicts of development and to solve problems.

Play Patterns

Peer Groups

Peer groups, including the gang and the close chum, provide companionship with a widening circle of persons outside the home and are extremely important to the school-age child. Between the ages of 7 and 9, children usually form close friendships with peers of the same sex and age. Later in this age group, peers are not necessarily of the same age. Children must earn their membership in the peer group, and being accepted by one's peers and belonging to a peer group are major concerns for this age group. Many factors determine a child's acceptance, including attractiveness and friendliness. Peer groups provide companionship and a chance for children to compete and to compare themselves with others their own age. Peer groups develop their own sets of values and goals, and each group member will have a specific status or role. These groups provide the child an opportunity to test mastery in a world parallel to adult society, with rules, organization, and purposes (58, 211, 233).

Play Activities

Play activities change with the child's development. From 6 to 8 years he or she is interested chiefly in the present and in the immediate surroundings. Because he or she knows more about family life than any other kind of living, the child plays house or takes the role of various occupational groups with which there is contact: mailcarrier, nurse, storekeeper, teacher. Although the child is more interested in playing with peers than parents, the 6- or 7-year old will occasionally enjoy having the parent as a "child" or "student." This allows the child to have imaginary control over the parent and also allows the parent to understand how the child is interpreting the parent or how the child perceives the teacher.

Both sexes enjoy some activities in common such as painting, cutting, pasting, reading, collecting items such as baseball cards or stamps, simple table games, television, digging, riding a bicycle, construction sets or models, puzzles, kites, running games, skating, and swimming. Again, the parent can sometimes enjoy these activities with the child, especially if the parent has a special talent the child wishes to learn. The child imitates the roles of his or her own sex and becomes increasingly realistic in play. By age 8, collections, more advanced models, the radio, art materials, "how to" books, farm sets, and train sets are favorite pastimes, and loosely formed, short-lived clubs with fluctuating rules are formed.

The schoolchild, usually near 8 or 9 years of age, enjoys computerized and electronic games, which give a sense of control and power; of being a peer with, or even superior to, the adult; of challenge and inventiveness; and an enjoyment of complexity and expandability. The computer can be a tool for robot thinking or for development of thought; for passivity or releasing aggressive impulses or creativity; for play or for learning. Computer toys can help the schoolchild understand the nature of systems and control of information—skills needed in the adult world. Let the child take the lead in when to move into computer games. There is no need to rush the child. He or she can pick up the skills and the enjoyment at any age. Further, some schoolchildren will prefer reading, painting, playing an instrument, doing crafts, camping, or playing sports to working with computers. These skills and what these activities teach are as essential to the workplace as the ability to operate a computer.

From 9 to 12 years the child becomes more interested in active sports but continues to enjoy quieter activity. He or she wants to improve motor skills. The child may enjoy carpentry or mechanic's tools, advanced models or puzzles, camera and film, and camping. Adult-organized games of softball, football, or soccer lose their fun when parents place excessive emphasis on winning. The hug from a teammate after hitting a home run means more than just winning. Further, adults' taking over the games robs the child of independence (211).

Creative talents appear; the child may be interested in more complicated arts and crafts, carpentry and other tools, advanced models and puzzles, science projects, music, or dance. At approximately age 10, sex differences in play become pronounced. Each sex is developing through play the skills it will later need in society; this is manifested through the dramatizing of real-life situations. The child's interest in faraway places is enhanced through a foreign pen pal and through travel (80).

Gang Stage

In preadolescence the gang becomes important. A **gang** is a *group whose membership is earned on the basis of skilled performance of some activity, frequently physical in nature. Its stability is expressed through formal symbols such as passwords or uniforms.* Gang codes take precedence over almost everything. They may range from agreement to protect a member who smoked in the boys' restroom at school to boycotting a school dance. Generally, gang codes are characterized by collective action against the mores of the adult world. In the gang, children discharge hostility and aggression against peers rather than adults and begin to work out their own social patterns without adult interference. Unfortunately, some gangs do turn their hostility against other youths or adults. When this occurs, the pattern is laid for delinquent behaviors (211, 233); however, these groups are not necessarily offenders against the law. Gang formation is loosely structured at first, with a transient membership that cuts across all social classes. Early gangs may consist of both boys and girls in the same groups. Later, gangs separate by sex (233).

Chum Stage

The chum stage occurs around 9 or 10 years of age and sometimes later when affection moves from the peer group and gang to a **chum,** a *special friend of the same sex and age.* This is an important relationship because it is the child's first love attachment outside the family, when someone becomes as important to him or her as self. Initially, a person of the same sex and age is easier than someone of the opposite sex to feel concern for and to understand. The friend becomes an extension of the child's own self. As he or she shares ideas and feelings, the child learns a great deal about both self and the chum. The child discovers that he or she is more similar to than different from others and learns to accept self for what he or she is. Self-acceptance of uniqueness increases acceptance of others so that the child of this age is very sociable, generous, sympathetic, enjoys differences in people, and is liberal in ideas about the welfare of others. He or she learns that others can do things differently but that they are still all right as people. It is also through the chum relationship that the child learns the syntaxic mode of communication described earlier, for he or she learns to validate word meanings in talking with the chum. Thus ideas about the world become more realistic. Loyalty to the chum at this age may be greater than loyalty to the family (205). **Altruism,** a *concern for others in various situations,* and an ability to respond to others' happiness and distress, to develop intimate associations, including with individuals of the opposite sex, and a sensitivity and concern for all humanity result from high-level chumship (188, 205).

The chum stage has homosexual elements, but it is not an indication of homosexuality. It provides the foundation for later intimacy with an individual of the opposite sex and close friends of both sexes. If the child does not have a chum relationship, he or she has little capacity for adolescent heterosexuality or adult intimacy. According to Sullivan, fixation at this level results in homosexuality (205). Other theories regarding causation of homosexuality have also been proposed (see Chapter 12).

Help parents understand the importance of the gang and chum stages.

Tools of Socialization

Competition, compromise, cooperation, and beginning collaboration are progressive tools the schoolchild uses in accomplishing satisfying relationships with peers. **Competition** *comprises all activities that are involved in getting to a goal first, of seeking affection or status above others.* When the child is competing, he or she has rigid standards about many situations, including praise and punishment. For example, regardless of the circumstance, the child believes that the same punishment should be given for the same wrongdoing. He or she cannot understand why a 3-year-old sibling and he or she should not be punished similarly for spilling milk on the kitchen floor. Similarly, the child thinks he or she should be praised for dressing self as is the 3-year-old. *The child accepts adult rules as compulsory and rigid; he or she experiences a* **morality of constraint** (164).

Compromise, a *give-and-take agreement,* is gradually learned from peers, teachers, and family. The child becomes less rigid in standards of behavior. **Cooperation,** an *exchange between equals by adjusting to the wishes of others,* results from the chum relationship with its syntaxic mode of communication (205). Through the **morality of cooperation** the *child begins to understand the social implications of acts.* He or she learns judgment through helping make and carry out rules (164). **Collaboration,** *deriving satisfaction from group accomplishment rather than personal success,* is a step forward from cooperation and enables experimentation with tasks and exploration of situations (129, 205).

If a child does not learn how to get along with others, future socialization will be inhibited. For example, if a person is fixated at the competition level and does not learn how to compromise or cooperate, he or she is hard on self and is a hard person with whom to live. Eventually the person derives satisfaction only from competing but fails to enjoy the accomplishment, the end product. If a child is not relating well with peers, a group assertiveness training program can effectively increase social and assertive behavior through reinforcement procedures, relaxation techniques, guided imagery, and behavior contracts (125).

Guidance and Discipline

In guidance, parents should invite confidence of the child as a parent, not as a buddy or pal. The child will find pals among peers. In the adult he or she needs a parent! The atmosphere should be open and inviting for the child to talk with the parents, but the child's privacy should not be invaded. The parents should see the child as he or she is, not as an idealized extension of themselves.

The schoolchild has a rather strict superego and also uses many rituals to maintain self-control. He or she prefers to initiate self-control rather than be given commands or overt discipline, and stability and routine in his or her life provide this opportunity. You can talk with parents about methods of guidance and the importance of not interfering with behavior too forcefully or too often. The child needs some alternatives from which to choose so that he or she can learn different ways of behaving and coping and be better able to express self later. If development has been normal during the preschool years, the child is now well on the way to absorbing and accepting the standards, codes, and attitudes of society. He or she needs ongoing guidance rather than an emphasis on disciplinary measures. Parents that are too controlling or punitive contribute to fearfulness in the child. If the parent is perceived as supportive and encouraging of autonomy, the child is less likely to be fearful. Research indicates that preadolescent girls perceive their mothers as more supportive but also more punitive than their fathers. Upper-middle-class parents are perceived by their daughters as less punitive and more autonomy granting than are lower-middle-class parents, and lower-class parents are perceived as even more punitive and less autonomy granting by their daughters (211). Boys who are less warmly treated by their parents are more responsive to social or peer influences than girls, which has implications for later antisocial behavior (129).

For some parents, guiding a child can be a problem. They will ask, "When, what kind, and how much should you punish a child?" "How do you handle guilt or hostile feelings that often accompany discipline?" You are in a position to help parents learn the value of positive guidance techniques (16, 37, 43, 121, 129, 136, 211).

When expressing anger to children, describe what you see, feel, and expect. Do not lower the child's self-esteem by humiliating him or her, especially in front of others. The child's dignity can be protected by using "I" messages: "I am angry. I am frustrated." Such statements are honest and are safer than "What's your problem? You are stupid!" If repeated frequently, the child may believe that he or she is stupid and carry that self-image for years. Although shouting is not recommended, the parent who shouts displeasure at the danger or inconvenience *only* is probably harming the child much less than the parent who quietly and continually verbalizes personal assaults against the child. Ideally, the limit should be set with firm conviction and should deal with only one incident at a time. More than one message can confuse the child.

Our grandparents are reputed to have disciplined their children with authority and certainty. By contrast, some of today's parents seem afraid of their children. The child needs an understanding authority and a good example. He or she needs to know what constitutes unacceptable behavior and what substitute will be accepted. For instance, say, "Food is not for throwing; your baseball is." He or she will not obey rules if parents do not. Inconsistent discipline, or the "Do as I say, not as I do" approach, will lead to maladjustment, conflict, and aggression. The suggestions about guidance listed in Chapter 9 are applicable to the schoolchild as well.

Guidance at this age takes many other and less dramatic forms. A mother can turn the often harried "getting back-to-school clothes" experience into a pleasant lesson in guidance. She can accompany the child on a special shopping trip in which he or she examines different textures of material, learns about color coordination, understands what constitutes a good fit, and appreciates how much money must be spent for certain items. This principle can be carried into any parent–schoolchild guidance relationship such as learning responsibility for some household task or earning, handling, and saving money.

Emotional Development

The schoolchild consolidates earlier psychosocial development and simultaneously reaches out to a number of identification figures, expands interests, and associates with more people. Behavioral characteristics change from year to year. Table 10–10 summarizes and compares basic behavior patterns, although individual children will show a considerable range of behavior. Cultural, health, and social conditions may also influence behavior (47, 58, 79, 80, 129).

Developmental Crisis

The psychosexual crisis for this period is industry versus inferiority. **Industry** is *an interest in doing the work of the world, the child's feeling that he or she can learn and solve problems, the formation of responsible work habits and attitudes, and the mastery of age-appropriate tasks.* (64). The child has greater body competence and applies self to skills and tasks that go beyond playful expression. The child gets tired of play, wants to participate in the real world, and seeks attention and recognition for effort and concentration on a task. He or she feels pride in doing something well, whether a physical or cognitive task. A sense of industry involves self-confi-

dence, perseverance, diligence, self-control, cooperation, and compromise rather than only competition. There is a sense of loyalty, relating self to something positive beyond the moment and outside the self. Parents, teachers, and nurses may see this industry at times as restlessness, irritability, rebellion toward authority, and lack of obedience.

The danger of this period is that the child may develop a sense of **inferiority,** *feeling inadequate, defeated, unable to learn or do tasks, lazy, unable to compete, compromise, or cooperate,* regardless of his or her actual competence (64). See Consequences of Inferiority for a summary of behaviors and traits of the child, and later the adult, if this stage is not resolved. If the child feels excessively ashamed, self-doubting, guilty, and inferior from not having achieved the developmental tasks all along, physical, emotional, and behavioral problems may occur. Sometimes opposite behavior may occur as the person tries to cope with feelings of being no good, inferior, or inadequate. The person might immerse self in tasks. If work is all the child can do at home and school, he or she will miss out on a lot of friendships and opportunities in life, now and later, and eventually

► **CONSEQUENCES OF INFERIORITY**

- Does not want to try new activities, skills
- Is passive, excessively meek, too eager to please others
- Seeks attention; may be "teacher's pet"
- Is anxious, moody, depressed
- Does not persevere in tasks
- Is very fearful of bodily injury or illness
- Does not volunteer to do tasks alone, always works with another on tasks
- Isolates self from others, withdraws from peers
- Tries to prove personal worth, a "good worker" with directives or assistance
- Lacks self-esteem unless praised considerably
- Is overcompetitive, bossy
- Insists on own way, experiences difficulty with cooperation or compromise
- May immerse self in tasks to prove self, gain attention
- Acts out to prove self: lying, stealing, fire setting
- Displays extreme antisocial behavior, destructive or aggressive acts
- Manifests illnesses associated with emotional state: enuresis, complaints of fatigue
- In adulthood, is unable to pursue steady work or become involved in life tasks as expected
- May become "workaholic"; in adulthood, is unable to engage in leisure

TABLE 10–10. ASSESSMENT OF CHANGING BEHAVIORAL CHARACTERISTICS IN THE SCHOOLCHILD

6 Years	7 Years	8 Years
Self-centered	Self-care managed	Expansive personality but fluctuating behavior
Body movement, temper outbursts release tension	Quiet, less impulsive, but assertive	Curious, robust, energetic
Behavioral extremes; impulsive or dawdles, loving or antagonistic	Fewer mood swings	Rapid movements and response; impatient
Difficulty making decisions; needs reminders	Self-absorbed without excluding others; may appear shy, sad, brooding	Affectionate to parents
Verbally aggressive but easily insulted	Attentive, sensitive listener	Hero worship of adult
Intense concentration short time, then abruptly stops activity	Companionable; likes to do tasks for others	Suggestions followed better than commands
Security of routines and rituals essential; periodic separation anxiety	Good and bad behavior in self and others noted	Adult responsibilities and characteristics imitated; wants to be considered important by adults
Series of three commands followed, but response depends on mood	High standards for self but minor infractions of rules: tattles, alibis, takes small objects from others	Approval and reconciliation sought; feelings easily hurt
Self-control and initiative in activity encouraged when adult uses counting to give child time (I'll give you until the count of 10 to pick up those papers")	Concern about own behavior; tries to win over others' approval	Sense of property; enjoys collections
Praise and recognition needed	Angry over others' failure to follow rules	Beginning sense of justice but makes alibis for own transgressions
		Demanding and critical of others
		Gradually accepts inhibitions and limits

9 Years	10 Years
More independent and self-controlled	More adultlike and poised, especially girls
Dependable, responsible	More self-directive, independent
Adult trust and more freedom without adult supervision sought	Organized and rapid in work; budgets time and energy
Loyal to home and parents; seeks their help at times	Suggestions followed better than requests, but obedient
More self rather than environmentally motivated; not dependent on but benefits from praise	Family activities and care of younger siblings, especially below school age, enjoyed
More involved with peers	Aware of individual differences among people, but does not like to be singled out in a group
Own interests subordinated to group demands and adult authority	Hero worship of adult
Critical of own and others' behavior	Loyal to group; chum important
Concerned about fairness and willing to take own share of blame	Some idea of own assets and limits
More aware of society	Preoccupied with right and wrong
	Better able to live by rules
	Critical sense of justice; accepts immediate punishment for wrongdoing
	Liberal ideas of social justice and welfare
	Strong desire to help animals and people
	Future career choices match parents' careers because of identification with parents
	Sense of leadership

11 Years	12 Years
Spontaneous, self-assertive, restless, curious, sociable	Considerable personality integration; self-contained, self-competent, tactful, kind, reasonable, less self-centered
Short outbursts of anger and arguing	Outgoing, eager to please, enthusiastic
Mood swings	Sense of humor; improved communication skills
Challenges enjoyed	More companionable than at 11; mutual understanding between parents and child
On best behavior away from home	Increasingly sensitive to feelings of others; wishes good things for family and friends; caught between the two
Quarrelsome with siblings; rebellious to parents	Others' approval sought
Critical of parents, although affectionate with them	Childish lapses, but wishes to be treated like adult
Chum and same-sex peers important; warm reconciliation follows quarrels	Aware of assets and shortcomings
Secrets freely shared with chum; secret language with peers	Tolerant of self and others
Unaware of effect of self on others	Peer group and chum important in shaping attitudes and interests
Strict superego; zeal for fairness	Ethical sense more realistic than idealistic
Future career choices fantasized on basis of possible fame	Decisions about ethical questions based on consequences
Modest with parents	Less tempted to do wrong; basically truthful
	Self-disciplined; accepts just discipline
	Enthusiastic about community projects

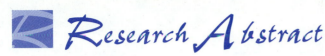

Pelletier, L., G. Godin, L. Lepage, and G. Dussault, *Social Support Received by Mothers of Chronically Ill Children*, Child Care, Health, and Development, *20, no. 2 (1994), 115–131.*

A study was conducted of 213 urban and rural mothers in outpatient clinics of a major hospital in Canada. Their children, ages 6 to 18 and more often boys, had been diagnosed with either asthma or juvenile diabetes. Interviews and questionnaires were used over a 12-month period to gather data about the social support network of mothers. During the year, 30% of the offspring had to be hospitalized and more than 40% had to visit the emergency room at least once because of their illness.

Results indicated that mothers wanted more support than they received, particularly emotional and informational. Spouses, professionals, and immediate family members were identified by mothers as important sources of support. The mother was less likely to receive support when the chronically ill child was of adolescent age, possibly because adolescents are perceived to be more autonomous; however, this is a time of grave adjustment problems. Mothers were also less likely to be supported if the father had a higher level of education and if family income was lower middle level. If the father had an occupation, based on education, that took him out of the home, he was less available. Lower-income mothers often had smaller networks.

Mothers need to be able to share their feelings and worries about what it means to have a sick child. Mothers need to be encouraged and praised in their ability and manner of taking care of their child and given information about how to handle daily care. Professionals should encourage spouses to share more of the responsibilities in daily child care, because mothers as the primary caregivers are heavily burdened psychologically and socially. Both parents should be present not only when they are informed of the diagnosis but also when they are taught specific care requirements. Professionals should also be supportive in development of self-help support groups for parents.

become the adult who is a slave to technology: he or she cannot stop working.

Stress is experienced by the school-age child. Often stress response occurs from the demands placed on the child in relation to school achievement or for extracurricular performance, or the fear of violence during transportation or at school may predominate. One study indicated three major areas of stress (108):

- Actual or anticipated loss of loved ones, pets, or space, such as home, school, and neighborhood
- Threats to self; situations of anger, fear, aggression, or violence against self or personal belongings; threats to personal safety
- Feelings of being hassled; extra responsibility or restrictions; sibling relations; peer relations; other stresses: violence in the home; abuse; divorce

The Life Stress Scale for Children, adapted from the Holmes and Rahe Life Change Scale (98), can be used to assess stress level in children (Table 10–11). Another scale developed by Coddington (40) can be used to assess stress levels in specific age groups of children or adolescents (Table 10–12).

Another kind of stressor for the child, as well as for family, is chronic illness. The Coping Health Inventory for Children (CHIC) is an instrument designed to assess coping behaviors of chronically ill schoolchildren. A total of 45 coping behaviors were identified and categorized into five patterns of coping: (1) develops competence and optimism; (2) feels different and withdraws; (3) is irritable, moody, and acts out; (4) complies with treatment; and (5) seeks support (12).

Relaxation methods and stress management can be taught to children through individual and group counseling (121), play therapy, and use of art and music. Several authors are helpful resources (16, 88, 93, 149 150, 151, 158, 229, 238, 239).

There are sharp differences in how children bear up under such stress as abuse or divorce. Some children are **vulnerable** to stressors; *they are sensitive to or drawn in by the events around them. They become nervous, withdrawn and feel inferior. Some are illness-prone* and slow to develop. Other children are **resilient:** *They shrug off the stressors, thrive, and go on to be industrious, have high self-esteem, and as adults lead highly productive lives.* Still other children have protective factors that buffer against risks. True, some children

TABLE 10–11. THE LIFE CHANGE TEST

Item No.	Item Value	Happened ( )	Your Score	Life Event
1.	100	_____	_____	Death of parent
2.	73	_____	_____	Divorce of parent
3.	65	_____	_____	Marital separation
4.	63	_____	_____	Incarceration
5.	63	_____	_____	Parent travels as part of his/her job
6.	63	_____	_____	Death of close family member
7.	53	_____	_____	Personal injury or illness
8.	50	_____	_____	Parent remarries
9.	47	_____	_____	Parent fired from job
10.	45	_____	_____	Parents reconcile
11.	45	_____	_____	Mother goes to work
12.	44	_____	_____	Change in health of family member
13.	40	_____	_____	Mother becomes pregnant
14.	39	_____	_____	School difficulties
15.	39	_____	_____	Birth of sibling/stepsibling
16.	39	_____	_____	School readjustment (new teacher or new class)
17.	38	_____	_____	Change in family's financial condition
18.	37	_____	_____	Death of close friend
19.	36	_____	_____	Starts a new (or changes) extracurricular activity
20.	35	_____	_____	Change in number of fights with siblings
21.	31	_____	_____	Threatened by violence at school
22.	30	_____	_____	Theft of personal possessions
23.	29	_____	_____	Change in responsibilities at home
24.	29	_____	_____	Brother or sister leaves home
25.	29	_____	_____	Trouble with grandparents
26.	29	_____	_____	Outstanding personal achievement
27.	28	_____	_____	Move family home (another city or another part of town)
28.	26	_____	_____	Begin or end school
29.	25	_____	_____	Change in living conditions
30.	24	_____	_____	Changes in personal habits
31.	23	_____	_____	Trouble with teacher
32.	20	_____	_____	Change in work hours or conditions
33.	20	_____	_____	Move to new house
34.	20	_____	_____	Change to a new school
35.	19	_____	_____	Vacations with family
36.	19	_____	_____	Change in church activities
37.	18	_____	_____	Change in friends
38.	17	_____	_____	Attend summer camp
39.	16	_____	_____	Change in sleeping habits
40.	15	_____	_____	Change in number of family get-togethers
41.	15	_____	_____	Change in eating habits
42.	13	_____	_____	Changes amount of TV viewing
43.	12	_____	_____	Birthday party
44.	11	_____	_____	Punished for not telling the truth
Total score for 12 months			_____	

Adapted from Elkind, D., The Hurried Child: Growing Up Too Fast Too Soon. Reading, MA: Addison-Wesley, 1981.

TABLE 10–12. LIFE EVENT SCALES FOR CHILDREN

Rank	Life Event	Life Change Units	Rank	Life Event	Life Change Units
Preschool Age Group			15	Change in child's acceptance by peers	51
1	Beginning nursery school	42	16	Increase in number of arguments between parents	51
2	Increase in number of arguments with parents	39	17	Death of a close friend	53
3	Change in parents' financial status	21	18	Birth of a brother or sister	50
4	Birth of a brother or sister	50	19	Pregnancy in unwed teenage sister	36
5	Decrease in number of arguments between parents	21	20	Serious illness requiring hospitalization of brother or sister	41
6	Change of father's occupation requiring increased absence from home	39	21	Loss of job by a parent	38
7	Death of grandparent	30	22	Failure of a grade in school	57
8	Outstanding personal achievement	23	23	Divorce of parents	84
9	Serious illness requiring hospitalization of parent	51	24	Suspension from school	46
10	Brother or sister leaving home	39	25	Addition of third adult to family	41
11	Serious illness requiring hospitalization of brother or sister	37	26	Marital separation of parents	78
12	Mother beginning to work	47	27	Serious illness requiring hospitalization of child	62
13	Change to a new nursery school	33	28	Marriage of parent to stepparent	65
14	Change in child's acceptance by peers	38	29	Having a visible congenital deformity	60
15	Decrease in number of arguments with parents	22	30	Acquiring a visible deformity	69
16	Increase in number of arguments between parents	44	31	Death of a brother or sister	68
17	Serious illness requiring hospitalization of child	59	32	Discovery of being an adopted child	52
18	Loss of job by a parent	23	33	Becoming involved with drugs or alcohol	61
19	Death of a close friend	38	34	Jail sentence of parent 30 days or less	44
20	Having a visible congenital deformity	39	35	Jail sentence of parent for 1 year or more	67
21	Addition of third adult to family	39	**Junior High Age Group**		
22	Marital separation of parents	74	1	Outstanding personal achievement	45
23	Discovery of being an adopted child	33	2	Breaking up with a boyfriend or girlfriend	47
24	Jail sentence of parent for 30 days or less	34	3	Increase in number of arguments with parents	46
25	Death of parent	89	4	Beginning junior high school	45
26	Divorce of parents	78	5	Beginning to date	55
27	Acquiring a visible deformity	52	6	Brother or sister leaving home	33
28	Death of brother or sister	59	7	Decrease in number of arguments between parents	29
29	Marriage of parent to stepparent	62	8	Suspension from school	54
30	Jail sentence of parent for 1 year or more	67	9	Not making an extracurricular activity he or she wanted to be involved in	24
Elementary Age Group			10	Becoming a full-fledged member of a church	28
1	Beginning another school year	27	11	Death of a grandparent	35
2	Outstanding personal achievement	39	12	Death of a close friend	65
3	Beginning school	46	13	Increase in number of arguments between parents	48
4	Move to a new school district	46	14	Becoming involved with drugs or alcohol	70
5	Increase in number of arguments with parents	47	15	Mother beginning to work	36
6	Change in parents' financial status	29	16	Decrease in number of arguments with parents	29
7	Death of a grandparent	38	17	Change in parents' financial status	40
8	Decrease in number of arguments between parents	25	18	Move to a new school district	52
9	Mother beginning to work	44	19	Serious illness requiring hospitalization of parent	54
10	Becoming a full-fledged member of a church	25	20	Serious illness requiring hospitalization of brother or sister	44
11	Brother or sister leaving home	36	21	Failure of a grade in school	62
12	Serious illness requiring hospitalization of parent	55	22	Change in child's acceptance by peers	68
13	Decrease in number of arguments with parents	27	23	Change in father's occupation requiring increased absence from home	42
14	Change in father's occupation requiring increased absence from home	45	24	Pregnancy in unwed teenage sister	60

(continued)

TABLE 10–12. LIFE EVENT SCALES FOR CHILDREN (continued)

Rank	Life Event	Life Change Units	Rank	Life Event	Life Change Units
25	Loss of job by a parent	48	13	Increase in number of arguments between parents	46
26	Birth of a brother or sister	50	14	Death of grandparent	36
27	Divorce of parents	84	15	Mother beginning to work	26
28	Addition of third adult to family	34	16	Suspension from school	50
29	Serious illness requiring hospitalization of child	59	17	Becoming a full-fledged member of a church	31
30	Marital separation of parents	77	18	Serious illness requiring hospitalization of parent	55
31	Marriage of parent to stepparent	63	19	Change in child's acceptance by peers	67
32	Death of a parent	94	20	Move to a new school district	56
33	Having a visible congenital deformity	70	21	Change in father's occupation requiring increased absence from home	38
34	Fathering an unwed pregnancy	76	22	Failure of a grade in school	56
35	Acquiring a visible deformity	83	23	Serious illness requiring hospitalization of brother or sister	41
36	Jail sentence of a parent for 30 days or less	50	24	Loss of job by a parent	46
37	Death of a brother or sister	71	25	Being accepted at a college of his or her choice	43
38	Unwed pregnancy of child	95	26	Pregnancy in unwed teenage sister	54
39	Discovery of being an adopted child	70	27	Birth of a brother or sister	50
40	Jail sentence of a parent for 1 year or more	76	28	Marital separation of parents	69
			29	Serious illness requiring hospitalization of child	58
Senior High Age Group			30	Divorce of parents	77
1	Breaking up with boy- or girlfriend	53	31	Fathering an unwed pregnancy	77
2	Increase in number of arguments with parents	47	32	Addition of third adult to family	34
3	Beginning senior high school	42	33	Marriage of parent to stepparent	63
4	Beginning to date	51	34	Unwed pregnancy of child	92
5	Outstanding personal achievement	46	35	Having a visible congenital deformity	62
6	Becoming involved with drugs or alcohol	76	36	Getting married	101
7	Brother or sister leaving home	37	37	Death of parent	87
8	Not making an extracurricular activity he or she wanted to be involved in	55	38	Discovery of being an adopted child	64
9	Decrease in number of arguments with parents	26	39	Death of a brother or sister	68
10	Decrease in number of arguments between parents	27	40	Jail sentence of a parent for 30 days or less	53
11	Change in parents' financial status	45	41	Acquiring a visible deformity	81
12	Death of a close friend	63	42	Jail sentence of a parent for 1 year or more	75

Reprinted with permission from Coddington, R.D., The Significance of Life Events as Etiologic Factors in the Diseases of Children, Journal of Psychosomatic Research, 16 (1972), 7–18, 205–213. Copyright 1972, Pergamon Press Ltd.

are born with an innately easy-going temperament and handle stressors better than do children with a nervous, overreactive disposition, but even highly reactive children can acquire resilience if they have a stabilizing, attentive parent or mentor (5, 62, 77, 82, 189, 190, 224, 225).

Vulnerable children, if placed in the right environment, become productive and competent adults. Children who have robust, sunny personalities are lovable and readily win affection, which further builds self-esteem and an identity. Robust children are flexible but persistent and will continue to look for a solid relationship—neighbor, teacher, relative—until they find at least one such adult. Then they distance self from the conflictual or abusive home, at least emotionally (5, 77, 82, 190, 224, 225).

Resilient children are likely to have personality characteristics similar to both traditional male and female characteristics—outgoing and autonomous, nurturant and emotionally sensitive. Resilient children are likely to have a number of protective factors, but the key is a basic, consistent, lasting, trusting relationship with an adult who is supportive and who is a beacon presence from infancy on. Then the child's ability to cope improves naturally as he or she develops and gains experience (5, 77, 190, 224, 225).

Research Abstract

Gloss, E., Children and Drug Education: The P.I.E.D. Pipers, Nursing Outlook, 43, no. 2 (1995), 66–70.

The P.I.E.D. Pipers—People Involved in Education About Drugs—was a project initiated in Spring 1990, to determine ways to prevent and decrease use and abuse of illicit or over-the-counter drugs. In contrast to studies of adolescents, little research had been done on preadolescent children and substance abuse. Biological, cultural, family, and psychosocial factors have been cited as influencing children to try and rely on drugs. Strategies to prevent or reduce drug use include education, treatment, and law enforcement. Yet, a majority of campaigns have not been successful; the problems continue.

Education at the primary level of education became the major strategy for the P.I.E.D. Pipers project; it was hypothesized that knowledgeable children would become positive examples for their peers.

Project participants were preadolescent and adolescent children in an underserved health care area in New York City who were exposed to drug users and abusers. A school system was selected as the community site for the project. The primary goals were for junior high and elementary schoolchildren, nurses, and drug counselors to share their time and knowledge to (1) assist children to develop positive coping skills and a sense of self-control, (2) to develop collective control in the community, and (3) to promote interactions and role modeling among peers and between older and younger children to prevent and decrease substance use and abuse.

Fifteen junior high students were selected as trainees for the 10-hour drug education program, based on their academic status, leadership potential, and willingness to assume responsibility. A variety of teaching methods and tests were used in the training. After completion, trainees were placed in one of three grammar schools where they were known.

Nurses, school drug counselors, and the trainees formed teams to educate fourth-, fifth-, and sixth-grade students, conduct exhibits, and present Drug Awareness Day.

The trainees were perceived as peers; teachers evaluated the project favorably. It was estimated by Spring 1991 that 400 persons had received educational information.

Implications include the need for further study to promote drug-free health and development of coping mechanisms in children to deal with the drug culture on a daily basis.

When the child's environment is overwhelmingly stressful, extra support and love are especially important. If the child is facing multiple stressors, it is more difficult for outside intervention to help the child. The more the risk factors, the worse is the outcome for the child, regardless of the intervention. Basic health, social, and educational programs must be provided to assist the child to adapt to the extent possible, now and in future adult life (5, 62, 73, 74, 77, 190, 224, 225).

Teach parents that they can contribute to a sense of industry and avoid inferiority feelings by not having unrealistic expectations of the child and by using the suggested guidance and discipline approaches. They can encourage peer activities and home responsibilities, help the child meet developmental crises, and give recognition to his or her accomplishments and unique talents. They must remember that part of the time their child may regress to jumping on the couch, drumming nervously on the table with fingernails, and insisting that keeping clean is only for parents. At other times they will marvel at the poised, contented child who is visiting so nicely with their guests.

Self-Concept, Body Image, and Sexuality Development

Until the child goes to school, self-perception is derived primarily from the parents' attitudes and reactions toward him or her. The child who is loved for what he or she is learns to love and accept self. If parental reactions have been rejecting, if he or she has been made to feel ugly, ashamed, or guilty about self or his or her behavior, the child enters school feeling bad, inadequate, or inferior. A positive self-concept is imperative for happiness and personality unity.

The child with a positive self-concept likes self and others; believes that what he or she thinks, says, and does makes a difference; believes he or she can be successful and can solve problems; has a realistic estimate of personal abilities and limitations; and expresses feelings of pleasure and enjoyment (58, 130).

A negative self-image causes the child to feel defensive toward others and self and hinders adjustment to school and academic progress. Children with a low self-concept show more social withdrawal, academic difficulties, and inappropriate attention seeking than children with a high self-concept (16, 58, 129).

At school the child compares self with and is compared by peers in appearance, and motor, cognitive, language, and social skills. If he or she cannot perform as well as other children, peers will perceive the child negatively, and eventually he or she will perceive self as incompetent or inferior because self-image is more dependent on peers than earlier. Schoolchildren are frequently cruel in their honesty as they make derogatory remarks about peers with limitations or disabilities.

Unattractive children may receive discriminatory treatment from parents, teachers, and babysitters because adults have learned the social value of beauty. Unattractive children are judged more antisocial and less honest than attractive children. Thus if an unattractive child expresses innocence, he or she is less likely to be believed. Attractive children are better liked by peers and adults and are judged to have a higher IQ and to be more likely to attend college. Because people tend to act as others expect them to, the prophecy is likely to become true (129, 233). It is important for you to avoid this kind of reaction.

Self-concept and body image are affected by cultural or ethnic/racial background, sex, and grade level of the child, father's education, history of illness, and type of illness, if any. Williams (226) found that American and Filipino boys did not score significantly different in body image, whereas Filipino girls scored lower than American girls. Third-grade American children had a better understanding of the body than Filipino third graders, but fifth graders in both cultures did not score significantly different from each other. American and Filipino children whose fathers had a college education did not score significantly differently; however, Filipino children whose fathers had less education scored lower in body organ knowledge than American children whose fathers were not college educated. Regardless of these variables, ill Filipino children did not score significantly lower in body image and concept of illness than American children. More research is needed on the child's concept of self, body, and illness, both in this and in other cultures.

Biracial children are increasing in number, and their special racial status affects racial identification, self-concept, self-esteem, and school adjustment. They must deal with overt racism affecting children of color, cope with outsiders who view their families as abnormal, and sometimes cope with the loyalty issues and negative feelings from the extended family of each parent. Positive parental feelings about racial identification and positive extended family relationships are critical to sound emotional adjustment of the child and a positive self-concept. The child may have difficulty identifying with either parent because of racism, and these feelings and issues must be discussed (29).

Parents, teachers, and health care professionals can contribute to a positive self-esteem and competence in performance by emphasizing the child's positive, healthy characteristics and reinforcing the child's potential. You can be instrumental in fostering a healthy relationship. Then the child, especially a girl who is competent in many activities, retains this competence in the teen years. Studies show girls can be as excellent as boys in a wide variety of activities (88).

The perception and reaction of the teacher, nurse, and parent are extremely important. The parent and nurse should listen carefully to the child's own estimate of self, school progress, and relationship with peers. The teacher should be informed if the child questions his or her adequacy. The nurse can assess and help correct physical or emotional problems.

The teacher (or nurse) can intervene when derogatory remarks are made among classmates. Teacher may move a child into another work or play group appropriate for his or her ability or explain to peers in simple language the importance of accepting another who is at a different developmental level. Meanwhile, teacher should encourage the child who has the difficulty. In turn, the nurse supports the teacher in such action. Thus the school experience may either reinforce or weaken the child's feeling about self as a unique, important person, with specific talents or abilities. If he or she is one of 30 children in a classroom and receives little attention from the teacher, self-concept may be threatened.

The child's body image and self-concept are very fluid. Schoolchildren are more aware of the internal body and external differences. They can label major organs with increasing accuracy; heart, brain, and bones are most frequently mentioned, along with cardiovascular, gastrointestinal, and musculoskeletal systems. The younger child thinks that organs change position, and organ function, size, and position are poorly understood. Organs such as the stomach are frequently drawn at the wrong place (this may reflect the influence of television ads). Children generally believe that they must have all body parts to remain alive and that the skin holds in body contents. Consider the impact of injury or surgery on the child. This is an excellent age to teach about any of these inaccuracies (76, 174).

The child is changing physically, emotionally, and socially. Physique is changing. Sexual identity is strengthening. He or she is learning how to get along with more people, both peers and adults, and is developing academic skills. Table 10–13 shows how aspects of the child's view of self change through the school years (16, 42, 43, 54, 76, 79, 80, 174).

Self-concept, body image, and sexuality development are interrelated and are influenced by parental and societal expectations of and reactions to each sex. You can assist parents in promoting a positive self-concept and body image. During latency boys and girls are similar in many ways, but differences are taught. Girls reportedly are less physically active, but they have greater verbal, perceptual, and cognitive skills than boys. Girls supposedly respond to stimuli—interpersonal and physical, including pain—more quickly and accurately than boys.

They seem better at analyzing and anticipating environmental demands; thus their behavior conforms more to adult expectations, and they are better at staying out of trouble. Girls are encouraged to depend on and to rely on others' appraisals for self-esteem more than boys. Girls are not usually forced to develop internal controls and a sense of independent self in the way that boys are because of the difference in adult reactions to each sex. Innate physiologic differences become magnified as they are reinforced by cultural norms and specific parental behaviors. Stereotypes are changing, however. Girls can cope with aggression and competition just as boys can (16, 88, 129, 233).

Research shows that fears about the girl's harming her childbearing functions or her feminine appearance

TABLE 10–13. ASSESSMENT OF CHANGING BODY IMAGE DEVELOPMENT IN THE SCHOOLCHILD

6 Years	7 Years	8 Years
Is self-centered	Is more modest and aware of self	Redefines sense of status with others
Likes to be in control of self, situations, and possessions	Wants own place at table, in car, and own room or part of room	Subtle changes in physical proportion; movements smoother
Gains physical and motor skills	Has lower-level physical activity than earlier	Assumes many roles consecutively
Knows right from left hand	Does not like to be touched	Is ready for physical contact in play and to be taught self-defense mechanisms
Regresses occasionally to baby talk or earlier behavior	Protects self by withdrawing from unpleasant situation	Is more aware of differences between the sexes
Plays at being someone else to clarify sense of self and others	Dislikes physical combat	Is curious about another's body
Is interested in marriage and reproduction	Engages less in sex play	Asks questions about marriage and reproduction; strong interest in babies, especially for girls
Distinguishes organs of each sex but wonders about them	Understands pregnancy generally; excited about new baby in family	Plays more with own sex
May indulge in sex play	Concerned he or she does not really belong to parents	
Draws a man with hands, neck, clothing, and six identifiable parts	Tells parts missing from picture of incomplete man	
Distinguishes between attractive and ugly pictures of faces		

9 Years	10 Years
Has well-developed eye–hand coordination	Is relatively content with and confident of self
Enjoys displaying motor skills and strength	Has perfected most basic small motor movements
Cares completely for body needs	Wants privacy for self but peeks at other sex
Has more interest in own body and its functions than in other sexual matters	Asks some questions about sexual matters again
Asks fewer questions about sexual matters if earlier questions answered satisfactorily	Investigates own sexual organs
Is self-conscious about exposing body, including to younger siblings and opposite-sex parent	Shows beginning prepubertal changes physically, especially girls

11 Years	12 Years
States self is in heart, head, face, or body part most actively expressing him or her	Growth spurt; changes in appearance
Feels more self-conscious with physical changes occurring	Muscular control almost equal to that of adult
Mimics adults; deepening self-understanding	Identifies self as being in total body or brain
Masturbates sometimes; erection occurs in boys	May feel like no part of body is his or hers alone but like someone else's because of close identity with group
Discusses sexual matters with parents with reticence	Begins to accept and find self as unique person
Likes movies on reproduction	Feels joy of life with more mature understanding

as a result of normal rigorous activity are unfounded. Traditionally, girls and women in rural areas have worked very hard physically with no ill effects. In addition, primarily the male hormones, not vigorous exercise, produce big bones, muscle mass, and a masculine appearance. Early physical education activities teach general coordination, eye–hand coordination, and balance, basic movements that carry over into all movement and sports. Rigorous conditioning activities such as gymnastics are suggested for achieving high levels of physical fitness for prepubertal girls and will improve agility, appearance, endurance, strength, feelings of well-being, and self-concept.

Sexuality Education

Sexuality education, *learning about the self as a person who is a sexual being,* has begun by the school years. The child can learn that both sexes have similar feelings and behavior potential, which can instill attitudes about maleness and femaleness for adulthood. The traditional stereotypes of the aggressive, competitive, intelligent, clumsy, brave, and athletic man and the passive, demure, gentle, graceful, domestic, fearful, and emotional woman must be discarded by parents, teachers, and other adults so that they will not be learned by the schoolchild. At this age both sexes are dependent and independent, active and passive, emotional and controlled, gentle and aggressive. Keeping such a range of behavior will contribute to a more flexible adult who can be expressive, spontaneous, and accepting of self and others.

You will have to work through your own stereotypes to help the parents, child, and child's peers avoid sex typing.

Sex education, *factual information about anatomy, physiology, and birth control methods,* should begin now for both sexes. By 7 or 8, children usually know that both sexes are required for childbirth to occur, but they are not sure how.

Almost all parents will experience at least some anxiety and embarrassment when they discuss sex with their children. Remember that these parents have come from a generation taught that the discussion of sex was at least partially taboo. Ideas about sexual behavior and what should be taught vary with socioeconomic level and age group.

Following are some guidelines for parents, teachers, or yourself when handling this subject:

- Know the facts.
- Do not lecture or preach.

- Do not skip anything because the youngster says, "I already know." Chances are the child has some twisted facts.
- Answer all questions as honestly as possible.
- Do not force too much at one sitting. Aim the information at the child's immediate interest. Do not pry into the child's feelings and fantasies. Try to make the conversation as relaxed as possible.

Many elementary schools introduce basic sex education in the fourth grade. Usually parents are asked to preview the film or presentation and give permission for their child to participate. Ideally this procedure will stimulate a bond among parents, child, and teacher so that all focus on accurate and positive education. In planning a sex education program, realize that there probably will be parents both in favor of and opposed to sex education classes. It is important to explore and clarify the attitudes of parents and teachers during the early planning phases.

Self-concept and sexuality can be traumatized by sexual advances from adults, sometimes family members. Burgess and her colleagues (22–26) and other authors (92, 131, 233, 238, 239) provide useful references for gaining additional information.

Burgess and Holmstrom (22) describe a study of school-age children who were sexually molested; feelings about the traumatic event; stages of resolution; defense mechanisms used by the children and parents; the issues; feelings of and difficulties for the parents in the community who joined together to prosecute the offender (a busdriver); other community issues; and the therapist's role with the children and parents over a period. Swanson and Biaggio (207) discuss the dynamics of and consequent problems of father–daughter incest. Other references discuss factors that contribute to sexual abuse, the trauma to the child and family members, treatment, and legal implications (22–26, 68, 102, 171, 233, 236, 238, 239). Refer also to Chapter 9.

Adaptive Mechanisms

The schoolchild is losing the protective mantle of home and early childhood and needs order and consistency in life to help cope with doubts, fears, unacceptable impulses, and unfamiliar experiences. Commonly used adaptive mechanisms include ritualistic behavior, reaction formation, undoing, isolation, fantasy, identification, regression, malingering, rationalization, projection, and sublimation (129, 211).

Ritualistic behavior, *consistently repeating an act in a situation,* wards off imagined harm and anxiety and provides a feeling of control. Examples include stepping on cracks in the sidewalk while chanting certain words, always putting the left leg through trousers before the right, having a certain place for an object, or doing homework at a specific time.

Reaction formation, undoing, and isolation are related to obsessive, ritualistic behavior. **Reaction formation** is used frequently in dealing with feelings of hostility. The child may unconsciously hate a younger brother because he infringes on the schoolchild's freedom, but such impulses are unacceptable to the strict superego. To counter such unwanted feelings, the child may become the classic example of a caring, loving sibling.

Undoing is *unconsciously removing an idea, feeling, or act by performing certain ritualistic behavior.* For example, the gang has certain chants and movements to follow before a member who broke a secret code can return. **Isolation** is a *mechanism of unconsciously separating emotion from an idea because the emotion would be unacceptable to the self.* The idea remains in the conscious, but its component feeling remains in the unconscious. A child uses isolation when he or she seems to talk very objectively about the puppy who has just been run over by a truck.

Fantasy *compensates for feelings of inadequacy, inferiority, and lack of success* encountered in school, the peer group, or home. Fantasy is necessary for eventual creativity and should not be discouraged if it is not used excessively to prevent realistic participation in the world. Fantasy saves the ego temporarily, but it also provides another way for the child to view self, thus helping him or her aspire to new heights of behavior.

Identification is seen in the hero worship of teacher, scoutmaster, neighbor, or family friend, someone whom the child respects and who has the qualities the child fantasizes as his or her own.

Regression, *returning to a less sophisticated pattern of behavior,* is a defense against anxiety and helps the child avoid potentially painful situations. For example, he or she may revert to using the language or behavior of a younger sibling if the child feels that the sibling is getting undue attention.

Malingering, *feigning illness to avoid unpleasant tasks,* is seen when the child stays home from school for a day or says he or she is unable to do a home task because he or she does not feel well.

Rationalization, *giving excuses when the child is unable to achieve wishes,* is frequently seen in relation to schoolwork. For example, after a low test grade, the response is, "Oh well, grades don't make any difference anyway."

Projection is seen as the child says about a teacher, "She doesn't like me," when really the teacher is disliked for having reprimanded him or her.

Sublimation is a major mechanism used during the school years. The child increasingly *channels sexual and aggressive impulses into socially acceptable tasks* at school and home. In the process, if all goes well, he or she develops the sense of industry.

Use of any and all of these mechanisms in various situations is normal, but overuse of any one can result in a constricted, immature personality. If constricted, the child will be unable to develop relationships outside the home, to succeed at home or school, or to balance work and play. Achieving a sense of identity and adult developmental tasks will be impaired.

Help parents understand the adaptive mechanisms used by the child and how to help the child use healthy coping mechanisms.

Child in Transition

American families are on the move. Moving from one part of the country to another, or even from one community and school system to another, brings a special set of tasks that should be acknowledged and worked through. Some families, because of the military or other career or as part of an exchange program, may live in another country for a number of years or move from country to country. This poses another kind of adjustment and set of tasks. Children who were born in a foreign country and then return with their parents to the United States undergo culture shock. They feel like citizens of another country and visitors in the land of which they are citizens. Lykins (135) describes the feelings of children of the "Third Culture" who have seen much of the world, know more than one language, are cognizant of and accepting of various lifestyles, and speak, dress, eat, and behave as if they were still in another land. He also describes family and employment dynamics. Educational considerations that must be made in school are also discussed. These students usually want to return to the country in which they had lived for some time, although they feel patriotism for the United States.

The school-age child is especially affected by a geographic move if he or she is just entering or is well settled into the chum stage. The child cannot understand why he or she cannot fit into the new group right away. Because routines are so important to the schoolchild, he or she is sometimes confused by the new and different ways of doing things. The parents will need to consult with the new school leaders about their child's adjustment.

If a family can include the schoolchild in the decision about where to move, the transition will be easier. If not, then the following ideas can still be used. Share them with parents. Ideally, the whole family should make at least one advance trip to the new community. If possible, the new home and town should be explored, and the child should visit the new school so that he or she can establish mentally where he or she is going. Writing to one of the new classmates before the actual move can enhance a feeling of friendship and belonging. If the child has a special interest such as gymnastics or dancing, a contact with the new program can form another transitional step.

When parents are packing, they are tempted to dispose of as many of the child's belongings as possible, especially if they seem babyish or worn. *Do not do this.* These items are part of the child, and they will help him or her feel comfortable and at home during adjustment to a new home and community.

Sometimes parents in the new community are reticent about letting their children go to the new child's house. The new parents should make every attempt to introduce themselves to the new playmates' parents, assuring them that the environment will be safe for play; or parents can have a get-acquainted party for the few children who are especially desired as playmates or chums.

Just as the family initiated some ties before they moved, so should they keep some ties from the previous neighborhood. If possible, let the child play with old friends at times. If the move has been too far for frequent visits, allow the child to call old friends occasionally. If possible, plan a trip back so that some old traditions can be revived and friends can be visited. The trip to the old neighborhood will cement in the child's mind that "home" is no longer there but in the new location.

The parents must accept as natural some grieving for what is gone. Letting the child express his or her feelings, accepting these feelings, and continuing to work with the above suggestions will foster the adjustment.

The nurse can foster the above through noticing the new child, watching his behavior, working with the teacher and peers, and contacting parents if necessary.

Moral–Spiritual Development

You can assist parents in understanding the importance of their role and that of peers, school, and even literature and the media in moral and spiritual development (41, 73, 149, 150, 151, 181, 187). If you care for a child over a period, you will also contribute to this development.

In the school years the child usually moves from the fairy tale stage of God's being like a giant to the realistic or concrete state of God's being like a human figure. For the Christian child, Jesus is an angelic boy growing into a perfect man.

The child is learning many particulars about his or her religion such as Allah, God, Jesus, prayer, rites, ancestor worship, life after death, reincarnation, heaven, and hell, all of which are developed into a religious philosophy and used in interpretation of the world. These ideas are taught by family, friends, teachers, church, books, radio, and television.

The child of 6 can understand God as creator, expects prayers to be answered, and feels the forces of good and evil with the connotation of reward and punishment. The 6-year-old believes in a creative being, a father figure who is responsible for many things such as thunder and lightning. The adult usually introjects the natural or scientific explanation. Somehow the child seems to hold this dual thinking without contradiction. The adult's ability to weave the supernatural with the natural will affect the child's later ability to do so. Coles discusses his studies of spiritual development in children. Most children, even those from an atheistic background, develop a concept of God and are likely to believe in God; however, children may not discuss their views if they fear ridicule or rejection from a secular society (41).

The developing schoolchild has a great capacity for reverence and awe, continues to ask more appropriate questions about religious teaching and God, and can be taught through stories that emphasize moral traits. The child operates from a simple framework of ideas and will earnestly pray for recovery and protection from danger for self and others. The child believes that a Supreme Being loves him or her, gives the earth and a house, and is always near. He or she may ask, "How does God take care of me when I can't see Him?" "Allah's here, but where?" "I don't know how to love God like I love you, Mommy, because I've never touched Him."

In prepuberty the child begins to comprehend disappointments more fully and realize that his or her answers to problems or desires to change the world quickly are not always possible (197). He or she realizes that self-centered prayers are not always answered and that no magic is involved. The child can now accept totally the scientific explanation for thunder and lightning. He or she may drop religion at this point; or because of strong dependence on parents, the child may continue to accept the family preference. Yet the blind faith that previously existed is gradually replaced by reason (129).

The schoolchild can be in the Conventional Stage of moral development, according to Kohlberg (228, 231, 232). (See Chapter 5, Table 5–12). Beliefs about right and wrong have less to do with the child's actual behavior than with the likelihood of getting caught for transgression and the gains to derive from the transgression. Other factors that influence moral development include the child's intelligence, ability to delay gratification, and sense of self-esteem. The child with high self-esteem and a favorable self-concept is less likely to engage in immoral behavior, possibly because he or she will feel more guilty with wrongdoing. Thus, moral behavior may be more a matter of strength of will or ego than of strength of conscience or superego. Morality is not a fixed behavioral trait but rather a decision-making capacity. The child progresses from an initial premoral stage, in which he or she responds primarily to reward and punishment and believes rules can be broken to meet personal needs, through a rule-based highly conventional morality, and finally to the stage of self-accepted principles (116–118).

Part of moral development is the ability to follow rules. Unlike the preschooler who initiates rules without understanding them, the 7- or 8-year-old begins to play in a genuinely social manner. Rules are mutually accepted by all players and are rigidly followed. Rules come from some external force such as God and are believed timeless. Not until the age of 11 or 12, when the formal operations level of cognition is reached, does the child understand the true nature of rules—that they exist to make the game possible and can be altered by mutual agreement (164).

Piaget (164) also identified stages of moral development as he studied the child's pattern of reasoning to think about moral issues:

1. *Premoral:* The child has no regard for rules.
2. *Heteronomous:* The child obeys rules because of fear of authority or powerful figures.
3. *Autonomous:* The child follows rules freely, expressing mutual rights and obligations. The person is increasingly able to distinguish between principles and rules, and at more advanced stages the person applies principles to guide behavior in specific situations instead of automatically following established rules.

Moral development is related to self-discipline and empathy, and how this is taught varies with the culture.

► SELECTED NURSING DIAGNOSES RELATED TO THE SCHOOL-AGE CHILD*

Pattern 1: Exchanging
Altered Nutrition: More than Body Requirements
Altered Nutrition: Less than Body Requirements
Altered Nutrition: Potential for More Than Body Requirements
Risk for Infection
Risk for Injury
Risk for Trauma
Impaired Skin Integrity

Pattern 2: Communicating
Impaired Verbal Communication

Pattern 3: Relating
Impaired Social Interaction
Social Isolation

Pattern 4: Valuing
Spiritual Distress

Pattern 5: Choosing
Ineffective Individual Coping
Impaired Adjustment
Health-Seeking Behaviors

Pattern 6: Moving
Impaired Physical Mobility
Fatigue
Sleep Pattern Disturbance
Diversional Activity Deficit
Bathing/Hygiene Self-Care Deficit
Dressing/Grooming Self-Care Deficit
Altered Growth and Development

Pattern 7: Perceiving
Body Image Disturbance
Self-Esteem Disturbance
Sensory/Perceptual Alterations
Hopelessness
Powerlessness

Pattern 8: Knowing
Knowledge Deficit

Pattern 9: Feeling
Pain
Dysfunctional Grieving
Anticipatory Grieving
Anxiety
Fear

*Other NANDA diagnoses are applicable to the ill school-age child.
From *North American Nursing Diagnosis Association, NANDA Nursing Diagnoses Definitions & Classification 1995–1996. Philadelphia: North American Nursing Diagnosis Association, 1994.*

For example, a study showed that Japanese and American mothers approach the task of discipline and moral development differently. For instance, reactions of Japanese mothers to the child's public misbehavior is to ask, "How do you think this makes the storekeeper feel when you run around the store? How do you think it makes me feel?" From an early age the Japanese child is taught to consider the feelings of others, to think out the consequences of his or her behavior and not just obey rules, which fosters discipline and thoughtfulness that facilitate academic performance later. In contrast, the Western child is told what to do and often is spoken to with an anger level that arouses rebellion rather than self-restraint and a selfishness rather than a spirit of cooperation (16).

A study of children ages 10 to 14 in seven cultures, including the United States, Europe, and Asia, revealed that this era is a crucial time for learning moral views and to obey rules. Almost all children in all cultures realized that laws and rules are norms that guide behavior and require obedience from all, and they realized that chaos would result without them (129, 187). In five of the seven cultures children accepted that rule breaking might be permissible for higher moral reasons. In six of the seven cultures parents were seen as most able to make children follow rules. Only in Japan did the teacher rank higher than the parents. Police ranked at least fourth in all cultures except India. Thus affiliative, nurturant strategies rather than punitive ones were seen as most effective in inducing compliance and assuring the stability of systems (129, 187).

Developmental Tasks

Although the schoolchild continues working on past developmental tasks, he or she is confronted with a series of new ones (57):

- Decreasing dependence on family and gaining some satisfaction from peers and other adults
- Increasing neuromuscular skills so that he or she can participate in games and work with others
- Learning basic adult concepts and knowledge to be able to reason and engage in tasks of everyday living
- Learning ways to communicate with others realistically
- Becoming a more active and cooperative family participant
- Giving and receiving affection among family and friends without immediately seeking something in return

- Learning socially acceptable ways of getting money and saving it for later satisfactions
- Learning how to handle strong feelings and impulses appropriately
- Adjusting the changing body image and self-concept to come to terms with the masculine or feminine social role
- Discovering healthy ways of becoming acceptable as a person

---

► CONSIDERATIONS FOR THE SCHOOLCHILD AND FAMILY IN HEALTH CARE

- Family and cultural background and values, the school, the support systems available, community resources
- Parents' ability to guide the child, to help the child develop coping skills and gain necessary competencies
- Relationships between family members
- Behaviors that indicate a parent(s) or another significant adult, such as a relative or teacher, is perpetuating abuse, neglect, or maltreatment
- Relationships between the family, school, and other community organizations (church, clubs) and resources
- Physical growth patterns, characteristics and competencies, nutritional status, and rest/sleep and exercise patterns that indicate health and are within age norms for the school-age child
- Growth spurt and secondary sex changes in prepubescence that indicate normal development in the boy or girl; self-concept and body image development related to physical growth
- Nutritional requirements greater than those for the adult
- Immunizations, safety education, and other health promotion measures
- Cognitive characteristics and behavioral patterns in the preschool child that demonstrates curiosity and Concrete Operations (concept formation, realistic thinking, and beginning social and moral value formation)
- Educational/school programs, demonstration of development of cooperation, compromise, and collaboration as well as competition
- Communication patterns; effect of television, computer, or other media on communication, learning, and behavior
- Overall appearance and behavioral patterns at home, school, and in the community that indicate development of industry, rather than inferiority
- Use of adaptive mechanisms that promote a sense of security, assist the child with relationships, promote realistic control of anxiety and age-appropriate emotional responses in the face of stressors
- Behavioral patterns that indicate ongoing superego development and continuing moral–spiritual development
- Behavioral patterns and characteristics that indicate the child has achieved developmental tasks
- Parental behaviors that indicate they are achieving their developmental tasks

- Developing a positive attitude toward his or her own and other social, racial, economic, and religious groups

The accomplishment of these tasks gives the schoolchild a foundation for entering adolescence, an era filled with dramatic growth and changing attitudes. Your support, teaching, and guidance can assist the child in this progression.

► HEALTH CARE AND NURSING APPLICATIONS

Your role in caring for the school-age child and family has been described in each section of the chapter. Assessment, using knowledge about this era that is presented in this chapter, is the basis for *nursing diagnosis*. Nursing diagnoses that may be applicable to the schoolchild are listed in Selected Nursing Diagnoses Related to the School-Age Child. Interventions may involve measures that promote health (e.g., immunization or control of hazards); teaching, support, counseling, or spiritual care with the child or family; or direct care measures to the ill child. Your understanding of the child developmentally will enable you to give holistic care—care that includes physiologic, emotional, cognitive, social, and spiritual aspects of the person.

SUMMARY

The schoolchild grows at a steady pace and continues physical growth and cognitive, emotional, social, and moral–spiritual development. The growth spurt at prepuberty or preadolescence accelerates and influences development in all dimensions. Relationships with parents, siblings, peers, and other adults change and influence development in all dimensions. Family is important as a base as peer relations become more important. The chum of the same sex is a major support and is vital in psychological, self-concept, and social development. The child meets many challenges, faces and overcomes insecurities, and develops competence that indicates industry and development of Concrete Operations. School, home, and community provide the avenues for development in all dimensions.

Considerations for the Schoolchild and Family in Health Care and Chart 3 in Appendix IV summarize what you should consider in assessment and health promotion with the schoolchild. The family is included in Considerations. Chart 3 presents the American Academy of Family Physicians Periodic Health Examination for Children Ages 7 to 12 Years. It includes guidelines for screening and parent and child health counseling. It summarizes the immunization schedule and categorizes risks to health (4).

REFERENCES

1. Adler, J., Kids Are Growing Up Scared, *Newsweek,* January 10 (1994), 43–50.
2. Allard, R., Beliefs About AIDS as Determinants of Preventive Practices and of Support for Coercive Measures, *American Journal of Public Health,* 78, no. 4 (1988), 448–452.
3. Amato, P., Life-span Adjustment of Children to Their Parents' Divorce, *The Future of Children: Children and Divorce,* 4, no. 1 (1994), 143–157.
4. American Academy of Family Physicians, *Age Charts for Periodic Health Examination.* Washington, DC: Author, 1995.
5. Anthony, E.J., and B. Cohler, *The Invulnerable Child.* New York: Guilford, 1987.
6. Aronsen, D., *Teaching Tolerance in the Classroom,* 4, no. 1 (Spring 1995), 1–64 (published by Southern Poverty Law Center, Montgomery, AL).
7. As TV Grows, So Does the Rate of Depression, *St. Louis Post Dispatch,* August 31 (1994), Sect. F, p. 5.
8. Atkins, F., An Uncertain Future: Children of Mentally Ill Parents, *Journal of Psychosocial Nursing,* 30, no. 8 (1992), 13–16.
9. Attention Deficit Disorder—Part I, *The Harvard Mental Health Letter,* 11, no. 10 (1995), 1–4.
10. Attention Deficit Disorder—Part II, *The Harvard Mental Health Letter,* 11, no. 11 (1995), 1–3.
11. Attitudes of Safety Preserve Young Lives, *Farm Week,* April 1 (1991), 7.
12. Austin, J., J. Patterson, and T. Huberty, Development of the Coping Health Inventory for Children, *Journal of Pediatrics,* 6, no. 3 (1991), 166–174.
13. Baker, S., and R. Henry, *Parents' Guide to Nutrition: Healthy Eating From Birth through Adolescence.* Reading, MA: Addison-Wesley, 1987.
14. Barker, P., and D. Lewis, The Management of Lead Exposure in Pediatric Populations, *Nurse Practitioner: American Journal of Primary Health Care,* 15, no. 12 (1990), 8–10.
15. Bates, B., *A Guide to Physical Examination and History Taking* (4th ed.). Philadelphia: J.B. Lippincott, 1987.
16. Bettelheim, B., and A. Freedgood, *A Good Enough Parent: A Book on Child-rearing.* New York: Random, 1988.
17. Black, J., AIDS: Preschool and School Issues, *Journal of School Health,* 56, no. 3 (1986), 93–95.
18. Boals, B., C. Tyree, and R. Barker, Promoting Quality Education for Children in Poverty, *Kappa Delta Pi Record,* 30, no. 3 (1994), 109–112.
19. Boy Soldiers, *Newsweek,* August 14 (1995), 44–46.
20. Boynton, R., E. Dunn, and G. Stephens, *Manual of Ambulatory Pediatrics* (3rd ed.). Philadelphia: J.B. Lippincott, 1994.
21. Brazelton, T., What Parents Need to Say (Children's Fears of War), *Newsweek,* February 26 (1991), 52.
22. Burgess, A., and L. Holmstrom, Sexual Trauma of Children and Adults, *Nursing Clinics of North America,* 10, no. 3 (September 1975), 551–563.
23. ———, C. Hartman, and S. Kelley, Assessing Child Abuse: The TRIADS Checklist, *Journal of Psychosocial Nursing and Mental Health Services,* 28, no. 4 (1990), 6–14.

24. ———, M. McCausland, and W. Wolbert, Children's Drawings as Indicators of Sexual Trauma, *Perspectives in Psychiatric Care,* 19, no. 2 (1981), 50–58.

25. ———, et al., Child Molestation: Assessing Impact in Multiple Victims (Part I), *Archives of Psychiatric Nursing,* 1, no. 1 (1987), 33–39.

26. Burgess, A., Sexually Abused Children and Their Drawings, *Archives of Psychiatric Nursing,* 2, no. 2 (1988), 65–73.

27. Busch, C., P. Zybem, and S. Shea, 5-A-Day: Dietary Behavior and the Fruit and Vegetable Intake of Latino Children, *American Journal of Public Health,* 84 (1994), 814–818.

28. Butler, W., V. Segreto, and E. Collins, Prevalence of Dental Mottling in School-aged Lifetime Residents of 16 Texas Communities, *American Journal of Public Health,* 75 (1985), 1408–1412.

29. Buttery, T., Biracial Children: Racial Identification, Self-esteem, and School Adjustment, *Kappa Delta Pi Record,* 23, no. 2 (Winter 1987), 50–53.

30. Butz, A., and C. Alexander, Use of Health Diaries with Children, *Nursing Research,* 40 (1991), 59–61.

31. Cacha, F., How Safe Are Students in School?, *Kappa Delta Pi Record,* 18, no. 3 (Spring 1982), 72–73.

32. Center for Disease Control and Prevention General Recommendations on Immunization: Recommendations of the Advisory Committee on Immunization Practices (ACIP). *Morbidity and Mortality Weekly Report,* 43 (January 28, 1994), 23.

33. Center for the Future of Children *The Future of Children, Children and Divorce,* 4, no. 1 (1994), 1–247.

34. Center for the Study of Social Policy, *Kids Count Data Book: State Profiles of Child Well-Being.* Washington, DC: A.E. Casey Foundation, 1991.

35. Childhood Sexual Abuse and Eating Disorders, *The Harvard Mental Health Letter,* 11, no. 10 (1995), 7–8.

36. Children and Divorce: Overview and Analysis, *The Future of Children, Children and Divorce,* 4, no. 1 (1994), 4–14.

37. Children Really Want Guidance in the Evolving Process of Self-Discovery, *Possibilities,* January–February (1989), 12–13.

38. Clore, E., Dispelling the Common Myths About Pediculosis, *Journal of Pediatric Health Care,* 3, no. 1 (1989), 28–33.

39. ———, Pediculosis Screening and Treatment, *School Nurse,* 6, no. 3 (1990), 14–18.

40. Coddington, R., The Significance of Life Events as Etiologic Factors in the Diseases of Children, *Journal of Psychosomatic Research,* 16 (1972), 7–18, 205–213.

41. Coles, R., *The Spiritual Life of Children.* Boston: Houghton Mifflin, 1990.

42. ———, Children of Crisis, *The Privileged Ones, the Well Off, and the Rich in America,* Vol. 5. Boston: Little, Brown, 1978.

43. Comer, J., and A. Pouissant, *Black Child Care.* New York: Simon & Schuster, 1975.

44. Common, R., and M. MacMullen, Home Schooling—A Growing Movement, *Kappa Delta Pi Record,* 23, no. 4 (Summer 1987), 114–117.

45. Conroy, M., Is Perfectionism Killing Your Kid? *Better Homes and Gardens,* November (1987), 79–80.

46. Cutright, M., What Parents Can Do, *Newsweek,* Special Section, March 12 (1990), 18.

47. Dacey, J., and J. Travers, *Human Development Across the Lifespan* (3rd ed.), Madison: Brown & Benchmark, 1996.

48. Dagenais, R., and R. Morris, A Gifted Program That Is Making a Difference, *Kappa Delta Pi Record,* 25, no. 1 (Fall 1988), 24–27.

49. Daley, S., Little Girls Lose Their Self-Esteem on Way to Adolescence, Study Finds, *New York Times,* January 8 (1991).

50. Davidson, L., M. Durkin, L. Kirby, P. O'Connor, B. Barlow, and M. Heagarty, The Impact of the Safe Kids/Healthy Neighborhoods Injury Prevention Program in Harlem 1988 through 1991, *American Journal of Public Health,* 84 (1994), 580–586.

51. Davis, R., Protect Your Family from Cults, *Home Life,* 47, no. 7 (April 1991), 32–33.

52. DeMoss, B., Do You Know What Your Children Are Watching? *Focus on the Family,* August (1994), 2–4.

53. De Santis, L., and J. Thomas, The Immigrant Haitian Mothers' Transcultural Nursing Perspective on Preventive Health Care for Children, *Journal of Transcultural Nursing,* 2, no. 1 (1991), 2–15.

54. DiLeo, J., *Young Children and Their Drawings.* Springfield, IL: Springer, 1971.

55. Duncan, B., A. Smith, and F. Briese, A Comparison of Growth: Spanish-Surnamed With Non-Spanish Surnamed Children, *American Journal of Public Health,* 69, no. 9 (1979), 903–907.

56. Duncan, G., Racism as a Developmental Mediator, *The Educational Forum,* 57 (Summer 1993), 360–370.

57. Duvall, E., and B. Miller, *Marriage and Family Development* (6th ed.). New York: Harper & Row, 1984.

58. Dworetzky, J., *Human Development: A Life Span Approach* (2nd ed.). St. Paul/Minneapolis: West, 1995.

59. Edelson, E., *Food & Your Child.* New York: Time-Life Books, 1988.

60. Edmiston, H., Attacking Asthma: Intervention Identifies Disease Triggers: Cockroach Allergen, Dust Mites and Others, *Outlook,* Winter (1994), 9–11.

61. Effects of Violence on Children's Ability to Learn Highlighted in New Report from NHEC, *The Nation's Health,* 25, no. 10 (1995), 23.

62. Elkind, D., *The Hurried Child: Growing Up Too Fast Too Soon.* Reading, MA: Addison-Wesley, 1981.

63. Ennett, S., N. Tobler, C. Ringwalt, and R. Flewelling, How Resistant Is Drug Abuse Resistance Education? A Meta-analysis of Project D.A.R.E. Outcome Evaluations, *American Journal of Public Health,* 84 (1994), 1394–1401.

64. Erikson, E., *Childhood and Society* (2nd ed.). New York: W.W. Norton, 1963.

65. Exposure to Violence Adversely Affects Children, *Journal of Psychosocial Nursing,* 31, no. 8 (1993), 45.

66. Farrand, L., and C. Cox, Determinants of Positive Health Behavior in Middle Childhood, *Nursing Research,* 42 (1993), 208–213.

67. The Fate of Violent Boys, *The Harvard Mental Health Letter,* 11, no. 11 (1995), 7–8.

68. Federation, S., Sexual Abuse: Treatment Modalities for the Younger Child, *Journal of Psychosocial Nursing,* 24, no. 7 (1986), 21–24.

69. Filipovic, Z., *Zlata's Diary: A Child's Life in Sarajevo,* New York: Viking Penguin/Penguin Books, 1994.

70. Flynn, B., J. Worden, R. Secker-Walker, P. Pirie, G. Badger, J. Carpenter, and B. Geller, Mass Media and School Interventions for Cigarette Smoking Prevention: Effects 2 Years After Completion, *American Journal of Public Health,* 84 (1994), 1148–1150.

71. Fordiani, T., Have You Read a Fairy Tale Lately? *Kappa Delta Pi Record,* Spring (1995), 116–119.

72. Frank A., *The Diary of A Young Girl.* New York: Doubleday. 1967.

73. Frederick, S., Ready for the Battle, *Believers' Voice of Victory,* 17, no. 6 (June 1989), 6–7.

74. Friar, L., and P. Grenoble, *Teaching Your Child to Handle Peer Pressure.* Chicago: Contemporary Books, 1988.

75. Garbarino, J., E. Guttmann, and J. Seeley, *The Psychologically Battered Child: Strategies for Identification, Assessment and Intervention.* San Francisco: Jossey-Bass, 1987.

76. Gelbert, E., Children's Conceptions of the Content and Functions of the Human Body, *Genetic-Psychologic Monographs,* 65 (1962), 293–411.

77. Gelman, D., The Miracle of Resiliency, *Newsweek Special Issue,* Summer (1991), 44–47.

78. The Gender Equation, *American Association of University Women Outlook,* 88, no. 3 (1995), 28–29.

79. Gesell, A., and F. Ilg, *The Child From Five to Ten* (rev. ed.). New York: Harper Collins, 1977.

80. ——, F. Ilg, and L. Ames, *Youth: The Years from Ten to Sixteen.* New York: Harper & Brothers, 1956.

81. Goldman, J., The Taming of the Tube, *Health,* July–August (1990), 42–47.

82. Goleman, D., Thriving Despite Hardship: Key Childhood Traits Identified, *The New York Times,* October 15 (1987), Sect. Y, p. 19ff.

83. Gloss, E., Children and Drug Education: The P.I.E.D. Pipers, *Nursing Outlook,* 43, no. 2 (1995), 66–72.

84. Greenberg, M., et al., Cigarette Use Among Hispanic and Non-Hispanic White School Children, Albuquerque, New Mexico, *American Journal of Public Health,* 77, no. 5 (1987), 621–622.

85. Grossman, D.S., Circadian Rhythms in Blood Pressure in School-Age Children of Normotensive and Hypertensive Parents, *Nursing Research,* 40, no. 1 (1991), 28–34.

86. Grube, J., and L. Wallach, Television Beer Advertising and Drinking Knowledge, Beliefs, and Intentions Among School Children, *American Journal of Public Health,* 84 (1994), 254–259.

87. Hager, R., L. Tucker, and G. Selfaas, Aerobic Fitness, Blood Lipids, and Body Fat in Children, *American Journal of Public Health,* 85 (1995), 1702–1706.

88. Hancock, E., *The Girl Within.* New York: Ballantine, 1990.

89. Haugaard, J., and N. Reppucci, *The Sexual Abuse of Children.* San Francisco: Jossey-Bass, 1989.

90. Hayman, L., J. Meininger, P. Coates, and P. Gallagher, Nongenetic Influences of Obesity in Risk Factors for Cardiovascular Disease During Two Phases of Development, *Nursing Research,* 44 (1965), 277–282.

91. A Head Start Does Not Last, *Newsweek,* January 27 (1992), 44–45.

92. Heindle, M.C., Symposium on Child Abuse and Neglect: Foreword, *Nursing Clinics of North America,* 16, no. 1 (1981), 101–102.

93. Heiney, S., Helping Children Through Painful Procedures, *American Journal of Nursing,* 91, no. 11 (1991), 20–24.

94. Hickie, K., School's Just Too Boring for Many of Our Gifted Children, *Sydney Morning Herald,* December 18 (1991), 3.

95. HIV and Children: A Growing Problem, *American Nurse,* November/December (1990), 21.

96. Hockenberry-Eaton, M., Family-Centered Care for Children with Chronic Illnesses, *Journal of Pediatric Health Care,* 8 (1994), 196–197.

97. Hoier, T., Child Sexual Abuse: Clinical Interventions and New Directions, *Child and Adolescent Psychotherapy,* 4, no. 3 (1987), 179–185.

98. Holmes, T. H., and R. H. Rahe, The Social Readjustment Rating Scale, *Journal of Psychosomatic Medicine,* 11, no. 8 (1967), 213–218.

99. Home Schooling Offers a Viable Alternative for Many Families, *Cappers,* 115, no. 6 (March 16, 1993), 12.

100. Home Schools Can Provide Personalized Education, *Cappers,* 115, no. 6 (March 16, 1993), 11.

101. Hoole, A., C. Pickard, R. Ouimette, J. Lohr, and R. Greenberg, *Patient Care Guidelines for Nurse Practitioners* (4th ed.). Philadelphia: J.B. Lippincott, 1995.

102. Hubbard, G., Perceived Life Changes for Children and Adolescents Following Disclosure of Father–Daughter Incest, *Journal of Child and Adolescent Psychiatric and Mental Health Nursing,* 2, no. 2 (1989), 78–82.

103. Human Nutrition Information Service, *Making Bag Lunches, Snacks, and Desserts Using the Dietary Guidelines.* Washington, DC: U.S. Government Printing Office, 1988.

104. Igoe, J.B., Beyond Green Beans and Oat Bran: A Health Agenda for the 1990s for School-Age Youth, *Pediatric Nursing,* 16, no. 3 (1990), 289–292.

105. Ikpa, V., What Educators Must Know About Children With HIV/AIDS, *Kappa Delta Pi Record,* 30, no. 3 (1994), 121–124.

106. Inclusion of Students with Disabilities Helps the Whole Classroom, *Cappers,* August 29 (1995), 12.

107. Injury-proofing the School-age Child, *Patient Care,* 23, no. 15 (1989), 178.

108. Jacobson, G., The Meaning of Stressful Life Experiences in Nine-to-Eleven-Year-Old Children: A Phenomenological Study, *Nursing Research,* 43 (1994), 95–99.

109. Jenkins, A., When Your Child Searches for a Birth Parent, *Home Life,* May (1991), 37–40.

110. John, E., D. Savitz, and D. Sandler, Prenatal Exposure to Parents' Smoking and Childhood Cancer, *American Journal of Epidemiology,* 133, no. 2 (1991), 123–125.

111. Jolley, J., and M. Mitchell, *Lifespan Development: A Topical Approach.* Madison, WI: Brown & Benchmark, 1996.

112. Karp, S., A 10-point Program for Bicycle Safety, *Contemporary Pediatrics,* 4, no. 6 (1987), 16–21, 24, 26–27.

113. Kempe, C., Sexual Abuse: Another Hidden Pediatric Problem, *Pediatrics,* 62 (1978), 582.

114. Kleinsasser, A.M., Equity in Education for Gifted Rural Girls, *Rural Special Education Quarterly,* 8, no. 4 (1988), 27–30.

115. Klug, R., Children with AIDS, *American Journal of Nursing,* 86, no. 10 (1986), 26–31.

116. Kohlberg, L., Development of Moral Character and Moral Ideology, in Hoffman, M.L., ed., *Review of Child Development Research,* Vol. 1. New York: Russell Sage, 1964, pp. 383–432.

117. ——, *Recent Research in Moral Development.* New York: Holt, Rinehart & Winston, 1971.

118. ——, Stages of Moral Development as a Basis for Moral Education, in Beck, C.M., Crittenden, B.S. and Sullivan, E.V. eds., *Moral Education: Interdisciplinary Approaches.* New York: Paulist Press, 1972, p. 23ff.

119. Kozinetz, C., Two Noninvasive Methods to Measure Female Maturation, *Journal of School Health,* 56, no. 10 (1986), 440–442.

120. Lamb, M., The Emergent Father, in Lamb, M.E., ed., *The Father's Role: Cross-cultural Perspectives.* Hillsdale, NJ: Lawrence Erlbaum, 1987, pp. 1–26.

121. Lamontagne, L., K. Mason, and J. Hepworth, Effects of Relaxation on Anxiety in Children: Implications for Coping with Stress, *Nursing Research,* 34 (1986), 389–392.

122. LaRossa, R., Fatherhood and Social Change, *Family Relations,* 37 (1988), 451–457.

123. Laskin, D., Safety at Home: An Ounce of Prevention Is Worth a Pound of Cure, *Parents,* 65, no. 9 (1990), 111–112.

124. Leland, J., Violence Reel to Real, *Newsweek,* December 11 (1995), 46–48.

125. Leone, S., and J. Gumaer, Group Assertiveness Training of Shy Children, *School Counselor,* 27, no. 2 (1979), 134–141.

126. Lepsoh, J., Confronting Sexual Harassment in America's Schools, *American Association of University Women Outlook,* 86, no. 3 (1993), 10–12.

127. Leshan, E., *When Grownups Drive You Crazy.* New York: Macmillan, 1988.

128. Levine, M., Childhood Neurodevelopmental Dysfunction and Learning Disorders, *The Harvard Mental Health Letter,* 12, no. 1 (1995), 5–6.

129. Lidz, T., *The Person: His and Her Development Throughout the Life Cycle* (2nd ed.) New York: Basic Books, 1983.

130. Liebert, R., and J. Spraskin, *The Early Window: Effects of Television on Children and Youths* (3rd ed.). New York: Pergamon Press, 1989.

131. Lieske, A., Incest: An Overview, *Perspectives in Psychiatric Care,* 19, no. 2 (1982), 59–63.

132. Lost, C., and C. Strauss, School Refusal in Anxiety-disordered Children and Adolescents, *Journal of American Academy of Child and Adolescent Psychiatry,* 29, no. 1 (1990), 31–35.

133. Lovrin, M., Interpersonal Support Among 8-Year-Old Girls Who Have Lost Their Parents or Siblings to AIDS, *Archives of Psychiatric Nursing,* 9 (1995), 92–98.

134. Lutz, M., The Effects of Family Structure and Regular Places of Care on Preventive Health Care for Children, *Health Values: Achieving High Level Wellness,* 14, no. 1 (1990), 38–45.

135. Lykins, R., Children of the Third Culture, *Kappa Delta Pi Record* (Winter 1986), 39–43.

136. Mackey, W., *Fathering Behaviors: The Dynamics of the Man–Child Bond.* New York: Plenum Press, 1985.

137. Manning, M., and L. Barath, Appreciating Cultural Diversity in the Classroom, *Kappa Delta Pi Record,* 27, no. 4 (1991), 104–110.

138. Markham, L., and J. Smith, Nickelodeon: An Alternative to Usual Television Fare? *Kappa Delta Pi Record,* 19, no. 4 (Summer 1983), 125–128.

139. Mason, J.O., Forging Working Partnerships for School Health Education, *Journal of School Health,* 59, no. 1 (1989), 18–20.

140. Mayer, S., and C. Jenicks, Growing Up in Poor Neighborhoods: How Much Does It Matter? *Science,* 243 (March 1989), 1441–1445.

141. McCormick, J., and P. Wingert, Whose Child Am I Anyway? *Newsweek Special Issue,* Summer (1991), 58–60.

142. McCoy, K., Help Your Child Beat Peer Pressure, *Reader's Digest,* May (1991), 67–70.

143. McKee, A., *The AAUW Report: How Schools Short-Change Girls.* New York: American Association of University Women, 1992.

144. Media, Violence May Be Linked, *University News,* September 21 (1990), 1, 8.

145. Mennger, J., et al., Genetics or Environment? Type A Behavior and Cardiovascular Risk Factors in Twin Children, *Nursing Research,* 37, no. 8 (1988), 341–348.

146. Miller, S., Children's Fears: A Review of the Literature With Implications for Nursing Research and Practice, *Nursing Research,* 29, no. 4 (1979), 217–223.

147. Morse, S., Growing Smart, *American Association of University Women Outlook,* 88, no. 3 (1995), 17–19.

148. ———, Why Girls Don't Like Computer Games, *Association of University Women Outlook,* 88, no. 4 (1995), 16–19.

149. Murphy, E., *God Cares When I Don't Feel Good.* Elgin, IL: David C. Cook, 1987.

150. ———, *God, You Fill Us Up With Joy: Psalm 100 For Children,* Elgin, IL: David C. Cook, 1987.

151. ———, *The Early Development of Sibling Relationships in Child-bearing Families.* San Francisco: University of California, 1989.

152. National Center for Health Statistics, *Health,* No. PHS 84-1232. Washington, DC: U.S. Government Printing Office, 1987.

153. National Institute of Nursing Research, *Health Promotion for Older Children and Adolescents.* Besthesda, MD: U.S. Department of Health and Human Services, 1993.

154. Nicklas, T., et al., Racial Contrasts in Hemoglobin Levels and Dietary Patterns Related to Hematopoiesis in Children: The Bogalusa Heart Study, *American Journal of Public Health,* 77, no. 10 (1987), 1320–1323.

155. Oakley, M., School Phobia, *Res Medica,* 3, no. 2 (1986), 11–14.

156. Oh, To Be Young and Gifted, *Newsweek,* February 23 (1987), 63–65.

157. Orbach, I., *Children Who Don't Want to Live: Understanding and Treating the Suicidal Child.* San Francisco: Jossey-Bass, 1988.

158. Orenstein, P., *School Girls: Young Women, Self-esteem, and the Confidence Gap.* New York: Doubleday, 1994.

159. Parke, R., and R. Slaby, The Development of Aggression, in Hetherton, E., and Mussen, P. eds., *Handbook of Child Psychology, Vol. 4: Socialization, Personality, and Social Development.* New York: Wiley, 1983.

160. Perkins, J., Television Must Begin to Curb Violent Programming, *Capper's,* July 20 (1993), 4.

161. Phillips, A., *The Trouble with Boys.* New York: Basic Books, 1995.

162. Phillips, S., and S. Lobar, Literature Summary of Some Navajo Child Health Beliefs and Rearing Practices Within a Transcultural Nursing Framework, *Journal of Transcultural Nursing,* 1, no. 2 (1990), 13–20.

163. Piaget, J., *Judgment and Reasoning in the Child.* New York: Humanities Press, 1928.

164. ———, *The Moral Judgment of the Child.* New York: Harcourt, Brace, 1932; Free Press, 1965.

165. ———, *The Growth of Logical Thinking From Childhood to Adolescence.* New York: Basic Books, 1958.

166. ———, *The Origins of Intelligence in Children.* New York: W.W. Norton, 1963.

167. ———, *The Child's Conception of Numbers.* New York: W.W. Norton, 1965.

168. ———, and B. Inhelder, *The Psychology of the Child.* New York: Basic Books, 1969.

169. ———, and B. Inhelder, *Memory and Intelligence.* New York: Basic Books, 1973.

170. ———, Introduction, in Schwebel, M., ed., *Piaget in the Classroom.* New York: Basic Books, 1973.

171. Polk-Walker, G., What Really Happened? Incidence and Factor Assessment of Abused Children and Adolescents, *Journal of Psychosocial Nursing,* 28, no. 11 (1990), 17–22.

172. Pontious, S., Practical Piaget: Helping Children Understand, *American Journal of Nursing,* 82, no. 1 (1982), 115–117.

173. Poponoe, D., The Controversial Truth, *New York Times,* December 26 (1992), A–21.

174. Porter, C., Grade School Children's Perceptions of Their Internal Body Parts, *Nursing Research,* 23, no. 5 (September–October 1974), 384–391.

175. Price, R., Are We Educators Ready for Inclusion and Goals 2000? *Kappa Delta Pi Record,* 30, no. 3 (1994), 138–139.

176. Raffa, J., Television and Values: Implications for Education, *The Educational Forum,* 49, no. 2 (1985), 189–198.

177. Rakestraw, J., and D. Rakestraw, Home Schooling: A Question of Quality, an Issue of Rights, *The Educational Forum,* 55, no. 1 (1990), 67–77.

178. Reek, J. van, M. Drop, and J. Joosten, The Influence of Peers and Parents on the Smoking Behavior of Schoolchildren, *Journal of School Health,* 57, no. 1 (1987), 30.

179. Richards, W., Allergy, Asthma, and School Problems, *Journal of School Health,* 56, no. 4 (1986), 151–152.

180. Richoux, D., A Look at Home Schooling, *Kappa Delta Pi Record,* 23, no. 4 (Summer 1987), 118–121.

181. Ritchie, A., Learning to Share: A Moral Necessity, *The Educational Forum,* 33, no. 4 (1989), 365–378.

182. Robertson, P., Helping Students Who Are Abused, *Kappa Delta Pi Record,* 30, no. 3 (1994), 129–133.

183. Rosenberg, M., *Growing Up Adopted.* New York: Bradbury Press, 1989.

184. Rubenstein, E., Television and Behavior: Research Conclusions of the 1982 NIMH Report and Their Policy Implications, *American Psychologist,* 38 (1983) 820–825.

185. Rubenstein, R., Raising Civilized Sons, *St. Louis Post Dispatch,* August 31 (1994), Sect. F, p. 5.

186. Scholl, T., et al., Ethnic Differences in Growth and Nutritional Status: A Status of Poor Schoolchildren in Southern New Jersey, *Public Health Reports,* 102, no. 3 (1987), 278–283.

187. Schulman, M., *Moral Development Training: Strategies for Parents, Teachers, and Clinicians.* Menlo Park, CA: Addison-Wesley, 1985.

188. Sandhu, D., and J. Rigney, Culturally Responsive Teaching in U.S. Public Schools, *Kappa Delta Pi Record,* 31, no. 4 (1995), 157–162.

189. Saunders, A., and B. Remsberg, *The Stress-proof Child: A Loving Parent's Guide.* New York: Holt, Rinehart, & Winston, 1984.

190. Scalza, A., Keeping Kids Safe: Parenting—Part 2, *Glennon: Magazine of Cardinal Glennon Children's Hospital,* 4, no. 2 (1991), 3–7.

191. Scheidt, P., Y. Hurel, A. Trumble, D. Jones, M. Overpeck, and P. Bijur, The Epidemiology of Nonfatal Injuries Among U.S. Children and Youth, *American Journal of Public Health,* 85 (1995), 932–938.

192. Schenker, M., R. Lopez, and G. Wintemute, Farm Related Fatalities Among Children in California, 1989, *American Journal of Public Health,* 85 (1995), 89–92.

193. School Health: Policy Issues, *Nursing and Health Care,* 15 (1994), 178–184.

194. Schraeder, B., M. Heverly, C. O'Brien, and K. McEvoy-Shields, Finishing First Grade: A Study of School Achievement in Very-Low-Birth-Weight Children, *Nursing Research,* 41 (1992), 354–361.

195. Schwartz, J., Early Identification of Gifted, Talented, and Creative Children, *Kappa Delta Pi Record,* 20, no. 1 (Fall 1983), 24–28.

196. ———, Portrait of a Generation, *Newsweek Special Supplement,* Summer (1991), 6–9.

197. Sexism in the Schoolhouse, *U.S. News and World Report,* March 9 (1992), 22.

198. Sheline, J., B. Skipper, and W. Broadhead, Risk Factors for Violent Behavior in Elementary School Boys: Have You Hugged Your Child Today? *American Journal of Public Health,* 84 (1994), 661–663.

199. Sherman, J.B., and M.A. Alexander, Obesity in Children: A Research Update, *Journal of Pediatric Nursing: Nursing Care of Children and Families,* 5, no. 3 (1990), 161–167.

200. Sieving, R.E., and S.T. Zirbel-Donisch, Development and Enhancement of Self-esteem in Children, *Journal of Pediatric Health Care,* 4, no. 6 (1990), 290–296.

201. Singer, J.L., and D.E. Singer, Implications of Childhood Television Viewing for Cognition, Imagination, and Emotion, in Bryant, J., and Anderson, D. eds., *Children's Understanding of Television: Research on Attention and Comprehension.* New York: Academic Press, 1983.

202. Spradley, B.W., *Community Health Nursing: Concepts and Practice* (3rd ed.). Glenview, IL: Scott, Foresman/Little Brown, 1990.

203. Stedwitz, U., C. Lariviere, and V. Rogers, What Do Kids Do When They're Not in School? *Kappa Delta Pi Record,* Winter (1988), 44–47.

204. Strickland, D., Friendship Patterns and Altruistic Behavior in Preadolescent Males and Females, *Nursing Research,* 30, no. 4 (1981), 222, 228, 235.

205. Sullivan, H.S., *The Interpersonal Theory of Psychiatry.* New York: W.W. Norton, 1953.

206. Sullivan, L., The Biological Message for Models of Learning, *Kappa Delta Pi Record,* Fall (1993), 29–32.

207. Swanson, L., and M.K. Biaggio, Therapeutic Perspectives in Father–Daughter Incest, *American Journal of Psychiatry,* 142, no. 6 (1985), 667–674.

208. Thompson, D., et al., A Case–Control Study of the Effectiveness of Bicycle Safety Helmets in Preventing Facial Injury, *American Journal of Public Health,* 80, no. 12 (1990), 1471–1474.

209. Top 25 in Children's Multicultural Literature, *Kappa Delta Pi Record,* Fall (1992), 30–31.

210. Tripp-Reimer, T., Retention of a Folk-healing Practice (Matiasma) Among Four Generations of Urban Greek Immigrants, *Nursing Research,* 32, no. 2 (1983), 97–101.

211. Turner, J., and D. Helms, *Lifespan Development* (5th ed.). New York: Harcourt & Brace, 1995.

212. Uphold, C., and M. Graham, *Clinical Guidelines in Family Practice* (2nd ed.), Gainesville, FL: Barmarrae Books, 1994.

213. U.S. Department of Health and Human Services, *Office of Maternal and Child Health USA '89,* No. HRS-MCH 8915. Washington, DC: Bureau of Maternal and Child Health Resources Development, 1989.

214. Vallbona, C., Importance of Immunization in Child Care and Prevention, in *Proceedings of Fourth National Health Policy Forum, April 24–25, 1992.* Washington, DC: National Academies of Practice, 1993, pp. 20–30.

215. Vasquez, J., Context of Learning for Minority Students, *Educational Forum,* 52, no. 3 (1988), 243–253.

216. Vessey, J., Comparison of Two Teaching Methods on Children's Knowledge of Their Internal Bodies, *Nursing Research,* 37, no. 5 (1988), 262–267.

217. Violent Crimes Linked to Early Childhood Factors, *The Menninger Letter,* 3, no. 7 (1995), 7.

218. Wadsworth, B., *Piaget's Theory of Cognitive and Affective Development* (5th ed.). New York: Longman, 1996.

219. Wallerstein, J., and S. Blakeslee, *Second Chances: Men, Women, and Children a Decade After Divorce.* New York: Ticknor & Fields, 1989.

220. What's TV Doing to Our Children? *Home Life,* December (1990), 37.

221. We Kill Too Many Farm Kids, *Successful Farming,* February (1989), 18A–18P.

222. Webb, P., Piaget: Implications for Teaching, *Theory Into Practice,* 19, no. 2 (1980), 93–97.

223. Weinberg, A., et al., A Pilot Study on Cholesterol Screening in the School Environment, *Journal of School Health,* 58, no. 8 (1988), 62.

224. Werner, E. *Vulnerable but Invincible.* New York: Adams-Bannister-Cox, 1989.

225. ———, *Against the Odds.* New York: Adams-Bannister-Cox, 1990.

226. Williams, P., A Comparison of Philippine and American Children's Concepts of Body Organs and Illness in Relation to Five Variables, *International Journal of Nursing Studies,* 15 (1978), 193–203.

227. Williams, S. *Nutrition and Diet Therapy* (10th ed.). St. Louis: C.V. Mosby: 1995.

228. Wilson, M., and M. Lagerborg, The Best Part of Dinner, *Focus on the Family,* August (1994), 12–14.

229. Winkelstein, M.L., Fostering Positive Self-Concept in the School-Age Child, *Pediatric Nursing,* 15, no. 3 (1989), 229–233.

230. Winpisinger, K., et al., Risk Factors for Child Homicides in Ohio: A Birth Certificate-Based Case-Control Study, *American Journal of Public Health,* 81, no. 8 (1991), 1052–1054.

231. Wintemute, G., et al., Drowning in Childhood and Adolescence: A Population-Based Study, *American Journal of Public Health,* 77, no. 7 (1987), 830–832.

232. Wolf, A., S. Gortmaker, L. Cheung, H. Gray, D. Herzog, and G. Coldin, Activity, Inactivity and Obesity: Racial, Ethnic, and Age Differences Among School Girls, *American Journal of Public Health,* 83 (1993), 1625–1627.

233. Wong, D., *Whaley and Wong's Nursing Care of Infants and Children* (5th ed.). St. Louis: C.V. Mosby, 1995.

234. World Bank Says Eradicating Macronutrient Deficiencies Would Be Cheap, Save Many Lives, *Nation's Health,* January (1995), 20.

235. Yoos, L., Chronic Childhood Illnesses: Developmental Issues, *Pediatric Nursing,* 13, no. 1 (1987), 25–28.

236. Yorker, B., The Prosecution of Child Sexual Abuse Cases, *Journal of Child Psychiatric Nursing,* 1, no. 2 (1988), 50–57.

237. The Zap Generation, *Newsweek,* February 26 (1990), 56–57.

238. Zimmerman, M., W. Wolbert, A. Burgess, and C. Hartman, Art and Group Work: Interventions for Multiple Victims of Child Molestation (Part I), *Archives of Psychiatric Nursing,* 1 (1987), 33–39.

239. ———, W. Wolbert, A. Burgess, and C. Hartman, Art and Group Work: Interventions for Multiple Victims of Child Molestation (Part II), *Archives of Psychiatric Nursing,* 1 (1987), 40–46.

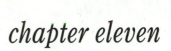
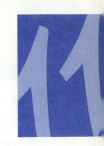

chapter eleven

Assessment and Health Promotion for the Adolescent and Youth

For some, adolescence is short; for others, adolescence extends many years.

—*Ruth Beckmann Murray*

Key terms

Puberty	Bulimia	Teen runaway	AIDS
Spermatogenesis	Obesity	Musculoskeletal chest pain	Vaginitis
Menstruation	Sexual harassment	Strain or Sprain	Candidal
Pubarche	Peer group	Minor ankle sprain	Trichomonal
Menarche	Peer-group dialect	Hordeolum (stye)	Nonspecific
Adolescence	Identity	Epistaxis	Chlamydia trachomatis
Preadolescence	Identity formation	Acne vulgaris	Genital warts
Early adolescence	Personal or real identity	Dental caries	Phthirus pubis
Middle adolescence	Ideal identity	Gingivitis	Contraception
Late adolescence	Claimed identity	Aphthous stomatitis	Abortion
Sperm production	Identity diffusion	Tinea cruris	Incest
Nocturnal emissions	Identity moratorium	Tinea pedis (athlete's foot)	Drug abuse
Sex hormones	Identity foreclosure	Infectious mononucleosis	Drug
Androgens	Sexuality	Hepatitis	Drug dependence
Estrogens	Masturbation	Rocky Mountain spotted fever	Addiction
Progesterones	Ego	Lyme disease	Tolerance
Ovulation	Frustration	Postvention	Cocaine
Primary dysmenorrhea	Conversion	Sexually transmitted diseases (STDs)	Kindling effect
Anorexia nervosa	Teen walkaway		Crack or rock

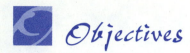

Objectives

1. Discuss the impact of the crisis of adolescence on family life and the influence of the family on the adolescent.

2. Explore with the family its developmental tasks and ways to achieve them while giving positive guidance to the adolescent.

3. Correlate the physiologic changes and needs, including nutrition, exercise, and rest, of early, middle, and late adolescence to those that occurred in preadolescence.

4. Discuss with parents the cognitive, self-concept, sexuality, emotional, and moral–spiritual aspects of development of the adolescent and ways in which the family can foster their healthy progress.

5. Identify examples of adolescent peer-group dialect and use of leisure time in your region, and discuss how knowledge of them can be used in your health-promotion activities and teaching.

6. Explore the developmental crisis of identity formation with the adolescent and the parents, the significance of achieving this crisis for ongoing maturity, and how to counteract influences that interfere with identity formation.

7. Describe the developmental tasks of adolescence and how the adaptive mechanisms commonly used assist the adolescent in achieving them.

8. Assess and work effectively with an adolescent with instructor supervision.

9. Discuss the challenges of the transitional period to young adulthood and your role in assisting the late adolescent into young adulthood.

10. Discuss common health problems of the adolescent, factors that contribute to them, and your role in contributing to the adolescent's health.

How can I best describe my son? He is 13 years old but could pass for 16 physically and mentally. He has the physique of a football player and appears to grow taller each day. His general knowledge is superior because he watches television for at least 2 hours a day, scans the morning and evening papers, and listens to the radio periodically during the day. He is full of contradictions; for example, he talks about love, but a hug or sign of affection from his mother will send him running to his room.

HISTORICAL AND CULTURAL PERSPECTIVES

Adolescence has long been considered a critical period in human development, and the search for an understanding of the adolescent can be traced historically. Early writers such as Rousseau, Francke, and Froebel directed their interest toward the education of the adolescent and his or her characteristics. In the late 19th century psychologists molded the Darwinian concepts into psychological terms and firmly established adolescence as an inevitable stage in human development. Before the 20th century, however, most people thought of themselves as young adults after puberty.

Adolescence is a long developmental stage, and because it differs cross-culturally, it is the most difficult to define. It is like old age in the United States, for each population is considered something of a burden and un-

able to contribute much to society. In the United States children are physiologically maturing at an earlier age. The increase in adult height and the change in age at which physical maturation occurs are called a secular growth trend. This trend is attributed to improved nutrition and health practices. Along with early maturation, the developmental era is being extended because of social, economic, employment, industrial, and family changes. For some people adolescence ends in the teens, but for most the period ends in the midtwenties (38, 50, 104, 121, 140, 145); however, adolescence is not so prolonged in all countries or cultures. Certainly in some cultures when puberty occurs, rites of passage signal adulthood. Some cultures practice female circumcision, which mutilates the external genitalia and carries a number of health risks. Others encourage the male to perform acts of bravery. Some cultures expect different behavior at a specific age (3, 70).

DEFINITIONS

In the past many people equated puberty and adolescence; they are now considered separate components. Puberty is preceded by prepuberty (discussed in Chapter 10).

Puberty is the *state of physical development between 10 and 14 years for females and 12 and 16 years for males when sexual reproduction first becomes possible with the* onset of **spermatogenesis** (*production of spermatozoa*) *and* **menstruation** (*onset of menses.*) Common law usually fixes puberty at 12 years for females and 14 years for males. **Pubarche** refers to the *beginning development of certain secondary sex characteristics that precedes the actual onset of physiologic puberty.* Some define puberty as a process involving a number of physical changes over a period that culminate in menstruation and spermatogenesis. The female may be unable to conceive for 1 to 2 years after **menarche,** the *first menstrual period,* and the male is usually sterile for a year or more after ejaculation first occurs. Some studies, however, have shown that some males become fertile at the onset of pubertal development (38, 46, 50, 104, 144, 185).

Adolescence is the *period in life that begins with puberty and extends for 8 to 10 years or longer until the person is physically and psychologically mature, ready to assume adult responsibilities and be self-sufficient because of changes in intellect, attitudes, and interests* (104, 121, 185, 197). Exceptions occur; some people never become psychologically mature. This definition does not reflect the individuality of the adolescent. Generalizations should be avoided as much as possible to prevent unjustified expectations from the adolescent.

Keniston (109) has delineated this period further between puberty and young adulthood by calling the period from 20 to 25 years *youth.* He believes that the affluent culture, especially in urban areas, has often created additional time before adult responsibilities must be assumed. For the purpose of this chapter, however, the adolescent period is divided into the subperiods of preadolescence, early, middle, and late adolescence. (The term *youth* is used interchangeably with adolescence.) Although age ranges are assigned to each subperiod, they are approximate; each adolescent may vary as to when and how he or she proceeds through the various stages.

Preadolescence, the *stage of prepuberty,* is discussed in Chapter 10, as these children are a part of the school-age population in America.

Early adolescence *begins with puberty and lasts for several years* (11 or 12 to 13 or 14 for females and 12 or 14 to 16 for males). The growth spurt focuses attention on self and the task of becoming comfortable with body changes and appearance. The teen tries to separate from parents; the dependency–independency struggle is shown by less involvement in family activities (and chores, if possible), criticism of the parents, and rebellion against parental and other adult discipline and authority. Conformity to and acceptance of peer-group standards and peer friendships are gaining in importance. The peer group usually consists of same-sex friends; however, the adolescent has an increased interest in the opposite sex. Group activities with peers are popular (38, 50, 104, 140, 185).

Middle adolescence *begins when physical growth is completed and usually extends from age 13 or 14 to 16 for females and 14 or 16 to 18 or 20 for males.* The major tasks during this period are achievement of ego identity, attainment of greater independence, interest in the future and career planning, and establishment of a heterosexual relationship. Peer-group allegiance, at a peak in 15- to 16-year-olds, is manifested by clothing, food, and other fads, preferred music, and common jargon. Experimentation with adultlike behavior and risk taking is common in an attempt to prove self to peers. Sexual experimentation often begins now (or earlier) as a result of social exploration and physical maturation. Changes in cognitive functioning may first be evident in that the person moves to more abstract thinking, returning to more concrete operations during times of stress (50, 185, 197).

Some teens are expected to move into the tasks of young adulthood at this point. Although they may be employed or independent in other ways, developmentally the person probably is in late adolescence.

Late adolescence *may occur from approximately 18 to 25 years of age.* The person has usually finished adolescent rebellion, formed his or her views, and established a stable sense of self. The youth is not fully committed to one occupation and questions relationships to existing social, vocational, and emotional roles and lifestyles. He or she may be a student or an apprentice (50, 110, 140, 185). Lack of economic freedom may be a concern and prolong dependence on parents. The value system is being clarified; issues of philosophy, religion, life and death, and ethical decisions are being analyzed. The peer group has lost its primary importance, and the youth may take the final step in establishing independence from parents by moving away from home. More adultlike friendships begin between late adolescents and their parents as the earlier family turbulence subsides. At the same time there is more individual dating and fewer group activities with friends; often the first emotionally intimate relationship develops with a member of the opposite sex. At that point the person is developmentally a young adult, having made the transition from adolescence. He or she is more realistically aware of strengths and limits in self and others (121).

FAMILY DEVELOPMENT AND RELATIONSHIPS

Developmental Tasks

The overall family goal at this time is to allow the adolescent increasing freedom and responsibility to prepare him or her for young adulthood.

Although each family member has personal developmental tasks, the family unit as a whole also has developmental tasks. They include the following (49):

- Provide facilities for individual differences and needs of family members
- Work out a system of financial responsibility with the family
- Establish a sharing of responsibilities
- Reestablish a mutually satisfying marriage relationship
- Strengthen communication within the family
- Rework relationships with relatives, friends, and associates
- Broaden horizons of the adolescent and parents
- Formulate a workable philosophy of life as a family

Discuss the developmental tasks and how to achieve them with the family. Generally speaking, the developmental tasks for a family at this time involve maintaining a grasp on these facets of life that continue to have meaning while striving for a deeper awareness and understanding of the present situation.

Family Relationships

During early adolescence the teen remains involved in family activities and functions. Gradually family relationships change, and the adolescent develops social ties and close relationships outside the family. The family's beliefs, lifestyles, values, and patterns of interaction influence the development of these relationships, as can socioeconomic level of the parents. The media report that one of every five children less than 18 years old lives in poverty. Poverty affects all spheres of family and individual development (71, 79, 82, 130).

It is during middle and late adolescence that the most severe changes occur in the parent–child relationship. The relationship must evolve from a dependency status to mutual affection, equality, and autonomy. This process of achieving independence usually creates family turmoil, conflict, and ambivalence as both parents and adolescent learn new roles. The emancipation process must be gradual. Parents should gradually increase the teenager's responsibilities and allow privileges formerly denied. The adolescent wants to make independent decisions and to have increased freedom of movement. At the same time, he or she wants financial support, food, and safe sanctuary. Parents must resist granting instant adult status when the child reaches teen years and instead remember that the adolescent needs to be independent yet dependent. Although he or she protests, the teen values parental restraints if the restraints are reasonable. The adolescent feels more self-confident in exploring the environment if reasonable limits are imposed. Parents should listen to their adolescent's viewpoints concerning restrictions. Views may offer hints about the readiness for more independence and freedom (15, 121, 140, 146, 197).

Most ambivalence and negative behavior in the adolescent stems from self-perceived external restrictions. Teenagers may fight for grownup privileges that they never use—the actual battle is more important than the privilege. Disagreements and conflicts about sexual behavior, dress, drugs, school performance, homework, friendship, family car, telephone privileges, manners, chores and duties, money, and disrespectful behavior frequently disrupt family harmony (15, 121, 123).

In addition to other conflicts, the youth must also work through feelings for the parent of the opposite sex and unravel the ambivalence toward the parent of the same sex. He or she reworks some of the sex identity and family triangle problems that remain from the preschool era. In an attempt to resolve this ambivalence, the adolescent may strive to be as different as possible from the parent of the same sex. Frequently affection is turned to an adult outside the family—teacher, relative, family friend, neighbor, mentor, clergy person, or someone in public life. "Crushes" of this nature are very common; they are usually brief and may occur once, twice, or on numerous occasions. Idolizing another adult person causes the adolescent to want to please that person; therefore the adolescent's actions and language may change when the idolized person is present. Frequently the adolescent identifies so completely with this person that he or she absorbs some of the person's adult characteristics into the personality. These relationships are not harmful to the adolescent unless the person who is chronologically an adult still feels confused and rebellious toward society and fosters immaturity. On the contrary, an adult outside the family usually will be more objective than the parent and can help the adolescent grow toward psychological maturity. Parents are experiencing sexuality changes at the same time. They are facing midlife and menopause and are concerned with self-perceived decreased sexual attractiveness and potency.

During this period parents may believe they are not as important to the adolescent as before. The adolescent complains that parents are old-fashioned and "out of it." He or she may appear hostile and resent parental authority and guidance. The teen seeks to find flaws in parental behavior and may try to build barriers between self and the parents to prove independence. The adolescent is critical, argumentative, and generally remote with both parents; a previously close and confiding relationship with the parents is lost. In their presence the adolescent may ridicule parents. This rejection is not consistent; response to parents varies with mood changes. At times the relationship can be close and positive; the adolescent may actually support the parents in the presence of peers (15, 116, 118, 132, 140, 185).

In addition to dealing with a loss of authority, parents are faced with other stresses. They are forced to redefine past child–parent relations and rethink their own values. Parents may also be forced to evaluate their own career choices as their adolescent begins vocational pursuits. Competition between parents and the teen may exist; parents may actually admit to not liking the adolescent. They may be anxious to relinquish financial, physical, and emotional childrearing responsibilities to increase their own freedom (1, 121, 185).

Stresses that frequently produce family discord grow out of conflicting value systems between the parent and child generations. Today's adolescents are a generation born with technology (and less emphasis on people skills) that has brought remote corners of the world into their homes and minds and has fostered questioning of instead of reliance on authority. Parents need help to see that the adolescent is a product of his or her time and the teen is reflecting what is happening socially. Further, teens may be confused by their parents' behavior. Some grow up with little parental supervision. Some are in single-parent or stepparent families. In some families, a parent may announce that he or she is bisexual or homosexual, or the teen may turn to another sexual orientation. Several references are relevant (11, 43, 68, 79, 101, 131, 132, 155, 162, 190).

Youngs' book (202) is a practical reference for parents and professionals on the teenager's behavior, factors that contribute to stress response, signs and symptoms that the youth and the family are having problems, and how to manage tense situations and teenage behavioral problems.

Parental and adolescent response to the ambivalence and conflicts of this period varies. Parents may adhere to rules and the status quo to bolster their own security or cultural traditions rather than change for the offspring's benefit. Parents may overprotect. Others may be reluctant to admit that their child is establishing an independent lifestyle; they may dread facing the empty-nest stage (1, 146). If the adolescent has come from a family that has provided past opportunities to learn responsibility, self-reliance, skills, and self-respect, he or she will make a smoother transition from childhood dependency to adulthood independence. If parents have been too liberal, overly permissive, or uninterested, the adolescent will have more difficulty adjusting because the past lacked structure and a system of standards or values. He or she has no point of reference to determine if the behavior is suitable and decisions appropriate (64, 116, 121, 146).

Fortunately some parents trust their offspring to live the basic values they taught, although at times behavior may appear differently. They realize that today's adolescent is growing up in a different historical era than when they were young, and they can accept the changes that result. They work at being communicative and flexible, yet supportive, following suggestions in Communicating with Your Teen. They accept that the adolescent may be as large as an adult but still behave childishly at times. The parents' behavior is adultlike so that they are a model for their offspring. They feel enough self-confidence that they do not have to belittle the adolescent. They are not threatened by his or her sexuality, and they maintain a balance of closeness and distance so that the adolescent can rework sex identity. If the parent–child relationship has been close in the past, it can remain close now in spite of superficial problems and responses.

Adolescence is not a period of conflict between parents and offspring in all cultures. For example, in Oriental and Indian cultures, some African groups, the Arabian countries, and certain European countries, behavior norms and role expectations provide the basis for a smoother transition from child to adult than is expected in the United States. Nontechnologic societies have less adolescent–parent conflict because there is less choice in occupations and lifestyles and less variance between generational behavior.

Discuss the above information and the points in Communicating with Your Teen with parents. Help them understand the interaction between parents and offspring. The home should provide an accepting and emotionally stable environment for the adolescent, as the home situation affects later marital adjustments and the type of parent he or she will become.

A factor that may affect parent–adolescent communication and relationships is the stepfamily or adoptive family structure. Often, adopted adolescents struggle with whether they really belong to the family. (Refer also to Chapter 4.) The adopted child may search for the birth parent(s). Adoptive parents should cooperate rather than feel threatened (101). Because of the proliferation of divorce, single-parenting, and stepfamilies, adoptive children have plenty of company; parents can assure the adolescent he or she is not alone in feeling different. Parents and the adopted adolescent may wish to attend group sessions organized by Minnesota-based Adoptive Families of America, which has 260 chapters nationwide. The organization plans activities by nationality. Adoptive parents learn about the child's native culture, and adopted children are with others who share

► COMMUNICATING WITH YOUR TEEN

- Make time for listening and talking.
- Create a beginning and an ending to the day.
- Respect the teen's privacy; do not insist on her or his disclosure.
- Do not judge or shame; state facts and recognition of differences.
- Say "thank you" and "please" as appropriate.
- Be generous with honest praise.
- Apologize when it is appropriate.
- Let the teen make choices and the inevitable mistakes.
- Talk about ways to cope with the consequences of unwise decisions.
- Avoid lectures, preaching, talking down, or sarcasm.
- Use open-ended questions, such as "How was your day?"
- Speak to feelings, "you look frustrated," or reflect back feelings that were disclosed.
- Nurture mealtime conversation; turn off the television, radio, computer, and stereo.
- Plan family times that emphasize casual talk.
- Take advantage of driving time, especially when you are alone with the teen, to talk. The need for the parent who is driving to keep "eyes on the road," avoiding eye contact, often helps exploration of sensitive issues.
- Welcome their friends; engage them in conversation, often through activity.
- Use "I" statements. If you have a plan, be open about it (e.g., a shopping trip).
- Keep the teen and self in perspective.
- Criticize the behavior, not the person.
- Talk about one issue at a time; do not bring in past events or behavior unrelated to the current topic.
- Make requests in a neutral, kind tone of voice, assertively but not ordering.

► PARENTAL BEHAVIOR CHARACTERISTICS OF PSYCHOLOGICAL MALTREATMENT OF THE ADOLESCENT

Rejecting

- Refuses to acknowledge changing social roles and to move to autonomy and independence
- Treats adolescent like a young child
- Subjects adolescent to verbal humiliation and excess criticism
- Expels youth from family

Isolating

- Tries to prevent youth from participating in organized and informal activities outside the home
- Prohibits adolescent from joining clubs or after-school activities
- Withdraws youth from school to work or perform household tasks
- Punishes youth for engaging in normal social activity such as dating

Terrorizing

- Threatens to expose youth to public humiliation such as undressing youth, forcing encounter with police or stay in jail
- Threatens to reveal intensely embarrassing characteristics (real or fantasized) to peers or adults
- Ridicules youth in public regularly

Ignoring

- Abdicates parental role
- Shows no interest in youth as person or in activities; refuses to discuss adolescent's activities, plans, interests
- Concentrates on activities or relationships that displace adolescent from affections

Corrupting

- Involves youth in more intense or socially unacceptable forms of sexual, aggressive, or substance abuse behavior; forces youth into prostitution
- Rewards aggressive or scapegoating behavior toward siblings, peers, or adults
- Encourages trafficking in illicit drug use or alcohol use or in sex rings

From Garbarino, J., E. Guttmann, and J. Seeley, *The Psychologically Battered Child: Strategies for Identification, Assessment, and Intervention.* San Francisco: Jossey-Bass, 1987. Copyright 1986 by Jossey-Bass, Inc., Publishers.

their heritage, ethnicity, and appearance. Thus, identity and self-esteem can be strengthened. Adopted children statistically fare better than would have been predicted from their socioeconomic roots.

Abuse, Neglect, and Maltreatment

Abuse, neglect, and maltreatment occur to millions of adolescents, although health care professionals may not be alert to physical and psychological cues. The adolescent who is physically abused may be present in the emergency room with some of the same kinds of injuries that are seen in the younger child (see Chapters 4, 6, 7, and 9). Sometimes bruises and lacerations are concealed from peers, teachers, and health care providers by cosmetics and clothes. Careful screening and astute communication skills are essential. You must establish a relationship and interview the adolescent alone. Then you are more likely to learn of physical, sexual, and psychological abuse (maltreatment) or neglect.

Maltreatment of the adolescent is demonstrated by the behaviors described in Parental Behavior Characteristics of Psychological Maltreatment of the Adolescent. Other references describe physical, psychological, and sexual abuse (23, 24, 25, 38, 41, 60, 67, 71, 81, 92, 97, 139, 153, 197, 201).

PHYSIOLOGIC CONCEPTS

Influences on Physical Growth

The precise physiologic cause for the physical changes characteristic of this period is unknown. It appears that the hypothalamus, probably in some way related to brain maturation, initiates the pubertal process through secretion of neurohumoral releasing factors. These neurohumors stimulate the anterior pituitary gland to release gonadotrophic hormones, somatotropic hormone (STH) or growth hormone (GH), thyroid-stimulating hormone (TSH), and adrenocorticotropic hormone (ACTH). The amygdala in the limbic system also apparently changes function and promotes hormonal production (38, 50, 185, 197).

Gonadotrophic hormones (follicle-stimulating hormone [FSH] and luteinizing hormone [LH]) stimulate the gonads to mature and produce sex hormones. FSH stimulates the ovaries in females to produce estrogen and the development of seminiferous tubules in males; LH stimulates the Leydig cells in the testes to produce testosterone. Growth and development of the adrenal cortex and stimulation of the secretion of androgens are promoted by ACTH. These androgens are responsible for producing secondary sex characteristics. Deoxyribonucleic acid (DNA) synthesis and hyperplastic cell growth, particularly of the bones and cartilage, are stimulated by STH. Under the influence of TSH, thyroxine secretion is slightly increased during the pubertal period. Thyroxine levels increase to meet body metabolic needs (38, 50, 185, 197).

Both male and female hormones are produced in varying amounts in both sexes throughout life. During the prepubescent years, the adrenal cortex secretes a small amount of sex hormones; however, it is the sex hormone production that accompanies maturation of the ovaries and testes that is responsible for the physiologic changes observed in puberty. Physiologic changes in the male are produced by androgens, whereas large amounts of estrogens produce the changes in the female. Both forms of gonadal hormones stimulate epiphyseal fusion by repression of the pituitary growth hormone, thus slowing physical growth at the end of puberty.

Physical Characteristics

Growth

Adolescence is the second major period of accelerated growth (infancy was the first). The adolescent growth spurt occurs approximately 2 years earlier in the female than in the male. During the years of the growth spurt, females grow $2\frac{1}{2}$ to 5 in. (6–12.5 cm) and gain 8 to 10 pounds (3.5–4.5 kg); males average 3 to 6 in. (7.5–15 cm) and gain 12 to 14 pounds (5.5–6.5 kg). In the initial phase of the growth spurt, the increase in height is due to lengthening of the legs; later, most of the increase is in the trunk length. The total process of change takes approximately 3 years in females and 4 years in males (38, 50, 185, 197).

Every system of the body is growing rapidly, but physiologic changes occur unevenly within the person. Variation exists in age of onset of puberty and rapidity of growth between different groups of people as well. For example, Chinese show an earlier height spurt and menarche and more advanced skeletal maturity than Europeans (197).

Sexual Development

Four physical characteristics define puberty for most adolescents as they observe themselves and each other (38, 50, 185, 197).

Females
- Height spurt: ages 8 to 17 years; peak age, 12
- Menarche: 10 to 16 years; average age, 12.5
- Breast development: 8 to 18 years
- Pubic hair: 11 to 14 years

Males
- Height spurt: 10 to 20 years; peak age, 14
- Penile development: 10 to 16 years
- Testicular development: 9 to 17 years
- Pubic hair: 12 to 16 years

Menarche is the indicator of puberty and sexual maturity in the female. Ovulation usually occurs 12 to 24 months after menarche. The onset of menarche varies among population groups and is influenced by heredity, nutrition, health care, and other environmental factors. In the United States the average age of onset is 12.3 to 12.6 years. Research on the onset of menarche has revealed conflicting results. Some researchers have shown a relationship between the height and weight of a girl and menarche (185). Onset of menarche also varies from country to country: in Sweden, 12.9 years; in Italy, 12.5 years; in Africa, 13.4 to 14.1 years (3, 70).

Secondary sex characteristics in the female begin to develop in prepuberty (see Chapter 10) and may take 2 to 8 years for completion. Breast enlargement and elevation occur; areola and papillae project to form a secondary mound. Axillary and pubic hair grows thicker, becomes darker, and spreads over the pubic area (38, 50, 185, 197).

Spermatogenesis (**sperm production**) and seminal emissions mark puberty and sexual maturity in the male. The first ejaculate of seminal fluid occurs approximately 1 year after the penis has begun its adolescent growth, and **nocturnal emissions,** *loss of seminal fluid during sleep,* occur at approximately age 14 (185, 197).

Secondary sex characteristics in the male also begin in prepuberty (see Chapter 10) and may take 2 to 5 years for completion. Changes in body shape, growth of body hair, and muscle development may continue until 19 or 20 or even until the late twenties. North American males complete growth in stature by 18 or 19 years, with an additional $\frac{1}{2}$ to 1 in. (1–2 cm) in height occurring during the twenties because of continued vertebral column growth. The penis, scrotum, and testes enlarge; the scrotum reddens; and scrotal skin changes texture. Hair grows at the axilla and base of the penis and spreads over the pubis. Body hair generally increases, especially facial hair. The voice deepens (38, 50, 185, 197).

Sex hormones are *biochemical agents that primarily influence the structure and function of the sex organs and appearance of specific sexual characteristics.* **Androgens** are *hormones that produce male-type physical characteristics and behaviors.* **Estrogens** are *hormones that produce feminine characteristics.* **Progesterones** are *female hormones that prepare the uterus to accept a fetus and maintain the pregnancy.* All three sex hormones are in both sexes. Androgens are in greater amounts in males; the other two hormones are in greater amounts in females (185, 197). More information about the function of sex hormones can be obtained in any physiology text.

The 28-day menstrual or reproductive cycle is controlled by an intricate feedback system involving (1) the hypothalamus, which audits the level of the hormones in the bloodstream; (2) the anterior lobe of the pituitary and its hormones, FSH and LH; (3) the ovaries and their hormones, estrogen and progesterone; and (4) the interplay between the ovarian hormones and FSH and LH (185, 197).

At the onset of the cycle, when the estrogen level is lowest, the shedding of the endometrium (lining of the uterus) occurs. The hypothalamus, because of the low estrogen level, stimulates the pituitary gland to release FSH, which causes maturation of one of the ovum-containing ovarian or graafian follicles and increased production of estrogen. This is the time of the highest level of estrogen in the bloodstream. In response to estrogen, the endometrium begins to thicken to prepare to receive the zygote if fertilization occurs (185, 197).

In response to the high level of estrogen, the anterior pituitary releases LH. The sudden increase in LH triggers **ovulation,** *release of the mature ovum,* from the follicle, which happens approximately 14 days after the onset of the cycle. The LH moves to the ruptured follicle, which causes development of the glandular corpus luteum. This produces both estrogen and progesterone, which, when acting together, cause the glands of the endometrium to prepare further for the nourishment of a possible zygote (185, 197).

If fertilization of the ovum by a sperm cell does not occur, the ovum deteriorates. The pituitary stops production of both FSH and LH, and the corpus luteum becomes dormant and atrophies. The resulting drop in estrogen and progesterone levels stimulates the shedding of the endometrial lining, which consists of blood, mucus, and tissues, or the menstrual discharge. Menstruation lasts 3 to 5 days. The cycle then begins anew (185, 197). **Primary dysmenorrhea,** *painful menstruation occurring without any evidence of abnormality in the pelvic organs,* may occur. The cause is unknown, but endocrine factors, natural pain processes, and psychological factors have all been considered. Various analgesics have been used for this condition through the years. More recently the nonsteroidal antiinflammatory agents have been used with some success. Some women find that adherence to a certain diet such as one with decreased caffeine and sugar and increased protein intake and exercise habits may decrease symptoms. Heat to the painful area may be palliative (197).

In the male the hormonal system for reproductive behavior is much simpler because there is no cyclical pattern. The male gonads, the testes, produce sperm continuously and secrete androgens. The major androgen is testosterone (185, 197).

Just as FSH promotes the development of the ovum in the female, FSH promotes the development of sperm in the male. A continuous level of sperm production takes place in the seminiferous tubules inside the testes. The secretion of LH (also called interstitial cell-stimulating hormone [ISCH]) stimulates the Leydig cells lying between these tubules to secrete the androgen (185, 197).

Musculoskeletal System

Structural changes—growth in skeletal size, muscle mass, adipose tissue, and skin—are significant in adolescence. The skeletal system grows faster than the supporting muscles; hands and feet grow out of proportion to the body; and large muscles develop faster than small muscles. Poor posture and decreased coordination result. Males and females differ in skeletal growth patterns; males have greater length in arms and legs relative to trunk size, in part because of a prolonged prepubertal growth period in boys. (Males are also more clumsy than females.) Males also have a greater shoulder width, a difference that begins in prepuberty. Ossification of the skeletal system occurs later for boys than girls. In girls, estrogen influences ossification and early unity of the epiphyses with shafts of the long bones, resulting in shorter stature. Muscle growth continues in males during late adolescence because of androgen production. Muscle growth in females is proportionate to growth of other tissue. Adipose tissue distribution over thighs, buttocks, and breasts occurs predominantly in females and is related to estrogen production (38, 50, 185, 197).

Skin

Skin texture changes. Sebaceous glands become extremely active and increase in size. Eccrine sweat glands are fully developed, are especially responsive to emotional stimuli, and are more active in males. Apocrine sweat glands also begin to secrete in response to emotional stimuli (197).

Cardiovascular System

The heart grows slowly at first compared with the rest of the body, resulting in inadequate oxygenation and fatigue. The heart continues to enlarge until age 17 or 18. Systolic blood pressure and pulse pressure increase; blood pressure averages 100 to 120/50 to 70. Pulse rate averages 60 to 68 beats per minute. Females have a slightly higher pulse rate and basal body temperature and lower systolic pressure than males. Hypertension is increasing in adolescents, both Caucasian and African-American, in males, in the obese, and in those with a family history of hypertension. Higher systolic pressure occurs in urban dwellers; higher diastolic pressure has been seen in those who smoked and lacked regular exercise. Routine hypertension screening should be done. The upper limit for normal blood pressure in individuals from 11 to 17 years old is 130/90 (64, 197).

Respiratory System

The respiratory system also grows slowly relative to the rest of the body, contributing to inadequate oxygenation. Respiratory rate averages 16 to 20 per minute. Males have a greater shoulder width and chest size, resulting in greater respiratory volume, greater vital capacity, and increased respiration. The male's lung capacity matures later than that of the female, which is mature at 17 or 18 years (197).

Blood Components

Red blood cell mass and hemoglobin concentration increase in both sexes because of increased hormone production. Hematocrit levels are higher in males; platelet count and sedimentation rate are increased in females, and white blood cell count is decreased in both sexes. Blood volume increases more rapidly in males. By late adolescence, males average 5000 mL and females 4200 mL of blood (197).

Gastrointestinal System

The gastrointestinal system matures rapidly from 10 to 20 years. By age 21 all 32 *teeth* have usually appeared. *Stomach capacity* increases to approximately 1 quart (more than 900 mL), up to 1500 mL, which correlates with increased appetite as the stomach becomes longer and less tubular; increased gastric acidity occurs to facilitate digestion of the increased food intake. *Intestines* grow in length and circumference. Muscles in the stomach and intestinal wall become thicker and stronger. Elimination patterns are well established and are related to food and fluid intake. The *liver* attains adult size, location, and function (185, 197).

Fluid and electrolyte balance changes reflect changes in body composition in terms of bones, muscle, and adipose tissue. Percentage of body water decreases, reaching adult levels. Approximately 60% of the male's total body weight is fluid, compared with 50% in the female; the difference is caused by the greater percentage of muscle mass in the male. Exchangeable sodium and chloride decline; intracellular fluid and body potassium levels rise with the onset of puberty. Again, because of their greater muscle mass, males have a 15% higher potassium concentration (185, 197).

Urinary System

Urinary bladder capacity increases; the adolescent voids up to 1½ quarts (1500 mL) daily. Renal function is like that of the adult (185, 197).

Special Sense Organs

The eyeball lengthens, increasing the incidence of myopia in early adolescence. Auditory acuity peaks at 13, and from that age on, hearing acuity gradually decreases. Sensitivity to odors develops at puberty; the female's increased sensitivity to musklike fragrances may be related to estrogen levels (185, 197).

Unique Differences

Racial differences in physical development exist, although adult statures are approximately the same. For example, African-American boys and girls attain a greater proportion of their adult stature earlier. Skeletal mass is greater in the African-Americans person; using Caucasian norms means that bone loss could go undetected. The normal value for hemoglobin concentration is 1 g less for African Americans. Thus, a low hemoglobin reading for African Americans has a different nutritional implication; the person may not be iron deficient (196, 197). Continued research is necessary to determine other differences that may exist.

Because of the changing body, the adolescent needs information about the normality of anatomic and physiologic changes in addition to sex education. Adults should be cautioned not to pass on superstitions and taboos (e.g., that girls must rest and not participate in social or sport activities or that they should not take showers during menstruation). The adolescent male must be told that the release of spermatic fluid through nocturnal emissions is *not* the result of disease or punishment for masturbation or sexual daydreaming.

If the parents are knowledgeable about pubertal growth changes, they can predict coming physical changes based on how the teen presently looks, which can be reassuring to the child whose onset of puberty is delayed. This may be more difficult in one-parent families, as the man or woman is less equipped to understand and help the opposite-sex child.

You can be very helpful in teaching the adolescent and in helping parents understand what they should teach their children. They both need realistic information about these subjects and an opportunity for discussion. Additional information can be obtained from the local library or health association, doctor, religious leader, counselor, or personal product companies. Having this knowledge can eliminate much fear and guilt and will help the adolescent understand his or her normal development.

Physical Assessment of the Adolescent

Regular physical examinations should be encouraged. See Appendix IV for a suggested schedule. Useful references to help you formulate a health history are Bates (12), Boynton et al. (22), Hoole et al. (94), Roye (161), and Sherman and Fields (171). Uphold and Graham is also a thorough reference (187).

The examination is conducted much as for the adult; however, it is crucial that the examiner knows and understands the special emotional needs, developmental changes, age and maturation level of the person, and physiologic differences specific to adolescence. Roye discusses methods for and barriers to communication with and education of the adolescent (161). Health assessment of the early adolescent is presented by Manning (124).

Honest and genuine interest in the adolescent and not "speaking down" as though the young person is a child are essential. Confidentiality and trust are key issues. Be sure to express honestly to the teen what part of the interview and examination can be kept in strict confidence and what may need to be shared. Specific age of the person and the nature of the findings determine these factors. Above all, do not say, "This is completely confidential," only to say later, "I believe we better share that."

Physical complaints and emotional symptoms may relate to underlying problems of drug abuse, alcoholism, sexual uncertainties and stress, pregnancy or fear of pregnancy, fear of or actual sexually transmitted disease, depression, family or peer adjustment problems, school problems, or concerns about future plans.

Because the adolescent may be extremely shy about his or her body, every effort must be made to protect privacy within the confines of the situation. With the advent of the female nurse practitioner and physician's assistant conducting examinations on male patients, the traditional "embarrassment roles" are switched. Much has been written on the conduct of the male examiner with the female patient but not on the reverse. The younger the adolescent male in terms of sexuality development, the more concern he has about a female examiner seeing and touching his body parts that are considered private. The female examiner ought to provide proper draping and emphasize the touching as little as possible. She may make the preliminary statement, "It is important that I palpate your scrotum to detect . . . . I know this is a tender area and I will proceed as quickly as possible while being thorough in my exam."

The blood pressure should be at adult levels. The athlete in training may have a slower pulse rate than his or her peers.

Pallor, especially in girls, should be a clue to check hemoglobin levels.

The teen needs frequent dental visits because most have caries. Many young adolescents whose parents have insurance for the service or have sufficient funds have orthodontic work in progress.

Because myopia seems to increase during these years, increased reading and study encourage eye strain. Many teens are now being fitted with contact lenses (171).

Although breast neoplasms are not common to this age group, females should be taught breast self-examination. Also, the girl should not be surprised if there is some asymmetric development. Some increase in breast tissue can also be expected in adolescent males. Excessive growth should be referred for evaluation. Both male and female breasts should be examined (171).

The heart should be found at the fifth left intercostal space as in the adult, and most functional murmurs should be outgrown. Serum cholesterol and triglyceride levels should be obtained if there is a family history of cardiovascular disease, and preventive dietary and exercise regimens should be discussed.

Striae may be found on the abdomen of females because of the rapid weight gain and loss experienced by fad diets followed by return to overeating (12, 171).

The examiner should be acutely aware not only of the pattern of sexual development of both males and females, but of the concerns and questions that may be voiced. The presence of the testes in the scrotum is of primary importance because undescended testicles at this age can mean sterility (171).

Papanicolaou (Pap) smears and pelvic examinations are done when the adolescent becomes sexually active. These procedures, done the first time with explanation and as much gentleness as possible, can set a positive tone for future examinations (171, 179).

Some have suggested that urine cultures be taken periodically on females between the ages of 15 and 18 because of the number of asymptomatic urinary infections (171).

Scoliosis is common in teenagers, so a close look for asymmetry of the musculoskeletal system is essential, and any severe, persistent pain in the long bone area should also be referred (171).

Nutritional Needs

Teach parents and teenagers the following information about normal nutrition. Refer also to Recommended Nutritional Intake for Adolescents, Uphold and Graham (187), and Appendix I. During this time of accelerated physical and emotional development the body's metabolic rate increases; accordingly, nutritional needs increase. Requirements peak in the year of maximum growth, between the 10th and 12th years in girls and approximately 2 years later in boys. Calorie and protein requirements during this year are higher than at almost any other time of life. The adolescent female's require-

► RECOMMENDED NUTRITIONAL INTAKE FOR ADOLESCENTS*

Food	Nonpregnant Adolescent (No. Servings)	Pregnant Adolescent (No. Servings)
Dairy products: one serving equals 1 cup milk, 1 oz hard cheese, 1¼ cups cottage cheese, ⅓ cup dry milk, or 1¾ cup ice cream (use low-fat milk)	4 (ages 12–18) 2–3 (ages 19–22)	4
Meat and meat alternatives: one serving equals 2 eggs, 2 oz lean meat, 1 cup beans or split peas, 4 tablespoons peanut butter, 2 oz cheddar cheese, or ½ cup cottage cheese	2–3	3
Fruits, vegetables, or juices: one serving equals ½ cup or 1 medium fresh fruit or vegetable	4–5	At least 5
Breads and cereals: one serving equals 1 slice of bread, ½ cup cooked cereal, ¾ cup ready-to-eat cereal, or ½ to ¾ cup cooked macaroni, spaghetti, rice, or grits, pasta	6–11 (6 servings for females)	6–11
Fats, oils, sweets	Use sparingly	Use sparingly

*Suggested amounts should support adequate weight gain

ments are equaled or surpassed only during pregnancy and lactation (see the box on nutritional intake). Even after the obvious period of accelerated growth has ended, nutritional intake must be adequate for muscle development and bone mineralization, which continue (196). The adolescent's nutritional status encompasses the life span; it begins with the nutritional experience of childhood and determines the nutritional potential of adulthood.

Both males and females have an increased appetite; they are constantly hungry. A fast-growing boy may never feel full. His stomach capacity may be too small to accommodate the amount of food he requires to meet growth needs unless he eats at frequent intervals. Adolescent females between 11 and 14 years of age may need 2200 kcal per day; males of the same age need 2700 kcal. Females between 15 and 18 years of age need 2400 kcal and males need 3000 kcal (163, 187, 196, 197); however, stage of sexual maturation, rate of physical growth, and amount of physical and social activity should be considered before determining exact caloric needs. In addition, the nutritional needs differ for the pregnant and nonpregnant adolescent.

Protein helps to maintain a positive nitrogen balance within the body during the metabolic process (196). Protein needs increase to between 45 and 56 g daily; approximately 15% of the total caloric intake should be derived from protein consumed in adequate quantities. Protein may be obtained from milk, cheese, eggs, meat, legumes, nuts, and whole grains. Today's teens often emphasize vegetarian diets rather than meat as a protein source (28). There is an additional need for iron and zinc during adolescence because of the increased muscle and soft tissue growth and the rapid growth demands of an expanding red cell mass. Girls may be especially susceptible to iron deficiency at menarche (196). Limit dietary fat to 30% or less of total calories (187).

Calcium is needed for bone growth and continued teeth formation; intake should be increased to 1200 mg daily. If the adolescent drinks a quart of milk daily, this dietary requirement can be easily met (196).

Underweight and overweight are probably the two most common but overlooked symptoms of malnutrition. Assess the adolescent; teach the adolescent and parents as indicated to foster health.

Underweight

Underweight can be caused by an inadequate intake of calories or poor use of the energy. It is often accompanied by fatigue, irritability, anorexia, and digestive disturbances such as constipation or diarrhea. Poor muscular development evidenced by posture and hypochromic anemia may also be observed. In children and adolescents growth and development may be delayed. Even with the recommended dietary intakes, malabsorption of protein, fat, or carbohydrate can result in undernutrition. Underweight may be a symptom of an undiagnosed disease (64, 197). The most severe form of underweight is seen in individuals with anorexia nervosa and bulimia. You may be the first person to assess these conditions in the adolescent.

Anorexia nervosa is a *syndrome,* occurring usually in females between the ages of 12 and 18, although onset may occur in the twenties and thirties, *in which the person voluntarily refuses to eat, presumably because of lack of hunger but related to distorted body image and conflictual relationships.* Refer to Signs and Symptoms of Anorexia Nervosa (15, 52, 63, 111, 126, 133, 202).

Men may also suffer from this disease but may be even more reticent than women to reveal symptoms or seek treatment (52, 111, 133).

Bulimia may be associated with anorexia nervosa and is a *syndrome characterized by voluntary restriction of food intake followed by extreme overeating and self-in-*

▶ SIGNS AND SYMPTOMS OF ANOREXIA NERVOSA

- Refusal to eat or eating only small amounts yet feeling guilt about eating; excuses about not eating; inability to tolerate sight or smell of food
- Denial of hunger (hunger becomes a battle of wills) but preoccupation with food (plays with food when eating; collects recipes)
- Intense fear of becoming obese, even when underweight; refusal to maintain body weight; compulsive exercise and weighing
- Large (at least 20–25%) weight loss with no physical illness evident
- Abuse of laxatives and/or diuretics; frequent trips to bathroom, especially after meals
- Distorted body image; perception of self as fat even when below normal weight
- Vital sign changes: bradycardia, hypotension, hypothermia
- Interruption of normal reproductive system processes in females: at least three consecutive menses missed when otherwise expected to occur
- Malnutrition adversely affecting (1) the skeleton, causing decalcification, decreased bone mass, and osteoporosis; (2) muscular development; and (3) cardiac and liver function, arrhythmia, and (4) body metabolic functions, which may decrease as a result of liver involvement
- Skin dry, pale, yellow-tinged skin; presence of lanugo; hair loss
- Enlargement of brain ventricles, with shrinkage of brain tissue surrounding them; depression, irritability
- Apathy, depression, low motivation, poor concentration
- Regular use of loose-fitting clothing

---

duced vomiting and laxative abuse. Refer to Signs and Symptoms of Bulimia (63, 126, 202).

Anorexia nervosa is more common than bulimia among adolescents, although the latter is increasing in incidence. Often both syndromes exist together (63). Impaired psychological functioning, disturbed body image, confused or inaccurate perceptions about body functions, and a sense of incompetence and helplessness are present in all anorectic and bulimic clients (50, 63, 64). There are several theories about causation and dynamics of anorexia nervosa (63, 64, 66, 111, 133, 196).

The person usually is treated on an outpatient basis; however, hospitalization, with nutritional support and intense psychotherapy, is recommended when loss of 25% or more of body weight leaves the person physically, emotionally, and socially compromised to the point of being in a life-threatening situation. The anorectic person should be hospitalized if there is a low serum electrolyte or fluid level; depression with suicidal thoughts or attempts; substantial disorganization of the family; or failure of outpatient treatment. These criteria

▶ **SIGNS AND SYMPTOMS OF BULIMIA**

- Binge eating—consumption of excessively large amount of food—followed by self-induced vomiting or laxative and/or diuretic abuse (at least twice weekly); secretive eating; frequent trips to bathroom, especially after eating
- Fear of inability to stop eating voluntarily
- Feeling of lack of control over the eating behavior during eating binges
- Preoccupation with food and guilt about eating
- Weight fluctuations and fluid and electrolyte imbalances due to binges, fasts, and vomiting/laxatives
- Use of crash diets to control weight
- Weakness, headaches, fatigue, depression, dizziness
- Orthostatic hypotension due to fluid depletion
- Scars on dorsum of hand from induced vomiting
- Loss of tooth enamel and esophageal and gastric bleeding in vomiters
- Chest pain from esophageal reflux or spasm
- Parotid gland enlargement in vomiters; swollen or infected salivary glands
- Increased peristalsis, rectal bleeding, constipation if laxative abuser
- Menstrual irregularities
- Bursting blood vessels in eyes
- Red knuckles from forced vomiting
- More time alone or cooking

also apply to the bulimic person; the additional criterion is spontaneous vomiting after binges. Hospitalization may also be helpful in diffusing parent–adolescent tensions and the resultant power struggle and in preventing suicide (5, 52, 63, 111, 133, 197).

The goals of treatment for the anorectic and bulimic client are to maintain normal weight, treat the hypokalemia and metabolic alkalosis, change attitudes toward food, and develop more effective coping skills to overcome the underlying conflicts. The approach is holistic. Treatment involves any of the following methods: behavior modification, insight-oriented, supportive, group, or family therapy. For further information refer to articles at the end of the chapter (5, 30, 52, 53, 63, 111, 126, 133, 134, 197).

Both the family and the adolescent need therapy. Goals of family therapy include reducing pathogenic conflict and anxiety within the family relationships, becoming more aware of and better meeting each other's emotional needs, promoting more appropriate role behavior for each sex and generation, and strengthening the capacity of the adolescent and family as a whole to cope with various problems (63, 64).

Overweight

Overweight is rarely the result of an endocrine, metabolic, or neurologic disturbance. Teach adolescents and parents the following information. Genetic predisposition to obesity may exist, as shown by studies that correlate parental weight more closely with the weight of their natural children than with those of adopted children (196). *Often weight status is a result of lifelong food and activity habits.* Children grow up associating food with much more than nourishment for their bodies. Food means celebration, consolation, reward, or punishment. People give and receive food as symbols of their love. Food and drink are chief forms of entertainment both at home and "on the town." We have learned to expect an offer of at least a beverage when we visit friends. This misuse of food, accompanied by a decrease in physical activity levels during the 20th century, has led to a steady increase in the prevalence of obesity. Energy input is greater than energy output.

Various theories are proposed regarding the deposition of fat in the body. Apparently obese persons have either more fat cells (hyperplastic obesity), or the fat cells are larger than those of normal-weight persons (hypertrophic obesity). Hyperplastic obesity is usually associated with early-onset obesity, and hypertrophic obesity is usually associated with adult-onset obesity. Critical times for proliferation of fat cells may be the last prenatal trimester, the first 3 years of life, and adolescence. Several references give more information about obesity in adolescence. Childhood obesity does not always lead to adult obesity. Early-onset obesity may be caused by a metabolic genetic defect that is compounded by excess caloric intake, with later-onset obesity caused by excess caloric intake. Onset of obesity in later life may have a situational basis; crises trigger fat cell hypertrophy or upset in appetite-control mechanisms (20, 42, 50, 63, 64, 94, 126, 187, 195, 196, 197).

According to most research, **obesity** *exists if more than 20% of the male's body weight and 30% of the female's body weight is adipose tissue.* (Normal values of adipose tissue are 12 to 18% for men and 18 to 24% for women.) Another means of determining the degree of obesity is to measure skinfold thickness near the midpoint of the upper arm with a skinfold caliper. Skinfold thickness exceeding 15 mm in males and 25 mm in females indicates obesity (20, 196).

It has been estimated that 10 to 30% of adolescents are obese and approximately 80% of these teens will remain obese as adults (196, 197). As with most abnormal states of health, prevention of obesity is better than treatment. A pound of body fat contains approximately 3500 calories. An intake in excess of need of even 100 calories a day will add up to 3000 calories a month, or almost 1 pound of body weight. With the obese adolescent, food intake and activity habits should be assessed with weight loss and/or control in mind. There are various approaches for treating obesity, including diet, exercise, medication, behavior modification, mechanical methods, and individual support (20, 196).

Both prescription and over-the-counter appetite depressants are available. Many of these contain caffeine, which can cause an elevated heart rate and high blood pressure. Many over-the-counter dietary aids contain bulk-producing agents and a sympathomimetic with anorectic action. The sympathomimetic agent in these aids (propanolamine) is capable of producing nervousness, restlessness, insomnia, and headaches; the bulk-producing agents have a laxative effect. Like other drugs, these appetite depressants can be addictive and have other side effects that might produce health problems. Thyroid hormone is beneficial only to persons who are in a hypometabolic state. Because thyroid hormone medication can inhibit thyroxine production in metabolically normal persons, it can be detrimental to their efforts at weight reduction. Thyroid hormones can also have adverse effects on the cardiovascular system. Similarly, the use of diuretics by a person who needs to lose fat is both misleading and dangerous. The person loses necessary fluid and electrolytes instead (196, 197).

Diet plans vary from balanced low-calorie diets to nutritionally poor fad diets. Some of the dietary plans encourage total fasting (therapeutic starvation); other plans change the type and amount of food, the frequency of eating episodes, and the speed at which food is eaten. Caloric restriction does not work well with adolescents. Teens want rapid, easy results. Eating also is an important part of the adolescent socialization pattern. Thus, limiting caloric intake or restricting foods eaten may alter their social interaction.

Mechanical methods, often advertised in popular magazines, include sauna suits, special exercise outfits, mechanical spot reducers, and steam baths. Because overweight is a problem of energy input and output, these methods have no long-term benefit.

Because obese people tend to gauge their eating according to external environmental cues rather than hunger, programs using behavior modification on eating habits have been used with some success (126, 195). By learning to change problem behaviors associated with eating or exercise, they can change habits and maintain their subsequent weight loss. Through daily school physical education classes, exercise programs should be designed.

An eating pattern assessment is described by White (195), as are areas for psychological, physiologic, and sociocultural assessment. Based on assessment, *the following suggestions, if followed, can help most obese adolescents lose weight:*

- Consciously ask self before eating, "Am I really hungry?"
- Eat only at mealtimes and at the table; avoid snacks. To lose 1 pound weekly, dietary intake must be reduced by 500 calories daily.
- Count the mouthfuls, cut food into small pieces, and eat slowly to eat less. Set down eating utensils between each bite of food.
- Keep a food diary, with the goal of reinforcing the adherence to the traditional food groups and avoid empty calories (20, 64).
- Engage in planned, regular exercise such as bicycle riding, walking the pet dog, gardening, yard work, calisthenics, or swimming.
- Maintain proper posture and an overall attractive appearance.

Families should be given the following suggestions to help the adolescent achieve weight loss:

- Limit purchases and cooking and baking of carbohydrate foods or snacks.
- Remove tempting snacks such as candy and cookies from the home.
- Ban eating in front of the television or reading while eating.
- Make dining at the table a pleasant time.
- Avoid using food as reward or punishment.
- Serve food in individual portions on the plate rather than in bowls on the table to avoid second helpings, and serve food on smaller plates.
- Praise even a small weight loss; avoid nagging (20, 64).
- Participate in physical activity with the adolescent when possible.

Further, you can reinforce the permanence of new food habits and achievement of weight loss through your continued guidance and realistic praise. The key to successful treatment may be in improving the adolescent's self-image. If emotional problems exist, you will need to counsel the adolescent or refer him or her to an appropriate source. Regardless of the methods of treatment used, parental understanding and cooperation are needed, and you are one member of the health team with whom both parents and the adolescent can discuss their concerns. Your listening, discussing, teaching, and referral when necessary can help the adolescent prevent or overcome the health hazard of obesity. You can also work with the school system to establish daily physical exercise programs that stimulate the teen to remain physically active, give dietary instructions, check weight, and provide low-calorie refreshments.

Obesity presents physical health hazards and problems with social and emotional adjustment. The obese adolescent is frequently rejected by the peer group and harassed by his or her parents. Many overweight teenagers withdraw from social interactions and develop feelings of inadequacy and inferiority. Physical health problems such as abnormal menstrual cycles, orthopedic difficulties, kidney stones, and gallbladder disease develop. If obesity persists into adulthood, the incidence of diabetes mellitus, cardiovascular diseases, and other illnesses increases.

Preventing adolescent obesity through education of the child and the parents and treating it when it occurs can eliminate future health problems. More information on types, effects, and treatment of obesity can be found in various references (20, 44, 45, 64, 65, 134, 187, 196, 197).

Adolescent Pregnancy

Adolescent pregnancy, discussed later in the chapter, presents another health problem related to nutrition as well as to other physical, social, and emotional factors. Clearly, many teenagers lack the physiologic maturity needed to withstand the stresses of pregnancy. The adolescent's nutritional intake may be only barely sufficient to support her own development, not adequate to satisfy two nutritional requirements (196).

Exercise, Play, and Rest

Exercise and rest must be balanced. Teach adolescents and parents the following information.

Exercise and Play Activities

Three types of play predominate in this age group: cooperative play, exemplified in games; team play, exemplified in sports; and construction play, exemplified in hobbies. All of these types of play can promote growth in the adolescent (185, 197).

Teenage boys are concerned with activities that require physical abilities and demonstrate their manliness. This age group probably spends more time and energy practicing and participating in sport-related activities than any other age group. Many boys attempt to participate in sports like basketball, football, baseball, hockey, and soccer, or work on cars or machines. There is growing acceptance, however, of the boy who wants to cook, garden, or do other activities that traditionally were not so popular or acceptable.

Some cultures still expect girls to develop the traditional interests in social functions and domestic skills such as cooking, cleaning, and serving. In the United States, adolescent girls are involved in swimming, gymnastics, volleyball, running, jogging, ice skating, dancing, and horseback or bicycle riding, as well as hockey, soccer, football or rugby teams, and weight lifting. Those who try out for and succeed on boys' teams are challenging long-accepted ideas about femininity, masculinity, strength and endurance of each sex, and competition. There is no physiologic reason why girls should not play aggressive sports (38, 50, 185).

Help parents and teens realize that competitive activities prepare young people to develop a process of self-appraisal that will last them throughout their lives. Learning to win and to lose can also be important in developing self-respect and concern for others. Physical activities provide a way for adolescents to enjoy the stimulation of conflict in a socially acceptable manner. Participation in sports training programs in junior and senior high schools can also help decrease the gap between biological and psychosocial maturation while providing exercise. Some form of physical activity should be encouraged to promote physical development, prevent overweight, formulate a realistic body image, and promote peer acceptance. Being an observer on the sidelines will not fulfill these needs.

As women join the labor force in growing numbers, the importance of the sports experience increases, because the working woman, like the working man, is involved in a structure in which rules are modeled on competitive sports teams. The worker must be able to play the game: follow rules, get along with all kinds of people, and not disparage colleagues or talk back to the boss (39). These attributes are increasingly important for the successful professional in the health care system.

Rest and Sleep

During adolescence bedtime becomes variable; the adolescent is busy with an active social life. The teen is expending large amounts of energy and functioning with an inadequate oxygen supply because the heart and lungs do not enlarge rapidly enough at the time of growth spurt. Both contribute to fatigue and need for additional rest. In addition, protein synthesis occurs more readily during sleep. Because of the growth spurt during adolescence, protein synthesis needs are increased (84, 197). Increased rest may also be needed to prevent illness.

Limit setting may be necessary to ensure adequate opportunities for rest. Rest is not necessarily sleep. A period spent with some quiet activity is also beneficial. Every afternoon should not be filled with extracurricular activities or home responsibilities, and when there is school the next morning, the adolescent should be in bed at a reasonable hour.

PSYCHOSOCIAL CONCEPTS

Cognitive Development

Formal Operations Stage

Tests of mental ability indicate that adolescence is the time when the mind has great ability to acquire and use knowledge. One of the adolescent's developmental tasks is to develop a workable philosophy of life, a task requiring time-consuming abstract and analytic thinking and inductive and deductive reasoning. Yet, according to media reports, many teens read at fourth-grade level or are functionally illiterate.

The adolescent uses available information to combine ideas into concepts and concepts into constructs, develop theories, and look for supporting facts; consider alternate solutions to problems; project his or her thinking into the future; and try to categorize thoughts into usable forms. He or she is capable of highly imaginative thinking, which, if not stifled, can evolve into significant contributions in many fields—science, art, music. The adolescent's theories at this point may be oversimplified and lack originality, but he or she is setting up the structure for adult thinking patterns, typical of the Period of Formal Operations. The adolescent can solve hypothetical, mental, and verbal problems; use scientific reasoning; deal with the past, present, and future; and understand causality. The Formal Operations Period differs from Concrete Operations in that a much larger range of symbolic processes and logic is used (152, 189).

Keniston (109, 110) describes cognitive development of youth or late adolescence as proceeding through a complex transition of dualism such as a simple understanding of right and wrong and either–or of an issue to an awareness of multiplicity, a realization of relativism, and a more existential sense of truth. An aspect of this stage of cognitive development is to think about thinking: the ability to achieve a new level of consciousness, an awareness of consciousness, and a decrease in self-consciousness that permits intellectual tricks, phenomenologic games, and a higher level of creativity. This stage involves being very aware of inner processes, focusing on states of consciousness as something to control and alter, and thinking about the ideal self and society (109, 110).

The abstract level of thinking described by Keniston can be considered a part of the Period of Formal Operations (109, 110, 152, 189). Even though there are no overall differences between female and male adolescents' intelligence, females have shown greater verbal skills, whereas males have shown more facility with quantitative and spatial problems. These differences are apparently the result of interest, social expectations, and training rather than different innate mental abilities (197).

In the United States the emphasis in education and the work world is on logical, analytic, critical, and convergent thinking. The goal of these linear thinking processes is precision, exactness, consistency, sequence, and correctness of response. The source of such thinking is the left hemisphere of the brain. Yet original concepts do not necessarily arise from logical thinking. Thinking that is creative or novel is marked by exploration, intentional ambiguity, problem solving, and originality. Creativity is a multivariate mental process, divergent, intuitive, and holistic in nature; its source is the right hemisphere of the brain. It is an intellectual skill in which the person creates new ideas rather than imitating existing knowledge.

Creativity can be encouraged when the educational process requires the following (185):

- Written assignments that necessitate original work, independent learning, self-initiation, and experimentation
- Reading assignments that emphasize questions of inquiry, synthesis, and evaluation rather than factual recall
- Group work to encourage brainstorming or exposure to creative ideas of others
- Oral questions that are divergent or ask for viewpoints during lectures
- Tests that include both divergent and convergent questions that engage the student in reflective, exploratory thought (questions should become increasingly complex in nature; ideally the questions are worded so that there is not just one right answer but answers that can be innovative and express thoughtfulness)
- A creative atmosphere, whereby the learner is autonomous, self-reliant, internally controlled, and self-evaluated (the curriculum emphasizes process, and the teacher provides a supportive atmosphere and recognizes creativity; in such an environment one would observe puzzlement and frustration but also eagerness, humor, laughter, and enjoyment related to the task at hand)

Parents sometimes underestimate the cognitive abilities of the adolescent. Help them work with the adolescent from an intellectual and creative perspective. Parents can learn from adolescents, just as adolescents learn from parents. Help the adolescent learn how to use cognitive skills in a way that will not antagonize parents.

The adolescent does not always develop intellectual potential by staying in school. Students drop out of school (about 1 million annually, with a rate of 50% for inner cities) for a variety of reasons, not just because of socioeconomic disadvantage (124, 132, 155). Dropping out has many negative consequences, including unemployment, welfare dependency, and problems with the law (155). Providing special classrooms for the teen during pregnancy and after delivery so that she can bring the baby for day-care while she attends class is one way to prevent school dropouts in that population (95).

Sexual Harassment in School and with Peers

Sexual harassment has occurred in the schools and workplace for decades but has only recently been a defined and illegal activity. **Sexual harassment,** or *troubling behavior toward the self as a sexual object from another,* has been endured from peers and adults in school because children did not know what to call it or do about it. Sexual harassment behavior has traditionally included:

- Uninvited touching from other students, teachers, or other adults at school
- Sexually provocative statements or sexual innuendos in conversation
- Rumors about sexual behavior or capacity of the person
- Rude, degrading, and wounding remarks toward a child who participates in classes not frequently enrolled in by others of their sex
- Activities called teasing, horseplay, or flirting. These include blocking the passage; grabbing, touching, pinching, or brushing against the person; spying on another; forcing a kiss or any unwanted sexual behaviors; calling another names or words with a sexual connotation; commenting about body parts, clothing, or looks; or whistling, howling, or lip smacking.

Schools no longer dismiss these behaviors because sexual harassment is a form of discrimination. It undermines self-confidence and denies the victim full educational opportunities (199). Feminists maintain that sexual harassment is part of a pattern of male persecution of females, which may appear as innocuous childish behavior. If this behavior is not corrected in childhood, it escalates into continuous oppression of women (199).

As public awareness of the problem grew during the 1970s and 1980s, the law evolved as well. In 1964, Title VII of the Civil Rights Act prohibited discrimination on the basis of sex, race, color, religion, or national origin. In 1980, the Equal Employment Opportunity Commission (EEOC), the agency responsible for implementing Title VII, issued guidelines that established criteria for sexual harassment. Two forms were defined (199):

1. *Quid pro quo:* the person's hiring, promotion, or wages conditioned on sexual favors.
2. *Hostile environment:* the pervasive, intrusive, unwelcome behavior that interferes with a person's job performance.

Sexual harassment exists on a continuum of unwanted behaviors ranging from the spoken or written comments and stares to actual physical assault and attempted rape. Sexual harassment is defined by the victim. If the individual finds the comments or physical contact to be unwelcome, it is sexual harassment. Title VII does not specifically apply to schools; it prohibits discrimination in the workplace. But courts have accepted EEOC guidelines as the legal definition of sexual harassment everywhere. School personnel have the kind of control that creates opportunity for harassment and for addressing it. Further, Title IX of the Education Amendment of 1972 also prohibits discrimination, and Title VII has been covered by it. Title IX is the law under which women athletes must have access to sports equipment and facilities equal to those provided for men, but the law is also used in the sensitive areas of relationships between teachers and students and students and peers. The Office of Civil Rights of the U.S. Department of Education enforces Title IX and has specified that schools must formulate policy opposing sexual harassment and procedures for handling complaints. The most common area of complaints has been harassment of students by other students, often on the school bus as well as on the school grounds. Children as young as 6 years can understand language and conduct that expresses hostility based on sex (199).

Title IX permits students to sue for damages suffered from sexual harassment in schools; however, legal remedies do not protect the student victim from the searing impact of sexual harassment in their lives. In addition, students who press charges suffer much humiliation and retaliation in the process from other students, teachers, school administrators, and staff. Some students switch schools or their parents move geographically, if they can, especially when complaints are ignored or denied, or legal proceedings are delayed.

Other students commit suicide because of the stress (199).

Sexual harassment in U.S. schools is pervasive; it occurs in all parts of the country, in big cities and small towns, in public, private, parochial, and vocational schools. Girls most often are the victims, as young as 6 years, but usually between ages 12 and 16; boys are sometimes also victims of harassment. As many as 39% of the students in some national surveys report harassment daily. Certainly education, as well as emotional and social development, is compromised in the process (199).

Students of both sexes report the same debilitating impact, but the effect on girls appears more profound and longer lasting. *Effects of harassment* include the following (199):

- Not wanting to go to school
- Talking less in class
- Difficulty with attention
- Feeling embarrassed
- Having difficulty with sleeping, eating, and daily activities
- Losing self-confidence, self-esteem, and trust in others
- Changing behavior, classes, routes home, and friends

Same-sex harassment may occur as well as harassment by the opposite sex, particularly against gay and lesbian students. Often adults who are nearby do not stop such harassment as calling someone a "homo" or "lesbo," and may even participate directly.

Students consistently state that when they report harassment to adults, they often encounter disbelief, find themselves blamed for the behaviors, and suffer much agony because of the lack of responsiveness of teachers and administrators. The lack of support for the students and their parents is demoralizing. Unfortunately, students who have been harassed often turn around and harass others. The behavior spirals (199).

Whether an action constitutes harassment depends on the area of the country. A teacher from the Rio Grande Valley may touch and hug students as part of caring or comradeship; in Austin that same behavior is likely to be called harassment. Terms of endearment vary between cultural groups. What may be appropriate for an African-American youth to call another African-American youth would not be appropriate to call a Hispanic, Asian, or Caucasian. Schools are part of the community and reflect the values and attitudes of the community. Others say that if behavior is wrong for one group, it is not right for members of any group (199).

A major issue is teachers who harass students. Incidence reports vary; however, there often appears to be a conspiracy of silence about student–teacher sex in high schools. Reports of harassment and sexual abuse can vary from misunderstanding a teacher's behavior (such as when a teacher stands too close to a student) to false accusation; yet, any student's report should be listened to seriously and investigated. False allegations can be detected when interrogated students back down or there are glaring inconsistencies in the reports. Girls who are abused by male members of the family may report a male teacher because it is too scary to report the real abuser. Some districts suspend students who falsely accuse teachers. Accused teachers who have been found innocent report a sense of betrayal, self-doubt, stigma, and rejection by colleagues and the wider community, and never again feel competent as teachers or acceptable as people. Yet, people who investigate these charges say that students are more likely to avoid reporting actual incidents than fabricating incidents (199).

Because teachers are vulnerable to charges of harassment or abuse, there has been a consequent chilling of classroom atmosphere. Teachers should make reasonable decisions. Teachers are told to teach, not touch, even if a child is hurt or crying. There should be two adults in any classroom ideally. The teacher should not hold a child in the lap. If a child needs help in the bathroom, two adults should accompany the child. Teachers are advised not to invite students to their homes. A teacher should never drive a student anywhere in a vehicle; parents should be called for transportation. Teaching, a personal and interactive profession, has been sterilized, as every pat on the back or congratulatory hug has become suspect at a time when there are even more emotionally needy children in the classroom. Teachers cannot be available to build a positive relationship with a child in an atmosphere of suspicion and fear. Teachers, as well as all school employees, are being given more assistance in complying with the law, eliminating sexual harassment, and being a positive role model to students. Teachers can effectively teach students how to identify unacceptable behavior and say "stop it, and don't do it again," when someone engages in harassing behavior. Teachers, administrators, and parents can work together to promote a safe learning environment. Schools must put a stop to sexual harassment because it is wrong, it is illegal, and it is expensive in every way (199).

In the United States, we live in a sex-saturated society, in which private behavior, public culture, and the media contradict traditional values and public pronouncements. Some heroes are convicted of rape while others boast of sexual exploits. Phrases of behavior that used to be a mark of respect (such as addressing someone as Mrs. or Ms. or holding open a door) may be interpreted as a mark of contempt. There is considerable confusion about appropriate behavior; even youth are having difficulty adjusting to changing sex behaviors. The battle over sexual harassment is occurring at a time when we rely less on individual restraint and more on official reminders of what is acceptable. The absence of concern for others is causing us to rely on the courts as a first, not last, resort (199).

Peer-Group Influences

The **peer group,** *friends of the same age,* influences the adolescent to a greater extent than parents, teachers, popular heroes, religious leaders, or other adults. Because peer groups are so important, the adolescent has intense loyalty to them. Social relationships take precedence over family and counteract feelings of emptiness, isolation, and loneliness. Significance is attached to activities deemed important by peers. Peers serve as models or instructors for skills not yet acquired. Usually some peers are near the same cognitive level as the learner; their explanations may be more understandable. When student peers of varying cognitive levels discuss problems, less advanced students may gain insights and correct inaccuracies in thinking. The more advanced students also profit; they must think through their own reasoning to explain a concept (189, 193).

The *purposes* of the peer group include to promote:

- A sense of acceptance, prestige, belonging, approval.
- Opportunities for learning how to behave.
- A sense of immediacy, concentrating on the here-and-now, what happened last night, who is doing what today, what homework is due tomorrow.
- A reason for *being* today, a sense of *importance right now,* and not just dreams or fears about what he or she might become in some vague future time (50, 121, 185, 197).
- Opportunities to learn behavior related to later adult roles.
- Role models and relationships to help define personal identity as he or she adapts to a changing body image, more mature relationships with others, and heightened sexual feelings.
- Experiences to integrate accepted masculine or feminine behavior although adults may not recognize the distinctions.
- Opportunities to try a variety of acceptable behaviors within the safety of the group.
- Incorporation of new ideas into the body image and self-concept. The adolescent who is rejected

by peers may be adversely affected, as he or she does not learn the high degree of social skill and ability to form relationships that are necessary for the adult culture (50, 140, 185).

Peer-group relations are beneficial, but they can also direct the adolescent into antisocial behavior because of pressure to conform and the need to gain approval. The adolescent may participate in drug and alcohol abuse, sexual intercourse, or various delinquent acts not because he or she wants to or enjoys them, but rather to prove self, to vent aggression, or to gain superiority over younger or fringe members of the group. He or she may even gain pleasure from sadistic activities toward others. Parents have reason to be concerned about their adolescent's peers and to guide their child into wholesome activities and groups that will reinforce the values they have taught. Help parents and teachers understand peer groups and work through crises related to peer relations (15).

Peer-Group Dialect

This dialect is a communication pattern seen in the adolescent period. Slang, or jargon, is one of the trademarks of adolescence and may be considered a **peer-group dialect.** *It is a highly informal language that consists of coined terminology and of new or extended interpretations attached to traditional terms.*

Slang is used for various reasons. It provides a sense of belonging to the peer group and a small, compact vocabulary for a teenager who does not want to waste energy on words. Slang also excludes authority figures and other outsiders and permits expression of hostility, anger, and rebellion. Unknowing adults do not understand the digs given with well-timed pieces of slang. Other adults sense the flippancy of underlying feelings but to their chagrin can do little other than try to understand. By the time they learn the meanings of the current terms, new meanings have evolved.

You can help parents understand the purposes of teenage dialect and the importance of not trying to imitate or retaliate verbally. In addition, encourage parents to enter into discussion with their teenager to understand more fully him or her and the teen-age dialect.

Use of Leisure Time

Leisure time with the peer group is important for normal social development and adjustment. The adolescent spends an increasing amount of time away from home, either in school, in other activities, or with peers, as he or she successfully achieves greater independence. School is a social center, even though abstract learning is a burden to some students. In school students seek recognition from others and determine their status within the group, depending on success in scholastic, athletic, or other organizations and activities.

Dating Pattern

Dating is one use of leisure time and is influenced greatly by the peer group but also varies according to the culture and social class and religious and family beliefs. Dating prepares the adolescent for intimate bonds with others, marriage, and family life. The adolescent learns social skills in dealing with the opposite sex, in what situations and with whom he or she feels least and most comfortable, and what is expected sexually.

In the United States dating may begin as early as age 10 or 11, especially with pressures from peers and family to attract the opposite sex. Generally, however, girls in junior high school are more mature than boys. Girls may seek male companionship, but boys frequently prefer activities with other males. Many fellows at this age are women haters. Near age 15, boys begin to catch up with girls in physical and emotional maturity, and their interests become better correlated. Social pursuits take on more meaning for boys.

Not all American adolescents assume this dating pattern. Some begin early to date one person and continue that pattern until marriage. Others do not date until young adulthood. A few prefer homosexual relationships. Isolated homosexual encounters are not unusual, especially among males, and do not mean the person will remain a homosexual. The dynamics behind homosexuality are more complex. Because the person is usually a young adult when homosexuality is declared the chosen sexual pattern, the topic is discussed in greater detail in Chapter 12; however, the adolescent may have always felt more comfortable with or more cared for by the same-sex person.

When dating begins, the emphasis is first on commonly shared activities. Later the emphasis includes a sharing, close relationship. Similarly, dating may start with groups of couples, move to double dates, and finally involve single couples. With each step, the adolescent learns more about and feels more comfortable with the opposite sex. He or she also learns personal acceptability to others. Going steady has become popular because it provides a readily available partner for social activities, but it can be detrimental if it stops the adolescent from searching for the qualities he or she wants in a future mate or involves date rape or sexual experimentation that he or she is unprepared to handle.

Further, the male is more likely to be the one to force regular sexual intercourse (7, 168).

As you work with adolescents, you should assess the stage of peer-group development and dating patterns. A few years will make a considerable difference in attitudes toward the opposite sex. You must be able to build your teaching on current interests and attitudes. The same age groups in different localities may also be in different stages. Adolescents from another culture may sharply contrast in pattern with American adolescents. For example, in Egypt the male is not supposed to have any intimate physical contact with the female until marriage. In the United States certain physical contact is expected.

Leisure Activities

Sports, dancing, hobbies, reading, listening to the radio or stereo, talking on the telephone, daydreaming, experimenting with hairstyles, cosmetics, or new clothes, and just loafing have been teenagers' favorite activities for decades. Motorcycle riding, driving and working on cars, using the computer, watching television, playing video games, and attending movies and concerts are also popular. Political activism draws some youth; various causes rise and then fade in interest as the youth matures. "Everybody's doing it" is seemingly a strong influence on the adolescent's interests and activities. Others participate in activities, such as camera club, Spanish club, or yearbook projects, because of personal talents or interests.

Socioeconomic and educational levels determine to some extent how youth use free time. Upper-class youths may travel extensively, go boating, and attend cultural events or debutante parties. Middle-class emphasis is on participation in activities. During adolescence these youths are involved in church- or school-related functions such as sports, theater, and musical events. Lower-class youths may spend more time in unstructured ways such as standing on the corner, talking to peers, or finding ways to earn extra money. In many homes, however, the absence of money does not mean the absence of healthy leisure activity. Smoking and using alcohol and drugs cannot be attributed primarily to lower-class youths, for a great deal of money is required to supply some of these habits. Shoplifting or burglary may be done for "kicks" or to obtain money for desired items.

Many parents consider a party in the home for a group of teenagers a safe use of leisure time. This is undoubtedly true if parents and other adults are on the premises and can give guidance as needed and if the parents are not themselves supplying the teens with alcohol and drugs. The latter sometimes happens; however, parents rationalize by saying they prefer their youngster to be at home (or at a friend's home) if they are using or abusing alcohol and drugs. They may even drive home teens who are unsafe to drive. Usually, however; drug and alcohol parties are hosted by teens when parents are out of town; teenagers chip in for beer for an "open" party (any number of people may attend). When behavior becomes boisterous, police are often called by the neighbors, but they find the situation difficult to handle because there is no responsible authority figure on the premises. The police in one community give the following *guidelines to help parents and teens host and attend* parties. You may wish to share these suggestions with parents (80):

- Parents should set the ground rules before the party to express feelings and concerns about the party, ask who will attend and whether adults will be present, and learn what is expected of their adolescent. The address and phone number of the host should be known by the parents of the teens who are attending.
- Notify neighbors that you will be hosting a party, and encourage your teen to call or send a note to close neighbors notifying them of the party and asking them to let the family know if there is too much noise.
- Notify the police when planning a large party. They can protect you, your guests, and your neighbors. Discuss with the police an agreeable plan for guest parking.
- Plan to have plenty of food and nonalcoholic beverages on hand.
- Plan activities with your teenager before the party so that the party can end before guests become bored (3 or 4 hours are suggested as sufficient party time).
- Limit party attendance and times. Either send out invitations or have the teenager personally invite guests beforehand. Discourage crashers; ask them to leave. Open house parties are difficult for parents and teenagers to control. Set time limits for the party that enable guests to be home at a reasonable time, definitely before a legal curfew. Suggested closing hours are: grades 7 and 8, 10:30 PM; grades 9 and 10, 11:30 PM; grades 11 and 12, 12:00 PM. Check curfew times for your locale. Transportation home for each teen who attends should be planned in advance by parents and the adolescent.

- A parent should be at home during the entire time of the party. The parent's presence helps keep the party running smoothly; it also gives the parent an opportunity to meet the teenager's friends. Invite other adults to help supervise.
- Decide what part of the house will be used for the party. Pick out where your guests will be most comfortable and you can maintain adequate supervision. Avoid having the bedroom area as part of the party area.
- Do not offer alcohol to guests under the age of 21 or allow guests to use drugs in your home. This sounds prudish in this permissive era; however, you may be brought to court on criminal charges or have to pay monetary damages in a civil lawsuit if you furnish alcohol or drugs to minors. Be alert to the signs of alcohol or drug use.
- Do not allow any guest who leaves the party to return to discourage teenagers from leaving the party to drink or to use drugs elsewhere and then return to the party.
- Guests who try to bring alcohol or drugs or who otherwise refuse to cooperate with your expectations should be asked to leave. Notify the parents of any teenager who arrives at the party drunk or under the influence of any drug to ensure his or her safe transportation home. Do not let anyone drive under the influence of alcohol or drugs.
- Teenagers frequently party at homes when parents are away. Typically, the greatest problems occur when parents are not at home. Tell your neighbors when you are going to be out of town.
- Many parties occur spontaneously. Parents and teens should understand before the party that these guidelines are in effect at all parties. If, despite your precautions, things get out of hand, do not hesitate to call the local police department for help.
- Emphasize to parents the importance of their being role models through minimum drinking of alcoholic beverages or use of drugs.

In some states there is legal parental responsibility in the home. A parent commits the crime of endangering the welfare of a child less than 17 years of age if he or she recklessly fails to exercise reasonable diligence in the care or control of a child to prevent him or her from behavior, environment, or associations that are injurious to the welfare of the child or to the welfare of others. In some states a person commits the crime of unlawful transactions with a child if he or she knowingly permits a minor child to enter or remain in a place where illegal activities in controlled substances are maintained or conducted. Parents have responsibility (possibly in all states) if a minor is killed or injured after leaving their home in which an illegal substance was consumed. Juvenile officers identify an adult doing an act "knowingly and recklessly" when a minor is involved as a criterion for possible prosecution. In the opinion of attorneys and judges, parents could be subject to suit for damages for careless or imprudent behavior (80).

The teenager may also feel more secure when the parent is actively interested in knowing where he or she will be and what he or she will be doing even though rebellion may ensue. Parents should be awake or have the teen awaken them when arriving home from a party. This is a good sharing time. Peers are important, but if peer activity and values are in opposition to what has been learned as acceptable, the adolescent feels conflict. Parental limits can reduce feelings of conflict and give an excuse to avoid an activity in which he or she does not want to engage. Parental limits appropriate to the situation and not unduly constraining develop ego strength within the adolescent.

Explore with parents the adolescent's need for constructive use of leisure time and the importance of participation in peer activities.

For some teenagers there is little leisure time. They may have considerable home responsibility, such as occurs in rural communities, or work to earn money to help support the family. Other youths are active in volunteer work. Ideally, the adolescent has some time free for personal pursuits, to stand around with friends, and to sit and daydream.

Emotional Development

Emotional Characteristics

Emotional characteristics of the personality cannot be separated from family, physical, intellectual, and social development. Emotionally, the adolescent is characterized by mood swings and extremes of behavior (Table 11–1) (57, 58, 69, 121, 129). Refer to Major Concerns of Teenagers; these concerns contribute to emotional lability and identity confusion (181). Emotional development requires an interweaving and organization of opposing tendencies into a sense of unity and continuity. This process occurs during adolescence in a complex and truly impressive way to move the person toward psychological maturity (69).

Share this information with parents and the adolescent. Through using principles of communication and crisis intervention and through your use of self as a role

TABLE 11–1. CONTRASTING EMOTIONAL RESPONSES OF ADOLESCENTS

Independent Behaviors	Dependent Behaviors
Happy, easygoing, loving, gregarious, self-confident, sense of humor	Sad, irritable, angry, unloving, withdrawn, fearful, worried
Energetic, self-assertive, independent	Apathetic, passive, dependent
Questioning, critical or cynical of others	Strong allegiance to or idolization of others
Exhibitionistic or at ease with self	Excessively modest or self-conscious
Interested in logical or intellectual pursuits	Daydreaming, fantasizing
Cooperative, seeking responsibility, impatient to be involved or finish project	Rebellious, evading work, dawdling, ritualistic behavior, dropout from society
Suggestible to outside influences, including ideologies	Unaccepting of new ideas
Desirous for adult privileges	Apprehensive about adult responsibilities

model, you will be able to help the adolescent work through identity diffusion and achieve a sense of ego identity and an appropriate sense of independence.

We regularly hear of the rebellious, emotionally labile, egocentric adolescent but do not stereotype all

► MAJOR CONCERNS OF TEENAGERS

- Their appearance
- Divorce of parents
- Having good marriage and family life
- School performance
- Choosing a career; finding steady employment
- Being successful in life
- Having strong friendships; how others will treat them
- Paying for college
- Making lots of money
- Finding purpose and meaning in life
- Contracting AIDS
- Drug and alcohol use by self, friends
- Hunger and poverty in United States and the world
- Societal violence

Data from Reference (181).

adolescents into that mold. Many, perhaps more than we know of, can delay gratification, behave as adults, and have positive relationships with family and authority figures.

Developmental Crisis

The psychosexual crisis of adolescence is identity formation versus identity diffusion: "Who am I?" "How do I feel?" "Where am I going?" "What meaning is there in life?" **Identity** means that an *individual believes he or she is a specific unique person;* he or she has emerged as an adult. **Identity formation** *results through synthesis of biopsychosocial characteristics from a number of sources, for example, earlier sex identity, parents, friends, social class, ethnic, religious, and occupational groups* (56, 57).

A number of influences can interfere with identity formation (56, 57, 58, 121):

- Telescoping of generations, with many adult privileges granted early so that the differences between adult and child are obscured and there is no ideal to which to aspire
- Contradictory American value system of individualism versus conformity in which both are highly valued and youth believe that adults advocate individualism but then conform
- Nuclear family structure (The adolescent perceives most adults as parent figures and has primarily parents as targets for conflicts and aggressions.)
- Middle-class cultural emphasis in childrearing, with inconsistencies between proclaimed and actual parental concern
- Emphasis on sexual matters and encouragement to experiment without frank talking about sexuality with parents
- Diminishing hold of Judeo-Christian traditions and ethics throughout society so that the adolescent sees that failure to live by the rules is not necessarily followed by unpleasant consequences
- Increasing emphasis on education for socioeconomic gain, which prolongs dependency on parents when the youth is physically mature
- Lack of specific sex-defined responsibilities (Blurring of the traditional male–female tasks has its positive and negative counterparts; although eventually allowing more individual freedom, it can be very confusing to the adolescent who must decide how to act as a male or female.)

- Rapid changes in the adolescent subculture and all society, with emphasis on conforming to peers
- Diverse definitions of adulthood (After 12 the adolescent pays adult airline fares; after 16 he or she can drive; after 18 he or she can vote.)

Identity formation implies an *internal stability, sameness, or continuity, which resists extreme change and preserves itself from oblivion in the face of stress or contradictions.* It implies emerging from this era with a sense of wholeness, knowing the self as a unique person, feeling responsibility, loyalty, and commitment to a value system. There are three types of identity, which are closely interwoven: (1) **personal**, or **real identity**—*what the person believes self to be;* (2) **ideal identity**—*what he or she would like to be;* and (3) **claimed identity**—*what he or she wants others to think he or she is* (56–58, 121).

Identity formation is enhanced by having support not only from parents but also from another adult who has a stable identity and who upholds sociocultural and moral standards of behavior (56, 57). If the adolescent has successfully coped with the previous developmental crisis and feels comfortable with personal identity, he or she will be able to appreciate the parents on a fairly realistic basis, seeing and accepting both their strengths and shortcomings. The values, beliefs, and guidelines they have given him or her are internalized. The adolescent needs parents less for direction and support; he or she must now decide what is acceptable and unacceptable behavior.

Students from different ethnic and racial backgrounds have unique needs and ways of adapting to stressors and unique aspects of the developmental crisis of identity formation. Some may feel isolated and alienated in relation to mainstream culture values. Parents, schoolteachers, and health care professionals can help these teens work through values and cognitive and emotional conflicts (3, 70).

Identity diffusion *results if the adolescent fails to achieve a sense of identity* (56, 57). He or she feels self-conscious and has doubts and confusion about self as a human being and his or her roles in life. With identity diffusion, he or she feels impotent, insecure, disillusioned, and alienated. Some researchers believe girls enter puberty and adolescence feeling self-confidence and high self-esteem and, because of classroom and socialization processes, are more likely than boys to enter their twenties feeling low self-esteem and insecure (39). Erikson (56, 57) believes such feelings exist in both males and females until identity formation occurs.

Identity diffusion is manifested in other ways as well, as listed in Negative Consequences of Identity Diffusion (56–58). The adolescent feels that he or she is

► NEGATIVE CONSEQUENCES OF IDENTITY DIFFUSION

- Feels she or he is losing grip with reality
- Feels fragmented; lacks unity, consistency, or predictability with self
- Feels impatient but is unable to initiate action
- Gives up easily on a task; feels defeated
- Vacillates in decision making; is unable to act on decisions
- Is unable to delay gratification
- Appears brazen or arrogant, sarcastic
- Is disorganized and inconsistent in behavior; avoids tasks
- Fears losing uniqueness in entering adulthood; displays regressive behavior; acts at behavioral extremes to attract attention
- Has low self-esteem, negative self-concept, low aspirations
- Is unable to pursue academic or career plans; may drop out of school
- Isolates self from peers; is unable to relate to former friends or significant adults
- Feels cynical, disillusioned, excessively angry or suspicious
- Engages in antisocial or illegal behavior; acts out sexually
- Seeks association with gang, cult, or negative community or media leader

losing grip with reality. He or she is impatient but unable to initiate action. The teenager vacillates in decision making; he or she cannot delay gratification and appears brazen or arrogant. Behavior at work, with peers, and in sexual contacts is distorted. The adolescent is apprehensive about and avoids adult behavior, fearing loss of uniqueness by entering adulthood. The real danger of identity diffusion looms when a youth finds a negative solution to the quest for identity. He or she gives up, feels defeated, and pursues antisocial behavior because "it's better to be bad than nobody at all." Identity diffusion is more likely to occur if the teenager has close contact with an adult who is still confused about personal identity and who is in rebellion against society (56–58).

In the process of achieving identity and committing to goals in life, the person may have experienced **identity moratorium,** a *time of making no decisions but a rethinking of values and goals,* which is part of identity crisis and a step beyond *identity diffusion,* when *the person has not begun to examine his or her own life's meaning and goals.* In some cultures, identity formation is not a task for the individual. Rather, **identity foreclosure** exists: *the goals, values, and life tasks have been established by the parents and the group, and the individual is not al-* *lowed to question or examine them. They are expected to follow the pattern set by the elders;* usually the roles are related to sex and socioeconomic or caste status.

Assist parents to work with the adolescent who feels identity diffusion. Most adolescents reach physical maturity before they achieve ego identity or the emotional maturity expected as a sign of having completed the adolescent era. One study showed that individuals between 17 and 20 years of age report significantly more ego diffusion than those between 21 and 24. Females report less ego diffusion in all age groups than males (57).

Norris and Kunes-Carroll (141) and Oldaker (142) describe nursing diagnoses pertinent to the adolescent who is having difficulty with identity formation.

Self-Concept and Body Image Development

Development of self-concept and body image is closely akin to cognitive organization of experiences and identity formation. The adolescent cannot be viewed only in the context of the present; earlier experiences have an impact that continues to affect him or her. The earlier experiences that were helpful enabled the adolescent to feel good about the body and self. If the youngster enters adolescence feeling negative about self or the body, this will be a difficult period.

Other factors influence the adolescent's self-concept, including (1) age of maturation, (2) degree of attractiveness, (3) name or nickname, (4) size and physique appropriate to sex, (5) degree of identification with the same-sex parent, (6) level of aspiration and ability to reach ideals, peer relationships, and (7) culture (3, 8, 15, 70, 77, 121, 136, 182).

The rapid growth of the adolescent period is an important factor in body image revision. Girls and boys are sometimes described as "all legs." They are often clumsy and awkward. Because the growth changes cannot be denied, the adolescent is forced to alter the mental picture of self to function. More important than the growth changes themselves is the meaning given to them. The mother who says, "That's all right, Tom, we all have our clumsy moments," is providing the understanding that a comment such as "Can't you ever walk through the room without knocking something down?" denies. The adolescent needs this understanding because he or she fears rejection and is oversensitive to the opinions of others. Physical changes in height, weight, and body build cause a change in self-perception and in how the adolescent uses his or her body. To some male adolescents, the last chance to get taller is very significant.

The body is part of one's inner and outer world. Many of the experiences of the inner world are based on stimuli from the external world, especially from the body surface. Therefore the adolescent focuses attention on body surface. He or she spends a great deal of time in front of mirrors and for body hygiene, grooming, and clothing. These are normal ways for the early adolescent to integrate a changing body image. If the teen does not seem to care about appearance, he or she may have already decided, "I'm so ugly, so what's the use?"

Growth and physical changes draw the adolescent's attention to the body part that is changing, and he or she becomes more sensitive to it. This can cause a distorted self-view. He or she may overemphasize a defect and underevaluate self as a person. The body acts as a source of acceptance or rejection by others. If the adolescent does not get much acceptance for self and his or her body, he or she may try to compensate for real or imagined defects through sports, vocational or academic success, a religious commitment, or a date or group of friends that enhances prestige. The adolescent is idealistic and may not be able to achieve an ideal body. Thus he or she may discredit self by seeing the body and self as defective, inferior, or incapable.

If the adolescent does have a disability or defect, peers and adults may react with fear, pity, repulsion, or curiosity. The adolescent may retain and later reflect these impressions, as a person tends to perceive self as others perceive him or her. If the adolescent develops a negative self-image, motivation, behavior, and eventual lifestyle may also be inharmonious and out of step with social expectations.

By late adolescence self-image is complete, self-esteem should be high, and self-concept should have stabilized. The person feels autonomous but no longer believes he or she is so unique that no one has ever experienced what he or she is currently experiencing. The late adolescent no longer believes everyone is watching or being critical of his or her physical or personality characteristics. Egocentricity has declined. Interactions with the opposite sex are more comfortable, although awareness of sex is keen.

Your understanding of the importance of the value the adolescent places on self can help you work with the adolescent, parents, teachers, and community leaders. Your goal is to avoid building a false self-image in the adolescent; rather, help him or her evaluate strengths and weaknesses, accept the weaknesses, and build on the strengths. You will have to listen carefully to the adolescent's statements about self and his or her sense of future. The adolescent who believes death will come by age 20 views self, others, available opportunities, and present experiences differently as someone who perceives the future extending to old age. You will have to sense when you might effectively speak and work with him or her and when silence is best. Share an understanding of influencing factors on body image and self-concept development with parents, teachers, and other adults so that they can positively influence adolescents.

You may wish to use a therapeutic group such as reality therapy or rational thinking group, using cognitive restructuring exercises to help adolescents think more positively about themselves and reduce anxiety. Small group sessions outside the regular classroom have been found effective in enhancing self-concepts of junior high students. Group sessions can focus on personal and social awareness and how to cope with age-related problems.

Sexuality Development

Sexuality *encompasses not only the individual's physical characteristics and the act of sexual intercourse but also the following: (1) search for identity as a whole person,* including a sexual person; (2) *role behavior of men and women;* (3) *attitudes, behaviors, and feelings toward self, each sex, and sexual behavior;* (4) *relationships, affection, and caring between people;* (5) *the need to touch and be touched;* and (6) *recognition and acceptance of self and others as sexual beings* (3, 136, 197). One of the greatest concerns to the adolescent is sexual feelings and activities. Because of hormonal and physiologic changes and environmental stimuli, the adolescent is almost constantly preoccupied with feelings of developing sexuality.

Sexual desire is under the domination of the cerebral cortex. Differences in sexual desire exist in young males and females, and desire is influenced by cultural and family expectations for sexual performance. The female experiences a more generalized pleasurable response to erotic stimulation but does not necessarily desire coitus. The male experiences a stronger desire for coitus because of a localized genital sensation in response to erotic stimulation, which is accompanied by production of spermatozoa and secretions from accessory glands that build up pressure and excite the ejaculatory response. The male is stimulated to seek relief by ejaculation (50, 121, 185, 197).

Menarche is experienced by the girl as an affectively charged event related to her emerging identity as an adult woman with reproductive ability. Menarche may be perceived as frightening and shameful by some girls; previous factual sex education does not necessarily offset such feelings. Often information in classes is not assimilated because of high anxiety in the girl during the class. The girl is likely to turn to her mother for instruction at the time of menarche, even if the two of them are not close emotionally.

Family and cultural traditions are needed to mark the menarche as a transition from childhood to adulthood. Menarche is anticipated as an important event, but in the United States no formal customs mark it, and no obvious change in the girl's social status occurs. The girl may get little help from her mother, other female adults, or peers in working through feelings related to menarche. Often menses is perceived as an excretory function, and advertisements treat it as a disease.

Nocturnal emissions are often a great concern for the boys but are also a sign of manhood.

Both sexes are concerned about development and appearance of secondary sex characteristics, their overall appearance, their awkwardness, and their sex appeal, or lack of it, to the opposite sex (15, 38, 50, 77, 121, 182, 185).

The most common form of sexual outlet for both sexes, but especially males, is **masturbation,** *manipulation of the genitals for sexual stimulation.* Public education about the normality of masturbation is reducing guilt about the practice and fears of mental or physical illness (50, 121, 185).

Intercourse is an increasing sexual activity among adolescents. Premarital sexual activity is often used as a means to get close, sometimes with strangers, and may result in feelings of guilt, remorse, anxiety, and self-recrimination. The feelings associated with the superficial act may be damaging to the adolescent's self-concept and possibly to later success in a marital relationship. Adolescent males and females often report that the initial coitus was not pleasurable. Despite overt sophistication and widespread availability of information on birth control devices, pregnancy or fear of pregnancy is the deciding factor in close to half of all high school marriages. The number of pregnant teenage females who are not marrying is significantly increasing, which has implications for the future care and well-being of the baby and implications for future intimate relations of the teenage girl. If teenagers do marry, the marriage is considerably more likely to end in separation and divorce than is true for the general population, which also has a high divorce rate, because of the unstable sense of self (77, 121).

You can teach parents and adolescents of both sexes that they and other people are not like disposable plastic cartons and that an intimate and important experience is cheapened and coarsened when it is removed from love. Some youths argue that sex can be pleasurable if one hardly knows or even loathes one's partner, but most youths are likely to get emotionally involved in the sexual act, and their feelings will be bruised when

the act leads nowhere. A wide variety of sexual experience before marriage may cause the person to feel bored with a single partner later (15, 121, 197).

Americans have to relearn the satisfaction of self-denial and anticipation. The adolescent will not be harmed by knowing about the body and sexuality and yet not engaging in intercourse. A certain amount of tension can be endured; in fact, it can be useful to become mature and creative. The values of self-discipline and self-denial with anticipation must be taught before adolescence begins, however (15, 121). Such teaching comes from how parents live more so than from sex education courses and is the most critical teaching. In fact, sex education should be directed toward the parents as much as toward their offspring, for what they teach—or do not teach—is the main factor in their child's eventual behavior (15, 121).

Other countries are also having their problems with teenage sexuality. In Kenya, East Africa, adolescent sexual development has for years been controlled by tribal customs. Recently, however, Western permissiveness has crept in, especially among the teenagers in the larger cities. Pregnancy among girls from 14 to 18, with a rash of self-induced abortions, has caused leaders to insist on some sex education for their youth. Small pilot programs, sponsored jointly by government and church groups in connection with African educators, are making some impact at the secondary education level (3, 70).

Adaptive Mechanisms

The **ego** is the *sum total of those mental processes that maintain psychic cohesion and reality contact; it is the mediator between the inner impulses and outer world.* It is that part of the personality that becomes integrated and strengthened in adolescence and has the following functions (121):

- Associating concepts or situations that belong together but are historically remote or spatially separated
- Developing a realization that one's way of mastering experience is a variant of the group's way and is acceptable
- Subsuming contradictory values and attitudes
- Maintaining a sense of unity and centrality of self
- Testing perceptions and selecting memories
- Reasoning, judging, and planning
- Mediating among impulses, wishes, and actions and integrating feelings

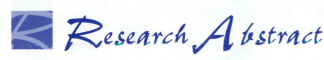
Research Abstract

Kelder, S., C. Perry, K. Klepp, and L. Lyttle, Longitudinal Tracking of Adolescent Smoking, Physical Activity, and Food Choice Behaviors, American Journal of Public Health, 84 (1994), 1121–1126.

A major assumption underlying youth health promotion has been that physiologic risk factors track from childhood and adolescence into adulthood. Few studies have systematically studied how cardiovascular disease-related behaviors change during adolescence or examined longitudinally the extent to which physiologic risk factors depend largely on initiation of health-compromising behaviors. It is assumed that early interventions prevent cardiovascular disease.

The purpose of this study was to do longitudinal tracking to determine stability of adolescent health behaviors over time in two Minnesota Heart Health Program communities.

The sample consisted of 2376 sixth graders enrolled in public schools in both communities in April 1983, who volunteered to participate in a baseline survey. This sample was followed annually in April until their graduation from high school in 1989. The students in the intervention group participated in 5 years of Minnesota Heart Health Program-sponsored behavioral health programs in schools from 6th through 10th grade. A control group did not receive the health programs but were given the usual health-related education in the curriculum. During this period, smoking behavior, healthy food choices, and exercise patterns were tracked by self-report.

Data analysis revealed, according to self-report, that students who participated in the intervention or education program were less likely to become smokers and were more likely to maintain healthy food choices and maintain more activity or hours of exercise per week. There was a progressive increase in the change to weekly smoking status. If students began to experiment with smoking, they were more likely to either begin to be or remain regular smokers. In food choices and exercises, individuals continued behaviors that were reported at baseline. These results indicate that there is consolidation and stability in physical activity, food preference, and smoking behavior, and behavioral patterns are resistant to change. Smoking results indicate that students experience difficulty with quitting smoking. Nicotine addiction begins early in use of tobacco and a large percentage of students who tried to quit returned to smoking unless they participated in a smoking cessation program.

Limitations to the study are that self-report was not verified with objective measurements, and these data do not include students who dropped out of school. Health care implications include the importance of early health education, preferably before 6th grade, and youth smoking cessation programs during the 9th and 10th years.

- Choosing meaningful stimuli and useful conditions
- Maintaining reality

When a strong ego exists, the person can do all these tasks. He or she has entered adulthood psychologically. Adolescence provides the experiences necessary for such maturity.

Ego changes occur in the adolescent because of broadening social involvement, deepening intellectual pursuits, close peer activity, rapid physical growth, and social role changes, all of which cause frustrations at times. **Frustration** is the *feeling of helplessness and anxiety that results when one is prevented from getting what one wants.* Adaptive mechanisms leading to resolution of frustration and reconciling personal impulses with social expectations are beneficial because they permit the self to settle dissonant drives and to cope with strong feelings. All adaptive mechanisms permit one to develop a self, an identity, and to defend the self-image against attack. These mechanisms are harmful only when one pattern is used to the exclusion of others for handling many diverse situations or when several mechanisms are used persistently to cope with a single situation. Such behavior is defensive rather than adaptive, distorts reality, and indicates emotional disturbance.

The adaptive mechanisms used in adolescence are the same ones used (and defined) in previous developmental eras, although they now may be used in a different way.

Compensation, a form of compromise, *sublimation,* and *identification* are particularly useful because they often improve interaction with others. They are woven into the personality to make permanent character changes, and they help the person reach appropriate goals.

Teach parents that adaptive abilities of the adolescent are strongly influenced by inner resources built up through the years of parental love, esteem, and guidance. The parents' use of adaptive mechanisms and general mental health will influence the offspring. Are the parents living a double standard? Has the teenager seen the parents enjoy a job well done or is financial reward the key issue? Do the parents covertly wish the teenager to act out what they could never do?

Even with mature parents, the adolescent will at times find personal adaptive abilities taxed. But the chances for channeling action-oriented energy and idealism through acceptable adaptive behavior are much greater if parents set a positive example.

Other factors influence ability to adapt to stress and the adaptive mechanisms that will be used. Adolescents from upper and middle socioeconomic levels report that the life events that were most stressful to them agreed with what adults consider the most stressful life change (129). Upper-class adolescents included "quitting school" and "parent losing a job" as more stressful than individuals of other ages and socioeconomic levels; and the importance of education and occupation are related to socioeconomic level. Middle-class adolescents viewed drug and alcohol abuse and hassling with parents as more stressful, which is reflective of middle-class moral values. Middle-class adolescents revealed more reliance on physical appearance than upper-class teenagers; the advantages of family status and more money for clothing and entertaining may make the upper-class adolescent less dependent on appearance for social acceptance. Items written in as stressful life events for both classes were "wrecking the car," "not getting selected for an activity," "brother getting someone pregnant," and "sister getting pregnant." Age in this sample was not a significant variable in scaling the events, but the number of events experienced increased with age. Girls perceive more events as more stressful than boys (129).

Moral–Spiritual Development

Refer to Kohlberg's Theory of Moral Development presented in Table 5–12. According to Kohlberg (113) the adolescent probably is in the Conventional Level most of the time; however, the adolescent may at times show behavior appropriate to the second stage of the Preconventional Level or the first stage of the Postconventional Level.

The early adolescent typically is in the conformist stage; structure and order of society take on meaning for the person, and rules are followed because they exist (analogous to Kohlberg's Conventional Level). The late adolescent is in the conscientious stage, in which the person develops a set of principles for self that is used to guide personal ideals, actions, and achievements. Rational thought becomes important to personal growth (analogous to Kohlberg's Post-Conventional Level, stage 1) (152). The young adolescent must examine parental moral and religious verbal standards against practice and decide if they are worth incorporating into his or her own life. He or she may appear to discard standards of behavior previously accepted, although basic parental standards likely will be maintained. In addition, he or she must compare the religious versus the scientific views. Although moral–spiritual views of sensitivity, caring, and commitment may be prevalent in family teaching, the adolescent in the United States is also a part of the scientific, technologic, industrial society that emphasizes achievement, fragmentation, and regimentation. Often youth will identify with one of the two philosophies (58). These two views can be satisfactorily combined but only with sufficient time and experience, which the adolescent has not had (15, 121).

Gilligan has found a difference between adolescent males and females in moral reasoning. Males organize social relationships in a hierarchical order and subscribe to a morality of rights. Females value interpersonal connectedness, care, sensitivity, and responsibility to others. Thus, adolescent males and females view the dating relationship differently and approach aggressive or violent situations from a different perspective (137). Other authors describe how our society interferes with development of moral standards or behavior (11, 82, 130, 194) so that neither Kohlberg's nor Gilligan's theory seems applicable.

If the adolescent matures in religious belief, he or she must comprehend abstractions. Often when he or she is capable of the first religious insights, the negativism tied with rebellion to authority prevents this experience.

Probably by age 16 the youth will make a decision. He or she will accept or reject the family religion. If the parents represent two faiths, the teen may choose one or the other or neither. He or she may be influenced by a friend or someone who is admired. He or she may have a religious awakening experience in the form of a definite crisis called, by some, **conversion,** or **getting saved.** *This connotes an emotional and mental decision to conform to some religious pattern.* The form may be a definite but not dramatic decision at a confirmation or first communion. Another form is the gradual awakening, one that is not completely accomplished in adolescence.

Help parents and adolescents realize that the adolescent who does find strength in the supernatural, who can rely on a power greater than self, can find much consolation in this turbulent period of awkward physical and emotional growth. If he or she can pray for help, ask forgiveness, and believe he or she receives both, a more positive self-image develops. In this period of clique and group dominance, the church is a place to meet friends, to share recreation and fellowship, and to sense a belonging difficult to find in some large high schools.

Adolescents whose faith is mixed with some God fearing are probably less likely to experiment in behavior they have been taught will bring them harm. Adolescents who have been taught that they are part of a divine plan and who have been given a specific moral code may better answer the essential questions, "Who am I?" "Where am I going?" "What meaning is there in life?" Adolescents who have been raised very strictly, however, may instead develop a reaction formation pattern of adjustment—rebelling and pursuing the previously forbidden activities.

The following methods of moral development have been most widely used: setting an example, persuading, limiting choices, dramatizing, establishing rules and regulations, teaching religious or cultural dogma, and appealing to conscience. Advice, approval, commands, lessons, sermons, warnings, criticisms, and interrogation have produced few results in the field of ethical development. Recent experiments show that a Socratic approach, which promotes moral development and clarifies values, produces fruitful results that have not been achieved by simply handing down rules of conduct. You can be instrumental in working with parents and teachers to use the Socratic approach and other value clarification exercises (113). Shelton (170) also discusses ways to promote moral decision making.

Late Adolescence: Transition Period to Young Adulthood

In some cultures parents select schooling, occupations, and the marriage partner for their offspring. In the United States the youth is usually free to make some or all of these decisions. Dobson writes about the dilemmas that face the teen as he or she moves through late adolescence into young adulthood (*Life On the Edge*, Word Publishing, Dallas, 1995).

By the time the youth is a junior or senior in high school, he or she should be thinking about the future: whether to pursue a mechanical or academic job; to attend some form of higher education; to live at home or elsewhere; to travel; to marry soon, later, or not at all; to have children soon, later, or not at all. Answers to these questions will influence the adolescent's transition into young adulthood.

Those who seem not to be making the transition into young adulthood—who continue to rebel against society, who wander from job to job or from college to college, who rely heavily on drugs and alcohol or sexual exploitation for emotional "highs," who cannot seem to make decisions about the future—may be the children of affluent parents and may not have had to become independent. The parents continue to dole out money and demands. The money is taken; the demands are ignored.

Establishing a Separate Residence

This step is one marker of reaching young adulthood. The late adolescent often spends less time at home and prepares for separation from parents. If there is intense intrafamily conflict, if the adolescent feels unwanted, or if the adolescent is still struggling with dependence on parents or identity diffusion, a different mode of separation may occur.

In an effort to find self and think about the future or to escape abuse, incest, or other home problems, the adolescent may become either a walkaway or a runaway. The **teen walkaway** *leaves home before finishing high school or before reaching legal age; however, parents generally know where the child is and are resigned to the child's new living arrangements.* The **teen runaway** *leaves home without overt notice and his or her whereabouts are unknown to parents, friends, or police.* Some walkaways may continue high school or get some type of job while living with relatives, friends, or a boyfriend or girlfriend. The problem with the walkaway is that the adolescent can achieve developmental tasks better in a stable family situation in which parents continue to give support and assist him or her as necessary while treating the offspring in an adult manner. If the newly found living situation is unstable or emotionally unsupportive or if the adolescent has no means of financial support, he or she may be forced into prostitution or juvenile offenses (23, 121).

You may have an opportunity to discuss residence situations with the adolescent. If you can get to the person before he or she walks or runs away, help him or her consider the intolerability of parental demands and the family situation. Discuss alternative ways of handling the problem. You may contact a high school counselor or potential employer. Although either the walkaway or runaway situation should be avoided if possible, the teen should be encouraged to report incest or abuse so that the teen's parents and other siblings can receive proper therapy and an appropriate, healthy living situation can be found for the teen.

Health care is a problem for adolescent runaways. Refer to the article by Manov and Lowther (125), which describes general health problems and sex-related health concerns such as pregnancy, sexually transmitted diseases, prostitution, alcohol abuse, and child abuse and incest. The following intervention strategies are described: (1) clarification of the health care provider's attitudes and values; (2) establishment of trust; (3) use of effective interviewing skills; (4) ability to provide maximum medical treatment and information when the client presents self for care; and (5) establishment of foundations for future interactions and care (125).

Career Selection

This selection has often been haphazard. High school counselors often do more record keeping than realistic guiding toward career choices. Often youth are influenced by parental wishes or friend's choices. Because of changes in societal role expectations for men and women, jobs or college study programs that were once considered exclusively "male" or "female" are now open to both. A woman may now comfortably major in mathematics, architecture, or medicine. A man may study home economics or nursing. A woman may be a lineman for the telephone company, and a man may be an operator.

Although these changes are positive, understand that the selection is more vast and thus more confusing to adolescents. You can guide them to testing centers in which their skills and interests are measured and jobs are recommended. You may direct them to members of various professions who can tell them about their jobs. You also must be aware of the national adolescent mood. Group biases and fads should not dictate career choices that do not coincide with the person's skills.

Occupation represents much more than a set of skills and functions; it is a way of life. Occupation provides and determines much of the physical and social environment in which a person lives, his or her status within the community, and a pattern for living. Occupational choice is usually a function or a reflection of the entire personality, but the occupation, in turn, plays a part in shaping the personality by providing associates, roles, goals, ideals, mores, lifestyle, and perhaps even a spouse.

For many youth the college years are a time to consider various careers, to decide what type of people he or she wishes to associate with and imitate, and to measure self against others with similar aspirations.

Although college attendance and pursuit of a profession are still the ideal of many, growing emphasis and opportunity exist for vocational and technical training. Many will enter jobs right out of high school.

You can be a key person in helping adolescents clarify values and attitudes related to occupational selection and in talking with parents about their concerns.

Moral–spiritual development may take on a special significance if the adolescent period is extended into the twenties because of college education or military duty. Instead of settling into the tasks coexistent with marriage, job, and family, the adolescent has a period in which a great deal of thinking can be accomplished. He or she has passed the physically awkward stage so that time and energy formerly spent in making the transition into physical adulthood can be turned toward philosophy.

The midtwenties apparently is the least religious period in life. College youth and late adolescents often reject affiliation with their childhood church. Perhaps it is part of their break from dependence to independence. They also are secure in pursuing their ambitions; they are not yet aware that their goals may not be met. They do not yet have children whom they want to educate to a religion; and they have not developed a perspective about the importance of their own upbringing. Yet these late adolescents are often altruistic: they wish to help others, defend a cause, and do not hesitate to devote many hours of the day to their goals.

Veterans, especially combat returnees or prisoners of war, are in a difficult position. The protective childhood religion of fantasy, left in some, is forcibly removed as they experience violence, torture, hatred—the worst of human nature. If they salvage a religious experience, it is one of maturity.

Explore moral–spiritual development with adolescents and parents. Your own behavior may be the best teacher.

Developmental Tasks

The following developmental tasks should be met by the end of adolescence (49, 87):

- Accepting the changing body size, shape, and function and understanding the meaning of physical maturity
- Learning to handle the body in a variety of physical skills and to maintain good health

- Achieving a satisfying and socially accepted feminine or masculine role, recognizing how these roles have similarities and distinctions
- Finding the self as a member of one or more peer groups and developing skills in relating to a variety of people, including those of the opposite sex
- Achieving independence from parents and other adults while maintaining an affectionate relationship with them
- Selecting an occupation in line with interests and abilities (although the choice of occupation may later change) and preparing for economic independence
- Preparing to settle down, frequently for marriage and family life or for a close relationship with another, by developing a responsible attitude, acquiring needed knowledge, making appropriate decisions, and forming a relationship based on love rather than infatuation
- Developing the intellectual and work skills and social sensitivities of a competent citizen
- Desiring and achieving socially responsible behavior in the cultural setting
- Developing a workable philosophy, a mature set of values, and worthy ideals and assuming standards of morality

Until these tasks are accomplished, the person remains immature, an adolescent regardless of chronologic age. How you interact with, or teach other adults to interact with, the adolescent will contribute to the adolescent's maturity.

► HEALTH CARE AND NURSING APPLICATIONS

Scope of the Health Care and Nursing Role

Your role in caring for the adolescent may be many faceted. Astute assessment is needed; knowledge from this chapter and relationship and communication principles described in Chapter 5 may be useful in gaining information from a client or family who may be hesitant to disclose about self. *Nursing diagnoses* that may be applicable to the adolescent are listed in Selected Nursing Diagnoses Related to the Adolescent. Interventions that may involve direct care to the ill adolescent or that involve various health promotion measures are described in the previous or following sections.

A mature and maturing body and an immature emotional state make the adolescent a source of misunderstanding, fear, and laughter. Mood swings, rebel-

lious behavior, and adherence to colorful fads baffle many adults, who then cannot look beyond the superficial behavior to identify health needs. Yet health care needs of today's adolescents are great.

Millions of teenagers in the United States between the ages of 13 and 19 are sexually active. Many adolescent girls from 13 to 19 years of age become pregnant each year. A number of adolescents will run away from home. A significant number of youths will die from motor vehicle and other accidents, unintended firearms injury, and homicide and suicide (197). Other health problems abound, including sexually transmitted diseases, substance abuse, chronic illness, and obesity and nutritional deficiency (the latter two previously discussed). Although the scope of this book does not allow discussion of needs assessment and intervention for adolescents with physical disabilities, you may wish to consult several references for information (22, 31 94, 171, 187, 197).

Health Promotion and Health Protection

Immunizations

Immunizations are a part of health protection to the adolescent, although they may be overlooked by that time of life. You should take a careful health history. If the immunizations discussed in relation to other age groups have not been received, they should be given as indicated. If the adolescent has been routinely immunized, combined tetanus and diphtheria toxiods (adult-type Td) should be given near 14 to 16 years of age and every 10 years thereafter. This preparation contains less diphtheria antigen than the DTP preparations given to children (27, 186).

The oral form of polio virus (POV) is recommended for all children younger than 18 years of age unless contraindicated. Influenza virus vaccine, pneumococcal polysaccharide vaccine, and hepatitis B vaccine should be given to adolescents in selected high-risk groups. Anyone who was not immunized for measles, rubella, or mumps should be immunized at this time. For clean wounds, no tetanus booster is needed by a fully immunized person unless more than 10 years has elapsed since the last dose. For dirty or contaminated wounds, a booster dose can be given if more than 5 years has elapsed since the last dose. Pertussis vaccine should not be given to anyone over 6 years of age. Periodic testing for tuberculosis should be included in all adolescent immunization programs (27, 197). See Chart 4 in Appendix IV.

Your actions and teaching in relation to immunizations are important for the teenager's health now and in the adult years.

SELECTED NURSING DIAGNOSES RELATED
TO THE ADOLESCENT*

Pattern 1: Exchanging
Altered Nutrition: More than Body Requirements
Altered Nutrition: Less than Body Requirements
Altered Nutrition: Potential for More Than Body Requirements
Risk for Infection
Risk for Injury
Risk for Trauma
Impaired Skin Integrity
Pattern 2: Communicating
Impaired Verbal Communication
Pattern 3: Relating
Impaired Social Interaction
Social Isolation
Altered Sexuality Patterns
Pattern 4: Valuing
Spiritual Distress
Pattern 5: Choosing
Ineffective Individual Coping
Impaired Adjustment
Defensive Coping
Ineffective Denial
Decisional Conflict
Health-Seeking Behaviors

Pattern 6: Moving
Fatigue
Risk for Activity Intolerance
Sleep Pattern Disturbance
Diversional Activity
Altered Growth and Development
Pattern 7: Perceiving
Body Image Disturbance
Self-Esteem Disturbance
Chronic Low Self-Esteem
Situational low Self-Esteem
Personal Identity Disturbance
Sensory/Perceptual Alterations
Hopelessness
Powerlessness
Pattern 8: Knowing
Knowledge Deficit
Pattern 9: Feeling
Pain
Dysfunctional Grieving
Anticipatory Grieving
Post-Trauma Response
Anxiety
Fear

*Other NANDA diagnoses are applicable to the ill adolescent.
From North American Nursing Diagnosis Association, NANDA Nursing Diagnoses Definitions & Classification 1995–1996. Philadelphia:North American Nursing Diagnosis Association, 1994.

Safety Promotion and Accident Prevention

Accidents, homicide, and suicide are responsible for approximately 75% of all deaths between the ages of 15 and 24. *Motor vehicle accidents* account for nearly half of the deaths of adolescents between the ages of 16 and 19 (32% of all deaths in persons 15 to 24 years) and are more common among young drivers who use alcohol, marijuana, and other drugs while driving (31, 59, 186, 197). One of the biggest adolescent–parent hurdles comes with learning to drive. The adolescent needs to learn this skill; yet the arguments between parents and their children concerning how to drive, what vehicle to drive, and where to go or not to go often keep parents in a state of anxiety and children in a state of rebellion.

Head and spinal cord injuries, skeletal injuries, abrasions, and burns may all result from an accident involving a car, motorcycle, motor scooter, moped, all-terrain vehicle, snowmobile, or minibike, or from the worksite as cited by Parker et al. (149). Sports-related accidents such as drowning, football, hockey, gymnastic and soccer injuries, and firearm mishaps are also common. Contusions, dislocations, sprains, strains, overuse syndromes, and stress fractures occur frequently (72). In the adolescent the epiphyses of the skeletal system have not yet closed, and the extremities are poorly protected by stabilizing musculature. These two physical factors, combined with poor coordination and imperfect sport skills, probably account for the numerous injuries (197).

Homicide is the second leading cause of death in the 15- to 24-year-old group and is the leading cause of death among non-Caucasian youths in this age group. Handguns are the most frequently used weapons (194, 197). Use of weapons in schools is a national concern, but intentional injury and death to others as a leisure activity, with no remorse involved, is a way of life for some adolescents (11, 82, 130, 194).

Suicide, the third leading cause of death, is discussed later in this chapter. (Non-motor-vehicle injuries are the fourth leading cause of death.)

As a group, adolescents represent one of the nation's largest underserved populations.

A review of the leading causes of mortality and morbidity among youth shows that nearly all contributory behaviors can be categorized in the following six areas (188):

1. Behaviors that result in unintentional and intentional injuries
2. Drug and alcohol use
3. Tobacco use
4. Sexual behaviors that cause sexually transmitted diseases, including HIV infection, and unintended pregnancies
5. Inadequate physical activity
6. Dietary patterns that cause disease

The Centers for Disease Control and Prevention (CDC) started a surveillance system in 1988, and in 1990 started offering each state and funded local education agencies assistance in conducting a Youth Risk Survey. The resultant program to cut down on high-risk behaviors will be offered through school health programs and through Guidelines for Adolescent Preventive Services (GAPS) developed by the American Medical Association (188).

Safety Education

Safety courses, including driver education, knowledge of safety programs in the community, instruction in water safety, routine safety practices, and emergency care measures should be required for every adolescent. Many accidents and deaths could be avoided if the adolescent were better equipped to handle the new freedom. As an informed citizen in the community or in relation to your job, you can initiate and teach in such programs with the school, church, clinic, industry, Red Cross, or other civic organizations. If you do not teach, you can insist on qualified and objective instruction. Parents and youths should be informed about the dangers and the exercise and prestige value involved with certain sports and privileges. A teenage safety checklist

can be obtained from the National Society for Crippled Children and Adults, 2023 W. Ogden Ave., Chicago, IL 60612, to help the adolescent be aware of how to improve safety behavior.

Because of the sports activities in which adolescents are involved, they may sometimes experience musculoskeletal chest pain, minor strains or sprains to a joint, and minor ankle strain. You should know how to advise for these conditions.

Musculoskeletal chest pain *arises from the bony structures of the rib cage and upper-limb girdle, along with the related skeletal muscles.* Age does not automatically rule out heart-related problems. Although musculoskeletal pain is usually aggravated by activity that involves movement or pressure on the chest cage rather than by general exertion (such as stair climbing), a thorough lung and cardiac examination is merited. Applying heat to the area (unless it is a fresh injury), resting the area, and taking an antipyretic can be recommended (94).

Minor strains and sprains to a joint involve a *mild trauma that results in minimal stretching of involved ligaments and contusion of the surrounding tissues.* The treatment is immobilization of the affected joint and use of an ice pack for 24 to 36 hours. Local heat can then be used if needed. Aspirin, if tolerated, can be used for its analgesic and anti-inflammatory effects (94).

A **minor ankle sprain** involving *stretching of the ligament without tearing* can be treated the same as minor strains and sprains with the addition of an Ace bandage and possibly keeping weight off the ankle longer than 24 to 36 hours through the use of crutches (94).

Common Health Problems: Prevention and Treatment

As you care for the adolescent, refer to the American Academy of Family Physicians Periodic Health Examination for ages 13 to 18 years (Table 11–7) for a schedule of health screening measures, immunizations, counseling, and high-risk categories (2). Several references describe how to conduct physical assessments with the adolescent (12, 22, 94, 124, 171, 197).

In addition to the hazards of accidents, health problems other than obesity, and teenage pregnancy, already discussed, are also apparent among adolescents. Table 11–2 summarizes definitions, symptoms and signs, and prevention and treatment for common conditions (12, 32, 94, 124).

Cardiovascular disease is the fifth leading cause of death. Although essential hypertension is consistently higher in African-American adults than in Caucasian adults, the same does not hold true for adolescents.

TABLE 11–2. COMMON HEALTH PROBLEMS OF ADOLESCENTS

Problem	Definition	Symptoms/Signs	Prevention/Treatment
Hordeolum (stye)	Localized infection of sebaceous gland on eyelid margin	Painful, reddened swelling on eyelid; sometimes drainage	Apply hot compresses. Administer antibiotic drops.
Epistaxis (nose bleed)	Spontaneous bleeding from nose caused by ruptured blood vessel	Bleeding from nose	Prevent dry and cracking nasal mucosa by keeping humidity level sufficient. If nose bleeds, sit with head slightly forward and pinch nostrils for at least 15 minutes. Use cold compresses.
Acne vulgaris	Comedones, pimples, and cysts formed from increased activity of sebaceous glands	"Blackheads," "whiteheads," and additional lesions, especially on face, chest, back	Use good hygiene techniques and cleansing agents. Apply topical preparations. Administer oral medications.
Dental caries and gingivitis	Decay of teeth and disease of gums	Broken, dark teeth; bleeding inflamed gums	Use good dental hygiene. Check periodically with a dental hygienist for education and treatment.
Aphthous stomatitis	Recurrent small painful ulcers in the oral mucosa, "canker sores"; unknown etiology, *not* herpes simplex	Burning and tingling before eruption; recurrent painful lesions from 1 to 10 mm; oval, shallow, light yellow or gray with erythematous border	Prevention: None is known. Use Kenalog in Orabase or other topical anesthetic. Use tetracycline/Benadryl mouthwash.
Tinea cruris	Ringworm of the groin, "jock itch," superficial fungal infection of the groin	Rash and soreness on groin and inner aspects of thighs; may include scrotum, gluteal folds, buttocks	Eliminate sources of heat and friction. Bathe daily; dry thoroughly. Wear cotton underwear. Use antifungal cream and Domeboro solution compresses.
Tinea pedis (athlete's foot)	Fungal infection affecting feet, especially toe webs	Intense itching; cracking; peeling	Soak feet and dry well. Apply antifungal agent. Wear clean cotton socks.
Infectious mononucleosis (mono)	Condition caused by Epstein–Barr virus	Fever, sore throat, enlarged lymph nodes; general malaise; enlarged spleen; sometimes jaundice	Treat symptoms: use rest, increased fluid intake, antipyretic, good nutrition.
Hepatitis A virus (HAV)	Inflammation of hepatocytes of liver caused by viruses, bacteria, drugs, chemicals; transmitted via fecal contamination of food or water with subsequent close person-to-person contact (25% of hepatitis cases)	Fatigue, anorexia, swollen glands; aversion to smoking (if smokes); short incubation period: 15–45 days	Prevention: stay in good physical condition. If condition develops, prevent transfer. Treat symptoms.
Hepatitis B virus (HBV)	Transmitted via blood, primarily parentally, although person-to-person contact possible (50% of hepatitis cases)	Prodromal stage: 2–20 days; jaundice phase: 2–8 weeks; recovery phase: 2–24 weeks	Vaccine is available; take recommended precautions. Treat symptoms. Avoid complications.
Hepatitis C virus (HCV) (non-A, non-B) and other types (D = HDV, E = HEV)	Diagnosed by deduction (25% of hepatitis cases)	Hepatitis symptoms; history of transfusion (HDV); history of fecal–oral route (HEV); some serologic markers	Treat symptoms.
Rocky Mountain spotted fever	Acute febrile disease caused by *Rickettsia rickettsii*; passed to human by bite of infected tick	Symptoms start in 2 days to 2 weeks: headache, fever, rash on hands and feet, pain in back and leg muscles	Prevention: Be aware of problem and appropriate removal of ticks. Treatment: Administer tetracycline.
Lyme disease	Tickborne disease introduced by the spirochete *Borrelia burgdorferi* from animal host to human (ticks are only 1–2 mm)	Early (3 or 4 days after bite): ringlike rash at bite site (approximately 4 in. in diameter) then secondary lesion, flulike symptoms, sometimes cardiac problems (10%); in 4 weeks neurologic problems (in 15%); in 6 weeks to 1 year, arthralgias and synovitis (in 50%)	Administer antibiotic (doxycycline). Provide rest and healthy diet. Treat symptoms. Prevent through education.

Neoplasms, both benign and malignant, are a major cause of death (197). Females exposed to diethylstilbestrol (DES) in utero should be watched closely for adenocarcinoma of the vagina. Males exposed to DES in utero have an increase in urinary tract abnormalities and a higher incidence of infertility (197). Dysplasia of the cervix, a precursor of cervical carcinoma, is a sexually transmitted disease that is occurring with increased frequency in adolescent females. Sexually active females should receive annual Pap smears. Testicular cancer, Hodgkin's disease, and certain bone cancers are not uncommon in this age group (187, 197).

Allergic dermatitis, cysts, and keloid formation of the earlobes are also seen with more frequency, as ear piercing has become popular. Inner ear damage from exposure to rock music is increasing and can be assessed by pure tone audiometry. The adolescent is also subject to postural defects, fatigue, anemia, and respiratory problems. Discuss prevention of these problems with adolescents.

Chronic Illness in Adolescents

It is estimated that 50% of Americans have one or more chronic conditions; about 15% of the population have chronic conditions that limit activity. Chronically ill children constitute 10 to 20% of those who are hospitalized, and advances in technology and medical practice also enable some children and adults to live longer with chronic conditions. With some chronic illnesses, such as diabetes, the issues may revolve around mealtime routines, adherence to medication or treatment schedules, daily bodily care, use of the family car, family rules, and being on one's own at parties. Death is not imminent; a change in lifestyle for the entire family will be. The family unit, with its unique parenting style, marital satisfaction, and parental self-esteem, will have an impact on the offspring. Illness brings the stress of pain, body mutilation, and body image changes and possible death. Chronic illness adds stressors: lifestyle changes, dependency on others, developmental delay, failure to master expected social roles and developmental tasks, a drain in emotional resources, disruption of the family system, and financial difficulties (86, 108).

Adolescents have a particularly difficult time dealing emotionally with chronic illness because they feel different than and set apart from peers, may have fewer peer relationships and activities in which they can participate, and thereby have a disruption of the social support system. Psychosocial problems can lead to social disabilities that far outweigh the effects of the physical illness (86, 108).

Positive coping in the ill adolescent is associated with independent behaviors, peer contact, school achievement, and participation in normalization activities. Negative coping centers around fear, withdrawal, regression, use of symptoms for secondary pain, and low self-esteem (86, 108).

Mothers tend to bear the brunt of caring for the chronically ill child. Usually mothers, rather than fathers, suffer loss of social life. Some fathers exclude themselves from care of the disabled child and from the family, which contributes to poor marital adjustment and relationship difficulties with the children (174).

Nurses are the health providers in the most critical position to assess coping strategies of the chronically ill individual and the family and to assist the family with the physical care, to cope with the impact of the chronic illness, and to practice stress management (86, 108).

Suicide

Suicide ranks as the third most frequent cause of death in adolescence (4, 19, 73, 78, 85, 88, 180, 186, 187, 197), and fourth as a cause of death, after cancer, in women ages 15 to 24 (89). Suicide in adolescents is frequently reported as an accidental death. Motor vehicle accidents, drug and alcohol overdose, firearm accidents, and even homicides can be disguised suicides (19). Psychological, social, and physiologic stressors are the apparent causes for the rising number of suicides. Television dramatizations on the nightly news or in movies of teenage suicides appear to contribute to an increased wave of teenage suicide attempts and successes (177).

Adolescents who attempt suicide often come from families who have nonproductive communication patterns, inconsistent positive reinforcement behaviors, and a high level of conflict or child abuse. Suicides occur in rich and poor, urban and rural families. Adolescent suicides occur most frequently in 15- to 25-year-old Caucasian males; African-American male incidence is lower. Females are now using forms of suicide usually associated with males. The males, however, are more successful, more violent, and less likely to give warning before the suicidal act (50, 78).

Frequently physical fatigue contributes to the emotional stress that precipitates a suicide attempt. Most adolescents have short bouts with suicidal preoccupations in the presence of these stresses. Sometimes even a small disappointment or frustration can lead to an impulsive suicidal attempt. Often the impulsive acts are committed to force parents to pay attention to the adolescent's pleas for help and get needs met. Because the adolescent often feels great ambivalence toward parents, he or she rejects parents and yet solicits love, sometimes by attempting suicide. In reality the parents may be giving all the love they can. In other situations

► WARNING SIGNS FOR SUICIDE AND INTERVENTIONS IN ADOLESCENTS

Loss of Someone or Something Important

- (The greater the number of losses in a short period, the higher the risk)
- Death
- Divorce
- Move to new school or geographic location
- Job
- Self-esteem related to poor relationship or loss of status
- Prolonged family disruption
- Pet
- Health

Feelings and Behaviors of Depression

- Change in daily habits
- Changed eating or sleeping patterns
- Lack of energy; fatigue; weakness; extreme lethargy
- Problems of concentration; slow speech or movements
- Drop in grades or work performance
- Neglecting appearance more so than usual
- Lack of friends or interests
- Truancy at school or poor work attendance
- Increase in drug or alcohol use; excessive smoking
- Appearing sad, angry, sullen, irritable most of time; mood swings
- Accident proneness
- Increase in promiscuity
- Continuous acting out that masks other behavior
- Negative self-concept; feeling unloved, rejected, guilty, hopeless

Statements About Suicide

- Direct or indirect statements about a plan
- Thought + Action = Suicide Attempt or Success

Behavioral Actions or Changes

- Subtle or abrupt, different than norm
- History of suicide attempt
- Giving away prized possessions
- Withdrawal from activities and friends
- Writing, art work, or talking about suicide and death
- Accident proneness
- Crying for no apparent reason
- Depressed mood quickly lifts
- Value physical complaints
- Listening only to music about death

High Risk Symptoms

- A clear plan with time and details, using a lethal method
- Intoxication with drugs or alcohol
- Anniversary of the death of a loved one by suicide
- Auditory hallucinations telling the teen to die
- Extreme isolation and no support systems
- Feelings of hopelessness, helplessness, and worthlessness
- A previous suicide attempt using a lethal method and continued suicide ideation

Interventions

- Determine lethality
- Encourage communication with family, teachers, or other supportive adults
- Encourage appropriate expression of feeling, especially guilt and anger
- Use self-esteem building activities
- Encourage positive statements about self
- Assist the child to cope with the situation that is causing despair or sense of helplessness

---

the adolescent may be experiencing (1) an intense sense of loss, external or internal, real or imagined, that is believed permanent, or (2) anger at parents, teachers, or another significant person, and hurting self is a way to get even and make the other sorry for not treating the person right. Death is not seen as irreversible. If there is a history of family suicide, the adolescent may attempt reunion with the deceased, often on the anniversary of the suicide. Other reasons for suicide are discussed in references at the end of the chapter (4, 35, 78, 85, 88, 120, 160, 172, 175, 197, 202).

Signs of suicide are often subtle to detect, but a composite of behaviors should be a clue that the teen is experiencing severe stress. See Warning Signs for Suicide and Interventions in Adolescents for a list of behaviors associated with or indicators of suicide at-tempts (35, 66, 85, 151, 197, 202). Do not be afraid to ask if the youth has thought of suicide. The stressed person welcomes this query and the fact that you are taking the statements and behavior seriously.

The suicidal adolescent may be a loner at school and feel unable to meet scholastic expectations of parents. School performance often drops; there may be frequent absences. If peers state that a friend is suicidal, investigate their concerns. No threat should be ignored. Depression is found in two-thirds of suicidal adolescents; depression may be masked by a variety of symptoms, signs, or behavior (19, 35, 50, 83, 85, 88, 197, 202).

Rarely does the adolescent plan a suicide because he or she really wants to die. At times, however, when death is desired, the adolescent is engaging in self-destructive behavior as a punishment for guilt over actions or thoughts that he or she has committed or experienced. Ten percent of adolescents who attempt suicide make further attempts within a year (4, 50, 78, 197).

Screen for emotionally distressed adolescents and be available to listen to and ask about their problems. Take a careful history to identify the underlying stresses. Refer to several references for guidelines in assessing family and school indicators, personality traits, and danger signs (31, 51, 83, 85, 88, 160, 197, 202). If you believe you are unable to handle the situation, discuss it with the teen and refer him or her to a guidance counselor, nurse therapist, clergy, school psychologist, or private or school physician or psychiatrist. Frequently the adolescent will turn to an adult with whom he or she has had a personal relationship or sees as an advocate for youth. This relationship may help the adolescent through the present crisis. You can accept, support, inform, and serve as an advocate for youth, working with parents and adolescents (35, 163, 197, 202).

Follow-up care with the family and adolescent after suicidal gestures is important. Some adolescents who attempt suicide ultimately do commit suicide.

If the adolescent makes a suicide attempt, crisis intervention is essential after the necessary medical and physical care is given. The goals, once life is assured, are to help the person work through feelings that led to and resulted from the suicide attempt, feel hope, identify the problem, see alternative ways of handling it, and mobilize supportive others to continue caring contact with the client. The family also needs your support and help in working through their feelings of anxiety, shame, guilt, and anger. Murray and Huelskoetter describe effective intervention for the suicidal person and **postvention,** *care of the surviving family, friends, and peers of a successful suicide victim* (136).

Alcoholism and Alcohol Abuse

Alcohol intake among adolescents also has greatly increased in recent years, and it is the most commonly used psychoactive drug used by adolescents. Statistics vary with the geographic area and researcher. Ten to 20% of adolescents are problem drinkers (50, 59, 61, 103, 138, 187, 192, 197). Frequent, heavy drinking patterns often begin in the eighth grade and peak between the ages of 18 and 22. More than a million Americans from the ages of 10 to 19 are addicted to liquor (59, 138, 192). Most states restrict the purchase and consumption of alcohol to people over 18 or 21 years of age, but this does little to prevent the underage drinker from acquiring alcohol when desired.

Adolescents drink because drinking is a widespread social custom in this country and drinking makes them feel more mature. The adolescent's drinking behavior is closely related to the drinking behavior of the parents and to peer-group pressure (59, 106, 136). The media also glamourize alcohol intake (6).

Adolescents who drink regularly generally start drinking at an unusually early age, and they use alcohol specifically for its mind-altering effects to participate in some activity that they would otherwise consider difficult or as a defense against depression, anxiety, fear, and anger. They become tolerant to the drug, and use of sedatives with alcohol is common. By the time they reach late adolescence, they may well be alcoholics (106, 127, 138, 183, 192, 197). (The person is often also abusing illicit drugs.) There are several programs in the United States for the rehabilitation of youthful alcoholics, such as Alateen.

The use of alcohol by adolescents has compounded the problem of motor vehicle injuries in youth. Overindulgence in alcohol impairs the ability of these inexperienced drivers and encourages risk taking while the adolescent is behind the wheel of the vehicle. The "rush" or "high" the teen feels from driving fast and alcohol intake is momentarily gratifying and stimulating but often fatal. Alcohol may also be involved in suicide attempts and drug-related deaths.

Medical hazards of alcohol abuse are numerous. All body systems may eventually become involved because of the toxic effects of alcohol, including the following conditions (48, 61, 136, 138, 197):

- Gastritis (nausea, vomiting, headache, gastric pain; may vomit blood or ropy, thick mucus)
- Pancreatitis (severe abdominal pain, nausea, vomiting)
- Hepatitis (fever, jaundice, abdominal edema, ankle and foot edema, tenderness in area of liver)
- Gastric and duodenal ulcers (vomiting of blood, severe pain, indurated abdomen; obstruction and perforation of stomach or intestine may occur)
- Impotency (inability to maintain or sustain erection)
- Neuritis (tingling, burning, itching, numbness, weakness, and finally paralysis of limbs if untreated)
- Fatty liver (enlarged liver on palpation; symptoms of hepatitis may persist)
- Cirrhosis (weight loss, chronic nausea, vomiting, weakness; impotency; abdominal pain; bloated, indurated abdomen; hemorrhage; seventh leading cause of death)

- Esophageal varices (varicose veins of the esophagus; internal hemorrhage may cause death)
- Degeneration of cerebellum (permanent loss of motor coordination, unsteady walk, tremors)
- Esophageal cancer (difficulty swallowing, sense of blockage behind sternum)
- Delirium tremens (withdrawal from alcohol causes tremors, sweating, nausea, insomnia, confusion, delusions, hallucinations, and convulsions; may be fatal 10% of the time)
- Birth defects (fetal alcohol syndrome; infant is underweight, has small brain and head size, may have cleft palate and congenital heart defect; slow growth in childhood; slower mental development)

Various other health problems, injuries, or death may result from alcohol abuse, including (1) automobile accidents; (2) suicide (more than 60% of fatal accidents and suicides involve alcohol); (3) fire deaths (50%); (4) choking on foods (25% of these deaths); (5) freezing to death (20% of these deaths); (6) drowning (20% of these deaths); (7) accidental asphyxiations (20%); and (8) falls (20% of all falls) (59, 61, 197).

Social problems, which may in turn cause physical and emotional health problems (and death), that arise from alcohol abuse include child and spouse abuse and homicide (a large percentage of violent crimes involve alcohol).

Avoid lecturing to adolescents about the hazards of drinking and driving and the medical effects of drinking. Help the person to clarify values about healthful activities and see the detrimental effects of drinking—physically, emotionally, mentally, and socially. Point out people who have suffered the ill effects of excessive alcohol intake. Teach adolescents how to identify hazards and to act responsibly to avoid injury to themselves and others.

Care of the alcoholic person and family is complex; specific measures vary with the stage of alcoholism and manifestations of the disease. For additional information on the needs of and nursing care for alcoholics, refer to references at the end of the chapter (6, 16, 60, 85, 91, 105, 106, 115, 136, 138, 183, 192, 197, 202).

Conditions Associated With Sexual Activity

Sexual decision making and premarital coitus were controlled in the past by family, social, and religious rules and restrictions. Today sexual activity is almost completely regarded as an individual responsibility. Because of the emotional and social characteristics of adolescents, the individual may have neither the readiness or desire to engage in sexual activity nor the decision-making skills *and* ego strength to behave counter to the peer group in order to abstain. Educationwise, there is not much to help the adolescent develop the necessary decision-making or value-clarification skills or the emotional strengths to be autonomous from the group or to avoid what is perceived as expected behavior. Add to that the stimulating influence of mass media, and the adolescent may feel caught. Growing up in poor neighborhoods seems to increase teenage pregnancy rates, especially for African Americans (128).

The areas related to the adolescent's sexual activity that influence health are those involving sexually transmitted diseases and the use of contraceptives, pregnancy, and abortion. A careful history is essential.

Sexually Transmitted Diseases. **Sexually transmitted diseases (STDs),** are *infections grouped together because they spread by transfer of infectious organisms from person to person during sexual contact, either through sexual intercourse, oral sex, or anal sex.* STD is currently replacing the term *venereal disease* (VD), defined as a *condition of the genital organs usually acquired through sexual intercourse.* The very words *venereal disease* produce responses of fear, shame, guilt, anger, and disgust in most individuals. These feelings may impede a person from seeking medical help or telling who his or her contacts were, even though the person may know rationally that treatment is needed for self and the contacts. The term *sexually transmitted disease* is broader in scope; it covers diseases not included in the traditional definition.

Sexually transmitted diseases are a public health epidemic and a major problem because of high communicability. Reports of new cases represent a percentage of those affected (50, 139, 185, 200). Enormous human suffering, the cost of hundreds of millions of dollars, and the tremendous demands on health care facilities all result. The problem is rooted in ignorance, apathy, and neglect. Women and children bear an inordinate share of the problem—sterility, ectopic pregnancy, fetal and infant deaths, birth defects, and mental retardation. Cancer of the cervix may be linked to the sexually transmitted herpes II virus. Some of the specific reasons for the increase in recent years include changing sexual patterns, changing attitudes and cultural mores regarding sexual behavior, lack of understanding about STDs, the feeling of "it can't happen to me," breakdown of the family unit, increased mobility within the population, and the widespread use of contraceptives. Adolescents have many reasons for wanting to be sexually active, including to (1) enhance self-esteem; (2) have someone care about them; (3) experiment; (4) be accepted by peers; (5) feel grownup; (6) be close and touched by another; (7) feel pleasure or have fun;

(8) seek revenge; (9) determine normality; (10) love and be loved; and (11) gain control over another (31, 38, 50, 121, 139, 157, 185, 200, 202).

In 1992, of the 1 million reported infectious diseases in the United States, one half were gonorrhea. Together, gonorrhea, syphilis (113,000 cases,) and **AIDS** (45,000 cases) accounted for two thirds of all reportable infections. Three of the most prevalent STDs are not even reported on a national level: chlamydia, 4,000,000 cases; papilloma infections, 500,000 to 1,000,000 cases; and genital herpes, 200,000 to 500,000 cases (200). It is probable that all cases of STDs are not reported. AIDS is discussed primarily in Chapter 12, although reference to AIDS is made in Chapter 10 and later in this chapter. Table 11–3 compares the causes, common symptoms, prognosis, and treatment of gonorrhea, syphilis, and herpes genitalis, to assist you as you assess and care for clients (22, 26, 29, 50, 75, 94, 139, 187). Other sexually transmitted diseases include vaginitis, chlamydia, genital warts, and pubic lice. **Vaginitis** can be grouped into four categories—candidal, trichomonal, nonspecific, and chlamydial—that may or may not be related to sexual activity (94). Other sexually transmitted diseases are described in Table 11–4 to assist you in assessment and treatment, as well as prevention (22, 26, 75, 76, 94, 171, 185, 187, 188, 200).

Contraceptive Practices

Contraception, or **birth control,** is the *use of various devices, chemicals, or abortion to prevent or terminate pregnancy.* The adolescent may choose contraception to avoid pregnancy while continuing sexual activity. Contraceptive practices are summarized in Table 11–5 and additional information may be obtained from various references at the end of this chapter (31, 34, 50, 84, 94, 119, 135, 187, 197). Although contraceptives may prevent pregnancy (and sexually transmitted diseases when the contraceptive device is the condom), they have unwanted side effects or disadvantages. *The only way to avoid both pregnancy and the unwanted side effects is sexual abstinence.* Your approach and the structure of the health care environment are critical to the teenage female's adherence to instructions about contraceptive practices or abstinence.

A large percentage of the teens in the United States report having had sexual intercourse by age 18; education and contraceptive services have not kept abreast of the changing sexual mores. Some youth, however, do not use contraceptives because of misconceptions or ignorance about them, inability to secure appropriate contraceptives, inability to plan ahead for their actions, a belief that using contraceptives marks them as promiscuous, or rebelliousness. Males are less likely to recognize risk of pregnancy as a result of sexual activity, have less information about contraceptives, and are less supportive of contraceptive use than females. The attitude of the male may indeed influence the female toward sexual activity without contraceptive use, even though she realizes the hazards and wishes to avoid them (50, 114, 121, 157).

Adolescent Pregnancy

Adolescent pregnancy is at epidemic proportions and may occur even in pre-teens; most of the pregnancies are unplanned. African-American teen pregnancy rates are higher, although rates for pregnancy in Caucasian adolescents are increasing. Many teenage mothers are unmarried. The United States has one of the highest teenage pregnancy rates in the Western world (50, 84).

Unintended pregnancy causes much human misery—for the pregnant teen and her family and often for the offspring. (Refer to Chapter 6 also for effects of teen pregnancy.) Effects on the teen father are less well known (31, 116, 118, 185, 197).

Various factors influence whether the adolescent becomes pregnant. Although some pregnancies may be accidental, four other themes may underlie the mask of "accident" (202):

1. Self-destruction or self-hate
2. Rebellion, anger, hate, reverse aggressiveness toward parents and authority
3. Lack of responsibility for self and personal behavior, related to identity diffusion or confusion
4. Plea for attention and help, either from parents, the boy involved, or others.

Other factors and combinations of factors may also contribute to the teenage girl's becoming pregnant. Factors Influencing Incidence of Adolescent Pregnancy (see page 535) summarizes these factors (18, 25, 31, 50, 114, 154, 158, 176, 197).

The early adolescent is not physically, socially, emotionally, educationally, or economically ready for pregnancy or parenthood. The late adolescent is physically mature but may not be ready for pregnancy emotionally, socially, or economically. These latter factors override the biological advantages of early pregnancy and may account, in part, for the lack of health care that is sought during pregnancy. In turn, health providers often do not understand the needs underlying adolescents' behavior and thereby fail to provide the necessary services.

TABLE 11–3. COMPARISON OF GONORRHEA, SYPHILIS, AND HERPES GENITALIS

	Gonorrhea	Syphillis	Herpes Genitalis
Cause	*Neisseria gonorrhoeae*	*Treponema pallidum*	Herpes simplex virus, type 2 (HSV-2)
Incubation	3–9 days	10–90 days; average, 3 weeks	Several days to 3 weeks
Symptoms	Male: asymptomatic at times, including when organism lodged rectally; urethritis—thin, watery, white urethral discharge, becoming purulent; dysuria Female: asymptomatic in 60 to 90% of cases, including when organism lodged rectally; dysuria and vaginal discharge common symptoms; trichomoniasis vaginalis present in 50% of cases Both sexes: gonococcemia, systemic gonorrhea, with skin lesions, malaise, fever, tachycardia Other names: GC, Clap, Drip, Dose	Male and female: Stage 1 (primary): chancre—solitary, indurated, painless, ulceration on genitalia 10–28 days after sexual contact; lesion occasionally on mouth, nipples, anus; lesion healing within 4 to 6 weeks; treponemes multiplying rapidly Stage 2 (secondary): rash covering skin, mouth, and genitalia (red-copper on white skin, gray-blue on black skin; red rash on palms and soles); hair loss; eyes and ears inflamed; lymphadenitis, low-grade fever; sore throat; pain from bone involvement; albuminuria; liver and spleen enlarged, jaundice, nausea; blood test positive after 5 weeks Stage 3 (latent): symptoms gone in 2–6 weeks; symptoms possibly absent from a few months to a lifetime; blood test positive; person is noninfectious, but possible for syphilitic pregnant woman to give birth to congenitally syphilitic child Stage 4 (tertiary): complications after 3 to 30 years in 30% of untreated cases; symptoms affecting heart, blood vessels, brain, spinal cord, eyes, skin, and bones; blood test positive *Note:* Symptoms from all stages may be present at once Other names: syph, the pox, bad blood	Male and female: Beginning infectious stage: after intercourse with infected partner, itchy, tingling, numb, when virus beneath skin Active infectious symptomatic stage: blisterlike sores that ulcerate on skin, mucous membranes, vagina, cervix, penis, anal area; fever, headache, muscle aches, general malaise, vaginal discharge, enlarged lymph glands; dyspareunia (painful intercourse); lesions heal in 5–7 days but are sites for secondary infection; symptoms last several weeks Infectious dormant stage: lesions heal; no symptoms; blisters within vagina or urethra may go undetected; may be transmitted sexually at this time Recurring symptomatic stage: usually recurrence of repeated painful attacks because virus remains dormant near base of spine between attacks; duration of time between attacks varies; may be precipitated by emotional stress, ovulation, onset of menses, poor diet, excess sun or wind, lack of sleep, friction from clothes
Prognosis	Male: usually treated successfully Female: sterility Both sexes: arthritis, endocarditis No immunity to future infections Reinfection common	Can be treated successfully; no immunity; transmitted to fetus via placenta unless mother treated before 16 weeks' gestation If untreated: aortic aneurysm, heart failure; complete or partial paralysis or crippling; personality changes; blindness, gumma, lesions of granulation tissue, causing tissue breakdown and impaired circulation; pain from bone involvement; convulsions Death: congenital syphilis or death for fetus	Incurable: one-half to 1 million new cases annually with several million recurrence Complications: herpes keratitis, eye infection (results from rubbing eye after touching herpes sore); repeated attacks and blindness possible Females: five times more likely to develop cervical cancer Pregnant women: pregnancy often ends in abortion, stillbirth, prematurity, neonatal infection, or death; fetal infection may occur in utero Infant: virus transmitted through placenta or by direct contact at birth; 50% chance of being born with disease unless delivered by cesarean section; 75% infected neonates blind or have brain damage; death may occur
Treatment	Aqueous penicillin Some drug-resistant strains of organisms developing	Penicillin G benzathine or procaine penicillin	Aseptic technique in care of patient; cleansing lesions with soap and water; use of drying medications Experimental drugs reported to reduce symptoms Antibiotics for secondary infection Incurable but zovirax suppresses signs and symptoms Psychological counseling Prevention of further spread by avoiding any contact with genitals and sexual intercourse while lesions are present unless male wears condom

TABLE 11–4. OTHER SEXUALLY TRANSMITTED DISEASES

Problem	Definition	Symptoms/Signs	Prevention/Treatment
Candidial vaginitis	Inflammatory process caused by a common skin fungus, *Candida albicans*	Copious cheesy vaginal discharge, intense vulval inflammation and itching or burning	May be related to diabetes, use of antibiotics, birth control pills, bath oil, lack of moisture-absorbing underpants, or sexual intercourse. Use cool compresses, vaginal cream
Trichomonal vaginitis (Trichomoniasis or Tric)	Inflammatory process caused by the common flagellate parasite, *Trichomonas vaginalis*	Frothy, bubbly, greenish-yellow, foul-smelling vaginal discharge; minimal inflammation, some itching	Oral medication if nonpregnant; vaginal cream if pregnant
Nonspecific or bacterial vaginitis	Inflammation caused by more than one bacteria, but especially *Gardnerella vaginalis*	Small amount of yellowish-white vaginal discharge with "fishy" smell; moderate itching	Douche; vaginal cream or oral medication with sexual partner also being treated
Chlamydia trachomatis	Infection caused by an intracellular parasite, *C. trachomatis*	Vaginal discharge or pelvic inflammatory disease in women. Can cause sterility, urethritis, epididymitis, painful and frequent urination or infertility in men. Conjunctivitis or pneumonia in infants	Antibiotic treatment
Genital warts	Growth caused by human papilloma virus, appearing 1–3 months, or longer, after contact	Seen on foreskin and penis in males and on perineum and vaginal mucosa in females	Repeated topical application followed by sitz bath
Phthirus pubis	Pubic lice or "crabs" infesting genital region after contact with a person, clothes, towels, or bedding that is infested	Intense itching; nits may be seen on hair shafts; small black dots (probably excreta) may be visible in pubic hair. Occurs 4–5 weeks after contact	Application of gamma benzene hexachloride 1% cream or lotion; repeat application in 7–10 days. Treat sexual contacts. Oral antihistamines for itching

Neonatal risks associated with teen-age maternity are not uniform but are high. The risks vary by age of the adolescent mother, amount of prenatal care, and racial identification. In the United States socioeconomically advantaged teenagers, with healthy and unimpaired physical growth and development, rarely bear children. Disadvantaged Americans, on the other hand, often initiate childbearing by their late teens and currently account for the majority of teenage births. Teenagers at highest risk of adverse pregnancy outcomes, specifically those less than 17 years old, are more likely to be African American, live in rural areas (especially if Caucasian), and receive inadequate prenatal care (especially if Caucasian) than older first-time mothers. Risks are highest for 11- to 14-year-old teens. Early fertility implies early menarche, which is associated with short stature, a risk factor for poor neonatal outcome. The excessive rates of short gestation, low birth weight, and neonatal mortality may result from a variety of physiologic consequences of environmental disadvantage, not primarily from inherent and intractable biological developmental limits (50, 197).

The late adolescent male is more likely to be involved in the pregnancy and be supportive to the girl than his younger counterpart. Urban teenage African-American fathers are more involved with their children and the children's mothers than stereotypes suggest (31, 116). The more mature the adolescent girl and boy when they become parents, the more likely they will manifest positive parenting characteristics described in Chapter 7. The younger the adolescent, the more likely it is that negative parenting behaviors will occur. Often the adolescent parent expects behavior beyond the developmental ability of the baby, which creates intense frustration and anger that result in child abuse or neglect. You may be able to assess these behaviors and intervene with support, teaching, and counseling. Agencies that have adolescent pregnancy programs should provide both teen fathers and mothers with parenting classes and child development information.

A major problem in adolescent parenting is that many teenage girls who become mothers have themselves come from single-parent homes or homes in which active participation by the father is lacking. Further, the teenage father often gives no real support—emotional or financial. The maternal grandmother is the one who is expected to raise the child; if she cannot, the adolescent single parent is likely to lack the emotional

TABLE 11–5. CONTRACEPTIVE MEASURES: EFFECTIVENESS AND DISADVANTAGES

Name	Description	Effectiveness	Disadvantages
Oral contraceptives	Pills used to suppress chemically ovaulation; new low-dose pill available, with one-tenth amount of hormones, thus fewer side effects	Highly effective, 2 pregnancies in 100	Fewer serious effects than previously seen; screen for nausea, edema, weight gain, depression, anemia, yeast infections, blood clots, myocardial infarction, liver cancer; smokers have increased triglycerides, total cholesterol, and lipoproteins and greater cardiovascular disease risk
Intrauterine device (IUD: Progestasert)	Metal coil inserted in uterus, preventing implantation of fertilized ovum	Very effective, 5 pregnancies in 100	Cramping and bleeding between periods, heavy periods, anemia, perforation of uterus, pelvic infection
Spermicidal chemicals	Chemical substances inserted in vagina before intercourse	Less effective, 5 to 24 pregnancies in 100; effective if used with diaphragm	Irritation of penis or vagina
Billings' ovulation method	Changes in cervical discharge show presence of ovulation	Very effective when followed and abstinence maintained during fertile time	Accurate observation by the woman is necessary
Diaphragm	Small occlusive device inserted over cervix before intercourse	Very effective when properly placed and checked often	Irritation of cervix; aesthetic objections
Condom	Occlusive device placed over penis before ejaculation or female intravaginal pouch	Effective when properly used, 9 to 10 pregnancies in 100	Aesthetic objections; possibly impaired sensation in male
Rhythm	Abstinence of intercourse before and during ovulation; increased body temperature during fertile days	Less effective, 5 to 24 pregnancies in 100	Pregnancy unless menstrual periods regular, ovulation closely observed, and abstinence adhered to
Prostaglandins	Chemicals that regulate intracellular metabolism administered parenterally or orally for contraception or to induce abortions	Effectiveness uncertain	Nausea, vomiting, diarrhea, and pelvic pain
Luteinizing hormone-releasing hormone (LHRH)	Daily injection of hormone decreases sperm; substance inhibits pituitary gland's release of hormone that controls ovulation and spermatogenesis	In women 98% effective; useful in men and women	Experimental; data on men still limited
Injections	150-mg injection of a progestogen, medroxyprogesterone acetate (Depo-Provera); 200-mg injection of a progestogen, Norigest	Injections 98% effective for 3 months	Intermittent vaginal bleeding
Implants	Levo-Norgestrel (progestin) inserted via silicone rubber, matchstick-size tubes into woman's arm	Implants last 5 years; continual release of synthetic hormone inhibits ovulation, thickens cervical mucus, and impedes sperm passage; removed if woman desires pregnancy	Contraindicated in women with liver disease, breast cancer, blood clots, unexplained vaginal bleeding. Headaches, dizziness, nervousness, nausea
Hysterectomy	Surgical removal of uterus; usually done for pathologic condition of uterus rather than for sterilization only	Completely effective; ovum and hormonal production unchanged; menstruation ceases	Mortality rate higher than after tubal ligation; possible postoperative complications; irreversible procedure
Tubal ligation	Surgical interference with tubal continuity and transport of an ovum	Effectiveness depending on type of procedure done, 0.5 to 3 pregnancies in 100; ovum maturation, menstruation, and hormonal production unchanged	Occasional recanalization (fallopian tube ends regrowing together) causing fertility; adhesions, infection, or swelling of tubes postoperatively
Vasectomy	Surgical severing of the vas deferens (sperm duct) from each testicle	Effectiveness depending on type of procedure done; failure rate low; less expensive and time consuming and easier to obtain than female sterilization; no risk to life; no effect on hormone production of testes or sexual functioning	Bleeding, infection, and pain postoperatively in 2–4%; occasional recanalization of severed ends of vas deferens causing fertility; uncertain reversibility

Note: A combination of contraceptive practices may be used by the couple.

► FACTORS INFLUENCING INCIDENCE OF ADOLESCENT PREGNANCY

Developmental Factors

- Low self-esteem
- Need to be close to someone; to relieve loneliness
- Recent experience of significant loss or change
- Early physical sexual maturation
- Egocentrism
- School dropout or truancy; school underachiever
- Personal fable (feeling that "it won't happen to me")
- Responsiveness to peers' sexual behavior
- Independence from family
- Need to prove own womanhood
- Denial of personal sexuality or sexual behavior
- Self-punishment for earlier sexual activity or pregnancy for which feels shame, guilt

Societal Factors

- Variety of adult sexual behavior values
- Implied acceptance of intercourse outside of marriage
- Importance of involvement in heterosexual relationships stressed by the media
- Inadequate access to contraception
- Access to public financial support for teen parents and offspring

Family and Friends

- Difficult mother–daughter relationship
- Desire to break symbiotic tie between self and mother
- Lack of religious affiliation
- Mother, sister, or close relative pregnant as teen
- Sexually permissive behavior norms of the larger peer group
- Sexually permissive values and behavior of close friends; immediate peer group sexually active
- Inadequate communication in heterosexual relationships
- Fulfillment of mother's prophecy if she expects such behavior
- History of sexual abuse or incest
- Few, if any, girlfriends
- Older boyfriend
- Substance abuse or use in family or peer group

maturity or knowledge to demonstrate positive parenting characteristics. If the teenage couple marries, divorce often occurs within the first or second year so that the baby is in a single-parent home (25, 116, 118, 176).

There are ways to help the teenage mother be a more effective and loving mother and also feel more secure and comfortable with parenting. Having a warm, caring woman visit the teen in her home during the infancy stage to assist with infant care, model nurturant child care, explain normal development, and encourage expression of the mother's feelings of frustration and anxiety improves the teen's parenting behavior. In addition, a drop-in center where the teen can take her baby for a few hours to be free of child care for a while and to gain emotional support and information is also a useful community support. The teen parent needs multiple support from family, school, peers, church, the media, the community, and legal system.

Abortion

Abortion is a *method of terminating a pregnancy through expulsion or extraction of the fetus,* usually for economic, emotional, or social reasons. Poor women who economically cannot take care of another child may resort to this drastic form of birth control when they believe they cannot possibly meet the demands of parenting. Abortion carries risks to the physical and psychological health of the female, although the legal abortion is statistically safer than the illegal abortion. More widespread use of abstinence or contraception, however, would reduce the need for abortion. You may be involved in helping the female who is pregnant, the parents, and even the father of the baby to determine their values and feelings about remaining pregnant versus having an abortion. The persons involved should decide (although future legislation may affect the choice); it is not appropriate for you to give advice. Give full information, including the effects of abortion and alternatives, be nonjudgmental, and listen. More people are choosing to keep the baby rather than have an abortion.

Incest

A universal taboo in all cultures is **incest,** *sexual intercourse between persons in the family too closely related to marry legally.* Incest has been present at epidemic levels for some time but is now being admitted more freely by victims as they speak of the resultant emotional and physical pain. (The woman may be in her thirties, forties, or fifties before she can talk about incest that occurred in early childhood.) In your assessment be aware that the adolescent, either male or female, is at risk for incest or for youth prostitution (23). The child and adolescent will tell you if you pick up the initial verbal cues or if you ask if he or she has been the victim of such activity. The risk to boys is not as well documented as that to girls but may be equally common, with either the mother or the father as the abuser. Incestuous relations usually begin when the child is young and continue through adolescence (92). The behavior and consequent signs and symptoms that occur are like those of the sexually abused child described in Chapter 10. Incest may involve stepparents or step siblings, grandparents, or the uncles or cousins.

In incestuous families the man is often the sole economic support. The woman often is isolated and may not drive a car. The family does not have visitors. The woman and other children are frequently beaten and abused; the daughter(s) singled out for the sexual relationship is usually spared the beatings, but she clearly understands what happens if she incurs her father's displeasure. Incestuous fathers are described as family tyrants but, when confronted with the behavior, will appear pathetic, meek, bewildered, and ingratiating. They are exquisitely sensitive to power and seldom try to intimidate anyone of equal or greater status. Instead, with the health care professional, the man will attempt to gain the professional person's sympathy and deny, minimize, or rationalize his behavior (23, 25, 92, 97, 153, 201).

Inexperienced professionals may incorrectly blame the mother for the incest; however, typically the mother is ill or disabled and unable to care for herself or her children. The mother usually cannot be independent and tries to preserve the marriage at any cost, including conscious or unconscious sacrifice of a daughter. Incestuous fathers do not assume maternal caretaking roles when wives are disabled. Rather they expect the eldest daughter to assume the "little mother" role for housework and child care responsibilities. The daughter's sexual relationship with the father often evolves as an extension of her other duties. When the oldest daughter becomes resistant, the father turns his attention to the next daughter or nieces, stepchildren, or grandaughters. The father continues to demand sexual activity with the wife during this time; it is his choice if he limits sexual activity only to the daughters (23, 92, 97, 201).

Father–daughter incest should be suspected in any family that includes (1) a violent or domineering and suspicious father, (2) a battered, chronically ill, or disabled mother, and (3) a daughter who appears to have assumed major adult responsibilities. If incest has been reported with one daughter, it should be suspected with all of the other daughters. Incest should also be suspected as a precipitant in the runaway, delinquent, drug abuse, sexual-acting-out/pregnancy, or suicidal behavior of adolescent girls. The main obstacle to obtaining a history of incest is the clinician's reluctance to ask about it. False accusations of sexual abuse or incest are rare; however, the girl commonly retracts a true allegation because of family pressure (23, 92, 97, 201).

Discovery of incest is a family crisis. *Immediate crisis intervention is essential.* Typically the behavior has been going on many years, and the family's defenses are organized around preservation of the incest secret. Disclosure interrupts patterns of functioning. The father faces loss of sexual activity, which has become an addiction, and the possible loss of a wife and family; social stigmatization; and possible criminal sanctions (these seldom are applied). The mother faces possible loss of a husband, social stigmatization, and the terrifying prospect of raising her family alone, which she is ill prepared to do. The man denies his behavior and maintains his innocence. The wife is torn between husband and daughter, and unless she is given rapid support, her initial belief of the daughter gives way to rallying to the husband's side in 1 or 2 weeks. The daughter then finds herself discredited, shamed, punished for bringing trouble on the family, and still unprotected from sexual abuse. Suicide and runaway behavior are likely at this time as the offspring is being segregated and driven out of the family (92, 97).

Professionals frequently accept the father's denial and rationalizations and support the family secret. They may believe that incest is harmless, consensual, with the daughter a willing or initiating participant, and the result of the man's being deprived of adult sexual expression. Traditional psychodynamic treatment will not be effective. An active, directive, even coercive approach is necessary. Treatment requires ongoing cooperation between the therapist and agencies of the state—both law enforcement and child protective services (92).

It may be necessary to remove the offspring from the home to ensure his or her safety. This intervention, however, is destructive because it (1) makes the adolescent (child) feel he or she has done something wrong and is being punished by banishment from the family, (2) reinforces the couple's bonding against the offspring, and (3) makes it difficult to find appropriate placement for him or her. If the safety of the adolescent (child) is in question, it is preferable to have the father leave during this period. Unfortunately, child protective services do not have legal authority to remove a parent, but a court order may be obtained, and the court can establish supervised visitation, mandated treatment, and family support.

All family members need intensive support. All too frequently this recommended approach is ignored or not implemented (92). *Crisis support for the offspring* involves the following (92):

- Reassure the adolescent (or child) that there are protective adults outside of the family that believe his or her story and will not allow further exploitation to occur.
- Praise the adolescent (child) for the courage to reveal the incest secret.
- Assure the offspring he or she is not to blame for the incest and that he or she is helping, not hurting, the family by seeking outside help.
- Tell the offspring explicitly that many children retract their initial complaint because of pressure or fear; encourage him or her not to do so, with the assurance he or she will not be abandoned by authorities if he or she does.

Crisis support for the mother involves encouragement and assistance to do the following (92):

- Continue to believe the offspring, even if this is painful.
- Resist the tendency to bond with the husband against the offspring.
- Talk about his or her feelings of shame, guilt, anger, fear, and inadequacy.
- Explore ways he or she can handle the issues of survival and seek needed help.
- Obtain treatment for health problems.

Crisis support for the father involves helping him face that the secret has been broken, that he must admit and give up his sexual relationship with his daughter before his problem can be resolved and the family restored (92).

Group treatment for the mother, father, and offspring is more effective than family or individual therapy alone, although individual therapy can be combined with group therapy. Family therapy may be used in the late stages of treatment. The best motivator for the offender to remain in therapy is the court mandate. Self-help activities can supplement other therapy. The family's intense need for support may be met by frequent peer contact such as through Parents United, Daughters and Sons United, or other such agencies (92, 97).

Restoration of the incestuous family centers on the mother–daughter relationship. Safety for the daughter comes not just from improving the marital relationship, but by helping the mother feel strong enough to protect herself and her children and by ensuring that the daughter feels sure she can turn to her mother for protection (92).

The father is ready to return to the family when he has admitted and taken full responsibility for the incest, apologized to the daughter(s) in the presence of all family members, and promised never to abuse the children or wife again. When he is ready to return to the family, they may or may not be ready to receive him. A decision for divorce may be as valid as family reunion. The best gauge for measuring successful treatment is the daughter's feeling of safety, the disappearance of her distress symptoms, and her resumption of normal development (92).

Destructive effects of incest continue into adult life, long after contact has ceased. Adult women have persistent and often severe impairments in self-esteem, intimate relationships, and sexual functioning. Incest victims also have a higher-than-normal risk for repeated victimization (battering and rape). Marriage to an abusive spouse, with potential repetition of abuse in the next generation, is a frequent outcome (23, 92). Of all the entanglements, incest between siblings apparently is the least psychologically harmful (23).

Rape and *other sexual abuse* may be part of the adolescent's experience as a victim. Burgess and co-workers (23, 24) describes three types of sex rings: child sex initiation rings, youth prostitution rings, and syndicated pornography and prostitution rings.

As you work with sexual assault victims, be aware of various types of assault and entanglements that exist so that you can better detect verbal and nonverbal cues, give immediate assistance, and refer the person (and parents) to receive the necessary medical and legal assistance. References at the end of the chapter are helpful (23, 24, 25, 41, 60, 79, 92, 97, 117, 136, 153, 197, 201).

Drug Abuse Problems

Drug abuse (illicit and prescription) is an epidemic adolescent health problem that is not new. The history of drug abuse is long throughout the world. The problem continues to intensify in the United States, a drug-conscious nation compared with other countries. It is an epidemic with serious consequences for future generations. A major problem is the increasing number of infants born with addiction to one or several drugs (36, 37, 96, 143, 197). Every age group takes a certain amount of medication at one time or another. Usually these drugs are taken for therapeutic reasons; however, reports show that schoolchildren, adolescents, and young adults are increasingly using drugs that cause dependence and toxicity (31, 50, 185).

Drug abuse is the *use of any drug in excess or for the feeling it arouses.* A **drug** is a *substance that has an effect on the body or mind.* Excessive use of certain drugs causes **drug dependence,** a *physical need or psychological desire for continuous or repeated use of the drug.* **Addiction** is *present when physical withdrawal symptoms* *result if the person does not repeatedly receive a drug and can involve* **tolerance,** *having to take increasingly larger doses to get the same effect.*

Reasons for drug abuse are many: curiosity; peer pressure; need to overcome feelings of insecurity and aloneness and to be a part of the group; need for acceptance; easy availability; imitation of family; rebellion, escape, or exhilaration; need for a crutch; unhappy home life; sense of alienation or identity problem; or an attempt at maturity or sophistication. Gradually the drug subculture replaces interest in family, school, church, hobbies, or other organizational activity. The beliefs and attitudes of the drug subculture are learned from experienced drug users and are fortified by certain rock-and-roll songs and stars (9, 35, 40, 50, 106, 121, 138, 185, 192, 197, 202).

Drug abuse and addiction affect all ethnic and racial groups. Entire communities are affected. In large cities much of the drug trade also involves street gangs, which have become ghetto-based drug trafficking organizations. Even rural communities are affected. Total community effort is needed to stop or prevent the problem.

Drug dependence is epidemic among the wealthy as well as among the middle class and poor. Children of wealthy parents may develop such traits as poor impulse control, poor frustration tolerance, depression, and poor coping ability. As a result, drugs may be used to cope. Predictably, these traits make children from wealthy homes a difficult population to treat. When drug abuse is the presenting problem, the financial ability to buy drugs of high quality, subcultural acceptance of their use, and at least a relative immunity from legal consequences do not motivate behavioral change.

Ingestion of alcohol and illicit drugs depresses the cerebral cortex, a still immature reasoning and intellectual center in the teens, and releases inhibitions in the limbic system, the center of love, pleasure, anger, pain, and other emotions. The limbic system seeks instant and constant gratification or stimulation and contributes to the adolescent's sense of boredom. Thus some adolescents go to extremes in seeking television, alcohol, hard drugs, hard rock, and aggressive video games. There is loosening of social controls and increase in aggressive and sexual behavior when the limbic system is stimulated. See Primary and General Signs and Symptoms of Drug Abuse Among Adolescents (36, 37, 40, 48, 50, 61, 96, 98, 99, 106, 138, 143, 173, 185, 192, 202).

Therapy is usually entered into as a result of family pressure—often in the form of threatened financial loss such as the withdrawal of allowance or inheritance—or a crisis event such as attempted suicide or arrest. The behavior and illness of the young drug abuser control the entire family, causing family illness. Parents must

► PRIMARY AND GENERAL SIGNS AND SYMPTOMS OF DRUG ABUSE AMONG ADOLESCENTS

- Decrease in quality of schoolwork without a valid reason (Reasons given may be boredom, not caring about school, or not liking the teachers.)

- Personality changes; lack of empathy; becoming more irritable, less attentive, less affectionate, secretive, unpredictable, uncooperative, apathetic, depressed, withdrawn, hostile, sullen, easily provoked, insensitive to punishment

- Less responsible behavior; not doing chores or school homework; school tardiness or absenteeism; forgetful of family occasions such as birthdays

- Change in activity; lack of participation in family activities, school or church functions, sports, prior hobbies, or organizational activities

- Change in friends; new friends who are unkempt in appearance or sarcastic in their attitude; secretive or protective about these friends, not giving any information

- Change in appearance or dress, in vocabulary, in music tastes to match those of new friends, imitating acid rock-and-roll stars

- More difficult to communicate with; refuses to discuss friends, activities, drug issues; insists it is all right to experiment with drugs; defends rights of youth, insists adults hassle youth; prefers to talk about bad habits of adults

- Rebellious, resistant to authority, antisocial behavior, persistent lying; seeks immediate gratification; feels no remorse

- Irrational behavior, frequent explosive episodes; driving recklessly; unexpectedly stupid behavior

- Loss of money, credit cards, checks, jewelry, household silver, coins in the home that cannot be accounted for

- Addition of drugs, clothes, money, albums, tapes, or stereo equipment suddenly found in the home

- Presence of whiskey bottles, marijuana seeds or plants, hemostats, rolling papers, drug buttons, and marijuana lead buttons; also may be unusual belt buckles, pins, bumper stickers, or T-shirts and magazines in the car, truck, or home

- Preoccupation with the occult, various pseudoreligious cults, satanism, or witchcraft; evidence of tattoo writing of 666, drawing of pentagrams on self or elsewhere, or misrepresentation of religious objects

- Signs of physical change or deterioration, including pale face, dilated pupils, red eyes; chewing heavily scented gum; using heavy perfumes; using eyewash or drops to remove the red; heightened sensitivity to touch, smell, or taste; weight loss, even with increased appetite (marijuana smoking causes the "munchies"—extra snacking)

- Signs of mental change or deterioration, including disordered thinking or illogical patterns, decreased ability to remember or to think in rapid thought processes and responses; severe lack of motivation

regain control of their home, forcing the youth to face the illness by seeking treatment. Love and care in a family are essential, but that alone will not cure the drug abuse problem or the craziness that results in a family in which a member is a drug abuser, nor will parental strictness solve the problems. Professional treatment should be obtained in a center that treats the whole person and family, using an interdisciplinary team approach, and that provides after-discharge care to the person and family. Intensive treatment over time to the entire family system creates the attitude change that is essential for remaining healthy and functional and for ongoing maturity. A combination of drug detoxification, methadone maintenance, and emotional, cognitive, didactic, and experiential therapies is helpful to reduce symptoms and work through underlying character and interactional pathology. Adolescent treatment centers typically prohibit use of stereo and rock music, television, video games, drugs, cigarettes, alcohol, and even rock-star T-shirts. Instead, the teens participate in a structured schedule that involves nutritious foods, jogging and other exercise, group discussions, individual therapy, reading, art and music therapy, school work, responsibility to follow rules, goal setting, and a milieu that builds a spiritual foundation similar to the 12 steps of Alcoholics Anonymous.

If after discharge the youth returns to his or her drug-using friends, there will be a return to drug abuse and all the consequences. It is not easy for the youth to give up drugs or to overcome the drug abuse reputation at school, among peers, or elsewhere. It may be very difficult to work into a new group of friends unless during the treatment program the youth and family were helped to establish new interests, new hobbies, new social ties and friendships, and new organizational connections. Remaining drug-free may mean giving up the prior boyfriend or girlfriend, certain favorite clothes or possessions, certain words in the vocabulary, and certain mannerisms or aspects of appearance. The change in attitudes, self-concept, and body image must be total enough so the person feels like a new person and is strong enough in that identity that the new self is maintained in the face of the inevitable peer, school, family, and other stressors. The ability to give up aspects of the old self and maintain the new identity begins in the treatment center, but can be accomplished only with love, support, and encouragement (not nagging) from family and other loved ones. *The person must feel that he or she is gaining more than what is being lost to maintain the changes begun in treatment and to move forward in maturity.* To remain drug-free involves more than just "saying no" or a one-time seminar. Support groups in the school, church, and community for teens who do not want to use alcohol or drugs are essential to prevent the loneliness and ostracism some teens feel when they go against peers. Illicit drug trade can be stopped best by community action, which reduces supply to individuals.

The Drug Abuse Resistance Education (DARE) program, developed by the police department in Los An-geles and adopted by about half of the local school districts in the United States, is the only federally funded drug abuse prevention program for elementary and junior high school students. The 17 weekly sessions are taught by specially trained police officers. The strongest outcome of DARE has been to impart knowledge about drugs. Effects on self-esteem and attitudes toward drug use have been statistically insignificant. The DARE programs that reduced drug use effectively in the short run were interactive; they encourged children to teach one another instead of relying on the adult authority teacher (47). Other studies show that building self-esteem is the most effective way, along with information, to reduce adolescent drug abuse (167).

Table 11–6 will assist you in assessing the **specific signs** (*objective evidence*) and **symptoms** (*subjective evidence*) **resulting from drugs commonly abused,** as well as give information pertinent to intervention. Often the youth is taking a mixture of these drugs, as use of any of them is likely to increase use of other drugs. Assessment becomes more complex. At times neither the person nor friends know for sure what drugs have been used. Various references at the end of this chapter give information on drug abuse (29, 31, 32, 33, 40, 47, 48, 50, 60, 91, 98, 106, 115, 136, 138, 185, 192, 197, 202).

Because the use of cocaine (or crack) is a serious health and social problem, a discussion in addition to the information under Stimulants in Table 11–6 is presented in the following pages.

Cocaine is an *alkaloid extracted from the leaves of the coca bush, which grows mainly in the eastern slope of the Andes mountains in Peru and Bolivia.* It is sold on the streets as a hydrochloride salt; it is a fine, white crystalline powder. Freebase cocaine resembles rock candy chunks. Street cocaine is diluted with cornstarch, talcum powder, sugar, amphetamines, and quinine. Its purity is usually 5 to 50%; it may be 80%. Cocaine is taken by (1) snorting (inhaled through a straw or a rolled-up dollar bill or coke spoon), (2) freebasing (smoked in a small water pipe filled with rum instead of water), or (3) mainlining (intravenously) (32, 33, 36, 50, 96, 185, 197).

Cocaine creates tolerance and is addicting because of the sense of stimulation (rush) that comes from activation of nerve cells in the brain that release dopamine. The sense of pleasure or good feeling is so great that the person develops a stronger compulsion for cocaine each time he or she uses it so that addiction results. Chronic cocaine use blocks the ability of the brain cells to release dopamine without increasing amounts of cocaine. The person feels terrible without the drug. Finally, there is the **kindling effect:** *a small amount of cocaine can trigger unexpectedly severe dopamine reactions,* resulting in seizures or bursts of psychotic behavior (32, 33, 115, 117, 143, 197).

TABLE 11–6. SUMMARY OF LEGAL AND ILLEGAL DRUGS RELATED TO NURSING ASSESSMENT AND INTERVENTION

Drug Type/Name	Street Names	Action & Duration of Action	Administration	Effect Sought by User	Physical & Emotional Effects/Complications
Narcotics Opiates opium, morphine, heroin, codeine Synthetic nonopi- ates Methadone, Demerol, Darvon, Percodan, Percoset	Snow, stuff, H, junk, smack, scag, dreamer	Central nervous system depressant: 3–24 hours Addicting	Oral; smoked; sniffed; injected under skin (skin popping); intramuscular (IM); intravenous (IV); cough medicine containing codeine	Euphoria Prevention of withdrawal discomfort	Drowsiness, sedation (nodding) stupor. Eye and nose secretions. Euphoria. Relief of pain. Impaired intellectual functioning and coordination. Constricted pupils that do not respond to light. Excessive itching. Poor appetite. Constipation. Urinary retention. Loss of sexual desire, temporary impotence or sterility. Slow pulse and respiration(s); hypotension. Death from overdosage caused by respiratory and cardiovascular depression and collapse. Severe infection at injection sites (needle marks and tracks)
Barbiturates Nembutal, Seconal, Amytal, Fiornal, Tuinal, Phenobarbital	Sleepers, downers, goofballs, redbirds, yellow jackets, heavens, red devils, barbs	Central nervous system depressant: 1–16 hours Can be lethal with alcohol	Oral, or injected IM or IV	Relaxation and euphoria	Relief of anxiety and muscular tension, relaxation, sleep. Respirations slow, shallow. Slowed reactions. Euphoria. Impaired emotional control, judgment, and coordination. Irritability. Apathy. Confused. Poor hygiene. Slurred, slow speech. Poor memory. Weight loss. Liver, brain, kidney damage from long-term use. Death from overdose. Psychosis, possible convulsions or death, from abrupt withdrawal of barbiturates
Sedatives Doriden Chloral hydrate, Methaqualone Placidyl		Central nervous system depressant 3–4 hours Can be lethal with alcohol	Oral	Sleep Relaxation	May be same effect as barbituates but not as severe
Minor tranquilizers Valium Librium Miltown Equanil		Central nervous system depressant: 3–4 hours	Oral, or injected IM or IV	Relaxation Sense of calm	Relieve anxiety. Varied onset and duration of effect according to preparation and administration
Inhalants (Glue sniffing, aerosols, airplane glue, amyl nitrate, nitrous oxide)		Central nervous system depressant: 1–3 hours	Inhaled through tubes, glue smears on paper or cloth	Intoxication, relaxation, euphoria	Excess nasal secretion. Watering of eyes. Tinnitus. Diplopia. Poor muscular control, lack of coordination. Appears dreamy, blank, or drunk. Impaired perception and judgment. Possibility of violent behavior. Sleepy after 35 to 45 minutes or unconscious. Damage to lungs, nervous system, brain, liver. Death through suffocation, choking, or overdose
Stimulants Amphetamines Dexedrine Methedrine	Pep pills, uppers, A, speed, crystal, dexies, bennies, lid poppers	Central nervous system stimulant. Varies in duration of action	Oral; or injected under skin or IV	Sense of well-being Alertness, feelings of activity and increased initiative.	Giggling, silliness, talkative. Rapid speech. Dilated pupils. Hypertension, dizzy, tachycardia. Loss of appetite, loss of weight. Diarrhea. Extreme fatigue. Dry mouth, bad breath. Chills, sweating, increased muscle tension; shakiness, tremors, restlessness. Irritability. Confused, grandiose thinking. Deep depression. Mood swings. Aggressive behavior. Paranoid ideas which may persist. Feelings of persecution. Delusions. Hallucinations. Panic. Toxic psychosis. Possible seizures. Tachycardia may cause heart damage or heart attack. Death from cardiac damage, hypertensive crisis, paralysis of respiratory center, fatigue or overdose
Cocaine	Leaf, snow, coke, speedballs, flake, gold dust, crack, smack, blow	2–4 hours Crack, immediate Depression and exhaustion can last several days	Cocaine sniffed, snorted, IV, or smoking (freebasing)	Excitation. Over confidence	
Crack Ice	Rock Fire				

Source: Refs. 33, 38, 48, 50, 60, 98, 104, 115, 136, 185, 187, 202

Tolerance Potential	Physical Dependence	Psychological Dependence	Withdrawal Characteristics	Nursing Care
Yes	High Controlled Substance	High	Abdominal pain. Muscle cramps, tremors, spasms. Nausea, vomiting, diarrhea. Lacrimation, watery eyes. Goose bumps, sweating, chills. Hypertension, tachycardia, increased respirations. Anxiety, irritability, depression. Craving for drugs	(1) Observe for symptoms of withdrawal and report to physician. (2) Give medications prescribed to suppress withdrawal symptoms. (3) Monitor for vital signs at least q.i.d. for first 72 hours following admission. (4) Carry out nursing measures to promote safety, general heatlh, and sense of security.
Yes	Moderate Controlled Substance	Moderate	Nausea, vomiting, diarrhea. Bleeding. Tremors. Diaphoresis. Hypertension or hypotension. Temperature above 99.6 F. Irritability, hostility, restlessness, agitation. Sleep disturbance. Impaired cognitive function. Acute brain syndrome. Seizures	(1) Observe for withdrawal symptoms and report to physician. (2) Give prescribed medication to suppress symptoms. (3) Provide calm, quiet, safe environment, as free of external stimuli as possible, for acute/severe withdrawal symptoms. (4) Observe for insomnia and nightmares and provide nursing measures to promote sleep. (5) Observe and take precaution for seizure activity. (6) Promote general health and sense of security
Yes	Controlled Substance	Yes	Anxiety. Insomnia. Tremors. Delirium. Convulsions.	(1) Observe and treat if taken in suicide attempt. (2) Provide environment for safety and sleep. (3) Teach measures to promote sleep and rest
Yes	Controlled Substance	Yes	Anxiety. Irritability. Poor concentration.	(1) Observe for withdrawal symptoms or if a suicide attempt and treat. (2) Provide calm safe environment. (3) Teach stress management. (4) Promote general health
Yes	No	Yes	Withdrawal symptoms have not been recorded	(1) Emergency care for respiratory damage or neurological complication. (2) Provide for safety. (3) Implement other nursing measures related to presenting symptoms, especially if this drug has been used in combination with others
Yes	Yes	High	Tremors. Neurological hyperactivity. Paranoia. Assaultive behavior. Irritability. Depression. Possible suicidal behavior or psychotic reaction. Tachycardia, hypertension. Oversensitivity to stimuli. Insomnia. Intense craving	(1) Observe for symptoms of withdrawal and report to physician. (2) Give medication as prescribed to suppress agitated state and prevent exhaustion. (3) Take precautions for staff and client safety according to client's paranoia and depression. (4) Monitor vital signs at least q.i.d. for first 72 hours following admission. (5) Provide calm, nonthreatening, quiet environment and sense of security. (6) Provide for sleep and nutrition. (7) Cocaine — observe for chronic nosebleed and perforated nasal septum. (8) Detoxification. (9) Teach stress management, alternate leisure activities

(continued)

Drug Type/Name	Street Names	Action & Duration of Action	Administration	Effect Sought by User	Physical & Emotional Effects/Complications
Caffeine (Found in tea, coffee, cocoa, cola and tablet form, including many over-the-counter drugs.)	Kiddie Dope (caffeine, ephedrine, phenylopropanolamine) Black beauty, speckled eggs, speckled birds, pink heart, 20-20's, blue and clears, green and clears	Central nervous system stimulant. Cardiac stimulant 2–4 hours High similar to amphetamines	Oral	A "pick-up"; to increase alertness and decrease fatigue. More rapid, clearer flow of thoughts	Restlessness. Disturbed sleep or insomnia. Nausea, abdominal distention. Myocardial stimulation, palpitation, and tachycardia. Large amounts have led to irrational or hysterical behavior and, very large doses, cardiac standstill. Stimulates gastric secretions. Raise BMR by 10%. Diuretic
Hallucinogens Synthetic D-lysergic acid (LSD) 4-methyl-2 (STP, DOM) Phencyclidine (PCP) Dimethyltryptamine (DMT) Natural Cactus (mescaline, peyote) Mushroom (psilocybin)	Acid, Big D, sugar, trips, cubes Serenity, tranquility, peace Businessman's special	Hallucinogenic Varies: LSD 10–12 hours; STP 6–8 hours Mescaline 12–24 hours	Primarily oral; some are inhaled or injected	Insight. Distortion of senses Exhilaration Increased energy	Severe hallucinations, feelings of persecution and detachment. Amnesia. Incoherent speech. Laughing, crying. Exhilaration, depression, or panic alternates with sense of invulnerability. Suicidal or homicidal tendencies. Suspicious. Impaired judgment. Cold, sweaty hands and feet; shivering, chills. Vomiting. Weight loss. Irregular breathing. Exhaustion. Dilated pupils. Hypertension. Brain damage from chronic use. Accidental death. Flashbacks. May intensify psychosis; long-lasting mental illness has resulted. Symptoms may persist for an indefinite period after discontinuation of drug
Marijuana (cannabis), *Indian hemp,* which produces varying grades of hallucinogenic material; *hashish,* pure canabis resin, the most powerful grade from leaves and flowering tops of female plants; *ganja,* less potent preparation of flowering tops and stems of female plant and resin attached to them; *bhang,* least potent preparation of fried mature leaves and flowering tops of male	Joints, reefer, pot, grass, weed Acapulco Gold The Sticks Hash	Mixed: central nervous system depressant and stimulant. Great variance in duration 2–12 hours THC is fat-soluble, absorbed especially by brain cells and reproductive organs. Builds in the brain; 2 cigarettes per week for 3 months causes personality change. Impairment during nonintoxicated state remains when smoking persists over months	Smoked or swallowed	Euphoria Relaxation Increased perception Escape	Nervous system Stored in fat portion of cells; remains in brain 6 weeks after cessation of smoking Speech comprehension, ability to express ideas, and ability to understand relationships impaired because of damage to the cerebral cortex Memory, decision making, handling complex tasks, ability to concentrate or focus impaired because of effects on cells in the hypocampus and cerebrum Emotional swings, depression, pessimism, irritability, low frustration tolerance, and temper outbursts because of cell damage in limbic system Does not learn adaptive skills or how to cope with stressors Lack of motivation, fatigue, moodiness, depression, inability to cope, loss of interest in vigorous activity or all previously enjoyed activities occur because of THC effects on various parts of the brain; fails to continue in emotional development Insomnia because of damage to cells in the hypothalamus

Tolerance Potential	Physical Dependence	Psychological Dependence	Withdrawal Characteristics	Nursing Care
Yes Develops quickly	Strongly possible	Yes	In moderate heavy users, there may be headache, irritability, nervousness, tremors, lethargy	(1) Introduce substitute decaffeinated beverage (2) Provide for general health needs and teaching (3) Observe for caffeinism: irritability, tremors, tics, insomnia, sensory disturbance, tachypnea, arrhythmias, diuresis, GI distress. (4) Teach cognitive methods and stress management techniques to reduce fatigue, promote alertness
Yes	No	Probable	Severe apprehension, fear, or panic. Perceptual distortions and hallucinations. Hyperactivity. Diaphoresis. Tachycardia	(1) Have someone who is close to client stay with client at all times to provide support and comfort. (2) Provide nonthreatening environment with subdued, pleasant stimuli. (3) Provide orientation and diversion to pleasant experiences. (4) Avoid use of sedative/tranquilizers, if possible. (5) Monitor vital signs. (6) Provide for general health needs. (7) Teach stress management and cognitive methods to increase energy, insight, feelings of health, and life satisfaction. (8) Teach alternate leisure activities.

See page 539 for information.

(continued)

Drug Type/Name	Street Names	Action & Duration of Action	Administration	Effect Sought by User	Physical & Emotional Effects/Complications
Marijuana (cont.) and female plants; *THC* in fat part of cell prevents nutrients from crossing cell membrane; RNA production and new cell growth reduced; *all* cell function interfered with					Vision blurred and irregular visual perception because of damage to cells in the occipital areas

Body coordination, maintenance of posture and balance, ability to perform sports or drive a car impaired because of damage to cells in the cerebellum

Respiratory system

Upper respiratory infections common because of destruction to mucosal cells from the smoke (more destructive than tobacco smoke)

Sinusitis, inflammation of the lining of one or more of the sinuses, from nasal infection

Bronchitis, with low-grade fever, chest pain, chronic cough, and yellow-green sputum, common because of inflammation to the bronchial tree caused by smoke inhalation

Lung cancer more likely because of the numerous chemicals in marijuana (smoking three to five joints a week is equivalent to smoking 16 cigarettes daily for 7 days a week)

Emphysema and chronic obstructive pulmonary diseases from long-time smoking and deep inhalation; lung function permanently damaged

Cardiovascular system

Cardiac arythmias and tachycardia related to the dose of THC absorbed (one joint immediately raises heart rate by as much as 50%)

Hypertension, which may contribute to aneurysm formation or cardiovascular accident, common

Myocardial infarction possible

Congested conjunctiva associated with hypertension

Reproductive system

Infertility in males from moderate to heavy use because production of testosterone is reduced and low sperm production or production of abnormal sperm occurs

Impotence, inability to ejaculate sperm

Gynecomastia, enlarged breast formation, in puberty when secondary sex characteristics are being developed (lower testosterone level causes fat deposits around the breast tissue)

Hirsutism in females, with increased androgen production resulting in male secondary sex characteristics (increased hair growth on face and arms, deeper voice), irregular menstrual cycles, serious acne, and lack of development of female secondary sexual characteristics

Tolerance Potential	Physical Dependence	Psychological Dependence	Withdrawal Characteriestics	Nursing Care
Yes	Yes	Yes	Heavy smokers report irritability, restlessness, loss of appetite, sleep disturbance, sweating, tremor, nausea, vomiting, and diarrhea, hyperactivity. Ability for memory, thinking, learning, concentration is impaired	(1) Not usually admitted to acute care settings unless this drug has been used in combination with others, so that a mixed effect occurs. (2) Implement nursing measures listed above under *Hallucinogens*. (3) Likely to see increasing number of children and adolescents with physical effects from chronic use or injuries from accidents; appropriate medical and surgical nursing care should be given. (4) Teach stress management and cognitive methods to relax, cope with stressors, and increase life satisfaction. (5) Explore alternate leisure activities

(continued)

TABLE 11–6. SUMMARY OF LEGAL AND ILLEGAL DRUGS RELATED TO NURSING ASSESSMENT AND INTERVENTION (continued)

Drug Type/Name	Street Names	Action & Duration of Action	Administration	Effect Sought by User	Physical & Emotional Effects/Complications
Marijuana (cont.)					Infertility in the female because of damage to the ova; menstrual cycle irregularity Pregnancy, if present when marijuana is smoked, endangers the embryo and fetus, increasing chance of congenital defects and fetal mortality because THC crosses the placental barrier Lactation, if breast-feeding while smoking marijuana, endangers baby's health because THC transfers through breast milk Immune system suppressed; prone to infections Endocrine system impaired for 11–16-year-olds Marijuana combined with PCP causes psychosis; if taken with other substances, effect of each drug multiplied
Nicotine (Found in cigarettes, cigars, pipe and chewing tobacco and snuff)		Variable action. Central nervous system toxin. Can act as stimulant or depressant: 15 minutes–2 hours	Smoked, sniffed, chewed.	Calmness, sociability	Can have stimulating and/or calming effect. Factor in lung cancer, coronary artery disease, circulatory impairment, peptic ulcer, and emphysema

Physical changes that occur from cocaine use are as follows (32, 33, 143):

- *Cardiovascular:* tachycardia, arrhythmias, hypertension
- *Respiratory:* nasal stuffiness, tachypnea, shortness of breath, runny nose
- *Musculoskeletal:* twitching, tremors, weight loss
- *Gastrointestinal:* nausea, constipation, anorexia
- *Genitourinary:* difficult urination, impotency
- *Dermatologic:* pallor, cold sweats
- *Ophthalmologic:* dilated pupils, blurred vision
- *Central nervous system:* fever, insomnia, fatigue, headache, seizures
- *Reproductive:* abnormal spermatozoa

Medical hazards that result from cocaine use include the following (29, 33, 36, 48, 115, 117, 143, 197):

- Nasal septum and mucous membrane destruction from inhalation
- Bronchitis, with infection, hemorrhage, and blocking of the respiratory tract from inhalation of foreign particles

- Respiratory failure from vasoconstriction of blood vessels in the lung, cyanosis, shortness of breath, dyspnea, pulmonary edema, respiratory collapse, and death
- Cardiac arrhythmias, tachycardia, myocardial infarction, cardiac arrest, sudden death
- Seizures from freebasing and mainlining, which cause strong, explosive stimulation; convulsions, which may result in death
- Phlebitis from repeated injections in the veins; resulting thrombus can cause an embolus, causing myocardial infarction, pulmonary embolus, renal embolus, or cerebrovascular accident
- Endocarditis from mainlining with bacteria-contaminated needles, causing infection of heart valves (fatality rate, 50%)
- Hepatitis from mainlining with blood-contaminated needles, causing tender, enlarged liver, jaundice (repeated attacks can be fatal)
- Brain abscess from mainlining with bacteria-contaminated needles, causing fever, convulsions, paralysis, and possible death
- AIDS from mainlining with blood-contaminated needles (75% of all intravenous addicts have

Tolerance Potential	Physical Dependence	Psychological Dependence	Withdrawal Characteriestics	Nursing Care
Yes	Possible to yes	Yes	Headache. Anorexia, irritability, nervousness. Decreased ability to concentrate. Craving for cigarette. Energy loss. Fatigue. Dizziness. Sweating. Tremor and palpitations	(1) Provide support. (2) Explore behavioral changes necessary to quit smoking as well as provide information as to available self-help groups. (3) Provide for general health needs (4) Teach smoking cessation program

been exposed to the virus, 5–10% or more will develop the fatal disease)

Crack or **rock** is an *extremely potent, highly addictive, inhalant form of cocaine.* It is beige or slightly brown, white or yellowish white, and it is sold in pellet-sized chips called "rocks" or in small plastic vials, in an envelope, or in foil wrap. It can be smoked using a glass pipe or a tin can; the user inhales the vapor from the heated crack. It may be mixed with marijuana or tobacco, or it may be mixed with PCP (angel dust), which is called "space blasting," or with other drugs. Some users smoke in a "base house," "crack house," or "rock house" in which the person pays a fee to use the house, pipes, and torches. The well-to-do individual may use crack in his or her suburban or urban home (32, 37, 117, 197).

The frightening aspect about *crack* is that *the person may become addicted the first time of use or in a matter of weeks.* The addiction is as powerful as heroin addiction. The intense high feeling is produced in 4 to 6 seconds and lasts 5 to 7 minutes. The high is followed by an intensely uncomfortable low feeling so that the person will do anything to get more crack. The person

may become violent toward friends or family; may become paranoid or psychotic, or may commit suicide. Death may occur because of heart or respiratory failure. The first dose may cost only a few dollars, but a binge that lasts 1 to 3 days and is repeated weekly may cost hundreds or thousands of dollars. Crack becomes the most, the only, important thing in life so that all other aspects of life suffer: family relations, friendship, jobs, emotional status, social status, ability to think or behave rationally, personal hygiene or self-care, activities of daily living. If the user is a pregnant woman, there is risk of miscarriage, stillbirth, an addicted baby, impaired physical and mental development in the child, or respiratory failure or strokes in the baby (32, 37, 138).

Nursing Role in Health Promotion

The adolescent is between childhood and adulthood. Allow him or her to handle as much personal health care and business as possible, yet be aware of the psychosocial and physical problems with which he or she cannot cope without help. Watch for hidden fears that may be expressed in unconventional language. For ex-

Case Situation: Adolescent Drug Abuse

Jess, 17, was taken for treatment to an adolescent chemical abuse unit. "My parents, when they put me in (the hospital), they thought I was just drinking and using pot. When they got my toxscreen back, my mom almost fainted."

The drug-screening analysis showed that marijuana, Valium, Demerol, Dilaudid, and codeine all had been ingested within a week. "All I did was live to get high—and, I guess you could say, get high to live," he said.

"I used to work at the home of a doctor who had a medicine cabinet full of everything anybody could dream of. He had a bunch of narcotics and stuff, and I thought I was in heaven. But I could go out right now and get drugs in about 15 minutes if I wanted. People, they're waiting for you to buy it. Around 10, I started drinking a little bit—just tasting it, and getting that warm feeling. The first time I got high, I was 12, and I loved it. There wasn't no stopping me then. I got high all I could. I used to wake up and think, "How can I get high today?"

His friends put pressure on him to try other drugs. "I told myself I'd never do any pills, never drop any acid, but those promises went by the wayside." He first took Quaaludes in the ninth grade and dropped acid that year at a concert. Soon he was drinking a lot and taking speed and Valium and other depressants.

"If I drank any beer, I'd want another one. If I got drunk, I'd want to get high; if I got high, I'd want to get pills. When I started out, I thought it was just cool, and that feeling was great. Instead of dealing with normal, everyday problems, I'd run off and get high. It got so I was picking fights just so I could stomp out of the house and get high."

He became a connoisseur. "I didn't buy dope at school. There's no good dope at school."

He also became more difficult to handle at home and at school.

"That period of time, I started fighting a lot with my parents. My grades dropped. I got into fistfights at school. I was real rebellious. I usually was high during class."

"I think it was real obvious to my teachers, because of the way I dressed and the way I acted in class. All the guys I hung around with had real long hair, moccasin boots, heavy metal T-shirts, and leather pants."

"I was pretty much an A student, and they (grades) dropped to low C's and D's. I was really withdrawing into myself."

"I wasn't myself when I was stoned. For years, I didn't even know how to feel (emotions). I've left home a few times."

"One time I was on LSD and I took a razor blade and cut my leg up. I still have the scars from that. I blanked out a lot. I'd come home beaten-up looking, and didn't know why."

Jess spent 8 weeks in treatment and now says he's been straight for over a year.

"It's a dependency," he said. "There's no way to eliminate it. You just try to control it. If I smoked a joint today or took a drink, I'd be right back."

Jess agrees with other former addicts: part of the problem is the naiveté of the parents.

"My parents, when I started getting in trouble, weren't going to admit it." Advice for parents who uncover a drug problem is simple: "Get some help. Not just for your kids, but for the parents and siblings also, because the whole family gets crazy. It's a family disease."

"I'll have to be on the lookout for the rest of my life to avoid falling back into drug use. I've learned just to be myself, and people will like me—and I never would have believed that before."

---

ample, the high school junior may state concern about her figure. Underlying this statement may be a fear that she will not adequately develop secondary sex characteristics. She may believe she is not physiologically normal or sexually attractive and will not be able to have children. With adequate assessment, you may discover that she is simply physically slow in developing. Explaining that not all adolescents develop at the same rate and that she is normal may rid her mind of great anxiety.

Today's adolescent, because of improved communications, knows more about life than did former generations. He or she is bombarded with information but does not have the maturity to handle it. Do not assume that because of apparent sophistication he or she understands the basis of health promotion. The adolescent may be able to discuss foreign policy but thinks that syphilis is caught from toilet seats.

Some teenagers, especially those with understanding and helpful families, go through adolescence with relative ease; it is a busy, happy period. But the increases in teenage suicide and in escape activities such as drugs and alcohol speak for those who do not have this experience. Adolescents are looking for adults who can be admired, trusted, and leveled with and who genuinely care. Parents are still important as figures to identify with, but the teenagers now look more outside the home—to teachers, community, and national leaders. They idealize such people, and if the leaders are found to be liars or thieves, their idealism turns to bitterness. As a nurse, you will be one of the community leaders with the opportunity, through living and teaching health promotion, to influence these impressionable minds.

Counseling the Adolescent for Health Promotion

Help the person clarify values, beliefs, and attitudes that are important and be more analytic in thinking as first steps in bringing behavior into congruence and to reduce a sense of conflict. Value clarification exercises may be helpful.

Teach the adolescent effective decision-making skills so that the person learns how to develop a plan of action toward some goal. The decision-making model involves (1) defining the problem; (2) gathering and processing information; (3) identifying possible solutions and alternatives of action; (4) making a decision about action; (5) trying out the decision; (6) evaluating whether the decision, actions, and consequences were effective or desirable; (7) rethinking other alternate solutions with new information; and (8) acting on these new decisions. Having the adolescent write out answers when setting goals, thinking of possible solutions, and analyzing consequences can help make an abstract process more concrete and more useful to the person who needs signs of structure.

Promote warm, accepting, supportive, nonjudgmental feelings, and honest feedback as the adolescent struggles with decisions. Help him or her make effective choices by fostering a sense of self-importance (he or she is a valuable and valued individual). Helping the person look ahead to the future in terms of values, goals, and consequences of behavior can strengthen a sense of what is significant in life and a resolve to live so the values and goals are fulfilled and positive consequences are achieved.

Both individual and group counseling are useful. In the group setting the adolescent may be asked to bring a close friend or parent to share the experience. Some concerns and conflicts, however, are best worked through with the individual. Group sessions are effective for the following reasons (136):

- The person realizes concerns, feelings, and sense of confusion are not unique to him or her.
- Experiences and successful solutions to problems can be shared with others who are at different points of development.
- Ideas and roles can be tried out in the group before being tried in real life.
- Values can be clarified and decisions made with support and feedback from others.

Care Related to Sexuality

Personal Attitudes. First examine personal attitudes toward yourself as a sexual being, the sexuality of others, family, love, and changing mores regarding sexual intercourse before you do any sex education through formal or informal teaching, counseling, or discussion. How objective are you? Can you talk calmly about biological reproduction and use the proper anatomic terms? Can you relate biological information to the scope of family life? Can you emotionally accept that masturbation, homosexuality, intimacy between unmarried persons, unwed pregnancy, sexually transmitted diseases, and unusual sexual practices exist? Can you listen to others talk about these subjects? If you cannot, let some other professional do sex education.

The adolescent may be trying to understand another kind of sexual experience in his or her own family. For example, a number of adolescents have to deal with the formerly hidden primary sexual orientation of their parents. Either parent may, during this time, announce a same-sex preference, so in addition to the adolescent's working out his or her own sexual identity, the identity of the parent must be reworked. If you cannot handle these issues, let some other appropriate professional provide sex education and counseling about being lesbian or gay (43).

Realize that no one can do all areas of intervention. Your astute assessment, case finding, and ability to refer the adolescent elsewhere are still major contributions toward helping him or her stay healthy. The rapport necessary to work with the adolescent in any area is highly sensitive, and if he or she has no rapport with the family, your attitudes are crucial.

Promoting Education. You can promote education about sexuality, family, pregnancy, contraceptives, and sexually transmitted diseases through your own intervention and by working with parents and school officials so that objective, accurate information can be given in the schools. Most adults favor sex education in school and on television as a way to reduce the problem of teenage pregnancy.

Teenagers need the opportunity to identify what they consider important problems and a chance to discuss their feelings, attitudes, and ideas and to obtain factual information and guidance with effective solutions (Fig. 11–1). The sex act should be discussed as part of a relationship between individuals requiring a deep sense of love, trust, and intimacy and not just as a means of biological gratification. Sexual behavior is not solely a physical phenomenon but one of great psychosocial significance. The consequences of sexual activity must be explored honestly. More progressive schools include this in the curriculum, and the teacher or school nurse must be comfortable, knowledgeable, and able to promote discussion. Sex education courses given outside the home supplement the influence of parental guidance and teaching. Such sex education and related discussions can also be offered through church youth groups, the Red Cross, local YMCA or YWCA, or other public organizations. Again, you can initiate and participate in such programs.

Perhaps most important, you can encourage the teenager and family to talk together and can teach the parents how and what to teach, where to get information, and the significance of formal sex education beginning in the home. References at the end of the chapter can be helpful in sexuality counseling (15, 31, 121, 136).

Care and Counseling. You may work directly with a pregnant teenager or one with a sexually transmitted disease as a school or clinic nurse or in your primary-care practice. That person needs your acceptance, support, and confidentiality as you do careful interviewing to learn his or her history of sexual activity, symptoms, and contacts. Effective interviewing, communication, and crisis intervention discussed in Chapter 5 and by Murray and Huelskoetter (136) are essential to reduce unwanted consequences of sexual activity. Because of the stigma and legal problems associated with unwed pregnancy, abortion, and sexually transmitted diseases, fear of reprisals, and the quixotic personality of the adolescent, your behavior at the first meeting is crucial. You may not get another chance for thorough assessment or beginning intervention.

The Department of Health and Human Services, U.S. Public Health Services, in its Put Prevention Into Practice program (1994), has provided excellent material for screening adolescents' sexual activity.

Basically, the teen with a sexually transmitted disease wants your help and comfort; he or she is a troubled person. Information is needed about the type of disease, symptoms, contagious nature, consequences of untreated disease, and where to get treatment. In all of these diseases, both male and female partners (along with any other person who has had sexual contact with these partners) should be treated by medication and use of hygiene measures and by counseling and teaching. You are in a key position to determine signs and symptoms and to help make a differential diagnosis. Refer to references at the end of the chapter that were cited earlier. You can also teach about the importance of continued body hygiene, avoiding unprescribed douching or other self-medication, the danger of continued reinfection from sexual intercourse, and the long-term damage to genital tissue from any sexually transmitted disease or repeated abortions. Remind your clients that the *symptoms* of the disease may go away, but the *disease* may not. Hence a complete round of treatment is essential. Further, there are two reliable ways to prevent infection or reinfection: abstinence or the male's use of a condom. One sexual contact is all that is necessary to acquire sexually transmitted diseases.

The girl wants to confirm whether pregnancy exists and talk about personal feelings, family reactions, and what to do next. Explain what services are available and answer her questions about the consequences of remaining pregnant, keeping or placing the baby for adoption, or terminating pregnancy.

Comprehensive maternity services for pregnant adolescents can reduce maternal and neonatal complications, including prematurity, low birth weight, congenital defects, and infant death so often found in this age group. Various references at the end of this chapter are helpful (31, 115, 117, 158, 196, 197, 202).

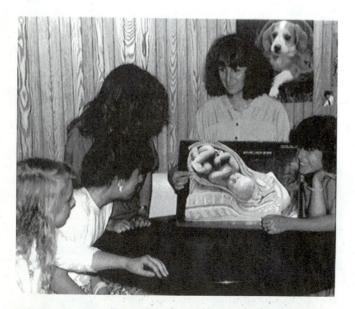

Figure 11–1. Nurses should encourage adolescents to discuss health concerns and provide teaching for the issues that are important to this age group. *(Courtesy of Mary Ann Scoloveno.)*

An adolescent girl may want to know about methods of abortion and services available. Reputable abortion clinics do counseling before the abortion so that the girl does not regret her decision, but you can begin counseling. The questions you raise and guidance you give can help her make necessary decisions (136).

Many states have the law that a minor can be treated for sexually transmitted diseases and other conditions without parental consent. Although this law prevents parents from being with their child in a serious situation, it does enable minors to receive treatment without fear of parental retribution and without having to wait until parents feel ready. Encourage the adolescent to confide in the parents if at all possible and to seek their support. In turn, encourage the parents to be supportive. Consent and confidentiality are key concerns in all areas of health care of the adolescent: emergency care and treatment for drug abuse, alcoholism, sexually transmitted disease, pregnancy, and other problems. Be familiar with local and state legislation and federal policies dealing with legal age and treatment of minors.

Reforming the Present Health Care System. Reforming the present health care system seems essential, as present public health services are frequently incapable of kindly or completely handling the problems resulting from adolescents' sexual activity, because of either policy, philosophy, understaffing, or underfinancing. You can participate in change by working through your professional organization and as an informed citizen. You can promote a deeper awareness of the adolescent as an individual with unique needs and work to extend education and counseling services, including peer-group counseling and teenage advisory boards. Further, you can help establish community services to work with the adolescent or youth in a health care crisis. The disabled adolescent also requires special care and teaching needs.

Working with the Drug Abuser and Alcoholic

Personal Attitudes. You must work through your attitudes about drug use and abuse to assess the person accurately or intervene objectively. Why does a drug problem exist? Do you believe drugs are the answer to problems? How frequently do you use drugs? Do you use amphetamines or barbiturates? Have you ever tried marijuana, LSD, or heroin? What are the multiple influences causing persons to seek answers through use of illegal drugs? What are the moral, spiritual, emotional, and physical implications of excessive drug use, whether the drugs are illegal or prescribed? What treatment do drug abusers deserve? How does the alcoholic differ from the drug abuser? Until you can face these questions, you will not be able to help the adolescent drug abuser or alcoholic.

An accepting attitude toward the drug abuser and alcoholic as a person is essential while at the same time you help him or her become motivated and able to cope with stresses without relying on drugs or alcohol. You will need to use effective communication and assessment, but because these problems are complex, you need to work with others. The treatment team should consist of other health care professionals, representatives from law enforcement and religious agencies, and self-help groups established in various cities by previous drug or alcohol abusers who have been rehabilitated and now seek to rehabilitate others.

Various references at the end of this chapter, which were cited previously, provide more detailed information to aid you in your care.

Members of society impose heavy responsibilities on the young adult. With your intervention, some adolescents who could not otherwise meet these forthcoming demands will exert a positive force in society.

Knowledge. Knowledge about drugs—current ones available on the street, their symptoms and long-term effects, legislation related to each—is necessary for assessment, realistic teaching, and counseling. Also learn about the effects of alcohol. Know local community agencies that do emergency or follow-up care and rehabilitation with drug abusers and alcoholics.

Help teenagers understand that problems of drug abuse and alcoholism can be avoided in several ways. They must get accurate information and make decisions based on knowledge rather than on emotion, have the courage to say "no," and know and respect the laws. They must also participate in worthwhile, satisfying activities, have a constructive relationship with parents, and recognize that the normal, healthy person does not need regular medication except when prescribed by an authorized practitioner. Help youths realize the unanticipated consequences of drug and alcohol abuse: loss of friends; alienation from family; loss of scholastic, social, or career opportunities; economic difficulties; criminal activities; legal penalties; poor health; and loss of identity rather than finding the self.

Every person with whom you work is a potential drug abuser or addict, and all drugs and chemical substances have a potential for harm from allergy, side effects, toxicity, or overdosage. Different drugs taken simultaneously may have an unpredictable or increased effect. In addition, taking unprescribed drugs may mask signs and symptoms of serious disease, thus postponing necessary diagnosis and treatment. Hence a major responsibility on your part is to teach others how to take drugs safely, the importance of taking only prescribed drugs as directed, and the hazards of drugs. Adolescents may not realize that drugs obtained illegally have an unknown purity and strength and are frequently produced under unsanitary conditions. They may not realize that when injections are given without sterile technique, infectious hepatitis, AIDS, tetanus, or vein damage may result. Help parents realize the impact their behavior and attitudes toward drug and alcohol use have on their children.

The Center for Substance Abuse Prevention (CSAP), in planning for drug-free communities by the year 2000, is currently conducting training systems that provide critical knowledge and skills to key people and organizations involved in preventing alcohol, tobacco, and other drug problems. For specific information on the Nurse Training Program, call (301) 572–0257. A one-day training session led by experts along with provision of resource material will provide an excellent foundation for action.

Two helpful resources are *Prevention Primer: An Encyclopedia of Alcohol, Tobacco and Other Drug Prevention Terms,* available from the Center for Substance Abuse Prevention (Rockville, MD: National Clearinghouse for Alcohol and Drug Information, 1993) and *The National Clearinghouse for Alcohol and Drug Information Publication Catalog, Summer 1995.* Call (800) 729–6686 for the U.S. Department of Health and Human Services, Substance Abuse and Mental Health Services Administration, to request your copy.

► ## CONSIDERATIONS FOR THE ADOLESCENT AND FAMILY IN HEALTH CARE

- Family, cultural background and values, support systems, and community resources for the adolescent and family
- Parents as identification figures, able to guide and to allow the adolescent to develop his or her own identity
- Relationship among family members or significant adults and its impact on the adolescent
- Behaviors that indicate abuse, neglect, or maltreatment by parents or other significant adults
- Physical growth patterns, characteristics and competencies, nutritional status, and rest/sleep and exercise patterns that indicate health and are within age norms for the adolescent
- Completion of physical growth spurt and development of secondary sex characteristics that indicate normal development in the male or female; self-concept and body image development and integration related to physical growth
- Nutritional requirements greater than for the adult
- Immunizations, safety education, and other health promotion measures
- Cognitive development into the Stage of Formal Operations, related value formation, ongoing moral–spiritual development, and beginning development of philosophy of life
- Peer relationships, use of leisure time
- Overall appearance and behavioral patterns at home, school, and in the community that indicate positive identity formation, rather than role confusion or diffusion, or negative identity
- Use of effective adaptive mechanisms and coping skills in response to stressors
- Behavioral patterns in late adolescence that indicate integration of physical changes; cognitive, emotional, social, and moral–spiritual development; effective adaptive mechanisms
- Behavioral patterns and characteristics that indicate the adolescent has achieved developmental tasks
- Parental behavior that indicates they are achieving their developmental tasks

SUMMARY

Adolescence is the final period of rapid physical growth, as well as considerable cognitive and emotional change. Relationships with the family remain basically important, but the peer group is dominant and exerts considerable influence on the adolescent's behavior. This is the time during which the individual works to develop his or her identity or sense of uniqueness, to become independent of and separate from parents while retaining basic ties and values. Because of the many available options, determining one's identity, value systems, and career or life path can be difficult, take time, and sometimes be detoured by various societal forces of acquired habits such as substance abuse. A number of health problems may arise in the physical, psychological, or social dimensions.

Considerations for the Adolescent and Family in Health Care and Chart 4 in Appendix IV summarize what you should consider in assessment and health promotion of the adolescent. The family is included in Considerations. Chart 4 presents the American Academy of Family Physicians Periodic Health Examination Ages 13 to 18 Years. It includes guidelines for screening, health counseling, an immunization schedule, and high-risk categories (2).

► ## REFERENCES

1. Acock, A., and J. Keicolt, Is It Family Structure or Socioeconomic Status? Family Structure During Adolescence and Adult Adjustment, *Social Forces,* 68, no. 2 (1989), 553–571.
2. American Academy of Family Physicians, *Age Charts for Periodic Health Examination.* Washington, DC: Author, 1995.

3. Andrews, M., and J. Boyle, *Transcultural Concepts in Nursing Care.* Philadelphia: J.B. Lippincott, 1995.

4. Andrus, J., et al., Surveillance of Attempted Suicide Among Adolescents in Oregon, 1988, *American Journal of Public Health,* 81, no. 8 (1991), 1067–1069.

5. Anorexia May Have Effect on Brain, Bones, Studies Show, *Health Scene,* Fall (1987), 3.

6. Atkin, C., Effects of Televised Alcohol Messages on Teenage Drinking Problems, *Journal of Adolescent Health Care,* 11, no. 1 (1990), 10–24.

7. Attachment Needs May Lead to Date Rape, *The Menninger Letter,* 3, no. 9 (1995), 2.

8. Austin, J., V. Champion, and O. Tzeng, Cross-cultural Relationships Between Self-concept and Body Image in High School Age Boys, *Archives of Psychiatric Nursing,* 3, no. 4 (1989), 234–240.

9. Bachman, J., et al., Racial/Ethnic Differences in Smoking, Drinking, and Illicit Drug Use Among American High School Seniors, 1976–89, *American Journal of Public Health,* 81, no. 3 (1991), 372–377.

10. Bailey, S., Adolescents Multi-substance Use Patterns: The Role of Heavy Alcohol and Cigarette Use, *American Journal of Public Health,* 82 (1992), 1220–1224.

11. Baker, S., and T. Gore, Some Reasons for Wilding, *Newsweek,* May 29 (1989), 8–9.

12. Bates, B., *A Guide to Physical Examination and Histroy Taking* (4th ed.). Philadelphia: J.B. Lippincott, 1987.

13. Batz, J., Casting Out the Sex Roles, *Universitas,* Spring (1990), 1–6.

14. Bess, C., *The Mayday Rampage.* Sacramento, CA: Lookout Press, 1993.

15. Bettelheim, B., and A. Freedgood, *A Good Enough Parent: A Book on Child-rearing.* New York: Random, 1988.

16. Bettes, B., et al., Ethnicity and Psychosocial Factors in Alcohol and Tobacco Use in Adolescence, *Child Development,* 61, no. 2 (1990), 557–565.

17. Blankenhorn, D., *Fatherless America: Confronting Our Most Urgent Social Problem.* New York: Basic Books, 1995.

18. Bloom, K., The Development of Attachment Behaviors in Pregnant Adolescents, *Nursing Research,* 44 (1995), 284–289.

19. Bolger, N., et al., The Onset of Suicidal Ideation in Childhood and Adolescence, *Journal of Youth and Adolescence,* 18, no. 2 (1989), 175–190.

20. Boyd, M., Living With Overweight, *Perspectives in Psychiatric Care,* 25, no. 3, 4 (1989), 48–52.

21. Broste, S., D. Hansen, R. Strand, and D. Stueland, Hearing Loss Among High School Farm Students, *American Journal of Public Health,* 79 (1989), 619–622.

22. Boynton, R., E. Dunn, and G. Stephens, *Manual of Ambulatory Pediatrics* (3rd ed.). Philadelphia: J.B. Lippincott, 1994.

23. Burgess, A., and H.J. Birnbaum, Youth Prostitution, *American Journal of Nursing,* 82, no. 5 (1982), 832–834.

24. ———, and L. Holmstrom, The Rape Victim in the Emergency Ward, *American Journal of Nursing,* 73, no. 10 (1973), 1741–1745.

25. Butler, J., and L. Burton, Rethinking Teenage Childbearing: Is Sexual Abuse a Missing Link? *Family Relations,* January (1990), 73–79.

26. Canadian Guidelines for the Treatment of Sexually Transmitted Diseases in Neonates, Children, Adolescents, and Adults, *Canadian Disease Weekly Report,* April (1988), 1452.

27. Centers for Disease Control and Prevention General Recommendations on Immunization: Recommendations of the Advisory Committee on Immunization Practices (ACIP), *Morbidity and Mortality Weekly Report,* 43 (January 28, 1994), 23.

28. Children of the Corn, *Newsweek,* August 28 (1995), 6a-6b.

29. Chirgwin, K., et al., HIV Infection, Genital Ulcer Disease, and Crack Cocaine Use Among Patients Attending a Clinic for Sexually Transmitted Diseases. *American Journal of Public Health,* 81, no. 12 (1991), 1576–1579.

30. Chitty, K., The Primary Prevention Role of the Nurse in Eating Disorders, *Nursing Clinics of North America,* 26 (1991), 789–801.

31. Clemen-Stone, S., D.G. Eigsti, and S.L. McGuire, *Comprehensive Family and Community Health Nursing* (4th ed.). St. Louis: Mosby–Year Book, 1995.

32. Cocaine, Glamorous Status Symbol of the "Jet Set," Is Fast Becoming Many Students' Drug of Choice, *Chronicle of Higher Education,* 31, no. 11 (November 12, 1985), 33–35.

33. Cocaine Toxicity, *National Institute of Drug Abuse Notes,* Washington, DC: U.S. Department of Health and Human Services, 1990, pp. 2, 3.

34. Condoms Work, But Many Don't Use Them, *American Journal of Nursing,* 94, no. 12 (1994), 12.

35. Conrad, N., Where Do They Turn? Social Support Systems of Suicidal High School Adolescents, *Journal of Psychosocial Nursing,* 29, no. 3 (1991), 14–20.

36. The Crack Children, *Newsweek,* February 12 (1990), 60–63.

37. *Crack: The New Cocaine.* Phoenix: DIN Publications, 1989.

38. Dacey, J., and J. Travers, *Human Development Across the Lifespan* (3rd ed.), Madison, WI: Brown & Benchmark, 1996.

39. Daley, S., Little Girls Lose Their Self-Esteem on Way to Adolescence, Study Finds, *New York Times,* January 9 (1991), p. 10.

40. Dangerous Alliance: Family Dysfunction, Adolescent Curiosity Leads Teens to Drugs, *West Citizen Journal* (St. Louis County), June 23 (1989), 1.

41. Davies, J., and M. Frawley, *Treating the Adult Survivor of Childhood Sexual Abuse: A Psychoanalytic Perspective.* New York: Basic Books, 1994.

42. Davis, J., and K. Sherer, *Applied Nutrition and Diet Therapy for Nurses* (2nd ed.). Philadelphia: W.B. Saunders, 1994.

43. Deevy, S., When Mom or Dad Comes Out: Helping Adolescents Cope with Homophobia, *Journal of Psychosocial Nursing,* 27, no. 10 (1989), 35–36.

44. Desmond, S.M., et al., Black and White Adolescents: Perceptions of Their Weight, *Journal of School Health,* 59, no. 8 (1989), 353–358.

45. Dietz, W.H., You Are What You Eat—What You Eat Is What You Are, *Journal of Adolescent Health Care,* 11, no. 1 (1990), 76–81.

46. Dorn, L.D., et al., Perceptions of Puberty: Adolescent, Parent, and Health Care Personnel, *Developmental Psychology,* 26, no. 2 (1990), 322–329.

47. Doubtful Dare, *The Harvard Mental Health Letter,* 11, no. 9 (1995), 7.

48. The Drug Advisory, St. Louis: National Council on Alcoholism and Drug Dependence, 1990.

49. Duvall, E., and B. Miller, *Marriage and Family Development* (6th ed.). New York: Harper & Row, 1986.

50. Dworetzky, J., *Human Development: A Lifespan Approach* (2nd ed.). St. Paul: West Publishing, 1995.

51. Earls, F., Studying Adolescent Suicidal Ideation and Behavior in Primary Care Settings, *Suicide and Life Threatening Behavior,* 19, no. 1 (1989), 99–107.

52. Eating Disorders—Not for Women Only, *Health Scene,* Fall (1987), 10.

53. Edmonds, M., Overcoming Eating Disorders: A Group Experience, *Journal of Psychosocial Nursing,* 24, no. 8 (1986), 19–25.

54. Elders, M., C. Perry, M. Eriksen, and G. Giovino, The Report of the Surgeon General's Preventing Tobacco Use Among Young People, *American Journal of Public Health,* 84 (1994), 543–547.

55. Engel, G., Reflections on the Next Generation, *The Courier,* 64, no. 5 (1993), 2.

56. Erikson, E.H., *Childhood and Society* (2nd ed.). New York: W.W. Norton, 1963.

57. ——, *Identity: Youth and Crisis.* New York: W.W. Norton, 1968.

58. ——, Memorandum on Youth, in Sze W., ed., *Human Life Cycle.* New York: Jason Aronson, 1975, pp. 351–359.

59. Escobedo, L., J. Chorba, and R. Waxweiler, Patterns of Alcohol Use and the Risk of Drinking and Driving Among U.S. High School Students, *American Journal of Public Health,* 85 (1995), 976–978.

60. Evans, K., and J. Sullivan, *Treating Addicted Survivors of Trauma.* New York: Guilford Press, 1995.

61. *Fact Sheet: Alcohol and Drug Use by Teenagers.* Jefferson City, MO: Missouri Department of Mental Health, 1991.

62. Farr, G., H. Gabelnick, K. Slurgen, and L. Dorflinger, Contraceptive Efficacy and Acceptability of the Female Condom, *American Journal of Public Health,* 84 (1994), 1960–1964.

63. Flood, M., Addictive Eating Disorders, *Nursing Clinics of North America,* 24, no. 1 (1989), 45–53.

64. French, S., C. Perry, G. Leon, and J. Fulkerson, Weight Concerns, Dieting Behavior, and Smoking Initiation Among Adolescents: A Prospective Study, *American Journal of Public Health,* 84 (1994), 1818–1820.

65. French, S., M. Story, B. Downs, M. Bronick, and R. Blum, Frequent Dieting Among Adolescents: Psychosocial and Health Correlates, *American Journal of Public Health,* 85 (1995), 695–701.

66. Fritz, T., and M. Barbie, What Are the Warning Signs for Suicidal Adolescents? *Journal of Psychosocial Nursing,* 31, no. 2 (1993), 37–40.

67. Garbarino, J., E. Guttman, and J. Seeley, *The Psychologically Battered Child: Strategies for Identification, Assessment, and Intervention.* San Francisco: Jossey-Bass, 1987.

68. Gelman, D., D. Rosenberg, V. Quade, E. Roberts, and D. Senna, Tune in, Come out, *Newsweek,* November 8 (1993), 70–71.

69. Gesell, A., F. Ilg, and L. Ames, *Youth: The Years from Ten to Sixteen.* New York: Harper Brothers, 1956.

70. Giger, J., and R. Davidhizar, *Transcultural Nursing: Assessment and Intervention* (2nd ed.). St. Louis: C.V. Mosby, 1995.

71. Gillis, A., Determinants of Health-Promoting Lifestyles in Adolescent Females, *Canadian Journal of Nursing Research,* 26, no. 2 (1994), 13–28.

72. Goldberg, B., Injury Patterns in Youth Sports, *Physician and Sports Medicine,* 17, no. 3 (1989), 174–176.

73. Gould, M., et al., Suicide Clusters: An Examination of Age-specific Effects, *American Journal of Public Health,* 80, no. 2 (1990), 211–212.

74. Glass, G.E., B.S. Schwartz, J.M. Morgan III, D.T. Johnson, P.M. Noy, and E. Israel, Environmental Risk Factors for Lyme Disease Identified With Geographic Information Systems, *American Journal of Public Health,* 85, no. 7 (1995), 944–948.

75. Graber, M.A., R.J. Allen, and B.T. Levy, *University of Iowa: The Family Practice Handbook* (2nd ed.). St. Louis: Mosby, 1994.

76. Greendale, G., S. Haas, K. Holbrook, B. Walsh, J. Schachter, and R. Phillips, The Relationship of *Chlamydia trachomatis* Infection and Male Fertility, *American Journal of Public Health,* 83, (1993), 996–1001.

77. Grieve, N., et al., Self-esteem and Sex-role Attitudes: A Comparison of Italian and Anglo-Australian Adolescent Girls, *Psychology of Women Quarterly,* 12, no. 6 (1988), 175–189.

78. Grossman, D., C. Milligan, and R. Deyo, Risk Factors for Suicide Attempts Among Navajo Adolescents, *American Journal of Public Health,* 81, 2 (1991), 870–874.

79. Growing up Against the Odds, *Newsweek,* September 11 (1989), 25.

80. Guidelines for Teenage Parties, *Olivette Advisory* (Olivette, MO.), 6, no. 4 (January 1983).

81. Guio, M.V., et al., Child Victimization, Pornography, and Prostitution, *Crime and Justice,* 3 (1980), 65–81.

82. Haberman, M., and V. Dill, Commitment to Violence Among Teenagers in Poverty, *Kappa Delta Pi Record,* 31, no. 4 (1995), 148–156.

83. Hall, J., and P. Stevens, AIDS: A Guide to Suicide Assessment, *Archives of Psychiatric Nursing,* 1, no. 2 (1988), 115–120.

84. Hatcher, R., et al., *Contraceptive Technology—1990–1992* (15th ed.). New York: Irvington, 1992.

85. Hatton, C., and S. Valente, *Suicide: Assessment and Intervention.* Norwalk, CT: Appleton-Century-Crofts, 1984.

86. Hauser, S., J. DiPlacido, A. Jacobson, J. Willett, and C. Cole, Family Coping With an Adolescent Chronic Illness: An Approach and Three Studies, *Journal of Adolescence,* 16, no. 3 (1993), 305–329.

87. Havighurst, R., *Developmental Tasks and Education* (3rd ed.). New York: David McKay, 1972.

88. Hawton, K., *Suicide and Attempted Suicide Among Children and Adolescents.* Beverly Hills, CA: Sage, 1990.

89. Health Risks, *Women's Health Advocate Newsletter,* 2, no. 11 (1996), 2–3.

90. Heiney, S., Helping Children Through Painful Procedures, *American Journal of Nursing,* 91, no. 11 (1991), 20–24.

91. Hemfelt, R., F. Minirth, and P. Meier, *Love Is a Choice.* Nashville, TN: Thomas Nelson, 1989.

92. Herman, J., Recognition and Treatment of Incestuous Families, *International Journal of Family Therapy,* 5, no. 2 (1983), 81–91.

93. Heroin's Use up Says U.S. Expert Drug Chief Lee Brown, *The Nation's Health,* May/June (1995), 17.

94. Hoole, A., R. Pickard, R. Ouimette, J. Lohr, and R. Greenberg, *Patient Care Guidelines for Nurse Practitioners* (4th ed.). Philadelphia: J.B. Lippincott, 1995.

95. Horwitz, E., World, Here We Come (An Alternate Public School for Pregnancy and Parenting Teens), *AAWW Outlook,* 85, no. 3 (1991), 14–19.

96. House, M., Cocaine, *American Journal of Nursing,* 90, no. 4 (1990), 41–45.

97. Hubbard, G., Perceived Life Changes for Children and Adolescents Following Disclosure of Father–Daughter Incest, *Journal of Child and Adolescent Psychiatric and Mental Health Nursing,* 2, no. 2 (1989), 78–82.

98. *Ice: Speed, Smoke, and Fire,* Phoenix: D.I.N., 1991.

99. *Inhalants: Just Say No.* Washington, DC: National Institute on Drug Abuse, 1986.

100. Jackson, M.M., and T. Rymer, Viral Hepatitis: Anatomy of a Diagnosis, *American Journal of Nursing,* 94, no. 1 (1994), 43–48.

101. Jenkins, A., When Your Child Searches for a Birth Parent, *Home Life,* May (1991), 37–39.

102. Joe, G., and D. Simpson, Mortality Rates Among Opioid Addicts in a Longitudinal Study, *American Journal of Public Health,* 77, no. 3 (1987), 347–348.

103. Johnson, C., L. Myers, L. Webber, S. Hunter, et al., Alcohol Consumption Among Adolescents and Young Adults: The

Bogalusa Heart Study, 1981 to 1991, *American Journal of Public Health,* 85 (1995), 979–982.

104. Jolley, J., and M. Mitchell, *Lifespan Development: A Topical Approach.* Madison, WI: Brown & Benchmark, 1996.

105. Jones, J., A Proposed Model of Relapse Prevention for Adolescents Who Abuse Alcohol, *Journal of Child and Adolescent Psychiatric and Mental Health Nursing,* 3, no. 4 (1990), 139–143.

106. Kafka, R., and P. London, Communication in Relationships and Adolescent Substance Use: The Influence of Parents and Friends, *Adolescence,* 26, no. 103 (Fall 1991), 587–597.

107. Kelder, S., C. Perry, K. Klepp, and L. Lytle, Longitudinal Tracking of Adolescent Smoking, Physical Activity, and Food Choice Behaviors, *American Journal of Public Health,* 84 (1994), 1121–1126.

108. Keller, C., and R. Nicolls, Coping Strategies of Chronically Ill Adolescents and Their Parents, *International Disability Studies,* 13, no. 4 (1991), 138–140.

109. Keniston, K., Youth: A New Stage of Life, *American Scholar,* 39 (1970), 631–654.

110. ———, Youth as a Stage of Life, in Sze, W., ed., *Human Life Cycle.* New York: Jason Aronson, 1975, 332–349.

111. Kiecolt-Glaser, J., and K. Davis, Post-adolescent Onset Male Anorexia, *Journal of Psychosocial Nursing,* 22, no. 1 (1982).

112. Knollmueller, R. (ed.), *Prevention Across the Life Span: Healthy People for the Twenty-first Century.* Washington, DC: American Nurses Association Council of Community Health Nurses, 1993.

113. Kohlberg, L., Moral Stages and Moralization: The Cognitive Development Approach, in Lickera, T., ed., *Moral Development and Behavior.* New York: Holt, Rineholt, & Winston, 1976.

114. Koniak-Griffin, D., and M. Brecht, Linkages Between Sexual Risk Taking, Substance Use, and AIDS Knowledge Among Pregnant Adolescents and Young Mothers, *Nursing Research,* 44 (1995), 340–346.

115. L'Abate, L., J. Farrar, and D. Serritella (eds.), *Handbook of Differential Treatments for Addictions.* Boston: Allyn & Bacon, 1992.

116. Lamb, M., The Emergent Father, in Lamb, M.E., ed., *The Father's Role: Cross-cultural Perspectives.* Hillsdale, NJ: Lawrence Erlbaum, 1987, pp. 1–26.

117. Landau-Stanton, J., and C. Clements, *AIDS, Health, and Mental Health: A Primary Sourcebook.* New York: Brunner/Mazel, 1993.

118. LaRossa, R., Fatherhood and Social Change. *Family Relations,* 37, (1988), 451–457.

119. Lethbridge, I., Post-tubal Sterilization Syndrome, *IMAGE: Journal of Nursing Scholarship,* 24, no. 1 (1992), 15–18.

120. Levy, J., and E. Deykin, Suicidality, Depression, and Substance Abuse in Adolescence, *American Journal of Psychiatry,* 146, no. 11 (1989), 1462–1467.

121. Lidz, T., *The Person—His and Her Development Throughout the Life Cycle* (2nd ed.). New York: Basic Books, 1983.

122. Lyme Borreliosis Foundation, *Up-to-Date Information Available on Lyme Disease.* Tolland, CT: Author, n.d.

123. Lynam, M. J., and L. Tenn, Communication: A Tool for the Negotiation of Independence in Families with Adolescents, *Journal of Advanced Nursing,* 14, no. 8 (1989), 653–660.

124. Manning, M., Health Assessment of the Early Adolescent: Challenges and Clinical Issues, *Nursing Clinics of North America,* 25, no. 4 (1990), 823–831.

125. Manov, A., and L. Lowther, A Health Care Approach for Hard-to-Reach Adolescent Runaways, *Nursing Clinics of North America,* 18, no. 2 (1983), 333–341.

126. Marchi, M., and P. Cohen, Early Childhood Eating Behaviors and Adolescent Eating Disorders, *Journal American Academy of Child–Adolescent Psychiatry,* 29, no. 1 (1990), 112–117.

127. Martin, M., and M. Pritchard, Factors Associated with Alcohol Use in Later Adolescence, *Journal of Studies on Alcohol,* 52, no. 1 (1991), 5–9.

128. Mayer, S., and C. Jencks, Growing Up in Poor Neighborhoods: How Much Does It Matter? *Science,* 241 (March 17, 1989), 242–246.

129. McBride, A., *How To Enjoy a Good Life With Your Teenager.* Tucson, AZ: Fischer Books, 1989.

130. McCoy, B., and G. Boutre, Excluding the Black Male in School and Society, *Kappa Delta Pi Record,* 31, no. 4 (1995), 172–176.

131. McGown, A., How to Help Your Lesbian Teenager, *Journal of Psychosocial Nursing,* 31, no. 8 (1993), 48.

132. McLanahan, S., and G. Sandefur, *Growing With a Single Parent.* Cambridge: Harvard University Press, 1994.

133. Melton, J., A Boy With Anorexia Nervosa, *American Journal of Nursing,* 74, no. 9 (1974), 1649–1651.

134. Mickley, D., Evaluating Common Eating Disorders: 10 Questions to Ask Your Patient, *Physician Assistant,* 13, no. 9 (1989), 147–148, 153, 156.

135. Mosely, C., and M. Beard, Norplant: Nursing's Responsibility in Procreative Rights, *Nursing & Health Care,* 15, no. 6 (1994), 294–297.

136. Murray, R., and M.M. Huelskoetter, *Psychiatric/Mental Health Nursing: Giving Emotional Care* (3rd ed.). Norwalk, CT: Appleton & Lange, 1991.

137. Muuss, R., Carol Gilligan's Theory of Sex Differences in the Development of Moral Reasoning During Adolescence, *Adolescence,* 23, no. 89 (1988), 229–243.

138. Myers, D., and A. Anderson, Adolescent Addiction: Assessment and Identification, *Journal of Pediatric Health Care,* 5, no. 2 (1991), 86–93.

139. Nettina, S., Syphilis: A New Look at an Old Killer, *American Journal of Nursing,* 90, no. 4 (1990), 68–70.

140. Newman, B., The Changing Nature of the Parent–Adolescent Relationship From Early to Late Adolescence, *Adolescence,* 24, no. 96 (1989), 915–924.

141. Norris, J., and M. Kunes-Carroll, Self-Esteem Disturbance, *Nursing Clinics of North America,* 20, no. 4 (1985), 745–761.

142. Oldaker, S., Identity Confusion: Nursing Diagnoses for Adolescents, *Nursing Clinics of North America,* 20, no. 4 (1985), 763–773.

143. Oswald, L., Cocaine Addiction: The Hidden Dimension, *Archives of Psychiatric Nursing,* 3, no. 3 (1989), 134–141.

144. Ott, M.J., and P.L. Jackson, Precocious Puberty: Identifying Early Sexual Development, *Nurse Practitioner: American Journal of Primary Health Care,* 14, no. 11 (1989), 21, 24–28, 30.

145. Otto, L., America's Youth: A Changing Profile, *Family Relations,* 37, no. 4 (1988), 385–391.

146. Pardeck, J., and J. Pardeck, Family Factors Related to Adolescent Autonomy, *Adolescence,* 25, no. 98 (1990), 311–319.

147. Parental Work Overload Affects Adolescents, *The Menninger Letter,* 3, no. 8 (November, 1995), 6.

148. Parish, T., Evaluations of Family by Youth: Do They Vary as a Function of Family Structure, Gender, and Birth Order? *Adolescence,* 25, no. 98 (1990), 353–356.

149. Parker, D., W. Carl, L. French, and F. Martin, Characteristics of Adolescent Work Injuries Reported to the Minnesota Department of Labor and Industry, *American Journal of Public Health,* 84 (1994), 606–611.

150. Pender, N.J., Expressing Health Through Lifestyle Patterns, *Nursing Science Quarterly,* 3, no. 3 (1990), 115–122.

151. Pfeffer, C., *The Suicidal Child.* New York: Guilford Press, 1986.

152. Piaget, J., *The Growth of Logical Thinking from Childhood to Adolescence.* New York: Basic Books, 1961.

153. Polk-Walker, G., What Really Happened? Incidence and Factor Assessment of Abused Children and Adolescents, *Journal of Psychosocial Nursing,* 28, no. 11 (1990), 17–22.

154. Poole, C., Adolescent Pregnancy and Unfinished Developmental Tasks of Childhood, *Journal of School Health,* 57, no. 7 (1987), 271–273.

155. Poponoe, D., The Controversial Truth, *New York Times,* December 26 (1992), A-21.

156. Public Health Reaches Out to Reduce Tobacco Use Among Teens, *The Nation's Health,* December (1995), 7.

157. Romer, D., M. Black, I. Ricardo, S. Feigebnan, et al., Social Influences on the Sexual Behavior of Youth at Risk for HIV Exposure, *American Journal of Public Health,* 84 (1994), 977–985.

158. Romig, C., and G. Thompson, Teen-age Pregnancy: A Family Systems Approach, *American Journal of Family Therapy,* 16 (1988), 133–143.

159. Rotheram-Borus, M.J., Ethnic Differences in Adolescents' Identity Status and Associated Behavior Problems, *Journal of Adolescence,* 12, no. 4 (1989), 361–374.

160. ———, Evaluation of Suicide Risk Among Youths in Community Settings, *Suicide and Life Threatening Behavior,* 19, no. 1 (1989), 108–119.

161. Roye, C., Breaking Through to the Adolescent Patient, *American Journal of Nursing,* 95, no. 12 (1995), 19–23.

162. Runyon, N., and P. Jackson, Divorce: The Impact on Children, *Perspectives in Psychiatric Care,* 24, nos. 3–4, (1987/1988), 101–105.

163. Rush, K.L., The School Nurse and Sport Nutrition for the Adolescent Athlete, *Journal of School Health,* 60, no. 8 (1990), 425–427.

164. Ryan, J., and A. Ryan, Courtship Makes a Comeback, *Focus on the Family,* November (1995), 9–12.

165. Ryerson, D., Suicide Awareness Education in Schools: The Development of a Core Program and Subsequent Modifications for Special Populations or Institutions, *Death Studies,* 14, no. 4 (1990), 371–390.

166. Scherer, P., How AIDS Attacks the Brain, *American Journal of Nursing,* 90, no. 1 (1990), 44–52.

167. School-based Prevention Program Reduces Adolescent Drug Abuse, *The Menninger Letter,* 3, no. 8 (1995), 3.

168. Self-esteem From Dating Differs by Gender, *The Menninger Letter,* 3, no. 6 (June, 1995), 7.

169. *Sexually Transmitted Diseases,* Jefferson City, MO: Missouri Family Health Council, 1995, pp. 1–6.

170. Shelton, C., Helping College Students Make Moral Decisions, *Conversations on Jesuit Higher Education,* Fall (1992), 2, 7–25.

171. Sherman, J., and S. Fields, *Guide to Patient Evaluation* (5th ed.). Garden City, NY: Medical Examination, 1987.

172. Slap, G.B., et al., Risk Factors for Attempted Suicide During Adolescence, *Pediatrics,* 84, no. 5 (1989), 762–772.

173. Spence, W., *Hallucinogens: Trip or Trap?* Waco, TX: Health Ed., 1988.

174. Steward, D., A. Stein, G. Forrest, and D. Clarke, Psychosocial Adjustment in Siblings of Children with Chronic Life-threatening Illness: A Research Note, *Journal of Child Psychology and Psychiatry,* 33, no. 4, 779–784.

175. Stiffman, A., Suicide Attempts in Runaway Youths, *Suicide and Life Threatening Behavior,* 19, no. 2 (1989), 147–159.

176. Strauss, S., and B. Clarke, Decision-making Patterns in Adolescent Mothers, *IMAGE: Journal of Nursing Scholarship,* 24, no. 1 (1992), 69–74.

177. Study Shows That TV Suicide Dramas May Contribute to Teen Suicide, *Journal of Child Adolescent Psychotherapy,* 4, no. 2 (1987), 139–140.

178. Suicides Among Black Men Double, *NAMI Advocate,* 16, no. 4 (1995), 8.

179. Szyalo, V., Approaching Adolescents About a Pelvic Exam, *American Journal of Nursing,* 88, no. 11 (1988), 1502–1506.

180. Teen Suicide Rate Up Sharply, *NAMI Advocate,* 16, no. 4 (1995), 7.

181. Teens Identify Worst Worries—Top 10, *Union Banner,* December 28 (1988), 10.

182. The Body of the Beholder, *Newsweek,* April 24 (1995), 66–67.

183. Thompson, K., Effects of Early Alcohol Use on Adolescents' Relations With Peers and Self-Esteem Patterns Over Time, *Adolescence,* 24, no. 96 (1989), 837–849.

184. Treatment of Drug Abuse and Addiction—Part II, *The Harvard Mental Health Letter,* 12, no. 3 (1995), 1–3.

185. Turner, J., and D. Helms, *Lifespan Development* (5th ed.). New York: Holt, Rinehart & Winston, 1995.

186. U.S. Department of Health and Human Services, *Office of Maternal and Child Health: Child Health USA '89,* No. HRS-MCH 8915. Washington, DC: Bureau of Maternal and Child Health Resources Development, 1989.

187. Uphold, C., and M. Graham, *Clinical Guidelines in Family Practice* (2nd ed.). Gainsville, FL: Barmarrae Books, 1994.

188. Vernon, M., Adolescent Risk Factors, lecture at Twentieth Annual NCAPA Conference, Myrtle Beach, SC, August 17, 1995.

189. Wadsworth, B., *Piaget's Theory of Cognitive and Affective Development* (5th ed.). New York: Longman, 1996.

190. Wallerstein, J., Children After Divorce: Wounds That Don't Heal, *Perspectives in Psychiatric Care,* 24, nos. 3–4 (1987/1988), 107–113.

191. Warren, J., F. Gary, and J. Moorhead, Self-reported Experiences of Physical and Sexual Abuse Among Runaway Youths, *Perspectives in Psychiatric Care,* 30, no. 1 (1994), 23–28.

192. Washburn, P., Identification, Assessment, and Referral of Adolescent Drug Abusers, *Pediatric Nursing,* 17, no. 2 (1991), 137–140.

193. Webb, P., Piaget: Implications for Teaching, *Theory Into Practice,* 19, no. 2 (1980), 93–97.

194. Webster, D., P. Gainer, and H. Champion, Weapon Carrying Among Inner-city Junior High Students: Defensive Behavior vs. Aggressive Delinquency, *American Journal of Public Health,* 85 (1995), 1604–1608.

195. White, J.H., Behavioral Intervention for the Obese Client, *Nursing Practice,* 11 (1986), 27–34.

196. Williams, S.R., *Nutrition and Diet Therapy* (10th ed.). St. Louis: Times Mirror/Mosby, 1995.

197. Wong, D., *Whaley and Wong's Nursing Care of Infants and Children* (5th ed.). St. Louis: C.V. Mosby, 1995.

198. Wright, D., ed., *Responding to the Needs of Today's Minority Students.* San Francisco; Jossey-Bass, 1987.

199. Yaffe, E., Expensive, Illegal, and Wrong: Sexual Harassment in Our Schools, *Phi Delta Kappa,* 77, no. 3 (1995), K1–K14.

200. Yankauer, A., Sexually Transmitted Diseases: A Neglected Public Health Priority, *American Journal of Public Health,* 84 (1994), 1894–1897.

201. Yorker, B., The Prosecution of Child Sexual Abuse Cases, *Journal of Child Psychiatric Nursing,* 1, no. 2 (1988), 50–57.

202. Youngs, B., *A Parent's Survival Guide: Helping Your Teenager Deal With Stress.* Los Angeles: Jeremy P. Tarcher, 1986.

IV

The Developing Person and Family: Young Adulthood Through Death

chapter twelve

Assessment and Health Promotion for the Young Adult

> When I was a child I spoke as a child, I understood as a child, I thought as a child, but when I became a man (an adult), I put away childish things.
>
> —I Corinthians 13:11

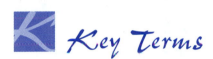

Key Terms

Average weight	Plateau phase	Circadian rhythm	Sleep onset
Basal metabolic rate	Orgasm	Chronopharmacology	Sleep maintenance
Sexuality	Resolution phase	Sleep	Terminal insomnia
Sex identity	Mittelschmerz	Electroencephalograms (EEGs)	Physical fitness
Sex role	Premenstrual syndrome (PMS)	Alpha rhythm	Vascularization
Absolutist (procreational) position	Dysmenorrhea	Delta rhythm	Substance abuse
Hedonistic (recreational sex) view	Premenstrual dysphoric disorder (PMDD)	Sleep spindles	Burnout
Relativistic (situational) position	Homosexuals	K-complexes	Stress burnout
Relational (person-centered) view	Homosexual man (gay)	NREM sleep	Leisure
Human sexual response cycle	Homosexual woman (lesbian)	NREM stage I sleep	Life structure
Vasocongestion	Transsexuals	NREM stage II sleep	Intimacy
Myotonia	Cohabitation	NREM stage III sleep	Homogamy
Four phases of the cycle	Biological rhythms	NREM stage IV sleep	Isolation (self-absorption)
Excitement phase	Exogenous rhythms	REM sleep	Body image
	Endogenous rhythms	Insomnia	Schema
		Primary insomnia	Singlehood

Announcement phase	Iron deficiency anemia	Acute pyelonephritis	Migraine headache
Moratorium period	Atopic dermatitis	Chronic fatigue syndrome	Aura
Focusing period	Folliculitis	Hepatitis B	Acquired immunodeficiency syndrome (AIDS)
Amniocentesis	Furuncle	Dental caries	
Infertility	Carbuncle	Periodontal disease	Biofeedback training
Surrogate parent	Urticaria	Lactose intolerance (milk malabsorption syndrome)	Stress reactions
Upper respiratory infection	Scabies		Battered woman syndrome
Influenza	Simple diarrhea	Anxiety	Incest
Essential hypertension	Cystitis	Tension headache	Divorce
Mitral valve prolapse			

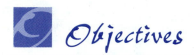

Objectives

Study of this chapter will enable you to:

1. Discuss young adulthood as a developmental crisis and how and why the present young adult generation differs from earlier generations.

2. Explore with middle-aged and older adults their feelings about and ways to be helpful to young adults.

3. List the developmental tasks of the young adult's family, and describe your role in helping families to meet these tasks.

4. Assess the physical characteristics of a young adult.

5. Explain facts from sex behavior research when asked for information about sexuality.

6. Teach nutritional requirements to the young adult male and female, including the pregnant and lactating female.

7. Identify various body rhythms, and give examples of body rhythms that maintain adaptation.

8. Describe factors that influence biological rhythms, illness, and dyssynchrony that may result.

9. Discuss nursing measures to assist the person's maintenance of normal biological rhythms during illness.

10. Compare the stages of the sleep cycle, effects of deprivation of the different stages of sleep, and sleep disturbances that occur.

11. Discuss with the young adult his or her need for rest, sleep, exercise, and leisure.

12. Assess emotional characteristics, self-concept and body image, and adaptive mechanisms of a young adult, and determine nursing implications.

13. Explore the meaning of intimacy versus isolation.

14. Contrast the lifestyle options of the young adult and their influence on health status and your plans for his or her care.

15. Discuss how cognitive characteristics, social concerns, and moral–spiritual–philosophic development influence the total behavior and well-being of the young adult.

16. State the developmental tasks of the young adult, and describe your role in helping him or her achieve them.

17. Assess a young adult who has one of the health problems described in this chapter, write a care plan, and work effectively with him or her to enhance health status.

When does young adulthood begin in the United States? A person must be 18 to vote, 30 to be a senator, and 35 to be president. A woman may have her first child at 15 or at 35, or she may have none. Even with these variations the generally accepted age range for young adulthood in America is about 25 to 45 years (182).

Childhood and adolescence are the periods for growing up; adulthood is the time for settling down. The changes in young adulthood relate more to sociocultural forces and expectations and to value and cognitive changes than to physical development. The young adult generally has more contact with people of different ages than previously. This experience tends to influence the young adult toward a more conservative, traditional viewpoint (94).

The young adult is expected to enter new roles of responsibility at work, at home, and in society and to develop values, attitudes, and interests in keeping with these roles. The young adult may have difficulty simultaneously handling work, school, marriage, home, and childrearing. He or she may work primarily at one of these tasks at a time, neglecting the others, which then adds to the difficulties (94).

The definition, expectations, and stresses of young adulthood are influenced by socioeconomic status, urban or rural residence, ethnic and educational background, various life events, and the historical era. This generation of young adults is unique. They have experienced economic growth and related abundance of material goods and technology, rapid social changes, and sophisticated medical care. They have never known a world without the threat of nuclear war, pollution, overpopulation, and threatened loss of natural resources. Instant media coverage of events has made the world a small and familiar place. Changes in the role of women, the decreasing birth rate, and increasing longevity are modifying the timing of developmental milestones in many people.

Generation X is a recently identified group of young adults in the United States. They are well educated and have the means to achieve the upper-middle-economic-level lifestyle; however, they differ from the dominant culture in some ways. They are concerned about the quality of family life and divorce rates, and want the job to accommodate to family values. They speak of promoting social equality, preserving parks, and improving the environment, but also want to get by with the status quo when possible. They say they want to "get back to basics." They desire to avoid risks and may feel paralyzed by the social problems around them. Older people may perceive this group as noncommitted, indecisive, lazy, and refusing to pay its dues because of the lack of active involvement in the community or civic affairs and a focus on self and family.

Overall, this young adult generation makes demands that may create discomfort and/or conflict for older generations (55, 129, 287).

Further, the person who is 25 or 30 (the young-young adult) works at developmental tasks differently from the person who is 35, 40, or 45 (the old young adult).

FAMILY DEVELOPMENT AND RELATIONSHIPS

The major family goal is the reorganization of the family into a continuing unity while releasing maturing young people into lives of their own. Most families actively prepare their children to leave home.

Family Relationships

In the United States the young adult is expected to be independent from the parents' home and care, although if the person has an extended education, he or she may choose to remain living with the parents to save expenses. Sometimes the young adult does not leave the parents' home as quickly as parents would like. With the increasing number of separations and divorces, the tight job market, and increasing apartment rental rates, the young adult child may move back home, sometimes with children. Emancipation from parents may not occur for years. Parents may resent the intrusion. As one mother said, "My son is 27, and I don't think he's ever going to leave home. I'm tired of being his cook, his cleaning maid, his laundress, his therapist, and his bank." If the young adult does live at home, he or she should expect, and be expected, to assume a share of the home responsibilities and to adjust lifestyle to that of the parents, to whom the home belongs. Sometimes the adult offspring can be a real help to the parents. Eventually the parents may have to ask the adult offspring to move out so that both parents and offspring can resume achieving their developmental tasks (94).

Some parents delay this emancipation process because of their own needs to hold onto their offspring. They may have a strong desire to be needed by or wish to continue living vicariously through their children; however, families have much less control over the lifestyle, vocational choice, and friends or eventual mate of their offspring than they did in earlier generations. For emancipation to occur, the parents must trust their offspring, and the offspring must feel the parents' concern, support, and confidence in his or her ability to work things through.

You can help parents understand that, although they are releasing their own children, new members are being drawn into the family circle through their offspring's marriage or close relationships. That the young adult is ready to leave home indicates the parents have done their job.

In a family with several children, the parents may anticipate having the older children leave. The parents then have less responsibility, and the remaining children get the benefit of a less crowded home and more parental attention. At the same time, the emancipated offspring can still use home as a place to return during times of stress.

Often family expenses are at a peak during this period as parents pay for education and weddings or finance their offspring while they establish their own home or profession. Young adults will earn what they can, but they may not be able to be financially independent even if they are no longer living at home. Both parents may work to meet financial obligations. As young adult offspring establish families, parents should take the complementary roles of letting go and standing by with encouragement, reassurance, and appreciation.

Often the main source of conflict between the parents and young adult offspring is the difference in philosophy and lifestyle between the two generations. The parents who sacrificed for their children to have a nice home, material things, education, leisure activities, and travel may now be criticized for how they look, act, and believe. In fact, the young adult may insist that he or she will *never* live like the parents.

Help the parents resolve within themselves that their grown children will not be carbon copies of them. The parents, however, can secretly take solace in knowing that usually the basic values they instilled within their children will remain their basic guidelines, although outward behavior may seem different. This becomes evident as the young adult becomes middle-aged. Help the parents to realize the importance of their acceptance and understanding of their offspring and of not deliberately provoking arguments over ideologies.

The parents need help in providing a secure home base, both as a model for the young adult and to reduce feelings of threat in the younger children. Although the parents are withstanding the criticism of their grown children, they must remain cognizant that younger children in the home will be feeling conflict, too. The parents are still identification models to them, but young children and adolescents value highly the attitudes and judgments of young adult siblings, who, in turn, can have a definite influence on younger children. The parents can help the younger children realize that there are many ways to live and that they will encourage each to find his or her own way when the time comes.

Gradually the parents themselves must shift from a household with children to a husband–wife pair again as the last young adult establishes a home. Family structure, roles, and responsibilities change, and use of space and other resources change.

Use the above knowledge to teach and counsel families as they work through concerns about family relationships.

Family Developmental Tasks

In summary, the following tasks must be accomplished by the family of the young adult (93). Your listening, teaching, and counseling may assist the family to meet these tasks.

- Rearrange the home physically and reallocate resources (space, material objects) to meet the needs of remaining members.
- Meet the expenses of releasing the offspring and redistribute the budget.
- Redistribute the responsibilities among grown and growing children and finally between the husband and wife or between the adult members living in the household on the basis of interests, ability, and availability.
- Maintain communication within the family to contribute to harmony and happiness while remaining available to young adult and other offspring.
- Enjoy companionship and sexual intimacy as a husband–wife team while incorporating changes.
- Widen the family circle to include the close friends or spouses of the offspring and the entire family of inlaws.
- Reconcile conflicting loyalties and philosophies of life.

PHYSIOLOGIC CONCEPTS

Although body and mind changes continue through life, most physical and mental structures have completed growth when the person reaches young adulthood. Changes that occur during adult life are different from those in childhood; they occur more slowly and in smaller increments.

Physical Characteristics

Weight and Height

Norms denote a set standard of development or the average achievement of a group; however, an average adult person has never really been described. Each person is an individual, and normal values cover a wide range in healthy individuals. Height and weight depend on many factors: heredity, sex, socioeconomic level, geographic area, food habits and preferences, level of activity, and emotional and physical environments. Weight loss or gain is unpredictable in this age group, and norms for height and weight are difficult to determine. Most height and weight tables do not consider the individual and specific influencing factors. Tables usually record either average weight for a given height and age or ideal or desirable weight for a specific height. The **average weight** is a *mathematic norm, found by adding the weights of many people and dividing by the number in the sample.*

The weight guidelines for American adults have been revised for the second time in five years by the Department of Agriculture and the Department of Health and Human Services. The new weight table (see Recommended Height and Weight for Adults) applies to men and women. Weights at the lower end of the range are recommended for individuals with low ratio of muscle and bone to fat; weights at the upper end are advised for people with muscular physiques. For example, the recommended weight for men who are not well-conditioned athletes would be at the lower end of the scale.

► RECOMMENDED HEIGHT AND WEIGHT FOR ADULTS

Height*	Weight† (pounds)
4'10"	91–119
4'11"	94–124
5'0"	97–128
5'1"	101–132
5'2"	104–137
5'3"	107–141
5'4"	111–146
5'5"	114–150
5'6"	118–155
5'7"	121–160
5'8"	125–164
5'9"	129–169
5'10"	132–174
5'11"	136–179
6'0"	140–184

*No shoes.
†No clothes.

Obesity-related health problems such as hypertension, diabetes, pulmonary problems, and cholesterol problems, increase with excess weight. Thus, the new guidelines do not allow a weight gain in the late thirties, early forties, or middle age. Weight increase with age may increase risk of premature death from heart disease, diabetes, and certain cancers.

Women tend to become overweight from 35 to 45 years. Overweight persons should not go on a crash diet to lose weight. Rather, they should start an exercise program and reduce fat intake to 30% of their total dietary intake. Exercise reduces the tendency toward pear-shape in women and maintains muscle mass. It is suggested that the weight of the mid-twenties be maintained as the baseline if that weight was normal (155, 331, 343).

Musculoskeletal System

Skeletal growth for the young adult is completed by age 25, or sooner, when the epiphyseal line calcifies and fuses with the mainshaft of the long bones. The vertebral column continues to grow until the individual reaches age 25; 3 to 5 mm may be added to an individual's height. Smaller leg bones, the sternum, pelvic bones, and vertebrae attain adult distribution of the red marrow by approximately 25 years of age. By the early forties, the bones will have lost some mass and density. The process begins earlier in women. With increasing age, the cartilage in all joints has a more limited ability to regenerate itself. Normally, posture is erect (94, 351).

Body systems are functioning at their peak efficiency, and the individual has reached optimum physiologic and motor functions and stamina. Muscle growth is complete at age 30. Peak muscle strength is attained, and maximum physical potential occurs between the ages of 19 and 30. It is during young adulthood that most athletes accomplish their greatest achievements. After this peak period, a 10% loss of strength occurs between the ages of 30 and 60; this loss usually occurs in the back and leg muscles. A person can maintain peak performance through the thirties and much of the forties, however, with regular exercise and dietary moderation (213, 351).

Skin

The skin of the young adult is smooth, and skin turgor is taut. Acne usually disappears because sex hormones have less influence on secretion of oils from sebaceous glands of the skin (276). The skin of the African American may manifest some conditions that are not seen or are manifested differently in Caucasians such as hypopigmentation, keloids, pigmentary disorders, pseudofolliculitis (razor bumps), and alopecia. Refer to the article on African-American skin problems for a pictorial and descriptive summary (337). In late young adulthood the skin begins to lose moisture, becoming more dry and wrinkled. Smile lines and lines at the corners of the eyes are usually noticeable (276).

Cardiovascular System

Maximum physical potential is reached in young adulthood so far as muscles and internal organs are concerned. **Heart** and **circulatory** changes occur gradually with age, depending on exercise and diet patterns. During young adulthood, the total *blood volume* is 70 to 85 mL/kg of body weight. Maximum *cardiac output* is achieved and peaks between 20 and 30 years of age. The male's heart weighs an average of 10 oz and the female's an average of 8 oz. Heart rate averages 72 beats per minute; the *blood pressure* gradually increases, reaching 100 to 120 mm Hg systolic and 60 to 80 mm Hg diastolic. Heart and blood vessels are fully mature, and cholesterol levels increase. Arteries become less elastic. Hemorrhoids and other varicose veins may become health problems, especially in the childbearing woman (147, 276). Maintaining normal blood pressure (120/80 to 129/84 or *below 120/80,* and not above 140/90) reduces risk for later heart disease and strokes (266, 276).

Respiratory System

Since birth, the lungs have increased in weight 20 times. Breathing becomes slower and deeper, 12 to 20 breaths per minute. The maximum breathing capacity decreases between ages 30 and 60. Breathing rate and capacity will differ according to the size of the individual. Larger people have a slower rate. Since birth, lungs have increased in weight 20 times (77, 351).

Gastrointestinal System

The digestive organs function smoothly during this period of life. Stomach capacity is 2000 to 3000 mL. The amount of ptyalin decreases after 20 years of age, and digestive juices decrease after 30 years of age. *Dental maturity* is achieved in the early twenties with emergence of the last four molars (wisdom teeth) (94, 351). Some people must have their wisdom teeth removed because they become impacted and cause pain.

Neurologic System

The **brain** continues to grow into adolescence and young adulthood and reaches its maximum weight and size during adulthood. Mature patterns of brain wave activity do not appear until age 20; maturation continues to age 30 (351). Nerve conduction velocity is at maximum functional capacity (77).

Visual and auditory sensory perceptions should be at their peak. Gradually during young adulthood the lenses of the eyes lose elasticity and begin to have difficulty changing shape and focusing on close objects; however, by age 30 the changes are seldom sufficient to affect function of the eye. Women in this age group can detect high auditory tones better than men (94, 351). Some young adults wear corrective glasses, contact lenses, or hearing aids. Assess for them when you are giving emergency care, especially if the person is unconscious, so that they are not lost or the person does not suffer eye or ear injury. Information on how to remove contact lenses from another person's eyes can be obtained from your local optometry association or optometrist.

Endocrine System

Adrenal secretion of cortisol (hydrocortisone) decreases approximately 30% over the entire adult life span. Because plasma cortisol levels remain constant, the person maintains good response to stress in young adulthood. **Basal metabolic rate** (*body's consumption of oxygen*) is at maximum functional capacity at age 30 and then decreases gradually, which is related to decrease in the mass of muscle tissue (primarily large oxygen-consuming tissue). A gradual decrease in thyroid hormone is an adjustment to the progressively slower rate at which it is broken down and removed from the blood. The blood level of thyroxine (T_4) falls approximately 15% over the adult life span. The blood level of triiodothyronine (T_3), the active thyroid hormone, declines only when the person is ill and not eating (77, 276).

Use the above knowledge in assessment or in health teaching with young adults.

Sexuality and Sexual Development

Sexual Maturity

Sexual maturity for men is usually reached in the late teens, but their sexual drive remains high through young adulthood. In healthy women menstruation is well established and regular by this time. Female organs are fully matured; the uterus reaches maximum weight by age 30. The woman is well equipped for childbearing. The optimum period for reproduction is between 20 and 30 years of age. Many of the dangers associated with adolescent pregnancy or pregnancy in the late thirties or early forties are not present. The Leydig cells, source of male hormones, decline in number after age 25 (94, 276).

Sexuality may be defined as a *deep, pervasive aspect of the total person, the sum total of one's feelings and behavior as a male or female, the expression of which goes beyond genital response.* Sexuality includes **sex identity,** *the sense of self as male, female, bisexual (feeling comfortable with both sexes), homosexual, or ambivalent (transsexual).* Sex identity also includes **sex role,** *what the person does overtly to indicate to self and others maleness, femaleness, bisexuality, or ambivalence* (377). Throughout the life cycle physiologic, emotional, social, and cultural forces condition sexuality. Today's society offers many choices in sexual behavior patterns.

You will encounter four basic values taken by young adults toward sexuality: absolutist, hedonistic, relativistic, and relational. The **absolutist** or **procreational position** *states that sexuality exists for the purpose of reproduction.* The **hedonistic** or **recreational sex view** *has pleasure and pursuit as its central value* and is interested in ultimate fulfillment of human sexual potentials. The **relativistic** or **situational position** is *based on research and has become the basis for the new morality, which says that acts should be judged on the basis of their effects.* The **relational** or **person-centered position** *views sexual activity as a natural extension of intimate relationships* (228, 351). You will have your private set of values, but you must recognize that others' values may be as valid as yours.

During adulthood a number of sexual patterns may exist, ranging from heterosexuality, bisexuality, and homosexuality to masturbation and abstinence. Few people are totally homosexual or heterosexual; most people feel attracted or sexually responsive at some time to both sexes. Within each of these patterns the person may achieve a full and satisfactory life ar be plagued with lack of interest, impotence, or guilt. Young adulthood is the time to reap the rewards or disasters of past sex education. Changes in sexual interest and behavior occur through the life cycle and can be a cause of conflict unless the partners involved can talk about their feelings, needs, and desires. Many misunderstandings arise because of basic differences between the male and female in sexual response. The more each can learn about the other partner, the greater will be the chance of working out a compatible relationship for successful courtship, marriage, and intimacy. The person cannot assume that the partner knows his or her wishes or vice versa. Each must declare his or her needs.

Sexuality Education

Often the popular literature promotes misinformation, and you should be prepared to give accurate information. Because people feel freer now to discuss sexual matters, you may be questioned frequently by the person recuperating from an illness, by the man or wife after delivery, or by the healthy young adult who feels dissatisfied with personal knowledge or sexual pattern. Various references provide in-depth information on this subject (29, 77, 94, 182, 305, 377). An organization that offers workshops and publications is the American Association of Sex Educators, Counselors, and Therapists (AASECT).

The following are facts based on current research that you can teach young adults (29, 77, 93, 94, 182, 215, 231, 324, 351; 377).

- Sexual mores and norms vary among ethnic groups, socioeconomic classes, and even from couple to couple. Sexual activity that is mutually satisfying to the couple and not harmful to themselves and others is acceptable.
- Sexual activity varies considerably among people in relation to sex drive, frequency of orgasm, or need for rest after intercourse.
- Various factors and feelings are as influential on men as on women in determining sexual expression. Sexual function, especially in men, is not an uninhibited, mechanical, automatic act requiring only appropriate stimulus and intact physical equipment.
- Heterosexual intercourse is a reproductive act, but people do not engage in sexual intercourse only for reproduction. *Many sexual acts are nongenital in nature but involve people sharing touch, affection, and pleasure.*
- The more sexually active person maintains the sex drive longer into later years.
- The human sexual drive has no greater impact on the total person than any other biological function. Sex is *not* the prevailing instinct in humans, and physical or mental disease does not result from unmet sexual needs.
- Erotic dreams that culminate in orgasms occur in 85% of all men at any age and commonly in women, increasing in older women.
- The woman is not inherently passive and the man aggressive. Maximum gratification requires that each partner is both passive and aggressive in participating mutually and cooperatively in sexual intercourse.
- Women have as strong a sex desire as men, sometimes stronger.
- Women have greater orgastic capacity than men with regard to duration and frequency of orgasm. The female can have several orgasms within a brief period.
- Female orgasm is normally initiated by clitoral stimulation, but it is a total body response rather than clitoral or vaginal in nature.

- The woman may need stimulation to the clitoris other than that received during intercourse to achieve orgasm. Some studies show that a large percentage of women regularly do not have orgasm in sexual intercourse. Overall sexual response is enhanced for the women when there is warm, loving behavior from the partner before, during, and after intercourse, when foreplay between partners increases arousal, and when she has worked through strict parental admonitions against touching self, enjoying her body, masturbation, or sexual intercourse.

- Simultaneous orgasm of both partners may be desired but is an unrealistic goal and occurs only in the most ideal circumstances. It does not determine sexual achievement or satisfaction.

- No physiologic reason exists for abstinence during menses as menstrual flow is from the uterus, no tissue damage occurs to the vagina, and the woman's sex drive is not necessarily diminished.

- No relationship exists between penile size and ability of the man to satisfy the woman, and little correlation exists between penile and body size and sexual potency. The women's reaction to penile size or her feelings with penile penetration, however, do affect the man's ability for orgasm and satisfaction.

- No single most accepted position for sexual activity exists. Any position is correct, normal, healthy, and proper if it satisfies both partners.

- Achievement of satisfactory sexual response is the result of interaction of many physical, emotional, developmental, and cultural influences and of the total relationship between man and woman.

- Chronically ill or disabled persons learn to live with physical changes and to adapt to express their sexual interests. Underlying fantasies, anxiety, guilt, attitudes toward self, and history of relationships with people affect sexual functioning.

- Decreased sexual desire may be related to physical or emotional illness, prescribed medications, use of alcohol or other drugs, changed behavior in the partner, or fatigue from the stress and demands of employment or professional life—for either men or women.

- Making love and having sex are not necessarily the same, although ideally they occur together.

Additionally, you may wish to share the following information. In the normal male spermatozoa are produced in optimum numbers and motility when ejaculation occurs two or three times weekly. A decreased or increased frequency of ejaculation is associated with decreased number of sperm (305).

Menstruation is a part of sexuality in women. Discomforts and disabilities associated with menstruation may be caused by social, cultural, and emotional factors and hard physical labor, not just by changing hormone levels. Many women learn to react to menstruation as "the curse" and treat it as an illness with medication and bed rest. Women of different sociocultural backgrounds may have different responses. Women who strongly identify with traditional sexual roles are more likely to experience menstruation as a disabling illness. Periods of emotional stress, either happy or upsetting, can cause irregular menses (221).

Human Sexual Response

The **human sexual response cycle** involves physiologic reactions, psychological components, and psychosocial influences or behavior. You may be asked to discuss the following information.

The two main physiologic reactions of the cycle are **vasocongestion,** *engorged blood vessels,* and **myotonia,** *increased muscular tension.*

The **four phases of the cycle** are *excitement, plateau, orgasm, and resolution,* and the phases vary with each person and from time to time. The **excitement phase** *develops from any source of body or psychic stimuli,* and if adequate stimulation occurs, the intensity of excitement increases rapidly. This phase may be interrupted, prolonged, or ended by distracting stimuli. The **plateau phase** *is a consolidation period that follows excitement, during which sexual tension intensifies.* **Orgasm** *is the climax of sexual tension increase* that lasts for a few seconds during which vasocongestion and myotonia are released through forceful muscle contractions. The **resolution phase** *returns the body to the preexcitement physiology.* The woman may begin another cycle immediately if stimulated, but the man is unable to be restimulated for approximately 30 minutes (231).

Physiologic requisites for the human sexual response include (1) an intact circulatory system to provide for vasocongestive responses and (2) an intact central and peripheral nervous system to provide for sensory appreciation and muscular innervation and to support vasocongestive changes. For a detailed account of changes that occur in both the genital system organs and other body systems during the four phases of the human sexual response, see references at the end of this chapter (231, 305, 377).

You may be asked subtly or directly about **sexual activity during pregnancy.** Be prepared to share the following information.

Intercourse can continue during pregnancy, although either partner may prefer other intimate behaviors: the woman because of comfort and fear that her appearance may be displeasing to the man and the man because of concern about discomfort to the woman or fetal distress or because he finds her body less attractive as pregnancy progresses. Although infection from intercourse is a possibility during pregnancy, this problem also applies to the nonpregnant state (305). Genital cleanliness is always an important measure in preventing infection. Concern for the partner's well-being is also an important concern. Signs of infection should always be reported early to a physician so that treatment can be given.

Sexual response during and after pregnancy varies slightly from the usual pattern. During orgasm, spasm of the third-trimester uterus may occur for as long as a minute. Fetal heart tones are slowed during this period, but normally there is no evidence of prolonged fetal distress. Vasocongestion is also increased during sexual activity in genital organs and the breasts. During the resolution phase the vasocongested pelvis often is not completely relieved; as a result, the woman has a continual feeling of sexual stimulation. Residual pelvic vasocongestion and pressure in the pelvis from the second- and third-trimester uterus cause a high level of sexual tension (231).

Teach couples that coital activity is prohibited if there is any threat to fetal viability throughout the pregnancy and during the postpartum period if there is concern about episiotomy breakdown or endometriosis. If there is potential aggravation by the physical nature of coitus with penile penetration, only that form of sexual activity should be avoided. If the problem is one of potential uterine contractility, abstinence from all orgasmic sexual activity, including masturbation by the female, should be recommended. If prostaglandins in semen contribute to the problem, the male should wear a condom during intercourse. If the problem is a combination of the above, all sexual activity with the female is contraindicated; however, sexual activity directed at the male may continue.

Couples should always receive specific instruction about continuing sexual intercourse during the last month of pregnancy, depending on the condition of the woman.

Teach couples that such orogenital sexual activity as blowing air into the vagina should be avoided during pregnancy and for at least 6 weeks postpartum. Inflation of air into the vagina may cause air embolism; death has occurred in minutes after air is blown into the vagina. (Air embolism is also the reason that douching is avoided during pregnancy and postdelivery) (305). By the fourth or fifth week postpartum, sexual tensions are similar to nonpregnant levels, but physiologically the woman has not returned to the nonpregnant state. By the third postpartum month, physiologic status has returned to prepregnancy levels (231).

Premenstrual Phenomena

Premenstrual syndrome (PMS) is a *group of signs and symptoms occurring approximately a week premenses and associated with hormonal changes and fluid retention:* mild cerebral edema and edema of fingers, feet, thighs, legs, hips, breasts, abdomen, and around the eyes. Common Signs and Symptoms of Premenstrual Syndrome (see next page) lists physiologic symptoms and signs and emotional reactions that are reported by some women. Symptoms are more likely to appear or increase as women enter the thirties or each age 40 (305). No simple etiology has been identified; several mechanisms for pathogenesis have been described (276, 353). PMS is not the same as **dysmenorrhea,** *painful or severely uncomfortable menstruation* (353).

Premenstrual syndrome is not the same as **Premenstrual Dysphoric Disorder (PMDD).** PMDD is rare (3–5% of menstruating women) and *involves a pattern of severe, recurrent symptoms of depression and other negative mood states in the last week of the menstrual cycle, and markedly interferes with daily living.* PMS occurs in 8 to 10% of women and is less disabling (13, 353).

Not all these signs and symptoms appear together; they are variable in degree, and they decrease after menses begins (158, 219, 248, 274, 276, 305, 353, 359, 377). Be empathic to the woman who describes these symptoms or feelings. Help the spouse and other family members recognize their significance, the importance of medical treatment, and that their caring and reduced stress may contribute to a decrease in symptomatology.

Estimates are that 10 to 20% of women have symptoms resulting from PMS, or menstruation that interfere with daily function. Five percent of women meet strict diagnostic criteria (274). (Recent media publicity would suggest that women are incompetent or commit crimes or suicide during this time of the menstrual cycle.) Recent studies show that PMS symptoms may appear because of how neurochemicals and hormones interact with estrogen and progesterone, and these interactions are affected by nutrition and stress. Other factors may be emotional conflicts related to femininity or other emotional stress (68, 248, 274, 276, 359). Woods (377) found that negative attitudes toward menstruation and a stressful social milieu increase PMS symptoms. Mitchell, Woods, and Lentz (248) found that women with PMS had more psychological distress,

► COMMON SIGNS AND SYMPTOMS
OF PREMENSTRUAL SYNDROME

Physiologic Symptoms and Signs

- Fatigue, increased need for sleep
- Appetite change, craving for salty or sweet foods
- Abdominal distention, swollen hands or feet, puffy eyes
- Headache or backache
- Breast tenderness
- Weight gain
- Nausea
- Constipation or diarrhea
- Acne or hives
- Dizziness
- Menstrual cramps
- Clumsiness
- Sex drive changes
- Thirst
- Proneness to infection
- Lower alcohol tolerance

Psychological Reactions

- Apprehension or anxiety
- Confusion
- Forgetfulness
- Frequent crying
- Indecisiveness
- Irritability
- Restlessness
- Mood swings
- Sadness or depression
- Suspiciousness
- Tenseness
- Withdrawal
- Difficulty with concentration

No consistent relationship between premenstrual mood and cognitive function has been found although some women describe difficulty with concentration. The magnitude of the premenstrual mood change is not great enough to affect intellectual functioning (274, 304, 353).

Treatment for PMS may be symptomatic, with hormones to curtail production of estrogen and progesterone, diuretics, antidepressants, antianxiety medications, and serotonin-reuptake inhibitors (e.g., fluoxetine [Prozac]). Some of the time these drugs are not necessary. Dietary measures and exercise are also suggested (274, 276, 353).

Teach women that the following measures can offset symptoms (158, 274, 305, 353, 359):

- Consume less caffeine in beverages, colas, and over-the-counter drugs and less sugar, alcohol, and salt, especially during the premenstrual period.
- Eat four to six small meals a day rather than two or three meals to minimize the risk of hypoglycemia that accompanies PMS.
- Snack on complex carbohydrates such as fresh fruits, vegetable sticks, and whole wheat crackers, which provide energy without excessive sugar.
- Drink six to eight glasses of water to help prevent fluid retention by flushing excess salt from the body.
- Limit fat intake (especially in red meats), which builds hormones that cause breast tenderness and fluid retention. Choose dairy products low in fat.
- Eat more whole grains, nuts, and raw greens, which are high in vitamin B, magnesium, and potassium, and add vitamin B_6 and calcium to reduce symptoms.
- Develop a variety of interests, including maintaining exercise routines, so that focus is not on self and body symptoms during this period.
- Walk and perform other physical exercise at least four times weekly to reduce symptoms of mood swings, increased appetite, crying, breast tenderness, craving for sweets, fluid retention, and depression (exercise raises beta-endorphin levels, which in turn increase feelings of well-being and improve the glucose tolerance curve).
- Get extra rest and use relaxation techniques, meditation, and massage. Treat yourself to a relaxing and creative activity.
- Discuss your feelings with family and friends so that they can be more understanding of your behavior.

more education, and a mother with premenstrual symptoms. Regardless of cause, symptoms are not evidence of biological or emotional inferiority. For the majority of women, the menstrual cycle is an ongoing but insignificant part of their lives—one that causes little discomfort.

- Join a self-help group to gain other ideas on how to more effectively cope with symptoms.

Ovulation

Share the following information about ovulation, especially with couples who desire **natural family planning** (276, 305, 377). Ovulation normally occurs in every menstrual cycle but not necessarily midcycle. The ovum is capable of being fertilized for 24 hours postovulation.

The mucous cycle by which to predict ovulation is as follows. It begins with menstruation. The period is usually followed by a few "dry days," variable in number, when no mucus is seen or felt. As the ovum begins to ripen, some mucus is felt at the vaginal opening and can be seen if the woman wipes the vaginal area with toilet tissue. This mucus is generally yellow or white, but definitely opaque and sticky. When the blood estrogen level (derived from the ripening ovum) reaches a critical point, the glands of the cervix respond with a different mucus. This fertile mucus starts out cloudy and is not sticky and becomes very clear, like raw egg white. After ovulation, progesterone causes the abrupt cessation of the clear, slippery, fertile mucus and produces its own mucus, which is sticky, much less preponderant, and sometimes not present at the vagina. Progesterone prepares the uterine lining for the reception of the egg if the egg has been fertilized. *Usually the egg is ovulated within 24 hours of the peak of wetness,* but this interval may be as long as 48 hours. Although the sticky mucus does not allow a sperm to live very long, the sperm could possibly survive long enough to reach a freshly ovulated egg through a lingering fertile mucous channel. If this method will be used to avoid pregnancy, there should be abstinence from intercourse from the beginning of the slippery fertile mucus until the height of wetness ("peak day" when there may be so much wetness that mucus is not seen but moisture is noted on the underclothing) *plus a full 72 hours* to ensure that the ovum will not be impregnated (145).

Because the lifetime of the sperm depends on the presence of the fertile mucus, all genital contact between the partners must be avoided. The first drop of semen (the one that escapes before ejaculation) has the highest concentration of sperm. A woman can conceive even if only one drop of semen touches her external genital organ; sperm are powerful, and the mucus is equally potent.

Teach that spotting or bleeding may occur between menses and may be associated with ovulation, a cervical polyp, postintercourse in the presence of cervicitis, or carcinoma. Any abnormal pattern of bleeding should be investigated by a gynecologist.

Sexual Dysfunctions

Sexual dysfunctions affect both male and female for various reasons. Several references provide additional information on sexual dysfunctions (13, 29, 231, 232, 253, 276, 305, 377). Your education and referral can assist couples in obtaining effective diagnosis and treatment.

Female Circumcision

Female circumcision may be appalling to you, but it is a widespread culturally and religiously based practice in some parts of the world such as some countries in the Middle East, Africa, Indonesia, and Malay. The circumcision may occur the eighth day after birth, the tenth day after birth, at 3 or 4 years, or at 8 or 10 years as part of prepuberty rites to womanhood. You may care for circumcised women, especially in maternity and gynecologic services, who have migrated to this country. There are several types of circumcisions, classified on the basis of severity. All types of this practice usually are followed by a variety of complications. Initially there is shock, hemorrhage, sepsis, and lacerations to surrounding tissue. Shortly thereafter retention of urine and tetanus may occur. Dysmenorrhea, urinary tract infections, pelvic inflammatory disease, and infertility are common. After marriage, painful intercourse, forceful cutting of the circumcision scar, perineal lacerations, infections, hemorrhage, frigidity, and severe anxiety occur. During childbirth the scar tissue must be cut during the second stage of labor, or mother and baby may die because of obstruction to delivery, sepsis, or hemorrhage (137, 301).

In most countries where female circumcision occurs, it is a way to control women sexually, economically, and religiously and to control the heritage line and inheritance. The tradition is practiced among Christians, Muslims, and Jews in some parts of Africa.

Some nurses in Kenya report their efforts to stop this practice. They report that Western approaches will not work in eliminating this problem because the practice is so traditional. It is accepted by women because in countries where it is practiced, the uncircumcised woman would not be considered for marriage. These nurses report that as the population becomes generally better educated, traditional practices, including circumcision, decline. Thus the nurses are heavily committed to promoting general and health education so that a better educated population will pass legislation prohibiting the practice.

When you care for women from the non-Western part of the world, assess for circumcision and its effects; be nonjudgmental of the woman. Focus on care that will prevent further complications. Help her gain understanding why this practice may be harmful to her daughter(s). As the male is the decision maker in these cultures, you will have to establish a working relationship with him if any changes are to be made for the female children. Be aware that female circumcision may be being practiced in this country outside of the traditional health care system. You may encounter the woman after her circumcision in the emergency room, the maternity service, the clinic, or the home. Work through your own feelings with a supervisor or counselor. This woman needs a sensitive caretaker. Refer to the article by Shaw (301) for greater detail in the maternity care needed by circumcised women.

Variations in Sexual Behavior

The identity crisis that occurs during adolescence may not be completely resolved by the time the person enters young adulthood chronologically. Identity confusion may lead to confusion over sexual identity and may precipitate homosexual and heterosexual experimentation and arouse homosexual fears and curiosity.

Homosexuality. **Homosexuals** are *people who are regularly aroused by and who engage in sexual activity with members of their own sex.* Being a **homosexual man** (*gay*) or a **homosexual woman** (*lesbian*) is becoming more socially acceptable in the United States, although persons with this sexual orientation may still suffer rejection and discrimination (164, 189, 352, 382). Members of some religious groups believe homosexuality is a sin; however, homosexuality was accepted by some ancient cultures. Studies show that these individuals love and care for each other, and are friends with and care for those who are straight. They are responsible citizens to the same extent as are straight or heterosexual people.

Many theories attempt to explain the causes of homosexual behavior: genetics, biochemistry, developmental, and emotional. A number of factors may be involved (4, 77, 94, 127, 179, 249, 351, 352, 382, 383). However, *homosexual experiences are a part of normal growth and development in childhood and early adolescence* (335). Most people can report having had a close emotional attachment, with or without sexual contact, with a peer or adult that involved sexual feelings (29). Sullivan (335) theorized that the normal homosexual period in life is the chum stage in preadolescence (see Chapter 10) when the person first cares for someone as much as he or she cares for self. Although the chum stage involves a very close emotional experience, it may include some fondling or exploration between the two

chums. Sullivan (335) believed that if the person did not have a chum in preadolescence or adolescence, he or she would enter young adulthood still seeking a chum of the same sex. At this point, however, the societal expectation is heterosexuality, and the person's behavior is interpreted in a sexual rather than emotional way. If the person is rejected by, or is uncomfortable with, persons of the opposite sex, he or she may receive the greatest acceptance (friendship) from other of the same sex. That reinforces the homosexual preference.

Research by Masters and Johnson (232) showed that the sexual response in homosexuals is the same as that of heterosexuals. Family interactions of homosexual partners and heterosexual partners without children are similar (29). Developmental tasks for the couple during the childbearing and childrearing experience are also similar to those of heterosexual couples, although there may be more planning for the child and their relationship (376). Gays and lesbians can be nurturing parents to their children if at some point they decide to leave a heterosexual marital relationship (or mixed-orientation relationship) for a stable gay or lesbian relationship (43).

Bell, Weinberg, and Hammersmith (29) found in their studies that homosexual men and women can be categorized as follows:

- *Close coupled:* involved in a marriage-like, affectionate relationship with a same-sex partner
- *Open coupled:* involved in marital relationships, with interest in sexual contacts other than with the partner and feelings of regret about the homosexuality
- *Functional:* single individuals with a large number of partners and high level of sexual activity and little regret about homosexuality
- *Dysfunctional:* single individuals with a large number of partners, many sexual problems, and much regret about their homosexuality
- *Asexual:* single, uncoupled individuals, with little interest in sexual activity, few partners, and significant regret about their homosexuality

It is important to realize that people who identify themselves as homosexual evidence a complexity and diversity of lifestyles, interests, problems, and relationships comparable to those of heterosexuals. There is also a wide spectrum of emotional experience on the homosexual–heterosexual continuum. Contrary to the stereotype, sexual intercourse is not the predominant concern; meaningful relationships are the key (29, 43, 179).

Both male and female homosexuals vary widely in their emotional and social adjustment, just as heterosexuals do. Some people demonstrate a homosexual orientation only under extreme conditions such as imprisonment. Some have their total life adjustment dominated by homosexuality and live in a homosexual subculture. For some, sexual behavior is only an aspect of their total life experience; they may remain discrete and secretive about their homosexuality. Others seek out heterosexual activity, marry, and have families (43, 163, 179, 215).

The lesbian has not been studied as much as the gay man. It is still more socially acceptable for two women to live together in one dwelling than for two men. There may also be less societal fear of gay women than of gay men. As a result, less is known about their feelings, reactions, lifestyles, or health problems (164, 324, 376).

The occurrence of sexually transmitted diseases such as pediculosis, gonorrhea, syphilis, urethritis, anorectal warts and infection, herpes genitalis, AIDS, intestinal infections, shigellosis, and hepatitis has been publicized. The rapidly increasing incidence of AIDS has caused some homosexuals to change their sexual practices, to limit the number of sexual partners, or to increase use of condoms. Heterosexual partners also get these diseases through sexual intercourse, and all homosexuals do not get them (36, 63, 208, 311, 353, 370). Refer to Chapter 11; sexually transmitted diseases do not occur only in adolescence but are likely to occur first in those years. Refer also to the section on health problems in this chapter.

It is essential that you convey a nonjudgmental attitude toward the person who is gay or lesbian. This person needs your respect and acceptance as a human being who is more than a bundle of sexual activity. This person may be a business executive, minister, inventor, health care professional, delivery person, artist, homemaker, or parent. The person may be contributing as much, or more, to society's betterment as any heterosexual person. If this person indicates a desire to change to a heterosexual identity or to relate more comfortably to people of both sexes, refer the person to a counselor who can help the person grow in ability to relate or acquire a new identity, if desired, without labeling, moralizing, rejecting, or becoming impatient as the person works through emotional and spiritual pain (36, 75, 77, 164, 189, 249, 382, 383). Further, assist lesbians and gays to obtain needed health care (324).

Parents of homosexual offspring are often not considered, but they may also need help in coping with the homosexuality. Parents of gay or lesbian offspring may feel too embarrassed to talk about their feelings; some believe that they have lost a child; some grieve at the prospect of not having a grandchild; some fear meeting a same-sex lover. Acceptance of the fact that their child is a homosexual may be a long time in coming, but most parents eventually reach that point. Listen to their feelings and concerns; help them focus on a wholesome relationship; caution against punitive behavior toward the offspring, and refer them to a counselor to work through spiritual and emotional conflicts related to the situation. You can refer parents to the Parents of Gays organization. A list of local chapters is available by writing 201 W. 13th Street, New York, NY 10011, or Box 24528, Los Angeles, CA 90024. You may also refer parents to the Federation of Parents and Friends of Lesbians and Gays, Inc. (Parent's FLAG), P.O. Box 20308, Denver, CO 80220. This organization has a booklet entitled *About Our Children,* published in several languages simultaneously. The organization also sponsors a newsletter, national projects, and regional meetings. In turn, adult children of homosexual parents may also need an opportunity to discuss concerns or issues (4).

Transsexuality. **Transsexuals** are *people who lack harmony between their anatomic sex and their psychological sex.* A disorder of sex identity occurs. Hormone therapy and surgery are used as treatment. Both therapies are directed at making the anatomic sex compatible with the psychological sex (253).

To care for persons with sexual identity different than your own, you must first determine your own feelings toward yourself as a sexual person and then your feelings toward them. These people need someone to listen to their fears and insecurities and a consistent, accepting approach. You may not be able to work with these people, but you can make appropriate referrals. If problems of sex identity related to genetic conditions are assessed in a child, you should encourage early treatment. Without intervention, the majority of people will become more deeply frustrated by their lack of sex identity.

Sexual Experimentation Outside Marriage. Sexual activity outside marriage may include homosexuality, group sexual experiences, premarital intercourse, cohabitation, or infidelity.

The moral, emotional, and psychological aspects of premarital sexual behavior have been widely discussed. Sexual intimacy without a sense of commitment and love, responsibility, and care for the other means using another to meet one's needs, taking the other as an object rather than as a person. Such activity and attitudes can be poor preparation for marriage and establishing a lasting relationship and personal maturity. Compatibility between two people is in the head, not the pelvis.

The rationalization of finding a compatible partner through premarital sexual intimacy is unfounded.

Yet **cohabitation,** *two persons of the opposite sex living together without being married,* is not unusual. Sometimes the arrangement of the young adult man and woman living together is asexual. They are friends and for economic, companionship, or convenience reasons wish to share an apartment. They may perceive themselves as androgynous, not tied to traditional sex roles. Sometimes the person may have had no siblings or no siblings of the opposite sex, and the person wants the experience of living with someone of the opposite sex who would be like a sibling. In such a situation both work to keep the relationship asexual. Most decide to marry or separate within 2 years (93, 175, 322).

Young adults sometimes live together in an effort to avoid some of the problems they saw in their parents' marriage or to test the degree of the partner's commitment before actually becoming married. Those goals may be achieved for some, but the danger is that one partner may take the commitment very seriously and the other may use the situation only as a convenient living arrangement. The uncaring person may suddenly decide to leave, an easy process because no legal ties are involved, and the other person is left with much the same hurt as a married person going through a divorce (20, 175).

American society probably expects too much of marriage. The partners in the ideal marriage are supposed to stay passionately and exclusively in love with each other for the rest of their lives. Yet infidelity is a growing problem in an increasingly liberal society.

Various factors contribute to infidelity: the need to prove masculinity or femininity; difficulty in maintaining a steady and continuing relationship; feelings of insecurity, rejection, or jealousy; and a sense of loss when heightened passions of the initial stages of love do not remain constant. Believing that one can love two people simultaneously, getting great satisfaction from doing something forbidden and secretly, or wishing to recapture one's youth may also be involved.

Staying married to one person and living with the frustrations, conflicts, and boredom that any close and lengthy relationship imposes requires constant work by both parties. Couples are unrealistic when they think that marriage will suddenly shield them from further attraction to members of the opposite sex. The mature couple will expect to feel physically attracted to others at times and will have to resolve the feelings within themselves through discussion with and understanding from their partner or with the help of a counselor. Stevens describes ways for the couple to build an enduring relationship (323). Others may choose to remain single.

American society offers no alternative to the family unit. Although society as a whole is in a state of flux, the family unit seems fundamental. The strains that infidelity places on it are damaging for most people.

Personal Attitudes

To incorporate human sexuality into health care and nursing practice, you must accept your own sexuality and understand sexuality as a significant aspect of development. Then you can acknowledge the concerns of the clients, recognize your strengths and limits in working with people who have sexual concerns, help these people cope with threats to sexuality, and counsel, inform, or refer them as indicated.

Supporting, caring, and nurturing are nursing behaviors. But at times you will have other feelings and may feel guilty about being sexually attracted to (or repulsed by) a client. These are honest feelings to acknowledge. After all, every thought and behavior will not result in intimacy or rejection. Feeling positively toward someone can help you give effective care. If you have negative feelings about someone, you can deal with these feelings if you can recognize the possible reasons for your feelings. Actually, when you begin to understand another person, most likely you will find that person interesting, even if that person might not be an individual you would choose for a friend. When someone is perceived as unique and interesting, it becomes easier to give effective care and form a relationship.

The patient may express sexual behavior by brushing against you, trying to feel breasts or hips, or referring to sexual topics in conversation. Recognize the behavior as an energy outlet or as a way to validate himself or herself as a person. If the patient is observed masturbating, do not make a joke of this discovery. Realize that this is an acceptable sexual release and provide privacy; however, if a patient becomes obnoxious in either words or actions, you must tell him or her what behavior is appropriate in the particular situation.

Sexual History

If you feel comfortable and if there is sufficient rapport between you and the client, take a sexual history, especially with clients who have conditions that interfere with sexual activity. Follow these guidelines when you are taking a sexual history:

- Ensure privacy and establish confidentiality of statements.
- Progress from topics that are easy to discuss to those that are more difficult to discuss.

- Ask the person how he or she acquired sexual information before asking about sexual experience.
- Precede questions by informational statements about the generality of the experience, when appropriate, to reassure the person and reduce anxiety, shame, and evasiveness.
- Observe nonverbal behavior while you listen to the person's statements.
- Do not ask questions just to satisfy your curiosity.

The following are topics to include in the sexual history:

- How sex education was obtained
- Accuracy of sex education
- Menstrual history if female or nocturnal emission history if male
- Past and present ideas on self as a sexual being, including ideas on body image, masturbation, coitus, childbirth, parenting
- Sexual experiences—with men, women, or both
- Number of partners in past year
- Use of condoms: when started, consistency of use
- Ability to communicate sexual needs and desires
- Partner's (if one exists) sexual values and behavior
- Sexual partners who have developed AIDS
- History of sexually transmitted disease of self or partner(s)

If necessary, use several interviews to obtain information and be sure to include any specific questions or concerns that the person voices. Respect the person's desire not to talk about sexual matters and moral, spiritual, or aesthetic convictions. Know the terminology and have a nonjudgmental attitude when the person talks about sexuality concerns. Your matter-of-fact attitude helps the adult feel less embarrassed. Be aware of how illness and drugs can affect sexual function. Do not assume that chronic or disabling disease or mutilating surgery ends the person's sexual life.

Give accurate information and counseling when the person or family asks questions or indicates concerns. You may wish to prepare instructional units for a specific teaching plan to share with patients with various conditions, especially chronic diseases, and with their families to help them better understand how to meet sexual needs. Give gentle encouragement related to pursuit of sexual activity rather than personal advice

or judgment. Know community resources for consultation or referral when necessary.

References at the end of the chapter will also be helpful on how to work with rape victims (5, 166, 253).

Nutritional Needs

As the nutrition of childhood set the stage for the health of the young adult, so now the stage is being set for health in middle and old age. Growth is essentially finished by young adulthood. Activity level may stabilize or diminish. Caloric intake should be based on occupation, amount of physical activity or mental effort, emotional state, age, body size, climate, individual metabolism, and presence of disease. (A *calorie* or *kilocalorie* [kcal] is a unit of measure of the amount of energy required to raise 1 kg of water 1°C.) Women have a 5 to 10% lower metabolism than men of comparable height and weight; thus in the healthy, nonpregnant state women need lower caloric intake. The greater the body surface, the higher is the basal metabolic rate. The obese person, however, requires fewer calories for size because adipose tissue consumes less oxygen than muscles; thus less energy is expended comparatively. Table 12–1 shows caloric expenditure for activity. Actual caloric consumption depends not only on type of activity but also on duration of activity and weight of the person (371).

TABLE 12–1. ENERGY EXPENDITURE FOR ACTIVITY

Type of Activity	Energy (kcal/h)	
	Men	Women
Sedentary Sitting, working on leisurely activity with little arm movement	100	80
Light House or office work, sitting and standing, some arm movement	160	110
Moderate Housecleaning, gardening, laundry, carpentry, walking moderately fast, vigorous arm movement with sitting activity	240	170
Vigorous Heavy housecleaning, walking fast, golfing, bowling	350	250
Strenuous Swimming, athletic games, running, dancing, skiing	>350	>350

Normal Nutrition

There are five major food groups, and some foods from each group should be consumed every day. Overall the diet should (1) have plenty of grain products, fruits, and vegetables; (2) contain a moderate amount of protein (about 12% of total calories; (3) contain moderate amounts of sugar and salt; and (4) be low in fat, saturated fat, and cholesterol. The Food Guide pyramid depicts suggested daily food choices (Fig. 12–1) (117, 155, 200, 259, 260, 318, 331, 341). Eight 8-oz glasses of water should be ingested daily. The latest nutritional guidelines include physical exercise as a key ingredient (260).

Table 12–2 lists the recommended daily number of servings for each food group for young adults and for pregnant and lactating women (77, 155, 371, 372). Appendix I shows the requirements for vitamins and minerals, comparing adults with children (371). Appendix II lists the functions and sources of the various nutrients (117, 155, 200, 259, 268, 331, 340, 341, 371, 372).

Theoretically, a man between the ages of 25 and 45, living in the United States under the usual environmental stresses, weighing 154 pounds (40 kg) and standing 69 inches (172 cm) tall, will consume approximately 2700 calories daily to maintain nutritional status and weight (120).

A woman between the ages of 25 and 45, living in the United States under the usual environmental stresses, weighing 128 pounds (58.2 kg), and standing 65 in. (162 cm) tall, will consume approximately 2000 calories daily to maintain nutritional status and weight. That same woman when *pregnant* should increase her calories by at least 300 daily and her protein by 30 g. Vitamin and mineral supplements are necessary and should contain 30 to 60 mg of elemental iron and 0.2 to

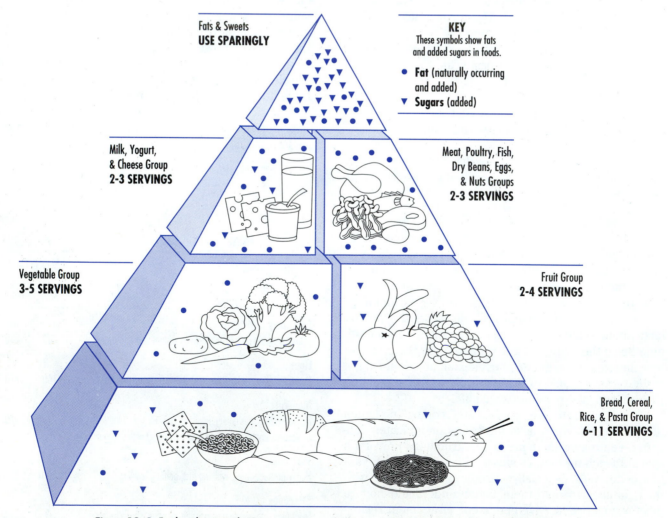

Figure 12–1. Food guide pyramid. (*Source: Department of Agriculture and Department of Health and Human Services.*)

TABLE 12–2. RECOMMENDED NUTRITIONAL INTAKE FOR YOUNG ADULTS

Foods	Young Adult	Pregnant Woman	Lactating Woman
Traditional Basic Four			
Milk and milk products	2 or more cups	3 or 4 cups	4 or more cups
Meat, fish, or protein equivalent	2 (2 or 3 ounce) servings	3 (2 or 3 ounce) servings	3 or 4 (2 or 3 ounce) servings
Fruits and vegetables (including a high vitamin C source)	4 ($\frac{1}{2}$ cup) servings	4 or 5 ($\frac{1}{2}$ cup) servings	4 or 5 ($\frac{1}{2}$ cup) servings
Grain, bread, and cereals	4 servings	4 or more servings	4 or more servings
Suggested Change			
Milk and milk products	2 or 3 cups	3 or 4 cups	4 or more cups
Meat, fish, poultry, dry beans, eggs, nuts	2 or 3 (2 or 3 ounce) servings	3 (2 or 3 ounce) servings	3 or 4 (2 or 3 ounce) servings
Fruits	2–4 ($\frac{1}{2}$ cup) servings	2–4 ($\frac{1}{2}$ cup) servings	2–4 ($\frac{1}{2}$ cup) servings
Vegetables	3–5 ($\frac{1}{2}$ cup) servings	3–5 ($\frac{1}{2}$ cup) servings	3–5 ($\frac{1}{2}$ cup) servings
Breads, cereal, rice, pastas	6–11 servings	6–11 servings	6–11 servings
Fats, Oils, Sweets			
Use sparingly for all age groups			

0.4 mg of folacin (353). Weight gain during pregnancy should be 22 to 28 pounds. Rigid calorie restriction may be dangerous. When *lactating,* her calorie intake should increase by 500, her protein intake by 30 g, and calcium intake should be 1200 mg for optimum health (77, 371, 372). Refer to Chapter 6 for additional information.

Nutrition Assessment

Incorporate nutritional status into nursing assessment and the health history. Ask questions related to the following list to guide your assessment with the person or family (371):

- Knowledge of nutrients, food groups, balanced diet, and their relationship to health
- Knowledge of nutrient requirements at present level of growth and development and whether nutrient needs are being met
- Associations with food and how they influence food and eating patterns
- What increases or decreases appetite
- Cultural background, including religious beliefs, ethnic patterns, and geographic area, and how these beliefs influence food intake and likes and dislikes
- Relationship of lifestyle and activity to food intake
- Income level and food buying power; influence of income on dietary habits
- Knowledge of alternatives to high-cost foods

- Usual daily pattern of intake: times of day, types, amounts
- Which is main meal of day
- Eating environment
- Special diet requirements
- Food allergies
- Relationship of eating patterns of family or significant others to individual's habits and patterns
- Medications and methods used to aid digestion and nutrition intake; influence of other medications on nutritional intake
- Condition of teeth and chewing ability
- Use, condition, and fit of dentures
- Types of food individual has difficulty chewing or swallowing
- Condition of oral cavity and structures
- Disabilities that interfere with nutritional intake
- Assistance or special devices needed for feeding

The oral cavity should be included in a nutritional assessment and at other times of nursing care (241, 305, 371).

Nutrition–Disease Relationships

Although overt clinical symptoms of *vitamin or mineral deficiencies* are seldom observed in most Americans, you will see individuals and families in whom you suspect inadequate nutrition. Pallor; listlessness; brittle, dull nails and hair; dental caries; complaints of constipation and poor resistance to common infections; and over-or underweight suggest a need for a complete diet history (371).

Laboratory evaluations of blood and urine supply meaningful information for a nutritional assessment. Hemoglobin, hematocrit, serum proteins and lipids (including cholesterol), glucose, sodium, and potassium levels are all important diagnostic tools.

One glaring deficiency you may find, however, is the lack of iron in women. A sizable percentage of women do not ingest sufficient dietary iron daily. The male can suffice with 10 mg of iron daily, but the female needs 18 mg (371, 372).

Your assistance will be sought when dietary problems occur during early pregnancy, usually the transitory nausea and vomiting, commonly called *morning sickness*. Physiologic and psychological factors contribute to this condition. Small frequent meals of fairly dry, easily digested energy foods such as carbohydrates are usually tolerated. Separating intake of liquids and solids and drinking flavored or carbonated beverages instead of plain water may also help. Constipation resulting from pressure of the expanding uterus on the lower portion of the intestine occurs in later pregnancy. Increased fluid intake and use of dried fruits, fresh fruits and juices, and whole-grain cereals should induce regularity of elimination. Laxatives should be avoided unless prescribed by a physician.

Americans have a vast array of food from which to pick, yet malnutrition may result from being overfed but undernourished. Additionally, *6 of the 10 leading causes of death in the United States are connected to eating habits:* heart disease, cancer, stroke and hypertension, diabetes, arteriosclerosis, and cirrhosis of the liver. Formerly thought of as middle-aged diseases, some of these diseases are taking the lives of young adults (156, 371).

Many Americans are more aware of the need for a nutritional diet, yet many other Americans eat too few fruits, vegetables, and grains and too much salt, fat, and sugar. The result is a big drop in vitamin and mineral intake. Television advertises heavily in the sugar, fat, and salt areas. Young adult working wives and single individuals may do less cooking and use instant, often less nutritious foods. In fact, some young adults have grown up on the junk food they have seen advertised on television and on the ever-growing "instant" dinners prepared by their parents or bought at fast-food restaurants.

Because of the claim that saturated fat and cholesterol are related to cardiovascular disease, some manufacturers have responded with low-cholesterol and polyunsaturated products. Fish, poultry, shellfish, and the leanest red meat have the lowest cholesterol–saturated fat index. Some African tribes consume enormous amounts of animal fats but rarely show signs of coronary disease, but the African tribal lifestyle differs drastically from the American lifestyle. Eating the recommended food groups, exercising, and losing weight are ways to increase the level of high-density lipoproteins that remove cholesterol from the arterial walls and to decrease low-density lipoproteins that contribute to disease (250, 371). In American society you can be helpful in recommending that young adults avoid too much sugar, excess salt, an abundance of animal products and red meats, and a steady diet of foods in which there are additives and preservatives (especially nitrates and nitrites).

Other diseases thought to be related to diet are diverticular disease of the colon and colon cancer, appendicitis, hiatus hernia, hemorrhoids, and varicose veins, again diseases affecting young adults. One theory relates these diseases to lack of fiber in the diet. Fiber (found mainly in plant foods) increases stool weight and transit time. Pressure is thus relieved all along the gastrointestinal tract so that these problems are not so likely to arise. Possibly potential carcinogens formed in the gastrointestinal tract do not have a chance to reach the harmful level (155, 259, 371). You can suggest an increase in fiber through eating bran or other foods (whole wheat bread, whole grain cereals, raw fruits or vegetables) so that young adults can cut down on disease proneness and improve their elimination pattern.

Obesity

Obesity is a persistent problem and is usually related to restricted activity (more than 3 hours of sitting daily was associated with obesity in one study) (260, 349, 350) psychological and body image problems, worry, diabetes, hypertension, cardiovascular disease, pain, and premature mortality (371). However, overweight people in Laffrey's study (206) perceived themselves as healthy as their normal weight peers. Often the active adolescent becomes the sedentary young adult but does not lower caloric intake. Thus more calories are eaten than are needed for energy. Those who have less education and lower family income and are married are also more likely to be obese, especially African-American women (186, 222, 365). In an attempt to lose weight, the young adult may try a variety of approaches.

You can help dieters by insisting that any special diet must be analyzed for its nutritional value and overall effect on the body. Additionally, you might suggest a group approach and behavior modification techniques. Many people can lose weight, but they gain it back as soon as they abandon their diets. Often an increase in exercise is recommended rather than a continual decrease in calories for the following reasons:

- Appetite is decreased after exercise because of lowered blood supply to the gastrointestinal tract.
- Exercise may decrease tension and stress, resulting in less frequent eating for nonnutritive purposes.
- Adequate energy or caloric intake is necessary for efficient use of protein for growth and tissue maintenance.
- Basal metabolic rate decreases after a period of caloric restriction.
- Caloric restriction combined with mild exercise can result in greater fat loss and reduced loss of lean body mass than caloric restriction alone.
- Nutritional adequacy of diets low in energy value (less than 1800–2000 kcal) is questioned, as many of the essential nutrients, especially minerals, are found in relatively low concentrations in foods.

Generally, a low-potency vitamin–mineral supplement is recommended for persons on calorie-restricted diets (371). Treatments for the obese person are discussed by several authors (47, 262, 276, 353).

Vegetarianism

In contrast to the obese person, the vegetarian is seldom obese. Vegetarianism has grown popular with young adults, but it is not new. Certain religious groups (e.g., the Seventh-Day Adventists) have been effectively practicing a form of vegetarianism for years. In addition to religious reasons, people are vegetarians for moral reasons (opposed to killing animals for food), for economic reasons (cannot afford animal protein), and for health reasons (may believe that a significant amount of animal food is detrimental or that a large amount of plant food is beneficial). Young adults probably fall mainly into the last category.

People who consider themselves vegetarians range from those who eat limited amounts of meat, milk products, or fish and animal products to vegetarians who eat only vegetables, fruits, legumes, nuts, and grains. Ovovegetarians consume eggs, and lactovegetarians consume milk products in addition to plant foods.

Depending on the extent of the vegetarian's dietary restrictions, certain precautions must be taken to maintain an adequate intake of required nutrients. If animal proteins, eggs, or milk is inadequate in the diet, the person may need supplementary calcium, iron, zinc, and vitamins B_2 and B_{12}. Soy milk fortified with vitamin D can supply that vitamin. Iron supplements may be needed, even if enriched grain products are used. If caloric and protein intake is minimal, serum albumin and total serum protein may be low (270, 371).

Eight amino acids are essential nutrients that must be obtained daily in the diet: isoleucine, tryptophan, threonine, leucine, lysine, methionine, valine, and phenylalanine. Cystine and tyrosine are quasi-essential. In addition, infants must have arginine and histidine. The bioavailability of protein depends on proper balance of essential amino acids. Dietary deficiency of any substance may enhance our vulnerability to herpes, anxiety, overeating, high blood pressure, insomnia, and other disorders. There is increasing evidence that specific amino acids play important roles in central nervous system function and therefore behavior. Some medical disorders such as a few of the many types of schizophrenia may be helped through dietary manipulations of amino acids (270, 371).

A wide variety of legumes, grain, nuts, seeds, vegetables, milk, and eggs can supply adequate amounts of required nutrients. Although the proteins in these foods are considered incomplete (in contrast to the complete proteins—meat, fish, poultry, and dairy products—which contain all essential amino acids) certain proteins such as those found in cereals (lysine) and those in legumes (methionine) complement each other when eaten together (270, 371). For example, peanut butter or chili beans (high in lysine but low in methionine) can be served with whole wheat bread or corn bread (low in lysine but high in methionine). Other complementary combinations are beans and wheat in baked beans and brown bread or refried beans and rice or corn tortillas; lentil and rice in soup; beans and rice in casserole or bean curd and rice or lentils and rice; peas and rye in split pea soup and rye bread; and peas and rice in black-eyed peas and rice. Further, amino acids in milk products and eggs complement plant proteins. Such combinations are cereals and milk in breakfast cereal with milk; pasta and cheese in macaroni and cheese or pizza; bread and cheese in a cheese sandwich; rice and milk in rice cooked in milk instead of water; bread and egg in poached egg on toast; peanuts and milk in a peanut butter sandwich and yogurt (270). Pure vegetarians who consume no milk and no eggs will need vitamin B_{12} supplements. A helpful guide in complementing proteins can be found in several references (270, 371).

Nutrition Education

You may be able to advise young adults about nutrition in a variety of settings. Keep in mind the basic foods as you suggest a diet pattern, and adjust your information to the vegetarians or those who have allergies or specific ethnic or cultural preferences. These suggestions, if followed, will contribute to nutritional health (156, 270, 353, 371, 372):

- Keep a specific record of intake for one week to determine eating patterns (Fig. 12–2).
- Increase consumption of fruits, vegetables, and whole grains (see Fig. 12–1). Eat a variety of foods.
- Decrease consumption of foods or beverages high in refined sugars; instead drink more water and fruit juices.
- Do not add salt to foods during cooking or at the table and avoid snack foods with visible salt or foods prepared in brine; instead use herbs, spices, and lemon for seasoning.
- Decrease consumption of foods high in total fat and animal fat and partially replace saturated fats (beef, pork, butter, fatty meats), whether obtained from animal or vegetable sources, with polyunsaturated fats (fish, poultry, veal, lean meats, margarine, vegetable sources). Keep fat total intake to no more than 30% of daily calories. Limit saturated fats to less than 10% of total fat calories.
- Substitute low-fat and nonfat milk for whole milk and low-fat dairy products for high-fat products (except for young children). Limit cholesterol intake to less than 300 mg daily.
- Reduce use of luncheon or variety meats (e.g., sausage, salami).
- Use skim or low-fat milk and cheeses instead of whole milk and cream.
- Avoid deep fat frying; use baking, boiling, broiling, roasting, and stewing, which help remove fat.
- Avoid excessive intake of any nutrient or food as excess consumption of, and in turn deficiency of, any substance can contribute to disease.
- Avoid more than a minimum intake of alcohol.

Suggest that young adults take vitamins and mineral supplements only with a practitioner's sanction and after a complete blood and urine analysis has been done. Suggest that exercise is as important as food in-

Record all foods and drinks that you had during the day and during the night.

Day of Week (Circle) Mon Tues Wed Thurs Fri Sat Sun

Breakfast

Foods/Amounts (cup, tbsp) Drinks/Amounts (cup, glass)

____

____

Lunch

Foods/Amounts (cup, tbsp) Drinks/Amounts (cup, glass)

____

____

Dinner

Foods/Amounts (cup, tbsp) Drinks/Amounts (cup, glass)

____

____

Snacks

Time Foods or Drinks Amount (cup, glass, tbsp, or pieces)

____

____

Do you take vitamin or mineral supplements? Yes___ No___
If yes, please list kind and how many per day.

____

____

Do you take any other nutritional supplement? (e.g., yeast, protein bran) Yes___ No___
If yes, please list and describe.

____

____

Figure 12–2. Form for assessing eating habits and nutritional state.

take when considering the number of calories needed. Suggest exercise not only to burn off calories but to maintain muscle tone, elimination, and circulation, to regulate sleep, and to release tension.

Keep in mind the young adult who may need suggestions on economical but nutritious foods. Using powdered skim milk, less expensive cuts of meat, and home-cooked cereals does not sacrifice nutrition but does save money.

Teach about the need for fiber in the diet, which can prevent constipation and help reduce the incidence of cancer of the colon, diverticulosis, appendicitis, gallstones, and heart disease. Using only one source of fiber such as bran while excluding the fiber from vegetables and fruits can produce problems, however. Some fibers contribute to constipation if they are not diluted with substantial amounts of water (156, 250, 276, 371).

Teach about the adverse effects of caffeine. Effects of caffeine can be detrimental to health (see Table 11–6). Warn also that herbal teas may contain strong drugs that can cause severe problems. Those containing catnip, juniper, hydrangea, jimson weed, lobelia, nutmeg, and wormwood can be toxic to the central nervous system and can cause severe reactions, including hallucinations. People with allergies should stay away from teas containing camomile, goldenrod, marigold, and yarrow. Also be aware that some herbal teas have as much as twice the caffeine as a regular cup of coffee.

Hospitalized young adults may be suffering from nutritional deficiencies resulting from a specific diet. Be aware that hospital-induced malnutrition exists. Patients whose meals are withheld because they are undergoing various diagnostic tests or treatments, especially over a long period, are candidates for this problem.

Biological Rhythms

Rhythms occur throughout the life cycle of each individual. From the time of birth different body structures and functions develop rhythmicity at different rates. By the time the individual reaches young adulthood, biological rhythms are established by body chemistry and by the suprachiasmatic nucleus, a tiny cluster of cells buried deep in the brain. **Biological rhythms** are *self-sustaining, repetitive, rhythmic patterns found in plants, animals, and man.* The rhythms are found throughout our external and internal environment and can be exogenous or endogenous.

Exogenous rhythms *depend on the rhythm of external environmental events,* such as seasonal variations, lunar revolution, and the night-and-day cycle that function as time givers. These events help to synchronize internal rhythms with external environmental stimuli and establish an internal time pattern or biologic clock.

Endogenous rhythms such as sleep–wake and sleep–dream cycles arise *within the organism.* Endogenous and exogenous rhythms are usually synchronized. Many internal rhythms do not readily alter their repetitive patterns, however, even when the external stimuli are removed. For instance, when a person shifts to sleeping by day and waking at night, as frequently happens with nurses, a transient or temporary desynchronization occurs. Body temperature and adrenal hormone levels are usually low during the sleep cycle. With the shift in sleep and waking, the person is awake and making demands on the body during the usual sleep period. Three weeks may be needed before internal rhythms adapt to the shift. A similar period of desynchronization occurs when a person makes a flight crossing time zones (8, 9, 28, 88, 96, 135, 183, 220, 278, 289, 308, 358).

Within any 24-hour period, physiologic and psychological functions reach maximum and minimum limits. When a physiologic function approaches a high or low limit, the body's feedback mechanisms attempt to counterregulate the action. *This form of endogenous rhythm that reoccurs in a cyclic pattern within a 20- to 28-hour period is a* **circadian rhythm.** Body temperature, blood pressure, pulse, respirations, urine production, and hormone, blood sugar, hemoglobin, and amino acid levels demonstrate this rhythmic pattern. Similar variations or rhythms in the levels of alertness, fatigue, tenseness, and irritability can also be demonstrated.

In humans mental efficiency and performance apparently are related to the rhythms of body temperature and catecholamine excretion in the adult. The body temperature rises and drops by approximately 2° over each 24-hour period. The body temperature begins to decline near 10 PM, is lowest on awaking, gradually rises during the morning, levels off in the afternoon, and then drops again in the evening (Fig. 12–3). The level of adrenocortical hormone secretion appears correlated with body temperature rhythms and the individual's state of alertness and wakefulness. The level of adrenocortical hormones rises early in the morning, peaks around the time we typically awaken, and then drops to a low point by late evening (96, 111, 183, 317). Usually the best mental and physical performances coincide with peak temperature, and the least desirable performances coincide with intervals of lowest body temperature. In addition, studies have shown that the lowest excretory rates of epinephrine in day-active people correlate with the time of maximum fatigue and poorest performance. Physical strength crests at different times of the day (72, 183, 289, 339).

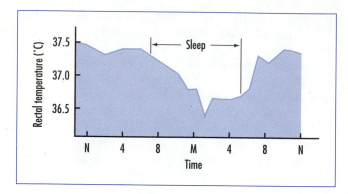

Figure 12–3. Diurnal cycle of temperature variations. *(From Berger, K.J., and M.B. Williams,* Fundamentals of Nursing: Collaborating for Optimal Health. *Stamford, CT: Appleton & Lange, 1992, p. 446.)*

Researchers have theorized that many disasters have resulted from failure to consider human biology. For example, at the nuclear accident at Three Mile Island, the three young men in the control area worked on a shift system called slow rotation—days for a week, evenings for a week, and late nights for a week. At the time of the disasters at Bopal and Chernobyl, people were working unusual shifts. Work schedules with changing shift rotation causes a desynchronization of circadian rhythms, altering performance levels (136, 183).

Circadian Rhythms in Illness

An interrelationship exists between circadian rhythms and mental or physical illness. The pattern of living taught by the culture also affects body rhythms. A few examples of how circadian rhythms influence the health of young adults are presented next. (For more extensive discussion, refer to References 9, 79, 96, 111, 122, 288, 295, and 308.)

Diagnostic cues are influenced by biological rhythms. Observing the integration of the body's rhythms (or lack of such integration) can be used to determine the person's health status. Diagnosis and treatment of some illnesses can be determined from the study of circadian rhythms or biological time. In some instances the illness alters the pattern of circadian rhythm. Other illnesses show exaggerated or decreased symptoms at a particular biological time. Blood pressure and temperature values, laboratory findings, and biopsy specimens for cell study differ according to the biological time of day. For instance, growth hormone levels in the blood are highest during the night hours; therefore routine blood values taken at 8 AM will

not give a total picture. The percentage of red blood cells drops approximately 4½% late at night; a decrease in red blood cells of 5% prompts blood transfusions in some hospitals. Concentrations of white blood cells peak in the morning and early afternoon (82, 151, 205). Ambiguous laboratory findings, the need for repeated medical tests, and the potential for unnecessary medical therapies can be avoided if the person's normal biological rhythms are considered first.

Rhythmic time cycles appear to influence many aspects of human life. Births and deaths occur more frequently at night and during the early morning. Persons with ulcers and allergies suffer more in the nighttime and in spring; allergic responses, including asthmatic attacks, occur more frequently at night and in the early morning hours. There are certain yearly peaks in the number of suicides, psychotic episodes, and accidents. Eventually knowledge about circadian rhythms and biological time may serve as a major tool in preventive health programs.

Depression has a number of causes but may be directly related to biological rhythms of depressed people. Altered biochemical rhythms, diurnal (daytime) mood swings, and altered sleep cycles have been noted. Researchers have hypothesized that abnormalities of sleep patterns in some types of depression are due to abnormal internal phase relationships of circadian rhythms. The circadian rhythm of rapid eye movement (REM) sleep may occur abnormally early (95, 183, 255, 280, 308). Depressed persons usually experience insomnia or periods of predawn wakefulness. Their sleep cycles are shortened and fragmented, and they are easily disturbed by environmental changes. Successful treatment frequently comes in the form of antidepressant drugs that slow biological clocks (i.e., lithium carbonate) or speed biological clocks (i.e., imipramine) (253).

Various mental functions and the emotion, behaviors, and autonomic responses associated with them depend on certain chemicals secreted at the synapses of the neurons in specific pathways of the brain. Several brain neurotransmitters (norepinephrine, dopamine, serotonin, and acetylcholine) undergo cyclic changes in amount of chemical present. These fluctuations are thought related to factors concerned with periodicity and emotion (133, 289, 339).

Cells in almost every tissue of the body divide or reproduce in circadian rhythm. Normal cells show intervals of accelerated reproductive activity. In human beings, for example, skin and liver cells are more active at night. Cancer cells do not reproduce at the same rate as normal cells; abnormal mitosis (cell reproduction) rhythms and, in many instances, a complete lack of circadian rhythms have been reported. Further, timing has been found crucial for surgical treatment or chemotherapy of cancer patients; recovery is linked to time of day of the treatment (133, 289).

Research suggests that people who are desynchronized or constantly consuming foods and drugs that change the phase of their circadian rhythms may be a high-risk group for cancer (133). Health teaching should include the need to decrease the intake of coffee, tea, and certain barbiturates that may be carcinogens.

Adrenal hormone production is cyclic in humans. The blood and urine concentrations of adrenocorticosteroid hormones in persons on schedules of diurnal activity and nocturnal sleep drop at night and rise to highest levels in early morning. The course of the adrenal cycle may also be followed by measuring the eosinophil (white blood cell) level; eosinophils decrease as the blood level of adrenal hormones increases (289).

Light is probably the synchronizer of the adrenocorticosteroid rhythm. This factor has implications for people who are night workers or who have varying degrees of blindness. Because adrenal hormones control other circadian rhythms within the body, knowledge of their cycle is important in the study and treatment of numerous conditions (289).

Low blood levels of adrenal hormones affect the nervous system and cause increased sensitivity to sounds, tastes, and smell. Sensory acuity reaches its maximum at the time of lowest steroid levels. A sudden drop in acuity occurs in the early morning as steroid levels begin to rise. A person is therefore better able to detect taste, smell, or sound at the end of the day. Daily fatigue from lack of sleep and neurologically related symptoms associated with adrenal insufficiency (Addison's disease) may be related to low levels of adrenal hormones (289).

Adrenal rhythm is also important in handling certain allergies. Sensitivity to histamine follows a circadian rhythm: it peaks near evening or night when adrenocorticosteroids are reaching their lowest levels. Nasal congestion from hayfever, skin reactions from drug sensitivity, and breathing crises in asthma patients occur more frequently during the evening or night. Suggest to individuals with hayfever and asthma that they do their gardening and weeding in the morning when their adrenocorticosteroid levels are at their highest.

Nursing Assessment and Intervention

Nursing care should be planned with biological rhythms in mind. Because our cyclic functioning is synchronized with environmental stimuli, physiologic disequilibrium occurs whenever we are confronted with environmental or schedule changes. Transient desynchronization may occur whenever a person is exposed to the hospital or nursing home stimuli. New noise levels; lighting patterns; schedules for eating, sleeping, and personal hygiene; and unfamiliar persons intruding on the person's privacy may all contribute to this desynchronization. Disturbed mental and physical well-being and increased subjective fatigue reflect the conflict between the internal time pattern and external events. Several days usually are required before the person adapts to the environment and thereby regains synchronization—normal biological rhythms.

You can control some external factors such as meals, baths, and various tests, make them more nearly similar to the patient's normal (outside) routine, and lessen the stress to which the patient is subjected. Obtaining and using a nursing history constitutes one method of lessening this stress.

Your *nursing history* should be directed at getting information about the patient's preillness or prehospitalization patterns for sleep, rest, food and fluid intake, elimination, and personal hygiene. The questionnaire developed by Alward and Monk (9) is a useful guide. Do you consider yourself a "day" person or a "night" person? Do you feel cheerful when you first wake up? What time of day do you feel most alert? What hours do you prefer to work? Why do you prefer these hours? How do you feel when something causes you to change your routine? Answers to these questions will provide you information about the patient's daily patterns (9, 37, 273, 279, 289). Once this information has been obtained, nursing actions can be initiated that support these established patterns and possibly prevent total disruption of body rhythms during hospitalization.

After the patient has been hospitalized for a few days, certain objective data are available that will assist you in determining a rough estimate of the person's circadian patterns. The routine graphic record supplies information about the patient's vital signs. Using this source, you might be able to identify peaks and lows in blood pressure, pulse, or temperature curves. Also, an intake and output record that shows both the time and the amount voided will aid in determining the patient's daily urinary–excretory pattern. In addition to the postadmission nursing history, a daily log of sleep and waking hours, mealtimes, hunger periods, voiding and defecation patterns, diurnal moods, and other circadian rhythms recorded for 28 days before hospitalization can help determine the person's cyclic patterns. Diagnostic tests and certain forms of medical and nursing therapy can then be appropriately prescribed by using the person's own baseline rhythm measurements. Determination of each patient's rhythms before, during, and after hospitalization or illness eventually will be possible when more simplified, economic, and accurate measurement devices are available.

The client's *medication schedule* can also reflect your understanding of biological rhythms. Drug effectiveness can be altered by the time of day that the particular drug is administered. Aspirin administered at 7 AM will remain in the body 22 hours; aspirin ingested at 7 PM will last 17 hours. Some antihistamines last only 6 to 8 hours if taken at night but are effective 15 to 17 hours when taken at 7 AM. Digitalis (a cardiac glycoside) is several times more effective when administered in the early morning than when administered at other times. The dosage of analgesics needed to relieve pain during the evening or dark hours is higher than that needed during the daytime. Sensitivity to pain increases in the evening (214, 361, 374).

One area of **chronopharmacology** (*study of cellular rhythms in relationship to drug therapy*) that has been researched extensively is the relationship of adrenocortical function and corticosteroid drug administration. The secretion of corticosteroids by the adrenal cortex has a 24-hour rhythm, with the highest corticosteroid values expected after the usual time of awakening. When corticosteroids are administered either daily or on alternate days, adrenal suppression and possibly growth disturbance can be minimized by timing to the circadian crest in adrenocortical function. Morning doses of prednisolone (a glucocorticoid) are less likely to cause alterations in the rhythmic pattern of urinary excretion than twice-daily divided doses or a single dose in the late evening (19, 110, 214).

Circadian rhythms are also important factors in determining drug toxicity. A distinct 24-hour rhythm of vulnerability or resistance to drugs has been identified. Before setting a drug's toxic level, both the person's biological clock and the drug dosage must be considered. At present, problems exist in determining toxicity levels. Federal research guidelines do not consider the circadian rhythms of the animals being tested. Nocturnal animals are tested in the daytime; animals are tested before they have had time to adjust to a new laboratory environment; animals are tested in light and dark cycles that are not regulated; and animals whose feeding schedules are not fixed and recorded are tested. All these factors can cause altered rhythms in animals and altered vulnerability or resistance to the drug being tested (111, 214).

Without the aid of suitable measurement devices, it is impossible to determine a person's biological clock. Drug administration is therefore usually based on other factors. Most medications are given before or after meals, at bedtime, or at the convenience of the nursing personnel and patients. In the future, as knowledge of the internal clock increases, you, the nurse, will find yourself altering drug administration times to suit the person's biological time. Perhaps you will be in charge of a master computer that, after analyzing information about each person's biological clock, will send the appropriate medication dose at the appropriate time.

Vital signs routine should be based on circadian rhythm patterns rather than on tradition or convenience of the agency staff. Both internal and skin temperatures show a systematic rise and fall over a 24-hour period, a cycle difficult to alter in normal adults. Body temperature usually peaks between 4 and 6 PM and reaches its lowest point around 4 AM in people who are active by day and sleep by night. When the internal temperature is normally peaking, other body functions such as pulse rate, blood pressure, and cardiac output (volume of blood pumped by the heart) are also changing. Pulse rate is high when the temperature is highest and drops during the night. The human heart rate will vary as much as 20 or 30 beats per minute in 24 hours. Blood pressure shows a marked fall during the first hour of sleep, followed by a gradual rise throughout the daily cycle, with a peak between 5 and 7 PM. Cardiac output reaches minimum levels between 2 and 4 AM, the period of lowest temperature findings (79, 118, 288, 295).

Work Schedules

Work schedules should be developed with biological rhythms in mind. You can also establish your own circadian patterns to help you gain insight into physical feelings and behaviors and can use this information to plan your days to advantage. You might choose to cope with the most difficult patient assignment during the time of peak mental and physical performance, for example.

Nurses and many industrial and law enforcement personnel are frequently required to change shifts every week or month. Night and rotating shift workers are at excessive risk for accidents and injuries on the job because of disrupted circadian rhythms. Sleep cycles are interrupted. There is difficulty in falling asleep, a shorter duration of sleep, poorer quality of sleep, and persistent fatigue. Alertness and other physiologic processes suffer. Eating habits are disrupted; diets are poorer; and digestion is interfered with. Constipation, gastric and peptic ulcers, and gastritis are more common. Social activities and interactions, essential to physical and mental health, are interrupted. Family life and relationships are interfered with; shift workers have difficulty fulfilling family and parental roles. Rotating shift assignments are thus relevant to worker's health and quality of work performance (9, 122, 135, 183, 198, 220, 308, 358). Altering the sleep–wake sequence requires time for the person to make adjustments and regain synchrony.

If shift rotation cannot be eliminated, individuals should be required to rotate no more frequently than once a month. Consistently working at night allows a person to acquire a new sleep–wake rhythm. Therefore night work should be made more attractive to persons who can adapt to the shift and are willing to remain on it permanently. Those who cannot adapt should be exempt from rotation.

Health teaching of any rotating-shift worker concerning the possible consequences of such a routine should not be overlooked. Night workers taking medications should be aware that the effects of medications may vary somewhat from those they usually experience when working days. The susceptibility to various degrees of drug metabolism occurs throughout the day but even more when a person is experiencing jet lag or the early phase of shift rotation. Individuals with a chronic illness such as diabetes, epilepsy, or hypertension and cardiac problems must consider these factors when they plan their medication regimen.

Rest and Sleep

Sleep is a *complex biological rhythm, intricately related to rest and other biological rhythms.* Help clients realize that such factors as emotional and physical status, occupation, and amount of physical activity determine the need for rest and sleep. For example, workers who alternate between day and night shifts frequently feel more exhausted and may need more sleep than people who keep regular hours. Surgery, illness, pregnancy, and the postpartum state all require that the individual receive more sleep. Mothers of infants, toddlers, and preschoolers may need daytime naps.

Some young people find themselves caught in a whirlwind of activities. Jobs, social activities, family responsibilities, and educational pursuits occupy every minute. The young adult can adjust to this pace and maintain it for a length of time without damaging physical or mental health. The person may think he or she is immune to the laws of nature and can go long periods without sleep. If the person finds that he or she is not functioning well on a certain amount of sleep, the schedule should be adjusted to allow for more hours of rest. He or she also must be cognizant of the biological rhythms for rest and activity. Setting aside certain periods for quiet activities such as reading, sewing, watching television, and various hobbies is restful but not as beneficial as sleep.

Each person has his or her own sleep needs and cycle, and research is helping us better understand the different stages of sleep and the importance of sleep to well-being. The tradition that young adults should have 7 to 8 hours of sleep seems valid, although some get along fine with less. When left to the body's natural pace, the person is likely to sleep every 25 hours (276).

Normal Sleep Pattern

Sleep is a complex phenomenon (35, 37, 42, 65, 113, 177, 202, 238, 276, 280, 309, 310). The functional component of the brain stem that exerts influence on consciousness and the wake–sleep cycle is called the *reticular activating system (RAS)*. The RAS activates the state of consciousness and functions as a deactivation mechanism to decrease alertness and to produce sleep. **Electroencephalograms (EEGs),** *recordings of brainwave activity,* vary with the awake and asleep states and at different intrasleep cycles (Fig. 12–4). When a person is wide awake and alert, the EEG recordings show rapid, irregular waves. High-frequency beta and alpha waves predominate. As he or she begins to rest, the wave pattern changes to an **alpha rhythm,** *a regular pattern of low voltage, with frequencies of 8 to 12 cycles per second.* During sleep a **delta rhythm,** a slow pattern of high voltage and 1 to 2 cycles per second, occurs. At certain stages of sleep, **sleep spindles,** sudden short bursts of sharply pointed alpha waves of 14 to 16 cycles per second, and **K-complexes,** *jagged tightly peaked waves,* occur.

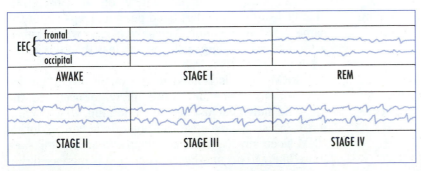

Figure 12–4. Changes in electroencephalogram during sleep.

Sleep is divided into **NREM** (*non-rapid eye movement*) and **REM** stages. NREM sleep is divided into four stages—light to deep. REM sleep follows the deepest NREM sleep as the person ascends to stage II sleep and occurs before repeated descent through stages II, III, and IV. In **NREM stage I sleep**, the *person makes a transition from wakefulness to sleep* in approximately 5 minutes. The alpha rhythm is present, but the waves are more uneven and smaller than in later stages. The person is drowsy and relaxed, has fleeting thoughts, is somewhat aware of the environment, can be easily awakened, and may think he or she has been awake. The pulse rate is decreased. **NREM stage II sleep** is the *beginning of deeper sleep* and fills 40 to 50% of total sleep time. The person is more relaxed than in the prior stage but can be easily awakened. Sleep spindles and K-complexes appear in the brain waves at intervals. **NREM stage III sleep** is a *period of progressively deeper sleep* and begins 30 to 45 minutes after sleep onset. EEG waves become more regular; delta waves appear; sleep spindles are present; muscles are more relaxed; vital signs and metabolic activity are lowered to basal rates; and the person is difficult to awaken. **NREM stage IV sleep** is *very deep sleep, occurs approximately 40 minutes after stage I, and rests and restores the body physically.* This stage is of as great importance as REM sleep. Delta waves are the dominant EEG pattern. The person is very relaxed and seldom moves, is difficult to arouse, and responds slowly if awakened. Physiologic measures are below normal. Sleep walking and enuresis may occur during this stage. After strenuous physical exercise, this stage is greatly needed.

REM sleep is called *active or paradoxic sleep* and is the *stage of rapid eye movements and dreaming that occurs before descending to the deeper sleep of stages II, III, and IV.* This stage is of great importance. In REM sleep the EEG readings are active and similar to those of stage I sleep, but various physiologic differences from other sleep stages are present. These differences, in addition to rapid, side-to-side eye movements, are:

- Muscular relaxation and absent tendon reflexes, with occasional twitching, so that the body is in immobility-like paralysis
- Respiratory rate increased 7 to 20% alternating between rapid and slow with brief apneic periods
- Pulse rate irregular and increased 5%
- Blood pressure fluctuations up to 30 mm Hg
- High oxygen consumption by the brain
- Increased production of 17-hydroxycorticosteroids, posterior pituitary hormones, and catecholamines
- Increased gastric secretions
- Penile erections in men of all ages

REM sleep occurs in 70- to 90-minute cycles that increase as the night progresses. It rests and restores mentally and is important for learning and psychological functioning. It allows for review of the day's events, categorizing and integrating of information into the brain's storage systems, and problem solving. During psychological stress this stage is vital. Dreams that occur during REM sleep allow for wish fulfillment and release of potentially harmful thoughts, feelings, and impulses so that they do not affect the waking personality.

In a 7- or 8-hour period the person will have 60- to 90-minute cycles of sleep descending from stage I to IV and back to REM sleep. After 10 to 15 minutes of REM sleep, the person again descends to stage IV. The person may ascend to REM sleep three or five times a night, but each time he or she spends a longer period in it. In the first third of the night he or she spends more time in stage IV sleep; in the last third of the night more time is spent in REM sleep. Dreams in the early REM stages are shorter, are less interesting, and contain aspects of the preceding day's activities. As the night progresses, the dreams become longer, more vivid and exciting, and less concerned with daily life. Stages III and IV together constitute approximately 20% of sleep time until old age, when deep sleep almost disappears.

Variations in Sleep Patterns

The percentage of time a person spends in sleep differs with age and with body temperature at the time of falling asleep. If the person's body temperature is at its high point in the biological rhythm, he or she will sleep two times longer than if the temperature is at a low point in the biological rhythm. REM sleep remains constant throughout adult life, constituting 20 to 25% of sleep, in contrast to 40 to 50% of sleep for babies. But the percentage of time spent in stage IV sleep decreases 15 to 30% with age so that the aged person sleeps less time and awakens more frequently. Elderly women's sleep patterns change approximately 10 years later than men's patterns. The aged person's adjustment to sleep seems dependent on arteriosclerotic changes so that the alert aged person sleeps about the same as the young adult. The aged person with cerebral arteriosclerotic changes sleeps 20% less than the young adult (42, 177, 276, 309, 310).

REM sleep is related to the onset of certain diseases. Convulsions are more likely to occur in the epileptic individual just before awakening, which is during REM sleep. Because the pulse is irregular during REM sleep, myocardial infarctions and arrhythmias are more likely to occur. Gastric secretion is increased during the REM state. The person with a peptic ulcer has more pain at these times (177, 276).

Sedatives, antidepressants, and amphetamines significantly decrease REM sleep. If the person continually takes a sedative, there is a gradual return to the usual amount of REM sleep. But when the drug is withdrawn, REM sleep is markedly withdrawn, causing insomnia and nightmares, irritability, fatigue, and sensitivity to pain, all of which persist up to 5 weeks. Thus sedatives should be given sparingly, including to the young adult, although different sedatives cause different effects, and effects differ from person to person. You should learn from the person if he or she is regularly on sedatives. If the person is, he or she must continue them to avoid withdrawal symptoms while receiving health care (42, 177, 214, 276, 316, 353).

If REM deprivation and the rebound of more REM sleep later occur because of administration of sedatives, the patient with any health problem, but especially cardiovascular disease, should have sedative administration stopped before discharge. At home the person will not have the close observation needed during the prolonged periods of REM sleep when myocardial infarction is more likely to occur. Further, in contrast to popular belief, alcoholic beverages should not be used to promote sleep. Alcohol speeds the onset of sleep but interferes with REM sleep, which may contribute to hangover feelings.

Sleep Deprivation

Sleep deprivation should be avoided by the young adult. The person may feel rested if he or she awakens after 4 or 5 hours of sleep, but there has been insufficient time for REM sleep. If the person is awakened frequently, the sleep cycle must be started all over again. See Physical and Psychological Changes with Sleep Deprivation for more information (42, 202, 269, 276, 309, 310, 353).

When the person decides to recover lost sleep by sleeping longer hours, he or she will spend more time in REM sleep. Twelve to 14 hours of sleep help to overcome brief periods of sleep deprivation. Studies indicate a minimum of 5 hours sleep daily is needed and for most people 7 to 8 hours are needed to avoid sleep deprivation (202). After 48 hours of sleep loss, the body produces a stress chemical related structurally to LSD-25, which may account for behavioral changes. After 4 days of sleep deprivation, the body does not produce adenosine triphosphate (ATP), the catalyst for energy release, which may be a factor in fatigue. With total sleep deprivation, confusion, hallucinations, and psychosis occur (42, 309, 310, 332).

> ### ► PHYSICAL AND PSYCHOLOGICAL CHANGES WITH SLEEP DEPRIVATION
>
> #### Physical Changes
>
> - Lack of alertness
> - Feeling pressure on head
> - Nystagmus; ptosis of eyelids
> - Uncoordination; tremors
> - Slowed reflexes
> - Fatigue
> - Bradypnea
> - Cardiac arrhythmias
> - Poorer performance
> - Increased errors
> - Physical discomfort; hypochondriasis
>
> #### Psychological Changes
>
> - Anxiety; insecurity
> - Introspective; unable to respond to support from others; irritable
> - Apathy; withdrawal
> - Depression
> - Increased aggressiveness
> - Suspicious
> - Decreased mental agility
> - Illusions
> - Decreased concentration
> - Loss of creativity
> - Poor judgment
> - Memory failure
> - Confusion; disorientation
> - Hallucinations
> - Bizarre behavior; psychosis

Thus the client, who needs all stages of sleep for physical and psychological restoration, *should not be awakened during the night if at all possible.* Observe the person before awakening by studying eye movements under the lids. If he or she is in REM sleep, wait a few minutes for it to end before awakening the person, as this is a short and important stage. Sleep has priority over taking vital signs, especially because the vital sign measurement is affected by the stage of sleep and therefore cannot be compared accurately to daytime measurements. As steroids are released during REM sleep, disturbance of REM sleep causes steroid release to be out of synchrony with other biological rhythms, affecting all areas of function in the person.

Being frequently awakened during the night such as happens to young parents with young children produces the same effects as sleeping fewer hours, even if the total length of time asleep is the usual amount. Blocks of uninterrupted sleep are a definite physical and psychological need.

Help parents work out a system that responds to baby's needs but also allows each parent to get as much uninterrupted sleep as possible. Use the above information on sleep stages and effects of sleep interruption and deprivation to teach the young adults.

Sleep Disturbances

Millions of people in the United States do not get normal sleep daily. They either sleep too much or not enough, suffer night terrors, or stop breathing for a minute or two during sleep. The cost of sleep disorders is enormous; some people pay a great deal for pills and potions to maintain normal sleep.

Insomnia, a *disorder of initiating and maintaining sleep,* is sometimes a problem for young adults. **Primary insomnia** is a *sleep problem that exists in the absence of any major medical or psychiatric condition.* Other types of insomnia are **sleep onset** (*difficulty falling asleep*), **sleep maintenance** (*awakening in the middle of the night*), and **terminal insomnia** (*early-morning awakening*). Factors that may lead to insomnia include (1) disturbed circadian rhythms, (2) physical symptoms such as pain, dyspnea, and fever, (3) environmental disturbances, (4) emotional stress, and (5) stimulant drugs (42, 276, 309, 310, 353).

Knowing the quantity and quality of sleep is useful in determining the existence of insomnia. Individual sleep requirements vary, and an individual's satisfaction with the length and quality of sleep is the basis for assessing the presence of insomnia.

You can help the insomniac by being an interested, calm listener and by suggesting that the following measures be tried (42, 113, 177, 276, 280, 309, 310, 353).

- Maintain a regular schedule of pre-bedtime relaxation, sleep, and wakefulness to keep biorhythms in synchrony.
- Avoid strenuous activity in the evening before retiring; instead rely on soothing but enjoyable stimuli such as a backrub for muscular and emotional relaxation, quiet music, warm bath, pro- gressive relaxation to loosen tight muscles, or a nonstimulating book or hobby.
- Try a glass of warm milk, which contains 1-tryptophan, a chemical that increases brain serotonin and induces sleep.
- Improve the sleeping environment: make the bedroom dark, quiet, and as comfortable as possible so it is associated only with pleasurable feelings.
- Purposefully relax after going to bed. Stretch out, get comfortable, let the body become heavy and warm.
- Use pleasant imagery; let the mind "float."
- Sleep on your back on a firm mattress. When sleeping on your side, tuck a small pillow between your waist and the mattress to provide proper support. Sleeping on the abdomen is not recommended because the head is turned sharply to one side all night, affecting neck joints and the lower back. In addition, pressure on one side of the face can irritate the jaw. Sleeping with one arm under the pillow stresses the jaw and may interfere with circulation or pinch a nerve in the wrist.
- If not asleep in 20 minutes, get out of bed and go to another room. Stay calm. Do something boring or relaxing until you are sleepy.

Tranquilizers and sedatives are a last resort. For the ill person, first try a monotonous, rhythmic stimulus such as a backrub, quiet music, a dim light, eyeshades and earplugs, a wrinkle-free bed, or reading a dull book that is conducive to sleep if it does not irritate the person, as the cerebral cortex has nothing for which to stay alert. In effect, with monotony or boredom, the cerebral cortex does not respond to the reticular formation.

Assess the ill person's sleep pattern and help him or her adhere to the normal pattern. The hospital routine of "pass the pills at 9:00 and be asleep by 9:30" fits very few individuals.

If the person does complain of sleep problems, the problems should be explored with the goal of eventual correction. Refer the person to a sleep research center so that, through electronic monitoring of the sleep cycle and close surveillance, the problem can be identified and treated.

Physical Fitness—Exercise

Physical fitness is a *combination of strength, endurance, flexibility, balance, speed, agility, and power* and reflects ability to work for a sustained period with vigor and pleasure, without undue fatigue, and with energy left for enjoying hobbies and recreational activities and for meeting emergencies. Fitness relates to how the person looks and feels, both physically and mentally. Basic to fitness are regular physical exercise, proper nutrition, adequate rest and relaxation, conscientious health practices, and good medical and dental care.

Recommendations for exercise are as follows: After the person has had a thorough physical examination and has been cleared by a physician, daily sessions of 30 minutes of moderate-intensity exercise (no sweating, walking, stairs) is recommended for maintaining health, muscle tone, and strength (Fig. 12–5). For conditioning the cardiovascular system, improving lung capacity, or raising metabolic rate, 20 minutes of aerobic exercise three times a week is necessary (106, 174, 176, 266). Very fast walking that increases heartbeat to 70 to 85% of maximum heart rate (MHR) is considered the best exercise of all; people who cannot jog or run can usually walk 20 to 30 minutes on alternate days. Exercise intensity is monitored by assessing MHR during exercise. MHR is calculated by subtracting the person's

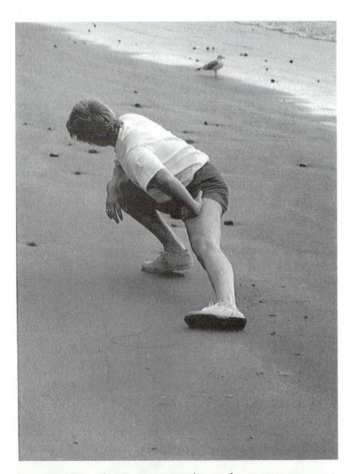

Figure 12–5. Stretching is an important element of any exercise program. *(From Berger, K.J., and M.B. Williams,* Fundamentals of Nursing: Collaborating for Optimal Health. *Stamford, CT: Appleton & Lange, 1992, p. 1422.)*

► LEVELS OF EXERCISE

Light-Intensity Activities

- Bowling
- Fishing
- Boating or sailing
- Horseback riding
- Gardening indoors
- Pet care
- Swinging

Moderate-Intensity Activities

- Walking briskly 3–4 mph
- Golfing
- Playing frisbee or catch
- Exercises or yoga
- Hunting
- Fishing (casting)
- Vacuuming
- Bicycling up to 10 mph
- Swimming
- Carpentry
- House painting
- Gardening outdoors (weed, use of power mower)
- Grounds improvement
- Social dancing
- Ping-pong
- Canoing 2–4 mph

Heavy-Intensity Activities

- Team sports
- Racquet ball
- Skating or skiing
- Jogging
- Jumping rope
- Lessons in body movements, calisthenics
- Aerobic dance
- Swimming vigorously
- Tennis

age from 220. During exercise the pulse should be 60 to 80% of that level. For example, the 40-year-old should have a pulse rate of 108 to 144 during exercise. Listed in Levels of Exercise are various activities based on intensity of the activity and time of participation, which indicates an index energy expenditure (106, 174, 176, 266, 270, 276).

Pregnant women can continue exercise routines unless they are contraindicated medically. The guidelines are as follows (276, 351):

- Avoid competitive exercise; do not push excessively.
- Avoid workouts in hot, humid weather.
- Strenuous exercise should not last longer than 15 minutes.
- Pulse rate should not exceed 140 beats per minute.

- Body temperature should not rise above 100.4°F (38°C) during exercise.
- After the fourth month of pregnancy, no exercises should be performed while lying on the back.

A health self-appraisal questionnaire and program can help the person determine the present state of health and fitness and implications for the years ahead (56, 190, 270, 273).

Jogging makes joints in good condition stronger. Jogging as a regular form of exercise can aggravate old injuries of the back, hips, knees, and ankles because it puts as much as five times normal body weight on lower joints and extremities. Jogging can cause abnormal wear on joints and muscles. The person who jogs must also engage in exercise for the upper extremities and other muscles. Weight lifting can strengthen. Aerobic exercise, brisk walking, jumping rope, and bicycling may actually be better exercise than jogging. These activities stress bone to promote bone building, thickness, and strength and increase circulation throughout the body (270, 351).

Swimming is probably the best overall activity because it increases strength and endurance and stimulates heart and blood vessels, lungs, and many muscle groups without putting excess stress on the person because of less gravity pull in the water. Further, swimming keeps joints supple, aids weight loss or weight control, and reduces hypertension. Perhaps more important, it is an enjoyable activity, either alone or with others.

Regular physical activity has been viewed as a natural tranquilizer, for it reduces anxiety and muscular tension. Some studies show that regular physical exercise improves a number of personality characteristics, correlating with composure, extraversion, self-confidence, assertiveness, persistence, adventuresomeness, and superego strength (94, 270).

Exercise periods are frequently not planned by young adults. Some will get abundant exercise in their jobs, but many will not. Those who do not can check with the local YMCA or YWCA organizations, community recreation departments, continuing education departments of 2-year colleges, or commercial gymnasiums and health salons for exercise programs appropriate to their lifestyles and physical conditions. Refer to Suggestions for an Exercise Program and Principles of Body Mechanics.

Sex Differences

Women and men sometimes share the same physical exercise activities; sometimes interests and energy levels are different, and partners may engage in exercise

> ### ► SUGGESTIONS FOR AN EXERCISE PROGRAM
>
> - Make exercise a part of your lifestyle.
> - Start in small increments, keep it fun, and avoid injury.
> - Avoid exercising for 2 hours after a large meal and eating for 1 hour after exercising.
> - Include at least 10 minutes of warmup and cool-down exercises in an exercise program.
> - Use proper equipment and clothing when exercising.
> - Post goals, pictures of the ideal self, and notes of encouragement in a readily seen place for self-encouragement.
> - Use visualization daily to picture successful attainment of exercise benefit (e.g., looking toned or graceful, ideal weight).
> - Keep records of weekly measures of weight, blood pressure, and pulse.
> - Focus on the rewards of exercise; keep a record of feelings and compare differences in relaxation, energy, concentration, and sleep patterns.
> - Work with a peer or join a structured exercise class, running club, or fitness center. Spend more time with people dedicated to wellness.
> - Stop exercising or at least slow down and consult with a practitioner if any unusual, unexplainable symptoms occur.
> - Reward self for working toward exercise goals and for attaining them. For example, after a month in an exercise program, buy a new pair of running shoes or treat yourself to a special wish.
>
> Taken from References 98, 99, and 270.

activities separately. Women may have as much endurance as men, especially with training, but there are some physiologic differences that account for differences in performance in physical exercise activities or athletic events.

Men have greater upper-body strength primarily because of their longer arms, broader shoulders, and higher muscle fiber counts. Muscle can be conditioned by exercise, but muscle fiber count cannot be increased. Whether men exercise or not, their muscle fibers gain bulk from the hormone testosterone. In men the heart and lungs, which average 10% larger than those of women, provide more powerful and efficient circulation. The delivery of oxygen to men's muscles, a factor crucial to speed, is further enhanced by the higher concentration of hemoglobin in the blood. Finally, the longer limbs provide them with greater leverage and extension.

The aspects of female physiology that result in women's athletic advantages are not as self-evident as in males. A woman's body contains an average of 9% more adipose tissue than a man's body. This tissue is deposited not only on the thighs, buttocks, and breasts,

► PRINCIPLES OF BODY MECHANICS

- The wider the base of support and the lower the center of gravity, the greater is the stability of the object.
- The equilibrium of an object is maintained as long as the line of gravity passes through its base of support.
- When the line of gravity shifts outside the base of support, the amount of energy required to maintain equilibrium is increased.
- Equilibrium is maintained with least effort when the base of support is broadened in the direction in which movement occurs.
- Stooping with hips and knees flexed and the trunk in good alignment distributes the work load among the largest and strongest muscle groups and helps to prevent back strain.
- The stronger the muscle group, the greater is the work it can perform safely.
- Using a larger number of muscle groups for an activity distributes the work load.
- Keeping center of gravity as close as possible to the center of gravity of the work load to be moved prevents unnecessary reaching and strain on back muscles.
- Pulling an object directly toward (or pushing directly away from) the center of gravity prevents strain on back and abdominal muscles.
- Facing the direction of movement prevents undesirable twisting of spine.
- Pushing, pulling, or sliding an object on a surface requires less force than lifting an object, as lifting involves moving the weight of the object against the pull of gravity.
- Moving an object by rolling, turning, or pivoting requires less effort than lifting the object, as momentum and leverage are used to advantage.
- Using a lever when lifting an object reduces the amount of weight lifted.
- The less the friction between the object moved and surface on which it is moved, the smaller is the force required to move it.
- Moving an object on a level surface requires less effort than moving the same object on an inclined surface because the pull of gravity is less on a level surface.
- Working with materials that rest on a surface at a good working level requires less effort then lifting them above the working surface.
- Contraction of stabilizing muscle preparatory to activity helps to protect ligaments and joints from strain and injury.
- Dividing balanced activity between arms and legs protects the back from strain.
- Variety of position and activity helps maintain good muscle tone and prevent fatigue.
- Alternating periods of rest and activity helps prevent fatigue.

but in a subcutaneous layer that covers the entire body. It is this adipose tissue that makes the women more buoyant and better insulated against cold, both of which are advantages in long-distance swimming. (The record for swimming the English Channel—7 hours 40 minutes—is held by a woman, Penny Dean.) Body adipose tissue may also be one of the reasons few female runners report the pain and weakness that most male runners encounter. The body is conditioned to call on stored fats once its supply of glycogen, which fuels the

muscles, has been exhausted. As women have greater reserves of body fat, they are able to compete in athletics longer. Females perspire in smaller amounts and less quickly than males. Perspiring is the body's way of avoiding overheating. Yet women may tolerate heat better than men. Not only can body temperature rise in a women several degrees higher before she begins to sweat, but women sweat more efficiently because of the even distribution of their sweat glands. In women **vascularization,** *capacity for bringing blood to the surface for cooling,* is also more efficient. The female has certain structural advantages for all types of running and swimming events. In swimming, narrower shoulders offer less resistance through water. Even at identical heights (and ideal weights), female bodies are lighter than male bodies, leaving them with less weight to carry while running (270).

Foot Care

Foot care is not considered often enough in an exercise program. The feet, during walking, will meet the surface at $1\frac{1}{2}$ to 2 times the body weight and up to 3 times its weight when running. Proper shoe fit, which includes heel height, stability, and cushion, wedge support, and forefoot cushion, must be considered. Also, proper fitting and absorbent socks are important, along with proper washing and careful drying of feet after exercise (89).

PSYCHOSOCIAL CONCEPTS

Cognitive Development

Different learning abilities are required in different life stages. Youth is the time for acquisition; young adulthood is the time for achievement; middle age is the time for responsibility; and old age is the time for reintegration (101, 221).

Theories About Cognitive Development

Cognitive theories are described here; refer also to Chapter 5. Erikson (100) theorized that the basis for adult cognitive performance is laid during the school years when the child accomplishes the task of industry, learns how to learn and win recognition by producing and achieving, and learns to enjoy learning. The child learns an attitude that lasts into adulthood: how much effort a task takes and how long and hard he or she should work for what is desired or expected. The sense of industry is useful in adult life, both in coping with new experiences and in functioning as a worker, family member, citizen, and lifelong learner.

Current researchers and theorists propose that learning continues throughout the adult years. Longitudinal studies indicate that the brain continues to change in structure and complexity until age 40 or 50. The brain shows increasing myelinization until middle age, which permits more integrated modes of social response and stable or increasing intellectual functions (77, 94, 351).

Becoming mature in young adulthood involves intellectual growth, becoming more adaptive and knowledgeable about self, forming values, and developing increasing depth in analytic and synthetic thinking, logical reasoning, and imagination. There are multiple and different intelligences besides academic aptitude, including leadership ability, creative and performing arts abilities, and ability to manage self, others, and a career. Further, developing social and interpersonal skills and personal friendships may have a powerfully maturing effect on intellectual skills (101, 221).

Table 12–3 summarizes ego functions of the adult based on the Analytic Theory discussed in Chapter 5. Table 12–4 will assist you in testing reality processes (30, 251).

Influences on Learning

Influences differ somewhat from childhood to adulthood and include (1) level of knowledge in society generally, (2) personal values and perceptions and previously learned associations, (3) level of education, (4) available life opportunities, (5) interests, (6) participation by the person in the learning activity, (7) the learning environment, and (8) life experiences (18, 77, 221, 351). As a result of these influences, the person develops a preferred way of learning or cognitive style—a characteristic way of perceiving, organizing, and evaluating information (185, 254, 345).

Formal Operations Stage

The young adult remains in the Formal Operations Stage, according to Piaget. The adult is creative in thought. He or she begins at the abstract level and compares the idea mentally or verbally with previous memories, knowledge, or experience. The person combines or integrates a number of steps of a task mentally instead of thinking about or doing each step as a separate unit. He or she considers the multiplicity and relativism of issues and alternatives to a situation, synthesizing and integrating ideas or information into the memory, beliefs, or solutions so that the end result is a unique product. Adult thought is different from adolescent thought in that the adult can differentiate among many perspectives and the adult is objective, realistic, and less egocentric. Thinking and learning are problem centered, not just subject centered. Reality is considered only a part of all that is possible. The person can imagine and reason about events that are not occurring in reality but that are possible or in which he or she does not even believe. Hypotheses are generated; conjectures are deduced from hypotheses, and observations are conducted to disconfirm the expectations. The thought system works independent of its context and can be applied to diverse data. The person can evaluate the validity of a train of reasoning independent of its factual content. A concrete proposition can be replaced by an arbitrary sign of symbolic logic such as p or q. Probability, proportionality, and combining of thought systems occur (94, 362).

Arlin (18) cites Gruber as proposing that some people continue to develop cognitively beyond the formal operations proposed by Piaget into a *fifth stage* of cognitive development that progresses through adulthood. The Stage of Formal Operations describes strategies used in problem solving. The *problem-finding stage* goes beyond the problem-solving stage and is characterized by creative thought in the form of discovered problems, the formation of generic problems, the raising of general questions from ill-defined problems, use of intuition and hunches, and the development of significant scientific thought.

The person may use different thinking for scientific operations, business transactions, artistic activities, and intimate interpersonal interactions. Thus mature thinkers can accept and live with contradictions and conflicts and engage in a number of activities. At times, however, the adult will of necessity do thinking typical of Concrete Operations. At times the adult may regress to the Preoperational Stage (some never get beyond this period), as shown by superstitious, egocentric, or illogical thinking. The adult may not have the ability to perform Formal Operations.

A further distinction in types of adult thinking separates the *managers,* those who have a better developed right brain and who synthesize data to see the overall picture, from the *planners,* those who have a better developed left brain and who analyze sequentially and look closely to the minute details. Women tend to have a better integrated brain and usually combine both manager and planner thinking (77, 345, 351).

The young adult continues to learn both formally and informally to enhance cognitive and job skills and self-knowledge. Learning may be pursued on "on-the-job training," job-sponsored orientation courses, trade schools, college studies, or continuing education

TABLE 12–3. MAJOR EGO (CEREBRUM) FUNCTIONS OR TASKS OF THE ADULT

1. **Reality testing**
   a. Distinguishes inner and outer stimuli
   b. Perceives accurately—time, place, and events that relate to self or are familiar
   c. Is psychologically minded and aware of inner states
   d. Has accurate sense of body boundaries

2. **Judgment**
   a. Anticipates probable dangers, legal limits, and social censure or disapproval of intended behavior
   b. Is aware of appropriateness and consequences of behavior
   c. Behaves in a way that reflects the above

3. **Sense of reality of the world and self**
   a. Distinguishes external events that are real and those that are embedded in familiar context, such as déjà vu, trance-like states
   b. Experiences the body and its functions and one's behavior as familiar, unobtrusive, and belonging to the self
   c. Develops a sense of individuality, uniqueness, self, self-esteem
   d. Develops a sense that the self is separate from the external environment

4. **Regulation and control of drives, affects, and impulses**
   a. Directs impulse expression to indirect forms of behavioral expression
   b. Balances delay and control behavior
   c. Demonstrates frustration tolerance
   d. Maintains self-esteem independent of daily occurrences and other's opinions
   e. Does minimal acting out

5. **Interpersonal relationships**
   a. Relates to and invests in others, taking account of one's own needs
   b. Relates to others in an adaptive way and based on present mature goals rather than past immature goals
   c. Perceives others as separate rather than as an extension of self
   d. Sustains relationships over long period and tolerates absence of the person
   e. Lists own assumptions against objective data or other's opinion

6. **Thought processes**
   a. Sustains processes for attention, concentration, anticipation, concept formation, memory, and language
   b. Controls unrealistic, illogical, loose, or primitive thinking
   c. Thinks clearly
   d. Has no association or communication problems

7. **Adequate regression in the service of the ego**
   a. Relaxes perceptual and conceptual acuity and other ego controls with concomitant increase in awareness of previously preconscious and unconscious contents
   b. Increases adaptive potentials as a result of creative endeavors

8. **Defensive functioning**
   a. Uses adaptive mechanism for ideation and behavior effectively
   b. Controls anxiety, depression, or other behavioral affects of weak defensive operations

9. **Stimulus barrier**
   a. Maintains a threshold for, sensitivity to, or awareness of stimuli that impinge on senses
   b. Uses active coping mechanisms in response to levels of sensory stimulation to prevent or minimize disorganization, avoidance, withdrawal

10. **Autonomous functions**
    a. Maintains function or prevents impairment of sight, hearing, intention, language, memory, learning, or motor function
    b. Maintains function or prevents impairment of habit patterns, learned skills, work routines, and hobbies

11. **Synthetic-integrative functioning**
    a. Reconciles or integrates potentially contradictory attitudes, values, affects, behavior, and self-representations
    b. Relates together and integrates psychic and behavioral events, whether or not contradictory
    c. Identies chronologic order of events
    d. Integrates good and bad aspects of self

12. **Mastery–competence**
    a. Is motivated with sufficient energy to meet daily demands
    b. Plans goal-directed behavior
    c. Performs in relation to existing capacity to interact with and master the environment
    d. Expects success in performance of tasks
    e. Maintains autonomy
    f. Evaluates self and resources, as well as expectations of others
    g. Is open to and capable of change
    h. Has diversity of interests

courses. Environmental stimulation is important in continued learning. Increasingly young adults are changing their minds about their life work and change directions after several years of study or work in the original field. Formal Operations or abstract thinking appears linked to the content areas in which the person has extensive training. After Concrete Operations, a person may acquire abstract thinking in behavioral, symbolic, semantic, or figural content areas, depending on experience (77, 94, 345, 351). There are some age differences between younger and older adults according to research findings, but the influences on learning described earlier may be major factors in those differences (77, 83, 94, 345, 351).

Sex Differences

Sex differences may be the result of sex bias in research. Cognitive ability in men and women has been considered unequal and has been described on the basis of different functions in each cerebral hemisphere, although brain structure is the same in men and

TABLE 12–4. ASSESSMENT OF REALITY TESTING FUNCTION OF EGO (CEREBRUM): DISTINCTION BETWEEN INNER AND OUTER STIMULI

1. **Maximal impairment**
   a. Hallucinations and delusions pervade
   b. Minimal ability to distinguish dreams from waking life
   c. Inability to distinguish idea, image, and hallucination
   d. Perception disturbed, e.g., moving objects appear immobile and vice versa

2. **Severe impairment**
   a. Hallucinations and delusions severe but limited to one or more content areas
   b. Difficulty distinguishing events as dream or reality

3. **Medium impairment**
   a. Illusions more common than hallucinations
   b. Aware of experiencing illusions and that others do not
   c. Projects inner states onto external reality more so than have hallucinations or delusions

4. **Minimal impairment**
   Possible confusion about inner and outer states when awakening, going to sleep, or under severe stress

5. **No impairment**
   a. Distinguishes inner and outer stimuli accurately
   b. Denies external reality occasionally as part of adaptive behavior
   c. Is aware whether events occurred in dreams or waking life
   d. Identifies source of thoughts and/or perceptions as being an idea or image and from internal or external source
   e. Distinguishes between inner and outer prescriptions even under extreme stress
   f. Checks prescriptions against reality with high degree of automaticity

women. The left hemisphere is dominant in 97% of people for language, logical reasoning, and mathematical calculation. The right hemisphere is nonverbal and mute: it knows but cannot tell what it knows without processing the knowledge through the left hemisphere. The right hemisphere processes spatial and visual abstractions, recognition of faces, body image, music, art forms, and intuitive, preconscious, and fantasy processes. At birth asymmetry in the left hemisphere is more marked in the male. Female infants have a somewhat larger area of visual cortex in the right hemisphere than male infants, which implies an anatomic advantage for nonverbal ideation. The female's brain matures earlier; thus the two hemispheres are more integrated in the female as indicated by less impairment of intellectual function in women who have suffered either right or left hemisphere damage. Males are more vulnerable to brain damage. On tests women use verbal strategies to solve spatial problems because of the greater interplay between the two hemispheres. In adulthood women are better able to coordinate activities of both hemispheres; thus they can think intuitively and globally. Men are better at activities in which the two hemispheres do not compete such as problem solving and determining spatial relationships (26, 27, 60, 77, 94, 351).

Nonconformity to sex-role stereotypes is positively related to IQ. The more assertive and active woman has greater intellectual ability and more interests. The less aggressive man focuses less on developing physique and develops intellectual ability and interests to a greater extent (26).

Cognitive abilities have often been related to personality traits and interpersonal orientation. Sex-role socialization has been related to cognitive style. Some researchers believe the level of information processing a person attains exerts a profound influence on personality and on ability to integrate and differentiate in problem solving (27, 60).

Claims about sex differences in other cognitive abilities such as creativity, analytic ability, and reasoning also apparently are the result of differences in verbal, quantitative, or visual–spatial abilities or in opportunity to develop such abilities—in either sex (27, 60, 235).

Both female and male young adults who are in formal education are causing shifts in the educational system. They are more vocal, persuasive, and determined about what they consider pertinent. They are stimulating diversity and quality in the higher-education patterns. The young adult wants to learn more about something or learn to do something better and wants a voice in planning education. The nontraditional education offered by some colleges is more an attitude than a system; the students' needs are first and the institution's convenience second. Competent performance and concern for the learner of any age rather than just obtaining degrees are being emphasized in adult education, including noncollegiate programs. Full educational opportunity through life is the goal of many young adults, enabling each to meet potential personally and as a citizen. The young adult is concerned about the most important principles or concepts to learn to provide the balance between the timely and timeless in this modern world.

The confident young adult takes pride in being mentally astute, creative, progressive, and alert to events. He or she normally has the mental capacity to make social and occupational contributions, is self-directive and curious, and likes to match wits with others in productive dialogue.

Both men and women have similar basic needs, their own unique cognitive abilities and talents, and often unspoken ideas and feelings longing for self-expression. From young childhood on, both females and males should be considered cognitively capable to their maximum potential and should have the opportunity, including in the adult years, to meet that maximum potential.

Teaching the Adult

Information on cognitive development should be considered whenever you are teaching adults. Table 12–5 presents principles of learning. See also Table 1–19 for suggestions on teaching methods, and References 14, 22, 34, 40, and 194. Avoid "canned" audiovisual presentations. Emphasize a sharing of ideas and experiences, role play, and practical application of information. In some cases you will be helping the person to unlearn old habits, attitudes, or information to acquire new habits and attitudes.

If you teach illiterate young adults, you must compensate for their inability to read and write. Slow, precise speech and gestures and the use of pictures and audiovisual aids are more crucial than with literate adults. *Demonstration* and *return demonstration* ensure learning. Do not underestimate the importance of your behavior and personality as a motivating force, especially if some members of the person's family do not consider learning important.

TABLE 12–5. PRINCIPLES OF THE LEARNING PROCESS

1. Learning is an active, self-directed process.
2. Learning is central to ongoing development and behavioral changes.
3. Learning is influenced by readiness to learn, abilities, and potential to learn, and the emotional state.
4. Learning is facilitated when the content or behaviors to be learned are perceived as relevant.
5. Learning proceeds from simple to complex and known to unknown.
6. Learning is facilitated when the learner has opportunities to take risks, test ideas, make mistakes, and be creative.
7. Learning is facilitated when the person has knowledge of progress and feedback that serves as a measure for further learning.
8. Learning transfer occurs when the person can recognize similarities and differences between past experiences and the present situation.
9. Learning is effective when it can be immediately applied.
10. Learning occurs best when the teaching methodology is relevant to the content to be learned.
11. Learning occurs best in an environment that is nonthreatening, comfortable, and free of distractions.
12. Learning occurs best and is continued when the learner feels satisfied and successful.

Work and Leisure Activities

Although the following discussion focuses on work outside of the home, implying paid employment, we do not demean or overlook the young adult woman or man who chooses to stay at home and rear a family. *Homemaking and childrearing are essential and important work;* each is fatiguing and stressful in its own way. In fact, staying at home can be hazardous to health. The many noise and air pollutants or chemical toxins that come from appliances, building materials, cleaning products, and combinations of materials or supplies used in a home should be discussed. (See Chapter 2.)

Work Options and Attitudes

There are many work options and attitudes. For example, the young adult "workaholic" executive may put in 70 to 80 hours weekly at the job, think about the job most of the remaining hours, feel guilty when not working, and channel much anger and aggression through work. In contrast, a factory worker while feeding a certain part into the assembly line, may be planning what he or she will do after work—to this person work is only a means of livelihood. The blue-collar worker may have more stress than the executive. The young adult, may after several years, lose interest in the job and has to decide whether to "stick it out" 35 more years to retirement or risk going into another field that appears challenging. There are also completely opposite attitudes about the same kind of work. For example, one young adult will choose to be a police officer or fire department employee because he or she cares more about adventure and challenge than money. Another will say, "Why should I put my life on the line when the public does not think enough of me to pay decent wages?" Then there are those people who work long hours and who are highly involved in their work but who are not workaholics. They feel exhilarated about the flow of work, the challenge, their goals, and the use of skills involved, and they feel creative, active, and motivated. These feelings are more likely to come from work than leisure. These people contribute a great deal to the advancement of their vocation or profession generally and to the individuals they serve.

In addition to agricultural, skilled and semiskilled workers, blue-collar and white-collar workers, managerial or executive personnel, and professionals, a new classification exists—the knowledge worker. Because of expanding technology, rapid change, the burgeoning size of industries and megaindustries, and the knowledge explosion, some people are hired to do job planning and to create, innovate, and make decisions within the organization. The ultimate goal of the knowledge worker is cost containment for the company, improved efficiency of the worker, a more marketable product, and a more willing buyer. If you are a knowledge worker, your task is less well defined. For example, you might be helping the health care agency develop long-range plans and goals; you might be a consultant; or you might be observing nurses or other health care providers at work to determine a more effective way to deliver care. You must cope with unanticipated changes, predict changes, and collaborate with others.

You may find the worker—all the way from the executive level to the delivery person—a victim of **substance abuse,** *ingesting excessive alcohol or drugs or engaged in pushing illicit drugs* on the job. Substance abuse is a response to stress, often job related. The implications of substance abuse are grave, including job errors, accidents to self or others, poor job performance, a product that does not meet standard results, and increased insurance and worker's compensation benefits to employees, all of which increases the cost of the product to the consumer. In addition, the lives of family, friends, and co-workers are affected. Work with the personnel director, safety director, employee assistance programs, administrative personnel, and the affected individual (and family, if possible) to help the person get the necessary medical treatment. A recovered employee saves the company money. The employee keeps a job, and it is more expensive to hire and train a new worker in many situations.

Nurses may also suffer from substance abuse, but they are no more likely to have such problems than are other employees. Several references are pertinent to understanding and assisting the colleague who is chemically dependent (107, 141, 333, 334). Refer also to the discussion of alcoholism and drug abuse later in this chapter.

The majority of young adult women are in the work force. Sometimes the job is a necessity (e.g., if she is single, divorced, and with children or if her husband has only seasonal work or a low-paying job). Many women are working to maintain occupational skills, self-esteem, and independence. If a woman is trying to work in addition to carrying on the traditional wife–mother–housekeeper roles, she will likely feel conflict. Finding day-care facilities for young children can be a problem. If the family can learn to work together on various home roles, the working wife–mother can be a real asset to the family because she will bring home her attitude of self-confidence and satisfaction. Also, the children will probably be more adaptive as they mature if they learn various household responsibilities and see their mother and father in a variety of roles instead of those stereotyped by traditional society (i.e., Mom sews, cooks, cleans; Dad mows the lawn, paints the house, repairs the car). Further, the children will learn that it is essential to become well prepared for adult work roles (26, 271).

Balancing work and family life responsibilities is often stressful for the woman who is a single parent, a divorced parent, or member of a two-career family. There is never enough time and often too much to do (21, 90, 91, 135, 271, 327). Shift work compounds the problems (6, 21, 135, 271, 327, 346). The American Nurses Association has published *The Nurse's Shift Work Handbook* to address needs of nurses and nurse managers. The book would be applicable to people in other disciplines as well who must work shifts (12). Employers are beginning to confront these dilemmas. Some employers, to attract and keep competent workers, are offering flexible work schedules, job sharing, on-the-site day-care, and both paternity leave and extended maternity leave. These suggestions can be shared with the parent who has the greatest responsibility for balancing home and work (12, 21, 327):

- Identify priorities. Discuss with the spouse, or the children if they are old enough, what tasks must be done, what can be delegated (either on the job or to a service company in the home), and who can take on which responsibilities to even the load.
- Allocate tasks. Design a system for assigning tasks, based on skill, age, availability, and fairness. Rotate tasks, if possible, or assign tasks that are especially requested.
- Speak up for yourself at home and on the job. Explore grievance channels if necessary.
- Use a support network. Family, friends, neighbors, and child care providers can be asked for assistance on a regular basis or for help in emergencies.
- Rechannel emotional investments. Having multiple roles gives an opportunity to excel in one realm if you have problems in another.
- Assess progress. Plan frequent review sessions to discuss effectiveness of the plan and problem areas to avoid resentments or rebellions or someone's taking advantage.

Fellow employees must be aware that women often look differently at the same work situation and respond to different rewards in the workplace than men and that they bring a perspective and judgment level that is not based solely on competition and aggressiveness. Further, equipment or protective clothing that fits men may well be hazardous to women because of size, weight, muscle stretching involved, or poor fit. The employer can benefit from the qualities and expertise women bring to the work force. Technologic change will increasingly compete with a rising demand for human services, especially in health, law, and recreation. Technology can help free people for service work; however, in a technologic age, skills related to caring for or serving others are often neglected. Colleges are already preparing for computer-addicted students with few human relation skills, as human relation skills will be as essential in the future as technologic ones.

Regardless of the various attitudes about work, it remains a central part of the adult self-concept in most Americans, and a close relationship exists between occupational and family satisfaction (Fig. 12–6). If the person is dissatisfied in one, either work or family life, he or she will try to compensate in the other (101, 221).

Because the nurse views the person holistically, you may be asked for assistance by the manager, executive level employees, or the employers. They may find it difficult to understand the young adult worker who acts differently than the middle-aged or older worker; the behavior of the young adult worker who has newly achieved an executive position may be poorly understood by employees who are middle-aged and near retirement. Help them understand that each generation of worker has a different value system and responds to different values and different motivational stimuli (101, 221).

As a nurse, others will seek you out as someone who can assist with safety and health problems, listen to and counsel about job problems, help another make decisions pertinent to occupation, and assist in resolving conflicts related to the work setting or homemaker, career woman, and mother roles. Through your counseling and education role, you can assist both the individual employee and administrative or management personnel to realize the importance of feelings of self-respect in relation to employment. Management consultants have learned that low self-esteem in the worker lowers productivity, morale, and profits. You can be instrumental in helping the work system promote workers' feelings of self-esteem and about the importance of their work.

You may also become an advocate for the woman who is undergoing sexual harassment on the job. Increasingly women workers are gaining the courage to talk publicly about and to seek legal aid for sexual harassment in factories, mines, offices, migrant farm fields, and health care facilities. Harassment can range from a passing caress to threats of or actual rape. Yet women or men who are harassed on the job may not complain, whether it is about the hug that the supervisor gives everyone daily—wanted or not—or about actual body contact, because of fear of lack of confidentiality, fear of greater or more subtle harassment or retaliation, and fear of poor evaluations, loss of pay raises, or actual job loss (12).

Each workplace must have policies and procedures established to handle complaints of harassment on the job. Ideally the work atmosphere should be such that, first, harassment would not occur, and second, everyone would be concerned about the problem and know how to handle it. The article by Heinrick (157) suggests how to cope with sexual harassment from clients.

The problems of sexism and sexual harassment in the workplace and in society in general is not limited to the United States. Black (39) describes how Japanese feminists are challenging the apathetic attitudes to sexism and consequent harassment in their society.

You must resolve your own job-related conflicts before you can help others. By using the above information and insights you gain from being a professional who works with and learns from many other people, you are indeed in a key position to assist the worker—whether you work in an occupational health setting, a clinic, or the emergency room or in a psychiatric–mental health, obstetric, medical, or surgical unit.

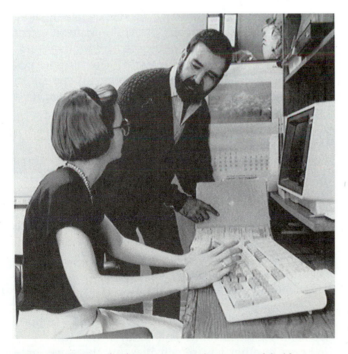

Figure 12–6. Career development is a central component of the life structure for many individuals. *(From Berger, K.J., and M.B. Williams,* Fundamentals of Nursing: Collaborating for Optimal Health. *Stamford, CT: Appleton & Lange, 1992, p. 266.)*

Burnout

Burnout, the *feeling of stress, worthlessness, of not being appreciated, a sense of hopelessness, or loss of creativity,* is discussed primarily in relation to a job. The person who continually stays at home, with or without child care, can also suffer burnout. Some people propose that the homemaker's or mother's work should be assigned monetary worth, as our society equates one's worth with earning power. Certainly the wife, husband, homemaker, mother, and father roles are each work and worthy, and the worth of each has not yet been calculated. A look at history and all cultures tells us we cannot survive without these roles, regardless of how they are acted out.

Work can create feelings of happiness, pleasure, and fulfillment or feelings of being frustrated, blocked, and dehumanized. Job satisfaction increases with the level of job skill, variety of work, and opportunity for decision making. Job dissatisfaction increases with automation, lack of attention to the individual worker, and controlled decisions. Income and comfort factors, although important, do not play as big a role as challenge factors in job satisfaction. McCloskey (234) found that women nurses believed that autonomy, social integration, and connectedness related to their employment were major factors for job contentment.

Stress response (*burnout*) *to the unrewarding, demanding work situation may become so great that the person undergoes physiologic and psychological changes in response to work. There is inadequate emotional and physical energy for tasks, responsibilities, and roles.* The physical and emotional exhaustion is accompanied by a sense of frustration and loss of control; a sense of tedium and apathy about first the job and then other aspects of life; anger about what is perceived as excessive work demands; guilt about not doing a good job or neglecting the family; depression; a number of somatic complaints; reduced productivity; disillusionment about the job; increased absenteeism; job turnover; low self-esteem; and poor morale. Although at first these feelings are related to the job, later they are also directed toward the family, home, friends, and other interests (12, 253, 327).

Health care professionals may suffer from burnout, especially if employed in a high-stress area, in one that is regularly understaffed, or if frequent shift rotation is required. Personal motivation toward work and the physical effort of work should be considered in determining the impact of the job on the health of the worker, including the pregnant woman (12, 167, 327, 351, 373).

It is important to assess yourself in relation to work satisfaction and response to the stresses at work. Several references assist in job self-assessment and ways to overcome job stress (6, 21, 178, 252, 271, 327).

Each of us must realize that every job has stresses and that stress can be viewed as a challenge. We all must realize, too, that every job, no matter how exciting it appears, has boredom and repetitive and noncreative aspects; it is unlikely that those aspects can be eliminated entirely. Thus each of us must be continually mindful of the satisfaction obtained from all pursuits of life; healthy ways to expand interests, hobbies, or social contacts; and ways to make the job more satisfying or interesting, if possible. Further, developing a sense of humor and a philosophic, spiritual outlook can give a balance to life that results in positive feelings about self, work, and others.

Leisure

Some young American adults are in pursuit of leisure (6, 271, 300). As job hours per week are being cut (especially in automated jobs), the time for leisure increases. Additionally, the work ethic is decreasing. Socialization of the current young adults has fostered a leisure ethic.

Leisure is *freedom from obligations and formal duties of paid work and opportunity to pursue, at one's own pace, mental nourishment, enlivenment, pleasure, and relief from fatigue of work.* Leisure may be as active as backpacking up a mountain or as quiet as fishing alone in a huge lake. Some people never know leisure, and others manage an attitude of leisure even as they work. Various factors influence the use of leisure time: sex; amount of family, home, work, or community responsibilities; mental status; income and socioeconomic class; and past interests.

Some people have never learned to pursue a hobby or an activity just for the "fun of it." Others have learned hobbies or have pursued recreational interests but use the same competitive spirit in the hobby or recreation as in work. Others pursue hobbies as the "current thing to do" but feel no real sense of pleasure.

Leisure gadgetry has invaded the marketplace. Electronic games have replaced household appliances as America's favorite gadgets. Technology affects leisure through changes in both products and values. As technology dictates specialized work, the games increasingly create specialized players and skills. The electronic games that reward aggressive and competitive behavior teach values and behavior that will be carried over to other leisure activities and the work force. The result may be contradictory to the meaning of leisure and even to meaning in life.

The real answer to the work–leisure dilemma is that the worker and the player are one. The unhappy worker will not automatically become the happy player. Challenging work makes leisure a time of refreshment. Successful leisure prepares the worker for more challenge.

Maintaining friendships is a healthy use of leisure time. It takes time, self-disclosure, and sharing of interests to form friendships. Gradually, a sense of reliability and confidentiality grows as a core to the friendship. Some conflict may surface and is natural as intimacy deepens. Getting closer to friends, rather than making more friends, is the way to reduce loneliness. Avoid developing all the friendships at the workplace. In today's competitive world people at work may not be able to be close. It is wiser to start out being more formal and distant until the trusting relationship evolves. In a world in which women juggle career, love, and family, time may limit the size of the friendship circle. Several close friendships should be made. Successful friendship combines the freedom to depend on one another with the freedom to be independent. If free time is too limited, fewer friendships can be formed, because you will have little to give to anybody emotionally.

Doing volunteer work with a favorite charity or community group is a way to use nonwork time that can promote a sense of leisure and enjoyment while simultaneously using skills and talents to improve life for others. The rewards are dual—to the self and to society.

Help the client realize the importance of leisure as a part of balanced living. The young adult needs to develop a variety of interests as preparation for the years ahead to maintain physical and mental health.

Emotional Development

Emotional development in young adulthood is an ongoing, dynamic process, an extension of childhood and adolescent developmental influences and processes. Development is still influenced by the environment, but the environment is different. The fundamental developmental issues continue as central aspects of adult life but in an altered form. Thus trust, autonomy, initiative, industry, and identity all are reworked and elaborated, based on current experiences (100, 101, 221).

Young adulthood is a time when there is increased clarity and consistency of personality, a stabilization of self and identity, established preferences of interests and activities, increased coping ability, less defensiveness, decrease in youthful illusions, fantasy, and impulsiveness, more responsiveness to and responsibility for self and others, more giving than taking, and more appreciation of surroundings. It is a time to develop expanded resources for happiness. There are restrictions and continuities not previously experienced, some sac-

rifice of freedom and spontaneity, and less opportunity for variety, novelty, and impulsive adventure. However, there is more challenge to develop empathy (i.e., a depth of feeling and understanding), to learn in detail how systems work, and to reevaluate self and the world. If behavior is not too heavily bound by defenses against anxiety, it becomes more varied as experience accumulates (100, 101, 221).

Certainly adult experiences, lifestyle, and geographic changes can contribute to personality development and change. Yet the psychosocial development of the adolescent maintains a pattern or direction into young adulthood, as shown in a study of youth activists in the 1960s and others (94). In a longitudinal study of psychosocial development, it was found that most behavior and personality characteristics of the school-age child 6 to 10 years old were good predictors of early adult behavior and personality; however, various life experiences modify behavior and personality in adulthood. A major modifying variable is gender. Degrees of childhood passivity and dependency remained continuous for women but not for men. The longitudinal study by Maas and Kuyper (225) also shows the influence of childhood experiences on adult personality and the continuity of adult personality characteristics over the years. Expression of one emotion such as anger has also been consistently manifested across the life span of the person (344).

Theories of Emotional Development

Various theorists referred to in Chapter 5 also have research findings on which to base their beliefs about adult personality development. The findings of Jung, Vaillant, Gould, Sheehy, Levinson, Sullivan, and Erikson are discussed in the following pages.

Jung (185) believes that the personality develops along different lines during the first and second halves of the life cycle. The first period, until approximately age 40 or 45, is a time of outward expansion. Maturational forces direct the growth of the ego and the unfolding of capacities for dealing with the external world. Young people learn to get along with others and try to win as many of society's rewards as possible. They establish careers and families, and they do what they can to advance up the social ladder of success. To do so, it is usually necessary for women to develop their feminine traits and skills and men their masculine ones, although in present society women who are successful must combine the traditional feminine and masculine traits into a unique, nonthreatening whole. During this phase a certain amount of one-sidedness is necessary and even valuable, for the young person needs to dedicate self to the task of mastering the outer world. It is not especially advantageous for young people to be too preoccupied with their self-doubts, fantasies, and inner nature. The task is to meet the demands of the external environment confidently and assertively. As one can imagine, extroverts, rather than introverts, may have an easier time in adjusting during this period.

From his longitudinal study of adult men, **Vaillant** (356, 357) proposes that development continues through adulthood in a number of ways; emotionally, mentally, socially in relationships, and in career. Simultaneously, the developing and successful adult also demonstrates what Freud calls the psychopathology of everyday life. All have special adaptational problems and mechanisms. Vaillant believes that emotional health and development are evolutionary, not static. Isolated traumatic events rarely mold individual lives; rather development comes from continued interaction between choice of adaptive mechanisms and sustained relationships with others. Poor adaptation, which lowers the threshold for perceiving or handling stress, leads to anxiety, depression, and physical illness. Vaillant's study identifies mature defenses—altruism, humor, suppression or minimization of discomforts, anticipation, sublimation—that promote adaptation. Successful adapters have had good relationships with parents, are energetic and alert, feel good about themselves, love their work, have very close relationships with wives and friends, and sublimate aggression into enthusiastic pursuits of projects, work, or competitive sports. His findings seem applicable to adult women as well.

Gould (138) describes life stages and key issues or tasks in late adolescence and young adulthood. Gould believes there is an increasing need throughout adulthood to win permission from the self to continue development. The direction of change through adulthood is becoming more tolerant of self and more appreciative of the surrounding world. Although Gould does not list specific assumptions about adult development, he sees adulthood as a time of thoughtful confrontation with the self—letting go of an idealized image, the desire to be perfect, and acknowledging the realistic image of self and personal feelings. Conflicts between past and present beliefs are resolved. Through constant examination and reformulation of beliefs embedded in feelings, the person can substitute a conception of adulthood for childhood legacy and fantasies. Whereas children mark the passing years by their changing bodies, adults change their minds, deepen their insights about self, and mature emotionally.

Sheehy (302–304) believes that development occurs throughout adulthood and is influenced by external events or crises, the historical period, membership in the culture, and social roles and by the internal realism of the person—values, goals, and aspirations. Sheehy ties developmental stage in late adolescence and young adulthood to Erikson's development stage.

Levinson (217, 218), like Vaillant, studied only men in formulating a concept of adult developmental stages; however, he believes the stages are age linked and universal and, thus should be applicable to women. In each period biological, psychodynamic, cultural, social, and other timetables operate in only partial synchronization, which makes for developmental difficulties. The organizing concept of **life structure** *refers to a pattern of the person's life at a specific time* and is used to focus on the boundary between the individual and society. In its external aspects life structure *refers to roles, memberships, interests, conditions or style of living, and long-term goals.* In its *internal aspects,* life structure includes the *personal meanings of external patterns, inner identities, core values, fantasies, and psychodynamic qualities that shape the person.*

Sullivan (335) believes young adulthood is normally the time when the sexuality of human development is powerful, and there is a need to find adequate and satisfying expression. Now is the time of expanding experiences with people. If for some reason the person is thwarted in expression or sublimation of sexual feelings, perhaps because of illness or injury that causes a felt or imagined change in body, sexual concerns may become paramount.

Developmental Crisis

According to Erikson (100), the psychosexual crisis is in intimacy versus self-isolation. **Intimacy** is *reaching out and using the self to form a commitment to and an intense, lasting relationship with another person or even a cause, an institution, or creative effort* (100). In an intimate experience there is mutual trust, sharing of feelings, and responsibility to and cooperation with each other. The physical satisfaction and psychological security of another are more important than one's own. The person is involved with people, work, hobbies, and community issues. He or she has poise and ease in the life style because identity is firm. There is a steady conviction of who he or she is, a unity of personality that will improve through life. Intimacy is a situation involving two people that permits acceptance of all aspects of the other and a collaboration in which the person adjusts behavior to the other's behavior and needs in pursuit of mutual satisfaction (335).

A person's mental health is dependent on the ability to enter into a relationship and experience self-disclosure; in so doing, the support and maintenance of the relationship alleviates feelings of loneliness. Women, more so than men, are concerned with relationships and are interested in the process rather than the product of something. They also recognize their vulnerability and can acknowledge the need to change more readily than men. Women self-disclose more easily than men (60, 235). Such people are less lonely. Interpersonal dependency, an element of the normal adult personality, encompasses attachment and dependency. Anxious or insecure attachment develops when a natural desire for a close relationship with another is accompanied by apprehension that the relationship will end. If anxiety is transferred to the other person, the response may be a withdrawal from the relationship, contributing to feelings of loneliness. If a healthy balance between dependence and independence exists, social relationships and intimacy are maintained more easily, and the risk of experiencing loneliness and isolation decreases (100, 101, 221).

Although intimacy includes orgasm, it means far more than the physical or genital contact so often described in how-to sex manuals. With the intimate person, the young adult is able to regulate cycles of work, recreation, and procreation (if chosen) and to work toward satisfactory stages of development for all offspring and the ongoing development of self and the partner. Intimacy is a paradox. Although the person shares his or her identity with another for mutual satisfaction or support (via self-abandon in orgasm or in another shared emotional experience), he or she does not fear loss of personal identity. Each does not absorb the other's personality.

Young adults may think that intimacy can be obtained primarily though sexual intercourse, and that cohabitation (living together) or having intercourse with a number of partners will ensure finding the right partner. Research studies show otherwise. Sexual intercourse is more satisfying for those who wait until marriage, and that also lessens the chance of contracting sexually transmitted disease (86). Surveys at the University of Chicago and State University of New York at Stony Brook found that of all sexually active people, married couples reported more physical and emotional satisfaction than did unmarried partners, and that it was best to have only one sexual partner in a lifetime because satisfaction declined as the number of partners increased (245). Married people have healthier unions than couples who live together and score higher on all measures of well-being than cohabitating couples (322). People who had been in a cohabitive relationship, compared with noncohabitators, experienced more difficulty in subsequent marriages with adultery, use of alcohol and drugs, abuse of the woman, and eventual breakup of the marriage; most marriages preceded by cohabitation are likely to end in divorce (20, 76, 322). Further, those people in satisfying marital relationships are less likely to experience depression than never married, cohabitating, or divorced people (285), as well as better physical health (282).

Many in late adolescence or early young adulthood do fear a loss of personal identity in an intimate relationship. So do identical twins (181). You can explore intimacy issues with young adults. In an increasingly complex society the search for self-definition is a difficult one. Identity is not always solidly possessed by the time one is 20 or even 25 years old. Achieving a true sense of intimacy seems very illusive to many of this generation. The media encourage self-seeking sexual gratification. Movies, novels, plays, and pornographic books glorify sex for kicks, and peer groups may pressure each other into sexual activity before they are ready for it. Many are puzzled, hurt, or dismayed when they find such sexual encounters are very disappointing. It is easy to *say* that understanding or insight into one's own sexuality is possible only when the self is fully defined. It is much more difficult to *act* on this principle. To come to the realization that sex is not a synonym for sexual intercourse may be a long and painful road.

Love

Love is the feeling accompanying intimacy (100, 335), and love and intimacy change over time (175). (Fig. 12-7). The young adult often has difficulty determining what love is. A classic description of love as stated by the Apostle Paul in I Corinthians 13:4–7 has been the basis for many statements on love by poets, novelists, humanists, philosophers, psychiatrists, theologians, and common people:

> *Love is patient and kind; love is not jealous or boastful; it is not arrogant or rude. Love does not insist on its own way; it is not irritable or resentful; it does not rejoice at wrong, but rejoices in the right. Love bears all things, believes all things, hopes all things, endures all things.*

One of the most important things the person can learn within the family as a child and adolescent is to love. By the time the person reaches the midtwenties, the person should be experienced in the emotion of love. If there was deprivation or distortion of love in the home when he or she was young, the adult will find it difficult to achieve mature love in an intimate relationship. By this time, the person should realize that one

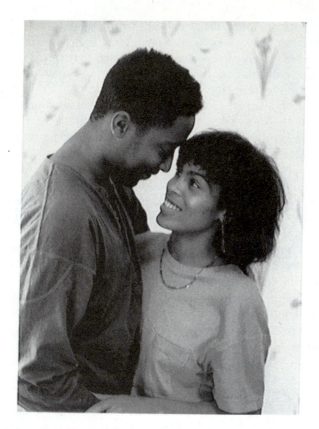

Figure 12–7. The principal developmental task of young adults is the formation of close relationships with significant others. *(Courtesy of Carol Toussie Weingarten.)*

does not *fall* in love; one *learns* to love; one *grows* into love.

Intimacy and love are usually considered from an emotional perspective, with an expression in physical closeness. Michael Liebowitz, a psychiatrist at New York State Hospital Psychiatric Institute, studied the effect of love on brain chemistry. He divided love between men and women into two stages: (1) the attraction stage, characterized by giddiness, euphoria, optimism, and energy; and (2) the attachment stage, characterized by peaceful, secure, comfortable feelings. These two phases are caused by increased brain activity, he believes. In the attraction stage, phenylethylamine causes euphoria and increased sexual attraction. Eventually the brain's tolerance for this natural aphrodisiac dulls; less infatuation is felt. Then the attachment stage, with increased production of endorphins and feelings of well-being, occur. This is an example of how the interpersonal situation influences brain chemistry and, in turn, influences behavior (115).

As a nurse, you will have many opportunities for discussions, individual and group counseling, and education on marriage, establishing a home, the relationship between spouses, and the relationship between parents and children. When you help people sort through feelings about life and love, you are indirectly making a contribution to the health and stability of them and their offspring.

Marriage

Attachment is a concept that applies across the lifespan and is manifested in several layers of relationship in adulthood (317). The socially accepted way for two people in love to be intimate is in marriage, a social contract or institution implying binding rules and responsibilities that cannot be ignored without some penalty. Marriage is endorsed in some form by all cultures in all periods of history because it formalizes and symbolizes the importance of family. Social stability depends on family stability. Marriage is more than getting a piece of paper.

There are norms in every society to prevent people from entering lightly into the wedded state (e.g., age limits, financial and property settlements, ceremony, witnesses, and public registration and announcement). One of the major functions of marriage is to control and limit sexuality and provide the framework for a long-term relationship between a man and a woman. Marriage gives rights in four areas: sexuality, birth and rearing of children, domestic and economic services, and property.

Most young people recognize that marriage is a decisive commitment. It marks the start of a new way of living and achievement of a different status in life. A bride and groom have reason to experience anxiety. Marriage is both a special commitment and a voluntary choice made by them, and the consequences must be accepted in advance. But the potential sources of disturbance and danger are overshadowed by the recognition of marriage as a new source of strength and support in which the well-being of each is bound with the fate of the other.

The pattern and sequence of a person's life history influence whom, when, and why he or she marries. Apparently many people do not really know the person they are marrying and do not realize how greatly the partner's personality will influence their own. The problems of marital adjustment and family living have their roots and basis in the choice of the partner (221).

Mates often choose each other on the basis of unconscious needs, which they strive to meet through a mate whose personality complements rather than replicates their own, or out of fear and loneliness or on the basis of physical attraction. The person chooses someone for an intimate relationship whose lifestyle and personality pattern strengthen and encourage personal development.

Although the person tends to marry an individual who lives and works nearby and has similar social, religious, and racial backgrounds, in the United States, an increasing number of mixed marriages are occurring, an outgrowth of more liberal social attitudes. A number of factors influence the success of the marriage that crosses religious, ethnic, socioeconomic, or racial boundaries:

- Motive for marriage
- Desire, commitment, and effort to bridge the gulf between the couple and their families
- Ability and maturity of the two people to live with and resolve their differences and problems
- Reaction of the parental families, who may secretly or openly support **homogamy** (*marriage between a couple with similar or identical backgrounds*)

In the United States every married couple belongs to three families: to each other, to his family, and to her family. If the young adults are to establish a strong family unit of their own and avoid inlaw interference, their loyalties must be to their *own* family before his or hers. The following guidelines may be helpful:

- Inlaws should not take priority over the spouse and home of the couple. If friends of either husband or wife are offensive to the partner, be prepared to minimize this friendship. Husband and wife together build new friendships.
- Be faithful to the spouse. If one person engages in an extramarital affair, it is possible to repair the brokenness, but a feeling of mistrust may remain and is difficult to overcome.
- Be mindful of sensitive areas, those that are sources of irritation in each other's life. Each needs to *work* at coping with the other's idiosyncrasies or habits and try to meet the other's preferences to keep love in the relationship.
- Manage money and material possessions or they will manage the couple. Money and things are important, but the focus in a relationship should be on the person.
- Maintain a spirit of courtship, spontaneity, and freshness to keep love in a marriage.

Marriage is becoming recognized as a close and loving partnership between two people rather than only a social institution in which the husband is the undisputed head of the house and the wife a childbearer. The current concept of companionship suggests intimacy and affection in a free and equal relationship. This concept imposes high standards. The success of the marriage depends ultimately on each feeling self-worth, each respecting the other, and on the two discovering and being able to fulfill mutual physical and psychological needs.

Whether the young couple is going through the regular channels of engagement and marriage or through less traditional ways of living together, the following tasks must be accomplished if the couple will remain a viable, intimate unit:

- Establishing themselves as a collaborative pair in their own eyes and in the eyes of mutual friends and both families; spending time together
- Working through intimate systems of communications that allow for exchange of confidences and feelings and an increased degree of empathy and ability to predict each other's responses
- Planning ahead for a stable relationship and arriving at a consensus about how their life should be lived; being committed to each other
- Giving each other positive reinforcement, expressing appreciation and affection, to release love rather than focus on problems
- Dealing with crises in a positive way

You may ask certain questions to ascertain readiness for marriage in the young adult or self. Can you take responsibility for your own behavior? Are you emotionally weaned from your parents? Have both of you thought about what lies ahead: both the disagreements and the agreements, days of sickness and health, periods of depression and happiness, financial difficulties? Have you considered whether or not to have children? Have you had any education about childrearing to know what it entails? Do you understand female and male sexuality—the differences and the similarities? What do you each want out of marriage? What can you each give to marriage? Do you have mutual agreement on boundaries? Does it include group sex, nonmarital play, or complete monogamy? You can explore these and other questions in premarital counseling or courses in family living.

Isolation, or **self-absorption,** is the *inability to be intimate, spontaneous, or close with another, thus becoming withdrawn, lonely, and conceited and behaving in a stereotyped manner* (100). The isolated person is unable to sustain close friendships. The person may not marry; there is avoidance of a need for a bond with another. If he or she does marry, the partner is likely to find personal emotional needs unmet while giving considerably of the self to the isolated, self-absorbed person (100, 221). See (p. 607) Consequences of Isolation (100, 101).

You may counsel the self-absorbed person and help him or her achieve the tasks of intimacy. You may

Case Situation: Young Adult Development—Marriage and Commitment

James Chaney, 26 years old, received his bachelor's degree in nursing this year after combining full-time employment as an attendant at a local hospital and part-time school attendance for 5 years. He has recently accepted a position at the hospital as a nurse in the surgical intensive care unit. James and his wife, Mary, have been married for 2 years. Mary, 25 years old, is finishing her bachelor's degree in accounting while she continues employment with an insurance firm. James and Mary plan to wait a few years before starting a family as both realize the importance of graduate education in their fields. They would also like to move from their apartment to a home with more space and a yard.

To save money to achieve their future plans, both James and Mary work extra hours when asked. This has frequently interfered with their studies. They also find they have little time for leisure activities and less time together. Communication is sometimes in the form of memos posted on the refrigerator. Increasingly, the stresses of balancing school, work, and home demands have resulted in arguments, often over minor issues.

When a long-anticipated vacation must be canceled because of unexpected expenses, James and Mary are disappointed and angry; however, they decide to plan a week of inexpensive activities in the local area that will allow them to spend time together uninterrupted. They decide to tell no one that they have remained at home. The resulting vacation is truly restful and meaningful, as they share favorite activities and explore their dreams and goals for the future.

---

also be a role model of commitment to serving others. Use the principles of communication and relationship described by Murray and Huelskoetter (253). Also see Consequences of Isolation for further description of behaviors and traits associated with isolation.

Moral–Spiritual Development

The young adult may be in either the Conventional or the Postconventional Level of moral development (see Chapter 5). In the Postconventional Level he or she follows the principles defined as appropriate for life. There are two stages in this level. In both stages the person has passed beyond living a certain way just because the majority of people do. Yet in stage I of this level the person adheres to the legal viewpoint of society. The person believes, however, that laws can be changed as people's needs change, and he or she is able to transcend the thinking of a specific social order and develop universal principles about justice, equality, and human rights. In stage II the person still operates as in stage I but is able to incorporate injustice, pain, and death as an integral part of existence (195).

Kohlberg (195) espouses that the reason for the behavior indicates the level of moral development and that for a person to be at any level, the reasons for behavior should be consistent to the stage 50% of the time.

Therefore it would appear difficult for the average young adult, concerned about family, achieving in a career, paying the bills, and so on, to be in the Postconventional Level. Although the person may follow principles some of the time, conflicting situations and demands arise. To be consistently in the Postconventional Level takes considerable ego strength, a firm emotional and spiritual identity, and a willingness to stand up to societal forces. It may take years of maturing before the adult can be that courageous and consistent in Western society. For example, how does the young adult handle the dishonesty seen on the job? How does the mother handle the child viewing violence on television or demanding that clothes be the same designer outfits the other children are wearing? How does the couple react when a friend brags that he is having extramarital sexual experiences?

Probably only a few adults ever get to the second stage: 5 to 10% may reach stage I of the Postconventional Level; 20 to 25% stay in the Conventional Level; and the rest stay locked into the Preconventional Level described in Chapters 5 and 11 (195). Moral judgment, however, can change during adulthood, depending on life situations and the person's maturing.

Today's young adults have grown up with the influence of science and technology. As early as World War II some prophesied that the children born then would be postreligious, disinterested in other worlds, and con-

► CONSEQUENCES OF ISOLATION

- Is pessimistic, distrustful, ruthless
- Is lonely; may rationalize why being alone is enjoyed
- Avoids close relationships, especially with person of the opposite sex
- Lives a facade
- Has experienced a number of unsuccessful relationships
- Insists on having own way in a relationship
- Lacks empathy for others; cannot see another's perspective
- Is naively childlike
- Is easily disillusioned, embittered, cynical
- Overextends self without any real interest or feeling
- Is unable to reciprocate feelings or behavior in a relationship; makes demands but cannot give in a relationship
- Participates readily in encounter groups or forced fellowship to temporarily relieve loneliness, alienation
- Avoids real issues in life
- May be overtly friendly but drops a relationship when it becomes intimate; unable to sustain a relationship; may become engaged but never marry

cerned only in the secular existence of the present. Although some young adults fit this description and others are rejecting the institutional church, many have retained a desire and ability to apply spiritual and moral principles in this world. Increasingly parents with young children are joining a church or synagogue, seeking religion and a way to instill values in the child(ren).

In young adulthood there is a humanizing of values and a trend toward relativism as conflicts are encountered. The person increasingly discovers the meaning of values and their relation to achievement of social purposes, and he or she brings both personal experiences and motives to affirm and promote a value system. The person's values, whatever they are, become increasingly his or her own and a part of a unified philosophy of life. At the same time, there is expanding empathy for others and their value systems (221).

The spiritual awakening often experienced during adolescence, which might have receded with seeking of success, may now take on a more mature aspect as the young adult becomes firmly established in another life stage. If the person has children, he or she must rear them with some underlying philosophy. Their moral–spiritual questions must be answered. The young adult's religious teaching, perhaps previously rejected, may now be accepted as "not so bad after all." Or the young adult may build a new version of it.

Several qualities contribute to a spiritually mature disposition. The disposition is:

- *Individualized and integrated:* The person translates the abstract knowledge into practical action. It helps him or her reach goals and attain harmony in various aspects of living.
- *Consistent:* It produces basic standards of morality and conduct.
- *Comprehensive, dynamic, and flexible:* It never stops searching for new attitudes and ideas. The person can hold ideas tentatively until confirmed or until evidence produces a more valid belief.

Because new and different ideas are always available, the mature disposition can continue for a lifetime. The person realizes that there is always more to learn (101, 221). Easum (97), Roof (287), and Woodward et al. (378, 379) discuss spiritual development in the current young adult generation and how they differ from parental generations.

One of the dilemmas for the interfaith or interculture couple is what values and religion, if any, to follow in the home and to teach the children; how to celebrate holidays; what rituals and traditions to follow (e.g., Hanukkah or Christmas). Even when the couple makes a choice, there may be conflicts with relatives. Grandparents often have difficulty accepting that their child married someone of another faith or culture. Such marriages can work, and the children can have a firm moral and spiritual development. It is important for both spouses and families to discuss their feelings openly from the beginning. The couple should learn as much as possible about each other's religion or culture and talk to their families and friends about their experiences. It is critical that each family group remain open and accepting of the other. In turn, the children can learn deeper dimensions of spirituality, moral values, and their cultural background.

Although spiritual development and moral development follow sequential steps and are often thought of simultaneously, there is no significant link between specific religious affiliation or education and moral development. Moral development is linked positively with empathy, the capacity to understand another's viewpoint, and the ability to act reciprocally with another while maintaining personal values and principles. Being with people who are at a higher moral level stimulates the person to ask questions, consider his or her actions, and move to a higher moral level (195).

Adaptive Mechanisms

The young adult seeks stability while he or she is adapting to new or changing events. When the young adult is physically and emotionally healthy, total functioning is smooth (101, 221, 265). Adaptation to the environment, satisfaction of needs, and social interaction proceed relatively effortlessly and with minimum discomfort. The young adult behaves as though he or she is in control of impulses and drives and in harmony with superego ideals and demands. He or she can tolerate frustration of needs and is capable of making choices that seem best for total equilibrium (221). The person is emotionally mature for this life stage.

Emotional maturity is not exclusively related to physical health. Under stress, the healthiest people might momentarily have irrational impulses; in contrast, the extremely ill have periods of lucidity. Emotional health and maturity have an infinite gradation of behavior on a continuum rather than a rigid division between healthy and ill. Concepts of maturity are generated by culture. What is normal in one society may be abnormal in another.

In coping with stress in the environment, the young adult uses any of the previously discussed adaptive mechanisms. Use of these mechanisms, such as *denial* and *regression,* becomes abnormal or maladaptive only when the person uses the same mechanism of behavior too frequently, in too many situations, or for too long a duration.

Self-Concept and Body Image Development

Self-concept and body image, defined in Chapters 5 and 7 and discussed in each developmental era, are now redefined and expanded to fit the young adult perspective.

The persons' perception of self physically, emotionally, and socially, based on reactions of others that have been internalized, self-expectations, perceived abilities, attitudes, habits, knowledge, and other characteristics affects how that person will handle situations and relate to others. How the person behaves depends on whether he or she feels positively or negatively about self, whether the person believes others view him or her positively or negatively, and how he or she believes others expect the person to behave in this situation. The reactions of the family members, including spouse, and the employment situation, are strong influences on the young adult's self-concept. Additionally, the person discloses different aspects of self to various people and in various situations, depending on needs, what is considered socially acceptable, reactions of others, and past experience with self-disclosure (87, 216, 221, 252, 277).

Body image, a *part of self-concept, is a mental picture of the body's appearance integrated into the parietotemporal area of the cortex. Body image includes the surface, internal, and postural picture of the body and values, attitudes, emotions, and personality reactions of the person in relation to the body as an object in space, separate from others.* This image is flexible, subject to constant revision, and may not be reflective of actual body structure. Body image shifts back and forth at different times of the day and at different times in the life cycle (216, 221, 252).

Under normal conditions the body is the focus of an individual's identity, and its limits more or less clearly define a boundary that separates the person from the environment. One's body has spatial and time sense and yields experiences that cannot be shared directly with others. A person's body is the primary channel of contact with the world, and it is a nucleus around which values are synthesized. Any disturbance to the body influences total self-concept (252).

Contributing Influences

Many factors contribute to the body image (216, 221, 252, 277):

- Parental and social reaction to the person's body
- The person's interpretation of others' reactions to him or her
- The anatomic appearance and physiologic function of the body, including sex, age, kinesthetic and other sensorimotor stimuli, and illness or deformity
- Attitudes and emotions toward and familiarity with the body
- Internal drives, dependency needs, motivational state, and ideals to which the person aspires
- Identification with the bodies of others who were considered ideal (a little bit of each person significant to the person is incorporated into the self-concept and personality)
- Perception of space and objects immediately surrounding the body such as a chair or car; the sense of body boundaries
- Objects attached to the body such as clothing, a wig, false eyelashes, a prosthesis, jewelry, makeup, or perfume
- Activities the body performs in various roles, occupations, or recreations

The kinesthetic receptors in the muscles, tendons, and joints and the labyrinth receptors in the inner ear inform the person about his or her position in space. By means of perceptual alterations in position, the postural image of the body constantly changes. Every new posture and movement is incorporated by the cortex into a **schema** (*image*) in relation to or association with previously made schemata. Thus the image of the body changes with changing movements—walking, sitting, gestures, changes in appearance, and changes in the pace of walking (216, 221).

Self-produced movement aids visual accuracy. When a person's body parts are moved passively instead of actively (e.g., sitting in a wheelchair instead of walking), perceptual accuracy about space and the self as an object in space is hindered. Athletes, ballet dancers, and other agile people are more accurate than most in estimating the dimensions of the body parts that are involved in movement (216, 221). Activity appears to enhance sensory information in a way that passive movements do not. If a person undergoes body changes, he or she must actively explore and move the involved part to reintegrate it (216, 221, 277).

Self-knowledge. How do you visualize your body as you walk, run, stand, sit, or gesture? How do you feel about yourself as you go through various motions? What emotions are expressed by your movements? How do you think others visualize you at that time? Movement of the body parts, gestures, and appearance communicate a message to the observer (e.g., the client, or family member) that may or may not be intended. The message you convey about yourself to another may aid or hinder the establishment of a therapeutic relationship. You must be realistically aware of the posture and movement of your body and what they may be conveying to another.

Self-knowledge is not necessarily the same as knowledge gained about the self from others. Each person sees self differently from how others see him or her, although the most mature person is able to view self as others do. New attributes or ideas are integrated into the old ones, but all ideas received are not necessarily integrated. Before any perception about the self can affect or be integrated into one's self-concept, the perceptions must be considered good or necessary to the self. If the person believes that he or she is competent, a statement about incompetence will not be integrated into the self-image unless he or she is repeatedly told about being incompetent. If, however, the person has a negative self-image, it will also take many statements of his or her worth before they can be accepted and integrated into the self-concept.

A person has definite ideas and feelings about his or her own body, what is satisfying and what is frustrating. The person discovers that he or she has certain abilities and disabilities, likes and dislikes. He or she thinks of self as shy or outgoing and irritable or calm and learns something of how he or she affects others. What the person thinks of self has remarkable power in influencing behavior and the interpretation of other's behavior, the choice of associates, and goals pursued.

Feelings about certain self-attributes vary according to the importance placed on them and how central or close they are to the essence of self. Events such as illness or injury involving the face and torso are usually more threatening than those involving the limbs, as the face and the torso are integrated first into the young child's self-perception. The extremities are seen as part of the self later and are therefore usually less highly valued in comparison (216, 221, 252, 277).

One's feelings about one's characteristics also depend on whether a characteristic or body part is viewed as a functional tool for living or as a central personal attribute. For example, teeth can be viewed as a tool for eating or as central to the face, smile, youth, and personality. Dentures can be accepted and integrated as part of the body image more easily if they are viewed as a tool rather than if they are thought of as a sign of decline and old age. The person's work may also be viewed as a tool, function, or way to earn a living and help others or as central to the self. For example, is your image that of a woman or man who works as a nurse and does other things as well, or is your whole image primarily that of being a nurse? Age and sex are also characteristics that differ in degree of centrality or importance to the person (216, 221).

Also involved in self-concept and body image are the body parts supposedly considered strategically important in the character of the ethnic group or race (e.g., the German backbone, the Jewish nose, or the dark skin of the black person). The body part with special significance, which would also include the afflicted limb in a disabled person, is believed heavier, larger, or more conspicuous and seems to the bearer of it to be the focus of others' attention, although it may not be.

The location and history of family residence, religion, socioeconomic background, and even attempts at climbing to another social class level are integrated into the adult self-concept but not the body image (221).

Body image in the adult is a social creation. Normality is judged by appearance, and ways of using the body are prescribed by society. Approval and acceptance are given for normal appearance and proper behavior. Self-concept continually influences and enlarges the person's world, mastery of and interaction with it, and ability to respond to the many experiences it offers. This integration, largely unconscious, is constantly evolving and can be identified in the person's values, attitudes, and feelings about self. The experiences with the body are interpreted in terms of feelings, earlier views of the self, and group or cultural norms (119, 216, 221, 252, 277). In the adult there is a close interdependence between body image and personality, self-concept, and identity. Women have a more clearly defined and stable body concept than men. Girls seem to have an earlier realistic appreciation than boys of the smallness of their own bodies in relation to adults and of a sexual definition of self and a more realistic concept of the body thereafter. The difference between male and female body images seems related partly to different anatomic structure and body functions but also to the contrasts between males and females in their upbringing, style of life, and role in culture (119, 221).

You need to remember and use information about self-concepts and body image; your feedback to others is important. If you are to help another elevate self-esteem or feel positively about his or her body, you must give repeated positive reinforcement and help the person overcome unrealistic guilt and shame. Saying something positive or recognizing abilities once or twice will not be enough. The self-concept, whether wholesome or not, is difficult to change, as the person perceives others' comments and behavior in relation to an already established image to avoid conflict and anxiety within self. The person with a sense of trust, self-confidence, or positive self-concept is less threatened by others' ideas, remarks, or behavior. He or she is more flexible, able to change, and admit new attributes to self.

Body Image Change in Illness

A wide variety of messages about the body are constantly fed into the self-image for rejection, acceptance with integration, or revision. You will see disturbances in the person's body image after loss of a body function, structure, or quality—teeth, hair, vision, hearing, breast, internal organs, or youth—that necessitate adjustment of the person's body image. Because the body image provides a base for identity, almost any change in body structure or function is experienced as a threat, especially in the United States, where wholeness, beauty, and health are highly valued.

A threat to body image is related to the person's pattern of adaptation. Some behavior patterns may depend heavily on certain organs of the body. If these organs become diseased or must be removed, the threat is greater than if an organ unimportant to the person is affected. The degree to which this loss of body control creates loss of customary control of self, physical environment, time, and contacts with others is very closely related to the degree of threat felt. To understand the nature of the threat, you must assess the pattern of adaptation, the value of this pattern for the person, and the usual coping mechanisms. The person with limited adaptive abilities, who easily feels helpless and powerless, will experience greater threat with a change in body structure or function.

The Adult Undergoing Body Changes

Assessment. Assessment during illness, injury, or disability that necessitates eventual changes to self-image is often difficult because of the abstractness of self-image. But if you listen closely to the person, validate statements for less obvious meanings, and explore feelings with him or her you can gain considerable information for worthwhile intervention. Direct or probing questions about the following items do *not* obtain any information, but through open-ended questions you should gradually be able to obtain information about the aspects that relate to body image. Assessment could include determining the person's response to the following (119, 252, 253):

- Feelings about the self before and since the condition occurred
- Values about personal hygiene
- Values on beauty, self-control, wholeness, and activity
- Value of others' reactions
- Meaning of the body part affected
- Meaning of hospitalization, treatment, and care
- Awareness of extent of condition
- Effect of condition on person, roles, daily activities, family, and use of leisure time
- Perception of others' reaction to person with this condition
- Problems in adjusting to condition
- Mechanisms used in adapting to condition and its implication

Observation of the client must be combined with purposeful conversation. Observe movements, posture, gestures, and expressions as he or she answers your questions or talks about self to validate the consistency between what is said and what is meant.

Nursing Intervention. Measures to help someone with a threat to or change of body image involve assisting the person to reintegrate the self-view and self-esteem in relation to his or her condition. You can help the person in the following ways (246, 252, 253):

- Encourage talking about feelings in relation to the changed body function or structure. Talking about feelings is the first step to reintegration of body image.
- Assist client, without pressure, to become reacquainted with self by looking at the dressing or wound, feeling the cast, bandage, or injured part, or looking at self in mirror. The client who wants to "show the scar" should be allowed to do so. Reaction from you and the family can make a difference in how the person accepts the changed body.
- Provide opportunity for gaining information about the body, both the intact and changed parts, and its strengths and limits.
- Provide opportunity to learn mastery of the body, resume activities of daily care and living routines as indicated, move about, become involved with others, resume roles, and handle equipment.
- Give recognition for what the person can do. Avoid criticism, derogation, or a nonverbal reaction of disgust or shame.
- Help him or her see self as a whole person despite losses or changes.
- Encourage talking about unresolved experiences, distortions, or fears in relation to body image.

You will be encountering many young adults with body image distortions or changes as a result of accidental or war injuries, disease, weight gain or loss, pregnancy, or identity problems. You can make a significant contribution to the health of this person for the remainder of life by giving assistance through physical care, listening, counseling, teaching, and working with the people important to his or her life.

Be aware that health care professionals and certain treatment practices contribute to a negative self-concept and sexual stereotypes, and often the health care system treats the client (well or ill) as an unthinking, incompetent object. Although there may be some attitudinal changes occurring, many men and women still hold traditional stereotyped beliefs about sex-related behavior.

You will encounter health professionals in every field who are influenced by a sexist orientation when working with you and clients. By your behavior, use of problem solving, verbal facility, and nonverbal messages you can work to change sexist attitudes. Your efforts are important for your own positive self-concept and for unbiased care of each person, thus promoting a positive self-concept.

Lifestyle Options

The increased pace of life in the United States has brought people an unparalleled degree of social alienation at all levels of society. Choosing a lifestyle very different from one's childrearing experiences is an attempt to ward off alienation and organize one's life around meaning. The young adult has many options. He or she may decide to base the style of living around age (the youth cult); work (the company man or woman executive); leisure (the surf bum); drugs; or marriage and family.

Singlehood, *remaining unmarried and following a specific lifestyle,* is not new. Maiden aunts, bachelors, and single schoolteachers are traditional, as are those whose religion calls for singlehood. But remaining unmarried is increasingly an option, either as an end in itself or as a newly prolonged phase of postadolescence.

The single person may be in emotional isolation, unable to establish a close relationship and alienated from self and others or may feel depressed about the life situation; however, not all singles fit this description. The single person can accomplish the task of intimacy through emotional investment of self in others. Many are extroverts, have several very close friends with whom they share activities, have a meaningful career, and have a harmonious rather than conflictual relationship with parents. If they marry, they want to feel that they have chosen the right partner and have spent time living just for themselves so that they do not resent the responsibilities of marriage.

Many prefer to remain single as they pursue prolonged education and strive to become established in their occupational field. Others find that being free of relationships and to sample a variety of lifestyles and travel as they please before settling down to raise a family is an important part of establishing a comfortable identity. They avoid living out their lives in the same manner and location as their parents and may live in apartment complexes for singles only, following a lifestyle that is supposed to convey freedom. For whatever reasons, the number of single people in this country is on the rise, especially in the 20 to 34 age group.

Trends suggest that young people are marrying later than they did in the 1960s. There still exists a great deal of cultural and family pressure for this age group to marry by the midtwenties. Americans so value family life that unmarried adults sometimes have been treated as immature and incomplete or even as failures and willful renegades who cannot or will not take up a respectable and responsible family role. Single adults have had to take reduced credit ratings and higher insurance rates just because they are single. Pressure from "embarrassed" families and friends leads many of these individuals to marry prematurely lest they be considered lifetime misfits.

The single person may need help in understanding that lifestyle choice is not irresponsible, that he or she can make significant contributions as a citizen, and that marriage and parenthood are only one way to demonstrate emotional maturity. If the person is single because of isolation and self-absorption, psychiatric counseling may be needed, not for singlehood, but because of feelings about self and others. Several references give suggestions for managing alone (91, 166, 253, 270, 351, 377). Haber (146) describes family therapy with single young adults. For additional information on singlehood, refer to Chapter 4.

Family Planning: The Expectancy Phase and Parenthood

Parenthood is an option for either the couple or a single person. It was not until the early 1960s that people felt in control of family planning. Birth control methods were often not successful either aesthetically or mechanically. But today oral contraceptives for the female and more skilled vasectomy procedures for the male make it possible for couples to say "We don't want children now." "We don't want children ever." "We want to try to have two children spaced 3 years apart."

Information presented in Table 11–5 that summarizes contraceptives and various references at the end of this chapter will help you teach about all aspects of family planning. Chapter 4 prevents information useful for understanding the family with whom you are working.

Reasons for Childbearing

The couple may have a child for a variety of reasons: (1) extension of self; (2) to offset loneliness; (3) sense of pride or joy; (4) psychological fulfillment of having a child; (5) having someone to love self; (6) attempt to hold a marriage together; (7) feeling of power, generated by ability to create life; (8) representation of wealth; (9) to secure replacements for the work force; (10) to have an heir for family name and wealth; and (11) religious convictions (305). Whether the couple chooses to have only one child or more children is related to more than fertility and religious background. Lifestyle, finances, career, available support systems, and emotional maturity are factors. End-of-chapter references give several perspectives on this decision (5, 166, 167, 305, 307, 315).

Developmental Tasks for the Couple During the Expectancy Stage

You are in a position to assist the couple in understanding the changes that childbearing will create and the following developmental tasks for this stage of family life (93, 292, 305):

- Rearrange the home to provide space, facilities, and supplies for the expected baby.
- Rework the budget and determine how to obtain and spend income to accommodate changing needs and maintain the family unit financially.
- Evaluate the changing roles, division of labor, how responsibilities of child care will be divided, who has the final authority, and whether the woman should continue working outside the home if she has a career or profession.
- Adapt patterns of sexual relationships to the pregnancy.
- Rework the communication system between the couple; explore feelings about the pregnancy and ideas about childrearing, and work to resolve the differences.
- Acquire knowledge about pregnancy, childbirth, and parenthood.
- Rework the communication system and relationships with family, friends, and community activities, based on the reality of the pregnancy and their reactions.
- Use family and community resources as needed.
- Examine and expand the philosophy of life to include responsibilities of childbearing and childrearing.

Developmental tasks that must be mastered during pregnancy and the intrapartum period to ensure readiness for the maternal role are as follows (292):

1. *Pregnancy validation:* accepting the reality of the pregnancy, working through feelings of ambivalence
2. *Fetal embodiment:* incorporating the fetus and enlarging body into the body image
3. *Fetal distinction:* seeing the fetus as a separate entity, fantasizing what the baby will be like
4. *Role transition:* after birth, an increasing readiness to take on the task of parenthood

A number of authors have researched transition to parenthood, feelings, symptoms, body image changes, and needs for social support during pregnancy. Events during pregnancy affect family functioning and child care after birth. References at the end of the chapter

Research Abstract

Ferketich, S., and R. Mercer, Predictors of Role Competence for Experienced and Inexperienced Fathers, Nursing Research, 44 (1995), 89–95.

The purpose of this study was to explore differences in paternal confidence between inexperienced and experienced fathers. Parents' perceptions of their competence in the parenting role reflect their confidence in their skills and abilities to care for their child(ren). This confidence affects their interactions with the child, achievement of parental role identity, attachment to the infant, and sense of harmony with other roles. Seeking information is a major way to prepare for a new role, but information for fathers is secondhand through the partners or health professionals.

The sample included 79 experienced and 93 inexperienced fathers between the 24th and 34th weeks of their partner's pregnancy; these fathers were part of another study of high- and low-risk parents. All were 18 years or older, and if unmarried, they lived with the pregnant woman. Experienced fathers, with one to eight children, were older than inexperienced fathers but did not differ on other demographic characteristics. Partners of experienced fathers had higher pregnancy risk scores. Infant health status at birth and birth weights did not differ.

Several instruments were used to measure the parents' perceptions of their abilities to meet parenting demands, self-esteem, sense of mastery or control over one's life, partners' relationships with each other, family functioning and relationships between family and other social systems, depression and anxiety levels, support received during the prior 4 weeks, stress of negative life events, and attachment to the baby. Interview questions sought information about the man's feelings related to the wife's labor and delivery experience and relationship with his own parents.

Results indicated some differences and some similarities between the two groups. Experienced fathers reported higher paternal role competence than inexperienced fathers during the first week, but no differences were found between the two groups at 1, 4, or 8 months after birth. No differences were observed for experienced fathers at the first week, or 1-, 4-, or 8-month testings for self-esteem, partner relationships, family function, or health status. Experienced fathers reported lower fetal attachment than inexperienced fathers. Experienced fathers reported a higher sense of mastery and receiving less support during the first week than inexperienced fathers. Experienced fathers were less anxious and depressed at 4 and 8 months than inexperienced fathers. Having a sense of control over life and satisfactory family relationships were critical for first-time fathers.

The stages of father role identity achievement may be viewed as follows:

1. **Formal stage:** During the first month the man adheres rigidly to opinions and advice of experts.
2. **Informal or role-making stage:** Beginning at 4 months, the father responds to the uniqueness of the child in his own creative way.
3. **Personal or identity stage:** Father is comfortable with decisions and responses in caring for the child.

After the initial transition to parenthood, the birth of a second or later child leads to insignificant change in the father's parental identity, according to the instruments used. The range of parenting experience extends, however, and new skills are required at each developmental stage.

The nurse can provide an environment to help fathers explore their feelings and goals, to negotiate to secure social support, to participate in childbearing activities, and to learn about childrearing.

provide more information (3, 58, 87, 108, 243, 244, 258, 305, 363).

Father's Response. Some research indicates that attachment of the father to baby begins during pregnancy, rather than after birth, and that a strong marital relationship and vicariously experienced physical symptoms resembling pregnancy (and sometimes the couvade syndrome) strengthen attachment (71, 77, 94, 108, 148, 149, 207, 209, 351).

Studies indicate a characteristic pattern of development of subjective emotional involvement in pregnancy among first-time expectant fathers. Three phases occur: announcement phase, moratorium, and focusing period (233).

The **announcement phase** is *when pregnancy is suspected and confirmed.* If the man desired the pregnancy, he shows desire and excitement. If he did not want the pregnancy, he shows pain and shock (233).

During the **moratorium period,** the *man suppresses thoughts about the pregnancy.* This period can last from a few days to months and usually ends when the pregnancy is obvious. This period is characterized by emotional distance, a feeling the pregnancy is not real, concentration on himself and other life concerns, and sometimes leaving home. The man's emotional distance allows him to work through ambivalence and jealousy of the woman's ability to bear a child, but his distance causes her to feel unloved, rejected, angry, and uncared for. Marital tension exists. Pregnancy often emphasizes the disparity in the couple's life pace and focus. Gradually the man faces the financial and lifestyle implications of the pregnancy. If he feels financially insecure, unstable with his partner, or wishes to extend the childless period, he resents pregnancy and spends a longer time in the moratorium stage. Most men eventually become enthusiastic about the pregnancy and baby when they feel the baby move or hear the heartbeat. If the man does not become enthusiastic and supportive, the couple may then be at risk for marital and parenting problems (233).

The **focusing period** occurs *when the man perceives the pregnancy as real and important in his life.* This begins at approximately 25 to 30 weeks' gestation and extends until labor onset. The man redefines himself as father; he begins to feel more in tune with and is more helpful to his wife. He begins to read or talk about parenting and child development, notices other children, and is willing to participate in childbirth classes and purchasing baby supplies. He constructs a mental image of baby, sometimes different from the woman's mental image of the baby. The circle of friends may change to those who have children. He may feel fear about the coming labor and birth and feel responsible for a successful birth (233). The man who participates in pregnancy and birth experiences greater closeness with the infant and spouse and heightened self-esteem and esteem for the spouse. The man's readiness for pregnancy may significantly influence emergence of father involvement. The man's unconscious feelings and his earliest memories of childhood play an important role in his emotional reaction and adjustment to pregnancy and childbirth (149, 184, 207, 209).

Mother's Response. Certainly one would expect that an even stronger attachment would occur in the woman as she physically experiences the fetus and physical symptoms related to pregnancy and that her feelings for the child are stronger if she has a loving, supportive partner. Be aware also that some men have difficulty accepting the responsibility implied by a pregnant partner and do not want to be involved in child care (77, 184, 207, 209, 305, 351).

Nursing Roles

An important decision for the expectant parents is whether to attend childbirth education classes. Encourage the pregnant woman and her partner to attend childbirth education classes during pregnancy that are taught by American Society for Prophylaxis in Obstetrics (ASPO) certified childbirth educators. Insist that they be allowed to use the techniques and practical suggestions they learned during the labor and delivery process. The woman who is well supported during pregnancy experiences fewer complications during labor and delivery. The woman who has had childbirth education during pregnancy and can practice Lamaze techniques during labor uses less medication and is more likely to choose rooming-in with the baby.

Your support, acceptance, flexibility, helping the couple to use what they learned and practiced in prenatal classes, letting them assume responsibility for decisions when possible, assistance to mother, and teaching during the postpartum period are crucial to family-centered care. Cultural considerations are important as well (173).

Refer to a maternity nursing book for specific information on prenatal care, the labor and delivery process, and postpartum care—for both the normal and high-risk pregnancy and delivery. Helpful references are found at the end of Chapter 7 and at the end of this chapter (77, 93, 114, 207, 209, 243, 244, 305, 329, 351).

Be aware that in contrast to the societal romanticized view of pregnancy and care of the pregnant woman, the pregnant woman may be a victim of battering. Helton and colleagues (159–161), Hoff (165), O'Campo (263), and Stets (322) describe assessment, how to assist the woman in the decision to leave her partner, and resources. Sonkin, Martin, and Walker (313) described assessment of and intervention with the male batterer. Later in this chapter general information is given on spouse abuse and male batterer.

Other Approaches to Parenthood

Some couples delay childbearing until they are in their thirties or early forties. The woman may wish to pursue her education, a career, or a profession; the couple may choose to travel, start a business, become financially established, or have a variety of experiences before they settle down with one or two children. With genetic counseling, the surgical ability to undo vasectomy and tubal ligation, improved prenatal and neonatal care, and reduced risk of maternal or neonatal complications, pregnancy is safe for the mother in her thirties and even early forties (152, 305). Many of the risks of late parenthood are related to preexisting disease, if any, rather than to late conception. Of equal concern are the emotional and social implications, especially after birth when the couple's life revolves around baby rather than work or earlier interests (305).

Maternal age does not affect maternal role behaviors, and the sense of challenge, role strain, and self-image in the mother role is similar during the first year for childbearing women of all ages. Mercer's study (243) of the process of maternal role attainment in three age groups (15–19, 20–29, and 30–42) over the first year of motherhood found that love for the baby, gratification in the maternal role, observed maternal behavior, and self-reported ways of handling irritating child behaviors remained the same over the year.

The single person may desire to be a parent. The single woman may, through pregnancy or adoption, choose to have a child(ren). More is being written about the single woman who decides to become a mother and remain single. Some are well-educated, professional women in their late thirties or forties who believe they have no chance of becoming married, for various societal reasons, but who wish to have the experience of motherhood. Some single men who will not be biological fathers are also choosing to experience fatherhood through adoption (43). The number of both African-American and Caucasian single women who are choosing to be mothers and heads of the family is increasing. The decision to parent without a father or mother figure for the child should be carefully considered, for the child needs both female and male caregivers and the characteristics, responses, and relationships that each can give. The woman may choose to remain single but maintain a relationship with the biological father or with a man who can act as father to the child. The man may have a close relationship with a woman who can assist in mothering, or he may decide to nurture alone.

You are in a key position to help the person as he or she thinks through why there is a wish to have a child and remain single. Who the support system will be, who can act in the father or mother role to the child, the consequences of a single mother or father to the child during school years or adolescence, and the social, familial, and economic consequences of single parenthood should be discussed. Implications related to the cultural and religious background of the person must also be considered.

Family planning is sometimes made difficult by **infertility,** *inability to achieve pregnancy after 1 year of reg-*ular, *unprotected intercourse or the inability to carry a pregnancy to a term, live birth,* which is a health problem for 15% of women of childbearing age. Both partners should be given diagnostic tests together, as 50% of infertility factors are in women and 50% are in men. Infertility can create great psychological problems for the woman and man, between the couple, and between families of each partner. The problem becomes compounded by the increasing difficulty in adopting a local healthy baby in most communities, as 90% of single mothers retain their babies. Artificial insemination and a surrogate mother are alternatives that may not always be acceptable to the couple (77, 305, 351, 353).

References listed at the end of the chapter describe fertility and diagnostic and treatment procedures for the woman and man (77, 305, 351, 353). You may refer your client to local infertility clinics or the American Fertility Society, 1688 13th Avenue South, Birmingham, AL 35256. Another organization, Resolve, formed by people with infertility problems, gives counsel and support to people in 26 metropolitan areas. You may obtain more information by writing Resolve, Department P, Box 474, Belmont, MA 02178.

The couple who cannot biologically have a child may consider a **surrogate parent,** a *woman who, for a fee, will conceive through insemination, carry, and deliver a child for the woman who cannot conceive.* Many ethical concerns arise with this practice: the meaning of family, psychological effects on the surrogate and contracting parents, relationship between fetus and pregnant woman, the possibility that the child who is born may not meet the desires of the contracting parents, care of the deformed child, and effect on the child when he or she learns about the surrogate parent. Does the couple have a right to children by any means? What are the cultural, moral, and religious implications? Further, legal aspects are also tenuous. As of now, there are no answers, just many questions. You can help a couple considering the surrogate parent method work through the above issues and questions according to their spiritual, cultural, and family values and beliefs and their personal philosophies, values, and beliefs.

Developmental Tasks

The specific developmental tasks of the youth as he or she is making the transition from adolescence into young adulthood are discussed in Chapter 11 and can be summarized as choosing a vocation, getting appropriate education, establishing a residence, and formulating ideas about selection of a mate or someone with whom to have a close relationship.

For the young adult in general, the following tasks must be achieved, regardless of the station in life (93, 101):

- Accepting self and stabilizing self-concept and body image
- Acknowledging and resolving conflicts between the emerging self and conformity to the social order
- Establishing independence from parental home and financial aid
- Becoming established in a vocation or profession that provides personal satisfaction, economic independence, and a feeling of making a worthwhile contribution to society
- Learning to appraise and express love responsibly through more than sexual contacts
- Establishing an intimate bond with another, either through marriage or with a close friend
- Establishing and maintaining a home and managing a time schedule and life stresses

- Finding a congenial social and friendship group
- Deciding whether or not to have a family and carry out tasks of parenting
- Resolving changed relationship with the parental families
- Formulating a meaningful philosophy of life and reassessing priorities and values
- Becoming involved as a citizen in the community
- Achieving a more realistic outlook about other cultures, mores, and political systems

McCoy (236), using the stages of development proposed by the life-stage theorists discussed earlier, formulated similar developmental tasks for each stage. These tasks are depicted in Table 12–6.

You can assist young adults in meeting these developmental tasks through use of therapeutic communication principles, counseling, teaching, and crisis intervention. An in-depth source of information to help you understand and work with the married and young adult

TABLE 12–6. DEVELOPMENTAL TASKS AND OUTCOMES FOR THE STAGES OF YOUNG ADULTHOOD

Developmental Stage	Developmental Task	Outcome Sought
Becoming adults, ages 23–28	1. Select mate	1. Successful marriage
	2. Settle in work; begin career ladder	2. Career satisfaction and advancement
	3. Parent	3. Effective parents; healthy offspring
	4. Become involved in community	4. Informed, participating citizen
	5. Consume wisely	5. Sound consumer behavior
	6. Own home	6. Satisfying home environment
	7. Socially interact	7. Social skills
	8. Achieve autonomy	8. Fulfilled single state, autonomy
	9. Problem solve	9. Successful problem solving
	10. Manage stress accompanying change	10. Successful stress management; personal growth
Catch-30, ages 29–34	1. Search for personal values	1. Examined and owned values
	2. Reappraise relationships	2. Authentic personal relationships
	3. Progress in career	3. Career satisfaction, economic reward, a sense of competence and achievement
	4. Accept growing children	4. Growth-producing parent–child relationship
	5. Put down roots; achieve "permanent" home	5. Sound consumer behavior
	6. Problem solve	6. Successful problem solving
	7. Manage stress accompanying change	7. Successful stress management; personal growth
Midlife reexamination, ages 35–43	1. Search for meaning	1. Coping with existential anxiety
	2. Reassess marriage	2. Satisfying marriages
	3. Reexamine work	3. Appropriate career decisions
	4. Relate to teenage children	4. Improved parent–child relations
	5. Relate to aging parents	5. Improved child–parent relations
	6. Reassess personal priorities and values	6. Autonomous behavior
	7. Adjust to single life	7. Fulfilled single state
	8. Problem solve	8. Successful problem solving
	9. Manage stress accompanying change	9. Successful stress management; personal growth

Modified from McCoy, V., Adult Life Cycle Tasks Adult Continuing Education Program Response, Lifelong Learning in the Adult Years, October (1977), 16.

family and with families across generations is the text by Kramer (199).

► HEALTH CARE AND NURSING APPLICATIONS

Health Promotion and Health Protection

Your role in caring for the young adult may be many faceted. Assessment based on knowledge presented throughout this chapter is the basis for for-mulating *nursing diagnoses*. Nursing diagnoses that may be applicable to the young adult are listed in Selected Nursing Diagnoses Related to the Young Adult. Health promotion interventions to assist the young adult and the family to meet physical, cognitive, emotional, social, and spiritual needs are described in the following, and in the previous, sections.

In your assessment and care of the person, it is impossible to calculate the exact probability of anyone developing disease. The following principles are a guide (284):

► SELECTED NURSING DIAGNOSES RELATED TO THE YOUNG ADULT*

- **Pattern 1: Exchanging**
- Altered Nutrition: More than Body requirements
- Altered Nutrition: Less than Body requirements
- Altered Nutrition: Potential for More Than Body Requirements
- Risk for Infection
- Risk for Injury
- Impaired Skin Integrity
- **Pattern 2: Communicating**
- Impaired Verbal Communication
- **Pattern 3: Relating**
- Impaired Social Interaction
- Social Isolation
- Altered Role Performance
- Altered Parenting
- Risk for Altered Parenting
- Alcoholism
- Altered Family Process: Alcoholism
- Parental Role Conflict
- Altered Sexuality Patterns
- **Pattern 4: Valuing**
- Spiritual Distress
- **Pattern 5: Choosing**
- Ineffective Individual Coping
- Impaired Adjustment
- Defensive Coping
- Ineffective Denial
- Ineffective Family Coping: Disabling
- Ineffective Family Coping: Compromised
- Family Coping: Potential for Growth

- Decisional Conflict
- Health-Seeking Behaviors
- **Pattern 6: Moving**
- Fatigue
- Risk for Activity Intolerance
- Sleep Pattern Disturbance
- Diversional Activity Deficit
- Impaired Home Maintenance Management
- Altered Health Maintenance
- **Pattern 7: Perceiving**
- Body Image Disturbance
- Self-Esteem Disturbance
- Chronic Low Self-Esteem
- Situational Low Self-Esteem
- Personal Identity Disturbance
- Sensory/Perceptual Alterations
- Hopelessness
- Powerlessness
- **Pattern 8: Knowing**
- Knowledge Deficit
- **Pattern 9: Feeling**
- Pain
- Chronic Pain
- Dysfunctional Grieving
- Anticipatory Grieving
- Potential for Violence: Self-directed or Directed at Others
- Post-Trauma Response
- Rape-Trauma Syndrome
- Anxiety

*Other NANDA diagnoses are applicable to the ill young adult.
From North American Nursing Diagnosis Association, NANDA Nursing Diagnoses Definitions & Classification 1995–1996. Philadelphia: North American Nursing Association, 1994.

1. *Genetic makeup or family history* is the strongest single determinant of risk. The Human Genome Project, an effort to identify and locate each of our 50,000 to 100,000 genes within the next decade, may help better predict risk profile in the future.
2. *Magnitude* or a *slight elevation* (10–30%) in risk for a given disease has a minor effect on the person. A *marked increase* in risk (100%) would serve as an alarm.
3. *Repetition,* or *independently researched risk factors,* such as cigarette smoking, excess alcohol intake, obesity, sedentary lifestyle, and diet high in saturated fats, must be taken seriously as risks for everyone.

Immunizations

The young adult, depending on her or his history, may need immunizations. The Centers for Disease Control and Prevention recommend that colleges and universities require student documentation of immunity (including tuberculin testing) to preventable diseases as a prerequisite to registration. Adults should be vaccinated each fall against influenza. Hepatitis B, rubella (German measles), regular measles, and polio immunizations should be given if not received earlier. A tetanus booster is needed every 10 years. Mumps vaccine is especially recommended for adult males. Pregnant women and the chronically ill should be vaccinated for pneumonia (64). (See Chart V in Appendix IV.)

Common Health Problems: Prevention and Treatment

Physical Problems

More than 2 billion people are sick at any one given time globally; many die from preventable illnesses, and for millions of people survival is a daily battle. The challenge is to prevent the world from heading toward a health catastrophe. Worldwide, in 1993, killers were (1) ischemic heart disease (4.3 million); (2) acute lower respiratory infections, mainly pneumonia, in children under 5 (4.1 million); (3) cerebrovascular disease (3.9 million); (4) diarrhea and dysentery (3 million); (5) chronic obstructive pulmonary disease (2.9 million); (6) tuberculosis (2.7 million); (7) malaria (2 million);

TABLE 12–7. COMMON HEALTH PROBLEMS FOR YOUNG ADULTS

Problem	Definition	Symptoms/Signs	Prevention/Treatment
Upper respiratory infection (URI or common cold)	Acute infection of the upper respiratory tract lasting several days	General malaise; nasal stuffiness and discharge, mild sore throat, watery eyes; sometimes ear discomfort	If bacterial: antibiotic; otherwise, symptomatic treatment—antipyretic, antihistamine, decongestants
Influenza	Acute contagious viral illness often occurring in epidemics	Fever, malaise, myalgia, and respiratory symptoms; sometimes cough, rhinitis, and scattered rales	Prevention: immunization Treatment: antipyretic, increase fluid intake, rest; for influenza: amantadine hydrochloride
Hypertension (uncomplicated), **essential**	Pertinent elevation of arterial blood pressure >150/100 but <200/110 present on three weekly determinations, without secondary cause found	Sometimes none; sometimes headache, dizziness, lightheadedness	Appropriate lab workup along with other testing; diet; weight reduction; exercise; possibly medication
Mitral valve prolapse	Insufficiency of valve to open and close appropriately	Usually in young adult female; chest pain, arrhythmias, palpitations, tachycardia, sense of fullness in neck and head, feeling faint, anxious	Medication, adequate rest; reduction of stress in life to extent possible
Iron deficiency anemia	Blood hemoglobin level ≤ 10 g/dL, compared with normal value of 12–16 g/dL (for women)	Usually caused by menses; sometimes no signs; fatigue, irritability, depression, weakness, dizziness, headache, pallor of skin and conjunctivae, brittle nails	Prevention: blood screen, iron-rich foods Treatment: iron preparation (ferrous sulfate)
Atopic dermatitis of adulthood	Dry, thickened skin, accentuating normal folds (different appearance than in infancy)	Hyperpigmentation, especially on flexor areas of extremities, eyelids, dorsi of hands and feet, and back of neck	Keeping skin dry in humid conditions; mild, nondrying soap; hydrocortisone cream

(continued)

TABLE 12–7. COMMON HEALTH PROBLEMS FOR YOUNG ADULTS (continued)

Problem	Definition	Symptoms/Signs	Prevention/Treatment
Folliculitis	Localized infection of hair follicle	Irritated area around hair follicle	Washing well; hot compresses
Furuncle (boil)	Infected area that has draining point	Raised red area with exudate	Hot compresses; antibiotics; sometimes incision and drainage
Carbuncle	Large group of furuncles with several draining points	Raised red areas with multiple exudate areas	Hot compresses; antibiotics; incision and drainage
Urticaria (hives)	Allergic reaction, usually to drugs, food, inhalants, or insect bites	Itching, red raised welts, usually on trunk or extremities	Cool compresses; sometimes antihistamine or epinephrine; attempt to find offending agent
Scabies	Dermatitis caused by mite burrowing into skin and consequent allergic reaction	Severe itching; punctate excoriation	Lindane (Kwell) treatment (all sexual and household contacts too)
Simple diarrhea of adulthood	Gastrointestinal upset caused by viral infection, psychological disturbance, dietary changes, laxatives	Frequent loose, watery stools that are not greasy, bloody, or purulent	Clear liquid diet; antidiarrhea preparation (e.g., loperamide hydrochloride [Imodium])
Cystitis	Inflammation of bladder (often seen in young, adult women)	Dysuria, frequency, bladder spasms	Appropriate antibiotics after clean-catch urinalysis and culture; increased water intake (at least eight 8-oz glasses daily); sometimes antispasmodic medication
Acute pyelonephritis	Cystitis plus inflammation of kidneys and collection system	Dysuria, frequency, flank pain, chills, nausea, vomiting	Appropriate antibiotic treatment plus antipyretic and antinausea medicine if necessary
Chronic fatigue syndrome (CFS)	Debilitating fatigue that lasts at least 6 months	Eight of the following must persist or recur over 6 months: chills or low-grade fever; sore throat; tender lymph nodes; muscle pain and weakness; extreme fatigue; headaches; joint pain without swelling; neurologic problems (confusion, memory loss); sleep disorders	Prevention: none known. Treatment: adequate rest, nutritious diet, small amounts of exercise; rationing of energy; dealing emotionally with disease; possibly tricyclic antidepressants
Hepatitis B	Type of liver inflammation	Jaundice, malaise, may lead to liver cancer, cirrhosis, or death; some are carriers only	Immunization (series of 3 injections) rest, nutritious diet
Dental caries and periodontal disease	Tooth decay and bleeding, hypertrophied gums	Gradual receding of gums and bones and loss of teeth	Early dental checks and personal mouth care; proper diet
Lactose intolerance or milk malabsorption syndrome	Lactose (milk sugar) not hydrolyzed because of lack of appropriate amounts of the enzyme lactose	Severe abdominal discomfort and flatulence following digestion of milk products	Use of Lactaid or Say Yes to Dairy, concentrated forms of the enzyme; also *Lactobacillus* milk; avoid foods made with milk or milk products
Anxiety	Combination of fearfulness, nervousness, apprehension, and restlessness, often associated with family or personal crisis and sometimes with physical or mental illness	Loss of appetite, increased appetite, lack of sleeping ability; increased perspiration, "thumping of heart," headaches, weakness, fatigue, trembling	Supportive therapy, crisis intervention, some medicines for short term
Tension headache	Bandlike pressure across forehead and around back of skull	Dull, aching pain with a feeling of tightness; tension in neck muscles	Reassurance, mild analgesics, occasionally a muscle relaxer, massage, manipulation, elimination of tension
Migraine headache	Vascular in origin: arterial spasm followed by dilation	Throbbing unilateral pain, sometimes preceded by **aura** (*inherent warning, usually visual*); sometimes nausea and vomiting	Try to rest when aura first appears, various medications such as anti-inflammatory drugs and caffeine; rest in a dark room; nutrition; chiropractic care; biofeedback

(8) measles (1.2 million); and (9) other heart diseases (1.1 million). At least 10 million people in the world were disabled by polio in 1993 (226).

Many diseases could have been prevented by access to health care and adequate nutrition as well as immunization against six serious childhood diseases: polio, tetanus, measles, diphtheria, pertussis, and tuberculosis (226).

In the United States, health problems and risks, preventive behavior, and response to illness are influenced by sex and lifestyle, as well as other factors. The references at the end of the chapter provide specific information on sex-related health issues (7, 121, 188, 267, 305, 311, 327). Table 12–7 summarizes common health problems encountered by the young adult (2, 45, 125, 153, 154, 169, 188, 262, 276, 305, 336, 353, 370, 373, 384).

Acquired Immunodeficiency Syndrome. **AIDS** was defined by the Centers for Disease Control and Prevention (CDC) is 1987 *as a disabling or life-threatening illness caused by human immunodeficiency virus (HIV) and characterized by HIV encephalopathy; HIV wasting syndrome, or certain diseases resulting from immunodeficiency in a person with laboratory evidence for HIV infection or without certain other causes of immunodeficiency* (208).

AIDS was first reported in the United States in 1981 but more likely occurred in 1977. Currently the World Health Organization (WHO) predicts up to 30 million world AIDS cases by the year 2000. With 10 million of these predicted infections expected in children by the year 2000, AIDS will be a major global cause of death, if not the biggest killer in some countries (369).

Since 1988, 40,000 new cases of HIV infection have been reported annually in the United States. In January 1995, there were 441, 528 reported AIDS cases in the United States (70, 286, 354).

AIDS has evolved from a disease of gay men in a few large cities to a major killer of young disadvantaged Americans. Everyone is at risk, regardless of sexual orientation or economic level (370). Among African-Americans, the transmission pattern is heterosexual as well as homosexual. AIDS is now the No. 1 killer of African-American women between the ages of 25 and 44 (70, 286, 354)! Other countries, such as Kenya and Rumania, are reported by the media to have a large number of babies with AIDS.

AIDS is a devastating disease to the already disadvantaged who are often carrying other sexually transmitted diseases (STDs) and who are often in the crack-cocaine culture. These young adults have a resigned attitude about their diagnosis and a mistrust of the conventional medicine system. Thus, they often will not take the medicine suggested or will not cooperate in informing past or current sexual partners of their diagnosis (70, 286).

For those who are cooperating with the health care system, the following treatment approaches are available. Treatment with AZT is still ongoing. Sometimes it is combined with 3TC (lamivudine). Protease inhibitors are being used, along with Ganciclovir for opportunistic infections. Vaccines are being tried in research trials and those "long-term nonprogressors," who are persons with AIDS who have lived 8 to 10 years and are being studied as to why they, against all odds, remain alive and well (70, 286). As of mid-June 1993, 315,390 cases of AIDS have been reported in the United States since reporting started. Over that same period, 194,334 deaths were reported (70,286).

Health care professionals are not immune; in fact, it is imperative that they take protective measures constantly and always follow Universal Precautions published by CDC.

Despite the action taken by the U.S. Public Health Service to isolate the causative virus, screen the nation's blood supply, and educate the public, the available data appear ominous. HIV infects and destroys white blood cells known as helper T cells. These particular cells regulate the body's immune system, and if they are destroyed, the capacity to fight disease is gone. In addition, HIV can affect the cells in the central nervous system (298, 299).

Infection with HIV does not always lead to AIDS, but if the person tests positive for HIV he or she can transmit the virus to another human being. Transmission of the bloodborne virus occurs through the following ways:

- Sexual intercourse with an infected person, male or female
- Contact with contaminated blood equipment such as sharing equipment for IV drug abuse
- From a mother to her unborn fetus during pregnancy or during birth or while breastfeeding

The virus has been isolated in semen, vaginal secretions, blood, saliva, and tears. Even though the virus has been found in saliva and tears, there are no known documented cases of transmission other than by the ways just listed (208, 298, 299).

In an individual more than 4 months of age, the AIDS antibody test can determine whether or not a person has been exposed to HIV. This does not mean that the person will necessarily develop AIDS. Unfortunately, the antibodies are not protective to the person like the antibodies to other disease organisms. It is not yet understood why this is so, but research is seeking an answer. It is also suggested that large amounts of virus are required to cause the infection and possibly cofactors are necessary for invasion to occur. The cofactors that have been suggested are an already decreased immune system, alcohol use, recreational drugs, poor nutrition, inadequate rest or exercise, severe stress, and other infections (208, 298, 299).

HIV disease appears to have four relatively distinct stages in the young adult: early or acute period with flu-like and respiratory symptoms lasting a few weeks; middle or asymptomatic period of minor or no clinical problems lasting months or sometimes years; transitional, symptomatic period lasting an intermediate length of time; and late or crisis period lasting months or occasionally years. Mean time from infection to disease is 8 years, and from disease to death, 18 months (24, 298, 299).

Public education is the only way of dealing with this public health menace. The incubation period of the virus varies from months to as many as 10 years; thus preventive education is the key factor. New approaches to education must be tried, including teaching groups at schools, occupational sites, churches, gay bars, gay or lesbian organizations, and developing organizations for Latinos and African Americans, as they may not attend general meetings. Television could be used to promote responsible sexual behavior, including abstinence and use of condoms to prevent sexually transmitted diseases. Further, some cities distribute free needles and syringes to drug users, using a monitoring system that is designed to prevent the spread of AIDS. This action appears to reduce sharing of needles between infected and noninfected drug users and provides a time for education (24, 63, 104, 143, 208, 286, 311, 370, 373). However, educational programs that emphasize hope and not just fear and include social and community issues and disease facts are most effective (104).

The prevention of AIDS is dependent on behavior that reduces or eliminates the possibility of contracting or transmitting the disease. *The Public Health Service recommends these behaviors* (63, 104, 208, 353):

- Do not have sexual intercourse with multiple persons or with persons who had multiple partners (including prostitutes). The more partners you have, the greater your risk.
- Avoid sexual intercourse with persons with or at risk for AIDS or HIV infection or persons who have had a positive result on the HIV antibody test; however, if you do have sexual intercourse with a person you think may be infected, protect yourself by taking precautions to prevent contact with that person's body fluids. (*Body fluids* include blood, semen, urine, feces, saliva, and vaginal secretions.) *Use of a condom* will reduce

the chances of spreading the virus. The intact, correctly applied rubber condom is effective against transmission of sexually transmitted disease. Landau and Clements (208) discuss types and their use; directions should be given clients so that the condom will be used correctly. Avoid practices such as anal intercourse that may injure body tissues and make it easier for the virus to enter the bloodstream. Oral–genital contact should also be avoided, as should open-mouthed, intimate kissing.
- Do not use IV drugs. If you do, do not share needles or syringes.
- Consult your doctor for counseling if you believe that you may be at increased risk for HIV infection. Consider taking the HIV antibody test, which will enable you to know your status and take appropriate action.

Persons in the following groups are at increased risk for infection with HIV (208, 286, 311, 353, 369, 370):

- Homosexual and bisexual men (or men who have had sexual intercourse with another man since 1977)
- People who inject illegal IV drugs or who have done so in the past
- Persons with symptoms of AIDS or AIDS-related illnesses
- Persons from Haiti and Central African countries, where heterosexual transmission is believed more common than in the United States
- Male or female prostitutes and their sex partners
- Sexual partners of persons infected with the AIDS virus
- Persons with hemophilia who have received clotting factor products
- Infants of high-risk or infected mothers

If hospital infection control practices are followed when health care providers care for patients with AIDS or work with their biological specimens, there is low risk of occupationally acquiring the opportunistic infections associated with AIDS: (1) HIV through serum conversion, (2) cytomegalovirus (CMV), or (3) hepatitis B virus (HBV) or herpes simplex virus type 2 (HSV-2). Seroconversion to HIV is most likely to follow a contaminated needle-stick injury. Health care professionals who use rubber gloves are effectively protected against transmission of HIV when the gloves are correctly fitted and worn and are intact. In addition, thorough hand-washing is mandatory. A face mask should be worn when required. Sharp objects, if contaminated, should be carefully handled. Contaminated instruments should be sterilized or disposed of properly (104, 208, 356).

The 10 warning symptoms of HIV infection in adults are as follows:

1. Swollen glands, especially in neck, armpits, or groin
2. Blotches or rashes, usually pink to purple, that grow in size, are harder than surrounding areas, and may appear under skin, in the mouth, nose, rectum, and at other body sites
3. Unexpected weight loss of more than 10 pounds within 2 months
4. Fever persisting longer than 1 week and night sweats
5. Persistent, dry cough
6. Diarrhea
7. Malaise and persistent fatigue
8. Thrush or white coating on tongue
9. Easy bruising
10. Blurred vision or persistent headaches

These symptoms may indicate early stages of various diseases that may lead to death such as Kaposi's sarcoma and *Pneumocystis carinii* pneumonia (208, 298, 299).

You may care for the person with AIDS in the hospital, in his or her home, or in a special home designated for AIDS clients and families. You will be a resource to relatives, partners, and friends of AIDS clients. Care will be determined by body parts affected, mind set, and neurologic and other physical and emotional symptoms and signs. Remember the extreme isolation and loneliness that most clients will experience as they deal with a disease with such stigma. Seek various educational tools (104, 197, 208, 264, 311, 348). A toll-free hotline has been set up by the Public Health Service. Publications are issued by public health organizations and agencies such as the American Red Cross. Information written in the appropriate language and at appropriate learning levels is essential to affect any person's attitude and behavior.

The following references provide additional information on all aspects of HIV and AIDS: 24, 44, 63, 104, 109, 143, 197, 264, 348, 353, and 370. Refer also to Chapter 11 for information on other sexually transmitted diseases that can be contracted by the adult.

Tuberculosis. Recent resurgence of tuberculosis in the United States and other countries, with emergence of multidrug-resistant strains, has reawakened interest in tuberculosis control. Tuberculin screening to detect infected persons and beginning treatment with isoniazid before disease emerges have been recommended for all health care practitioners, residents of mental and cor-

rection facilities, medically underserved populations, and immigrants on entry to the United States. A study in Canada indicated that such a tuberculin screening program would be less cost effective than anticipated because of high rates of patient and provider noncompliance (69, 226).

Tuberculosis is reemerging according to WHO because "deteriorating social conditions are now ruthlessly exposing weaknesses in many of the regions' TB control programmes." We are warned to follow TB control guidelines. If drug-resistant strains develop, the disease will be expensive and incurable (*The Nation's Health,* August [1994], 14).

Accidents. Accidents are a leading cause of death for young adult men and the second leading cause of death for young adult women, with motor vehicle accidents producing the most deaths in both sexes. Among the young male population, industrial accidents and drownings also rank high as major causes of accidental death. Other injuries typical in young adulthood are fractures, dislocations, lacerations, abrasions, and contusions (169, 360). These injuries require restriction of activity, which also presents the young adult with social and economic problems.

Because accidents and their resultant injuries are serious health hazards for the young adult, safety education should be a prime concern for you in all occupational settings. You should initiate and actively participate in safety programs in various settings: employment, school, or recreation. Young adults should be reminded of the safety rules for swimming and other sports and be encouraged to drive defensively. The groundwork in safety education should be established when the individual is young. Old habits and patterns are difficult to change.

Malignancies. Cancer is a major cause of death in the United States. Table 12–8 summarizes the types, incidence, risks, signs and symptoms, and prevention and treatment measures for cancers found in young adults.

Breast cancer is rare under the age of 25, but the risk increases steadily after the age of 30. All young women should be taught and encouraged to do breast self-examinations, as most breast cancers are first detected by the individual. In addition, examination by a physician or nurse practitioner should be done annually. Many women are hesitant to do breast self-examinations; fear, lack of knowledge, modesty, health orientation, education level, and age contribute to this reluctance. Women are likely to practice self-examination of the breasts if they have a positive self-concept, if they are aware of the benefits, if barriers are minimized, and if they perform other preventive health measures.

TABLE 12–8. TYPES OF CANCER FOUND IN YOUNG ADULTS

Type and Impact*	Risks, Symptoms, Signs	Prevention, Teaching
Oral cancer or cancer of mouth 29,000 diagnosed in 1994 with an estimated 7929 deaths	Twice as high in men as in women; highest incidence in African-American males Color changes in mouth; a sore in mouth that does not heal	Avoid smoking, alcohol, smokeless tobacco; have a thorough exam by a professional including lips, gingival, buccal mucosa, palate, floor of mouth, tongue, and pharynx
Cervical cancer 15,000 diagnosed in 1994 with an estimated 4600 deaths	Risk factors include early age at first intercourse, multiple sex partners, smoking, human papillomavirus infection, diethylstilbestrol exposure Abnormal vaginal bleeding or abnormal discharge	Avoid risk factors listed; avoid smoking; have a Pap smear at recommended intervals
Breast cancer 182,000 diagnosed in 1994 with an estimated 46,000 deaths	Risk factors include age > 50 and first-degree relative history of breast cancer, first child born after age 30, never had children Breast lump or thickening, bleeding from nipple	Breast self-exam, clinical breast exam and mammography as indicated for age and time interval
Cancer of the testes 6800 diagnosed in 1994 with an estimated 325 deaths	Increased incidence in males with history of cryptorchidism, gonadal dysgenesis, Klinefelter's syndrome or in utero exposure to diethylstilbestrol Any mass in testicle	Teach person proper self-exam technique and recommend regular checks as part of periodic health exam
Skin cancer 700,000 new cases of basal and squamous cell carcinoma as well as 32,000 cases of malignant melanoma diagnosed in 1994 with an estimated 6900 deaths from malignant melanoma and 2300 deaths from other skin cancers	Increased incidence in fair skin, sun exposure, severe sunburn in childhood, and familial conditions like dysplastic nevus syndrome A change in a mole or sore that does not heal	Advise against overexposure to sun by using appropriate sunscreens (at least a 15 protective value); wear protective clothing; examine skin for any changes; have periodic skin exam as part of regular health exam

All impact figures are for United States.

Media coverage of someone who has successfully recovered from a mastectomy increases the incidence of self-examination (74, 169, 353). You should teach the information about breast self-examination described and depicted in Table 12–9.

During young adulthood the man should be taught to examine his scrotum and penis regularly since **cancer of the testes** may occur and may be detected by palpating unusual nodules (256). Table 12–10 describes the examination procedure. Teach the information about the examination.

Teach clients the *warning signs* of cancer as shown in Seven Warning Signs of Cancer (see next page). Teach also signs that should be considered *suspicious* and reported to a physician (168, 353):

- Changes in a dark-colored mole or spot
- Pink or flesh-colored nodule that slowly grows larger
- Open or crusted sore that does not heal
- Red, rough patch or bump that persists
- Mole that grows, changes, hurts, bleeds, or itches

- Mole that is larger in size than a pencil eraser and has irregular borders or variegated colors with shadings of red-white or blue-black
- Elevation or bulge in a mole that was flat
- Mole on the bottom of the feet or in an area of repeated trauma

Daily habits may contribute to risk for cancer in other ways. For example, risks for lung and hematopoietic cancers apparently are increased in adulthood after childhood exposure to parental smoking. Tell women that the incidence of breast cancer of fibrocystic disease is higher in those who consume increased amounts of caffeine. Consuming two or more cups of caffeinated coffee a day may be associated with increased risk of colon or bladder cancer. Realize that some cultural groups are more prone to cancer. Environmental and cultural factors (e.g., diet, lifestyle stress, exposure to pollutants) contribute significantly to increased incidence of cancer (see Chapter 2). American Indians, in comparison to Caucasians, have lower rates for cancer of the lung, breast, and colon and higher rates for gallbladder, kidney, and cervical cancer, possibly related to genetics, diet, or lifestyle. American Indians have a

TABLE 12–9. BREAST SELF-EXAMINATION

There are many good reasons for doing breast self-examination (BSE) each month. One reason is that breast cancer is most easily treated and cured when it is found early. Another is that if you do BSE every month, it will increase your skill and confidence when doing the exam. When you get to know how your breasts normally feel, you will quickly be able to feel any change. Another reason, it is easy to do.

The best time to do BSE is about a week after your period, when breasts are not tender or swollen. If you do not have regular periods or sometimes skip a month, do BSE on the same day every month.

1. Lie down and put a pillow under your right shoulder. Place your right arm behind your head.
2. Use the finger pads of your three middle fingers on your left hand to feel for lumps or thickening. Your finger pads are the top third of each finger.
3. Press firmly enough to know how your breast feels. If you're not sure how hard to press, ask your health care provider. Or try to copy the way your health care provider uses the finger pads during a breast exam. Learn what your breast feels like most of the time. A firm ridge in the lower curve of each breast is normal.
4. Move around the breast in a set way. You can choose either the circle (A), the up and down line (B), or the wedge (C). Do it the same way every time. It will help you make sure that you've gone over the entire breast area, and remember how your breast feels each month.
5. Now examine your left breast using right-hand finger pads.
6. If you find any changes, see your doctor right away

Remember: BSE could save your breast — and save your life. Most breast lumps are found by women themselves, but, in fact, most lumps in the breast are not cancer. Be safe, be sure.

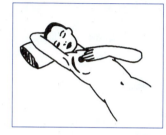

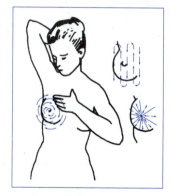

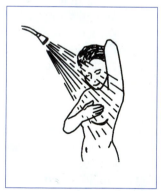

Three BSE techniques.

From How To Do Breast Self-Examination. *No. 2674, Atlanta: American Cancer Society, 1995.*

TABLE 12–10. PROCEDURE FOR EXAMINATION OF THE SCROTUM AND PENIS

1. Perform the examination immediately after shower or a warm bath. Both the scrotum and examiner's hands should be warm.
2. Hold the scrotum in the palms of the hands and palpate with the thumb and fingers of both hands.
3. Examine each testicle individually.
4. Locate the epididymis (found on top of and extending down behind the testicle); it should be soft and slightly tender.
5. Examine the spermatic cord next; it ascends from the epididymis and has a firm, smooth, tubular texture.
6. Become familiar with the consistency of normal testicular structures so that changes can be detected.

higher rate of alcoholism than Caucasians. Although Asian populations have low rates of breast and colon cancer, those who have migrated to Western countries experience a higher frequency of carcinoma of each anatomic site than prevails in their original country.

Lifestyle and Physical Illness. Life is rooted in and organized around a person's changing culture and society, whether the changes are dramatic or subtle. Coping with extreme change taxes the person physically and psychologically and may be responsible for physical disease. Research shows relationships between physical adaptation and illness and sociocultural experiences. Death rates from cancer, diabetes, tuberculosis, heart disease, and multiple sclerosis for urban populations are inversely proportional to income, implying that stresses of poverty may be a cause of disease (169, 253).

► ## SEVEN WARNING SIGNS OF CANCER

- **C**hange in bowel or bladder habits
- **A** sore that does not heal
- **U**nusual bleeding or discharge
- **T**hickening or lump in breast or elsewhere
- **I**ndigestion or difficulty in swallowing
- **O**bvious change in wart or mole
- **N**agging cough or hoarseness

Used by permission, American Cancer Society, Inc., *Cancer Facts and Figures—1991.*

The adult is most likely to fall ill when he or she is experiencing the "giving up–given up complex": feelings of lowered self-esteem, discouragement, despair, humiliation, depression, powerlessness to change or cope with a situation, imagined helplessness, loss of gratifying roles, sense of uncertain future, and memories of earlier periods of giving up. Apparently such feelings modify the capacity of the organism to cope with concurrent pathogenic factors. Biologically, the central nervous system fails in its task of processing the emergency defense system so that the person has a higher statistical tendency toward illness or death. Conversely, contentment, happiness, faith, confidence, and success are associated with health (240, 270).

One lifestyle that involves geographic mobility, transient and inadequate housing, hard work, poor nutrition, and inadequate immunizations or other health promotion measures is that of the **migrant farm worker.** The migrant worker has unique and numerous health care needs because of the following: (1) the opportunity for prevention of certain illnesses is nonexistent; (2) prenatal and maternal care is lacking; (3) chronic health problems are numerous; (4) economic resources are scant; and (5) contacts with the health care system are sporadic and temporary. **Homeless** individuals and families also have similar health care needs and problems. Refer also to Chapter 1. Be attuned to cultural differences, including language difficulties, definitions of health and illness, food preferences, lines of authority, health practices, job-related diseases, and general lifestyle of your clients.

Biofeedback. The young adult is likely to be interested in and benefit from **biofeedback training,** *learning to control body functions once considered involuntary* such as heartbeat, blood pressure, breathing, and muscle contractions (see Chapter 5 for further discussion). Learning biofeedback is much like learning other skills of muscular coordination and physical activity. Involved is controlled production of alpha waves, the brain waves typical of relaxation and reverie, the fringe of conscious-

Research Abstract

Ireys, H., S. Gross, L. Werthamer-Larrson, and K. Kolodner, Self-esteem of Young Adults With Chronic Health Conditions: Appraising the Effects of Perceived Impact. Journal of Developmental and Behavioral Pediatrics, *15, no. 6 (1994), 409–415.*

A community-based sample of 1200 young adults, ages 20 to 24, with chronic illnesses and disabilities who had been in state programs for Children With Special Health Care Needs in Illinois and Ohio were randomly selected for telephone interview. A total of 424 persons consented to be interviewed; of these, 138 were parents of offspring who were unable to communicate for themselves because of mental retardation or severe speech or language impairments. Of the 286 who could speak for themselves, all had a serious health problem that was treated on a regular basis and required special diet or equipment for care.

Data from the two-state sample were combined because there was little difference between the samples in Illinois and Ohio. Most respondents were unmarried, unemployed, and living with parents. About 40% were receiving entitlements (Supplemental Security Income or welfare). The Rosenberg Self-Esteem Scale reflected a relatively high esteem level in the sample as a whole. More than 25% of the respondents had low self-esteem scores, and these individuals were more likely to have:

• A history positive for mental health problems
• Mothers who completed less than a high school education
• No employment; relying on entitlements financially
• More severe or unpredictable conditions, more restricted activity, or unsure prognosis
• Hearing or speech problems, especially with concurrent learning disabilities

The Rosenberg Self-Esteem Scale may be a useful inventory to detect young adults with chronic health problems who are at risk for serious emotional problems. Within this high-risk group, interventions to reduce perceived impact of the chronic condition should be investigated.

ness. Biofeedback has been used to treat a variety of conditions (253, 270, 332).

Emotional Health Problems

Stress reactions, *physiologic and psychological changes resulting in unusually or disturbed adaptive behavior patterns,* result when the young adult is unable to cope with the newly acquired tasks and responsibilities. Mate selection, marriage, childrearing, college, job demands, social expectations, and independent decision making are all stressors that carry threats of insecurity and possibly some degree of failure. Some of these stress reactions take the form of physical illnesses just described. Others take the form of self-destructive behavior such as suicide, alcoholism, drug abuse and addiction, eating disorders, and smoking. Other stress reactions include abuse of spouse. Appendix III presents information and references pertinent to a stress management program. See also the section on Cognitive Theory in Chapter 5.

Self-destructive behavior, in the form of death by suicide, is increasing despite the many religious, cultural, and moral taboos. Thousands of people take their own lives or attempt suicide yearly.

Suicide. Suicide is the fourth leading overall cause of death among young adults in the United States and contributes to many physical, emotional, and social health problems for those who survive. Although medicine has decreased the threat of many physical illnesses, the present-day lifestyle has increased the physical, mental, and emotional stress on individuals. Suicide statistics might actually prove higher if all accidental deaths were investigated more closely for clues of suicidal intent. Many people deliberately conceal their suicide under the guise of an accident: driving their car off the road, combining alcohol and barbiturates, or discharging a gun while cleaning it (5, 150, 153, 332).

Women make the majority of unsuccessful suicide attempts, whereas men complete suicide more frequently. Both physiologic and psychological factors influence the choice of method for suicide. Women tend to use less lethal methods such as aspirin or barbiturate overdose, poisoning, or cutting the wrists. Men usually use the more lethal methods: gunshot wounds of the head or hanging. Women may see attempted suicide as a means of expressing aggression or manipulating relationships or events in the environment; therefore they select the less lethal methods. Degree of physical strength and the subconscious fear of disfigurement may also influence women's choice of methods (5, 166, 253, 332). Most of the time the person does not really desire death but rather a way out of an apparently hopeless or intolerable situation.

Statistics indicate that suicide occurs less frequently among married persons. Suicide is higher among single (especially males) and widowed individuals and highest among the divorced. Apparently married persons do not suffer from the social isolation and total lack of someone with whom to communicate as do the single, divorced, or widowed individuals. But the suicide rate for married persons less than 24 years of age is higher than for single persons. Perhaps these people sought marriage as an attempt to escape from their unmanageable situations. When marriage does not immediately solve their problems or creates new stresses, they end their lives (5, 166, 332).

Occupation is also an important factor in suicide rates. Professional groups such as dentists, psychiatrists, and physicians are considered high-risk groups, although the underlying causes for this are undetermined. The required strenuous educational courses or the stressful demands and responsibilities of their positions may be factors.

Consider three factors when planning primary prevention of suicide among young adults. Educate the public about emotional needs of the person and early signs of suicide so that high-risk persons can be more easily identified by family and friends. To compensate for the effects of separating from home and encountering a variety of stressors, a close and significant relationship should be established between the high-risk person and a caring person. The person needs opportunity to talk through frustration, anger, and despair and to formulate life plans. Finally, encourage young adults to participate in group and extracurricular activities that prevent social isolation.

Nursing responsibility for the suicidal person extends to the industrial setting, clinic, general or psychiatric hospital, and general community. You are in contact with and in the position to identify persons who may be potential candidates for suicide: unwed mothers, divorcees, widows and widowers, alcoholics, the terminally ill, and depressed people. Watch for signs of depression:

1. Expressions of overwhelming sadness, worthlessness, hopelessness, or emptiness.
2. Complaints of sleep and gastrointestinal disturbances, lack of energy, or chronic illness.
3. Decreased muscle tone with slumped shoulders, slowed gait, drooped faces.
4. Decreased interest in work, personal appearance, religion, family and friends, or special events.
5. Preference for being alone; self-preoccupied.

6. Unable to carry out ordinary tasks or make simple decisions.

Once identified, these signs of depression must be communicated to others: friends, relatives, a physician, or other persons concerned with the potentially suicidal person.

The person is more prone to attempt suicide *when the depression is lifting* and energy is greater. Listen closely to the person who speaks of being alienated, in an impossible situation, or of the future looking bleak and unchangeable, even after saying the situation is improving. He or she is a high-risk suicidal candidate, as is the person who talks of suicide, who has made an attempt, who is in crisis, or who is an alcoholic or a drug abuser (5, 166, 253, 332).

Your responsibility in individual suicide prevention varies according to the setting, the source, and extent of distress. You will need to protect the person against self-destructive behavior by reducing environmental hazards; but *emotional support is of greater importance while the person works through problems.* The principles of crisis intervention, therapeutic communication, and nurse–client relationship are discussed in psychiatric nursing texts (253, 332). Show the person verbally and non-verbally that someone—you—understands, respects, and cares about him or her.

You must know your own feelings about suicide and other self-destructive behavior. If you have more than transient depression, you cannot help another. You must see yourself and each person as an individual who possesses dignity and worth. Acceptance, understanding, and respect must be shown each person. Above all, you must be available and willing to listen. You can always listen long enough to assess and refer, even if you cannot work with the situation.

Alcoholism. Alcoholism, a complex disease, is also a form of self-destructive behavior. One suicide in every five is that of an alcoholic (5, 144, 166). In addition, many alcoholics literally drink themselves to death or die as a result of physical debilitation or injuries sustained while under the influence of alcohol.

In the United States there is much ambivalence about drinking. Some states prohibit the purchase and consumption of alcohol until the age of 21; other states have lowered the age to 18. Drinking frequently starts during preadolescence or early adolescence, is introduced by the parents, and follows the pattern of the person's parents. Thus with drinking behavior and expectancies poorly defined during the young years, lack of cultural norms of alcohol consumption, and individual biochemical predispositions, the state is set for alcoholism in later life.

Alcoholism may occur during any life period. Male alcoholics outnumber female alcoholics; however, identification of female alcoholics is increasing yearly. The alcoholic's life span is shortened approximately 12 years, and most alcoholics show physical and cognitive complications because of their prolonged drinking. In addition, millions of dollars are lost yearly in business as a result of absenteeism, lowered work efficiency, and accidents.

Alcoholism is a disease with physiologic, psychological, and sociologic aspects. Excessive drinking causes physiologic addiction and psychological dependence. Not drinking causes mild to severe withdrawal symptoms. Alcohol is used to relieve worry and guilt, and it falsely leads to an increased sense of adequacy and sociability. In turn, the person becomes more anxious and guilty when learning of his or her behavior while drinking. He or she drinks again to forget and deny. The vicious cycle becomes worse; behavior, performance, and health deteriorate until he or she is forced to seek help or dies. References at the end of this chapter give more information on the causes, psychodynamics, symptoms, and treatment of alcoholism (15, 105, 123, 162, 191, 204, 253, 299, 332). Alcoholism in nurse colleagues is a concern. Several references give more information (17, 107, 141, 332, 333, 347, 375).

The same stress-producing situations that led to suicide may also promote alcoholism in the young adult. Early case finding and early treatment are important in alcoholism, both for the ill individual and for the family members. A growing concern is the effect of the alcoholic parent on the development of the child(ren) (105, 162, 204, 227, 332). You can be active in both case finding and treatment.

Acceptance of the alcoholic as a sick person and providing support for those close to him or her are as important as the technical care you give during or after detoxification. You might write for the self-administered test for alcoholism that is available through the National Council for Alcoholism or Alcoholics Anonymous. A certain score indicates alcoholic tendencies.

Drug Abuse and Addiction. These are other forms of self-destructive behavior. Drug use and the nurse's responsibility are discussed in Chapter 11. The same information is applicable to the young adult. Drug abuse is increasing in the young adult, including all levels of workers, and abuse and addiction contribute to a number of other physical, emotional, and social health problems.

As with alcoholism, male addicts are more numerous than female ones. Symptoms of drug addiction differ with the type of drug, amount used, and personality of the user (see Table 11–6). Symptoms may also differ

> ### ► SIGNS AND SYMPTOMS OF DRUG ABUSE IN THE YOUNG ADULT
>
> • Late to work frequently; late in producing assignments
>
> • Increased absenteeism (Abusers miss twice as much work as nonabusing employees.)
>
> • Increased productivity in work for a short period (Cocaine will cause some people to perform better than normal or more creatively for a short time; overachievement can be used to compensate for or cover up initial stages of abuse.)
>
> • Falling productivity, poorer quality work, disorganized thinking and work outcome, missed deadlines
>
> • Forgetfulness, failure to follow instructions properly and to carry out usual steps of a procedure
>
> • Personality change, increasing irritability, depression, suspicion
>
> • Chronic runny nose from cocaine inhalation or sniffing glue or other chemicals that cause irritation of the nasal mucous membrane; regular complaints of a cold
>
> • Nodding or sleeping on the job
>
> • Accident proneness, clumsiness at work, poor gross or fine motor coordination on the job, reports of accidents in the auto or at home
>
> • Clandestine meetings and discussions with other employees (Users become dealers for fellow employees and withdraw from supervisory staff.)

for the young adult at work; see Signs and Symptoms of Drug Abuse in the Young Adult for a listing.

Treatment for drug abuse and addiction involves helping the person work through emotional problems, seeing that he or she has proper medical and nutritional regimens, helping him or her return to a community where the dangers of becoming addicted again are not too great, and helping him or her get involved in worthwhile work or activities. Several references cover the many facets of multiple addictions and their assessment and intervention (15, 17, 66, 105, 128, 162, 191, 204, 227, 253, 332, 375).

Eating Disorders. Eating disorders (anorexia and bulimia) currently are identified more frequently in young adults. Refer to Chapter 11 for information also pertinent to the young adult who has this condition. Several references provide helpful information (204, 224, 247, 252, 283).

Smoking. Smoking is considered self-destructive behavior because nicotine causes many harmful physiologic effects and is habit forming. Many people, even some with serious respiratory and vascular disorders, continue to smoke heavily despite the warnings from their physicians and reports from the Surgeon General's of-

fice about the harmful effects of smoking. Various reasons are given for smoking: smoking is relaxing; it prevents nervousness and overeating; and it gives the person something to do with his or her hands in social gatherings. All these reasons may stem from internal tensions and may well be the young person's way of dealing with stress. If the pattern of smoking is not altered during the stage of young adulthood, it may be impossible for changes to be made later in life.

More women than men now smoke cigarettes. Smoking in younger women has significantly increased the number of cardiac deaths and the incidence of lung cancer in women. Other health problems are also attributed to smoking. Smoking more than 10 cigarettes a day during pregnancy can cause low-birth-weight babies, premature births, spontaneous abortions, bleeding, fetal and neonatal deaths, and abnormal sperm and chromosomal damage in the newborn. Additional problems are periodontal disease, carcinoma in situ of the cervix, chronic respiratory disease, and shortened life expectancy. Offspring of the person who smokes are subject to more respiratory infections and allergies (132, 180, 294, 347).

Less well known, but equally dangerous, is that chemicals found in cigarette smoke are also commonplace in many work environments. Thus the person who smokes may suffer double jeopardy. Further, the person who smokes has more occupational accidents and injuries and uses more sick time and health benefits (49, 293).

Work with the young adult to reduce or stop cigarette smoking. To achieve this goal, you will have to do more than give information about morbidity and mortality rates. Explore his or her ideas of health and personal vulnerability to adverse effects from smoking. The social dynamics of smoking must also be considered. It is important not to ridicule the smoker or interpret his or her behavior and smoking norms. Realize that to give up smoking represents a loss. Help the person who is trying to stop smoking to acknowledge feelings of loss and grief related to giving up a part of self and social lifestyles. Instead of emphasizing that the person is "giving up" smoking, help the person verbalize feelings and identify what is being gained by a smoking cessation program. Give the person positive feedback for not smoking. Give the person time to change habits. If the person has smoked for many years, it is not easy to stop (134, 204, 270, 281, 291). See Smoking Cessation Suggestions for tips on the initiation, maintenance, and successful completion of a smoking cessation program (98, 204, 270, 332).

Battered or Abused Women. Battering is a social and emotional health problem of all socioeconomic levels that

► SMOKING CESSATION SUGGESTIONS

- Keep a notebook of current and past successes. Use the list as a reminder of your ability to succeed in new ventures.
- Identify a personal reason for quitting smoking other than because "it's bad for me."
- Make a list of things that are personally pleasurable; choose one as a reward (instead of a cigarette) when feeling uncomfortable or bored.
- Make a list of reasons smoking began and compare it with a list of current reasons for smoking.
- Keep a log of each cigarette lit, including the purpose; focus on smoking the cigarette and sensations occurring during and after smoking.
- Put cigarettes in an unfamiliar place.
- Every time you reach for a cigarette, ask "Do I really want this cigarette?," "Do I really need a cigarette?," "What can I do instead of smoking this cigarette?"
- Develop and prepractice responses to peer pressure to smoke.
- Smoke with the hand opposite that usually used.
- Buy cigarettes only by the pack, not by the carton.
- Buy different brands of cigarettes and avoid smoking two packs of the same brand in a row.
- Stay away from friends who smoke and from places where people smoke.
- End all meals with foods not associated with smoking (e.g., a glass of milk or half a grapefruit rather than a cup of coffee or a drink).
- Switch to noncaffeinated coffee or tea or bouillon.
- When using cigarettes as an energizer, substitute six small high-protein meals, sufficient sleep, a glass of milk, a piece of fresh fruit, or vegetable juice, exercise or movement, or a relaxation exercise.

- Have carrot sticks, celery, or sunflower seeds ready to chew instead of smoking a cigarette.
- Eat more foods that leave the body alkaline such as vegetables, seeds, and fruits and reduce the urge to smoke.
- Write a list of stress enhancers; learn structured relaxation and stress reduction approaches to deal with each stressor.
- Use affirmations such as, "I no longer smoke," "I can quit," "It's getting easier and easier to quit smoking," or "It's getting easier and easier to think about quitting smoking." Tell six people.
- Use deep breathing or breath for centering when the urge for a cigarette appears.
- Work with a peer who can be called for positive feedback when the urge for a cigarette occurs. Be sure the peer is positive about ability to quit and does not nag or induce guilt.
- Ask friends and co-workers not to leave cigarettes around or offer them.
- When the urge for a cigarette occurs, picture the word "STOP" in big red letters.
- Ask for a hug instead of having a cigarette.
- Choose a time to stop smoking when peak mental or physical performance is not expected.
- Write a contract and sign it with a trusted person so continuing to smoke will prove embarrassing or will result in great loss.
- Read articles and books by people who have successfully quit smoking or helped others to do so.
- When feeling depressed, talk with people who have successfully quit smoking and ask for information about why they are glad they quit.
- Reward self at specified intervals for not smoking.

has gained increasing public attention. Wife beating has always been a problem: woman was the man's property and beating was accepted behavior in some cultures. Traditionally the woman was too ashamed or too helpless to admit the problem or seek help. Further, no help existed. Efforts are being made in cities to make the police and legal system more aware of the **battered woman syndrome,** *a symptom complex of violence in which a woman has received deliberate and severe injury more than three times from the husband or a man with whom she has a close relationship.* Further, attempts have been made to make the police and legal system more protective of the woman who has been treated violently and more punitive to the violent man. Emergency shelters for battered women and their children are increasingly being established in urban areas so that the woman who seeks help does not have to return home or be at home when the man who was released shortly after arrest returns home even more violent than before. Crisis telephone lines have been established and publicized by the media, and hundreds of women have

memorized these numbers. In some communities rap sessions and referrals are available for battered women. Assistance to women seeking divorce is inadequate in most cities because of the cost and bureaucratic red tape (5, 165, 166).

You can work with other health and legal professionals to identify and overcome the problem of abused women. *Assessment of a family and woman* suffering adult abuse often reveals the following typical characteristics (54, 116, 142, 159–161, 165, 166, 212, 263, 313, 321, 332):

- The family and the woman are isolated socially or physically from neighbors, relatives, and friends.
- The woman feels increasing helplessness, guilt, isolation, and low self-esteem. She feels trapped and has been forced to be dependent on the man.
- The woman may range in age from 17 to 76 and may suffer violent injury for months or years.

- The woman's educational and occupational status is often higher than that of the man.
- Most beatings begin early in marriage and increase in frequency and intensity over the decades.
- Most violence occurs in the evening, on weekends, and in the kitchen.
- Generally there are no witnesses.
- The woman is frequently unable to leave the home because of lack of money, transportation, a place to go, support people, or support agencies in the community. Further, she has learned helplessness behaviors and feels unable to try to escape.
- The injuries from abuse may not be visible, but if abuse is present, the woman usually talks about the problem freely when asked directly if abuse is occurring.
- With increasing incidence of abuse and the physical and emotional consequences of abuse, the woman becomes more passive, less flexible, less able to think logically, more apathetic, depressed, and possibly suicidal.
- Eventually the frustration, stress, and anger may be externalized into physical behavior that is more than protective of the self or the child(ren); she may in turn become violent to the point of killing the battering partner.

Women remain in a threatening situation for many complex and interrelated reasons, as described in Reasons Why Women Are Unable to Leave a Violent Situation (165, 192). An astute assessment will uncover at least some of these characteristics and factors if present. Identification of Wife Abuse in the Health Care Setting describes some "red flags" that can help you identify a battered adult in an emergency room or intensive care, occupational, or other medical setting (5, 52, 62, 116, 142, 159–161, 165, 166, 228, 380).

Several authors present helpful information on assessment and treatment of the rape victim (54, 211, 212, 332). Increasingly the literature is discussing *marital* (not just date) *rape* as a problem in young adulthood. Marital rape meets the criteria for criminal sexual conduct. The difference is that the rapist and his victim are married; thus the man may be immune from prosecution. Often the women have been child victims of sexual abuse or incest, and there are physical, psychosomatic, and emotional effects. Some of the content related to the abused or battered women applies in this situation. Often children in these marriages are also raped or molested (5, 61, 62, 165, 166, 172, 263, 322, 366).

Incest, *sexual intercourse between biologically related persons,* is another form of battering that may af-

► REASONS WHY WOMEN ARE UNABLE TO LEAVE A VIOLENT SITUATION

- Lacking economic independence and being without money
- Being forbidden to leave the house or visit or call others
- Fearing being alone, being unable to support self and children, or the man's finding and harming her after she left him (Personal safety is a continual issue.)
- Lack emotional or social support (Often parents encouraged her to return to the abusive partner.)
- Believing that she is unworthy of anything better
- Having nowhere to go or being turned away from a public shelter
- Believing traditional norms related to women's role, marriage, religion, and violence; believing the woman is less than human
- Believing there are positive aspects of the relationship that the woman believes are worth preserving; emotional dependency in the relationship
- Desiring a father for her children; wanting to protect the children from greater harm
- Feeling disbelief, sense of horror, and shock about the man's violent behavior to her and denial or rationalizations that it would happen again
- Believing the man's promise that he will not hit again; thinking she can change him
- Finding the police unresponsive to calls for help (Many women have kept extensive records of the number of times legal action was taken with unsatisfactory results.)
- Taking responsibility for the violence, feeling guilty and that this behavior is her fault (Often the man would say, "Look what you made me do.")
- Feeling helpless; being unable to counter the power, authority, and threats of the man (Often the women were forced out or locked out of the home in the middle of the night in winter without clothing or money.)
- Increasing force or violence, which was condoned by police or society, from failing to comply with the husband's wishes or demands
- Relying on the sexual relation to punish him, to prevent battering, and to prove self-worth (Sexual enjoyment lessened as battering increased.)
- Wanting to protect the man's reputation in the community or in the job
- Having several small children and the related child care responsibility, often coupled with need to protect the children against the man's violence
- Fearing what would happen after leaving the home and man (welfare, homelessness, unemployment, single parenting) (Often there is a predictability about his behavior versus the unpredictability of the future.)
- Introjecting the societal attitude that the victim is to blame
- Believing that all marriages are like this (violent), especially if the woman grew up in a violent home

fect either the man or the woman, but more commonly the woman. Women victims of incest outnumber men 10 to 1. Incest is considered one form of sexual abuse, although adult family members may convey that incestual behavior is normal.

Symptoms and problems in adulthood resulting from childhood sexual abuse and incest are:

- Chronic depression, hopelessness related to shame and guilt
- Drug and alcohol abuse
- Various physical complaints, including symptoms of panic attacks, headaches, hysterical seizures
- Problems with trusting or intimate relationships with the opposite sex
- Character disorders such as borderline or narcissistic states
- Multiple personality disorders
- Sexual dysfunction and gynecologic problems

This problem is expected to affect more young adults in the future, based on the statistics currently of childhood sexual abuse and incest (5, 142, 166, 201).

Why do women leave the violent situation? Often the woman leaves when she feels suicidal but does not want to kill herself because of concern about the children's welfare; or the woman may fear for the life of the unborn child, if pregnant, or for the lives of her other children. Fear of being killed may be a motivator; acknowledging that the situation will never improve is important. The shock of a particular beating or the horror of being beaten while pregnant may be the turning point (an estimated 25–45% of pregnant women are battered). She realizes she has no power to make him change. At some point the woman may have received enough subtle or overt encouragement to leave or a new vision of what marriage and family life should be, coupled with a renewed sense of self-worth and the feeling she "doesn't have to take it anymore." The woman realizes the point at which the man no longer asks for forgiveness, shows no remorse (as he might have after the first beating), and usually denies he behaved violently. There comes a decision point, and then a plan may be made. Some women, however, leave abruptly to avoid being murdered (165). O'Campo et al. (263) also presents information about male violence against childbearing women.

Women may or may not be in acute distress when they leave. Despite the desperate situations and the difficulty in finding aid, these women are not typically helpless. Generally, they continually scheme how to stop the battering, either by examining personal behavior or planning ways to escape and how to get and keep some money. They take steps to please their partners and to satisfy their demands while protecting and caring for the children. Often they are the primary wage earner in the home. They may describe how they actively defended themselves; if they did not, it was not because they felt helpless but because other negative consequences or a worse beating would ensue (165).

► IDENTIFICATION OF WIFE ABUSE IN THE HEALTH CARE SETTING

Multiple Injuries

- Multiple abrasions and contusions to different anatomic sites should alert health care providers. There are relatively few ways of sustaining such injuries.

Body Map

- Many incidents of abuse involve injury to the face, neck, chest, breasts, or abdomen, whereas most accidents involve the extremities.

Rape

- Most women are raped by a male intimate, and many times rape is yet another incident of ongoing physical abuse.

Severity of Injury

- Severity varies among abused victims. Presentation of medically insignificant trauma to the emergency service may alert medical personnel that ongoing assault and impending danger constitute the real emergency for which she is seeking aid.

Pregnancy

- Abused women are more likely to be beaten when pregnant. There is a higher rate of miscarriage among battered women.

Trauma History

- A history of trauma can be the key indicator! Both asking about previous injuries and looking at her medical records are important. Records may indicate repeated visits and injuries to the same site.

Suicide Attempts

- Studies indicate that battering is a frequent precipitant of female suicide attempts; conversely, women who attempt suicide are likely to have a history of domestic violence.

Inconsistent Description of Injuries

- Injuries do not fit with the woman's description of the genesis of injury.

Vague and Nonspecific Complaints

- Complaints include, for example, anxiety, depression, and sleeplessness and many indicate intrafamilial crisis.

Heavy Use of Alcohol and Drugs

- Victims are more likely than nonvictims to use alcohol and drugs, and partners are much more likely to use alcohol and drugs excessively.

The *typical adult and parental behavior of the male batterer,* in order of incidence, according to the research by Sonkin, Martin, and Walker (313) is as follows:

1. Has battered a previous partner
2. Is employed, frequently under stress at work
3. Has children who have viewed the domestic violence and his battering behavior
4. Was under the influence of alcohol or drugs at the last battering incident
5. Uses physical punishment on his children
6. Has been violent with others not in their family, outside the home
7. Has been violent both when and when not under the influence of drugs and alcohol
8. Has a family history of suicide (attempted and completed)
9. Has been violent only when under the influence of alcohol and drugs
10. Has been violent only when not under the influence of alcohol or drugs
11. Lacks close friends or someone with whom to talk

Psychological violence by the man against the woman can be categorized as follows (313):

- Explicit threats
- Extreme controlling type of behavior, taking her everywhere; saying when she must come home; knowing her whereabouts, companions, and life activities
- Pathologic jealousy; continually questioning her about her behavior; making accusations without cause; highly suspicious
- Mental degradation; calling her names or telling her she is incompetent, stupid, and no good
- Isolating behavior (Because of his jealousy, suspicion and dependence, he controls the woman's behaviors so that she in turn becomes extremely isolated and dependent on him.)

The man who batters the female partner has the following typical childhood history, in order of incidence, according to research by Sonkin, Martin, and Walker (313):

1. Received physical punishment as a child
2. Saw his mother abused or treated violently by his father
3. Attacked one of the parents
4. Was physically abused as a child
5. Was sexually abused as a child

The male batterer comes from all walks of life and cultures. Personality characteristics of the male batterer that are typical include:

- Denying of or minimizing the violent behavior and its effects (The batterer may actually lose memory of the event because of his rage.)
- Blaming the behavior of the woman or others as the cause of the violent scenes
- Periodic uncontrollable anger and rage, which is externalized into physical and verbal behavior
- Dependency on the partner as sole source of love, support, intimacy, and problem solving, resulting from the controlling and isolating behavior that entwined him and the partner and children
- Sense of alienation from others and society (He considers himself a loner and therefore his "own boss"—means he can do whatever he wants in his home.)
- Jealousy of and suspiciousness of his partner, children, and finally everyone else
- Low self-esteem; lack of confidence in his ability to keep his partner; lack of skill or ability to ask for what is wanted in a nonthreatening way

Some stresses predispose to family violence and male battering of the woman and children. These stresses are listed in Stresses that Predispose to Family Violence.

You are in a position to (1) make a thorough and holistic assessment, using the prior content; (2) provide

▶ STRESSES THAT PREDISPOSE TO FAMILY VIOLENCE

- Financial pressures, low pay, high cost of living
- Family separation
- Geographic mobility; loss of friends, social supports, and familiarity
- Isolation and communication barriers
- Cultural differences; living in a strange environment or with unfamiliar customs, creating higher mutual dependence
- Lack of family support
- Living abroad such as in military families
- Inability to separate administrative or work roles from home life (Behavior that is functional at work may not be at home.)
- Lack of privacy at work or at home
- Job pressures or competitiveness; lack of support from supervisor

necessary crisis and emergency care; (3) encourage the battered woman to share her secret with you, another nurse, a social worker, confidante, or religious leader; (4) educate the public and abused women about the myths of abuse, as described in the Myths and Realities About Battered Women (see p. 634). (165, 166, 192); help her secure help from social service agencies, legal aid societies, counselors, health centers, and the welfare office; and (5) encourage separation from her husband if her life is in danger. Work with the individual woman to the extent possible for her to talk through her feelings of shame, guilt, embarrassment, anger, and fear. Help her gain courage to make decisions, including decisions on how to protect herself and her children, how to leave her husband, and where to go.

Group therapy and individual therapy are effective for the woman victim (61, 62, 142, 161, 165, 166, 192, 253). Group therapy may be more effective than individual therapy for the man as it helps him recognize angry and frustrated feelings in self, realize it is not acceptable to vent feelings through violent behavior to the spouse, and learn alternate coping and behavior patterns (31, 257, 313). Intervention must take into account incest, marital rape, and battering. Work also with the children, if possible. Research shows that children (ages 2–12) of battered women have deep feelings of fear about safety and abandonment, anger, confusion, social isolation, and aggression. The children's play reveals conflicts about overpowering adults and identification with the same-sex parent; children are learning abnormal behavior and roles that could be carried into their adult relationships and lifestyle (165). You can also work with others to establish emergency centers or crisis phone lines for the woman and to exert pressure to reform the current legal and judicial system so it will be more equitable to women.

Social support and the meaning a person attaches to stressful events can influence whether the person becomes ill or remains healthy—physically and emotionally—in a situation. The battered woman who extricates herself from her violent situation has strengthened her ability to survive, to resolve crisis, and to move forward (165).

The problem of spouse abuse, like that of child abuse discussed in Chapters 6 and 9, violent television programming discussed in Chapter 10, and elder abuse discussed in Chapter 14, is part of overall societal violence. Each professional, as a citizen and health care provider, must work in whatever way possible to decrease violence, its cause, and its effects. Several references provide additional information (53, 61, 116, 142, 161, 165, 166, 192, 201, 228, 381). Check also with the legal services of your area for information.

Hoff (165) describes the shelter experience for battered women and their children, the difficulties of poor and homeless women and children, the struggles of moving to a life without violence, the complexities of starting new relationships, and the effects on the children. Hoff calls the battered woman who removes herself from a violent situation not just a victim, but also a survivor. A 5-year follow-up study of the women showed their continued resilience despite hardships. Most still felt shock that someone who supposedly loved them beat them, but they also sensed victory, self-mastery, and recognition of their survival ability.

Social Health Problems

Divorce. **Divorce** is the *termination of marriage, preceded by a period of emotional distress in the marriage, separation, and legal procedures.* Divorce is a *crisis* for those involved and can affect society in general as well as the physical and emotional health of the persons involved (5, 25, 50, 77, 94, 146, 166, 351).

Some young people enter marriage to escape the problems of young adulthood. Marriage provides them with a ready-made role, and it supposedly solves the problem of isolation. If marriage takes place before the individual has developed a strong sense of identity and independence, however, intimacy cannot be achieved.

Most divorces (one in two marriages) occur in the first 3 to 5 years of married life and involve persons less than 29 years of age. These couples are frequently from lower economic groups and have married at an early age. They tend to have less education and money and fewer personal resources than couples from higher economic groups. Approximately one in four children lives with a single parent as a result (187, 203).

Marriage often breaks down because of the partners' inability to satisfy deep mutual needs in a close demanding relationship. One of the partners may be overly dependent and seek in the other a mother or father. Dependent behavior may at first meet the needs of the more independent partner. But as the dependent person matures, the relationship is changed. If the stronger partner neither understands nor allows this change, divorce may follow.

Emotional deprivation in childhood is also a poor foundation for marriage. The deprived person grows up without sufficient experience of feeling acknowledged, wanted, appreciated, or loved. He or she has low self-esteem and is too sensitively tuned to rejection and not adequately responsive to acceptance and approval. He or she can easily misinterpret the partner's behavior, feel exploited, and have difficulty accepting any form of appreciation and love. The person from a home in

► ## MYTHS AND REALITIES ABOUT BATTERED WOMEN

Myth 1: Battered Women Are a Small Percentage of the Overall Population.

- **Fact:** Domestic violence is the most underreported crime in the United States. The Federal Bureau of Investigation estimates that 60% of all married women experience physical violence by their husbands at some time during their marriage. There are an estimated 2 to 6 million female victims of family violence each year.

Myth 2: Battered Women Are Masochistic.

- **Fact:** Battered women are *not* masochistic. The prevailing belief has always been that only women who "liked it and deserved it" were battered; that women experienced some pleasure, often akin to sexual pleasure, from being beaten by the men they love. Because this is such a prevailing stereotype, many battered women begin to wonder if indeed they are masochistic.

Myth 3: Battered Women Are Crazy.

- **Fact:** Battered women are not crazy, although battering may contribute to mental illness. This myth places the blame for battering on the woman's negative personality characteristics and takes the focus off the batterer. Further, being abused and beaten may result in what apparently is abnormal behavior — the woman's attempt to adapt.

Myth 4: Middle-Class Women Are Not Battered as Frequently or as Violently as Poorer Women.

- **Fact:** Women from lower socioeconomic classes are more likely to come in contact with community agencies, so their problems are more visible. Middle- and upper-class women often fear that disclosure will result in social embarrassment and harm to their own or their husband's career or that people will not believe them. This is often true when the husband is held in high esteem in the community.

Myth 5: Women From Ethnic or Racial Minority Groups Are Battered More Frequently Than Caucasian Women.

- **Fact:** Studies show that battering crosses all ethnic lines, with no one group suffering more than another.

Myth 6: Battered Women Are Uneducated and Have Few Job Skills.

- **Fact:** Educational levels of battered women range from grade school through completion of professional and doctoral degrees. Many successful career women would be willing to give up their careers if to do so would eliminate battering. Changing jobs or staying home to ease the situation usually has no effect on their partner's behavior, and sometimes battering worsens.

Myth 7: Batterers Are Unsuccessful and Lack Resources to Cope With the World.

- **Fact:** It has been suggested that men who feel less capable than women resort to violence. Contrary findings were reported in England, where the highest incidence of wife beating was among physicians, service professionals, and police. Affluent batterers include attorneys, professors, and salesmen. Many of these men donate a great deal of their time to community activities and could not maintain their involvement in these projects without the support of their wives.

Myth 8: Batterers Are People With Personality Disorders.

- **Fact:** If batterers could simply be considered antisocial personalities, individual therapy could be used to differentiate batterers from other men. Unfortunately, it is not that simple. One trait they share is the ability to use charm as a manipulative technique. Manipulation, acting out of anger, exhilaration felt when they dominate and beat the woman, and denial of the behavior are characteristic of people with personality disorders.

Myth 9: Police Can Protect Battered Women.

- **Fact:** At most, only 10% of battered women call the police. Of those who did, many believe the police officers were ineffective. When the police left, the men continued the assault with vigor. In St. Louis a pro-arrest policy is improving police response to domestic violence. Several thousand women are murdered annually by male partners, often as a part of the battering act. At least one-half of the injuries presented by women at an emergency room are the result of battering. Battering may also be the basis for a suicide attempt.

Myth 10: Batterers Are Violent in All Their Relationships.

- **Fact:** Most men who batter their wives are generally not violent in other aspects of their lives. Although being violent in public has definite, negative consequences, there are few consequences in domestic cases.

Myth 11: The Batterer Is Not a Loving Partner.

- **Fact:** Batterers are often described by women during the honeymoon phase of the cycle of violence as fun-loving, playful, attentive, sensitive, exciting, and affectionate. The woman may describe some very positive characteristics in the man that cause her truly to love him.

Myth 12: Long-standing Battering Relationships Can Change for the Better.

- **Fact:** Relationships that have rested on the man's having power over the woman are stubbornly resistant to an equal power-sharing arrangement. Even with the best of help, such relationships usually do not become battering-free.

(continued)

> ## ► MYTHS AND REALITIES ABOUT BATTERED WOMEN (continued)
>
> ### Myth 13: Once a Batterer, Always a Batterer.
>
> - **Fact:** Batterers can be taught to change their aggressive responses; however, very few batterers are willing to get help. If the batterer does not get treatment and if he is divorced and then remarries, he is likely to batter the next woman he marries.
>
> ### Myth 14: Battered Women Can Always Leave Home.
>
> - **Fact:** Many battered women have no place to go and no means of survival outside the framework of their marriage. They also may have small children to care for, whom they would not want to leave home alone with the father. Because battering weakens a woman's self-esteem, she may believe she is incapable of managing on her own.
>
> ### Myth 15: Battered Women Are Weak and Come From a Bad Background.
>
> - **Fact:** Typically the battered woman in Hoff's study (166) had a warm, loving relationship as a child with the mother and a negative, destructive relationship with the father. Not all battered women were abused as children. Women who experienced violence before they were battered by their mates showed resilience and strength. But long-standing abuse breeds self-degradation and despair so that a women feels unworthy of the continued love of even her mother and unable to reach out for help. The battered woman should be considered a survivor type of person.
>
> ### Myth 16: Battering May Occur Only Once or Infrequently and Could Be Predicted, and Thus Prevented, by the Woman.
>
> - **Fact:** For most of the battered women in several studies, the violence was frequent, extended over time, and often unexpected and included many similar incidents. Often violence occurred concomitantly with the man's rages, drunkenness, and/or financial insecurity and during the woman's pregnancy. Often each beating was worse than the previous one. Women consistently report doing everything possible to avoid violence; they try to second-guess the husband. "It's like walking on eggshells." Women have been socialized into the nurturing role, so they doggedly try to succeed in it as wife and mother, regardless of the circumstances. Further, society and medical and psychiatric services and professionals reinforce the belief that the woman's troubles are the result of her own inadequacies and failures (men are taught that the source of stress is other than self). Although the battered woman may think of hurting or killing the man as a punishment, the woman is often inhibited from such action by concern for the children, if present, and fear of consequences for self. Yet there have been times that the women retaliated; most women found that if they fought back, the man became even more violent.

which the parents' marital relationship was one of detachment, disharmony, or conflict or in which abuse or divorce occurred is poorly prepared for marriage. He or she has no healthy or loving marital model to follow. The person may try to model the marriage after another's happy marriage; however, the person learns most thoroughly that which is lived during childhood.

The divorce rate reflects the ease with which a divorce can be obtained. The lack of commitment to people and relationships when the going gets tough, seen also in other areas of life, and the dichotomy between the romanticized ideal of marriage and the reality of married life contribute to separation and divorce. Further, our youth are not educated for family life in any formal sense, and what they learn in the home may be poor preparation for marriage and good preparation for the divorce court.

When marriage fails and bonds are broken, aloneness, anger, mistrust, hostility, guilt, shame, a sense of betrayal, fear, disappointment, loss of identity, anxiety, and depression, alone or in combination, can appear both in the divorcee and the one initiating the divorce. Eventually there may be a feeling of relief. There must be an interval of adjustment to the physical and emotional loss. Often the second marriage is a rebound affair: a partner is selected as soon as possible to help assuage the feelings from the divorce and relieve the loneliness. Second and subsequent remarriages can be successful, but they carry a higher risk of instability and are more likely to end in divorce because of (1) the person's lack of ability to form a mutually satisfactory new relationship; (2) the past experiences, vulnerability, guilt, and insecurity that cannot be easily removed; (3) the hassles of her kids, his kids, and their kids; (4) child and wife support; and (5) interference from the ex-spouse. Psychological effects of divorce vary because of the following factors: (1) family psychodynamics before divorce; (2) nature of the marital breakup; (3) relationship between the ex-spouses after the divorce; (4) developmental age and coping skills of the children, if any, during the time of marital disharmony and divorce; and (5) coping skills of each ex-spouse. If the offspring are adolescents, expression and control of aggressive and sexual impulses, dependency–independency issues, deidealization of the parents, peer acceptance and social approval, and premature responsibilities of adulthood may intensify.

Children, even 15 or more years later, suffer from the consequences—emotional and social—of divorce. The problems of low self-esteem, depression, anxiety about intimacy and relationships, mistrust of others and close relationships, depression, guilt, and fantasies about the parents' reunion remain strong for many years (187, 240, 364). Thus some researchers believe it is critical for parents to work at resolving marital conflicts, to recommit to each other, and ultimately to improve the relationship and gain greater maturity. Health care professionals and society must provide support systems so that parents can work out their stresses in other than divorce courts (187, 240, 364).

If the divorce cannot be prevented, the parents and children should be given emotional support. (Mothers and children may also have to struggle to meet physical needs and may need help in getting financial support.) The losses must be resolved, a new identity must be formed, and the children involved should have the option of continued close relationships with both parents (25, 73, 77, 91, 94, 146, 187, 351, 364).

If the person embarks on a second marriage with an understanding of how he or she has matured and of the reasons the first marriage failed, the second marriage may be satisfactory. If the mistakes of the first marriage are repeated in finding a partner, the second marriage is also likely to fail. The person may meander from one relationship to another, hoping for satisfaction, but always finding frustration and disappointment because he or she carries within self the seeds of failure. Ideally, the second marriage should be entered into with time (at least 1 year) and thought. The success of the second marriage depends on finding another person with whom common needs can be met and whose personality development matches that of the divorcee (25, 77, 91, 94, 146, 166, 253, 351).

Recently more emphasis has been given to helping people through the emotions involved in divorce. Divorce has been likened to death except that contact is often maintained, especially if small children are involved (73, 91, 94, 146, 166, 253, 364).

Helping divorced women identify and pursue personal goals is important. Primary needs of divorced women are economic independence, education, managing parenting, maintaining friendships, establishing a partner relationship, and obtaining adequate housing, school, and environment for self and children. Mental health goals are a low priority, although the theme of accepting the divorce and establishing a happy lifestyle as a single-parent family would encompass mental health. Support groups for the divorced woman can assist her in meeting needs and securing goals. Such groups can also assist the woman with custody rights and with obtaining child support.

Groups for children of divorcing and divorced parents can help the child work through the feelings of loss, anger, guilt, and ambivalence about relationships with parents and often, eventually, stepparents and stepsiblings. The key is for the parents to continue showing love to their child(ren) and to maintain open communication between them about the offspring.

The ideal situation is for the departing parent to be pictured in the best possible light by the one with whom the child remains and for unimpeded contact to be maintained. The child should be given honest information at whatever level he or she can understand. The child must know that he or she did not cause the divorce. Delinquency, lack of sex identification, and eventually inability to form a lasting relationship may result in the child unless he or she is handled with care.

Abortion. Changing legislation and changing social attitudes toward women's rights, sexual mores, and human life are present in the United States. The trend is pro-life. Many young adult women, married and unmarried and of all socioeconomic classes, are having abortions to terminate unwanted pregnancies; many other unmarried women are choosing to keep their babies. Abortion should not be considered lightly. Abortion induces physical complications such as hemorrhage and later cervical incompetency. Emotional anguish, guilt, unhappiness, or self-directed anger sometimes follows the decision to have an abortion. The mature young adult must consider the consequences of sexual activity. *The Post-Abortion Review* published by the Elliot Institute, PO Box 9079, Springfield, IL 62791, presents information about the ethical and moral issues, the woman's reactions, the many consequences, and pre- and postabortion counseling and avenues of assistance.

As a nurse, you may experience considerable emotional turmoil unless you think through the abortion issue. Women or men seeking your counsel on this issue need to hear a professional presentation. If you feel incapable of this counsel, refer the person to someone who can counsel.

Continuing Health Promotion. As a nurse, realize that the health state of the young adult and the type of health care sought are influenced by the person's background, knowledge, experience, philosophy, and lifestyle. Young adults with health problems might more readily seek care and information if they could find programs compatible with their expectations and lifestyles. You can initiate programs that are specifically aimed at young adults, as they seem to accept the treatment plan more readily when they understand the rationale and expected effects. Keep the previously discussed health problems and unmet physiologic needs in mind as you talk with young adults and plan and give care.

Young adulthood ends in the forties when the person should have a stable position in society and the knowledge of what he or she can make out of life. Your

► CONSIDERATIONS FOR THE YOUNG ADULT
IN HEALTH CARE

- Cultural and family background, values, support systems, community resources
- Relationships with family of origin, extended family, family of friends or spouse
- Behaviors that indicate abuse by spouse or significant other
- Physical characteristics, nutritional status, and rest/sleep and exercise patterns that indicate health and are age-appropriate
- Integrated self-concept, body image, and sexuality
- Immunizations, safety education, and other health promotion measures used
- Demonstration of continued learning and use of Formal Operations and Concrete Operations competencies in cognitive ability
- Overall appearance and behavioral patterns that indicate intimacy rather than isolation
- Behavioral patterns that demonstrate a value system, continuing formation of philosophy of life, and moral–spiritual development.
- Established employment, vocation, or profession, including homemaking and child care
- Behavioral patterns that reflect commitment to parenting, if there are children
- Relationships with work colleagues, coping skills for work stress
- Demonstration of integration of work and leisure and avoidance of physical or emotional illness
- Behavioral patterns and characteristics indicating the young adult has achieved developmental tasks

SUMMARY

Young adulthood is a time of stabilization. Physical growth is completed. The person has established independence from parents but maintains a friendly relationship with them. The person is settling into a committed intimate relationship and friendships and into career or profession. The couple may choose to become parents or to remain single. Development continues in the cognitive, emotional, social, and moral–spiritual dimensions. The philosophy of life is being formulated. Behaviors, whether at home, on the job, at leisure, or with family, friends, or strangers, are adaptive in response to stressors. Stress effects may result in unhealthy habits or physical or emotional illness.

Considerations for the Young Adult in Health Care and Chart 5 in Appendix IV summarize what you should consider in assessment and health promotion of the young adult. The family is included in Considerations. Chart 5 presents the American Academy of Family Physicians Periodic Health Examination Ages 19–39 Years. It includes guidelines for screening, health counseling, immunization schedules, and high-risk categories (10).

efforts at teaching and counseling can enhance the young adult's awareness of health promotion and establish a program to make that position more stable.

Continuing Adjustments. One couple invited others to a celebration of their 25th wedding anniversary with the following words (385):

We continue to adjust to each other, an adjustment that started 25 years ago, and will never stop because we each continue to grow and change. We will always be different.

Don't mistake it for a solid marriage. There is no such thing. Marriage is more like an airplane than a rock. You have to commit the thing to flight, and then it creaks and groans, and keeping it airborne depends entirely on attitude. Working at it, though, we can fly forever. Only the two of us know how hard it has been or how worthwhile.

Celebrate with us . . .

► **REFERENCES**

1. A Change in the Women's Health Initiative, *Harvard Women's Health Letter*, 2, no. 11 (1995), 7.
2. A Genetic Key to Breast Cancer, *Harvard Women's Health Watch*, 3, no. 4 (1995), 1.
3. Aaronson, L., Perceived and Received Support: Effects on Health Behavior During Pregnancy, *Nursing Research*, 38, no. 1 (1989), 4–9.
4. Adult Children of Lesbians, *The Harvard Mental Health Letter*, 12, no. 6 (1995), 1.
5. Aguilera, D., and J. Messick, *Crisis Intervention: Theory and Methodology* (6th ed.). St. Louis: C.V. Mosby, 1989.
6. Alderman, L., How to Tell the Boss You're Getting Worked to Death—Without Killing Your Career, *Money*, May (1995), 41–42, 44.
7. Allan, J., Identification of Health Risks in a Young Adult Population, *Journal of Community Health Nursing*, 4, no. 4 (1987) 225–233.
8. Alward, R., Are You a Lark or an Owl on the Night Shift? *American Journal of Nursing*, 88 (1988), 1337–1339.
9. Alward, R.R., and T.H. Monk. A Comparison of Rotating Shift and Permanent Night Nurses, *International Journal of Nursing Studies*, 27, no. 3 (1990), 297–302.
10. American Academy of Family Physicians, *Age Charts for Periodic Health Examination*. Washington, DC: Author, 1995.
11. American Cancer Society. *Cancer Facts and Figures—1994*. Atlanta: American Cancer Society, 1994.
12. American Nurses Association, *The Nurse's Shift Work Handbook*. Washington, DC: Author, 1994.

13. American Psychiatric Association, *Diagnostic and Statistical Manual of Mental Disorders* (4th ed.). Washington, DC: American Psychiatric Association, 1994.

14. Ammon-Gaberson, K., Adult Learning Principles, *AORN Journal,* 45, no. 4 (1987), 961–963.

15. Archer, L., B. Grant, and D. Dawson, What If Americans Drunk Less? The Potential Effect on the Prevalence of Alcohol Abuse and Dependence, *American Journal of Public Health,* 85 (1995), 61–66.

16. Antioxidants Re-Examined, *Harvard Women's Health Watch,* 1, no. 11 (1994), 1.

17. Antai-Otong, D., Helping the Alcoholic Patient Recover, *American Journal of Nursing,* 95, no. 8 (1995), 22–29.

18. Arlin, P., Cognitive Development in Adulthood: A Fifth Stage? *Developmental Psychology,* 11, no. 5 (1975), 602–606.

19. Aronson, J.K., Chronopharmacology: Reflections on Time and a New Text, *Lancet,* 335, no. 8704 (1990), 1515–1516.

20. Axinn, W., and A. Thornton, The Relationship Between Cohabitation and Divorce: Selectivity or Caused Influence, *Demography,* 29 (1992), 358.

21. Badgers, J., Tips for Managing Stress on the Job, *American Journal of Nursing,* 95, no. 9 (1995), 31–33.

22. Bailey, K., M. Hoepner, S. Jeska, S. Schneller, and C. Wolohan, The Nurse as an Educator, *Journal of Nursing Staff Development,* 11, no. 4 (1995), 205–209.

23. Bailey, W.T., Fathers' Involvement in Their Children's Healthcare. *The Journal of Genetic Psychology,* 152, no. 3 (1990), 289–293.

24. Barrick, B., Light at the End of a Decade, *American Journal of Nursing,* 90, no. 11 (1990), 37–40.

25. Barron, C., Causal Explanations and Emotional Health of Women During Divorce, *Archives of Psychiatric Nursing,* 3, no. 5 (1989), 266–271.

26. Basow, S., *Sex Role Stereotypes: Traditions and Alternatives.* Monterey, CA: Brooks/Cole, 1980.

27. Batz, J., Casting the Sex Roles, *Universitas,* Spring (1990), 5–9.

28. Beh, H.C., and P.J. McLaughlin, Mental Performance of Air Crew Following Layovers on Transzonal Flights, *Ergonomics,* 34, no. 2 (1991), 123–136.

29. Bell, A., M. Weinberg, and S. Hammersmith, *Sexual Preference: Its Development in Men and Women.* Bloomington, IN: Indiana University Press, 1981.

30. Bellak, L., and L. Goldsmith, *The Broad Scope of Ego Function Assessment.* New York: John Wiley & Sons, 1984.

31. Bennett, G., Group Therapy for Men Who Batter Women: Some Promising Developments, *Holistic Nursing Practice,* 1, no. 2 (1987), 33–42.

32. Benson, H., *Beyond the Relaxation Response.* New York: William Morrow, 1988.

33. Bentley, K.S., and R.B. Fox, Mothers and Fathers of Young Children: Comparison of Parenting Styles. *Psychological Reports,* 69 (1991), 320–322.

34. Berger, K.S., *The Developing Person Through the Life Span.* New York: Worth, 1988.

35. Bes, F., et al., The Distribution of Slow-wave Sleep Across the Night: A Comparison for Infants, Children, and Adults, *Sleep,* 14, no. 1 (1991), 5–12.

36. Bevier, P., M. Chiasson, R. Hefferman, and K. Castro, Women at a Sexually Transmitted Disease Clinic Who Reported Some Sex Contact: Their HIV Seroprevalence and Risk Behaviors, *American Journal of Public Health,* 85 (1995), 1366–1371.

37. Biddle, C., and T.R. Oaster, The Nature of Sleep. *AANA Journal,* 58, no. 1 (1990), 36–44.

38. Binkley, S., et al., Human Daily Rhythms Measured for One Year, *Physiological Behavior,* 48, no. 2 (1990), 293–298.

39. Black, A., Game of Life, *Elle,* January (1992), 62–63.

40. Bonheur, B.B., Creating a New Learning: The Story of Art and Prudent Art, *The Journal of Continuing Education in Nursing,* 25, no. 5 (1994), 209–212.

41. Boning up with Fluoride, *Harvard Health Letter,* 21, no. 2 (1995), 8.

42. Bootzin, R., H. Lahmeyer, and J. Lilie, eds., *Integrated Approach to Sleep Management.* Washington, DC: American Nurses Association, 1994.

43. Bozett, F., *Gay and Lesbian Parents.* New York: Praeger, 1987.

44. Bradley-Springer, L., Nutritional Support in HIV Infection: A Multilevel Analysis, *IMAGE Journal of Nursing Scholarship,* 23 (1991), 155–159.

45. Breast Cancer: Environmental Influences, *Harvard Women's Health Watch,* 1, no. 8 (1994), 1.

46. Breast Cancer: Invasive Disease, *Harvard Women's Health Watch,* 3, no. 2 (1995), 4–6.

47. Brentin, L., and A. Sieh, Caring for the Morbidly Obese, *American Journal of Nursing,* 91, no. 8 (1991), 41–43.

48. Brewer, M.J., To Sleep or Not to Sleep: The Consequences of Sleep Deprivation, *Critical Care Nurse,* 5, no. 6 (1985), 35–41.

49. Brigham, J., J. Cross, M. Stitzer, and L. Felch, Effects of a Restricted Work Site Policy on Employees Who Smoke, *American Journal of Public Health,* 84 (1994), 773–778.

50. Broom, B., Impact of Marital Quality and Psychological Well-being on Parental Sensitivity, *Nursing Research,* 43 (1994), 138–143.

51. Broverman, B., Eliciting Assessment Data From the Patient Who Is Difficult to Interview, *Nursing Clinics of North America,* 25, no. 4 (1990), 743–750.

52. Bullock, L., and J. McFarlane, The Birth-Weight/Battering Connection, *American Journal of Nursing,* 89, no. 9 (1989), 1153–1155.

53. ——, et al., The Prevalence and Characteristics of Battered Women in a Primary Care Setting, *Nurse Practitioner,* 14, no. 6 (1989), 47–56.

54. Burgess, A., W. Fehder, and C. Hartman, Delayed Reporting of the Rape Victim, *Journal of Psychosocial Nursing,* 33, no. 9 (1995), 21–29.

55. Burke, R., Generation X: Measures, Sex, and Age Differences, *Psychology Reports,* 74, no. 2 (1994), 555–562.

56. Burman, M., Health Diaries in Nursing Research, *IMAGE: Journal of Nursing Scholarship,* 27 (1995), 147–152.

57. Buxman, K., Make Room for Laughter, *American Journal of Nursing,* 91, no. 12 (1991), 46–51.

58. Cabral, H., et al., Foreign-born and US-born Black Women: Differences in Health Behaviors and Birth Outcomes. *American Journal of Public Health,* 80, no. 1 (1990), 70–72.

59. Caffeine and Health: The Caffeine Connection, *Harvard Women's Health Watch,* 1, no. 8 (1994), 2–3.

60. Campbell, A., ed., *The Opposite Sex: The Complete Illustrated Guide to Differences Between the Sexes.* New York: Salem House, 1989.

61. ——, and P. Alford. The Dark Consequences of Marital Rape, *American Journal of Nursing,* 89, no. 7 (1989), 846–849.

62. ——, and D.J. Sheridan, Emergency Nursing Interventions With Battered Women, *Journal of Emergency Nursing,* 15, no. 1 (1989), 12–17.

63. Cates, W., and S. Bowen, Education for AIDS Prevention: Not Our Only Voluntary Weapon, *American Journal of Public Health,* 79, no. 7 (1989), 871–874.

64. Centers for Disease Control and Prevention General Recommendations on Immunization: Recommendations of the

Advisory Committee on Immunization Practices (ACIP), *Morbidity and Mortality Weekly Report,* 43 (January 28, 1994), 23.

65. Chase, M., H. Morales, and R. Francisco, The Atonia and Myoclonia of Active (REM) Sleep, *Annual Review of Psychology,* 41 (1990), 557–584.

66. Chen, K., and D. Kandel, The National History of Drug Use from Adolescence to the Mid-thirties in a General Population Sample, *American Journal of Public Health,* 85 (1995), 41–47.

67. Chiropractic Manipulation, *Harvard Women's Health Watch,* 3, no. 4 (1995), 4–5.

68. Clare, A.W., Pre-menstrual Syndrome: Single or Multiple Causes? *Canadian Journal of Psychiatry,* 30 (1985), 474–480.

69. Clemen-Stone, S., D. Eigsti, and S. McGuire, *Comprehensive Family and Community Health Nursing* (4th ed.). St. Louis: C.V. Mosby, 1995.

70. "Clinical Guidelines," *The Nurse Practitioner,* 20, no. 2 (1995), 69.

71. Clinton, J., Expectant Fathers at Risk for Couvade, *Nursing Research,* 35, no. 5 (1986), 290–294.

72. Clodore, M., et al., Psychophysiological Effects of Early Morning Bright Light Exposure in Young Adults, *Psychoneuroendocrinology,* 15, no. 3 (1990), 193–205.

73. Cohen, M., *Long Distance Parenting: A Guide for Divorced Parents.* New York: Nal-Dutten, 1989.

74. Coleman, E.A., and H. Pennypacker, Evaluating Breast Self-examination Performance, *Journal of Nursing Quality Assurance,* 5, no. 3 (1991), 65–69.

75. Comiskey, A., *Pursuing Sexual Wholeness: How Jesus Heals the Homosexual.* Lala Mary, FL: Creation House, 1989.

76. Coombs, R., Marital Success and Personal Well-being: A Literature Review, *Family Relations,* 40 (1991), 97–102.

77. Dacey, J., and J. Travers, *Human Development Across the Lifespan* (3rd ed.). Madison, WI: Brown & Benchmark, 1996.

78. Davies, J., and M. Frawley, *Treating the Adult Survivor of Childhood Sexual Abuse: A Psychoanalytic Approach.* New York: Basic Books, 1994.

79. Davis, C., and M.J. Lentz, Circadian Rhythms: Charting Oral Temperatures to Spot Abnormalities. *Journal of Gerontological Nursing,* 15, no. 4 (1989), 34–41.

80. Dawson, D.A. (1991) Family Structure and Children's Health: United States, 1988, *Vital and Health Statistics,* Series 10: No. 178 (DHHS Publication No. (PHS) 91-1506).

81. Dawson, D.A. (1991) Family Structure and Children's Health and Well-being: Data From the 1988 National Health Interview on Child Health, *Journal of Marriage and the Family,* 53, 573–584.

82. Decousus, H., et al., Circadian Dynamics of Coagulation and Chronopathology of Cardiovascular and Cerebrovascular Events: Future Therapeutic Implications for the Treatment of These Disorders? *Annals of the New York Academy of Science,* 618 (1991), 159–165.

83. Denney, N., T. Tozier, and C. Schlotthauer, The Effect of Instructions on Age Differences in Practical Problem Solving, *Journal of Gerontology: Psychological Sciences,* 47 (1992), P142–P145.

84. DiClemente, R.J. "Confronting the Challenge of AIDS in the African American Community," *Ethnic Origins.,* 2, no. 4 (1992), 358–360.

85. Dobson, J., *Life on the Edge: A Young Adult's Guide to a Meaningful Future.* Dallas: World, 1995.

86. Donovan, P., A Prescription of Sexually Transmitted Diseases, *Issues in Science and Technology,* 9, no. 4 (1993), 40.

87. Drake, M., et al., Spouses' Body Image Change During and After Pregnancy: A Republican in Canada, *IMAGE: Journal of Nursing Scholarship,* 20, (1988), 88–92.

88. Drew, B.J., Cardiac Rhythm Responses: Review of 22 Years of Nursing Research, Part 2, *Heart and Lung Journal of Critical Care,* 18, no. 2 (1989), 184–191.

89. Drimmer, A., If the Shoe Fits, Wear It, *St. Louis Manager,* March (1986), 24–26.

90. Duffy, M., When a Woman Heads a Household, *Nursing Outlook,* 30, no. 5 (1982), 468–473.

91. ——, C. Mowbray, and M. Hudes, Personal Goals of Recently Divorced Women, *IMAGE: Journal of Nursing Scholarship,* 22, no. 1 (1990), 14–17.

92. Dugan, D., Laughter and Tears: Best Medicine for Stress, *Nursing Forum,* 24, no. 1 (1989), 18–26.

93. Duvall, E., and B. Miller, *Marriage and Family Development* (6th ed.). New York: Harper & Row, 1984.

94. Dworetzky, J., *Human Development: A Lifespan Approach* (2nd ed.). St. Paul: West, 1995.

95. Eastman, C.I., Natural Summer and Winter Sunlight Exposure Patterns in Seasonal Affective Disorder, *Physiological Behavior,* 48, no. 5 (1990), 611–616.

96. ——, and K.J. Miescke, Entrainment of Circadian Rhythms with 26-h Bright Light and Sleep–Wake Schedules, *American Journal of Physiology,* 259, no. 6 (1990), 1189–1197.

97. Easum, W., *How to Reach Baby Boomers,* Nashville: Abingdon Press, 1991.

98. Edelman, C., and C. Mandle, *Health Promotion Throughout the Lifespan* (3rd ed.). St. Louis: C.V. Mosby, 1994.

99. Edmunds, M., Strategies for Promoting Physical Fitness, *Nursing Clinics of North America,* 26, no. 4 (1991), 855–866.

100. Erikson, E., *Childhood and Society* (2nd ed.). New York: W.W. Norton, 1963.

101. ——, ed., *Adulthood.* New York: W.W. Norton, 1978.

102. Estrogen and the Heart, *Harvard Women's Health Watch,* 1, no. 12 (1994), 7.

103. *Evaluation and Management of Early HIV Infection, Clinical Practice Guideline, No. 7,* U.S. Department of Health and Human Service, Agency for Health Care Policy and Research, January 1994.

104. Evans, C., Reducing AIDS Anxiety on the Unit With Preventive Infection Control, *Journal of Psychosocial Nursing,* 28, no. 1 (1990), 36–39.

105. Evans, K., and J. Sullivan, *Treating Addicted Survivors of Trauma.* New York: Guilford Press, 1995.

106. Exercise: What Is Enough, *Harvard Health Letter,* 20, no. 11 (1995), 6.

107. Farley, P., and M. Hendrix, Impaired and Non-impaired Nurses During Childhood and Adolescence, *Nursing Outlook,* 41, no. 1 (1993), 25–31.

108. Fawcett, J., et al., Spouses' Body Image Changes During and After Pregnancy: A Replication and Extension, *Nursing Research,* 35, no. 4 (1986), 220–223.

109. Fedor, M.A., AIDS: Advocacy and Activism, *Nursing and Health Care,* 12, no. 4 (1991), 177.

110. Fehm, H.L., and J. Born. Evidence for Entrainment of Nocturnal Cortisol Secretion to Sleep Processes in Human Beings, *Neuroendocrinology,* 53, no. 2 (1991), 171–176.

111. Felton, G., Human Biologic Rhythms, *Annual Review of Nursing Research,* 5 (1987), 45–77.

112. Ferketich, S. and R. Mercer, Predictors of Role Competence for Experienced and Inexperienced Fathers, *Nursing Research,* 44 (1995), 89–95.

113. Finlay, G., Sleep and Intensive Care, *Intensive Care Nursing,* 7, no. 1 (1991), 61–68.

114. Fischman, S., et al., Changes in Sexual Relationships in Post-partum Couples, *Journal of Obstetric, Gynecologic, and Neonatal Nursing,* 15, no. 1 (1986), 58.

115. Fisher, H., The Four-Year Itch, *Natural History,* October, 1987, 22–33.

116. Fishwick, N., Getting to the Heart of the Matter: Nursing Assessment and Intervention With Battered Women in Psychiatric Mental Health Settings, *Journal of the American Psychiatric Nurses Association,* 1, no. 2.

117. Folic Acid: For the Young and Heart, *Nutrition Action,* 22, no. 7 (1995), 4–6.

118. Folkard, S., D.S. Minors, and J.M. Waterhouse, "Demasking" the Temperature Rhythm After Simulated Time Zone Transitions, *Journal of Biological Rhythms,* 6, no. 1 (1991), 81–92.

119. Fontaine, K., The Conspiracy of Culture: Women's Issues in Body Size, *Nursing Clinics of North America,* 26, no. 3 (1991), 669–676.

120. For Men Only, *Nutrition Action,* 22, no. 5 (1995), 4–5.

121. Forrester, D., Myths of Masculinity: Impact Upon Men's Health, *Nursing Clinics of North America,* 21, no. 1 (1986), 15–24.

122. Fossey, E., Shiftwork Can Seriously Damage Your Health! *Professional Nurse,* 5, no. 9 (1990), 476–480.

123. Frank, S., M. Tuer, and S. Jacobson, Psychological Predictors of Young Adults' Drinking Behaviors, *Journal of Personality and Social Psychology,* 59, no. 4 (1990), 770–780.

124. Friman, P.C., and J.W. Finney, Health Education for Testicular Cancer, *Health Education Quarterly,* 17, no. 4 (1990), 443–453.

125. Garrity, T., et al., The Association Between Type A Behavior and Change in Coronary Risk Factors Among Young Adults, *American Journal of Public Health,* 80, no. 11 (1990), 1354–1357.

126. Gelfand, D., and D. Teti, How Does Maternal Depression Affect Children? *The Harvard Mental Health Letter,* 12, no. 5 (1995), 8.

127. Genetically Determined Homosexuality? *Journal of Psychosocial Nursing,* 30, no. 5 (1992), 45.

128. Gfroerer, J., and M. Brodsley, Frequent Cocaine Users and Their Use of Treatment, *American Journal of Public Health,* 83 (1993), 1149–1154.

129. Giles, J., Generations, *Newsweek,* June 8 (1994), 62–68.

130. Gillin, J., and W. Byerley, Medical Intelligence—Drug Therapy: The Diagnosis and Management of Insomnia, *New England Journal of Medicine,* 322, no. 4 (1990), 239–248.

131. Gillooly, P.B., et al., Circadian Variation in Human Performance Evaluated by the Walter Reed Performance Assessment Battery, *Chronobiology International,* 7, no. 2 (1990), 143–153.

132. Glantz, S.A., and W.W. Parmley, Passive Smoking and Heart Disease: Epidemiology, Physiology, and Biochemistry, *Circulation,* 83, no. 1 (1991), 1–12.

133. Glass, L., *From Clocks to Chaos: The Rhythms of Life.* Princeton, NJ: Princeton University Press, 1988.

134. Glynn, T., et al., Essential Elements of Self-help/Minimal Intervention Strategies for Smoking Cessation, *Health Education Quarterly,* 17, no. 3 (1990), 329–345.

135. Gold, D., S. Rogacz, N. Beck, T. Tosteson, T. Baum, F. Speizer, and C. Czeisler, Rotating Shift Work, Sleep, and Accidents Related to Sleepiness in Hospital Nurses, *American Journal of Public Health,* 82 (1992), 1011–1014.

136. Goldstein, I.B., and D. Shapiro, The Beat-to-Beat Blood Pressure Response to Postural Change in Young and Elderly Healthy Adult Males, *Journal of Behavioral Medicine,* 13, no. 5 (1990), 437–448.

137. Goodman, E., Female Mutilation Immigrates to the U.S., *St. Louis Post Dispatch,* October 23 (1995), Sect. B, p. 7.

138. Gould, R., Adult Life Stages: Growth Toward Self-tolerance, *Psychology Today,* 8, no. 7 (February 1975), 74–78.

139. Gray, M.E., Factors Related to Practice of Breast Self-examination in Rural Women, *Cancer Nursing,* 13, no. 2 (1990), 100–107.

140. Greaves, W.L., "AIDS and Sexually Transmitted Diseases," in Livingston, J.L., ed., *Handbook of American Health.* Westport, CT: Greenwood Press, 1994, pp. 158–168.

141. Green, P., The Chemically Dependent Nurse, *Nursing Clinics of North America,* 24, no. 1 (1989), 81–94.

142. Greenfield, M., Disclosing Incest: The Relationships That Make It Possible, *Journal of Psychosocial Nursing,* 28, no. 7 (1990), 20–23.

143. Gruen, S.M., et al., Setting Up a School-based Sexual Education Program to Help Prevent AIDS and Other Sexually Transmitted Diseases, *Nurse Practitioner,* 16, no. 8 (1991), 47–51.

144. Guohua, L., D. Smith, and S. Baker, Drinking Behavior in Relation to Cause of Death Among U.S. Adults, *American Journal of Public Health,* 84 (1994), 1402–1406.

145. Guyton, A., *Textbook of Medical Physiology* (9th ed.). Philadelphia: W.B. Saunders, 1995.

146. Haber, J., A Family Systems Model for Divorce and the Loss of Self, *Archives of Psychiatric Nursing,* 4, no. 4 (1991), 228–234.

147. Hahn, W.K., J.A. Brooks, and R. Hite, Blood Pressure Norms for *Healthy Young Adults:* Relation to Sex, Age, and Reported Parental Hypertension, *Research in Nursing and Health,* 12, no. 1 (1989), 53–56.

148. Hansen, S., Single Custodial Fathers and the Parent–Child Relationship, *Nursing Research* 30, no. 4 (1981), 202–204.

149. Hanson, S., and F. Bozett, The Changing Nature of Fatherhood: The Nurse and Social Policy, *Journal of Advanced Nursing,* 11, no. 6 (1986), 719–727.

150. Hatton, C., and S. Valente, *Suicide: Assessment and Intervention.* Norwalk, CT: Appleton-Century-Crofts, 1984.

151. Haus, E., et al., Circadian Variations in Blood Coagulation Parameters, Alpha-antitrypsin Antigen and Platelet Aggregation and Retention in Clinically Healthy Subjects, *Chronobiology International,* 7, no. 3 (1990), 203–216.

152. Having It All, *Elle,* January (1992), 42–47.

153. Health Risks: Perception and Reality, *Harvard Women's Health Watch,* 1, no. 10 (1994), 1.

154. Health Risks, *Women's Health Advocate Newsletter,* 2, no. 11, (January 1996), 2–3.

155. *Healthy People 2000: National Health Promotion and Disease Prevention Objectives.* Washington, DC: U.S. Dept of Health and Human Services, 1990 (DHHS publication PHS 91-50212).

156. Heart Disease: How to Lower Your Risk, *Nutrition Action Health Letter,* 22, no. 8 (1995), 4–7.

157. Heinrick, K., Effective Responses to Sexual Harassment, *Nursing Outlook,* 35, no. 2 (1987), 70–72.

158. Heitkemper, M., et al., GI Symptoms, Function, and Psychophysiological Arousal in Dysmenorrheic Women, *Nursing Research,* 40, no. 1 (1991), 20–28.

159. Helton, A., Battering During Pregnancy, *American Journal of Nursing,* 86, no. 8 (1986), 910–913.

160. ———, et al., Battered and Pregnant: A Prevalence Study, *American Journal of Public Health,* 77, no. 10 (1987), 1337–1339.

161. ———, and F.G. Snodgrass, Battering During Pregnancy: Intervention Strategies, *Birth,* 14, no. 3 (1987), 142–147.

162. Hemfelt, R., F. Minirth, and P. Meiser, *Love Is a Choice.* Nashville: Thomas Nelson, 1989.

163. Hill, I., ed., *The Bisexual Spouse.* McLean, VA: Barlina Books, 1988.

164. Hitchcock, J., and H. Wilson, Personal Risking: Lesbian Self-disclosure of Sexual Orientation to Professional Health Care Providers, *Nursing Research,* 41 (1992), 178–183.

165. Hoff, L., *Battered Women as Survivors.* New York: Routledge, 1990.

166. ———, *People in Crisis: Understanding and Helping* (4th ed.). Redwood City, CA: Addison-Wesley, 1995.

167. Homer, C., S. James, and E. Siegel, Work Related Psychosocial Stress and Risk of Preterm, Low Birthweight Delivery, *American Journal of Public Health,* 80, no. 2 (1990), 173–177.

168. Home Test Kits: Left to Our Own Devices, *Harvard Health Letter,* no. 11 (1995), 3–4.

169. Hoole, A., R. Greenberg, and C.G. Prickard, *Patient Care Guidelines for Nurse Practitioners* (3rd ed.). Boston: Little, Brown, 1988.

170. ———, C. Pickard, R. Ouimette, J. Lohr, and R. Greenberg, *Patient Care Guideline for Nurse Practitioners* (4th ed.). Philadelphia: J.B. Lippincott, 1995.

171. ———, *Clinicians' Handbook of Preventive Services: Put Prevention Into Family Practice.* Department of Health and Human Service, U.S. Public Health Service, 1994.

172. Holtzworth and Monroe, A., Marital Violence, *The Harvard Mental Health Letter,* 12, no. 2 (1995), 4–6.

173. Horn, B., Cultural Concepts and Postpartal Care, *Journal of Transcultural Nursing,* 2, no. 1 (1990), 48–51.

174. How Hard Do You Really Need to Exercise? *Tuft's University Diet and Nutrition Letter,* 13, no. 5 (1995), 4–6.

175. How Intimacy Changes, *Glamour,* January (1993), 27.

176. How Much Exercise Is Enough? *Harvard Women's Health Watch,* 2, no. 11 (1995), 1.

177. Intregrating an Understanding of Sleep Knowledge Into Your Practice, *The American Nurse,* November/December (1994), 24–25.

178. Intrinsically Rewarding Work Relieves Workplace Stress, *The Menninger Letter,* 3, no. 7 (1995), 3, 5.

179. Isay, R., *Being Homosexual: Gay Men and Their Development.* New York: Farrar, Strauss, Giroux, 1990.

180. John, E.M., D.A. Savitz, and D.P. Sandler, Prenatal Exposure to Parents' Smoking and Childhood Cancer, *American Journal of Epidemiology,* 133, no. 2 (1991), 123–132.

181. Johnson, E., and G. Johnson, Premature Developmental Jumps: The Effects of Early Intimacy on the Adult Lives of Identical Twins, *Perspectives in Psychiatric Care,* 20, no. 2 (1982), 87–90.

182. Jolley, J., and M. Mitchell, *Lifespan Development: A Topical Approach.* Madison, WI: Brown & Benchmark, 1996.

183. Jones, G., Biological Clocks: Testing Our Internal Timing, *Science: The Teacher,* 58, no. 3 (1991), 16–20.

184. Jordan, P., Laboring for Relevance: Expectant and New Fatherhood, *Nursing Research,* 39, no. 1 (1990), 11–16.

185. Jung, C., Psychological Types, in Adler, G., et al., eds., *Collected Works of Carl G. Jung,* Vol. 6, Princeton, NJ: Princeton University Press, 1971.

186. Kahn, H., D. Williamson, and J. Stevens, Race and Weight Change in US Women: The Roles of Socioeconomic and Marital Status, *American Journal of Public Health,* 81, no. 3 (1991), 319–323.

187. Kantrowitz, B., P. Wingert, D. Rosenberg, V. Quade, and D. Foote, Breaking the Divorce Cycle, *Newsweek,* January (1992), 48–53.

188. Kaplan, R., J. Anderson, and D. Wingard, Gender Differences in Health-related Quality of Life, *Health Psychology,* 10, no. 2 (1991), 86–93.

189. Kass, N., R. Faden, R. Fox, and J. Duley, Homosexual and Bisexual Men's Perceptions of Discrimination in Health Services, *American Journal of Public Health,* 82 (1992), 1277–1279.

190. Keep Your Own Medical History, *Women's Health Advocate Newsletter,* 2, no. 10 (1995), 3–8.

191. Kelleher, K., M. Chaffin, J. Hollenberg, and E. Fischer, Alcohol and Drug Disorders Among Physically Abusive and Neglectful Parents in a Community-based Sample, *American Journal of Public Health,* 84 (1994), 1586–1590.

192. King, M.C. and J. Ryan, Abused Women: Dispelling Myths and Encouraging Interventions, *Nurse Practitioner,* 14, no. 5 (1989), 47–58.

193. Knollmueller, R. (ed., *Prevention Across the Life Span: Healthy People for the Twenty-first Century.* Washington, DC: American Nurses Association Council of Community Health Nurses, 1993.

194. Knowles, M.S., *Androgogy in Action.* San Francisco: Jossey-Bass, 1984.

195. Kohlberg, L., *Recent Research in Moral Development.* New York: Holt, Rinehart & Winston, 1971.

196. Koons, C., and M. Anthony, *Single Adult Passages: Uncharted Territories.* Grand Rapids, MI: Baker Book House, 1991.

197. Korniewicz, D.M., M. O'Brien, and E. Larson, Coping with AIDS and HIV: Psychosocial adaptation, *Journal of Psychosocial Nursing,* 28, no. 3 (1990), 14–21.

198. Kostreva, M., and P. Genevier, Nurse Preferences Vs. Circadian Rhythms in Scheduling, *Nursing Management,* 20, no. 7 (1989), 50–51, 54, 56, 58, 60, 62.

199. Kramer, J., *Family Interfaces: Transgenerational Patterns.* New York: Brunner/Mazel, 1985.

200. Krebs-Smith, S., A. Cook, A. Subar, L. Cleveland, and J. Friday, U.S. Adults' Fruit and Vegetable Intakes, 1989 to 1991: A Revised Baseline for the Healthy People 2000 Objective, *American Journal of Public Health,* 85 (1995), 1625–1629.

201. Kreidler, M., and R. Carbon. Breaking the Incest Cycle: The Group as a Surrogate Family, *Journal of Psychosocial Nursing,* 29, no. 4 (1991), 28–32.

202. Kryger, M.H., R. Roth, and W.B. Dement. *Principles and Practice of Sleep Medicine.* Philadelphia: W.B. Saunders, 1989.

203. Kutner, L., *Parent and Child: Getting Through to Each Other.* New York: William Morrow, 1991.

204. L'Abate, L., J. Farrar, and D. Serritella, eds., *Handbook of Differential Treatments for Addictions.* Boston: Allyn & Bacon, 1992.

205. LaDou, J., Rhythmic Variations in Medical Monitoring Texts, *Occupational Medicine,* 5, no. 3 (1990), 479–489.

206. Laffrey, S., Normal and Underweight Adults: Perceived Weight and Health Behavior Characteristics, *Nursing Research,* 35, no. 3 (1988), 173–177.

207. Lamb, M., The Emergent Father, in Lamb, M.E., ed., *The Father's Role: Cross-cultural Perspectives.* Hillsdale, NJ: Lawrence Erlbaum, 1987, pp. 1–26.

208. Landau, Stanton, J., and C. Clements, *AIDS, Health, and Mental Health: A Primary Sourcebook.* New York: Brunner/Mazel, 1993.

209. LaRossa, R., Fatherhood and Social Change, *Family Relations,* 37 (1988), 451–457.

210. Lazarus, R., *Coping With the Stress of Illness,* WHO Regional Publications, European Series, no. 144, 1992, pp. 11–31.

211. Ledray, L., Counseling Rape Victims: The Nursing Challenge, *Perspectives in Psychiatric Care,* 26, no. 2 (1990), 21–27.

212. ———, and S. Arndt, Examining the Sexual Assault Victim: A New Model for Nursing Care, *Journal of Psychosocial Nursing,* 32, no. 2 (1994), 7–12.

213. Lefevre, J., et al., Motor Performance During Adolescence and Age Thirty as Related to Age at Peak Height Velocity, *Annals of Human Biology,* 17, no. 5 (1990), 423–435.

214. Lehne, R., *Pharmacology for Nursing Care* (2nd ed.) Philadelphia: W.B. Saunders, 1994.

215. Leland, J., Bisexuality, *Newsweek,* July 17 (1995), 44–49.

216. Lerner, R., and J. Jovanovic, The Role of Body Image in Psychosocial Development Across the Life Span, in Cash, T., and Pruzinsky, T. eds., *Body Images: Development, Deviance, and Change.* New York: Guilford Press, 1990.

217. Levinson, D., *The Seasons of a Man's Life.* New York: Ballantine Books, 1978.

218. ———, et al., Periods in the Adult Development of Men: Ages 18 to 45, *Counseling Psychologist,* 6, no. 1 (1976), 21–25.

219. Lewis, L., One Year in the Life of a Woman with Premenstrual Syndrome: A Case Study, *Nursing Research,* 44 (1995), 111–115.

220. Licopantio, E., Shift Work in Nursing and Circadian Rhythms, *Imprint,* 36, no. 2 (1989), 161, 163, 165.

221. Lidz, T., *The Person: His and Her Development Throughout the Life Cycle* (2nd ed.). New York: Basic Books, 1983.

222. Life Experiences May Prompt Onset of Obesity, *Journal of Psychosocial Nursing,* 31, no. 10 (1993), 45–46.

223. Loria, C., T. Bush, M. Carroll, A. Looker, et al., Macronutrient Intakes Among Adult Hispanics: A Comparison of Mexican Americans, Cuban Americans, and Mainland Puerto Ricans, *American Journal of Public Health,* 85 (1995), 684–689.

224. Love, C., and H. Seaton, Eating Disorders, *Nursing Clinics of North America,* 26, no. 3 (1991), 677–697.

225. Maas, H., and J. Kuyper, *From Thirty to Seventy.* San Francisco: Jossey-Bass, 1974.

226. Many Deaths Preventable, Says WHO's First Global Health Survey, *The Nation's Health,* May/June (1995), 17.

227. Martin, S., *Healing for Adult Children of Alcoholics.* Nashville: Broadman Press, 1988.

228. Martin, W., Sexual Wounds: Steps to Healing, *Journal of Christian Nursing,* 8, no. 4 (1992), 18–22.

229. Martin, S., and M. Burchinal, Young Women's Antisocial Behavior and the Later Emotional and Behavioral Health of Their Children, *American Journal of Public Health,* 82 (1992), 1007–1010.

230. Mason, J., and M. McGinnis, "Health People 2000": An Overview of the National Health Promotion and Disease Prevention Objectives, *Public Health Reports,* 105, no. 5 (1990), 441–446.

231. Masters, W., and V. Johnson, *The Human Sexual Response.* New York: Bantam, 1981.

232. ———, *Homosexuality in Perspective.* Boston: Little, Brown, 1979.

233. May, K., Three Phases of Father Involvement in Pregnancy, *Nursing Research,* 31, no. 8 (1982), 337–342.

234. McCloskey, J., Two Requirements for Job Contentment, *IMAGE: Journal of Nursing Schlarship,* 22 (1990), 140–143.

235. McCollum, E., Talking Man to Man, *New Choices,* June (1991), 87.

236. McCoy, V., Adult Life Cycle Tasks/Adult Continuing Education Program Response, *Lifelong Learning in the Adult Years,* October (1977), 16.

237. McLanahan, S., and G. Sandefur, *Growing up With a Single Parent.* Cambridge: Harvard University Press, 1994.

238. McNeil, B.J., et al., Sleep Questionnaire, *American Journal of Nursing,* 86, no. 1 (1986), 261.

239. Mead, G.H., *Mind, Self, and Society.* Chicago: University of Chicago Press, 1962.

240. Medved, D., *The Case Against Divorce.* Atlanta: Ivy Books, 1990.

241. Meissner, J., A Simple Guide for Assessing Oral Health, *Nursing '80,* 10, no. 4 (1980), 84–85.

242. Melatonin, *Newsweek,* August 7 (1995), 48–49.

243. Mercer, R., The Process of Maternal Role Attachment Over the First Year, *Nursing Research* 34, no. 4 (1985), 198–203.

244. ———, and S. Ferketich, Predictors of Family Functioning Eight Months Following Birth, *Nursing Research,* 39, no. 2 (1990), 76–81.

245. Michael, R., J. Gagnon, and E. Lauman, *Sex in America: A Definitive Study.* Boston: Little, Brown, 1994.

246. Miller, K., Body Image Therapy, *Nursing Clinics of North America,* 26, no. 3 (1991), 727–736.

247. ———, Compulsive Overeating, *Nursing Clinics of North America,* 26, no. 3 (1991), 699–705.

248. Mitchell, E., N. Woods, and M. Lentz, Differentiation of Women With Three Premenstrual Symptom Patterns, *Nursing Research,* 43 (1994), 25–30.

249. Moberly, E., Can Homosexuals Really Change? *Journal of Christian Nursing,* 8, no. 4 (1992), 14–17.

250. More to Life Than Just Lowering Your Cholesterol, *Taft's University Diet and Nutrition Letter,* 13, no. 8 (1995), 2–3.

251. Morris, M., and C. Myton, Ego Functions, *Journal of Psychosocial Nursing,* 24, no. 12 (1986), 17–22.

252. Murray, R., Self-Concept, in Potter, P., and Perry, A. eds., *Fundamentals of Nursing: Concepts, Process, and Practice* (2nd ed.). St. Louis: C.V. Mosby, 1989, pp. 722–747.

253. ———, and M.M. Huelskoetter, *Psychiatric/Mental Health Nursing: Giving Emotional Care* (3rd ed.). Norwalk, CT: Appleton & Lange, 1991.

254. Myers, I., and M. McCaulley, *Manual: A Guide to the Development and Use of the Myers–Briggs Type Indicator.* Palo Alto, CA: Consulting Psychologists Press, 1985.

255. Nadis, S., Rhythm and Blues, *Technology Review,* 94, no. 1 (1991), 22–25.

256. Neef, N., et al., Testicular Self-examination by Young Men: An Analysis of Characteristics Associated With Practice, *Journal of American College Health,* 39, no. 4 (1991), 187–190.

257. Nikstaitis, G., Therapy for Men Who Batter, *Journal of Psychosocial Nursing,* 23, no. 7 (1985), 33–36.

258. Norbeck, J., and N. Anderson, Psychosocial Predictors of Pregnancy Outcomes in Low Income Black, Hispanic, and White Women, *Nursing Research,* 38, no. 4 (1989), 204–209.

259. *Nutrition and Your Health: Dietary Guidelines for Americans* (3rd ed.). Washington, DC: Dept. of Agriculture, Dept. of Health and Human Services, 1990. Home and Garden Bulletin 232.

260. Nutrition Guidelines Incorporate Physical Activity, *The Nation's Health,* October (1995), 10.

261. Nyamathi, A., C. Bennett, B. Leake, and S. Chen, Social Support Among Impoverished Women, *Nursing Research,* 44 (1995), 376–378.

262. Obesity Insights, *Harvard Women's Health Watch,* 3, no. 2 (1995), 1.

263. O'Campo, P., A. Grelen, R. Faden, N. Xine, N. Kass, and N. Wang, Violence by Male Partners Against Women During the

Childbearing Year: A Contextual Analysis, *American Journal of Public Health,* 85 (1995), 1092–1097.

264. O'Donnell, T.G., and S.L. Bernicer, Parents as Caregivers: AIDS, *Journal of Psychosocial Nursing,* 28, no. 6 (1990), 14–17.

265. Oelbaum, C., Hallmarks of Adult Wellness, *American Journal of Nursing,* 74, no. 9 (1974), 1623–1625.

266. One Nation Under Pressure, *Nutrition Action,* 22, no. 6 (1995), 6–7.

267. Ossler, C., Men's Work Environments and Health Risks, *Nursing Clinics of North America,* 21, no. 1 (1986), 25–36.

268. Owens, M., Keeping an Eye on Magnesium, *American Journal of Nursing,* 93, no. 2 (1993), 66–67.

269. Parish, J.M., and J.W. Shepard, Cardiovascular Effects of Sleep Disorders, *Chest: The Cardiopulmonary Journal,* 97, no. 5 (1990), 1220–1226.

270. Pender, N., *Health Promotion in Nursing Practice* (2nd ed.). Norwalk, CT: Appleton & Lange, 1987.

271. Persuhn, P., Job Sharing: Two Who Made It Work, *American Journal of Nursing,* 92, no. 9 (1992), 75–76, 78, 80.

272. Physical Symptoms Result from Unspeakable Dilemmas, *The Menninger Letter,* November (1995), 4.

273. Pinnell, N., and M. deMeneses, *Nursing Process: Theory, Application and Related Processes.* Norwalk, CT: Appleton-Century-Crofts, 1986.

274. P.M.S.: It's Real, *Harvard Women's Health Watch,* 1, no. 11 (1994), 2–3.

275. Positive Life Events Enhances Women's Self-esteem, *The Menninger Letter,* 3, no. 7 (1995), 5.

276. Potter, P., and A. Perry, *Fundamentals of Nursing: Concepts, Process, and Practice* (2nd ed.). St. Louis: C.V. Mosby, 1989.

277. Pruzinsky, T., and T. Cash, Integrative Themes in Body Image Development, Deviance, and Change, in Cash, T., and Pruzinsky, T., eds., *Body Images: Development, Deviance, and Change.* New York: Guilford Press, 1990.

278. Regulating the Body's Rhythms, *Newsweek,* January 7 (1995), 48–49.

279. Reilly, T., Human Circadian Rhythms and Exercise, *Critical Review of Biomedical Engineering,* 18, no. 3 (1990), 165–180.

280. Reynolds, C.F., et al., Sleep, Gender, and Depression: An Analysis of Gender Effects on the Electroencephalographic Sleep of 302 Depressed Outpatients, *Biologic Psychiatry,* 28, no. 8 (1990), 673–684.

281. Richard, E., and A. Shepard, Giving Up Smoking: A Lesson in Loss Therapy, *American Journal of Nursing,* 81, no. 4 (1981), 755–757.

282. Riessman, C., and N. Gerstel, Marital Dissolution and Health: Do Males or Females Have Greater Risk? *Social Science and Medicine,* 20 (1985), 627.

283. Riley, E., Eating Disorders as Addictive Behavior, *Nursing Clinics of North America,* 26, no. 3 (1991), 715–726.

284. Risk: What It Means to You, *Harvard Women's Health Watch,* 3, no. 3 (1995), 3–4.

285. Robins, L., and D. Regier, *Psychiatric Disorders in America: The Epidemiologic Catchment Area Study.* New York: Free Press, 1991, p. 72.

286. Robinson, P., New Face of an Epidemic: HIV/AIDS in Minority Populations, in *HIV/AIDS Update '95: New Treatments and Therapies, Twentieth Annual NCAPA Conference, Myrtle Beach, SC,* lecture on August 17, 1995.

287. Roof, W., *A Generation of Seekers.* San Francisco: Harper, 1993.

288. Rosenthal, N.E., et al., Phase-shifting Effects of Bright Morning Light as Treatment for Delayed Sleep Phase Syndrome, *Sleep,* 13, no. 4 (1990), 354–361.

289. Rossi, E., *The 20 Minute Break: Using The New Science of Ultradian Rhythms.* Los Angeles: Jeremy P. Tarcher, 1991.

290. Rothenberg, K., and S. Paskey, The Risk of Domestic Violence and Women with HIV Infection: Implications for Partner Notification, Public Policy, and the Law, *American Journal of Public Health,* 85 (1995), 1569–1576.

291. Royce, J., N. Hymovitz, K. Corbett, T. Harwell, and M. Orlandi, Smoking Cessation Factors Among African Americans and Whites, *American Journal of Public Health,* 83 (1993), 220–226.

292. Rubin, R., Maternal Tasks in Pregnancy, *Maternal–Child Nursing Journal,* 4, no. 3 (Fall 1975), 143–153.

293. Ryan, J., C. Zwerling, and E. Orav, Occupational Risks Associated With Cigarette Smoking: A Prospective Study, *American Journal of Public Health,* 82, no. 1 (1992), 29–32.

294. Samet, J.M., New Effects of Active and Passive Smoking on Reproduction? *American Journal of Epidemiology,* 133, no. 4 (1991), 348–350.

295. Samples, J.F., et al., *Using Nursing Research Circadian Rhythms: Basis for Screening for Fever.* New York: UNLN Publication, No. 15-2232 (1989), pp. 92–96.

296. Sande, M., and P. A. Valberdin, eds., *The Medical Management of AIDS.* Philadelphia: W.B. Saunders, 1995.

297. Scavnicky-Mylant, M., The Process of Coping Among Young Adult Children of Alcoholics, *Issues in Mental Health Nursing,* 11, no. 2 (1990), 125–139.

298. Scherer, P., How AIDS Attacks the Brain, *American Journal of Nursing,* 90, no. 1 (1990), 41–52.

299. ———, How HIV Attacks the Peripheral Nervous System, *American Journal of Nursing,* 9, no. 5 (1990), 66–70.

300. Schoolman, J., Leisure Time: More Desirable Than Money? *St. Louis Post-Dispatch,* March 27 (1991), Sect. E, pp. 1, 4.

301. Shaw, E., Female Circumcision, *American Journal of Nursing,* 83, no. 6 (1983), 684–687.

302. Sheehy, G, *Passages: Predictable Crises of Adult Life.* New York: Bantam Books, 1976.

303. ———, Introducing the Postponing Generation: The Truth About Today's Young Men, *Esquire Magazine,* October (1979), 264–272.

304. ———, *The Silent Passage: Menopause.* New York, Random House, 1992.

305. Sherwen, L., M. Scoloreno, and C. Weingarten, *Nursing Care of the Childbearing Family.* Norwalk, CT: Appleton-Lange, 1991.

306. Shopland, D., S. Niermcryk, and K. Marconi. Geographic and Gender Variations in Tobacco Use, *American Journal of Public Health,* 82, no. 1 (1992), 103–106.

307. Single Mothers' Perceptions of the Newborns, *American Journal of Nursing,* 85, no. 12 (1985), 1397.

308. Skipper, J.K., F.D. Jung, and L.C. Coffey, Nurses and Shiftwork: Effects on Physical Health and Mental Depression, *Journal of Advanced Nursing,* 15, no. 7 (1990), 835–842.

309. Sleep Disorders—Part I, *The Harvard Mental Health Letter,* 11, no. 2 (1994), 1–4.

310. Sleep Disorders—Part II, *The Harvard Mental Health Letter,* 11, no. 3 (1994), 1–5.

311. Smeltzer, S., and B. Whipple, Women and HIV Infection, *IMAGE: Journal of Nursing Scholarship,* 23, (1991), 249–256.

312. Smith, H., *Positively Single: Coming to Terms with the Single Life.* Wheaton, IL: Vector Books, 1988.

313. Sonkin, D., D. Martin, and L. Walker, *The Male Batterer: A Treatment Approach.* New York: Springer, 1985.

314. Southwell, M., and G. Wistow, Sleep in Hospitals at Night: Are Patients Needs Being Met? *Journal of Advanced Nursing,* 21, no. 6 (1995), 1101–1109.

315. A Special Needs Child Affects Marriage, *Home Life,* 46, no. 2 (1991), 44–45.

316. Spencer, M.B., et al., Circadian Rhythmicity and Sleep of Aircrew During Polar Schedules, *Aviation and Space Environment Medicine,* 62, no. 1 (1991), 3–13.

317. Sperling, M., and W. Berman, *Attachment in Adults: Clinical and Developmental Perspectives.* New York: Behavioral Science Book Science, 1994.

318. Standards for Healthy Eating, *The Nation's Health,* May/June (1995), 6.

319. Stanton, G., *Twice As Strong: The Undeniable Advantages of Raising Children in a Traditional Two Parent Family.* Dallas; Word, 1994.

320. Steinberg, J., Living and Working in the Year 2000, *New Choices,* January (1991), 52–55.

321. Stets, J., Verbal and Physical Aggression in Marriage, *Journal of Marriage and the Family,* 52 (1990), 501–514.

322. ———, Cohabitating and Marital Aggression: The Role of Social Isolation, *Journal of Marriage and the Family,* 53 (1991), 669–670.

323. Stevens, R., *Married for Good: The Lost Art of Staying Happily Married.* Donners Grove, IL: Interuniversity Press, 1986.

324. Stevens, P., and J. Hall, Stigma, Health Beliefs, and Experiences With Health Care in Lesbian Women, *IMAGE: Journal of Nursing Scholarship,* 20, (1988), 69–73.

325. Stevensen, S., Heading Off Violence With Verbal De-escalation, *Journal of Psychosocial Nursing,* 29, no. 9 (1991), 6–10.

326. Stinnett, N., and J. DeFrain, *Secrets of Strong Families.* New York: Berkeley Books, 1985.

327. Stress and Work, *Harvard Women's Health Watch,* 2, no. 1 (1994), 1.

328. Stress Reactions to Auto Accidents Common, *The Menninger Letter,* November (1995), 5.

329. Strickland, O., The Occurrence of Symptoms in Expectant Fathers, *Nursing Research,* 36, no. 3 (1987), 184–189.

330. Strickland, S., Critical Health Issues in the Workplace . . . Alcohol and Substance Abuse, *American Association of Occupational Health Nursing,* 34, no. 9 (1986), 443–444.

331. Stricter Weight Guidelines in the Offing, *Tufts' University Diet & Nutrition Letter,* 13, no. 7 (1995), 3–5.

332. Stuart, G., and Sundeen, S. *Principles and Practice of Psychiatric Nursing* (5th ed.). St. Louis: Mosby, 1995.

333. Sullivan, E., A Descriptive Study of Nurses Recovering From Chemical Addiction, *Archives of Psychiatric Nursing,* 1, no. 3 (1987), 194–200.

334. ———, Is Campus Drinking an Antecedent to Professional Impairment? *Journal of Professional Nursing,* 11, no. 1 (1995), 4.

335. Sullivan, H.S., *The Interpersonal Theory of Psychiatry,* New York: W.W. Norton, 1953.

336. Swanson, J., S. Dibble, and C. Chenitz, Chemical Features and Psychosocial Factors in Young Adults with Genital Herpes, *IMAGE: Journal of Nursing Scholarship,* 27 (1995), 16–22.

337. Sykes, J.A., P. Kelly, and J.A. Kennedy, Jr., Black Skin Problems, *American Journal of Nursing,* 79, no. 6 (1979), 1092–1094.

338. Testosterone: Wimping Out? *Newsweek,* July 5 (1995), 61.

339. Testu, F., Diurnal Variations of Performance and Information Processing, *Chronobiologia,* 13, no. 4 (1986), 319–326.

340. The B Vitamins: Why Women Need Them, *Women's Health Advocate Newsletter,* 2, no. 9 (1995), 4–6.

341. *The Food Guide Pyramid.* Washington, DC: Dept. of Agriculture, Dept. of Health and Human Services, 1992. Home and Garden Bulletin 252.

342. The Morning-after Pill, *Harvard Women's Health Watch,* 1, no. 12 (1994), 7.

343. The New Weight Guidelines, *Harvard Women's Health Watch,* 3, no. 3 (1995), 1.

344. Thomas, S., and R. Williams, Perceived Stress, Trait Anger, Modes of Anger Expression, and Health Status of College Men and Women, *Nursing Research,* 40, no. 5 (1991), 303–307.

345. Tobias, C., How Do We Understand? *Focus on the Family,* October (1995), 13.

346. Toterdell, P., E. Spelten, and J. Pikorski, The Effects of Nightwork on Psychological Changes During the Menstrual Cycle, *Journal of Advanced Nursing,* 21, no. 5 (1995), 996–1005.

347. Trinkoff, A., W. Eaton, and J. Anthony, The Prevalence of Substance Abuse Among Registered Nurses, *Nursing Research,* 40, no. 3 (1991), 172–175.

348. Trudeau, M., Dark Nights and Bright Mornings: Caring for a Person with AIDS, *Journal of Psychosocial Nursing,* 29, no. 1 (1991), 32–33.

349. Tucker, L., and M. Bagwell, Television Viewing and Obesity in Adult Females, *American Journal of Public Health,* 81, no. 7 (1991), 908–911.

350. ———, and G. Friedman, Television Viewing and Obesity in Adult Males, *American Journal of Public Health,* 79, no. 4 (1989), 516–518.

351. Turner, J., and D. Helms, *Lifespan Development* (5th ed.). Ft. Worth: Harcourt Brace College, 1995.

352. Underword, A., and B. Shenitz, Do You, Tom, Take Harry . . . ,*Newsweek,* December 11 (1995), 82–84.

353. Uphold, C., and M. Graham, *Clinical Guidelines in Family Practice* (2nd ed.), Gainesville, FL: Barmarrae Books, 1994.

354. U.S. AIDS Cases Reported Through December, 1992. *HIV/AIDS Surveillance Report.* Atlantic: Centers for Disease Control and Prevention, 1993.

355. U.S. Bureau of the Census, *Statistical Abstract of the United States: 1989.* Washington, DC: U.S. Government Printing Office, 1989.

356. Vaillant, G., How the Best and the Brightest Came of Age, *Psychology Today,* 11, no. 9 (1977), 34ff.

357. ———, The Normal Boy in Later Life: How Adaptation Fosters Growth, *Harvard Magazine,* 55, no. 6 (1977), 234–239.

358. Van Cauter, E., and F. Turek, Strategies for Resetting the Human Circadian Clock, *New England Journal of Medicine,* 322, no. 18 (1990) 1306–1308.

359. Van Den Akker, O., and A. Steptoe, Psychophysiological Responses in Women Reporting Severe Premenstrual Symptoms, *Psychosomatic Medicine,* 51 (1989), 319–328.

360. Vegega, M.E., and T.M. Klein, Alcohol Related Traffic Fatalities Among Adolescents and Young Adults—United States, 1982–1989, *Journal of the American Medical Association,* 265, no. 15 (1991), 1930.

361. Von-Roemeling, R, The Therapeutic Index of Cytotoxic Chemotherapy Depends Upon Circadian Drug Timing, *Annals of the New York Academy of Science,* 618 (1991), 292–311.

362. Wadsworth, B., *Piaget's Theory of Cognitive and Affective Development* (5th ed.). New York: Longman, 1996.

363. Walker, L., H. Cran, and E. Thompson, Maternal Role: Attainment and Identity in the Postpartum Period: Stability and Change, *Nursing Research* 35, no. 2 (1986), 68–71.

364. Wallerstein, J., and S. Blakeslee, *Second Chances: Men, Women and Children a Decade After Divorce—Who Wins, Who Loses, and Why.* New York: Picknor & Fields, 1990.

365. Weight Control: Eating and Body Image, *Harvard Women's Health Watch,* 3, no. 4 (1995), 6.

366. Weingourt, R., Wife Rape in a Sample of Psychiatric Patients, *IMAGE: Journal of Nursing Scholarship,* 22, (1990), 144–147.

367. When Taking Supplements Is a Double-edged Sword, *Tuft's University Diet and Nutrition Letter,* 13, no. 6 (1995), 1–2.

368. WHO Calls Attention to TB, AIDS, and Aging Health Issues, *The Nation's Health,* August (1994), 14.

369. WHO Predicts Up to 30 Million World AIDS Cases by Year 2000, *Nation's Health,* January (1991), 1.

370. Williams, A., Women at Risk: An AIDS Educational Needs Assessment, *IMAGE: Journal of Nursing Scholarship,* 23, (1991), 208–213.

371. Williams, S., *Nutrition and Diet Therapy* (10th ed.). St. Louis: Times Mirror/Mosby, 1995.

372. ———, Nutritional Guidance in Prenatal Care, in Worthington-Roberts, B., S. Williams, and Vermeersch, J., eds., *Nutrition in Pregnancy and Lactation* (4th ed.). St. Louis: C.V. Mosby, 1989.

373. Williamson, K., et al., Occupational Health Hazards for Nurses—Part II, *IMAGE: Journal of Nursing Scholarship,* 20, (1988), 162–168.

374. Willis, J., Keeping Time to Circadian Rhythms, *FDA Consumer,* 24, no. 6 (1990), 18–21.

375. Wine, Women, and Health, *Harvard Women's Health Watch,* 1, no. 9 (1994), 1–2.

376. Wismont, J., and N. Reame, The Lesbian Childbearing Experience: Assessing Developmental Tasks, *IMAGE: Journal of Nursing Scholarship,* 21, no. 3 (1989), 137–142.

377. Woods, N., *Human Sexuality in Health and Illness* (3rd ed.). St. Louis: C.V. Mosby, 1984.

378. Woodward, K., et al., A Time to Seek, *Newsweek,* December 17 (1990), 50–56.

379. ———, et al., Religion: Talking to God, *Newsweek,* January 6 (1992), 39–44.

380. Wright, J., A.G. Burgess, A.W. Burgess, G. McCrary, and J. Douglas, Investigating Stalking Crimes, *Journal of Psychosocial Nursing,* 33, no. 9 (1995), 38–46.

381. Wright, L., and M. Leahey, *Nursing Families: A Guide to Family Assessment and Intervention* (2nd ed.). Philadelphia: F.A. Davis, 1994.

382. Yamamoto, J., ed., *The Crisis of Homosexuality.* Wheaton, IL: Victor Books, 1990.

383. Young, M., Leaving the Lesbian Lifestyle, *Journal of Christian Nursing,* 8, no. 4 (1992), 11–13.

384. Zlotnick, C., and M. Cassanego, Unemployment and Health, *Nursing and Health Care,* 13, no. 2 (1993), 78–90.

▶ INTERVIEW

385. Heuermann, P., and J. Personal Correspondence—Twenty-fifth Wedding Anniversary Invitation, August 1988, Des Moines, IA.

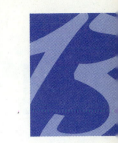

chapter thirteen

Assessment and Health Promotion for the Middle-aged Person

Forty is the old age of youth. Fifty is the youth of old age.

—*Victor Hugo*

Key Terms

Middle age	Presbyopia	Hyperthyroidism	Generativity
Generation gap	Foot balance	Hyperuricemia or gout	Mentor
Social mobility	Sleep apnea	Diabetes type II	Stagnation or self-absorption
Widow(er) hood	Sinusitis	Acute prostatitis	Maturity
Filial responsibility	Hiatal hernia	Chronic prostatitis	Adult socialization
Menopause	Duodenal peptic ulcer	Lumbosacral strain	Midlife crisis
Perimenopausal years	Angina pectoris	Foot callus	Midlife transition
Climacteric	Secondary hypertension	Sexual dysfunction	

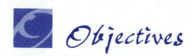

Objectives

Study of this chapter will enable you to:

1. Explore with a middle-aged person ideas about his or her generation, lifestyle, and the conflict between the generations.

2. Discuss the family relationships and sexuality development of the middle-aged adult, conflicts that must be resolved, and your role in helping the family work through concerns and conflicts.

3. List the developmental tasks for the middle-aged family, and give examples of how these can be accomplished.

4. Discuss the emotional, social, economic, and lifestyle changes usually encountered by the widow(er).

5. Describe the hormonal changes of middle age and the resultant changes in appearance and body image, physiologically and emotionally.

6. Discuss the nutritional, rest, leisure, work, and exercise needs of the middle-aged adult, factors that interfere with meeting those needs, and your role in helping him or her meet these needs.

7. Describe how the middle-aged adult's cognitive skills and emotional and moral development influence your nursing care plan.

8. State the developmental crisis of this era and its significance to social welfare.

9. Contrast the behavior of generativity, or maturity, and self-absorption, or stagnation, and related adaptive mechanisms.

10. Describe the developmental tasks for this person and your role in helping him or her accomplish these tasks.

11. Explore with a middle-aged adult ways to avoid injury and health problems.

12. Assess the body image, physical, mental, and emotional characteristics, and family relationships of a middle-aged person.

13. Plan and give effective care to a middle-aged person by using scientific principles and considering special needs and reaction to illness and hospitalization.

The next generation complains about what we are and do. They say they'll do better. They should! They're standing on our shoulders.

Middle age does not exist in every country; it is attributed to improved nutrition, control of communicable disease, discovery and control of familial disease, and other medical advances. In the United States, life has been stretched in the middle; what used to be old age is now middle age. Most non-Westernized and preindustrial cultures recognize only mature adulthood, from about 25 to 60 years, followed by old age. In some countries, the average lifespan is shorter than the age span that constitutes middle age in the United States (37).

Further, as the work structure and roles and technologic development become more complex, as family life and childrearing patterns change toward smaller families and a longer postparental period, the periods of childhood and youth are lengthened. Life is divided into more stages with more precise time periods and special developmental tasks for each age group. Thus, middle age has become a distinct life period. New concepts of adulthood involve a change in definitions of sex and age roles. Midlife development implies growth of the personality to encompass some characteristics that had

stereotypically in the past been assigned to the opposite sex. Thus, biology diminishes its influence on much of what had been held to be immutably biological characteristics. Individuals may also work out more flexible adaptations. Middle adulthood is a time of widening social interest in which the family becomes increasingly oriented to its responsibility to the greater society.

Defining middle age is a nebulous task. Chronologically, **middle age** *covers the years of approximately 45 to 65 and even 70, but each person will also consider the physiologic age condition of the body and psychological age—how old he or she acts and feels* (24, 88). Point of view alters definition: a child or an adult of 40 may think age 45 is old. The 45-year-old may consider himself or herself young. Many people today consider themselves young until nearly age 50 and middle-aged until around 70 years. Age assignment varies according to social class; the poorer person perceives the prime or midpoint of life to vary from the mid-twenties to mid-thirties to 40. Currently those people who are becoming 50 years of age in 1996 are called "the baby boomer generation." They have always lived in an affluence that has kept them young physically, and they perceive themselves as youthful and in control as they enter the second half of life.

Because of changing demographics (76 million born between 1946 and 1964), an increasing number of Americans are considered middle-aged. They earn most of the money, pay a major portion of the bills and most of the taxes, and make many of the decisions. Thus, the power in government, politics, education, religion, science, business, industry, and communication is often wielded not by the young or the old, but by the middle-aged.

Middle age is a time of relatively good physical and mental health, new personal freedom, and maximum command of self and influence over the social environment. At work the person has increasing ability to make decisions, hold high-status jobs, and earn a maximum income. The person has expanding family networks and social roles, and married life for postparental couples can be as harmonious and satisfying as the early married years.

In his book, *Time Flies,* Bill Cosby has popularized becoming middle-aged. Some of the toils and deficits may be exaggerated, but the book conveys a middle-aged adult's attitude—the ability to see his or her strengths and limits and to accept, with a sense of humor, those normal changes that are part of development (35).

In her book, *The Silent Passage: Menopause,* Gail Sheehy describes middle age and the postmenopause as a time of health and zest, a "second adulthood" for women (164). That also applies to middle-aged men.

FAMILY DEVELOPMENT AND RELATIONSHIPS

Relationship With Children

The **generation gap,** the *conflict between parents and adolescents,* may have always existed to some degree (106, 130). The experience of the parent generation, and therefore their values and expectations, differs from that of their offspring. Actually the generation lines are blurring. Some present middle-aged adults, perhaps out of fear of their own mortality, are looking and acting more like their children. These adults would rather think of themselves as carefree, innocent, and young ("the baby boomers"). The changing attitudes, values, behavior, and dress of middle-aged persons reflect our cultural emphasis on youth and beauty, versus wisdom, and our more informal society (32).

Carlson (27) and Kaplan (91), however, say the term *generation gap,* which was coined in the 1960s, is inaccurate. The generations are not really in conflict with each other; rather each generation is concerned about the other, although for different reasons. In fact,

the younger and older generations can successfully combine efforts to work for legislation, policy changes, or social justice.

There is a difference in values and lifestyle between the early and late middle-agers (see Table 1–2). In contrast to the baby-boomers, the late middle-aged adult was born sometime between the late 1920s and early 1940s, experiencing as a child or adolescent the Great Depression and World War II. He or she learned that interdependence of nations, economic security, and material possessions may be lost for reasons beyond personal control. Values and behavior have been influenced by growing up with inadequate material resources after the Great Depression and during World War II and by rapid social and technologic changes that occurred after World War II and during the 1950s.

The generation gap may be as much between early and late middle-agers as between middle-agers and their offspring.

The nuclear family is no longer prominent in the United States, and we discount learning from elders. The offspring cannot be fully prepared for the future by the parent generation. Youth must develop new patterns of behavior based on the changing world, their own experience, and that of peers. The present affluence, emphasis on age differences and independence, blurring of sex differences and independence, and insistence on a unique lifestyle of today's younger people add to the conflict for late middle-agers—both value conflicts and envy of the younger people. Youth's seeking of control over self and cultural institutions and living various lifestyle options may be better understood by younger middle-aged persons. Negative reactions of offspring to societal problems or to their parents' lifestyles reawaken in parents or late middle-agers some personal conflicts engendered by the remembrances of early personal commitments to ideals that became compromised over the years to fit narrower concerns. The addition of innate parental feelings of affection, admiration, and compassion for youth to the negative feelings produces an ambivalence (106).

Social mobility, *in which the child moves away from the social position, educational level, class, occupation, or ethnicity of parents,* causes offspring overtly to forsake parental teaching and seek new models of behavior. The mass media and societal trends help to set standards and expectations about behavior that may be counter to parental teaching or wishes. Rapid social changes and awareness that much about the future is unknown threaten established faiths and stimulate attraction to new ideologies and exceptional behavior.

You may discuss with middle-aged persons what they as adults have to offer their children. They are the only generation to ever know, experience, and incorporate such rapid changes into daily life and the job. They can give their offspring imaginative, innovative, and dedicated adult care, a safe and flexible environment in which children can be given support, feel secure, grow, and discover themselves and the world. Reaffirm that it is up to the parents to teach *not what* to learn but *how to learn, not what to be* committed to but the *value of commitment*. Tell parents that research shows the continuity of values from generation to generation within a family. Typically the values of young adults are more similar to their parents' values than to those of other adults or peers. Help youth to ask questions adults do not think of but yet to trust their parents enough to work on the answers together. The middle-aged parent can be encouraged to listen and exchange information and ideas honestly and with a sense of humor. The parent can accept youth's rejection of the faulty areas of society while supporting the values, principles, and institutions he or she knows are sound and necessary. As parent and offspring learn together to cope with the future, the parent will be able to assist youth to reach responsible, independent adulthood without a false maturity or alienation. The adult cannot abdicate the role of parent. If the parent works to maintain open communication, the generation gap may be minimal. Your work with families can promote greater harmony.

Divorce of offspring is an increasing area of concern for middle-aged parents. The parents may feel shock (or relief if they did not like the child's spouse). They may believe that their effort and help in getting the child "out of the nest" through marriage or helping the couple set up a home were to no avail. This feeling may be especially strong if the divorced family member decides to live at the parents' home again. The parents may blame their child or the inlaws and may criticize the couple for not working on the marital problems as the middle-aged parents have done (65).

If younger children are still at home, their needs and desires may be temporarily neglected because the emphasis is on the divorce crisis. Furthermore, the younger children may have to give back a room to the divorced brother or sister. The parents, in an attempt to make the divorced family member feel comfortable, may negate their own new patterns of freedom. Additionally, they may question their childrearing ability and be too embarrassed, guilt ridden, or depressed to talk about the situation with others. If the divorced son or daughter is in a financial crisis, the parents' money may also go to help him or her instead of as originally planned. If the divorcing couple has children, an additional strain will be added to the middle-aged grandparents, who wonder what their future relationship with their grandchildren will be. Relations may be strained between the inlaws as each family wonders

how to interact with the other. Recent cordiality and affection may turn to anger and criticism.

The divorce may not have a completely negative effect on the middle-aged parents. If the parents have a healthy self-esteem and an ability to proceed cautiously, they may help their offspring to gain the essential maturity that he or she was previously lacking; however, the crisis and stages of grief that accompany divorce and loss of a family member are still keenly felt.

Young adults may return home to live with parents for reasons other than separation or divorce. Some new college graduates cannot find a job of their choice or are finding that their first jobs are not paying enough for them to cover high rents along with other costs of living, so they are living with parents until they can accumulate some money or can move to higher-income jobs. Some young adult children return home more than once until they finally become independent (134).

This may cause stress, as most middle-aged parents look forward to having children leave the home—the so-called "empty nest" (129). The middle-aged adult wants space, time, and financial resources to pursue personal, organizational, and civic goals rather than to continue child care responsibilities. Prolonged dependence of young adult offspring may also create conflict with grandparents and other children who are still at home.

The **grandparent role** has a different dimension in middle age than in later maturity, although many people become grandparents during the middle-age era. If the offspring has established his or her own home and has a family, grandparenthood is a happy status and role. The relationship to the grandchild is informal and playful; the child is a source of fun, leisure activity, and self-indulgence. Emphasis is on mutual satisfaction, authority lines are irrelevant, and the child is seen as someone for whom to buy gifts (129).

If the adult offspring is divorced and brings young grandchildren into the middle-aged adult's home or if the offspring is unmarried and has children, the sense of responsibility and loss of independence are heightened. The middle-aged woman, especially, may resent the demands and constraints placed on her by having young children, including grandchildren, in the home full-time. The carefree relationship is less likely if the grandchild lives in the home with the middle-aged person. Further, having extra children and grandchildren in the home interferes with the relationship with the spouse. Normal developmental tasks cannot be met. The return of children to the home and the resultant demands may also serve to prevent the middle-aged woman from attempting to pursue new career goals, either because of a defensive withdrawal from an anxiety-producing new situation or because her conflict about roles prevents her from finding reasonable creative solutions to meet her own needs (106). The middle-aged person is not necessarily happy about being a grandparent because that may indicate old age.

A growing number of grandparents are raising their grandchildren because their children are dead, divorced, or incapacitated from drugs or another devastating habit. Two groups addressing this issue are Grandparents Raising Grandchildren, P.O. Box 104, Coffeyville, TX 76034, and Sylvie de Toledo, Grandparents as Parents, Psychiatric Clinic for Youth, 2801 Atlantic Inc., Long Beach, CA 90801. (Refer also to Chapter 4.)

Increasingly you will be caring for middle-aged parents who are being threatened emotionally or are having social or financial problems because of their children's separation or divorce. Use the principles of crisis intervention described in Chapter 5, as well as principles of communication and crisis intervention described in other texts (79, 124, 180). Parents should be cautioned to proceed carefully with financial assistance. Few young adults pay back family loans. Further, there seldom are tax benefits to giving such assistance. The middle-aged grandparents may also need encouragement in securing visitation rights when divorce or death has severed the relationship (65). Help the middle-aged couple regain a sense of self-esteem, a sense of confidence in setting limits so that they can pursue their own life goals, and a method of working through decisions and problems with the young adult offspring.

Relationship With Spouse

Equally important as rearing the children and establishing wholesome affectional ties with them, and later with the grandchildren, is the middle-aged adult's relationship with the spouse.

A *happy marriage* has security and stability, although there are also struggles. The couple knows each other well; they no longer have to pretend with each other. Children can be a source of pleasure rather than concern, as conflicts that arose between partners about rearing or disciplining children vanish when the children leave home. Each knows that his or her way of life and well-being depend on the other. Each has become accustomed to the way of the other. There is increased shared activity, and the sexual relationship can be better than before. Because the middle-aged adult is likely to have roots firmly implanted in the community of choice, he or she is able to cultivate warm friendships with members of the generation and with parents, the family of the spouse, and families of married children.

Marriage can be secure economically, for the median income usually is above the national average. Middle-aged adults generally have more money in savings accounts and proportionately less debt than other age groups. Economic influence begins to wane as retirement nears, but the middle-aged working wife helps to offset this. Nationally, many working women are over 45.

Although there has been much discussion in the literature about the crisis of menopause and the "empty nest," menopause and middle age may bring both men and women an enriched sense of self and enhanced capacity to cope with life. It may be a transition in that behavioral changes are necessary but not a crisis in the negative sense of incapacitation. In a study reported in 1972 of 54 middle- and lower-middle-class men and women whose youngest child was about to leave home, Lowenthal and Chiriboga (110) found that the parents anticipated the departure with relief, in contrast to earlier research about the "empty nest syndrome" (128); however, the "empty nest" may be felt more by single parents (79). The years before retirement are anticipated as promising, for responsibility for the children is over; adultlike peer relationships are sought with the children. Parents realize that if they have done their job as parents, the children should be ready to leave the nest. Their independence is what parenting is about.

Negative, critical feelings can gradually erode what was apparently a happy relationship. At some point the husband and wife may feel they are each living with a stranger, although the potential still exists for a harmonious marriage. With everything seeming to go well for them, the middle-aged couple may now feel that the zest has gone out of their love life. The wife and husband may have drifted apart instead of growing closer together with the years. The wife feels neglected; the husband feels nagged; and both feel bored with each other. Why has their relationship changed so suddenly? It has not! It only seems that way. Their relationship is changing because they are changing. Marital crisis may result from feelings of disappointment with self, feeling depleted emotionally because of lack of communication with the spouse, seeking rebirth or changing directions, or seeking escape from reality and superego pressures (51, 106, 164). In contrast, two factors are predictive of successful long-term marriages: (1) congruence of perceptions between spouses of the marriage and each other and (2) sexual satisfaction (36, 37).

Often the woman and man overlook that they still do really love each other. They simply have to become reacquainted. It may be difficult for the middle-aged man and woman to "tune in" to each other because both are encountering problems peculiar to their own sex. The woman may equate ability to bear children with capacity to enjoy sexual relationships, although they have nothing to do with each other. Whereas the woman needs the man's support to reinforce her femininity, he too is undergoing a crisis; he believes that he is losing his vigor, virility, and self-esteem, which are products primarily of psychological reactions rather than physiologic inabilities. In the fifties there may be a reduction of male potency triggered by fears of incompetence and feelings of inability to satisfy his wife, who may be sexually more active after menopause. He may equate success on the job with success as a husband, believe that he is losing both, and covet his son's potency and youth.

Society and health care professionals have until recently ignored the sexual needs or problems of the married middle-aged adult. But the middle-aged person is an active sexual being. Physical changes in appearance and energy and the multiple stresses of daily living may result in an increased desire for physical intimacy and the need for reassurance of continuing sexual attractiveness and competency. Intercourse is not valued for procreation but for body contact, to express love and trust, and to reaffirm an integral part of the self-concept. The person may fear loss of potency and rejection by the partner, but talking with the spouse about feelings and preferences related to sexual activity can promote increased closeness.

Men and women differ in their sexual behavior. Males reach their peak in their late teens and early twenties. Females peak in desire in the late thirties or forties and maintain that level of desire and activity past the menopause into middle age. The enjoyment of sexual relations in younger years, rather than the frequency, is a key factor for maintenance of desire and activity in the female, whereas frequency of relations and enjoyment are important factors for males (37, 78, 113, 185).

Disenchantment in any or all areas of life, with lack of enthusiasm for self and each other and for their physical relationship, may threaten the marriage in the middle years. Husband and wife are no longer distracted by daily activities of raising a family, and children are no longer present to act as buffers. There is increasing awareness of aging parents, aging friends, and signs of their own aging. Each becomes preoccupied with the self and anxious about losing youthfulness, vitality, sex appeal, and the partner's love. Each needs the other but may hesitate to reach out and demonstrate affection or intimacy. The end result may be for one or the other to reach outside the marriage to prove youthfulness, masculinity, or femininity.

The man who feels frustration in his marriage or that his wife is nagging or unattractive may pursue a younger woman to feel youthful, masculine, and ad-

mired. The woman may overcompensate for her felt loss of femininity by getting her face lifted, dressing more youthfully, acting like a teenager, and being flirtatious with her daughter's suitors.

Relationships with work colleagues may set the stage for an extramarital affair. This tendency is increased when the younger woman finds the company of an older man more interesting than that of the men in her own age group. Although divorce occurs during these years, the extramarital affair does not necessarily lead to the divorce courts. Divorce is major surgery, and the man may be reluctant to cut that much out of his life. Besides, he may find, having aroused the ardor of the younger woman, that he is no match for her physical demands. With increased consciousness of his age, he may return to his wife, particularly if she has in the meantime assessed her own situation and tried to change her behavior (37, 46, 78, 84, 106, 185). Midlife crisis is discussed further in another section.

Be aware that the number of over-40 divorces is increasing. The middle-aged man often remarries; fewer women are entering later maturity with the first marriage intact. (These women are also more likely to have a divorced daughter. Both generations have a lower standard of living as a result [187].) In the community mental health setting you will increasingly work with troubled families who are contemplating divorce or who have experienced separation and divorce.

Helping the couple regain closeness and happiness is worth the effort, for the mature years can be regarded as the payoff on an investment of many years together, many problems shared, and countless expressions of love exchanged. Each knows that his or her way of life and well-being depend on the other, so there is a willingness to change outlook, habits, and lovemaking, if necessary, to enhance their marriage. You can promote such changes.

You may teach or counsel the middle-aged adult who is having difficulty in relating to his or her spouse. Share the information in this chapter. Help the person determine, and then live out, the values of continuing to love and being patient and forgiving when the spouse has been unfaithful. Facilitate a desire to change behavior so that two people can grow together rather than apart. Work with the couple or refer them to counseling.

The following *guidelines for couples may help them reduce stress in the marriage:*

- Talk daily to each other about feelings so that small problems are solved continually, rather than allowing emotional tensions to accumulate, creating a breaking-point scene.

- Explore with each other feelings and ideas about possible, even if unlikely, life events that may occur—"what if" conversations. Such anticipatory worry helps the couple expand the repertoire of ideas and behavior so that if unexpected events occur, each will have more adaptive resources.
- Vary schedules and chores, family goals or expectations, and roles and rules or make other periodic changes just to stay comfortable with change and to be prepared to adapt if a crisis requiring flexibility occurs.
- Use each other as a resource. Talk to each other about individual problems, validate solutions, or ask each other about options for dealing with problems. Each must be willing to disclose about self to the other and be willing to support and help the other.
- Maintain contact with others, including the extended family, who can help during a crisis. Sometimes the family does not exist or cannot be supportive; seek other resources such as a church or other support group.
- In times of high stress or crisis, each should express the feelings of anger, grief, or helplessness to the other and to others who are caring. Expressing feelings about the circumstance, not about the spouse, allows conflict to surface and be handled.
- Keep active with each other and with others, which prevents feelings of either stagnation during routine times or helplessness during stressful times.

Refer also to the section on midlife crisis later in the chapter for ideas on how to assist the couple.

Widow(er)hood, the *status change that results from death of husband (or wife),* is a crisis in any life era, but it is more likely to occur first in middle age. The person who is about to become a widow(er) usually appreciates being able to participate in care of the spouse but must feel that the wife or husband will not suffer lack of care or support if a few hours are taken for rest. She or he needs someone to listen to feelings of anger, sadness, and guilt; nurses may be better able to listen, support, and encourage than family or friends. You can gently test reactions to determine if he or she is ready for the shock of death by offering to call a clergyman or by asking if family members need to be prepared for deterioration of the spouse's condition. If the person appears brave and strong, allow her or him to keep the veneer of courage if that is holding the person together. Realize the person may feel much ambivalence—not wanting the partner to suffer pain and yet wanting him

or her to be alert so that she or he can talk, or praying that death will relieve his suffering and yet hoping for his or her survival. After death the person may linger on the nursing unit—a place of support—rather than leaving for home, a very empty place.

The person's reaction to death of a spouse depends on personality and emotional makeup, the relationship between the couple (how long they have been married, how long the mate has been ill), and religious, cultural, and ethnic background. It will also be determined by other factors that existed in the relationship; for example, there may be less sorrow, or even relief, if the dead spouse was abusive, or severely or chronically disabled, either physically or mentally.

The loss of a spouse may mean many things: loss of a sexual partner and lover, friend, companion, caretaker, an audience for unguarded spontaneous conversation, accountant, plumber, or gardener, depending on the roles performed by the mate. Managing finances is often a major problem, especially for the widow. Secondary losses involve reduced income, which frequently means moving to a new residence and strange environment, change in lifestyle and social involvements, return to the work force, and giving up any number of things previously taken for granted. Widowhood is a threat to self-concept and sense of wholeness; now the person is seen as "only one." The woman's identity may be so tied to that of her husband that she feels completely lost, alone, and indecisive and as a nonperson after his death. If she has no one else close with whom to talk or from whom to receive help, she may believe she will lose her mind or become suicidal. The widow(er) misses having someone with whom he or she can share both happy occasions and sad news and problems. He or she can dial a crisis line to talk about a problem; it may be more difficult to tell about a source of happiness. The pet or houseplant is a poor substitute for a person. The emotional burden is increased if there are still children in the home to raise. The remaining parent has a hard time helping them work through their grief when she or he is in mourning. Friendship patterns and relations with inlaws also often change.

The widow is a threat to women with husbands; they perceive her as competition, and she is a reminder of what they might experience. With friends the widow is the odd person in number, so social engagements become stressful and are a constant reminder of the lost partner. The widow also becomes aware that she is regarded as a sexual object to men who may offer her their sexual services at a time when she has decreased sexual desires but a great need for companionship and closeness. Yet in contrast to assumptions, one study showed that many widows are quite competent in managing their lives (79, 132).

Although the widower is more accepted socially, he too will have painful gaps in his life. If the wife concentrated on keeping an orderly house, cooking regular and nutritious meals, and keeping his wardrobe in order, he may suddenly realize that what he had taken for granted is gone. Even more significant is the loss if his wife was a "sounding board" or confidante in business matters and if she was actively involved in raising children still in the home.

The bereavement of widowhood affects physical health; somatic complaints related to anxiety are not unusual. The widow(er) may experience symptoms similar to those of the deceased spouse.

Studies show that mortality rates, based on person-years at risk, were approximately the same for widowed and married women, but significantly higher for widowed than married men. Mortality rates among widowed males who remarried were very much lower than among those who did not remarry, but no significant difference was observable among widowed women who did or did not remarry (77, 79). Death, including from suicide, is more likely to occur during the first year of widowhood (79, 93).

Your contact with the widower(er) can help to resolve the crisis. Encourage the bereaved to talk about feelings as you provide a supportive relationship (or help the widow[er] to find one). Death of a husband in middle age is more common than that of wife; you will encounter more widows. Building up the widow's confidence and self-esteem, especially if she had lived a protected life, is essential. Help her identify people other than her children who can assist her with various tasks to avoid feelings of burden in any helper. Encourage her to try new experiences, expand interests, join community groups, do volunteer work, seek new friends, and become a person in her own right. Now is a good time to pursue activities formerly not done because the mate did not enjoy them. Encourage getting a medical checkup and following healthful practices in response to physical complaints, and help her recognize the somatic aspects of grief and mourning (42, 79, 124). You may want to offer group crisis intervention through the local Red Cross, a church, or school. Several books and articles can be useful to the widow(er) (22, 26, 42, 64, 79, 87, 121, 135).

Some national organizations that help the widow(er), are Naim, Parents Without Partners, THEOS, and the Older Women's League. Naim was founded by a couple in cooperation with a priest in Chicago. The chapters have well-planned monthly meetings about educational, spiritual, legal, and social needs of the widowed. Information can be obtained from Father Corcoran, Naim, St. Patrick's Roman Catholic Church, in Chicago (22).

Parents Without Partners, Inc., 8807 Colesville Rd, Silver Springs, MD 20010, is an international nonprofit, nonsectarian, educational, and social organization devoted to the welfare and interest of one-parent families and their children. Monthly meetings help the widow(er) get practical assistance and information and work through mourning (22).

They Help Each Other Spiritually (THEOS), 717 Liberty Avenue, Pittsburgh, PA 15222, is a national, nonsectarian organization designed primarily to help recently bereaved persons and young and middle-aged adults who need to resolve the grief related to the death of a loved one. Monthly meetings deal with various problem areas: reorganizing life, working through grief and loneliness, coping with the feeling of being a "fifth wheel," raising children alone, finances, dating and remarriage, expressions of bitterness, anger, and fear, and integrating loss and grief into belief in God and spiritual life (22).

Another organization that is an informational resource to help women adapt and plan for the future is Older Women's League, 730 11th Street NW, Suite 300, Washington, DC 20001. The middle-aged woman can get information about life insurance and Medicare and responses to other questions. Such information can help plan for later maturity.

Many of the problems that confront the widow(er) also confront the divorced person. Your intervention principles will be similar, although the words will be different.

Relationship With Aging Parents and Relatives

Because people are living longer, parents in later maturity and their adult offspring may expect more than 50 years of overlap; there is an increase in the number and duration of intergenerational linkages. The middle-aged person is in the middle in many ways, including in the middle of two demanding generations. Although child care responsibilities may be decreasing, considerable care of or involvement with offspring may remain at the same time there is increasing care of, involvement with, and responsibility for aging parents, aunts, uncles, or grandparents. The adult daughter and elderly mother may have remained in a close relationship through the years; if so, that daughter is likely to become more involved in that parent's life as the years pass. The friendship and interdependency of the younger years develop into a relationship with an increasingly dependent mother (87). The middle-aged woman may be in additional close relationships with elderly relatives more so than the middle-aged man or son.

The literature about middle-aged caregiving focuses on the caregiving to parents; however, sometimes the middle-aged adult is the caregiver for the grandparents or other elderly relatives, a disabled or chronically ill spouse, and the child (e.g., when the adult offspring has a chronic illness, an injury causing permanent loss of some function, or, increasingly, AIDS (33). More frequently, the middle-ager is carrying out these several caregiving roles simultaneously. Hainsworth et al. (70) discuss the chronic sorrow that women experience who care for a chronically mentally ill husband. Chronic sorrow may be felt by the other caregivers also.

Responsibility for Elderly Relatives

These cultural trends affect the dilemma of caring for older dependent relatives (30):

- Long-term societal emphasis on personal independence and social mobility of middle-aged and young adults, which creates physical separateness of generational households and new kinship patterns of intimacy at a distance
- Focusing on the dynamics of the marriage bond and socialization of young children, with the emphasis on affection, compatibility, and personal growth of each person in the nuclear family as the most important aspects of family life
- Longer life spans of older people and the problem of caring for the older generation when they become dependent

Filial responsibility is an *attitude of personal responsibility toward the parents that emphasizes duty, protection, care, and financial support,* which are indicators of the family's traditional protective function. Middle-class Caucasian culture in the United States believes that good relationships between the aged and their adult children are dependent on the autonomy of the parents. They believe that a satisfactory role reversal between generations is not possible because the mores of society do not sanction it and both children and parents resent it; however, older persons expect children to assume responsibilities when they can no longer maintain their independence. Families do in fact continue to provide nurturance and companionship through (1) visits and telephone calls, (2) information, (3) assistance in decision making, (4) transportation, (5) assistance with shopping, laundry, and household chores, (6) immediate response to crisis, (7) a buffer against bureaucracies, (8) help in searching out services, and (9) facilitation for continuity of individual–bureaucracy relations. In many ethnic or racial cultures, structure and style for the younger generation(s) have evolved through an extended family system to provide support, assistance, protection, and mobility. Often inadequate family economic reserves and inadequate health insurance necessitate the middle-aged adult's having to be caregiver (71, 103, 178).

Middle-aged children of various racial/ethnic groups are more likely than Caucasians to provide a home for elderly parents or other relatives. There are some differences within groups. For example, elderly Japanese are more likely to live with spouse or alone than other Asian groups. Elderly Southeast Asians are more likely to live with family members (71).

Many families have four or five generations; the young middle-aged person may have parents, grandparents, and great-grandparents. Further, elderly siblings, aunts, uncles, or cousins may also be living and need and expect help from the middle-aged adult. The person who is in his or her forties, fifties, or early sixties may be seen as possessing energy, free time, and money. Older relatives become more demanding just when the middle-aged adult believes he or she deserves time for self, a vacation, and an opportunity to pursue additional education or a social cause. The additional stress occurs when the older relatives want their needs met *right now;* they can create considerable guilt in the middle-aged adults.

Certainly the older and middle-aged generations can give a great deal to each other. The older generation(s) can share insights and wisdom about life. Sometimes they can give assistance financially or with various tasks. The older generation(s) can be a source of joy, pride, and inspiration. If they live long enough, however, the middle-aged adult will have someone who is increasingly dependent and in need of help. Sometimes the middle-aged adult realizes the dependence and need for help before the elderly person is ready to admit the need, and that can become a source of frustration and stress.

Caregiver Role

Care of a parent is a normative but stressful experience, although most people willingly help the parent and derive satisfaction from doing so. Various *factors that influence the caregiving role* include the following (10, 20, 21, 56, 58, 59, 60, 114, 115, 139, 141, 143, 150, 169, 177, 181, 182, 200, 207, 209):

- Seriousness of the elder's health status
- The caregiver–care recipient relationship and living arrangement
- Duration of the caregiving experience
- Other roles and responsibilities of the caregiver

- Overall coping effectiveness of the caregiver
- Caregiver sex and age
- Number of generations needing care
- Help and support from others—family or social agencies
- Information needed to carry out tasks related to physical care of the parent

Meeting parent's dependency needs may have many diverse effects (10, 20, 21, 28, 56, 58, 114, 122, 123, 143, 152, 156, 165, 169, 181, 209):

- Financial hardship
- Physical symptoms such as sleeplessness and decline in physical health, especially in the primary caregiver
- Emotional changes and symptoms in the caregiver and other family members, including frustration, inadequacy, anxiety, helplessness, depression, guilt, resentment, lowered morale, and emotional distance
- Emotional exhaustion related to restrictions on time and freedom and increasing responsibility
- A sense of isolation from social activities
- Conflict because of competing demands, with diversion from care of other family members
- Difficulty in setting priorities
- Reduced family privacy
- Inability to project future plans
- Sense of losing control over life events
- Interference with job responsibilities through late arrival, absenteeism, or early departure needed to take care of emergencies or even routine tasks
- Interference with lifestyle and social and recreational activities

Thus the whole family and its relationships are affected.

The dilemma of care for the elderly inevitably has an emotional impact on their grown children. The *caregiver role* is a major one, especially for the woman. In fact, the word *caregiver* is a euphemism for *unpaid female relative*. The middle-aged woman who is the older daughter is most likely to do the caregiving. Caregiving apparently is a woman's career; care of the dependent parent is only one phase of the woman's caregiving career. The woman often is caring for many people and several generations simultaneously either in her own home or in their homes. Caregiving may also be extended, finally, to the husband in old age. Interestingly, women who work provide as much caregiving as women who do not work outside the home. Nonemployed daughters provide more tangible help, but employed daughters contribute in other ways (56, 103, 115, 139, 150, 182). Some may reduce their working hours;

others quit their jobs, especially if the aged parent lives with them. For some, adult day-care services may be available for the woman to use with elderly parents or relatives during the day while she is at work (see Chapter 14.) Parent care makes the woman feel tied down and competes for time with the husband. Relations between husband and wife are affected because of financial or other help one person may give to the elderly parent(s), especially when done without consulting the other spouse. The needs of elderly parents may cause discord among their sons and daughters by recalling childhood rivalries and jealousies. A common phenomenon is when the middle-aged person resents those siblings who will not help care for the elderly parent(s) or other relatives. Further, if the middle-aged adult believes he or she was not well cared for by the parents as a child, continued resentment, anger, or hate may inhibit a nurturing attitude or even minimum assistance.

The meaning of caring for the dependent parent is different than for caring for the dependent child. The child's future holds promise for reducing dependency needs; the older parent will have increasing dependency needs. Parent care also stimulates anticipation of the final separation from the parent and of one's potential dependence on one's child. The way filial care is negotiated depends on the past and has implications for the future when the adult child is old.

Sometimes the adult child continues to care for the parent beyond physical and psychological means to do so rather than to use formal support systems. Various dynamics are at work: (1) symbiotic ties, (2) gratification from being the burden bearer, (3) a fruitless search for parental approval that has never been received, and (4) expiation of guilt for having been a favorite child. The middle-aged adult may perceive caregiving as an acceptable, permanent, full-time role that is altruistic and enhances self-esteem. Because this role gives meaning, a job or other roles may be discontinued, or this role may be a substitute for a failed marriage or for being widowed. Thus, successful resolution of this crisis may be acceptance of what cannot be done, as well as of what can and should be done. Refer to Danger Signals Indicating Caregiver Needs Assistance for more information. For the elderly, successful adaptation to dependence includes accepting what adult children cannot do (20, 56, 60, 114, 115, 141, 165, 181, 182).

The popular trend of expecting the middle-aged family to care for the dependent aged in their home assumes an emotional closeness and family cohesion that may not exist. The caregiving may instead contribute to a deterioration of relationships, even though a commitment to caring for family members is a value. Closeness may not be a basis for caregiving. Nor can we assume

► DANGER SIGNALS INDICATING CAREGIVER NEEDS ASSISTANCE

- Your relative's condition is worsening despite your best efforts.
- No matter what you do, it is not enough.
- You believe you are the only person in the world enduring this.
- You no longer have any time or place to be alone for even a brief respite.
- Things you used to do occasionally to help are now part of your daily routine.
- Family relationships are breaking down because of the caregiving pressures.
- Your caregiving duties are interfering with your work and social life to an unacceptable degree.
- You are going on in a "no-win situation" just to avoid admitting failure.
- You realize you are alone and doing all the work because you have shut out everyone who offered to help.
- You refuse to think of yourself because "that would be selfish" (even though you are unselfish 99% of the time).
- Your coping methods have become destructive; you are overeating or undereating, abusing drugs or alcohol, or being harsh or abrasive with your relative.
- There are no more happy times; loving and caring have given way to exhaustion and resentment; and you no longer feel good about yourself or take pride in what you are doing.

that satisfactory family relationships in early and middle adulthood will persist without change into late adulthood. Apparently there is a periodic rebalancing in family ties throughout life. Bonds may either loosen or grow closer with the conflicts and demands inherent in the caregiving role (60, 86).

A kind of psychological distancing between parents and caregiving children may occur. The adult children may feel little affection for the parent, feeling rather a kind of grief, and may hesitate to cancel the caregiving burden out of a sense of respect and loyalty to the parent. The adult child, often a married daughter, does not feel enough gratification from the caregiving to offset the sense of burden, yet the cultural expectation of closeness and love for family members leads her to feel guilt or despair. The person may question whether she can care for the parent if she does not feel love and may be concerned about the cost of caregiving to personal emotional stability (86, 143, 165).

Some of the impatience, aggravation, and desire to see less of the older person comes from the middle-aged adult's dawning realization that the older person is a picture of what the middle-aged person may become. The person who is in the prime of life may fear greatly the physical disabilities, illness, personality eccentrici-

ties, intellectual impairments, or social changes that old age brings.

Research findings document the strength of intergenerational ties, the continuity of responsible filial behavior, the frequency of contact between generations, the predominance of families rather than professionals in providing health and social services, the strenuous family efforts to avoid institutional placement of the old, and the central role played by families in caring for non-institutionalized impaired elderly (10, 20, 58, 86, 115, 139, 141, 150, 177, 207).

One of the most difficult decisions when parents become aged and dependent concerns the housing arrangement. The older daughter usually is the one to take the dependent parent into her home. Or the unmarried adult child may move into the parent's home. When the parent(s) cannot manage living alone, the middle-aged person may not have the room to take the parent(s) into his or her home. Even if there is adequate space, if all members of the household are working, finding someone to stay during the day may be difficult, although such an arrangement or the use of adult day care is less cost prohibitive than placing the parent who is in poor health in an institution. Most communities do not have adequate, or any, day-care facilities for elderly adults. Placing the parent(s) in an institution may be the only answer, but it is typically considered the last resort. Refer to Chapter 14 for more information on what to consider in that event.

Considerable research has been done on the middle-aged adult's caregiving role to parents, the tasks faced by and the effect on the caregiver and the middle-aged adult's family relations, physical and emotional health, and lifestyle. For additional information see References 10, 20, 21, 28, 56, 58, 59, 60, 71, 86, 103, 115, 122, 123, 139, 141, 143, 150, 152, 156, 165, 177, 178, 181, 182, 200, 207, and 209 at the end of the chapter.

Health Care Role

You are in a key position to help the middle-aged adult work through the conflicts, feelings of frustration, guilt, and anger about the increased responsibility and past conflicts or old hurts from parents or siblings. The middle-aged adult who verbally expresses great irritation typically also loves the older relative very much. Assist the middle-aged adult to gain a sense of satisfaction from the help he or she gives and a greater understanding of the person being helped. The generation gap and negative feelings that exist between the middle-aged adult and elderly person can be overcome with love, realistic expectations, a sense of forgiveness, and the realization that sometimes it is all right to say "No" to the

Research Abstract

Farran, G., et al., Finding Meaning: An Alternative Paradigm for Alzheimer's Disease Family Caregivers, Gerontologist, 31, no. 4(1991), 483–489.

Caregiving can be stressful; research shows that caregivers experience a sense of burden, depression, and decline in physical health. There are also caregivers who, although not intentionally seeking such a situation, may choose to make the best of the situation and to find positive outcomes.

Existentialism was the framework for this study. The purpose of this study was to understand how caregivers grow emotionally and spiritually and find meaning in the caregiving situation and in the suffering that is part of being a caregiver.

The sample comprised 94 caregivers—wives (34%), husbands (32%), daughters (24%), sons (3%), and other family members (6%)—who ranged in age from 30 to 78. All care receivers were diagnosed with an irreversible, progressive form of dementia and ranged in age from 49 to 92 years. The sample was middle class and primarily Caucasian (81%).

A 2-hour structured interview about caregiving was carried out in the home. Qualitative techniques were used to analyze the data. The data were grouped into four major themes: (1) loss and powerlessness; (2) values, choices, and provisional and ultimate meaning; (3) caregiving resources; and (4) responsibilities of caregiving.

Results indicated that these caregivers express existential themes. Finding meaning is an individual process, and spouses may differ from others in developing a caregiving attitude. Suffering is experienced at physical, psychological, social, and spiritual levels by caregivers. Suffering involves a sense of powerlessness—the inability to change one's circumstances.

Caregivers mourn their own losses as they experience changes in the relationship with the family member and realize their future plans have changed. Values form a basis for meaning. Experiential values focus on relationships and the feelings people have toward each other and are expressed as the caregiver focuses on who the person was in the past and enjoys the person for who he or she still is. Attitudinal values include philosophic or spiritual beliefs, and caregivers persevere in their efforts to provide care based on spiritual philosophy. Caregiving involves accepting the responsibility for making decisions about whether to be a caregiver and how to carry out these responsibilities. Caregivers may find provisional or short-term meaning from daily tasks, and ultimate meaning comes from exploring the deeper meanings in life.

Creative values are expressed in jobs, hobbies, or other creative activities. Caregivers are creative as they develop innovative approaches to daily problems. Each person must work through these values and meaning for self; this is an individual process not linked to race, sex, or relatedness to the care receiver. Caregivers can respond to the caregiving experience by making personal choices about life and caregiving, by valuing positive aspects of the caregiving experience, and by searching for meaning. Health care professionals can assist caregivers in these tasks. The caregiver spouse of a person with dementia must face the guilt of not caring for the impaired spouse and the guilt of not going forward with her or his own life. The caregiving role must be freely chosen, according to the Existential Framework.

demands of the elderly. Refer also to Chapter 14 for specific information you can share about physiologic, emotional, cognitive, and social needs, changes, and characteristics of the elderly person. One study indicated that teaching the caregiver stress management and time management techniques may reduce the sense of burden more so than participation in a support group (39). Encouraging the caregiver to maintain other roles outside of caregiving and family roles, although adding extra commitments to the sense of burden, may also increase the sense of caregiver well-being and health. Refer to a counselor or spiritual leader if necessary. Counseling can promote a resolution of feelings that in turn fosters a more harmonious relationship between the middle-aged adult and parents.

One way to help the adult child to continue the caregiving role, set aside guilt, and gain more positive feedback is to offer a *relabeled perspective*. The cultural mandate of affection for aging parents is of recent origin. Historically, aged parents have been cared for on the basis of obligation. Being a good child means not feeling great affection but showing concern for the well-being of the parent and giving care to the limits of one's ability. Helping the adult child internalize this perspective helps him or her begin to cope with the stresses without being overwhelmed. Thus, the parent cared for in the adult child's home has the advantage of a home environment. Further, outside resources can be used to support the adult child in the caregiving role. Often a little help will enable the person to make changes and use inner resources in a distressing situation. Having the caregiver keep a daily list of helping behaviors and of negative behaviors (not feelings) is a way of assisting the caregiver to see the role and behavior in a positive light and to gain reinforcement from the caregiving because almost always the helping behaviors far outnumber the negative behaviors. Such a log can provide a base for talking with the adult child about the interaction with the parent and ways to resolve feelings and improve the interaction (86).

Although some adult children are helped through this relabeling process, some ethnic or racial groups do not respond to this technique. For example, African-Americans have maintained a kind of behavioral closeness between generations that produces a different pattern of attitudes and less social and emotional distance between middle-generation adults and their parents.

Deaths of Parents in Adulthood

A critical time for the adult is when both parents have died, regardless of whether the relationship between parent(s) and offspring was harmonious or conflictual. The first death of a parent signals finiteness and mortality of the self and of the other parent and other loved ones. Memories of childhood experiences are recalled. The person may wish deeply, even though simultaneously realizing it is impossible, to be able to relive some of those childhood days with the parent, to undo naughty behavior, to be a good child just once more, to sit on the parent's lap and be cuddled one more time, to return to the relatively carefree days and to relive holidays. Further, more recent memories are recalled—the joys that were shared and the disharmonious times that are normal in any relationship but that are likely to engender guilt. There may be deep yearning to hold the parent one more time. Mourning may be done not only for the parent but for previously lost loved ones, and some mourning is in anticipation of future losses of the other parent, other beloved relatives and friends, and self. When the other parent dies, the adult is an orphan. Now he or she is no longer anyone's "little boy" or "little girl." The person may feel forlorn and alone, especially if there are few other relatives or friends. Sometimes there are no other living relatives and no sons so that the adult offspring represents the last of the family line. The person may question who and what will be remembered and by whom. This is a time of spiritual and philosophical searching whether or not the adult child is alone, has siblings, or has other relatives.

If there was conflict between the adult offspring and parents to the point of one-sided or mutual hate and unforgiveness, grief feelings may be denied or repressed or may be especially guilt laden. Consequently, the mourning process is delayed and not resolved as effectively. There is a yearning that life experiences with the parent(s) could have been better or different, a wish that harsh feelings could have been smoothed, and a sadness over what was never present more so than a sadness over what has been lost. The adult survivor may fear that he or she in turn may have similarly parented children, if any, and anxiety may arise about how the third or current child generation will feel when this parent dies. Will the scene and feelings be replayed? Can that be prevented? Certainly this can be a time for the adult to take stock, undo past wrongs with his or her children (and others), resolve old conflicts, and become motivated to move ahead into more harmonious relations with family members and others.

Throughout the period of parental loss, you may be a key person in helping the adult survivor or adult orphan relive, express, and sort out feelings; accept that any close relationship will not always go smoothly; and finally achieve a balance between happy, sad, and angry memories and feelings in regard to the parent(s). Finally, through such counseling the person can mature to accept and like self and other significant persons better and to change behavior patterns so that future relationships are less thorny.

Little is written specifically about bereavement experienced when the adult's parents die. One useful book is *The Orphaned Adult: Confronting the Death of a Parent,* by Marc Angel (31).

Developmental Tasks

In summary, the following developmental tasks must be accomplished for the middle-aged family to survive and achieve happiness, harmony, and maturity (45):

- Maintain a pleasant and comfortable home.
- Assure security for later years, financially and emotionally.
- Share household and other responsibilities, based on changing roles, interests, and abilities.
- Maintain emotional and sexual intimacy as a couple or regain emotional stability if death or divorce occurs.
- Maintain contact with grown children and their families.

- Decrease attention on child care tasks and adapt to departure of the child(ren).
- Meet the needs of elderly parent(s) in such a way as to make life satisfactory for both the parent(s) and middle-aged generations.
- Participate in community life beyond the family, recommitting energy once taken by child care.
- Use competencies built in earlier stages to expand or deepen interests and social or community involvement.

McCoy (116) has formulated developmental tasks and their outcomes for the stages of middle age (Table 13–1).

As a nurse you will have the opportunity and responsibility to help the middle-aged couple meet their developmental tasks.

PHYSIOLOGIC CONCEPTS

Physical Characteristics

The growth cycle continues with physical changes in the middle years, and different body parts age at different rates. One day the person may suddenly become aware of being "old" or middle-aged. Not all people decline alike. How quickly they decline depends on the stresses and strains they have undergone and on the health promotion measures that were maintained. If the person has always been active, he or she will continue with little slowdown. People from lower socioeconomic groups often show signs of aging earlier than people from more affluent socioeconomic groups because of their years of hard physical labor, poorer nutritional status, and lack of money for beauty aids to cover the signs of aging (46).

Now the person looks in the mirror and sees changes that others may have noticed some time ago. Gray, thinning hair, wrinkles, coarsening features, decreased muscular tone, weight gain, varicosities, and capillary breakage may be the first signs of impending age.

Because a number of your clients will be middle-aged, you are in a key position to help them understand the physiologic changes that occur in middle age, work through feelings about these changes, reintegrate the body image, and find specific ways to remain as healthy as possible. Use the following information to assist you in listening, teaching, reaffirming a positive self-concept, and counseling.

Hormonal Changes

Female Climacteric. This is the era of life known as the *menopause* for the woman or the *climacteric* for either sex. The terms are often used interchangeably. The

TABLE 13–1. DEVELOPMENTAL TASKS OF MIDDLE AGE AND THEIR OUTCOMES

Developmental Stage	Developmental Task	Outcome Sought
Restabilization, 44–55 years	Adjust to realities of work	Job adjustment
	Launch children	Letting go of parental authority
	Adjust to empty nest	Exploring new sources of satisfaction
	Become more deeply involved in social life	Effective social relations
	Participate actively in community concerns	Effective citizenship
	Handle increased demands of older parents	Better personal and social adjustment of elderly
	Manage leisure time	Creative use of leisure time
	Manage budget to support college-age children and ailing parents	Sound consumer behavior
	Adjust to single state	Fulfilled single state
	Solve problems	Successful problem solving
	Manage stress accompanying change	Successful stress management, personal growth
Preparation for retirement, 56–64 years	Adjust to health problems	Healthier individuals
	Deepen personal relations	Effective social skills
	Prepare for retirement	Wise retirement planning
	Expand avocational interests	Satisfaction of aesthetic urge; broadening of knowledge; enjoyment of travel
	Finance new leisure	Sound consumer behavior
	Adjust to eventual loss of mate	Adjustment to loss, fulfilled single state
	Use problem solving	Successful problem solving
	Manage stress accompanying change	Successful stress management, personal growth

Modified from McCoy, V., *Adult Life Cycle Tasks/Adult Continuing Education Program Response, Lifelong Learning in the Adult Years,* October (1977), 16.

menopause is the *permanent cessation of menstruation preceded by a gradually decreasing menstrual flow.* The term **perimenopausal years** denotes a *time of gradual diminution of ovarian function and a gradual change in endocrine status from before the menopause through 1 year after the menopause.* The **climacteric** is the *period in life when important physiologic changes occur, with the cessation of the woman's reproductive ability and the period of lessening sexual activity in the male.* Basic to the changing physiology of the middle years is declining hormonal production (137, 138).

Contrary to myth (see Table 13–2) depression or other symptomatology is neither inevitable nor clearly related to the perimenopausal or climacteric years (41, 145, 158, 164, 198). Most women feel relieved or neutral about menopause; only a small percentage view it negatively. Attitudes toward menopause improve as women move from pre- to postmenopause, and perception of health becomes more positive as menopause proceeds (41, 48, 145, 198). The worst part about the menopause or climacteric may be not knowing what to expect, as there is still a dearth of research and scientific knowledge about this normal period of life. Myths abound and there are several conceptual views of menopause.

In North American culture, menopause is viewed primarily as a biomedical or psychiatric event, but sociocultural and feminist views are found in the literature (Table 13–3) (41).

In the biomedical view, menopause is a cluster of symptoms or syndrome. The ovarian failure, with a hormone deficiency, is the cause of various physical and psychological symptoms, such as hot flashes, vaginal atrophy, and depression. The syndrome can be treated by hormone replacement (41).

In the psychiatric view, the changes of menopause cause anxiety and depression, which can be treated with psychotropic medication. Women who think of menopause primarily in these terms may feel negative about themselves during the climacteric period, because the emphasis is on the body's deficiency or loss. Thus traditional homemakers in the United States may experience greater difficulty with menopause because the reproductive role has passed (41).

In societies in which women rise in status after menopause or generally enjoy high status regardless of reproductive stage, a menopausal syndrome is nonexistent. A woman's perception of her menopause experience is largely her perception of the physical, social, and psychological changes she undergoes (41, 112).

The sociocultural view has emerged over several decades in reaction to the biomedical and psychiatric view, in response to the feminist movement, and especially in response to greater understanding of women from various cultures in the United States or of women

TABLE 13–2. MYTHS ABOUT THE MENOPAUSE

Myth	Fact
1. Menopause is a deficiency disease and catastrophe.	1. Menopause is a normal developmental process.
2. Most women have serious disability during the menopause.	2. Most women pass through it with a minimum of distress. Some have no noticeable symptoms or reactions and simply stop menstruation.
3. Menopause is the end of life.	3. The average life expectancy for today's 50-year-old woman is 81 years; one-third of her life is postmenopausal. Postmenopause is a time of new zest.
4. Menopausal women are more likely to be depressed than other people.	4. Menopausal depression in middle age is likely to be due to social stresses: a. The double standard of aging (older men are handsome, distinguished, and desirable; older women are worn out and useless) b. Caregiver demands c. Loss of loved ones d. Loss of roles e. Other health problems (the decreased level of estrogen affects neurotransmitters that regulate mood, appetite, sleep, and pain perception.)
5. Numerous symptoms accompany the menopause.	5. Predictable manifestations of menopause are: a. Change in menstrual pattern b. Transient warm sensations or vasomotor instability (hot flashes) to some degree (47–85% of women) c. Vaginal dryness in some women
6. Hot flashes are "in the woman's head."	6. Vasomotor instability results from hemodynamic compensatory mechanisms. Until the body adjusts to less estrogen, hypothalamic instability causes dips in body's core temperature. The flash is the body's adaptive response to equalize peripheral and core temperatures through dermal heat loss.
7. The woman may have a heart attack during a hot flash.	7. The tachycardia that occurs during a flush is the body's adaptive response to skin temperature changes.
8. The woman loses sexual desire during and after the menopause.	8. Vaginal changes may cause some discomfort, which would reduce libido. Psychosocial concerns about the empty nest, partner's loss of sexual capacity, or expectation of loss of libido are more likely the cause than reduced estrogen.
9. The indicators of the menopause are the various symptoms women experience.	9. Women may have regular menstrual cycles with decreased estrogen levels; hot flashes may occur before the menopause begins.
10. Only women have to worry about osteoporosis.	10. By age 70, osteoporosis risk is equal in men and women.

TABLE 13–3. ASSUMPTIONS ABOUT MENOPAUSE

Biomedical

1. Science, which is objective and precise, provides the true knowledge about a condition.
2. Women are products of their reproductive systems and hormones.
3. Women's behavior is caused by their biology and hormones.
4. Menopause can be studied as biomedical variables, treatments, and outcomes.
5. Menopause is a disease that causes psychological distress, an outcome of the handicap of menstruation.
6. Women are considered medically old and socially useless when menopause occurs.
7. Norms of the male are the baseline for considering norms for the woman.
8. Menopause can be treated as a disease of decreased hormones.
9. Treatment will restore the woman to the premenopausal, and desirable, state.

Sociocultural

1. Science is an important model for research, but view of women is less negative than in the biomedical model.
2. The world, and therefore women, is dynamic and cannot be fully understood from experimental studies.
3. Social and cultural variables are basic to understanding people, their behavior, and reactions to their bodies.
4. Attitudes, relationships, roles, and interactions are important variables in understanding people.
5. Positions of women and societal conditions contribute to women's reactions to the menopause.
6. The meaning of an event is critical to the person's reaction to the event.
7. There is no consistent relationship between the biochemical or physiologic processes and the person's perception of an event or behavior.
8. *Menopause is a natural developmental phase, not a disease process,* based on changes in the endocrine system.
9. *Menopause is a part of natural life transitions,* and views include cultural ideas about life and nature.

in other societies. In the sociocultural view, menopause has little or no effect on the woman. Instead, role changes or cultural attitudes toward aging are identified as the cause of any discomforts (41).

In the feminist view, menopause has been a taboo subject, veiled in secrecy and myths, in which womens' rights are suppressed in the name of biology. This view has become marginal, but in the late 1970s and early 1980s, the feminists were the force behind initiation of research on the perimenopausal years and on the menopause event (41).

The sociocultural view explains the difference between 2 million women in the United States with severe menopausal symptoms and the absence of incapacitation during the menopause in women in other cultures.

In other cultures, there is a role beyond the menopause (41). In the *United States,* most women and men, and a growing number of scientists, also see that *there are life and roles beyond the menopause!*

See Table 13–3 for assumptions about menopause from the biomedical and sociocultural perspectives (41).

Male Climacteric. This comes in the fifties or early sixties, although the symptoms may not be as pronounced as in the female climacteric. A man's "change of life" is passed almost imperceptibly, but he usually notices it when he makes comparisons with past feelings and performance. A few men may even complain of hot flashes, sweating, chills, dizziness, headaches, and heart palpitations. Unlike women, however, men do not lose their reproductive ability, although the likelihood diminishes as age advances. The output of sex hormones of the gonads does not stop; it is merely reduced. Testosterone level usually is lower in the middle-aged man who has high stress, lowered self-esteem, and depression. Testosterone therapy should be used cautiously because administration may increase prostatic hypertrophy and cancer development (84, 113).

Menopause. The average age for onset of menopause is 51; the usual range is between 45 and 55 years, although it may occur as early as age 35 for approximately 1% of women (188). In the woman the process of aging causes changed secretion of follicle-stimulating hormone (FSH), which brings about progressive and irreversible changes in the ovaries, leading to the menopause and loss of childbearing ability. The primordial follicles, which contain the ovum and grow into vesicular follicles with each menstrual cycle, become depleted, and their ability to mature declines. Finally, ovulation ceases because all ova have either degenerated or been released. Thus, the cyclic production of progesterone and estrogen fails to occur and levels rapidly fall below the amount necessary to induce endometrial bleeding. (The adrenal glands continue to produce some estrogen.) The menstrual cycle becomes irregular; periods of heavy bleeding may alternate with amenorrhea for 1 or 2 years, eventually ceasing altogether (69). Consistent or regular excessive bleeding may be a sign of pathology, not of the approaching menopause.

The pituitary continues to produce FSH and luteinizing hormone (LH), but the aging ovary is incapable of responding to its stimulation. With the pituitary no longer under the normal cyclic or feedback influence of ovarian hormones, it becomes more active, producing excessive gonadotropins, especially FSH. A disturbed endocrine balance influences some of the symptoms of menopause. Although the ovaries are producing less estrogen and progesterone, the adrenals may continue to produce some hormones, thus helping to maintain younger feminine characteristics for some time (69).

During the perimenopausal period (approximately 5 years) some discomforts may occur in a small percentage of women. Vasomotor changes cause hot flashes associated with chilly sensations, dizziness, headaches, perspiration, palpitations, water retention, nausea, muscle cramps, fatigability, insomnia, and paresthesia of fingers and toes. Many symptoms, including irritability, depression, emotional lability, and palpitations, are frequently attributed to menopause. Some women experience *no* symptoms, only a decrease, then cessation, of menses. The great majority of women experience no effect in their sexual relationships from the menopause. Most find menopause a time of integration, balance, liberation, confidence, and action (164, 198).

Difficulties experienced during menopause may be associated with concurrent life change or recent loss, or marital, psychological, or social stress. The cause of the symptoms apparently is more complex than simple estrogen deficit. Psychological factors such as anger, anxiety, and excitement are considered as important in precipitating hot flashes in susceptible women as conditions giving rise to excess heat production or retention such as a warm environment, muscular work, and hot food; however, the symptoms may arise without any clear psychological or heat-stimulating mechanism (41, 79).

Physical Changes. Table 13–4 summarizes physical changes that occur in middle age, physiological reasons for the changes and characteristics that are commonly seen, and implications for health promotion and client teaching (1, 37, 43, 46, 52, 69, 78, 80, 99, 100, 112, 113, 140, 145, 163, 164, 185, 188, 198, 199, 210).

Hormone Replacement Therapy. The benefits of hormone replacement therapy (HRT), as well as the side effects or drawbacks, have been widely discussed. HRT can reduce the intensity of menopausal symptoms and the risks of coronary heart disease, and osteoporosis. *Yet it must be prescribed on an individual basis,* and the woman should be started on the lowest possible dose (188, 198).

Estrogen deficiency, the cause of hot flashes, may cause a disturbance in the chemical messengers that regulate the body's thermostat through the autonomic nervous system. Estrogen supplementation is effective but has risks in combating hot flashes; side effects include irregular bleeding, depression, headaches, nausea, edema, breast swelling, and weight gain. Androgens or other synthetic medications or psychotropic medications also have uncertain benefit and may cause other side effects (43, 80, 158, 183, 188, 198).

Hormone replacement therapy *is appropriate* when a woman (43, 52, 61, 78, 80, 158, 188, 198):

- Has had ovaries removed before age 45 or experiences premature menopause (before age 40)
- Is at high risk of fractures, especially if the risk is due to medical factors such as removal of ovaries or use of corticosteroid or other medications that can cause bone loss
- Has extreme menopausal discomfort such as hot flashes and/or night sweats (Vaginal dryness usually responds to estrogen cream.) (158, 188, 198)

Avoid estrogen-only products for HRT, as they are associated with (1) higher risk of endometrial cancer (5–10 times higher than if not taking estrogen); (2) adverse reactions such as fluid retention, weight gain, headache, breast discomfort, nausea, leg cramps, thrombosis, hyper- or hypotension, gallbladder disease, and general malaise; (3) diabetes, as a result of lowered glucose tolerance; and (4) higher risk of breast cancer if taken long-term (43, 78, 83, 158, 188, 198).

When progestin is added to estrogen, unacceptable premenstrual symptoms and withdrawal bleeding may occur. Progestin may also increase the risk of breast cancer. When estrogen is given with progestin, unless it is for less than 5 years, the risk of breast cancer is 30 to 40% higher than in those who take no hormones (43, 83, 188, 198).

Hormone therapy should *not* be implemented even if any of the above circumstances apply, when a woman (43, 78, 83, 158, 188, 198):

- Has a history of any blood-clotting event (e.g., stroke, thrombophlebitis, pulmonary embolus, heart attack)
- Has breast cancer
- Has endometrial cancer
- Has active liver disease or chronic impairment of her liver function
- Experiences unexplained vaginal bleeding
- Is or may be pregnant

Risks and other drawbacks of hormone use include (1, 43, 78, 83, 158, 188, 198):

- Possible increased risk of breast cancer after long-term use
- Possible increased risk of gallbladder surgery

TABLE 13–4. PHYSICAL CHANGES AND CHARACTERISTICS OF MIDDLE AGE AND HEALTH PROMOTION IMPLICATIONS

Body System or Physical Parameter	Change/Characteristic	Implications for Health Promotion
Endocrine and Reproductive System	Decline in production of neurotransmitters that stimulate hypothalamus to signal pituitary to release sex hormones	
Women	Less estrogen synthesized	Reproductive cycle is ended; this may represent sexual liberation or loss of femininity.
	No estrogen produced by ovaries; menses stops	Counsel about meaning of femininity.
	Aging oocytes (eggs) destroy necessary genetic material for reproduction.	Support group may be helpful.
	Uterine changes make implantation of blastocyte unlikely	Instruct in Kegel exercises.
	Gradual atrophy of tissues:	Hormone replacement therapy may be prescribed.
	Uterus and cervix become smaller	Artificial (water-soluble) lubrication can be used during intercourse to reduce discomfort.
	Vulva epithelium thins	Regular sexual intercourse maintains lubrication and elasticity of tissue.
	Labia majora and minora flatten	
	Vaginal mucosal lining thinner, drier, pale (20–40% women; some never experience this)	
	Natural lubrication during intercourse decreases	
	Neuroendocrine symptoms, such as hot flashes and night sweats followed by chilling, fatigue, nausea, dizziness, headache, palpitations, and paresthesias may occur.	Avoid precipitating factors such as hot drinks, caffeine, alcohol, stress, and warm environment.
		Counsel to stop smoking.
		Hormone replacement therapy may reduce symptoms.
Men	Testosterone production gradually decreases, which eventually causes:	Sperm production continues to death, so man is capable of producing children.
	Degeneration of cells in tubules	
	Production of fewer sperm	Premature ejaculation is less likely, which may contribute to more enjoyable intercourse.
	More time needed to achieve erection	Practice Kegel exercises for firmer erections.
	Less forceful ejaculation	
	Testes less firm and smaller	
Basal Metabolism Rate (BMR) (minimum energy used in resting state)	BMR declines 2% per decade	If eating pattern is maintained, 3 to 4 pounds are gained per decade
	Gradually reduces as ratio of lean body mass to adipose tissue decreases (metabolic needs of fat is less than for lean tissue)	Fewer calories (2%) need to be consumed, even if the person exercises regularly, to avoid weight gain.
Weight	Gain should not occur; weight gain occurs if as many calories consumed as earlier: wider hips, thicker thighs, larger waist, more abdominal mass	Overweight contributes to a number of health problems; crash diets should be avoided.
Integumentary System		
Sebaceous oil glands	Produce less sebum secretions, skin drier and cracks more easily	Protect and lubricate skin with lotion or moisturizer.
	More pronounced in women after menopause than in men of same age	Avoid excess soap and drying substances on skin.
		Avoid excessive strong sun and wind exposure.
Sweat glands	Decrease in size, number, and function	Ability to maintain even body temperature is affected; dress in layers to maintain comfort.
Skin	Skin wrinkles, tissue sags, and pouches under eyes due to:	Wrinkles are less apparent with use of moisturizer or lotion.
	Epidermis flattens and thins with age, collagen in dermis becomes more fibrous, less gellike	Wrinkled appearance of skin is made worse by excess exposure to sun or sunburn; use sunscreen.
	Elastin loses elasticity, causing loss of skin turgor.	Skin is more prone to injury; healing is slower.
	Loss of muscle tone causes sagging jowls.	Use humidifier in home.
Women	Estrogen decrease gradually causes skin and mucous membranes to lose thickness and fluids; skin and mucous membranes thinner, drier, and begin atrophy	Avoid burns and bruises.
		Use lotions.
	Estrogen decrease gradually causes breasts to sag and flatten	Maintain support with correctly fitted brassiere.
		Maintain erect posture.
Hair	Progressive loss of melanin from hair bulb causes gray hair in most adults by age 50; hair thins and growth slows; hair rest and growth cycles change	Slow hair loss by gentle brushing, avoiding excess heat from hair dryer, and avoiding chemical treatment.

(continued)

TABLE 13–4. PHYSICAL CHANGES AND CHARACTERISTICS OF MIDDLE AGE AND HEALTH PROMOTION IMPLICATIONS (continued)

Body System or Physical Parameter	Change/Characteristic	Implications for Health Promotion
Women	Estrogen decrease may gradually cause increased growth of facial hair Hair loss not as pronounced as in male	Accept change. Manage cosmetically.
Men	Testosterone decrease causes gradual loss of hair Hereditary male-pattern baldness occurs with receding hairline and monk's spot area on back of head	Accept change. Manage with styling, hairpiece, or hair transplant.
Muscular System	Slight decrease in number of muscle fibers; about 10% loss in muscle size from ages 30 to 60 Gradual loss of lean body mass Muscle tissue gradually replaced by adipose unless exercise is maintained Most loss of muscle occurs in back and legs Grip strength decreases with age Gradual increase in subcutaneous fat	Physical exercise and fitness, proper nutrition, and healthy lifestyle can improve or sustain muscle strength during middle age. Variations in peak muscular activity depend on type of exercise.
Skeletal System	Gradual flattening of intervertebral disks and loss of height of individual vertebrae cause compression of spinal column	Maintain erect posture. Maintain adequate calcium intake (1000–1500 mg daily). Exercise maintains bone mass and joint flexibility, improves balance and agility, and reduces fatigue. Loss of height occurs in later life.
Men and women	At age 70, osteoporosis risk equal in men and women unless vitamin D has been taken to increase bone density	Vitamin D decreases risk of fractures.
Women	Estrogen reduction increases decalcification of bones, bone resorption, decreased bone density, and gradual osteoporosis Cultural differences: Caucasians and Asians more likely than Latinos and African-Americans to suffer bone porosity because their bones are less dense and they lose mass more quickly	Maintain exercise and calcium intake. Maintain erect posture. Maintain calcium and good nutrition intake. Teach safety factors; forearms, hips and spinal vertebrae are most vulnerable to fractures. Supplemental vitamin D and and regular small amounts of exposure to sunlight improve calcium absorption. Avoid smoking, high alcohol intake, and high caffeine intake, all of which interfere with nutrition. Caffeine causes calcium loss. Women may eventually be 3 in. shorter if they have vertebral osteoporosis. Dowager's hump will form in cervical and upper thoracic area if osteoporosis occurs. Women who have taken oral contraceptives for 6 or more years have higher bone density in lumbar spine and femoral neck.
Neurologic System	Speed of nerve conduction, nerve impulse traveling from brain to muscle fiber, decreases 5% by age 50, and only 10% through life cycle Brain structural changes minimal; gradual loss of neurons does not affect cognition	Sensation to heat and cold and speed of reflexes may be impaired. Teach safety factors. Functional abilities are maintained, and learning from life experiences enhances functional abilities.
Sensory *Vision*	Average 60-year-old requires twice the illumination of 20-year-old to do close work Eyes begin to gradually change at about 40 or 50, causing **presbyopia** (*farsightedness*) Lens less elastic, loses accommodation Cornea increases in curvature and thickness, loses luster Iris responds less well to light changes; pupils smaller Retina begins to lose rods and cones Optic nerve fibers begin to decrease	Wear brimmed hat and sunglasses that block UV rays to protect vision. Person eventually needs bifocals or trifocals to see small print or focus on near objects. Eyes do not adapt as quickly to darkness, bright lights or glare (implications for safety and night driving). More light is needed to see well.

(continued)

TABLE 13–4. PHYSICAL CHANGES AND CHARACTERISTICS OF MIDDLE AGE AND HEALTH PROMOTION IMPLICATIONS (continued)

Body System or Physical Parameter	Change/Characteristic	Implications for Health Promotion
Hearing	Auditory nerve and bones of inner ear gradually change Gradual decrease in ability to detect certain tones and certain consonants Loss of hearing from high-pitched sounds	Reduce exposure to loud work machinery or equipment; wear ear protectors. Reduce exposure to loud stereo, radio, or electronic music. Cross-culture studies show our high-tech culture contributes to increasing and earlier impairment. Hearing aids, correctly chosen, or surgery may correct hearing impairment.
Voice		
Women	Estrogen decrease gradually causes lower pitch of voice	
Men	Testosterone decrease gradually causes higher pitch of voice	
Cardiovascular System	Efficiency of heart may drop to 80% between 30 and 50 Decreased elasticity in muscles in heart and blood vessels Decreased cardiac output Cardiovascular disease risk for women equal to that of men by age 70 because reduced estrogen causes lipid changes, increase in low-density lipoproteins (LDLs), decrease in high-density lipoproteins (HDLs), and gradual increase in total serum cholesterol.	Regular aerobic exercise maintains heart function and normal blood pressure. Inactivity affects system negatively. Quit smoking. Maintain healthy diet. Take regular low doses of aspirin. Maintain low cholesterol diet.
Respiratory System	Gradual loss of lung elasticity Thorax shortens Chest cage stiffer Breathing capacity reduced to 75% Chest wall muscles gradually lose strength, reducing respiratory efficiency	Regular exercise enhances respiratory efficiency. Inactivity affects system negatively.
Urinary System	Glomerular filtration rate gradually decreases	Maintain adequate fluid intake; drink 8 glasses of water daily.
Women	Loss of bladder muscle tone and atrophy of supporting ligaments and tissue in late middle age causes urgent urination, possibly cystocele, rectocele, and urine prolapse.	Instruct in Kegel exercises as follows: Draw in perivaginal muscles (pubococcygeus muscle) and anal sphincter as if to control urination, without contracting abdominal, buttock, or inner thigh muscles. Maintain contraction for 10 seconds. Follow with 10 seconds of relaxation. Perform exercises 30–80 times daily.
Men	Hypertrophy of prostate begins in late middle age; enlarging prostate around urethra causes frequent urination, dribbling, and nocturia	Urinary stasis may predispose to infections. Drink adequate amount of water. Surgery may be necessary.

- Possible nausea, weight gain, breast tenderness, uterine bleeding, fluid retention, and depression
- Possible shifts in the insulin needs of a woman with diabetes
- Return of monthly bleeding when combined hormones are taken sequentially

The following are often reasons *not* to institute HRT, although special conditions may override them (43, 78, 83, 158, 188, 198):

- History of breast cancer
- History of endometrial cancer
- History of liver disease
- Large uterine fibroids
- Endometriosis
- History of thrombophlebitis or thromboembolism
- History of stroke or transient ischemic attack
- Recent heart attack
- Pancreatic disease
- Gallbladder disease
- Fibrocystic breast disease
- Hypertension that is aggravated by estrogen
- Migraine headaches aggravated by estrogen

Whenever a woman is on HRT, she needs to be fully informed about all aspects of the treatment. Regular monitoring is needed to determine dosage adjustment. If exogenous estrogen is given, the woman should have serial mammograms, annual gynecologic examinations, and careful assessment of bleeding. (Estrogen alone or unopposed estrogen is usually prescribed only for women who have had hysterectomies.) How long HRT must be continued to maintain benefits is unknown. When HRT is withdrawn, women again experience the symptoms of menopause and become subject later to reduced bone density (43, 188, 198).

Reinforce in the middle-aged woman that hormonal changes are normal, that they can be adapted to and lived with. Regular exercise (202) and relaxation methods reduce symptoms, as do meditation, biofeedback, and massage (1, 164, 198). Support groups may be helpful. Emphasize that estrogen products, whether facial and skin products or vaginal creams, should be purchased with medical guidance; likewise, HRT is done only when deemed by the physician as essential.

All women receiving estrogen replacement therapy because ovaries were surgically removed or to relieve menopausal symptoms should be seen every 6 to 12 months for a Papanicolaou test, breast examination, and blood pressure reading. Blood and liver function tests should also be done (188). All menopausal women should be taught that any abnormal bleeding (if receiving estrogen–progestin therapy) or spotting 12 months after cessation of menses indicates an increased risk of carcinoma and should be reported immediately to a physician.

Emotional Changes Related to Physical Changes. Depression, irritability, and a change in sexual desire may occur in response to physical changes and their meaning, but they do not automatically occur. Some women fear loss of sexual identity. Earlier personality patterns and attitudes are more responsible for the symptomatology than the cessation of glandular activity. Women who had previous low self-esteem and life satisfaction are more likely to have difficulties with menopause. Reactions to menopause are consistent with reactions to other life changes, including other reproductive turning points such as puberty. Women with high motherliness scores and heavy investment in childbearing react more severely to the menopause (106, 138, 164).

Reactions to menopause vary across social classes and according to the availability of alternate roles. Middle- and upper-class women appear to find the cessation of childbearing more liberating than lower-class women, perhaps because more alternatives are open to them. In the relatively advantaged social classes,

younger women anticipating menopause express the most concern. Postmenopausal women generally take a more positive view than premenopausal women, agreeing that the menopause creates no major discontinuity in life and, except for the underlying biological changes, women have a relative degree of control over their symptoms and need not inevitably have difficulties. In general, menopausal status is not associated consistently with measurable anxiety in any group (48, 163, 164).

Studies of women in middle age from working- and middle-class backgrounds who were in good physical health, married, and had at least one child have consistently indicated that these women saw the menopause as a normal life event rather than as a threat to feminine identity. They minimized the significance of the menopause and regarded it as unlikely to cause much anxiety or stress. Some believed health improved after menopause, and 65% believed there was no effect on sex life. Any changes in sexual activity during the climacterium was seen as a function of the woman's (or couple's) attitudes. Half reported sexual relations as more enjoyable because menstruation and fear of pregnancy were removed. Few reported having symptoms sufficient to seek medical treatment, although 75% reported minor discomforts. A majority believed change in health or emotional status during the menopause reflected individual differences in coping with stress or idiosyncrative factors. Only 4 of the 100 regarded the menopause as a major source of worry. Women who had difficulties with the menarche, menses, or pregnancy were more likely to have menopausal problems. More than half indicated that the death of the husband was the greatest concern; other concerns were fear of cancer and the implications of getting older. In general, 80% attributed little or no change in their lives to menopause. Most believed they had control over the symptoms and need not have symptomatic difficulties (48, 127, 129).

There are minimal cross-cultural studies of the male climacteric. A construction worker who gauges his age by physical strength may feel middle-aged or old before he reaches 40 or 45. The factory worker may not have as many frustrations of unattainable goals as a white-collar worker and thus may be less likely to undergo a midlife crisis. Another manual laborer who feels oppressed by his foreman and stifled by his job may fear the day when physical powers decline and he may lose his only source of security—his job. The African-American man apparently experiences a midlife crisis much like that of the Caucasian man. Bachelors and widowers who may be lonely and lack the warmth of family ties frequently suffer at least temporary loss of libido in the middle years and symptoms of midlife crisis related to fears of mortality and the meaninglessness of their life. Some men may experience again a long-dormant homosexual interest (84).

You are in a key position to help the middle-aged adult work through feelings about the meaning of midlife changes and ways to prevent or minimize their effects. Refer to Chapter 12 for ways to help the person work through self-concept and body image changes and for ways to enhance self-concept.

Nutritional Needs

Basal metabolic rate gradually decreases by 2% every decade after age 20. For each decade after 25 years, there should be a reduction in caloric intake proportionate to activity level and to the reduced basal metabolism rate (BMR) (78, 119, 203). The reduced basal energy requirements caused by losses in functioning protoplasm and the frequently reduced physical activity combine to create less demand for calories (2400 calories for men and 1800 calories for women).

Teach the intake of carbohydrate and foods with high fat, saturated fat, and cholesterol content should be reduced, including the foods with "empty" calories: rich desserts, candies, fatty foods, gravies, sauces, and alcoholic and nondiet cola beverages, substitute sparkling waters or reduced-calorie wines or beers; half the intake of alcoholic beverage is desired. Intake of salty food should be limited; herbs, spices, and lemon juice can be used for flavoring. Overweight is not just a genetic factor (78, 109, 131, 203) and should be avoided, because it is a factor in diabetes, cardiovascular and hypertensive disease, and problems with mobility such as arthritis.

Dietary intake will be imbalanced nutritionally if meals are not wisely planned. For the healthy person daily diet should contain all of the food groups found in a variety of foods, with emphasis on protein, minerals, vitamins, low-cholesterol and low-calorie foods, and fiber. Refer to Table 12–2 for recommended daily servings (78, 140, 203). Often the middle-ager does not eat enough of certain nutrients—vitamins A, B, C, and folate, and the minerals calcium, iron, magnesium, and fluoride (5, 78, 203). Plenty of fluids, especially water and juices, along with an adequate diet, will maintain weight control and vigor and help prevent "heartburn," constipation, and other minor discomforts caused by physiologic changes. Equally important, the person should chew food well, eat smaller portions, eat in a pleasant and unhurried atmosphere, and avoid eating when overtired.

Drinking too much coffee or tea can be a real problem in middle age. Intake should be limited to 1 or 2 cups daily, including decaffeinated forms, and drunk between meals. The tannins in coffee and tea at mealtime can reduce the body's ability to absorb nutrients such as calcium. There may also be an association between coffee and high blood cholesterol levels. Coffee and tea should be avoided if there is a family history of heart disease or if the person is overweight, eats a high-fat diet, and does not exercise (78).

There is no evidence that use of commercial vitamin–mineral preparations is necessary unless they are prescribed by a physician because of clinical signs of deficiency and insufficient diet. Adequate calcium intake is essential for both men (1000 mg/d) and women (1200–1500 mg/d; 2000 mg/d for the postmenopausal woman who is not treated with estrogen). Note that one glass of milk contains 300 mg of calcium, although there are many other sources of calcium (78, 198, 203) (see Appendix II). Calcium supplements should be avoided if there is existing kidney disease, as high calcium intake will increase the risk of kidney stones (203).

Teach younger women or adolescents in the middle-age family that regular milk consumption by female adolescents and young adults is associated with better bone density in the spine, hip, trochanter, but not femoral neck, in later middle age and old age (171). Further, vitamin D is necessary for calcium absorption; supplements are recommended but should not exceed 800 mg daily to avoid an overdose (199).

Considerable information is available to the public about healthful nutrition, yet the American diet remains overloaded with sugar-filled and fatty foods. Only as values change will diet change. Health teaching must begin with understanding cultural concepts and values before a significant trend toward wise eating habits can begin. Joining self-help groups such as Weight Watchers or Take Off Pounds Sensibly (TOPS) is effective for many people. It is possible to change habits of overeating and to lose weight in middle age.

Teach the middle-aged person to avoid using extreme diets to decrease weight quickly and to avoid repeatedly losing weight that is then regained. Each gain–lose cycle reduces the total muscle mass with weight loss and increases body fat, as regained weight is in the form of adipose tissue. Adipose tissue burns fewer calories than muscle, so each round of dieting makes it more difficult to lose weight and maintain weight loss. Extreme low-calorie diets should also be avoided because with them, the basic metabolic rate becomes lower so that, even with restricted calories, little weight is lost. Thus, to lose weight it is essential to exercise—at least moderately for 40 minutes a day—and eat a healthy high-fiber, low-fat diet. See Healthy–Eat-

► **HEALTHY-EATING PLAN FOR THE MIDDLE-AGED ADULT**

Go Nutrient Dense and High Fiber

- Buy cereals that give you a larger portion for the calories.
- Serve meals loaded with complex carbohydrates such as pasta, rice (brown for more fiber), barley, and potatoes.
- Be creative with your potato toppings — plain yogurt mixed with herbs, picante sauce, or melted low-fat cheese.
- Use meats such as lean beef and skinless turkey and chicken not as the biggest part of the meal but more as condiments. Serve them in 2- to 3-oz portions.
- Use romaine lettuce in salads instead of the pale, anemic-looking variety. Romaine lettuce has approximately eight times more vitamin A and double the iron of iceberg lettuce.
- Serve an iron-rich plant food such as a legume or dried fruit with a vitamin C-rich food such as citrus fruit. Vitamin C helps your body use the iron more efficiently.
- Chop fruits and vegetables as little as possible, cook them just a short time, and minimize standing time. A number of vitamins are destroyed by air, light, and heat.
- Choose dark green and bright orange vegetables and fruits. They tend to have more nutrients than the paler plant foods. One-half cup of cooked, chopped broccoli, for instance, has more than double the vitamin A and eight times more vitamin C than the same amount of lighter green beans.
- Choose plain, low-fat yogurt and add your own fruit.
- Steam foods rather than cook them in large amounts of water, which can leach away important nutrients.
- Select whole-grain products more often than refined ones.
- Try to avoid empty calories (those giving you few nutrients) such as those found in alcohol or in desserts such as cake and pie.
- Work more fiber into your meals with peas and beans: mix them with rice or pasta, use them in meatless chili, or sprinkle them on salads.

Ease More Fish Into Meals

- Try fish in your favorite meat and chicken recipes.
- Do not overcook fish. Cook fish for approximately 10 minutes per inch of thickness, be it on the grill, under the broiler, or in an oven preheated to 450°F.
- Be creative: serve fish and shellfish in soups, salads, stews, pasta, and stirfry dishes.

Cut the Fat

- Reduce fat in the diet by eating ordinary foods and cutting back on just four things: fat used in prepared foods and in cooking, oils, red meats, and whole milk dairy products. These measures will reduce fat intake to approximately 20% of caloric intake.
- Avoid fried foods. Simulate the crunch of fried foods by oven frying. For instance, dip fish or chicken in egg whites and then in bread or cracker crumbs and bake on a nonstick cookie sheet at 300°–350°F until done; or slice potatoes into spears and bake in the oven at 350°F for 30 minutes.
- Invest in a large nonstick frying pan that uses little or no oil when sautéing or pan frying. Lightly coat regular pans and casseroles with nonstick vegetable spray.
- Experiment with low-fat, low-calorie flavor enhancers such as Dijon mustard, horseradish, chopped green or red peppers, onions, and seasonings such as tarragon, dry mustard, dill, and curry powder.
- Chill sauces, gravies, and stews ahead of time so the hardened fat can be skimmed from the surface.
- Make sauces without fat by slowly mixing cold liquid directly into the flour or cornstarch. Stir until smooth and bring to a boil, stirring frequently.
- Use evaporated skimmed milk instead of cream in coffee and recipes.
- In place of sour cream, use nonfat sour cream, low-fat or nonfat yogurt, or lowfat cottage cheese that has been mixed in a blender with a little milk and lemon juice.

Boost Milk Intake (Without Drinking a Drop)

If your system is not lactose intolerant, but you prefer not to drink milk as a beverage:

- Sneak nonfat dry milk powder into anything you can: soups, sauces, casseroles, meat loaf, and stews. Add a few teaspoons of it to coffee; this blend will taste like café au lait.
- Treat yourself to low-calorie puddings made with skim or low-fat milk.
- Make milk-based soups with skim milk.
- Use a blender to make a low-fat milk shake with a few ice cubes, skim or low-fat milk, fresh fruit, and low-calorie sweetener.
- Experiment with fun flavorings in low-fat milk: vanilla, rum extract, or even cocoa with a little artificial sweetener.
- Have cold breakfast cereals with milk and fresh fruit.

ing Plan for the Middle–Aged Adult for some helpful suggestions. (78, 198, 203).

Rest and Exercise

Middle age need not be a time when a person's body fails, but it is a period that requires better maintenance than was necessary in the earlier years.

Exercise

Exercise and erect posture may not increase longevity but they will enhance quality of life by keeping people healthy and independent (Fig. 13–1). A combination of the following activities appears optimum: *consistent brisk walking,* stretching, weight bearing, bicycling, rowing, swimming, aerobics, and resistance activities. *Forty minutes daily of moderate exercise* maintains muscle mass and strength; improves coordination and agility; stimulates bone formation and increased bone size and density; improves cardiovascular function and circulation; maintains body flexibility and collagen tissue elasticity; promotes deeper respirations; and promotes weight loss. In fact, the more a person exercises,

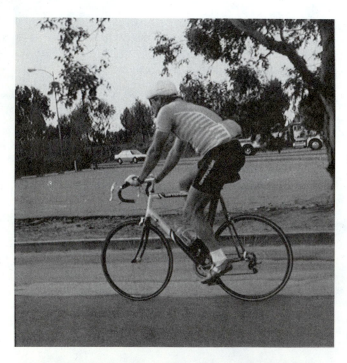

Figure 13–1. Middle-aged adults should be encouraged to participate in healthy behaviors such as exercising. *(From Berger, K.J., and M.B. Williams, Fundamentals of Nursing: Collaborating for Optimal Health. Stamford, CT: Appleton & Lange, 1992, p. 314.)*

the less will be his or her percentage of body fat, regardless of age (69, 78, 105).

Working with weights in a 12-week program can increase muscle size by about 11% and strength by 170%, as well as burn off calories (78, 105, 179). *Stretching* exercises can be helpful in maintaining flexibility; such exercise prevents shortening of connective tissue (78, 179). Strengthening abdominal muscles can improve posture, aid gastrointestinal function, and reduce chance of back injury, as well as improve self-image (78, 105, 179). Also refer to Lewis et al. for information on health counseling related to promoting an exercise regimen (105). Studies show that engaging in regular exercise decreases physical and psychological symptoms and increases self-esteem and life satisfaction (44, 74, 175, 176, 194, 202).

One of the most stable characteristics is *activity level.* Although there is a general and gradual decline in quickness and level of activity during the latter part of life, people who were most active among their age group during adolescence and young adulthood usually are the most active among their age group during middle and old age. It is almost as though each person has a physical and mental "clock" that runs at a fast or slow rate throughout life. The rate at which an individual's clock runs is reflected as well in various cognitive and personality charasteristic.

There is frequently a postmenopausal rise in energy and activity possibly for several reasons. Less time and energy go into childrearing. The children's leaving home allows time for self and pursuits in creative, social, or community projects. The person may feel more self-confident and satisfied with life achievements and less competitive. Less physical and psychic energy may be used in various internal conflicts or in worrying unnecessarily about the details in life. New self-awareness and flexibility can increase psychic and physical energy and a feeling of well-being. This new energy permits a developmental impetus and opportunities for personal growth.

The middle-aged adult invests considerable energy in occupational or professional, home, and organizational activity and in leisure time pursuits. He or she often has fine physical health. Although chronic disease is more prevalent than in the young, there is ordinarily good resistance to communicable diseases, superior emotional stamina, and a willingness to work despite minor illnesses. The person brings economy of effort, singleness of purpose, and perseverance to various roles.

Teach that, although physical changes do occur, adopting sedentary habits will not maintain health. Balanced with rest and sleep must be physical activity to keep the body posture and functioning at its optimum.

Capacity for intense and sustained effort diminishes, especially if engaged in irregularly, but judicious exercise may modify and retard the aging process. In addition to the physical benefits, regular and vigorous exertion is an excellent outlet for emotional tensions. For people with sedentary jobs, doing back exercises (Fig. 13–2) can prevent loss of muscle tone and discomfort (6).

Teach about the value of exercise. The type of exercise does not matter as long as the person *likes* it and engages in it *regularly,* and it is *suitable* for personal strength and physical condition. The middle-aged person should take certain precautions: (1) gradually increase the exercise until it is moderate in strenuousness, (2) exercise consistently, and (3) avoid overexertion. Ten minutes after strenuous exercise, the heart should be beating normally again, respirations should be normal, and there should be no sense of fatigue. If the person is overweight, has a personal or family history of cardiovascular disease, or has led a sedentary life, new exercise routines should not be started until after a thorough physical checkup (6, 78, 179). Using exercise as an overcompensation to prove youthfulness, health status, or prevent old age is pointless. The person may benefit from enrolling in an exercise program that is directed by a health professional.

Foot balance, the *ability to alter one's position so that body weight is carried through the foot with minimum effort,* is essential to prevent strain, foot aches, and pain during exercise as well as when walking or standing. Foot imbalance may result from contracted toes, improper position, size or shape of one or more bones of the foot, weak or rotating ankles, muscle strain, weak ligaments, poor body posture, overweight, arthritis, injuries, and improperly fitted or shaped shoes. Treatment by a podiatrist consists of careful assessment of the posture and provision of balance inlays for insertion into the shoes (208).

Foot problems may occur in middle age. Teach the person to observe for the following common signs

---

Given that back pain is unpredictable, a daily dose of preventive exercises will help keep your back strong. Here are several exercise you can do at home.

The first rule of exercising is to warm up. Shake out the arms and legs. Stretch the arms, reaching up with one, then the other. March in place for several minutes to circulate the blood and loosen leg muscles.

(1) The pelvic tilt can be done in any position. Lie on your back, knees bent, feet flat. Press your waist and lower back to the floor, tightening the abdominals, tucking the buttocks under the pelvis and relaxing the upper body. Release. Tuck again. Release. Repeat.

(2) Tightening the abdominal muscles will strengthen the back. Begin by lying on your back on a carpeted floor. Bend the knees and keep the feet flat on the floor. Arms are on the floor with palms down. Slowly bring one knee to your chest and face. Slowly return the leg, knee still bent, to the starting position. Repeat this exercise with each leg 5-10 times.

(3) Kneel on the floor on all fours. Extend the left leg out from the buttocks so that there is a straight horizontal line from the heel to the head. Now bend the knee so the bottom of the foot is facing the ceiling. Raise the leg carefully and evenly several times. Straighten the leg again and start over. Repeat with the opposite leg.

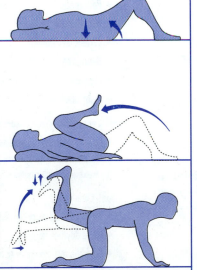

While the exercises illustrated here are considered comparatively safe, if you suffer from back or joint problems, extreme overweight or chronic heart, circulation or respiratory problems, check with your doctor of chiropractic before starting any exercise program. If any exercise selected becomes painful, ease off immediately.

Figure 13–2. Back exercises for daily sitters. *(From Back Protection for Daily Sitters, Staying Well Newsletter, May–June (1991), 2. Publication produced by The Foundation for Chiropractic Education and Research, Des Moines, Iowa.)*

of need for diagnostic evaluation and possible treatment (208):

- Swelling of the feet and ankles
- Cramps in the feet and the calf while walking or at night
- Inability to keep the feet warm
- Loss of the fat tissue on the padded surfaces of the feet
- Chronic ulcers on the feet that fail to respond to treatment
- Absence of or bounding pulse in the arteries of the feet
- Showing of arteries in the foot on routine x-ray film
- Burning in the soles of the feet

Foot care should include the following:

- Clean the feet with soap and water at least once daily; dust with foot powder or cornstarch.
- Exercise the feet, extend the toes, and then flex rapidly for 1 or 2 minutes. Rotate the feet in circles at the ankles. Try picking up a pencil or marble with toes.
- Walk barefoot on uneven surfaces, thick grass, or sandy beach.
- Walk daily and properly. Keep toes pointed ahead and lift rather than push the foot, letting it come down flat on the ground, placing little weight on the heel.
- Massage the feet to rest them after a tiring day.
- Lie down with feet higher than head for approximately ½ hour daily.
- Avoid wearing poorly fitted shoes or shoes with high heels and pointed toes.

Teach that the callus or other foot problems should be treated by a podiatrist. If the person scrapes or cuts a callus, there is risk of infection (208).

Sleep

Most middle-aged adults sleep without difficulty; 7 to 8 hours of sleep constitute a normal pattern. Refer to Chapter 12 for more information on normal sleep patterns; however, one kind of sleep disturbance—sleep apnea—in middle age is being studied to a greater extent.

Sleep apnea, *more than five episodes of cessation of air flow for at least 10 seconds each hour of sleep,* is a problem that is being increasingly recognized. This syndrome is found primarily in men over 50 and postmenopausal women, especially in people who are obese and have short, thick necks. Thirty-five to 40% of the el-

derly suffer sleep apnea. Often it is first detected because the person snores loudly or dozes during the daytime. Sleep apnea can be life threatening. There are three types (19, 161, 167, 168, 188):

- *Obstructive:* Respiratory effort continues despite pharyngeal obstruction to airflow.
- *Central:* There is no respiratory effort with airflow.
- *Mixed:* Episodes of no respiratory effort initially are followed by respiratory effort and then airflow.

The person may have the symptoms or manifestations listed in Table 13–5 (19, 161, 167, 168, 188). A sleep

TABLE 13–5. SLEEP APNEA

Pathophysiology

- Airway collapses or is restricted during sleep
- Continued effort to breathe, respiratory difficulty
- Hypoxemia due to intervals of not breathing
- Sleep disturbed

Manifestations

- Excessive daytime sleepiness
- Frequent nocturnal awakening
- Chronic heavy loud snoring
- Severe morning headaches, sleepiness
- Unrefreshed daytime sleep
- Irritability and personality changes
- Poor concentration, impaired memory
- Hypertension
- Cardiac arrhythmias
- Depression
- Impotence, sexual dysfunction
- Right-sided heart failure

Differential Diagnosis: Narcolepsy

- Manifestations of unexpected falling asleep, sudden loss of muscle tone, REM sleep disturbed, temporary paralysis of muscles when falling asleep or awakening, hallucinations

Client Care

- Maintain sleep diary, including hours in bed, hours slept, and sleep quality
- Avoid daytime napping
- Schedule rest time prior to bedtime
- Establish regular bed and wakeup times
- Avoid caffeine, nicotine, alcohol, and stimulants such as decongestants
- Avoid pharmacotherapy
- If no improvement, schedule sleep laboratory referral for evaluation

diary can be kept, on which treatment and teaching can be based (see Table 13–5). Refer also to Chapter 12 for more information on sleep.

Health Promotion and Health Protection

Immunizations

Middle-aged adults should have been immunized for tetanus/diphtheria, measles, mumps, and rubella. Tetanus toxoid should be administered every 10 years as a booster. Influenza, hepatitis B, and pneumonia vaccines are recommended for health workers and those with chronic disease or heart or lung disease (29).

Injury and Accidents

The gradually changing physical characteristics and preoccupation with responsibilities may contribute to the middle-aged person's having accidents.

Fractures and dislocations are the leading cause of injuries for both sexes, with more men affected than women, probably because of occupational differences. Because of the middle-aged adult's changing physical abilities, motor vehicle accidents are the most common cause of accidental deaths in the later years, especially for men. Occupation-related accidents rank second, and falls in the home rank third as causes of death; however, women suffer less than one-third as frequently as men from fatal falls during the middle years (112).

The middle-aged adult is a person at work in an industry, office, school, home, or out-of-doors. Accidents that disable for 1 week or more sharply increase for the worker after age 45 (75). Because of their interest in accident protection legislation, industries and other occupational settings are increasingly health and safety conscious. Efforts must continue in this direction.

You can teach about safety as it relates to remodeling a home, maintaining a yard, or establishing a work center. Handrails for stairways; a handgrip at the bathtub; conveniently located electric outlets; indirect, nonglare, and thorough lighting; and tools, equipment, and home or yard machines kept in proper working condition all provide ways to avoid an accident, especially in later middle age. Sensible middle-aged people plan for the gradual failing of their physical abilities by making the home as safe, convenient, and comfortable as possible as they rethink homemaking functions for the coming decades. Further, you can be instrumental in initiating or strengthening a safety program in an occupational or school setting.

Illness Prevention

Middle age is not automatically a period of physical or psychological hazard or disease. No single disease or mental condition necessarily is related to the passage of time, according to an American Medical Association Subcommittee on Aging, although the middle-aged person should be carefully assessed for signs of illness. Major health problems of this era are cardiovascular disease, cancer, pulmonary disease, diabetes, obesity, alcoholism, anxiety, depression, and glaucoma (140).

You can help the person maintain energy and improve health by teaching the information presented in this chapter. The person can learn moderate eating, drinking, or smoking habits and to use only medically prescribed drugs. Many measures promote health: regular physical examinations, pursuit of leisure activity, use of relaxation techniques, working through the emotional and family concerns related to middle age, affirming the worth of self as a middle-aged person, preparing for the later years, and confronting developmental tasks. The person also needs to prepare for possible accidents or illness.

Teach that the mounting statistical, experimental, and autopsy findings point to cigarette smoking as a causative factor in breast and lung cancer, cardiovascular disease, chronic obstructive pulmonary disease, and peptic ulcer. For the person who feels trapped, depressed, frustrated, or isolated, easily accessible escapes are alcoholism, drugs, and excess food intake. Assist the person in finding other ways to cope with stressors (124, 140).

The medicine cabinet may look like a pharmaceutical display if the self-absorbed person retreats into hypochondriasis. Old injuries may become bothersome, and new injuries do not heal as quickly. Illness or accident proneness can also be a means of resolving serious difficulties or of escaping responsibilities. If understanding and help from others is negligible or nonexistent and the possibility of recouping losses or rearranging one's life seems unlikely, the brief care and attention given during illness or after injury may not offer sufficient gratification. Suicidal thoughts and attempted or actual suicide is a call for help or an escape from problems (124). The prop of ill health should not be removed without study and caution, for removing one syndrome may only result in discharge of emotional tension through another physical or emotional syndrome. Thus nursing intervention and medical treatment must be directed toward both physical and emotional factors.

Because nursing care is holistic, you can meet emotional and spiritual needs of the person while giving physical care and doing health teaching related to common health problems discussed in the following pages.

Common Health Problems: Prevention and Treatment

A variety of health problems may occur, although many middle-aged adults remain healthy. Refer to Table 13–6 for a summary of diseases that are frequently experienced and to a medical–surgical nursing text for more information on the diseases summarized in the table. Health problems common in middle age, in addition to those listed on Table 13–6, are atherosclerosis, coronary artery disease, obesity (gaining 20 pounds in adulthood increases risk by 60%), arthritis, osteoporosis, and various kinds of cancer. (Cancer is the leading cause of death for women aged 45 to 64. In men the primary sites for cancer are the prostate, lung, colon, and rectum, and bladder. In women, the common sites are lung, breast, colon, and rectum (75, 149, 185).

Respiratory conditions, including acute as well as chronic pulmonary disease, are a frequent cause for days absent from work. Generally middle-aged women have more disability days from work because of respiratory and other acute disorders; men have more disability days from injuries (75, 140).

The Nurse's Health Study, which obtained information from 115,000 women over a 20-year period, has looked at a wide-ranging assortment of risk factors. Their findings indicate that 1 in 8 women will develop breast cancer and 1 in 2 will develop cardiovascular disease eventually. Long-term hormone replacement therapy increases the likelihood of breast cancer in women by 40% (149). Annual mammography screening has been found to reduce cancer deaths by one-third in women aged 50 to 60; mammography should not be eliminated on the basis of cost (149, 153).

The middle-ager may experience chronic illness in self or a family member. A number of references give information about reactions to as well as coping with chronic illness in this era (7, 8, 34, 42, 72, 102, 144, 146, 155, 157, 170, 172, 174, 175, 184, 186, 192, 201, 206).

Also useful are references on keeping a health diary, which can be useful for health promotion as well as in times of illness treatment (8, 78).

Sexual dysfunction, *severely diminished or absent orgasmic response,* may result from alcoholism, obesity, preoccupation with career or finances, mental or physical fatigue, boredom, fear of failing sexually, or chronic illness related to impaired circulation or neuropathy. For example, in one study of diabetic men, more than half of them were impotent, probably because of autonomic neuropathy involving the sacral parasympathetic fibers that supply the penis and bladder. Vascular disease affects potency because a high volume of blood flow is necessary to distend the vascular spaces or erectile tissue. Occlusion of the pudendal arteries or their tributaries may result in impotence. Hypertension with a blood pressure of 180/110 constitutes a contraindication to coitus because of increased risk of strokes. Antihypertensive drugs, other than diuretics, may cause impotence or inhibition of ejaculation. A past myocardial infarction may limit physical activity of any kind, but after a period of recovery most coronary patients resume sexual relations. Although hysterectomy does not affect sex drive, oophorectomy may because of the hormonal changes; however, hormone replacement may return sex drive. Adrenalectomy has a negative effect on libido because hormone production is diminished. Most men retain potency after prostatectomy unless the surgical approach has been through the sex-related nerve centers. If the prostate is malignant and surgery more radical, however, the man's possibilities of retaining potency are not as favorable (113). Increased expectations in this age of sexual liberation may also increase sexual problems along with other marital problems.

The middle-aged person may subtly, hesitantly, or openly discuss problems of sexual function with you. Listen carefully. Let the person know that such problems are not unusual. You may not know the answers, but your listening can help the person make a decision to seek medical care or counseling, realize the need to change behavior, or assist in attitude and value clarification about sexuality and sexual behavior. Refer the person or couple to a counselor who can help with physical and emotional problems. Your discussion with the physician of the person's problems with changed libido or impotence can also be helpful. Sometimes a change in medication dosage or modification in treatment regimen can reduce sexual dysfunction.

PSYCHOSOCIAL CONCEPTS

Factors That Influence Research Findings on Cognitive Ability

Because most studies on adult cognition have been cross-sectional, caution is necessary in interpreting the results, as many factors are influential. For the middle-aged person especially, the following can negatively influence test scores: (1) amount of education, (2) experiential differences, (3) fixed attitudes, (4) number of years since formal schooling was completed, and (5) general health status. The gradual neuron loss that occurs over the lifetime does not affect cognitive function. Because most intelligence tests are developed for children and adolescents, the kind of test given can influence the scores. The middle-aged adult scores higher on tests that require general information or vocabulary abilities. At age 60 intelligence quotient (IQ) test results

TABLE 13–6. COMMON HEALTH PROBLEMS IN MIDDLE AGE

Problem	Definition	Symptoms/Signs	Prevention/Treatment
Sinusitis, nonbacterial and bacterial	Inflammation of mucous membrane lining paranasal sinuses; may be caused by bacteria, viruses, irritants, or allergies	Normal sinus drainage prohibited Usually clear drainage in nonbacterial type Purulent drainage in bacterial type, with fever (headache and tenderness of frontal and maxillary sinus to palpation frequent with bacterial involvement)	Oral antihistimine and decongestant for nonbacterial type Addition of antibiotic for bacterial type
Hiatal hernia with esophagitis	Herniation of stomach through diaphragm with reflux of acid into esophagus	Substernal pain, usually worse when bending over or lying down Sometimes nausea and vomiting	Maintenance of ideal weight Avoidance of tight clothing Eat frequently in small amounts Elevation of head of bed
Duodenal peptic ulcer disease	Ulceration of duodenal mucosa	Pain in the epigastrum or right upper quadrant usually 1–2 hours after meals	Antacids or prescription drugs (e.g., cimetidine [Tagamet]) Small frequent meals Avoidance of caffeine, alcohol, and spices
Angina pectoris	Imbalance between oxygen needed by myocardium and oxygen supplied	Pain in substernal region but sometimes in neck, back, and arms	Workup to determine accurate diagnosis Nitroglycerin
Secondary hypertension	High blood pressure based on specific cause	Blood pressure >150/100 More common in men, but after 55 years, women likely to be affected	Following treatment plan based on cause of high blood pressure Reduction of sodium and cholesterol in diet Reduction of weight as needed Relaxation techniques
Hyperthyroidism (Graves' disease)	Too much secretion of thyroid hormone	Can mimic heart problems with accelerated or irregular heartbeat Feeling of agitation	Antithyroid medications or radioactive iodine therapy
Hyperuricemia or gout	High uric acid level, causing acute inflammatory arthritis (can also be chronic)	Usually red, hot tender joint; often in great toe but can be in other joints	Specific drugs Rest Elevation of joint(s) Cold compresses
Diabetes type II	Glucose intolerance corrected by means other than insulin	High blood sugar Thirsty Weight loss Frequent urination	Diet Exercise Oral medication
Prostatitis, acute	Acute infection of prostate gland; often caused by *Escherichia coli*	Low back and perineal pain referred sometimes to inguinal region and testes Extremely tender prostate	Sitz baths Appropriate antibiotics
Prostatitis, chronic	Prolonged inflammation of prostate	Only slightly tender and enlarged prostate	Prostatic massage Sitz baths Increased sexual activity
Lumbosacral strain, mild	Strain and inflammation of ligaments and musculature in lumbosacral region	Muscle spasm over region but no radiation No flank pain Negative result from straight leg raising	Cold packs Muscle relaxant medication Analgesic Bed rest Chiropractic treatment Education in bending and lifting techniques Use of firm mattress
Foot callus	Thickness of the outer layers of the skin on the sole of the foot	Pain when congestion and swelling press nerve endings and underlying bursa	Avoid shoes that put excess pressure and friction on the sole of the foot

Research Abstract

Anderson, J., C. Blue, A. Holbrook, and M. Ng, On Chronic Illness: Immigrant Women in Canada's Work Force—A Feminist Perspective. Canadian Journal of Nursing Research, 25, no. 2 (1993), 7–22.

People who migrate usually do so in search of a better life, but being uprooted from one's home country and re-establishing roots in another land often disrupts their life in every way and brings hardships. The difficulties are exacerbated by being in a country with different language and culture. Health problems may result, and the jobs they get may expose them to health hazards.

In Canada, as in the United States, the immigrant women are often subject to triple discrimination: sex, birth place, and class, and they occupy the lowest levels in the labor market hierarchy and have little job security or benefits. Even well educated women may be unable to obtain jobs similar to what they had in their home countries; their qualifications often are not recognized. When these workers must also deal with a chronic illness, their difficulties are compounded.

The immigrant woman is likely to be subordinate socially and in the workplace to both Caucasian and ethnic female citizens in the USA and Canada. Thus, her struggles are even more difficult and her plight different from those of other women.

Chronic illness invades all of life's activities and interactions. Non-English speaking immigrants, especially women, have great difficulty in finding jobs that allow them to attend to the needs that result from chronic illness. Health care providers must be aware that the chronically ill person must be cared for from both a social and clinical context. For example:

1. Chronic illness is a part of the marital relationship, child care, care of the home, employment, family finances, and all social interactions.

2. The person's willingness to disclose chronic illness in the work setting may be related to ethnicity, but even more so to position in the labor force and job security. Women who have a chronic illness may not tell the employer for fear of not being hired or of being fired.

3. Disclosure about chronic illness depends on the type of employment, how people in the place of employment are perceived, and if the chronically ill person believes people in the employment setting could give care if something happened (such as fainting from low blood sugar).

4. Immigrant women, even more so than men, may not be able to express their concerns to health care providers and obtain necessary services. Often they feel they are scolded and treated as children, and that health care providers do not understand practical difficulties with and limits to illness management.

5. Even when health care professionals give explanations to the person, the immigrant may be unable to understand it conceptually or in relation to their knowledge or beliefs about the body. People with limited English skills have even more difficulty; written materials, libraries, and support groups may not be helpful.

6. The hours for delivery of health services are often not available to people who do not have a flexible work schedule. If the person has to take off a day of work for treatment, income is lost. Further, the person may hesitate to reveal the illness to the employer.

7. Non-English speaking people are often expected to bring their own interpreter to the treatment facility. If a family member fills this role, both members must take off work and lose income.

8. Non-English speaking people may be perceived by providers as not complying to treatment or managing their illness. They may not understand our emphasis on self-care or share notions about what constitutes good management. They may not be able to reorganize work schedules or access resources. They may not be able to adjust their usual diet to the dietary changes required by the illness.

9. Ethnicity may not be the deciding factor in how someone manages the chronic illness. The history of colonialism and sense of oppression that has shaped subjective experiences, both in immigrants and poor citizens, may be major factors in how the person responds to and manages a chronic illness.

10. Knowledge of the person's day-to-day circumstances must be incorporated into clinical practice. Not following the treatment plan may not be the choice of the person but rather the result of life conditions.

Case Situation: Combating the Stresses of Disability — Becoming a Survivor

Until her car was wrecked in a snowstorm, Marlene was a healthy, divorced 57-year-old woman who led an active and rewarding life. Almost immediately after the accident she noticed difficulty using her hands but discounted this as "nerves." The car was hit on the driver's side at 50 mph, and although Marlene experienced severe pain in the neck and upper back area, she conscientiously returned to work as a medical secretary within a few days of the accident.

The back pain and weakness in Marlene's arms and hands continued to worsen, but nothing specific showed on the x-ray films. She consulted with an orthopedist, neurologist, rheumatologist, physical therapist, and internist; none was able to make a specific diagnosis related to the increasing pain and weakness.

After a year of misdiagnosis Marlene was becoming unable to live independently. She could not use her arms for preparing food, shopping, or doing laundry and was barely able to dress herself or comb her hair. At the age of 58, Marlene was afraid that she would have to move into a nursing home. Finally, after a year of frustration and despair she requested referral to a pain management program (PMP). She had decided that if the physicians could not cure the problem, she would have to learn to live with it. That was when life began to turn around for her.

At the PMP Marlene's pain and dysfunction were identified as probable results of the whiplash injury, which caused thoracic outlet syndrome, soft tissue injury in the cervical area, and chronic myofascial pain. The PMP team's opinion was that surgery was not a viable option.

Marlene was taught stress-reduction strategies such as relaxation techniques, biofeedback, and guided imagery. But most important, she learned to listen to her body and set appropriate limits on what she could make it do. Because the pain was not always constant and did not immediately follow action but sometimes occurred as much as 2 hours later, it became necessary to set limits and not do things that would increase pain.

Pacing and/or setting appropriate limits to accommodate the lack of physical strength was and remains the hardest thing Marlene had to learn. It was like living on a very strict budget of physical energy. If she expended too much energy in the morning, nothing was left for the rest of the day. It meant taking breaks, conserving energy, avoiding long shopping trips, resting up for big days, taking into consideration barometric changes, and practicing pain management techniques. She had to do a tremendous amount of planning, negotiating, and compromising.

One of the greatest causes of stress, especially for persons with chronic pain and/or various physical limitations, is feeling like a victim of life. Marlene felt powerless over much of her life, as if she were controlled by everyone and everything around her. When she learned how to control some of the physical problems, she felt she had more control of life and felt less like a victim. She made it a point to join organizations that could provide information and find people who could share areas of her disabilities. She found this was extremely rewarding. She learned she could not afford to waste energy on emotional problems from the past. Resolving them was necessary so that all available energy could be used with current physical problems. Becoming mentally healthy made a big difference in the quality of her life, although the past problems were not the cause of the disabilities.

Continued typing work as a secretary would eventually have caused Marlene to lose the use of her arms and hands, so she gave up her job of 18 years and started over at age 59. Fortunately, Marlene had been doing self-help counseling on a volunteer basis before the auto accident. She could not tolerate doing nothing and decided to enroll in school for a graduate degree in counseling. (One of the most important methods of controlling pain is keeping the mind occupied.) Her physical abilities were limited, but her brain and mouth still functioned with no impairment. To stay within her physical limitations, she was able to take only 6 graduate hours per semester. It took 4 years to complete a 2-year graduate curriculum in counseling services.

Marlene has had to discover and develop new and different ways of living, to change totally her previous methods of dealing with life, to accept her limitatioins, and to move beyond those limits. She had to learn not to be a victim of chronic illness and the value of sharing and caring for others. She has developed the following program for recovery and survival:

1. Let reality sink in slowly. Acceptance of disability is necessary before one can find happiness.
2. Expect a time of anger and denial.
3. Learn to use anger constructively rather than destructively. Fight for personal rights.
4. Let yourself experience the grief; do not be afraid to cry. It hurts in many, many ways. Tears are healing.
5. Become determined to accept the past and make the best of the present. Live one day at a time.

(continued)

Case Situation: Combating the Stresses of Disability — Becoming a Survivor

6. Be good to yourself and do not forget to pace activities. Try to look forward to a new future and new interests.

7. Learn to be flexible and trust in yourself. Do not let the world pass by; get more active in a personally satisfying way.

8. Start taking charge of small areas of life. Feeling in control is extremely important.

9. Find a support group and use it. Do not stand on the outside looking in. Participate.

10. Develop regular phone contacts, which will help you as others are helped.

11. Create meaning in life, develop new interests, and stay mentally active. Find goals that are consistent with limitations.

12. Look outward instead of inward. It is impossible to feel hateful and grateful at the same time.

---

are equal to or better than those of young adults. Only arithmetic reasoning shows a plateau through the adult years. Speed requirements of the test may mitigate against the IQ test scores; adults show a peak in speed of performance in the twenties and a gradual decrease in overall speed of performance through the years. Adults usually value accuracy and thoroughness more than speed (46, 97, 185). In fact, IQ tests may be irrelevant. What should be tested is how people identify problems and use reason and intuition to solve problems (46).

In various studies physically fit and active men were found to have a higher intelligence score than men who engaged in little physical activity (46, 97).

In the early 1970s Kangas and Bradway (46) did a 38-year follow-up study of people tested for intelligence as preschoolers, junior high school students, young adults, and early middle-aged adults. They found an increase in IQ across the four testing periods, indicating continued mental growth during middle age and possibly even beyond. Interesting sex differences emerged from these findings. Women whose IQs had been high as children gained less than those with medium or low preadult IQs and less than men with any level of preadult IQ. On the other hand, the higher the level of a man's preadult IQ, the greater was his adult gain. These findings have interesting implications in light of the theory that bright women fear success. Women who tested high as girls inhibited their intellectual potential later in life. The recent study by the American Association of University Women reveals the same results (46, 185). The phenomenon of different educational processes and expectations has meant that society in general and specific women both lost the benefit of talent and ability.

In the past decade more middle-aged women have returned to college for baccalaureate, graduate, doctoral, and postdoctoral degrees. They have shown themselves as capable as men scholastically and in applying intellectual ability in the workplace.

Cognitive Development

Cognitive processes in adulthood include reaction time, perception, memory, learning and problem solving, and creativity. These are performed through characteristics of both Concrete and Formal Operations, depending on the situation (195).

Reaction time or speed of performance is individual and generally stays the same or diminishes during late middle age. The speed of response is important primarily in test situations, as much of the problem solving necessary in adulthood requires deliberation and accuracy rather than speed. Reaction time is related to complexity of the task, the habitual pattern of response to stimuli, and familiarity with the task. Time for new learning increases with age, but adults in their forties and fifties have the same ability to learn as they did in their twenties and thirties (37, 46, 185).

Memory is maintained through young and middle adulthood; no major age differences are evident. Some quantitative changes may occur. For example, a person in early adulthood who could recite a 10-digit span of numbers as a series of discrete units may recite 8 digits grouped or categorized in late middle age. The ability to categorize or group information, to sharpen observational skills and give more attention to the phenomenon, to relate meaning to that to be remembered, and to use interactive imagery—imagining events in a story form with self in the interaction—are all ways to strengthen memory and aid learning (37, 46, 185). The middle-aged adult memorizes less readily material that is not well organized and seems to retain less from oral presentation of information than younger students (185).

There are different types of memory. *Sensory memory,* information stored in a sense organ, is transitory, a few seconds. *Short-term memory* may be based on recall for days or weeks. *Long-term memory* may last a lifetime. Memory is not reliable in the adult years or at any age. Most people forget or ignore episodes that do not fit the self-image or that are considered unimportant. People who think they remember an event from childhood or a number of years previously may be making up plausible scenarios, fantasies, or confabulations based on earlier reports or stories. The middle-aged adult who continues to use memory will retain a keen memory (37, 46, 97, 185).

Learning occurs in adults of all ages. The highly intelligent person becomes even more learned. The capacity for intellectual growth is unimpaired and is enhanced by interest, motivation, flexibility, a sense of humor, confidence, and maturity attained through experience. Learning means more; it is not just learning for learning's sake. Knowledge is applied; motivation to learn is high for personal reasons. Reluctance to learn occurs if the new material does not appear relevant or does not serve the person as well as current information (37, 46, 97, 185, 195).

Problem-solving abilities remain throughout adulthood. There are no significant differences between 20-, 40-, and 60-year-olds in learning a task. Generally, better educated people perform better than less educated people in any age group. When there is no time limitation, there are no task differences in complex task solutions because young and middle-aged adults use different strategies. Young adults, knowing they can function quickly, may be more likely to use less efficient reasoning strategies such as trial and error. In late middle age, because people know they are becoming slower, they tend to think a problem through first so they can solve it in fewer tries. Thus, they appear to be slower in grasping and solving a problem. But the wider life experiences prompt recognition of more variables in a situation and thus enhance problem solving (46, 185, 195).

The middle-aged adult is able to do all the cognitive strategies of **Piaget's Stage of Formal Operations** described in Chapters 11 and 12. Sometimes the practicality of a situation will call forth use of Concrete Operations; because not all problems in life can be solved by abstract reasoning, the middle-aged adult does both operations realistically in problem solving. He or she also uses the fifth stage of cognitive development, problem finding, described in Chapter 11. Societal, occupational, and general life experiences are crucial to cognitive operations of the middle-aged person. Thus, perceptions about the same situation, problem, or task can vary considerably in a group of middle-aged adults (195).

Cognitive characteristics that are developed in the young adult are used throughout middle age as well. Various patterns mark the development of **intellectual skills.** The mature adult can symbolize experience and behaves in a way that shows organization, integration, stability, and unity in the cognitive process. Representing experience symbolically as hunches, words, thoughts, or other symbols is part of becoming mature. The person can reflect on past and current experience and can imagine, anticipate, plan, and hope. The person develops an inner private world that gives him or her resources for happiness and potential for anxiety. The person can recall past defeats and triumphs and monitor ongoing thoughts for consistency and logic. When the person solves a problem, he or she can explain how it was solved. Because the mature adult is more imaginatively productive, he or she is capable of producing more images, thoughts, and combinations of ideas, is able to use reflection to gain perspectives about life, and is aware of personal beliefs, values, motives, and powers. The mature person is increasingly interested in other persons and warm, enduring relationships and is adaptable, independent, self-driving, conscientious, enthusiastic, and purposeful. The person can reflect about personal relationships, the ups and downs or contradictions in relationships, and their sources of strain and satisfaction and concomitantly understand why other persons feel and act as they do (46, 51, 97, 106, 185). These characteristics of cognition are part of *contextual intelligence* and *social* or *postformal intelligence* (46).

Buhler (24) implies cognitive development as she describes the *maintenance* and *change* tendencies in life. *Maintenance,* through the restitution of deficiencies (need satisfaction) and upholding of the system's internal order, is necessary for cognitive function to occur. *Change,* involving self-limited adaptation and creative expansion, is part of the cognitive development of the adult. Maintenance and change occur with different emphases in various life stages. The child develops self-limiting adaptation as he or she learns; the adolescent and adult move into creative expansion; after middle age the person assesses the past and self and wants to restore inner order; and in old age the person either continues to follow previous adaptive and creative drives or regresses to need-satisfying tendencies.

The intellectually curious have an increased need and ability to spin new syntheses and theories, to make meaningful that which seems meaningless, to coordinate hypothesis formation and testing, to be systematic at problem solving, to seek environmental diversity, and to become more subtle, differentiated, integrated, and complex. The mature person has a progressive integration; that is, he or she is continually open, flexible, curious, and actively engaged. If cognitive efficiency becomes disrupted, a mature person is able to recover from such disorganization more quickly than an immature person, even though the two do not differ in intelligence. The mature person becomes discriminating in decisions based on the facts at hand and can postpone, suppress, or ignore. The person can analyze and judge information, even that which is personally relevant, in terms of demands of the information itself without being influenced by either personal desires or persuasive opinions of others. Thought becomes objective and judgment independent (37, 46, 51, 106, 185).

Neugarten (129) believes that the person changes both cognitively and emotionally over time as the result of accumulated experience. The person abstracts from experiences and creates more encompassing and more refined categories for interpreting events. The middle-aged person differs cognitively from the young adult in that he or she was born in a different historical era and thereby has different formative experiences. The middle-aged adult thus has a greater apperceptive mass or store of past experience by which to evaluate events or make decisions. Through the adult years perspectives and insights broaden and deepen, and attitudes and behaviors change.

Although **Gould** (66) focuses more on personality than cognitive development, he sees adulthood as a time of thoughtful confrontation with the self—letting go of the idealized image, the desire to be perfect, and acknowledging the realistic image of self and personal feelings. The adult continues to gain new beliefs about self and the world. Conflicts between past and present beliefs are resolved.

Assist the middle-aged adult (and others) in understanding the cognitive changes and strengths of cognitive ability. Reinforce a positive self-image related to cognitive abilities.

Creativity

Dennis (40) found an age pattern for creative output. He found that scientists show a peak activity in early and middle adulthood. Unique, original, and inventive productions are more often created in the twenties, thirties, and forties than later in life. The more a creative act depends on accumulated experience, the more likely it is to occur in middle age or later life. People are less productive in total creative output in the twenties than in the thirties and forties. Poets, novelists, and scholars

gain in productivity in middle and old age, and, although quantity may decrease, quality increases as a greater proportion of contextual, intuitive, and social intelligence is used (37, 46). Some creative works cannot be produced without the benefit of years of experience and living, absorbing the wisdom of the culture, and the resultant development of new insights.

Creativity is seen not only in famous people or young people. The average middle-aged adult may have many responsibilities and stresses; however, typically he or she approaches a situation, task, or learning experience in a creative way.

You can encourage the middle-aged adult to pursue creative ideas and activities and to approach roles, responsibilities, and tasks in a creative way. Help the middle-aged adult overcome any self-consciousness about the unique cognitive response to a situation.

With increasing emphasis on continued learning, the middle-aged person is frequently enrolled in refresher courses, continuing education courses, or workshops related to occupation or profession. He or she takes college credit and noncredit courses to deal with specific problems; learn specific content; learn for fun; find an academic program necessary for changing a profession or occupation; gain more personal satisfaction; relieve boredom, loneliness, or an unhappy situation; or broaden the mind and learn for the sake of learning. Rapid technologic changes in business or the professions cause obsolescence of knowledge and skills, which also forces middle-aged persons to continue to learn.

When you are teaching, use methods that capitalize on the learning strengths of mature adults, including active discussion and role play. Deemphasize memorization and acquisition of large amounts of new information. Assist the learner to develop cognitive strategies that will help him or her synthesize, analyze, integrate, interpret, and apply knowledge. Your major role may be in convincing the middle-aged adult and others that he or she can learn, because myths to the contrary are prevalent. Further, you can enhance learning by providing a conducive environment, one that considers sensory changes. Your verbal and visual presentations must also consider the sensory changes discussed previously.

Work and Leisure Activities

Work

Work will be viewed differently by different middle-agers. Consider that the older middle-aged person grew up under the influence of the Depression and with the

Protestant ethic. Both stressed the economic and moral importance of work. Thus, work became respected and sought. Being without a job or idle was a harbinger of problems and meant being lazy and worthless. How has this middle-aged adult adjusted to mechanization, waning of the work ethic, the demise of a full day's work for a full day's pay? For the young middle-ager, what was a promising career or lifetime employment may have ended in being laid off permanently by the company, forced early retirement, or forced job hunting. Finding work could be difficult.

The person may be fortunate enough to be in a business or profession in which he or she works successfully for self or is allowed freedom within a specialized area of work. He or she will experience the dignity of being productive and will enjoy increasing self-esteem, autonomy, and sense of achievement; however, most middle-aged adults are employed in a system in which the value is on production, not the person. Often, in contrast to union-set rules, whereby no more than a specified amount can be done within a specified time, ever-greater output is demanded on the job. If the person is unemployed and job hunting, see Suggestions for Someone Who is Unemployed (136). Or you may want to explore career options described in Career Track Options in Late Middle Age (18).

Many middle-aged women work outside of the home; thus, they are especially in the middle in terms of the demands of various roles on their time and energy. The middle-aged woman is wife, mother, homemaker, grandmother, worker, and organization member. The women who are caregivers also have childcare responsibility; some may have quit their jobs or have work conflicts. The middle-aged woman is often in the middle in terms of two competing values: (1) that traditional care of the elderly is a family responsibility and (2) that women should be free to work outside the home if they wish. Each family member feels the repercussions as the balance of roles and responsibilities changes. Most middle-aged women are working today for a variety of reasons (11, 46, 185):

- Inflation and the rising cost of living
- Changes in attitudes about sex-appropriate roles as a result of the woman's movement
- The rising divorce rate that forces the woman to become economically independent
- Fewer children in the home
- Use of labor-saving devices for the home that results in free time
- Increasing educational levels that stimulate career interests or the desire to remain in the profession
- Expectancy of a higher standard of living

► **SUGGESTIONS FOR SOMEONE WHO IS UNEMPLOYED**

- Offer hope and encouragement, but guard against sounding "spiritually superior." This is a dark valley, emotionally, economically, philosophically, and spiritually.
- Remind the person that unemployment is a reflection of current economic conditions, not of personal worth.
- Seek opportunities to affirm the person's talents and positive attributes.
- Help him or her consider all the options, including launching a business from home, changing careers, and working part-time.
- Allow the person to express feelings, but do not encourage self-pity. Your time with the person should leave him or her feeling uplifted and hopeful. Pray with the person if he or she desires.
- Offer to hold him or her accountable to a specific job-hunting schedule. It is often hard to stay motivated and organized without a friendly nudge.
- Talk about subjects other than unemployment.
- Encourage the person/family to relax and have fun. If you are a friend, invite them to your home or give them a gift certificate for dinner and a movie.
- If the person is a friend or relative, provide practical, but discreet, help, including food, clothing, and finances.

- Assistance with costs of sending children to college

References at the end of the chapter provide more information about the middle-aged caregiver (and see pages 651 to 659).

Knowing the degree of work stability, extent to which work is satisfying, and emotional factors that have operated in the person's concept of work and in the self-concept is important in assessing how well the middle-aged person can function as a mentally and physically healthy person. As a professional person, you will have to resolve conflicts related to your work role. Hence, you are in a position to assist the middle-aged person in talking about and resolving feelings and values related to work and other activity.

Because the demands on middle-aged adults are often overwhelming—work, home, family, church, social and civic organizations—teach steps for effective *time management* (see Guidelines for Time Management).

Some people in this era *retire* early by plan; for some it comes after a layoff and no job is found, for years. For others, because of financial need, they will work as long as possible (111). But retirement will have to come eventually (see Suggestions for Planning for

► **CAREER TRACK OPTIONS IN LATE MIDDLE AGE**

Coast Into Retirement

- Do the job but no more; collect the paycheck; enjoy the final years.

Go for Last Promotion

- Campaign to obtain final reward for all that was contributed to receive public acknowledgment of the importance of work done.

Try for Great Achievement

- Work to outdo the present record and others' records so that others will see you saved the best for last.

Survive Difficult Period

- Recognize the company's difficult period; learn to survive and even prosper in the challenging time.

Retire Early

- Take the attractive package being offered by the company so that the years of later maturity can be enjoyed.

Start Your Own Business

- If tired of working for others, go into business for self (e.g., consulting in work arena, turning hobby into business).

► **GUIDELINES FOR TIME MANAGEMENT**

- Establish priorities; maintain a log if necessary. *Write goals.*
- *Do it now.* Do not procrastinate with small tasks; schedule large projects.
- *Recognize unpleasant tasks; work on them first.*
- *Clear the decks and desks.* Eliminate clutter; organize the workplace for efficiency.
- *Stick to the job.* Avoid distractions.
- *Do one thing at a time.* Finish one major task before beginning another; however, there are times you can do two things at once, e.g., planning while waiting in line.
- *Plan ahead.* Assemble what is needed for a task before initiating it; set aside relaxation time.
- *Consider limitations*—your own, equipment not available for a project, and other responsibilities that will interfere.
- *Learn to say "no" and suggest someone else* who would be able to handle the situation. Delegate low-priority jobs to others.
- *Anticipate delays* that are inevitable in every task; plan for interruptions and unforeseen events.
- *Plan an alternative way* to do the job; have backup activity if a selected task cannot be done as scheduled.
- *Use odd times.* Shop when stores are not crowded; carry a notebook to jot ideas while you wait.

- Have high job satisfaction
- Perceive retirement as unfeasible because they have not done advance financial (or emotional) planning
- Retain their health

Leadership Role

The middle-aged adult's cognitive stage is in favor of his or her being a designated or an informal leader if other factors are favorable. (Usually middle-aged leaders have developed necessary qualities from childhood on, but occasionally a person does not believe that he or she has this ability until there is a measure of success in the life work.)

The *leader* usually has the *following characteristics* (37, 46, 106, 185):

- Adequate socioeconomic resources
- Higher level of education or success than majority of group to be led
- Realistic self-concept
- Realistic goals and ability to encourage others toward those goals
- High frustration tolerance

Early Retirement) (111). Explore with the person various options to prepare for retirement—at 55, 62, 65, 70, or 75 years (18). Assist the person to examine risks or the worst possible scenario if an option is chosen. Examine what it will take in effort and ability to make the option happen, strategies to fall back on if the option is not successful, the support system (financial, emotional, and social) to ensure success, and personal willingness both to take the risks and to enjoy the benefits (18). A part of planning for retirement is to study the financial plans that go with each option to ensure, to the extent possible, financial security in old age (11, 18, 64, 73, 111, 148).

The decade of the fifties is a point of transition in development of consciousness about retirement. Middle-aged persons *least* likely to anticipate retirement include those who (94):

- Work in a company that is prospering
- Have unfinished agendas at work

► SUGGESTIONS FOR PLANNING
FOR EARLY RETIREMENT

- Start planning early. Most successful early retirees have long-range plans in place before they reach 40.

- Stay with a good employer. Unless you are sure you can strike it rich on your own, work for secure companies with generous pension plans. Avoid excessive job hopping so you can accrue substantial pension benefits.

- Make use of employer-sponsored investment programs. Place a percentage of your paycheck into tax-deferred plans. Participate to the maximum. You have to be $59\frac{1}{2}$ to begin withdrawing without penalty.

- Save and invest wisely in other plans — bonds, stocks, property, other annuities, IRAs. You cannot count on Social Security or a company pension. You may have to live off savings. You will need between 60 and 80% of preretirement income.

- Plan for medical bills. Unless you have an early retirement package that extends your health coverage, you will need to factor in high insurance premiums until Medicare begins at age 65.

- Scale back your lifestyle. There are many ways to do this. You might buy a smaller house, forgo extravagant vacations, or send your kids to public colleges instead of Ivy League schools.

- Explore career directions you can pursue later in life. You may want to work a few months a year or hours a week. Some individuals have turned a hobby into a way to make money.

- Mentally prepare yourself. Assess your values, goals, and aspirations and relate them to how you would like to live given more time and sufficient income.

- Ability to express negative thoughts tactfully
- Ability to accept success or failure gracefully
- Ability to delegate authority
- Understanding of group needs
- Flexibility in meeting group needs

The middle-aged person may demonstrate this leadership ability on the job or in community or church organizations. Women who are most successful in leadership careers are those who have little conflict in the multiple roles of career woman, mother, and wife. Their husbands' support and encouragement are major assets, but women are also becoming more assertive on their own behalf about their roles outside the home.

You can encourage or reaffirm the middle-aged person in the leadership role. You may also assist him or her in working through feelings or conflicts related to the work setting or the job itself.

Leisure

The middle-aged person, taught little about how to enjoy free time, is now faced with increasing amounts of

leisure because of advances in technology, earlier retirement, and increased longevity. The average middle-aged adult who has moved up the pay scale and whose children may be grown will have more money and more time to take trips or try new hobbies. Yet various *factors* hinder use of these new opportunities (106):

- Value of work learned in younger years
- Cultural emphasis on intellectual pursuits so that play is considered childish and a poor use of time and talents
- Conditioning to at least appear busy
- Fears of regression and not wanting to return to work
- Lack of previous opportunity to learn creative pursuits or hobbies
- Hesitation to try something new because of fear of failure

You can help the person avoid feelings of alienation that result from inability to use leisure time. Use the suggestions in Teaching Use of Leisure in the Daily Schedule with your middle-aged clients.

► TEACHING USE OF LEISURE
IN THE DAILY SCHEDULE

- Emphasize that play and recreation are essential to a healthy life.

- Stress the indispensability of leisure as a part of many activities, whether work or creative endeavors. Leisure is both a state of mind and use of time away from work. Have the person analyze leisure activities, whether they bring pleasure, work off frustration, make up deficits in life, or create a sense of pressure or competition.

- Help the person recognize the interplay of physical and intellectual endeavors and their contribution to mental health.

- Differentiate compulsive, competitive, and aggressive work and play from healthy, natural work and play. Intrinsic in play are spontaneity, flexibility, creativity, zest, and joy.

- Recognize the person's creative efforts to encourage further involvement in leisure activities.

- Educate the person about the importance of preparing for retirement.

- Inform the person of places, courses, or workshops at which he or she can learn new creative skills and use of talents.

- Encourage the person to enjoy change, to participate in organizations, and to initiate stimulating contacts with others.

- Encourage the person to stop the activity when it no longer meets personal needs.

Information taken from References 45 and 106.

Emotional Development

The middle years, the climacteric, are a period of self-assessment, and greater introspection—a transitional period. In middle age (and beyond) the person perceives life as time left to live rather than time since birth. Time is seen as finite; death is a possibility. Middle-aged adults clock themselves by their positions in different life contexts—changes in body, family, career—rather than by chronologic age. Time is seen in two ways: (1) time to finish what the person wants to do and (2) how much meaning and pleasure can be obtained in the time that is left (37, 46, 88, 106, 185). The person makes the often agonizing reappraisal of how achievements measure up against goals and of the entire system of values. He or she realizes that the choices of the past have limited present choices. He or she can no longer dream of infinite possibilities. The person is forced to acknowledge that he or she has worked up to or is short of personal capabilities. Goals may or may not have been reached; aspirations may have to be modified. The possibility for advancement becomes more remote. The person will have to go on with ever-brighter, ever-younger men and women crowding into the competitive economic, political, and social arena. In the United States success is highly valued and is measured by prestige, wealth, or power. To be without these by middle age causes stress, and the likelihood of achieving them diminishes with age. Contrary to an earlier trend, however, the middle-aged adult is again being perceived as a valuable worker because of the experience and knowledge he or she can contribute. Thus, he or she is less likely to be replaced on the job by a younger employee just on the basis of age. Federal legislation prohibiting age discrimination contributes to this later trend.

Developmental Crisis

The psychosexual crisis of middle age, according to Erikson (50), is generativity versus self-absorption and stagnation. **Generativity** is a *concern about providing for others that is equal to the concern of providing for the self.* If other developmental stages were managed successfully, the person has a sense of parenthood and creativity; of being vital in establishing and guiding the next generation, the arts, or a profession; of feeling needed and being important to the welfare of humankind. The person can assume the responsibility of parenthood. As a husband or wife, each can see the strengths and weaknesses of the other and combine their energies toward common goals.

A biological parent does not necessarily get to the psychosocial stage of generativity, and the unmarried person or the person without children can be very generative.

The middle-aged person who is generative takes on the major work of providing for others, directly or indirectly. There is a sense of enterprise, productivity, mastery, charity, altruism, and perseverance. The greatest bulk of social problems and needs falls on this person who can handle the responsibilities because of personal strengths, vigor, and experience. There is a strong feeling of care and concern for that which has been produced by love, necessity, or accident. He or she can collaborate with others to do the necessary work. Ideas about personal needs and goals converge with an understanding of the social community, and the ideas guide actions taken on behalf of future generations.

The generative middle-aged adult may be a mentor to a young adult. A **mentor** is an *experienced adult with patience and understanding who befriends, guides, and counsels a less experienced and younger adult in the work world or in a social or an educational situation.* The mentor is usually approximately 10 years older, is confident, warm, and flexible, enjoys sharing knowledge and skills, is trustworthy, and promotes psychosocial development and success of the younger person. The mentor is found in business, management, nursing, or other careers or professions, sponsoring the younger person as an associate, creating a social heir, teaching him or her as much as possible for promotion into a position, or recommending the one being mentored for advancement. Several references present more information on mentoring (9, 25, 37, 46, 120, 162, 193).

The person's adaptive mechanism and superego are strong but not rigid. There is an expansion of interests and investment in that for which the person is responsible. Youth and young adults usually are self-centered. With approaching middle age and the image of one's finite existence faintly in view, the person consciously reappraises and uses self. With introspection, the self seems less important, and the words *service, love of others,* and *compassion* gain new meaning. These concepts motivate action. In church work, social work, community fund drives, cultural or artistic efforts, the profession, or political work, the person is active and often the leader. The person's goal is to leave the world a better place in which to live. A critical problem, however, is coming to terms with accomplishments and accepting responsibility that comes with achievement. In addition, he or she must come to terms with violations of the moral codes of society (e.g., tax loopholes used by some adults) and, with superego and ego in balance, develop a constructive philosophy and honest method of operation.

Some middle-aged adults believe the most important work of the person begins after parenthood ceases and is cognitive and emotional in nature: preserving culture, maintaining the annals of history, keeping alive human judgment, maintaining human skills, preserving and skillfully contriving the instruments of civilization, and teaching all this to oncoming generations. Although young and middle-aged adults are involved in such functions, these qualities of the human mind are best manifested in the late middle years or thereafter.

The generative person feels a sense of comfort or ease in lifestyle. There is realistic gratification from a job well done and from what has been given to others. He or she accepts self and the body, realizing that although acceptance of self is originally based on acceptance from others, unless he or she accepts self, he or she cannot really expect acceptance from others.

The mature middle-aged person has tested ways of doing things. He or she can draw on much experience; thus, he or she may have deep sincerity, mature judgment, and a sense of empathy. He or she has a sense of values or a philosophy underlying the life, giving a sense of stability and causing him or her to be reflective and cautious. The person recognizes that one of the most generative things he or she can give to society is the life led and the way he or she lives it. Consider the following statement by a 50-year-old man:

> *Those were full years—raising the kids with all its joy and frustration. I'm glad they're on their own now. This is a new stage of life. I can go fishing; Mary can go out to lunch. We have more time together for fun, and now we have more time for working at the election polls and in volunteer activities.*

The middle years can be wise and felicitous, or they can be foolish and frantic, fraught with doubts and despair.

If the developmental task of generativity is not achieved, a sense of **stagnation,** or **self-absorption,** enshrouds the person (50). Thus, *he or she regresses to adolescent, or younger, behavior characterized by physical and psychological invalidism.* This person hates the aging body and feels neither secure nor adept at handling self physically or interpersonally. He or she has little to offer even if so inclined. Her or she operates on a slim margin and soon burns out (see Consequences of Self-absorption). Consider the following statement by a 50-year-old woman:

► CONSEQUENCES OF SELF-ABSORPTION

- Denial of signs of normal aging
- Unhappiness with advancing age, desire to stay young, fear of growing old
- Regression to inappropriate youthfulness in dress or behavior, rebelliousness, foolish behavior
- Preoccupation with self, self-indulgence
- Physical, emotional, social, and interpersonal insecurity
- Attempts to prove youthfulness with infidelity to spouse
- Resignation, passivity, noninvolvement with societal or life issues
- Isolation or withdrawal from others
- Despair about signs of aging (considers self old, life is over)
- Either overcompliance or excessive rigidity in behavior
- Intolerance, cynicism, ruthless attitude
- Lack of stamina, chronic health problems that are not coped with
- Chronic defeatism, depression

> *I spent all those years raising the kids and doing housework while Bob moved up the professional ladder. We talked less and less about each other, only about the kids or his job. Now the kids are gone. I should be happy, but I'm lost. I can't carry on a decent conversation with Bob. I don't have any training for a job. And I look terrible! I sit around and eat too much. I wear high collars to hide my wrinkled neck, and no cosmetics will hide the dark circles under my eyes.*

Immature adults have impaired and less socially organized intellectual skills and value systems; their intellectual skills are fused by personal emotions and are coordinated in strange and unrealistic ways. The immature person seeks private self-absorption and vicarious immersion in subjective problems of others (50, 51, 106). Yet the characteristics of the self-absorbed person are health-endeavoring attempts and reparative efforts to cope or adapt. They may or may not work well, depending on the intensity of personality characteristics and the social and physical environment.

Maturity

Because **maturity,** *being fully developed as a person,* is not a quality of life reached at any one age or for all time, the characteristics described as generativity are general guidelines. If the person is doing what is appropriate for age, situation, and culture, he or she is acting maturely for the age. Attaining feelings of maturity and independence come later for the professional than for technical workers or laborers because of prolonged education. Also, as the person grows older, the ideal level of maturity and autonomy may recede further into the future and never be fully achieved (51, 85). Maturity is the achievement of efficiently organized psychic growth predicated on integration of experiences of solving environmentally stimulated conflicts. The external environment is a potent force on the person; conflicts are primarily socially incurred. The psychosocial organization in maturity shows a cultural direction. As one ages, the psychic interests broaden and are less selfish. Part of maturity is staying power, the power to see it through, which is different from starting power. Seeing it through is to use faith and persistence, to continue even against great odds. Characteristics of staying power include (1) integrity of consciousness and personhood; (2) remaining loyal to values, faith, philosophy, beliefs; (3) holding to a cause greater than self; and (4) giving up something worthwhile rather than worrying about present risks.

In adulthood there is no one set of appropriate personality characteristics or any one characteristic such as inflexibility or intolerance that is bad. The great person is inflexible or stands firm in the face of opposition at a crucial moment in history. The great person is intolerant of the evils he or she is trying to combat. Each of us leads a particular life at a particular time, place, and circumstance and with a particular personal history. Success in leading that life depends on a *pattern* of qualities appropriate to that life. No person can lead everyone's life. The mature person is reflective, restructures or processes information in the light of experience, and uses knowledge and expertise in a directed way to achieve desired ends. No one will reach the ideal of self-actualization described by Maslow (Chapter 5), yet each can reach his or her own ideal and peak of well-being and functioning relatively free of anxieties, cognitive distortions, and rigid habits and with a sense of the individuality and uniqueness of the self and others (85, 129).

The following *characteristics of positive mental health and maturity* were described by Jahoda (85):

- Accepting personal strengths and limits, having a firm sense of identity, and living with the past without guilt
- Striving for self-actualization and living up to the highest potential

- Developing a philosophy of life and code of ethics, an ability to resist stress and tolerate anxiety, and an equilibrium of intrapsychic forces
- Having a sense of autonomy, independence, and ability for self-direction
- Having an adequate perception of reality and of factors affecting reality, having a social sensitivity, and treating others as worthy of concern
- Mastering the environment: working, playing, solving problems, and adapting to the requirements of life
- Valuing human relationships and feeling responsible to others.

Others authors have also identified criteria for emotional maturity (37, 50, 51, 101, 102, 129, 138). See Criteria of Emotional Maturity.

Personality Development

Emotional or personality development has also been described by the stage theorists Jung (89, 95), Sheehy (162–164), Gould (66–68), Levinson (104), and Vaillant (190, 191).

Jung divided personality development to correspond to the first and second halves of the life cycle. In the first half, until the age of 35 or 40, the person is in a period of expansion. Maturational forces direct the growth of the ego (the conscious or awareness of self and the external world); capacities unfold for dealing with the external world. The person learns to get along with others and tries to win as many of society's rewards as possible. A career and family are established.

► CRITERIA OF EMOTIONAL MATURITY

- Ability to deal constructively with reality
- Capacity to adapt to change
- Relative freedom from symptoms that are produced by tensions and anxieties
- Capacity to find more satisfaction in giving than receiving
- Capacity to relate to other people in a consistent manner with mutual satisfaction and helpfulness
- Capacity to sublimate, to direct one's instinctive hostile energy into creative and constructive outlets
- Capacity to love
- Ability to use intuition, the natural mental ability, associated with experience to comprehend life events and formulate answers

To achieve, it is usually necessary for men to overdevelop their masculinity and for women to overemphasize their feminine traits and skills. The young person dedicates self to mastery of the outer world. Being preoccupied with self-doubt, fantasy, and the inner nature is not advantageous to the young adult, for the task is to meet the demands of society confidently and assertively (89, 95).

Jung believed that during the forties the personality begins to undergo a transformation. Earlier goals and ambitions have lost their meaning. The person may feel stagnant, incomplete, depressed, as if something crucial is missing, even if the person has been quite successful, because success has often been achieved at the cost of personality development. The person begins to become introspective, to turn inward, to examine the meaning of life. Separating self from ordinary conformity to the goals and values of mass society and achieving a measure of psychic balance are accomplished through individuation—finding one's individual way (89, 95).

Jung recognized that, although middle-aged persons begin to turn inward, they still have much energy and resources for the generativity described by **Erikson** and for making personal changes. The person may begin new or long-forgotten projects and interests or even change careers. Men and women begin giving expression to their opposite sexual drives. Men become less aggressively ambitious and more concerned with interpersonal relationships. They begin to realize that achievement counts for less and friendship for more. Women tend to become more aggressive and independent. Such changes can create midlife marital problems. Although ongoing development may create tension and difficulties, Jung believed that the greatest failures come when adults cling to the goals and values of the first half of life, holding on to the glories and beauty of youth (89, 95).

Neugarten (126–130) found personality characteristics in middle age similar to those described by Jung (89).

Sheehy (162–164), **Gould** (66–68), **Levinson** (104), and **Vaillant** (190, 191) also describe midlife stages of development. These stage theorists confirm many of the characteristics already described and emphasize that this is a time of new stability and authenticity.

As you work with the middle-aged person, use the concept of generativity versus self-absorption in assessment of the client's developmental level, and promote achievement of this developmental task through your listening, support, encouragement of activities, teaching, and counseling. The self-absorbed person should be referred to a long-term counselor. The generative person or mentor needs to hear that what he or she is doing is indeed a worthwhile contribution. Your own generativity can be a positive model for others. Your reinforcement of another's strengths facilitates further emotional development and maturity.

Body Image Development

The gradually occurring physical changes described earlier confront the person and are mirrored in others. The climacteric causes realignment of attitudes about the self that cuts into the personality and its definition. Other life stresses cause the person to view self and the body differently. The person not only realizes he or she is looking older but subjectively feels older as well. Work can bring a sense of stress if he or she feels less stamina and vigor to cope with the task at hand. Illness or death of loved ones creates a concern about personal health, sometimes to excess, and thoughts about one's own death are more frequent. The person begins to believe that he or she is coming out second-best to youth, for the previous self-image of the youthful, strong, and healthy body with boundless energy becomes inadequate. Depression, irritability, and anxiety about femininity and masculinity result. In the United States, more so than in European or Asian cultures, youth and vigor are highly valued, a carryover from frontier days. The person's previous personality largely influences the intensity of these feelings and the symptoms associated with body image changes. Difficulties are also caused by fear of the effects of the climacteric, folklore about sexuality, attitudes toward womanhood, social and advertising pressures in our culture, and emphasis on obsolescence.

Whether a man or a woman, the person who lacks self-confidence and who cannot accept the changing body has a compulsion to try cosmetics, clothes, hairstyles, and the other trappings of youth in the hope that the physical attributes of youth will be attained. The person tries to regain a youthful figure and face, perhaps through surgery; tints the hair to cover signs of gray; and turns to hormone creams to restore the skin. These people are clients at times. There is nothing wrong with dressing attractively or changing the color of one's hair. But too few men or women realize that the color and texture of their skin have changed as the color of their hair faded and that their aging hands contrast considerably with the commercial coloring on the head. Women in the 18th century may have had a more realistic self-picture. They used white wigs or powdered their hair instead of dyeing it, perhaps because they recognized that white or gray hair softens the contours and flatters the face as the years go by.

Most people gradually adjust to their slowly changing body and accept the changes as part of maturity.

The mature person realizes it is impossible to return to youth. To imitate youth denies the mature person's own past and experience. The excitement of the middle years lies in using adeptly the experience, insights, values, and realism acquired earlier. The person does not need to downgrade or agree continually with everything youth say and do. The middle-aged person feels good about self. Healthy signs are that he or she prefers this age and has no desire to relive the youthful years.

You can promote integration of a positive body image through your communication skills and teaching. Reaffirm the strengths of being middle-aged to the client, using information presented in this chapter and emphasizing the specific strengths of the person.

Adaptive Mechanisms

The adult may use any of the adaptive mechanisms described in previous chapters. **Adult socialization** is defined as the *processes through which an adult learns to perform the roles and behaviors expected of self and by others and to remain adaptive in a variety of situations.* The middle-aged adult is expected and normally considers self to be adaptive. The emphasis is on active, reciprocal participation of the person; little preparation is directed to anticipating, accepting, or coping with failure. The ability to shift emotional investments from one activity to another, to remain open-minded, and to use past experience as a guide rather than as the rule is closely related to adaptive ability (51, 106, 163, 164).

The adult, having been rewarded for certain behaviors over the years, has established a wide variety of role-related behaviors, problem-solving techniques, adaptations to stress, and methods for making role transitions; they may not be adaptive to current demands or crises or to increasing role diffusion. There is a continuous need for socialization in adulthood, for a future orientation, for anticipating events, and for learning to respond to new demands (51, 106). Ongoing learning of adult roles occurs through observation, imitation, or identification with another, trial-and-error behavior, the media, books, or formal education.

Coping or adaptive mechanisms or ego defenses used in response to the emotional stress of the middle years depend on the person's capacity to adapt and satisfy personal needs, sense of identity, nature of interaction with others, sense of usefulness, and interest in the outside world.

The middle-aged adult must be able to channel emotional drives without losing initiative and vigor. During middle age the person is especially vulnerable to a number of disrupting events: physiologic changes and illness in self and loved ones, family stresses, changes in job or role demands or responsibilities, conflict between family generations, and societal changes. The person should be able to cope with ordinary personal upheavals and the frustrations and disappointments in life with only temporary disequilibrium. He or she should be able to participate enthusiastically in adult work and play and to experience adequate sexual satisfaction in a stable relationship. The person should be able to express a reasonable amount of aggression, anger, joy, and affection without undue effort, unnecessary guilt, or lack of adequate control (106, 164). Further, the middle-aged adult is a role model of maturity for the young adult.

The person can retain a sense of balance by recognizing that each age has its unique joys and charms, and the entire life span is valued as equally precious. He or she can appreciate what is past, anticipate the future, and maintain a sense of permanence or stability. The person can adapt successfully to the stresses of middle age by achieving the developmental crisis.

You can help the middle-aged adult prevent or overcome maladaptive mechanisms. As you extend empathy and reinforce a sense of emotional maturity and health, the person may feel more able to cope with life stressors and perceived failures. You may use principles and techniques of stress management and do and teach crisis intervention as described in *Psychiatric/ Mental Health Nursing: Giving Emotional Care* (124). If you feel unable to listen to or work with the problems of someone who may be twice your age, refer the person to a counselor.

Midlife Crisis

The midlife crisis was first described by Jung (89). He believed that at approximately age 40 or 45, the psyche begins to undergo a transformation. The individual believes that the goals and ambitions that once seemed so eternal have lost their meaning. Quite often, the person feels depressed, stagnant, and incomplete, as if something crucial is missing. Jung observed that this happens even among people who have achieved a good measure of social success, for rewards have been won at the cost of a diminution of personality. Middle age can be seen as a transition or a crisis.

Midlife crisis is a *major and revolutionary turning point in one's life, involving changes in commitments to career and/or spouse and children and accompanied by significant and ongoing emotional turmoil for both the individual and others.* The term **midlife transition** has a different meaning; it includes *aspects of crisis, process, change, and alternating periods of stability and transition* (64, 89, 142, 163, 164).

Case Situation: Midlife Crisis

Louise, a 48-year-old architect, had an uneasy feeling, about her relationship with her husband Charles, age 49, a teacher. The feeling had been there for some time, and she had tried a time or two to talk about it but had been rebuffed by Charles.

Louise believed that she and Charles were slowly drifting apart, each into his or her own profession. Yet the pronouncement by Charles seemed so sudden. As she joined him in the family room after dinner, he quietly looked at her and said, "I have something to tell you. I'm leaving. There's nothing here for me anymore. I'm almost 50. I've got to get on with things."

Louise was overcome with shock, grief, guilt, disbelief, helplessness, and worry. They had been married for 22 years. She had often thought about all they could do together when they retired. Because they were childless, they would be free to travel. She panicked as she thought of life and aging without him. For days she slept and ate little but managed to go to work.

In the following months Louise and Charles met to talk several times. She wanted them to see a marriage counselor and work out their differences. As Charles continued to move his clothes, belongings, and favorite items from the home, he revealed that he would be living with another woman, a colleague from his work, and they would marry as soon as both divorces were finalized.

The divorce proceedings took more than a year. During that time Louise sought counseling for herself. Gradually she revealed her situation to her family, other relatives, and friends. She often blamed herself for Charles' leaving and talked frequently of what a wonderful person he was. She maintained a hectic pace, caring for the home and yard and handling the responsibilities of her job; however, in the months after the initial separation, Louise also reestablished a daily exercise routine, which she had interrupted after Charles left home. She contacted a number of friends she had seen only occasionally in the past few years and began to attend the church of her childhood faith. She was pulling herself together—physically, emotionally, mentally, socially, and spiritually.

After the divorce was finalized, Louise continued to blame herself for several years. She worked hard, achieving recognition at the architectural firm where she was employed. She also maintained her home and neighborhood ties and became active in her church.

After 10 years Charles, who is remarried, still visits Louise occasionally and calls every few weeks. Louise has resolved the events of Charles' midlife crisis but has avoided opportunities to date or remarry. She believes the struggles and crises of the past decade, including various illnesses and the death of her parents, have prepared for for adaptation to her eventual retirement, aging, and dying. She still believes that she and Charles could reestablish a marriage and that it would be more love-filled and happy. Yet she remains fully committed to caring for a number of older friends; the responsibilities of her profession, home, and organizational and church membership; and to continuing to deepen her spiritual and emotional maturity.

For some, midlife is one of the better periods of life: it is a *transition* from youth to later maturity; life expectancy is longer; psychologically and physically, midlife is healthier than ever in history; and parental responsibilities are decreasing. Most people are in their late forties or early fifties when the last child leaves home, leaving a couple of decades for the spouses to be together without the obligations of childrearing. The couple realizes that the myth of decreasing sexual powers is not true. Women in midlife may begin or continue their education or a career. Men see midlife as a time of continuing achievement. Experience, assurance, substance, skill, success, and good judgment more than compensate for the disappearance of youthful looks and physical abilities.

Levinson (104), found in his study of men that the period of midlife transition is around ages 40 to 45. For a few, the sense of change even in relation to body changes was slight, not particularly painful, and a manageable transition. For approximately 80% of the men, however, the early forties evoked tumultuous struggles within the self and with the external world. This period involved for many a profound reappraisal. It involves false starts, emotional turmoil, and despair. At least one-third of the male population in the United States between the ages of 40 and 60 will experience some aspect of midlife crisis.

If the person has not resolved the identity crisis of adolescence and achieved mature intimacy in young adulthood, if the person fears the passage of time, physical changes, aging, and mortality, *if the person cannot handle the meaning of life's routines and changes, midlife is seen as a crisis.*

The person may declare he or she is bored. The nagging feeling that all is not right within the self and with the world can become a way to avoid facing the challenges presented by a deepening self-awareness and to avoid responsibility for personal immaturities or failures. Although many areas of life can be a source of boredom, the two most blamed as tedious and unsatisfying are marriage and work. Leaving either one may be a practical solution to a nagging expediency that was only partially satisfying. Often, however, the joblessness or job change or the affair or the divorce is a headlong flight from aging—an attempt to slow the passage of time by recapturing a lost sense of wholeness, by trying to gain total freedom to explore, and by changing goals and becoming a different sort of person. The new freedom may be found as equally stressful and full of rejection, competition, loneliness, meaninglessness, and personal dissatisfaction as the old routines. Often the structure and tedium of work or marriage look comfortable, pleasant, and meaningful only after either situation has been left behind. The identity crisis, when it is over, is seen to have been a denial of reality, not a new level of maturity. The "rational" goal seeking and need to change turn out to be compulsive and meaningless activity.

The psyche itself provides the way out of this crisis. It urges the person to turn inward and examine the meaning of his or her life. This turning inward is prompted by the unconscious, the region in which all the repressed and unlived aspects of the self have grown and now clamor to be heard. The unconscious calls out for recognition to bring about psychic balance and harmony. This often becomes apparent first in dreams. The unconscious speaks to us primarily through dreams. As middle-aged adults examine their lives and listen to unconscious messages, they sooner or later encounter images of the self, the symbols of wholeness and centeredness. The person must confront the negative aspects of self to become whole and find his or her true center (89).

The introspectiveness of middle age can cause a change in perceptions, felt needs, feelings toward others, and a heightened sense of disappointment without the balance of an increased awareness of achievements and positive aspects of life. The person may feel bitter, depressed, and desperate even though he or she has success, wealth, material possessions, and power.

Family experiences are undoubtedly integral to the direction of the midlife crisis. The midlife transition for men, often the husbands of menopausal women, brings new stresses. This period is often accompanied by sexual problems, sometimes leading to affairs, marital disruption, and the abandonment of the wife. Adolescent children may be sexually and aggressively provocative, challenging, or disappointing. Children leaving home for school or marriage change the family balance. Hav-

ing no children can be a keen disappointment when the man realizes he has no heirs. Some women view their children's leaving home and marrying as an extension or expansion of parenting to include the wider interests and loci of their children. Far-flung needs of family members and expanded interests and activities lead to a different kind of parenting. Some women are restored to themselves and to their own development. Restored to themselves does not mean alone: women depend much more on their relationships for their development—not only for their emotional comfort and security but also to express the acting-on-the-world component of their aggression. The potential for autonomy, changes in relationships, and the development of their occupational skills, contacts, and self-image may start after childbearing is completed (46, 51, 106, 164). The woman's new-found autonomy, role changes, and increased interaction with or demands on the husband may be very threatening to the man.

In essence, the midlife crisis involves internal upheaval that may or may not be precipitated by such external events as job crisis, children's maturation, and marital difficulty. Often these events are the symptoms, rather than the causes, of the upheaval. Midlife crisis is not always experienced consciously. The feelings of rebellion, meaningless, and depression and the need for change may lead instead to altered behavior or attitudes in several life areas, involvement with a variety of causes, or escape into psychosomatic illness, alcoholism, and psychiatric illness (64).

It is healthier in the long range for the person to acknowledge the disruptive feelings and the diffusion of identity and to work through them rather than to deny them, and to seek a healthy and constructive outlet for these feelings. Refer to references at the end of the chapter for more information on various issues in midlife for both men and women related to physical changes, changes in relationships with spouse, family, and children, the relationship of the parent with the same- and opposite-sex child, work relationships and dissatisfactions, and time perspectives.

You can be instrumental in assisting the person in working through this crisis. You will use principles of communication and crisis intervention (see Chapter 5). Refer the person to a counselor who can work with the individual and family. The following *guidelines may help the person who feels he or she is in midlife crisis.* Share and use them as you work with others, or use them in your own life.

- Do not be scared by the midlife crisis. Physical and psychological changes are normal throughout life; see them as opportunities for maturing.

- Face your feelings and your goals realistically. If you feel confused, see a counselor who can help you sort through your feelings and goals.
- See your age as a positive asset. Acknowledge your strengths, the benefits of middle age. Take steps to adjust to your liabilities or to correct them if you can. If a change in hairstyle or clothes makes you feel better, make that change.
- Reconcile yourself to the fact that some or many of your hopes and dreams may never be realized and may not be attainable. Remain open to the opportunities that are available; they may exceed your dreams.
- If the job is not satisfying, consider another job or another field after appraising yourself realistically; or be willing to relinquish some responsibility at work.
- If you dread retirement, plan for it financially, along with leisure and other activities.
- If job pressures are great, seek outlets through recreational activities or other diversions, become involved in community service, and renew spiritual study and religious affiliations.
- Renew old friendships; initiate new ones. Invest in others and in the process enhance personal self-esteem and emotional well-being.
- Try to be flexible and open-minded rather than dogmatic or inflexible in meeting and solving the problems you face.
- If you are concerned about sexual potency, realize that the problem is typically transient. The more you worry, the worse it gets. Talk about your sexual feelings and concerns with your spouse. The love and concern you have for each other can frequently overcome any impotency. It is important for the woman to perceive sexuality apart from childbearing and menstruation and for the man to perceive sexuality apart from having children and love affairs. If you are so inclined, together read how-to sex manuals. Seek a marriage counselor if together you cannot work out problems of sexual dysfunction.
- Share your feelings, concerns, frustrations, and problems with your spouse or confidante so that she or he can understand the changes you are experiencing. Keeping feelings to yourself can increase alienation and the difficulty of repairing the relationship.
- Examine your attitudes as a parent; strike a balance between care and protection of offspring. Realize their normal need for independence.
- Realize that frequently the middle-aged woman is becoming more assertive just when the middle-aged man is becoming more passive. Recognizing this as normal and talking about these changes can help the spouses better understand each other's needs and aspirations.
- Get a physical examination to ensure that physical symptoms are not indicators of physical illness. Do not think that vitamins or health foods alone will cause you to feel differently.
- Seek counseling for psychological symptoms. The counselor may be a nurse, religious leader, mental health therapist, social worker, marriage counselor, psychologist, or psychiatrist.

You can give some specific *suggestions to the spouse of the man in midlife crisis:*

- Recognize and acknowledge changes in him, but do not make value judgments. Do not say, "You look awful dressed in that. Who do you think you are, a young swinger?" Say instead, "I notice you're no longer wearing your regular suits and ties. Why is that?"
- Make it easier for him to talk about his feelings and fears by listening to verbal and nonverbal messages. Avoid telling him how he should feel, dress, or behave.
- Try not to make him feel guilty by hurling your fears or anger at him. His guilt about your fears will only cause him to withdraw and refuse to discuss his problems with you.
- Emphasize to him that he does not have to leave to find what he is looking for. Try to find new joint interests, friends, or hobbies. Be willing to see a marriage counselor with him.
- Focus on changing yourself. Become more alive by taking care of your appearance, keeping informed, and broadening your interests.
- Avoid threatening his self-concept by appearing too competent in managing all areas of life while he neglects his usual family and home roles. Encourage him to maintain roles. Be prepared to pick up loose ends, however.
- Try to reestablish the intimacy and closeness that you once shared. Be willing to compromise and change your own attitudes and behavior.
- Try to maintain a certain spontaneity in your sexual life. Allow a sense of adventure to rekindle the relationship. If you can reestablish an active and satisfying sexual life at this point, you can both be certain that it will continue for many more years.
- If he is coping with a midlife crisis symptom, focus on his strengths. But do not hand out empty praise. Instead find a real reason to praise him.

- Do not adopt a motherly role toward him. Whereas sympathy and compassion are constructive, constant mothering and giving advice tend to diminish his sexual interest and ability to relate as husband.
- Do not feel guilty when your husband develops any of the midlife crisis symptoms. It is not your fault. If handled with honesty and intelligence, the midlife crisis in men can be a positive turning point in a marriage, eventually creating a more constructive, satisfying, loving relationship.

Individuals considering midlife career or work changes must be able to assess their current job skills and applicability of them to new careers, explore alternatives within their current job position and external counseling services, and examine personal values. Career transition then becomes the response to seeking compatibility between self-image and the world of work (106, 164). How the career change is negotiated depends in part on whether it is forced by external forces such as job layoff and technologic advances or voluntarily pursued because of value conflicts or as a means to personal, creative, economic, or social advancement. The person considering career change in life structure needs time, opportunity to talk, and help in working through the various facets of the situation.

Benefits from the midlife crisis include personality growth and deepening maturity because of personal introspection and desire to change behavior to feel better and improve one's life. Further, if the person in crisis can accept assistance, affection, and acceptance from loved ones, he or she can grow closer to them, and relationships deepen as a result. Sometimes the changes made in relation to a second career can enhance social status, financial well-being, or a sense of independence. The concern about mortality can motivate the person to take better care of health and to take time to pursue new interests or reinitiate old relationships. The person can experience an invigorating rebirth, generating new energies and new commitments.

Moral–Spiritual Development

The middle-aged person continues to integrate new concepts from widened sources into a religious philosophy if he or she has gained the spiritual maturity described in Chapter 12. He or she becomes less dogmatic in his or her beliefs. Faith and trust in God or another source of spiritual strength are increased. Religion offers comfort and happiness. The person is able to deal effectively with the religious aspects of upcoming surgery and its possible effects, illness, death of parents, or unexpected tragedy.

The middle-aged person may have become alienated from organized religion in early adulthood or may have drifted away from religious practices and spiritual study because of familial, occupational, and social role responsibilities. As the person becomes more introspective, studies self and life from new perspectives, ponders the meaning of life, and faces crises, he or she is likely to return to study of religious literature, practices of former years, and organized religious groups for strength, comfort, forgiveness, and joy. Spiritual beliefs and religion take on added importance. The middle-aged adult who becomes revived spiritually is likely to remain devout and active in his or her faith throughout life. If the person does not deepen spiritual insights, a sense of meaninglessness and despair is likely in old age.

Moral development is advanced whenever the person has an experience of sustained responsibility for the welfare of others. Middle age, if it is lived generatively, provides such an experience. Although the cognitive awareness of higher principles of living develops in adolescence, consistent commitment to their ethical applications develops in adulthood after the person has had time and opportunity to meet personal needs and to establish self in the family and community. Further, the level of cognitive development sets the upper limits for moral potential. If the adult remains in the state of Concrete Operations, he or she is unlikely to move beyond the Conventional Level of moral development (law and order reasoning), as the Postconventional Level requires a deep and broad understanding of events and a critical reasoning ability (98).

Although Kohlberg's work (98) on moral development was done on men, women generally come out at Stage 3 of the Conventional Level (Table 5–12), which emphasizes an interpersonal definition of morality rather than a societal definition of morality or an orientation to law and order. Perhaps the stage of moral development often seen in women, with concern for the well-being of others and a willingness to sacrifice self for others' well-being, is an aspect of Stage 5 of the Postconventional Level.

Loevinger (108) sees middle age as the Autonomous Stage of Ego Development, when the person evolves principles for self apart from the social world. The person deals with the differences between personal needs, principles by which to live, and duties demanded by society.

Gilligan (62, 63), whose research centered on moral development in women, found that women define morality in terms of selfishness versus responsibility. Women subjects with high morality scores emphasized the importance of being responsible in behavior and of exercising care with and avoiding hurt to others. Men think more in terms of general justice and fairness; women think in terms of the needs of specific individuals. Gilligan's view of moral development is outlined in Table 13–7 according to three levels and the transition points from level I to level II and from level II to level III (62, 63).

Developmental Tasks

Each period of life differs from the others, offering new experiences and opportunities and new tasks to surmount. The developmental tasks of middle age have a biological basis in the gradual aging of the physical body, a cultural basis in social pressures and expectations, and an emotional origin in the individual lifestyle and self-concept that the mature adult has developed.

The following developmental tasks should be accomplished by middle-aged people (45, 51, 116, 126, 130). Through your care, counsel, and teaching, you can assist your clients to be aware of and to achieve these tasks.

- Maintain or establish healthful life patterns.
- Discover and develop new satisfactions as a mate, give support to mate, enjoy joint activities, and develop a sense of unity and abiding intimacy.
- Help growing and grown children to become happy and responsible adults and relinquish the central position in their affections, free the self from emotional dependence on children, take pride in their accomplishments, stand by to assist as needed, and accept their friends and mates.
- Create a pleasant, comfortable home, appropriate to values, interests, time, energy, and resources; give, receive, and exchange hospitality; and take pride in accomplishments of self and spouse.
- Find pleasure in generativity and recognition in work if employed; gain knowledge, proficiency, and wisdom; be able to lead or follow; balance work with other roles; and prepare for eventual retirement.
- Reverse roles with aging parents and parents-in-law, assist them as needed without domineering, and act as a buffer between demands of aging parents and needs of young adults; prepare emotionally for the eventual death of parents unless they are already deceased.
- Maintain a standard of living related to values, needs, and financial resources.
- Achieve mature social and civic responsibility; be informed as a citizen; give time, energy, and resources to causes beyond self and home. Work cooperatively with others in the common responsibilities of citizenship; encourage others in their citizenship; stand for democratic practices and the welfare of the group as a whole in issues when vested interests may be at stake.
- Develop or maintain an active organizational membership, deriving from it pleasure and a sense of belonging; refuse conflicting or too burdensome invitations with poise; work through intraorganizational tensions, power systems, and personality problems by becoming a mature statesperson in a diplomatic role, leading when necessary.

TABLE 13–7. MORAL DEVELOPMENT IN WOMEN

Level	Characteristics
I. Orientation of individual survival	Concentrates on what is practical and best for self
Transition 1: from selfishness to responsibility	Realizes connection to others; thinks of responsible choice in terms of another as well as self
II. Goodness as self-sacrifice	Sacrifices personal wishes and needs to fulfill others' wants and to have others think well of her; feels responsible for others' actions; holds others responsible for her choices; dependent position; indirect efforts to control others often turn into manipulation through use of guilt
Transition 2: from goodness to truth	Makes decisions on personal intentions and consequences of actions rather than on how she thinks others will react; takes into account needs of self and others; wants to be good to others but also honest by being responsible to self
III. Morality of nonviolence	Establishes moral equality between self and others; assumes responsibility for choice in moral dilemmas; follows injunction to hurt no one, including self, in all situations

Source: Ref. 62

- Accept and adjust to the physical changes of middle age, maintain healthful ways of living, attend to personal grooming, and relish maturity.
- Make an art of friendship; cherish old friends and choose new; enjoy an active social life with friends, including friends of both sexes and of various ages; accept at least a few friends into close sharing of feelings to help avoid self-absorption.
- Use leisure time creatively and with satisfaction without yielding too much to social pressures and styles; learn to do some things well enough to become known for them among family, friends, and associates; enjoy use of talents; share some leisure time activities with a mate or others and balance leisure activities with active and passive, collective and solitary, service-motivated and self-indulgent pursuits.
- Acknowledge and confront the psychological sense that the time left for cognitive, creative, emotional, social, and spiritual fulfillment is shorter and that fulfillment may never come.
- Continue to formulate a philosophy of life and religious or philosophic affiliation, discovering new depths and meanings in God or a creator that include but also go beyond the fellowship of a particular religious denomination; gain satisfaction from altruistic activities or the concerns of a particular denomination; invest self in significant causes and movements; and recognize the finiteness of life.
- Prepare for retirement with financial arrangements and development of hobbies and leisure activities, and rework philosophy and values.

The single or widowed middle-aged person will have basically the same developmental tasks but must find a sense of intimate sharing with friends or relatives (see Key Interpersonal Relationships for Never-married Women) (154).

Peck (138) sees the issues, conflicts, or tasks the person must work through in middle age as encompassing four aspects:

1. *Valuing wisdom gained from living and experience versus valuing physical powers and youth.* The person needs to accept his or her age, that youth cannot be regained, and that although physical strength and power may diminish, wisdom may accomplish more than physical strength anyway.
2. *Socializing versus sexualizing in human relationships.* The middle-aged adult, although still active sexually, now sees and relates to people as humans rather than just on the basis of men or women. The person relates to others without the sex self-consciousness of adolescence or young-young adulthood and sees the intrinsic dignity and worth of all people as social and spiritual beings.
3. *Emotional flexibility versus emotional impoverishment.* The middle-aged adult, although often accused of being rigid and unable to change, remains accepting of and empathic to others, open to people of different backgrounds, and open to changing personal behavior. The person becomes emotionally impoverished only if he or she withdraws from others, avoids learning from experience, refuses to change, or demonstrates the self-absorption described by Erikson (50).
4. *Mental flexibility versus mental rigidity.* The middle-aged adult, although accused of being closed to new ideas and excessively cautious, remains open to learning and flexible in problem-solving strategies. The person becomes mentally rigid if he or she avoids new experiences or learning opportunities or denies social, educational, or technologic changes.

► KEY INTERPERSONAL RELATIONSHIPS FOR NEVER-MARRIED WOMEN

Blood ties:	Nieces, nephews, siblings, aging parents. Often the woman gives assistance, which involves sacrifice.
Constricted ties:	Affiliation with a nonkin family; establishment of a quasi-parental tie with a younger person who is like a son or daughter; or a long-term relationship with a same-generation companion. These relationships are voluntary and positive, but there is no assurance of care from these individuals.
Quasi-parental relations:	Acting like a parent to younger nonrelatives. There is no biogenetic tie but the relationship is modeled on parent–child tie.
Companionate:	A marriagelike interdependency in which there is much involvement over time and a sense of obligation to care for each other.
Friendship:	A close relationship that endures and provides security. Depending on the duration and closeness, the friend may provide help in time of need.

► SELECTED NURSING DIAGNOSES RELATED TO MIDDLE AGE*

Pattern 1: Exchanging

- Altered Nutrition: More than Body Requirements
- Altered Nutrition: Less than Body Requirements
- Altered Nutrition: Potential for More than Body Requirements
- Risk for Infection
- Risk for Injury
- Risk for Trauma
- Impaired Skin Integrity

Pattern 2: Communicating

- Impaired Verbal Communication

Pattern 3: Relating

- Impaired Social Interaction
- Social Isolation
- Altered Role Performance
- Risk of Altered Parenting
- Altered Family Processes
- Parental Role Conflict
- Altered Sexuality Patterns

Pattern 4: Valuing

- Spiritual Distress

Pattern 5: Choosing

- Ineffective Individual Coping
- Impaired Adjustment
- Defensive Coping
- Ineffective Denial
- Ineffective Family Coping: Disabling
- Ineffective Family Coping: Compromised
- Family Coping: Potential for Growth
- Decisional Conflict
- Health-Seeking Behaviors

Pattern 6: Moving

- Impaired Physical Mobility
- Activity Intolerance
- Fatigue
- Risk for Activity Intolerance
- Sleep Pattern Disturbance
- Diversional Activity Deficit
- Impaired Home Maintenance Management
- Altered Health Maintenance

Pattern 7: Perceiving

- Body Image Disturbance
- Self-Esteem Disturbance
- Chronic Low Self-Esteem
- Situational Low Self-Esteem
- Sensory/Perceptual Alterations
- Hopelessness
- Powerlessness

Pattern 8: Knowing

- Knowledge Deficit

Pattern 9: Feeling

- Pain
- Chronic Pain
- Dysfunctional Grieving
- Anticipatory Grieving
- Risk for Violence: Self-Directed or Directed at Others
- Post-Trauma Response
- Anxiety
- Fear

*Other NANDA nursing diagnoses are applicable to the ill middle-aged adult.
From North American Nursing Diagnosis Association, NANDA Nursing Diagnoses: Definitions & Classification 1995–1996. Philadelphia: (rev.). St. Louis: North American Nursing Diagnosis Association, 1994.

► HEALTH CARE AND NURSING APPLICATIONS

Your role in caring for the middle-aged person and family has been described throughout the chapter. Assessment, using knowledge presented in this chapter, is the basis for formulating *nursing diagnoses*. Nursing diagnoses that may be applicable to the middle-aged adult are listed in Selected Nursing Diagnoses Related to Middle Age. Interventions may involve the health promotion or direct care measures described throughout the chapter to assist the person and family in meeting physical, emotional, cognitive, spiritual, and social needs.

TRANSITION TO LATER MATURITY

The middle-aged adult has developed a sense of the life cycle; through introspection, he or she has gained a heightened sensitivity to the personal position within a complex social environment. Life is no longer seen as an infinite stretch of time into the future. The person anticipates and accepts the inevitable sequence of events that occur as the human matures, ages, and dies. The middle-aged adult realizes that the course of his or her life will be similar to the lives of others. Sex differences between men and women diminish in reality and perception. Turning points affect all and are inescapable. Personal mortality, achievements, and failures and personal strengths and limits must be faced if the person is to be prepared emotionally and developmentally for later maturity and the personal aging process. The person realizes that the direction in life has been set by prior decisions related to occupation, marriage, family life, and having or not having children. Although occupation and lifestyle can be changed, at least to some extent, the results of other earlier decisions cannot be changed. The consequences must be faced and resolved. The middle-aged person realizes he or she may not achieve all dreams, but remaining open to opportunities along the way may enable the person to achieve accomplishments never fantasized that are equally meaningful.

For example, if the young adult woman focused on career and did not marry and have children, at age 50 she may still marry, but having children—or adoption—is less likely. Having no children means not being a grandparent in old age. The need to be a parent or grandparent or to nurture must be met in another way. In turn, the single or childless middle-aged woman may realize that she has been nurturing a larger number of people than some middle-aged women who focused their attention solely on the children.

The person in late midlife realizes that life's developmental markers and crises call forth changes in self-concept and sense of identity, necessitate incorporation of new social roles and behaviors, and precipitate new adaptations. But they do not destroy the sense of continuity within the person from youth to old age. This adaptability and a sense of continuity are essential for the achievement of ego integrity in the last years of life.

SUMMARY

The middle years are filled with challenge, pleasures, and demands. This is the prime of life, a time of generativity. For some, it is a time of struggle, crisis, loss, or illness. Considerations for the Middle–Aged Client in Health Care and Chart 6 in Appendix IV summarize what you should consider in assessment and intervention with the middle-aged client.

► CONSIDERATIONS FOR THE MIDDLE-AGED CLIENT IN HEALTH CARE

1. Family and cultural history
2. Personal history
3. Preexisting illness
4. Risk factors for disease in family (e.g., cardiovascular disease, cancer, osteoporosis, developmental disability, mental illness)
5. Psychosocial evaluation (age-related stresses, distress with partner, midlife crisis issues)
6. Caregiver responsibilities
7. Knowledge of normal changes in middle age and coping strategies—adaptive capacity
8. Nutrition history—weekly diet intake
9. Complete physical examination
10. For women:
    a. Menstrual history (age onset, pattern, current pattern)
    b. History of estrogen administration
    c. Reproductive history (number of pregnancies, at what age, miscarriages or abortions)
    d. Perimenstrual history (beginning of menopausal symptoms, response, whether menopause has occurred).
    e. Interest in or current administration of hormone replacement therapy; any side effects
11. Other members of household (review 1–9)

REFERENCES

1. Alternatives to Hormone Replacement, *Harvard Women's Health Watch,* 1, no. 12 (1994), 3–4.
2. American Academy of Family Physicians, *Age Charts for Periodic Health Examination.* Washington, DC: Author, 1995.
3. Angel, M., *The Orphaned Adult: Confronting the Death of a Parent.* New York: Human Sciences Press, 1987.
4. Arlin, P.K., Cognitive Development in Adulthood: A Fifth Stage? *Developmental Psychology,* 11 (1975), 602–606.
5. Ask the Experts, *Tufts University Diet and Nutrition Letter,* 13, no. 1 (1995), 8.
6. Back Protection for Daily Sitters, *Staying Well Newsletter,* May–June (1991), 1–2.
7. Badura, B., Health Promotion for Chronically Ill People, *WHO Regional Publications: European Series,* 37 (1991), 365–390.
8. Baert, H., P. Gielen, and M. Smet, A Health Diary for the Chronically Ill, *WHO Regional Publications: European Series,* 44 (1992), 328–331.
9. Bajinck, I., et al., Nurses as Colleagues and Mentors, *Canadian Nurse,* 84, no. 2 (1988), 16–17.
10. Baum, M., and M. Page, Caregiving and Multigenerational Families, *The Gerontologist,* 31, no. 6 (1991), 762–769l.
11. Beck, M., L. Denworth, and N. Christian, Finding Work After Fifty, *Newsweek,* March 10 (1992), 58–60.
12. Begley, S., and D. Glick, The Estrogen Complex, *Newsweek,* March 21 (1994), 76–78.
13. Belenky, M., B. Clinchy, N. Goldberg, and J. Tarule, *Women's Way of Knowing.* New York: Basic Books, 1986.
14. Bennett, C., Expanding the Mind–Body Connection: Working Women and Stress, *Capsules & Comments in Psychiatric Nursing,* 2, no. 4 (1996), 249–254.
15. Berg, B., I've Got a Hunch, *New Choices,* May (1991), 74–77.
16. Berglas, C., *Mid-Life Crisis.* Lancaster, PA: Technomic, 1987.
17. Bieber, L., M. Hendrix, C. Taylor, and M. Wykle, The Challenge of Diversity, *Journal of Psychosocial Nursing,* 31, no. 8 (1993), 23–29.
18. Bolles, R., The Decade of Decisions, *Modern Maturity,* March (1990), 36–45.
19. Bootzin, R., H. Lahmeyer, and J. Lilie, Eds., *Integrated Approach to Sleep Management.* Washington, DC: American Nurses Association, 1994.
20. Brackley, M. H., The Plight of American Family Caregivers: Implications for Nursing, *Perspectives in Psychiatric Care,* 30, no. 4 (1994), 14–20.
21. Brody, E. M., S. J. Litvin, C. Hoffman and M. H. Kleban, Marital Status of Caregiving Daughters and Co-residence With Dependent Parents, *The Gerontologist,* 35, no. 1 (1995), 75–84.
22. Buchaman, R., The Widow and the Widower, in Grollman, E., ed., *Concerning Death: A Practical Guide for the Living.* Boston: Beacon Press, 1974, pp. 287–311.
23. Bucher, H., and D. Ragland, Socioeconomic Indicators and Mortality From Coronary Heart Disease and Cancer: A 22-Year Follow-up of Middle-aged Men, *American Journal of Public Health,* 85 (1995), 1231–1236.
24. Buhler, C., The Developmental Structure of Goal Setting in Group and Individual Studies, in Buhler, C., and Massarik, F. eds., *The Course of Human Life.* New York: Springer, 1968.
25. Burnard, P., Mentors: A Supporting Act, *Nursing Times,* 84, no. 46 (1988), 27–28.
26. Caine, L., *Being a Widow.* New York: Arbor House, 1988.
27. Carlson, E., The Phony War, *Modern Maturity,* February–March (1987), 34–44.
28. Cattanach, L., and J. Tebes, The Nature of Elder Impairment and Its Impact on Family Caregivers' Health and Psychosocial Functioning, *The Gerontologist,* 31, no. 2 (1991), 246–255.
29. Centers for Disease Control and Prevention General Recommendations on Immunization: Recommendations of the Advisory Committee on Immunization Practices (ACIP), *Morbidity and Mortality Weekly Report,* 43 (January 28, 1994), 23.
30. Clark, N., and W. Rakowski, Family Caregivers of Older Adults: Improving Helping Skills, *The Gerontologist,* 23, no. 6 (1983), 637–641.
31. Clemens-Stone, S., D.G. Eigsti, and S. McGuire, *Comprehensive Community Health Nursing: Family, Aggregate, and Community Practice* (4th ed.). St. Louis: C.V. Mosby, 1995.
32. Colen, B., The Generation Blur, *Health,* October (1989). 30–31.
33. Collison, C., and S. Miller, Using Images of the Future in Grief Work, *IMAGE: Journal of Nursing Scholarship,* 19, (1987), 9–11.
34. Corbin, J., and A. Strauss, A Nursing Model for Chronic Illness Management Based Upon the Trajectory Frame Work, *Scholarly Inquiry for Nursing Practice,* 5, no. 3 (1991), 155–174.
35. Cosby, B., *Time Flies.* Garden City, NY: Doubleday, 1987.
36. Crowley, S., Much Ado about Menopause, *AARP Bulletin,* 35, no. 5 (1994), 2–3.
37. Dacey, J., and J. Travers, *Human Development Across the Lifespan* (3rd ed.). Madison, WI: Brown & Benchmark, 1996.
38. Deciding on Hormone Replacement Therapy, *American Journal of Nursing,* 95, no. 8 (1995), 57–59.
39. Dellasega, C., Coping With Caregiving: Stress Management for Caregivers of the Elderly, *Journal of Psychosocial Nursing,* 28, no. 1 (1990), 15–22.
40. Dennis, W., Creative Production Between the Ages of 20 and 80, *Journal of Gerontology,* 21, no. 1 (1966), 8.
41. Dickson, G., The Metalanguage of Menopause Research, *IMAGE: Journal of Nursing Scholarship,* 22, no. 3 (1990), 168–173.
42. Di Matteo, M., *The Psychology of Health, Illness, and Medical Care: An Individual Perspective.* Pacific Grove, CA: Brooks/Cole, 1991.
43. Doreso-Worters, P., and D. Siegal, Managing Menopause, *Modern Maturity,* May–June (1995), 40–42, 76.
44. Duffy, M., Determinants of Health Promotion in Midlife Women, *Nursing Research,* 37 (1988), 358–362.
45. Duvall, E., and B. Miller, *Marriage and Family Development* (6th ed.). New York: Harper & Row, 1984.
46. Dworetzky, J., *Human Development: A Lifespan Approach* (2nd ed.). St. Paul: West, 1995.
47. Early Retirement: A Disappearing American Dream, *Capper's,* March 14 (1995), 18.
48. Eastman, P., Life After Menopause Liberating, Women Say, *AARP News Bulletin,* July–August (1988), 4–5.
49. Edelman, C., and C. Mandel, *Health Promotion Throughout the Lifespan* (3rd ed.). St. Louis: C.V. Mosby, 1994.
50. Erikson, E., *Childhood and Society* (2nd ed.). New York: W.W. Norton, 1963.
51. Erikson, E., ed., *Adulthood.* New York: W.W. Norton, 1978.
52. Estrogen and Bone Loss: A Matter of Timing? *American Journal of Nursing,* 94, no. 2 (1994), 9.
53. Estrogen and Your Arteries, *Harvard Women's Health Watch,* 2, no. 11 (1995), 6.
54. Exercise: Strength Training, *Harvard Women's Health Watch,* 11, no. 9 (1995), 2–3.
55. Feet: Dressing for Distress, *Harvard Women's Health Watch,* 1, no. 7 (1994), 4–5.
56. Fink, S. V., The Influence of Family Resources and Family Demands on the Strains and Well-being of Caregiving Families, *Nursing Research,* 44, no. 3 (1995), 139–146.

57. Fitness Over 40, *Harvard Women's Health Watch,* 3, no. 5 (1996), 4–5.

58. Franks, M. M., and M. A. P. Stephens, Multiple Roles of Middle-generation Caregivers: Contextual Effects and Psychological Mechanisms, *Journal of Gerontology,* 47, no. 3 (1992), S123–S129.

59. ———, and M. A. P. Stephens, Social Support in the Context of Caregiving: Husband's Provision of Support to Wives Involved in Parent Care, *Journal of Gerontology,* 51B, no. 1 (1996), P43–P52.

60. Fredman, L., M. P. Daly, and A. M. Lazur, Burden Among White and Black Caregivers to Elderly Adults, *Journal of Gerontology,* 50B, no. 2 (1995), S110–S118.

61. Getting the Jump on Osteoporosis, *Harvard Women's Health Watch,* 3, no. 5 (1996), 1.

62. Gilligan, C., In a Different Voice: Women's Conceptions of Self and of Mortality, *Harvard Educational Review,* 47, no. 4 (1977), 481–517.

63. Gilligan, C., N. Lyons, and T. Hammer, eds., *Making Connections.* Cambridge, MA: Harvard University Press, 1990.

64. Golan, N., *Passing Through Transitions.* New York: Free Press, 1983.

65. Gottlieb, D., I. Gottlieb, and M. Seavin. *What To Do When Your Son or Daughter Divorces.* New York: Bantam Books, 1988.

66. Gould, R., Adult Life Stages: Growth Toward Self-tolerance, *Psychology Today,* 8, no. 7 (February 1975), 74–78.

67. ———, Transformation in Mid-life, *New York University Education Quarterly,* 10, no. 2 (1979), 2–9.

68. ———, Old Wine in New Bottles: A Feminist Perspective on Gilligan's Theory, *Social Work,* September–October (1988), 411–415.

69. Guyton, A., *Textbook of Medical Physiology* (9th ed.). Philadelphia: W.B. Saunders, 1995.

70. Hainsworth, M., P. Busch, G. Eakes, and M. Burkes, Chronic Sorrow in Women with Chronically Mentally Ill Disabled Husbands, *Journal of the American Psychiatric Nurses Association,* 1, no. 4 (1995), 120–124.

71. Hamon, R., and R. Blieszner, Filial Responsibility Expectations Among Adult Child–Older Parent Pairs, *Journal of Gerontology: Psychological Sciences,* 45, no. 3 (1990), P110–P112.

72. Handron, D., Denial and Serious Chronic Illness: A Personal Perspective, *Perspectives in Psychiatric Care,* 29, no. 1 (1993), 29–33.

73. Hardy, M., and J. Quadnagno, Satisfaction with Early Retirement: Makeup Choices in the Auto Industry, *Journal of Gerontology: Social Sciences,* 50B, no. 4 (1995), S217–S228.

74. Hartweg, D., Self-care Actions of Healthy Middle-aged Women to Promote Well-being, *Nursing Research,* 42, no. 4 (1993), 221–227.

75. Health Risks, *Women's Health Advocate Newsletter,* 2, no. 11, (January 1996), 2–3.

76. Health Risks: Perception and Reality, *Harvard Women's Health Watch,* 1, no. 10 (1994), 1.

77. Helsing, K., M. Szklo, and G. Comstock, Factors Associated With Mortality After Widowhood, *American Journal of Public Health,* 71, no. 8 (1981), 802–809.

78. High Health in the Middle Years, *Prevention,* July (1988), 35–47, 100–110.

79. Hoff, L., *People in Crisis: Understanding and Helping* (4th ed.). Redwood City, CA: Addison-Wesley, 1995.

80. Holm, K., S. Penckofer, and P. Chandler, Deciding on Hormone Replacement Therapy, *American Journal of Nursing,* 95, no. 8 (1995), 57–60.

81. Holmes, T. H., and R. H. Rahe, The Social Readjustment Rating Scale, *Journal of Psychosomatic Medicine,* 11, no. 8 (1967), 213–218.

82. Hoole, A., C. Pickard, R. Ouimete, J. Lohr, and R. Greenberg, *Patient Care Guidelines for Nurse Practitioners* (4th ed.). Philadelphia: J. B. Lippincott, 1995.

83. HRT and Breast Cancer Risk, *Harvard Women's Health Watch,* 2, no. 12 (1993), 1.

84. Irwin, T., *Male Menopause: Crisis in the Middle Years.* New York: Public Affairs Pamphlets, 1982.

85. Jahoda, M., *Current Concepts of Positive Mental Health.* New York: Basic Books, 1958.

86. Jarrett, W., Caregiving Within Kinship Systems: Is Affection Really Necessary? *The Gerontologist,* 25, no. 1 (1985), 5–10.

87. Johnson, K., and T. Ferguson, *Trusting Ourselves: The Sourcebook on Psychology for Women.* New York: Atlantic Monthly Press, 1991.

88. Jolley, J., and M. Mitchell, *Lifespan Development: A Topical Approach.* Madison, WI: Brown & Benchmark, 1996.

89. Jung, C., *Modern Man in Search of a Soul.* New York: Harcourt, Brace & World, 1955.

90. Kallman, D., C. Plato, and J. Tobin, The Role of Muscle Loss in the Age-related Decline of Grip Strength: Cross Sectional and Longitudinal Perspectives, *Journal of Gerontology: Medical Sciences,* 45, no. 3 (1990), M82–M88.

91. Kaplan, S., The New Generation Gap, *Common Cause Magazine,* March–April (1987), 13–15.

92. Kaplan, M., M. Adamek, and S. Johnson, Trends in Firearm Suicide Among Older American Males: 1979–1988, *The Gerontologist,* 34, no. 1 (1994), 59–63.

93. Kaprio, J., M. Koskenvuo, and H. Rita, Mortality After Bereavement: A Prospective Study of 95, 647 Widowed Persons, *American Journal of Public Health,* 77, no. 3 (1987), 283–287.

94. Karp, D., The Social Construction of Retirement Among Professionals 50–60 Years Old, *The Gerontologist,* 29, no. 6 (1989), 750–760.

95. Kelleher, K., The Afternoon of Life: Jung's View of the Tasks of the Second Half of Life, *Perspectives in Psychiatric Care,* 28, no. 2 (1992), 25–28.

96. Knollmueller, R., ed., *Prevention Across the Life Span: Healthy People for the Twenty-first-Century.* Washington, DC: American Nurses Association Council of Community Health Nursing, 1993.

97. Knowles, M., *The Adult Learner: A Neglected Species* (4th ed.). Houston: Gulf, 1990.

98. Kohlberg, L., *Recent Research in Moral Development.* New York: Holt, Rinehart & Winston, 1977.

99. Kritz-Silverstein, D., and E. Barrett-Connor, Bone Mineral Density in Postmenopausal Women as Determined by Prior Oral Contraceptive Use, *American Journal of Public Health,* 83 (1993), 100–102.

100. ———, Early Menopause, Number of Reproductive Years, and Bone Mineral Density in Postmenopausal Women, *American Journal of Public Health,* 83 (1993), 983–988.

101. Krueger, J., and J. Heckhausen, Personality Development Across the Adult Life Span: Subjective Conceptions vs Cross-sectional Contrasts, *Journal of Gerontology: Psychological Sciences,* 48, no. 3 (1993), P100–P108.

102. Lazarus, R., *Coping With the Stress of Illness.* World Health Organization, Regional Publications, European Series, no. 144. Geneva: WHO, 1992, pp. 11–31.

103. Lerner, M., et al., Adult Children as Caregivers: Egocentric Biases in Judgments of Sibling Contributions, *The Gerontologist,* 31, no. 6 (1991), 746–755.

104. Levinson, D., *The Seasons of a Man's Life*. New York: Alfred A. Knopf, 1986.

105. Lewis, J., L. Sperry, and J. Carlson, *Health Counseling*. Pacific Grove, CA: Brooks Cole, 1993.

106. Lidz, T., *The Person: His and Her Development Throughout the Life Cycle* (2nd ed.). New York: Basic Books, 1983.

107. Linderman, E., Symptomology and Management of Acute Grief, *American Journal of Psychiatry*. 101 (1944), 141–148.

108. Loevinger, J., *Ego Development*. San Francisco: Jossey-Bass, 1976.

109. Low Fat Mind Games, *Tufts University Diet and Nutrition Letter*, 13, no. 9 (1995), 1.

110. Lowenthal, M., and D. Chiriboga, Transition to the Empty Nest: Crisis, Challenge, or Relief? *Archives of General Psychiatry*, 26, no. 1 (1972), 8–14.

111. Marino, V., Early Retirement: A Disappearing American Dream, *Capper's*, March 14 (1995), 18.

112. Mastering Menopause, *Prevention*, April (1990), 46–55.

113. Masters, W., and V. Johnson, *Human Sexual Response*. Boston: Little, Brown, 1981.

114. Mathews, S. H., Gender and the Division of Filial Responsibility Between Lone Sisters and Their Brothers, *Journal of Gerontology*, 50B, no. 5 (1995), S312–S320.

115. Matthews, S., J. Werkner, and P. Delaney, Relative Contributions of Help by Employed and Nonemployed Sisters to Their Elderly Parents, *Journal of Gerontology: Social Sciences*, 44, no. 1 (1989), S36–S44.

116. McCoy, V., Adult Life Cycle Tasks/Adult Continuing Education Program Response, *Lifelong Learning in the Adult Years*, October (1977), 16.

117. Mead, M., *Culture and Commitment: A Study of the Generation Gap. The New Relationships Between the Generations in the 1970's*. Garden City, NY: Natural History Press/Doubleday, 1978.

118. Menopause: Alternatives to Hormone Replacement, *Harvard Women's Health Watch*, 1, no. 12 (1994), 2–3.

119. Middle-Aged Spread, *Harvard Women's Health Watch*, 11, no. 12 (1993), 6.

120. Million, S., Training Mentors and Proteges: The Key to Successful Mentoring, *Kappa Delta Pi Record*, Fall (1990), 21–26.

121. Morgan, D., Adjusting to Widowhood: Do Social Networks Really Make It Easier? *The Gerontologist*, 29, no. 1 (1989), 101–107.

122. Mui, A. C., Caregiver Strain Among Black and White Daughter Caregivers: A Role Theory Perspective, *The Gerontologist*, 32, no. 2 (1992), 203–212.

123. ———, Caring for Frail Elderly Parents: A Comparison of Adult Sons and Daughters, *The Gerontologist*, 35, no. 1 (1995), 86–93.

124. Murray, R., and M. Huelskoetter, *Psychiatric/Mental Health Nursing: Giving Emotional Care* (3rd ed.). Norwalk, CT: Appleton & Lange, 1991.

125. Natural Progesterone, *Harvard Women's Health Watch*, 11, no. 12 (1995), 1.

126. Neugarten, B., The Awareness of Middle Age, in Owen, R., ed., *Middle Age*. London: British Broadcasting Corporation, 1967.

127. ———, Women's Attitudes Toward Menopause, in Neugarten, B., ed., *Middle Age and Aging*. Chicago: University of Chicago Press, 1968.

128. ———, Dynamics of the Transition of Mid-Age to Old Age, *Journal of Geriatric Psychiatry*, 4 (1970), 71–87.

129. ———, Adaptation and the Life Cycle, *The Counseling Psychologist*, 6, no. 1 (1976), 16–20.

130. ———, and J. Moore, The Changing Age-Status System, in Neugarten, B., ed., *Middle Age and Aging*. Chicago: University of Chicago Press, 1968.

131. Newman, B., et al., Nongenetic Influences of Obesity on Other Cardiovascular Disease Risk Factors: An Analysis of Identical Twins, *American Journal of Public Health*, 80, no. 6 (1990), 675–678.

132. O'Bryant, S., and L. Morgan, Recent Windows' Kin Support and Orientations to Self-sufficiency, *Gerontologist*, 30, no. 3 (1990), 391–397.

133. O'Donnell, T., and S. Bernier, Parents as Caregivers: When a Son Has AIDS, *Journal of Psychosocial Nursing*, 28, no. 6 (1990), 14–17.

134. Okimoto, J., and P. Stegall, *Boomerang Kids*. Boston: Little, Brown, 1987.

135. Olson, T., and J. Hanover, Preparing Women to be Widows, *Health Values: Achieving High Level Wellness*, 9, no. 1 (1985), 8–11.

136. Parton, D., Out of Work: One Family's Journey, *Focus on the Family*, January (1994), 2–4.

137. Pearson, L., Climacteric, *American Journal of Nursing*, 82, no. 7 (1982), 1098–1102.

138. Peck, R.C., Psychological Developments in the Second Half of Life, in Neugarten, B., ed., *Middle Age and Aging*. Chicago: University of Chicago Press, 1968.

139. Penrod, J. D., R. A. Kane, R. L. Kane, and M. D. Finch, Who Cares? The Size, Scope, and Composition of the Caregiver Support System, *The Gerontologist*, 35, no. 4 (1995), 489–497.

140. Phipps, W., et al., eds., *Medical–Surgical Nursing: Concepts and Clinical Practice* (4th ed.). St. Louis: Mosby–Year Book, 1991.

141. Picot, S. J., Rewards, Costs, and Coping of African American Caregivers, *Nursing Research*, 44, no. 3 (1995), 147–152.

142. Pierson, J., and R. Pierson, Post-traumatic Stress Disorder or Midlife Crisis in Vietnam Veterans? *Social Work*, 39, no. 3 (1994), 328–330.

143. Pohl, J. M., C. Boyd, J. Liang, and C. W. Given, Analysis of the Impact of Mother–Daughter Relationships on the Commitment to Caregiving, *Nursing Research*, 44, no. 2 (1995), 68–75.

144. Pollock, S., B. Christian, and D. Sands, Responses to Chronic Illness: Analysis of Psychological and Physiological Adaptation, *Nursing Research*, 39, no. 5 (1990), 302–304.

145. Putting Polish on the Golden Years, *Postgrad: St. Louis University School of Medicine*, 17, no. 1 (1995), 8–12.

146. Raleigh, E., Sources of Hope in Chronic Illness, *Oncology Nursing Forum*, 19, no. 3 (1992), 443–448.

147. Rathbun, N., Giving–Gaining, *American Association of University Women Outlook*, 88, no. 2 (1994), 16–18.

148. Real Mid-life Crisis, *Newsweek*, June 26 (1995), 62–63.

149. Risk: What It Means to You, *Harvard Women's Health Watch*, 3, no. 3 (1995), 3–4.

150. Robison, J., P. Moen, and D. Dempster-McClain, Women's Caregiving: Changing Profiles and Pathways, *Journal of Gerontology*, 50B, no. 6 (1995), S362–S373.

151. Rolland, J., *Families, Illness and Disability: An Integrative Treatment Model*. New York: Behavioral Sciences, 1994.

152. Rosenthal, C. J., J. Sulman, and V. W. Marshall, Depressive Symptoms in Family Caregivers of Long-stay Patients, *The Gerontologist*, 33, no. 2 (1993), 249–257.

153. Routine Mammograms Found to be Cost-effective for Women Age 40–49, says UC—Davis Study, *The Nation's Health*, 25, no. 10 (1995), 12.

154. Rubenstein, R., et al., Key Relationships of Never Married, Childless Older Women: A Cultural Analysis, *Journal of Gerontology: Social Sciences*, 46, no. 5 (1991), S270–S277.

155. Schaefer, K., Women Living in Parodox: Loss and Discovery in Chronic Illness, *Holistic Nursing Practice*, 9, no. 3 (1995), 63–74.

156. Schulz, R., P. Visintainer, and G. Williamson, Psychiatric and Physical Morbidity Effects of Caregiving, *Journal of Gerontology: Psychological Sciences,* 45, no. 5 (1990), P181–P191.

157. Schussler, G., Coping Strategies and Individual Meanings of Illness, *Social Science Medicine,* 34, no. 4 (1992), 427–432.

158. Seligman, J., C. Friday, and P. Wingert, Menopause, *Newsweek,* May 25 (1992), 71–72.

159. Shanan, J., Who and How: Some Unanswered Questions in Adult Development, *Journal of Gerontology: Psychological Sciences,* 46, no. 6 (1991), P309–P316.

160. Shapiro, E., *Grief as a Family Process.* New York: Behavioral Sciences, 1994.

161. Shaver, J., and Rodgers, A., Screening for Sleep-related Disorders: Sleep Apnea and Narcolepsy, *The American Nurse,* November–December (1994), 24–25.

162. Sheehy, G., *Passages.* New York: Bantam Books, 1984.

163. ———, *Pathfinders.* New York: Wm. Morrow, 1991.

164. ———, *The Silent Passage: Menopause.* New York: Random House, 1992.

165. Skaff, M. M., and L. I. Pearlin, Caregiving: Role Engulfment and the Loss of Self, *The Gerontologist,* 32, no. 5 (1992), 656–664.

166. Sleep: Are You Getting Enough? *Harvard Women's Health Watch,* 1, no. 7 (1994), 2–3.

167. Sleep Disorders—Part I, *The Harvard Mental Health Letter,* 11, no. 2 (1994), 1–4.

168. Sleep Disorders—Part II, *The Harvard Mental Health Letter,* 11, no. 3 (1994), 1–5.

169. Smith, G., M. Smith, and R. Toseland, Problems Identified by Family Caregivers in Counseling, *The Gerontologist,* 31, no. 1 (1991), 15–22.

170. Snelling, J., The Effect of Chronic Pain on the Family Unit, *Journal of Advanced Nursing,* 19, no. 3 (1994), 543–551.

171. Soroko, S., T. Holbrook, S. Edelstein, and E. Barrett-Connor, Lifetime Milk Consumption and Bone Mineral Density in Older Women, *American Journal of Public Health,* 84 (1994), 1319–1322.

172. Sprangers, M., and N. Aaronson, The Role of Health Care Providers and Significant Others in Evaluating the Quality of Life of Patients with Chronic Disease: A Review, *Journal of Clinical Epidemiology,* 45, no. 7 (1992), 743–760.

173. Steinbaum, E., Tomorrow's Health Care, Baby Boomers Stack the Odds in Their Favor, *Arthritis Today,* March–April (1995), 38–42.

174. Stetz, K., F. Lewis, and G. Houck, Family Goals as Indicants of Adaptation During Chronic Illness, *Public Health Nursing,* 11, no. 6 (1994), 385–391.

175. Stewart, A., R. Hays, K. Wells, W. Rogers, K. Spritzer, and S. Greenfield, Long-term Functioning and Well-being Outcomes Associated With Physical Activity and Exercise in Patients With Chronic Conditions in the Medical Outcomes Study, *Journal of Clinical Epidemiology,* 47, no. 7 (1994), 719–730.

176. ———, A. King, and W. Haskell, Endurance Exercise and Health-related Quality of Life in 50–65 Year-old Adults, *The Gerontologist,* 33, no. 6 (1993), 782–788.

177. Stoller, E., Males as Helpers: The Roles of Sons, Relatives, and Friends, *The Gerontologist,* 30, no. 2 (1990), 228–235.

178. Strawbridge, W., and M. Wallhagen, Impact of Family Conflict on Adult Child Caregivers, *The Gerontologist,* 31, no. 6 (1991), 770–777.

179. Strength Training, *Harvard Women's Health Watch,* 2, no. 9 (1995), 2–3.

180. Stuart, G., and S. Sundeen, *Principles and Practice of Psychiatric Nursing* (5th ed.). St. Louis: C.V. Mosby, 1995.

181. Talbott, M. M., The Negative Side of the Relationship Between Older Widows and Their Adult Children: The Mothers' Perspective, *The Gerontologist,* 30, no. 5 (1990), 595–603.

182. Temple, A., and K. Fawdry, Resolving Filial Caregiver Role Strain, *Journal of Gerontological Nursing,* 8, no. 3 (1992), 11–15.

183. The Pill Until Menopause? *Harvard Women's Health Watch,* 1, no. 7 (1994), 1.

184. Titus, M., Dealing With Chronic Illness: A Family Concern, *The Menninger Letter,* 3, no. 6 (1995), p. 4.

185. Turner, J., and D. Helms, *Lifespan Development* (5th ed.). Ft. Worth: Harcourt Brace College, 1995.

186. Turner-Henson, A., and B. Holoday, Daily Life Experiences for the Chronically Ill: A Life Span Perspective, *Family–Community Health,* 17, no. 4 (1995), 1–11.

187. Uhlenberg, P., T. Cooney, and R. Boyd, Divorce for Women After Midlife, *Journal of Gerontology: Social Services,* 45, no. 1 (1990), S3–S11.

188. Uphold, C. and M. Graham, *Clinical Guidelines in Family Practice* (2nd ed.). Gainesville, FL: Barmarrare Books, 1994.

189. U.S. Bureau of Census, *Statistical Abstract of the United States: 1990* (110th ed.). Washington, DC: Government Printing Office, 1990.

190. Vaillant, G., How the Best and the Brightest Came of Age, *Psychology Today,* 11, no. 9 (1977), 34ff.

191. ———, The Normal Boy in Later Life: How Adaptation Fosters Growth, *Harvard Magazine,* 55, no. 6 (1977), 234–239.

192. Vamos, M., Body Image in Chronic Illness: A Reconceptualization, *International Journal of Psychiatry in Medicine,* 23, no. 2 (1993), 163–178.

193. Vance, C., Is There a Mentor in Your Career Future? *Imprint,* 36, no. 5 (1989–1990), 41–42.

194. Vitaliano, P., J. Russo, and R. Niaura, Plasma Lipids and Their Relationship With Psychosocial Factors in Older Adults, *Journal of Gerontology: Psychological Sciences,* 50B, no. 1 (1995), P18–P24.

195. Wadsworth, B., *Piaget's Theory of Cognitive and Affective Development* (5th ed.). New York: Longman, 1996.

196. Warda, M., The Family and Chronic Sorrow: Role Theory Approach, *Journal of Pediatric Nursing,* 7 (1992), 205–206.

197. Warshaw, R., Can Grandparent Caregivers Find Help? *Modern Maturity,* July–August (1995), 28.

198. Wasaha, S., What Every Woman Should Know About Menopause, *American Journal of Nursing,* 96, no. 1 (1996), 24–32.

199. Whipple, B., Common Questions About Osteoporosis and Menopause, *American Journal of Nursing,* 95, no. 1 (1995), 69–70.

200. Whitbeck, L., R. Simmons, and R. Conger, The Effects of Early Family Relationships on Contemporary Relationship and Assistance Patterns Between Adult Children and Their Parents, *Journal of Gerontology: Social Sciences,* 46, no. 6 (1991), S330–S337.

201. White, N., J. Richter, and C. Fry, Coping, Social Support, and Adaptation to Chronic Illness, *Western Journal of Nursing Research,* 14, no. 2 (1992), 211–224.

202. Wilbur, J., K. Holm, and A. Dan, The Relationship of Energy Expenditure to Physical and Psychologic Symptoms in Women at Midlife, *Nursing Outlook,* 40, no. 6 (1992), 269–275.

203. Williams, S., *Nutrition and Diet Therapy* (10th ed.). St. Louis: C.V. Mosby, 1995.

204. Willits, F., and D. Crider, Health Rating and Life Satisfaction in the Later Middle Years, *Journal of Gerontology,* 43, no. 5 (1988), S172–S176.

205. Woods, N., and F. Lewis, Women with Chronic Illness: Their Views of Their Families' Adaptation, *Health Care for Women International,* 16 (1995), 135–148.

206. Woog, P., ed., *Chronic Illness Trajectory Frameworks: The Corbin and Strauss Nursing Model.* Springfield, IL: Springer, 1991.

207. Young, R. F., and E. Kahana, The Context of Caregiving and Well-being Outcomes Among African and Caucasian Americans, *The Gerontologist,* 35, no. 2 (1995), 225–232.

208. *Your Feet After Fifty.* Miami Beach, FL: Foot Facts Publications, n.d.

209. Zarit, S., P. Todd, and J. Zarit, Subjective Burden of Husbands and Wives as Caregivers: A Longitudinal Study, *The Gerontologist,* 26, no. 3 (1986), 260–266.

210. Zhang, J., P. Feldblum, and J. Fortney, Moderate Physical Activity and Bone Density Among Perimenopausal Women, *American Journal of Public Health,* 82 (1992), 736–737.

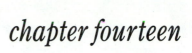

chapter fourteen

Assessment and Health Promotion for the Person in Later Maturity

Old age, to the unlearned, is winter: to the learned, it is harvest time.

—*Yiddish Proverb*

Key Terms

Aging

Biological age

Social age

Psychological age

Cognitive age

Senescence

Later maturity

   Young-old

   Mid-old

   Old-old

Gerontology

Geriatrics

Ageism

Nongenetic Cellular Theories

   Wear and Tear Theory

   Cross-linkage Theory

   Accumulation of Waste Theory

Accumulation of Errors Theory

   Free Radical Theory

   Deprivation Theory

Physiologic Theories

   Biological Clock (aging by program) Theory

   Neuroendocrine Theory

   Immune Theory

Gene Theory

Continuity Theory

Selective Perception

Situation Reinforcement

Erikson's Epigenetic Theory

Peck's Theory

Disengagement Theory

Finitude

Terminal Drop

Activity Theory

Symbolic Interaction Theory

Urban Ecologic Model of Aging

Interiority

Organ reserve

Presbyopia

Cataracts

Glaucoma

Arcus senilis

Sensorineural deafness

Presbycusis

Functional reach

Refractory time

Dyspareunia

Herpes zoster (shingles)

Parkinson's disease

Alzheimer's disease

Chronic obstructive pulmonary disease

Pernicious anemia

Secondary anemia

Chronic lymphocytic leukemia

Hodgkin's disease

Benign prostatic hypertrophy (BPH)

Osteoporosis

Osteoarthritis

Congestive heart failure

Chronic occlusive arterial disease

Stasis ulcer

Pitting edema

Brawny edema

Angina

Failure-to-thrive

Polypharmacy	Ego differentiation	Somatization	Perseverance
Crystallized intelligence	Body transcendence	Counterphobia	Self-reliance
Fluid intelligence	Ego transcendence	Rigidity	Meaningfulness
Intellectual plasticity	Regression	Sublimation	Existential aloneness
Reminiscence	Emotional isolation	Displacement	Leisure time
Life review	Compartmentalization	Projection	Prosumers
Ego integrity	Denial	Insight	Translocation syndrome
Despair or self-disgust	Rationalization	Equanimity	

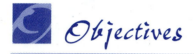

Objectives

Study of this chapter will enable you to:

1. Define terms and theories of aging related to understanding of the person in later maturity.

2. Explore personal and societal attitudes about growing old and your role in promoting positive attitudes.

3. Contrast relationships in the late years with those of other developmental eras, including with spouse, offspring, grandchildren, other family members, friends, pets, and other networks.

4. Contrast the status of either singlehood or widow(er)hood in later maturity to that status in early and midadulthood.

5. Describe signs of and factors contributing to elder abuse and contrast with child and spouse abuse.

6. Describe physiologic adaptive mechanisms of aging and influences on sexuality, related health problems, and assessment and intervention to promote and maintain health, comfort, and safety.

7. Discuss the cognitive, emotional, body image, and spiritual development and characteristics of the aged person, their interrelationship, and your role in promoting health and a positive self-concept.

8. Contrast the adaptive mechanisms used by the person in this period with those used in other periods of life.

9. Describe the developmental crisis of later maturity, the relationship to previous developmental crises, and your role in helping the person meet this crisis.

10. List the developmental tasks for this era, and describe your contribution to their accomplishment.

11. Identify changing home, family, social, and work or leisure situations of this person and your responsibility in helping the person face retirement, loss of loved ones, and changes in roles and living arrangements. Discuss selection of an adequate nursing home or residence for seniors.

12. Describe major federal, state, and local programs to assist the elderly financially, socially, and in health care, and describe your professional and personal responsibility in this regard.

13. Demonstrate remotivation technique and discuss the value, purpose, and use of this and other group processes with the elderly.

14. Summarize the needs of the elderly, standards of nursing care to assist in meeting those needs, and future trends in care of the person in later maturity.

15. Assess and work effectively with a person in later maturity, using the information presented in this chapter and showing empathy and genuine interest.

*I really don't like being labeled a golden-ager. I
acknowledge my age and my limits, but I certainly didn't
turn incompetent at 65.*

When does later maturity begin? Historically, it was the
designation of an eligible age for receipt of Social Security benefits that established 65 years old as the beginning age for this period in the life cycle. In reality, the
age span for this period is continually changing. Images
once associated with later maturity are no longer clear.
The chronologic age of 65 no longer determines or predicts behaviors, life events, health status, work status,
family status, interests, preoccupations, or needs. Individuals undergo aging at different rates, and their view
of the aging process is influenced by many factors—culture, generation, and occupation. Not everyone 65 or 70
years old and older considers himself or herself old, but
in the United States a person of that age is expected to
assume roles appropriate to later maturity. Some individuals, especially members of ethnic minorities and
lower socioeconomic levels, view the onset of old age as
taking place earlier than age 65 (46, 122). Younger generations may misperceive how the old view themselves.

In 1860, 2.7% of the population in the United States
was more than 65 years of age. This figure changed dramatically during the next 125 years. By 1985, there
were 28.5 million people in this age group, 12% of the
population. By 1988, the median age of people over 65
was approximately 73 years. In 1994, there were 3.2 million people over age 65 in the United States (279, 284).
At present in the United States, more than 5000 persons
reach their 65th birthday every day, and 55 reach 100
years daily. Those individuals reaching 65 live longer
than in the past. In fact, the fastest growing segment of
population in the United States is the group over 85
years old. It is projected that by the year 2000, there will
be more than 36 million Americans over 65, constituting
as much as 17% of the population, with 4.9 million over
85 and approximately 100,000 people over age 100
(there were 20,000 in 1980). By 2030, 65 to 70 million
people, or approximately 25% of the U.S. population, will
be 65 years of age or over (2½ times their number in
1980). This rapid increase between the years 2000 and
2030 reflects the aging of the baby boom generation
born in the 1960s (111, 284). As mothers of the post-
World War II baby boom reach old age, the current
trend of elderly women living alone will increase, according to a study in 21 European and North American
countries. Four-generation families will be the norm
(Fig. 14–1); five-generation families will be increasing in
number. Recently the elderly population has been growing faster among nonwhites than Caucasians. By 2025,
15% of the elderly is projected to be nonwhite, in con-

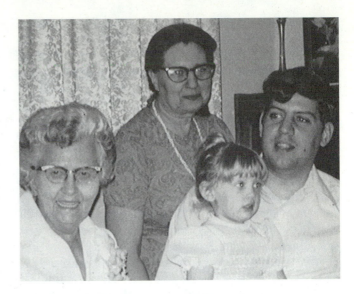

Figure 14–1. Four-generation families, once unusual, will become the norm
as the population ages.

trast to 10% in 1980 (11). This continued aging trend in
the population requires changes in all aspects of our
social structure—employment, housing, education,
leisure activities, transportation, industrial development, and health care.

DEFINITIONS

Because the terms describing this age group are not
clearly defined by the general public or health care professionals, it is important to clarify some of the terms
used in this chapter (85, 122, 140, 274, 279).

Aging, which *begins at conception and ends at
death, is a process of growing older, regardless of chronologic age.*

Biological age is the *person's present position with
respect to the potential life span, which may be younger or
older than chronologic age,* and encompasses measures
of functional capacities of vital organ systems.

Social age, which *results from the person's life
course through various social institutions,* refers to *roles
and habits of the person with respect to other members of
society.* Social age may be age-appropriate or older or
younger than that of most people in the social group.
Social age includes such aspects as the person's type of
dress, language usage, and social deference to people in
leadership positions.

Psychological age refers to *behavioral capacity of
the person to adapt to changing environmental demands
and includes capacities of memory, learning, intelligence,*

skills, feelings, and motivation for exercising behavioral control or self-regulation.

Cognitive age includes *the age the person feels and looks to self, plus the fit of behavior and interests to his or her chronologic age.* The person says, "I do most things as if I were _____ years old."

Senescence is the *mental and physical decline associated with the aging process.* The term describes a group of effects that lead to a decrease in efficient function.

Later maturity is the *last major segment of the life span; this stage begins at the age of 65 or 70.* The World Health Organization (WHO) divides this segment of life into the elderly (65–75), the old (76–90), and the very old (over 90). Some authors divide this group into **young-old,** *ages 65 to 74 or 65 or 70 to 80;* **mid-old,** *75 to 84;* and **old-old,** *80 or 85 and older.* The term **frail-old** is sometimes used instead of **old-old** or **very old** (85, 140).

Senility is a *wastebasket term still used to denote physical and mental deterioration often associated with old age. It is used when other options have not been carefully considered.* The correct term would be related to a specific disease, such as Senile Dementia, Alzheimer's Type (13). Yet what looks like senility or Alzheimer's disease may be the result of drug reactions; malnutrition; dehydration; delirium; hypothyroidism; microstrokes and hypertension; toxicity in the system; disorders resulting from lack of communication and experiencing sensory deprivation for physical reasons or because of institutionalization; or the expectations of caregivers (13, 85).

Gerontology is the *scientific study of the individual in later maturity and the aging process from physiologic, pathologic, psychological, sociologic, and economic points of view.*

Geriatrics is a *medical specialty concerned with the physiologic and pathologic changes of the individual in later maturity and includes study and treatment of the health problems of this age group.*

Later maturity is divided into three sequential segments. The first segment may be regarded as *a sociopolitical or cultural–organizational perspective.* Offspring are in a creative period, and the mature adult is in the ruling, protective stance as he or she assumes parental hierarchical leadership over the family of families. The older person becomes concerned with the creation, ordering, and maintenance of a larger society. The second segment is characterized by a *reaffirmation of social, moral, and ethical standards* necessary for establishment of pacific relationships among the oncoming generations as they are involved in rendering decisions, planning, erecting social guideposts, and se-

lecting subordinate leaders. The judgmental functions of the mind are most highly developed at this time, created out of actual and vicarious experience with conflict situations and from cultural learning and values. The last segment of psychic maturity involves *retrospective examination,* the need to correlate the present with the past to determine the true nature of accomplishments, errors, and rediscoveries. Cultural vision is at its broadest possible development, embracing one nearly complete life cycle and its interrelatedness with a multitude of other life cycles. The person compares and contrasts his or her values with cultural values and, through reasoning and intuition, evaluates meaning and purpose and has an increased interest in the history of human development. Values of the adolescent are movement, agility, quantitative productivity, exhibitionistic sexual attractiveness, and artfulness. In contrast, values of the older adult are deliberation, caution, equality, modesty, and loyalty. Whereas the adolescent views self as the ambitious master of a dimly concerned personhood, the older adult views self with real humility as at least a participant in, and at most a contributor to, the improvement of society (88, 174).

SOCIETAL PERSPECTIVES ON AGING

I may be old and wrinkled on the outside but I'm young and vulnerable on the inside.

Ageism refers to *any attitude, action, or institutional structure that discriminates against individuals on the basis of their age or that infers that elderly people are inferior to those who are younger.* Ageist attitudes toward older adults are not new in the United States. Even during colonial days, the elderly were categorized as unnecessary and burdensome. Of growing concern is the ageism of the aged; the attitudes of some older people are discriminatory toward others who are in their own age group. Generally, older women are judged more harshly than older men (116). Children appear most positive in their perception of elderly persons (27, 113, 178, 245).

In the United States old age frequently is characterized as a time of dependence and disease. Negative presentation of older adults, especially women, in movies, books, and magazines, in jokes, and on television contributes to negative beliefs and attitudes (83, 140). Society's fear of the changes associated with aging such as gray hair, hearing loss, wrinkles, loss of muscle tone, slowness, and approaching death also contributes to negative attitudes.

Numerous unproven *myths* and age-related *stereotypes* pervade American culture. One study revealed that of three age groups, young, middle-aged, and elderly adults, the elderly reported more stereotypes than did either of the other age groups. Interestingly, the young adults reported the fewest stereotypes (134). These myths and stereotypes obscure the truth and may prevent us from achieving our own potential as we grow older. Society stereotypes the older adult as being asexual, unemployable, unintelligent, and socially incompetent. Statements such as "You can't teach old dogs new tricks" and "dirty old men and women" typify the feelings of many. Instead of seeking the truth, most individuals accept myths that have been perpetuated through the years. Some of these myths and the contrasting realities are listed in Myths and Misconceptions and Their Realities for the Elderly Person (69, 83, 86, 140, 279).

Many of the myths and stereotypes associated with aging are culturally determined. The older adult in America lives in a culture oriented to youth, productivity, and rapid pace. Because of this orientation, older Americans may feel that they are not respected, valued, or needed.

There is no one criterion for successful aging. A study by Roos and Havens (246) of more than 3500 people in Manitoba, Canada, from 1971 to 1983 found few consistent predictors of successful aging. A book that provides suggestions for growing older and aging well is *Your Renaissance Years* by Robert Veninga, Little, Brown, 1991. As more people live longer, are healthy, and are aging successfully, attitudes are becoming more positive. The elderly are more and more perceived as powerful, admired, healthy, active, sexy, and even affluent (27, 170).

Culture, ethnicity, and socioeconomic level influence the role of the older adult in family relationships and determine health practices. Differences exist among cultural populations in how they esteem and care for the elderly, how the elderly stay involved in family matters, and the types of health care services used. Differences also exist among urban and rural families of the elderly (42, 58, 189, 200, 214). For example, with the African-American, aging and death are viewed as natural processes; the older family members are held in esteem. In Asian cultures the older adults have an important role, and the young are expected to respect and care for them. Westernized children may have difficulty accepting this role. Many older adults continue to follow health practices that are linked to their cultural heritage. Respect must be shown for these cultural aspects of aging and cultural influences on health practices and healing methods (3, 21, 42, 58, 68, 71, 130, 138, 157, 189, 200, 211, 214, 237, 248, 269, 276, 278).

THEORIES OF AGING

Although biological and psychosocial theories of aging have been proposed, the specific cause of aging is unknown. Evolutionists relate senescence to the lack of selection pressure in postproductive years; they believe there is no universal cause for aging (73, 101, 115, 274, 279).

Biological Theories

Biological theories can be categorized as nongenetic cellular, physiologic, and genetic. See Table 14–1 for definitions or explanations and limitations related to the theories (31, 69, 83, 86, 115, 140, 161, 247, 274, 277, 279).

Psychosocial Theories

Just as one biological theory does not adequately address biological aging, one single psychosocial theory of aging is not adequate to explain psychological or social aging. The **Continuity Theory** proposes that *an individual's patterns of behavior are the result of a lifetime of experiences, and aging is the continuation of these lifelong adjustments or personality patterns.* Personality traits remain stable, and early personality function is a guide for the retirement years (69, 83, 140, 279). Continuity Theory, as first proposed by Brim and Kagan, assumes neither a necessary reduction in activity levels (Disengagement Theory) nor the necessity of maintaining high activity levels (Activity Theory). They associated successful aging with the ability of the person to maintain patterns of behavior that existed before old age. Continuity in behavioral patterns and lifestyle exists over time, regardless of the actual level of activity present. Each of us has a powerful drive to maintain the sense of identity or continuity that allays fears of changing too fast or being changed against one's will by external forces. There is a simultaneous drive to develop and mature further, which fosters continuing change in at least small ways. Adult development is not in the genes but in the intricacies of life experiences. Two psychological mechanisms, selective perception and situational reinforcement, are used to maintain a sense of continuity. **Selective perception** means that *experiences are reacted to on the basis of their relative congruence with currently held values, beliefs, and attitudes.* Noncongruent ideas are screened out of awareness, ignored, or not attended to. **Situational reinforcement** means that the

MYTHS AND MISCONCEPTIONS AND THEIR REALITIES FOR THE ELDERLY PERSON

Myth 1: Age 65 Is a Good Marker for Old Age.

Fact: Factors other than chronologic age cause the person to be old. Many people are more youthful than their parents were at age 65. With increased longevity, perhaps 70 or 75 should be the chronologic marker (85).

Myth 2: Most Old People Are in Bed or in Institutions and Are Ill Physically and Mentally.

Fact: Approximately 5% are institutionalized; 95% are living in the community. Although 67% of older persons outside institutions have one or more chronic conditions, 14% do not. Chronic conditions range from mild and correctable to more severe. Approximately 81% of the aged living in the community have no mobility limitations; 8% have trouble getting around; 6% need the help of another person; and 5% are homebound. The average number of restricted activity days is only twice that for young adults. Some report no physical illness, and some with physical disease processes do not consider themselves ill (85).

Myth 3: All Old People Are Alike.

Fact: Each older adult is unique and *quite diverse*. This segment of the life span covers more years than any other segment—sometimes more than 35 years. The older people are, the more varied are their physical capabilities, personal style, economic status, and lifestyle preferences. From birth, physical and mental elaboration continues through life to make people more and more unlike one another (46, 83, 85).

Myth 4: The Next Generation of Older Adults Will Be the Same as This Generation.

Fact: The next generation will be better educated, healthier, more mobile, more youthful in appearance, more accustomed to lifestyle change and technology, and more outspoken. The world is changing so quickly that each successive generation is vastly *different* from the ones that came before (46, 140).

Myth 5: Old Age Brings Mental Deterioration.

Fact: Approximately 5% of older adults show serious mental impairment, and only 10% demonstrate even mild to moderate memory loss. Many professionals work past 65 to 70 years (46, 85).

Myth 6: Old People Cannot Learn and Are Less Intelligent.

Fact: Older adults *can* and *do* learn; however, they may need a longer period in which to respond to questions and stimuli. When learning problems occur, they are usually associated with a disease process. Intelligent people remain so (46, 85).

Myth 7: Most Older Adults Are Incompetent.

Fact: Older people may have a slower reaction time and take longer to do psychomotor tasks; however, they have more consistent output, less job turnover, greater job satisfaction, fewer accidents, and less absenteeism (85).

Myth 8: Most Older Adults Are Unhappy and Dissatisfied With Life.

Fact: How happy or sad the person feels reflects basic temperament throughout life, the adaptation to past and current life events, and social support. Positive social ties and realistic expectations buffer psychological distress. Older people tend to be as satisfied with their lives as middle-aged people, even when they have lower incomes and poorer health (46, 85, 237).

Myth 9: The Elderly Are Self-Pitying, Apathetic, Irritable, and Hard to Live With.

Fact: Research shows that mood is related to the present situation and past personality. The older person is as likely as a younger one to have an interesting and pleasant personality (46, 85, 140).

Myth 10: The Elderly Are Inactive and Unproductive.

Fact: Many young children have working grandparents. Thirty- sixpercent of men over 65 years are employed in some type of job. Older women often do their housework into their eighties or nineties. Older workers have a job attendance record that is 20% better than that of young workers, and they also sustain fewer job-related injuries (46, 85).

Myth 11: The Elderly Do Not Desire and Do Not Participate in Sexual Activity.

Fact: Recent research refutes this assertion. Sexual activity may decline because of lack of a partner or misinformation about sexuality in late life. The person who has been sexually active all along is able to continue sexual activity, and sexual activity involves more than intercourse between the partners (46, 85, 140).

Myth 12: The Elderly Are Isolated, Abandoned, and Lonely, and They Are Unlikely to Participate in Activities.

Fact: Many elderly prefer to live in a separate household. Many elderly live with someone and do not feel lonely. Approximately 10% of people over 65 years never married and have adjusted to living alone. Elderly people who do not have children often have siblings or friends with whom they live. Other elderly live in institutions or residences for the aged where they make friends. The percentage of purposefully abandoned elderly is small; often the person who is a loner in old age has always been alone (46, 83, 85).

Myth 13: Retirement Is Disliked by All Old People and Causes Illness and Less Life Satisfaction.

Fact: Although this may be true for some people, many older people look forward to retirement and are retiring before 65 so that they can continue other pursuits. Most are not sick from idleness and a sense of worthlessness. More than three-fourths of them have satisfying lives (46, 85, 140).

Myth 14: Special Health Services for the Aged Are Useless Because the Aged Cannot Benefit Anyway.

Fact: At age 65 the average person can look forward to 15 more years of life. The elderly have fewer acute illnesses and accidental injuries, and these conditions are correctable, although older people take longer to recover than younger people do. Common chronic conditions are cardiovascular disease, cancer, arthritis, diabetes, sensory impairments, and depression, which can be treated so that the person can achieve maximum potential and comfort (46, 85, 140).

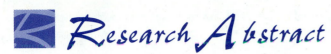

Research Abstract

Garfein, A., and A. Herzog, Robust Aging Among the Young-old, Old-old, and Oldest-old,
Journal of Gerontology: Social Sciences, 50B, no. 2 (1995), S77–S87.

Robust, successful, productive aging, vitality, aging well, or maintaining health into the older years is increasingly expected. Old age is not necessarily a time of declining health and resources. Older people compete in athletic events, are employed full- or part-time, and contribute their expertise to a variety of community, social, church, and political causes.

The purpose of this study was to examine interrelationships between four multicategorical definitions or predictors of robust aging: productive involvement, affective status, functional status, and cognitive status. The national sample included 1644 adults age 60 or older who participated in a survey. The sample comprised predominantly Caucasian (90%), female (59%), married (62%), or widowed (27%) persons who had at least a high school education (54%) and a family income of less than $25,000 annually (75%). Age range was divided into three categories: 60–69 years (52%), 70–79 years (36%), and 80 and over (12%).

Analysis of data revealed that productive involvement and affective, functional, and cognitive status were generally independent of each other. There was modest correlation between productive involvement and functional status and between functional and affective status. Aged persons who were most robust reported greater social contact by telephone, had more frequent visits with friends and relatives, rated their health and vision status as high, and experienced few life crises or changes in the past 3 years. There was essentially an absence of depressive symptoms. Although fewer of the oldest old were less robust, a substantial proportion remained so.

Health care implications include the need for more research and better indicators of robust aging and recognition of the heterogeneity in health status among elders. It is important not to focus only on pathology or negative aspects of function. Understanding the full range of possible trajectories in later life and challenging ageism and stereotypes about aging are essential for health maintenance, restoration, and management at all age levels in late adulthood.

behaviors used are those that are rewarded. Previously established behavior patterns tend to have a long history of reinforcement (174). Continuity Theory may explain why, when one spouse was relocated to a long-term institution, the other spouse did not appear to perceive the marriage much differently than before the move (104).

Developmental Theories

Several developmental theories have addressed psychosocial aging. **Erikson's Epigenetic Theory** (88, 89) suggests that *successful personality development in later life depends on the ability to resolve the psychosocial crisis known as integrity versus despair.* Erikson's theory is psychodynamic and is part of a life cycle approach that emphasizes that the developmental tasks of each stage must be met before the person can work through the next tasks. The theory is discussed in detail later in this chapter.

Peck's Theory (228) hypothesizes that *there are three psychological developmental tasks of old age: ego differentiation versus work-role preoccupation, body transcendence versus body preoccupation, and ego transcendence versus ego preoccupation* (see Chapter 13). Reed (236) also identified these tasks. These issues are an extension and further development of Erikson's stage, with emphasis on change and growth in later life. Havighurst (117, 118) presents several major developmental tasks that must be mastered or achieved to meet the developmental needs of later maturity (see Developmental Tasks later in this chapter). He uses an eclectic approach that combines previously developed concepts into one theory (118). According to all developmental theories, the older adult's behavior and response depend on how earlier developmental crises were handled.

TABLE 14–1. THEORIES OF PHYSICAL AGING

Theory	Definition/Explanation	Limitation to Theory
Nongenetic Cellular Theories		
Wear and Tear Theory	Body systems wear out because of accumulation of stress of life and effects of metabolism. Most general and obvious explanation of aging compares body to a machine.	Little scientific evidence. Theory does not consider self-repair mechanisms of body or differences of life span with the human species.
Cross-linkage Theory	Bonds or crosslinkages develop between molecules or peptides: these bonds change the molecules' properties physically and chemically. Thus collagen in intracellular or extracellular material is chemically altered and function affected. When collagen is cross-linked with other molecules, changes range from wrinkling, to atherosclerosis, to inelasticity of tissue. When cross-linkages occur with DNA molecules that carry genetic program, DNA is damaged and mutation or death of cell occurs. A viable theory.	
Accumulation of Waste Theory	Substances such as metabolic waste materials and lipofuscins, which interfere with cellular metabolism and cause cell death, accumulate in cells. Examples of accumulation of metabolic waste are cataracts on the eye, cholesterol in the arteries, and bone brittleness.	These substances may be a result rather than cause of senescence.
Accumulation of Errors Theory	As cells die, they must synthesize new proteins to make new cells; sometimes an error occurs. When enough errors occur, organ failure results.	Little scientific evidence.
Free Radical Theory	Free radicals (charged or unstable molecules) or chemicals that contain oxygen in a highly activated state and react with other molecules during normal metabolism cause damage to cells and aging. Exposure to radiation and certain enzymes may cause these reactions.	Little scientific evidence; not generally accepted.
Deprivation Theory	Aging is caused by deprivation of essential nutrients and oxygen to cells.	Little scientific evidence. It is likely that deprivation is the result of aging.
Physiologic		
Biological Clock or Aging by Program Theory	Each organism contains genes or evolutionary processes that govern or control speed at which metabolic processes are performed. These genes or processes act as a genetic clock dictating occurrence of aging and dying. Cells are genetically programmed to reproduce only a certain amount of time; human limit may be 100 to 120 years.	Humans may be able to outlive inner governing processes because of medical technology and improvements in lifestyle. Cells in nervous system and muscles do not reproduce themselves; all other cells do, at least to some extent.
	Hypothalamus may be the timer that keeps track of age of cells and determines how long they will keep reproducing.	
	Reproduced older cells do not appear to pass on information accurately through the DNA, which weakens functioning ability of older cells.	Cells are more likely to reproduce imperfectly as they get older.
Neuroendocrine Theory	Hormonal changes produce free radicals, cross-linkages, and autoimmunity.	Free radicals may be a special form of cross-linkage; may cause free radicals.
Immune Theory	Ability of immune system to deal with foreign organisms or processes diminishes with age. Greatest decline is observed in thymus-derived immunity (T-cell production reduced) Production of antibodies declines after adolescence. **Autoimmune responses** may occur, whereby normal cells are engulfed and digested, making person more vulnerable to disease. A viable theory.	Autoimmunity may result from production of new antigens caused by (1) mutations that cause formation of altered RNA or DNA; or (2) the new antigens may have been hidden in the body earlier in life and are not recognized by body in late life.
Genetic Gene Theory	Aging is programmed; the program exists in certain harmful genes. Genes that direct many cellular activities in early life may become altered in later years, which alters function and may be responsible for functional decline and structural changes associated with aging.	Genetic basis exists for longevity, although environmental factors such as vaccines, nutrition, pollutants safety factors, and medical care and technology can alter life span.

Levinson theorizes that late adulthood is characterized by a *transition period which occurs between 60 and 65 years of age; the person does not become suddenly old, but physical and mental changes increase awareness of aging and mortality* (173).

Sociologic Theories

Disengagement Theory, Activity Theory, and Interactionist Theory are sociologic theories. **Disengagement Theory,** proposed by Cumming and Henry (67), *suggests that all old people and society mutually withdraw, that the withdrawal is biologically and psychologically intrinsic and inevitable, and that it is necessary for aging and beneficial to society.* This voluntary withdrawal or separation from society is related to a decreased life space in the older adult, relinquishment of roles, decreased integration into society, fewer social interests, and increased preference for individual interactions and rewards. Cumming and Henry's Disengagement Theory suggests that society finds ways to minimize the social disruption that results from death of its members. In addition, individuals in a society undergo a self-disengagement process during the middle and later years of life. This process is characterized by a reduction in general energy levels, reduction in societal involvement, and increased preoccupation with one's own needs and desires. Studies do not support the Disengagement Theory. The older person may be alone but enjoy the solitude, be mentally alert, and be responsive socially (183, 224).

Cross-cultural studies show disengagement is not inevitable, and it is generally not applicable to family relationships. Thus, Disengagement Theory as proposed by Cumming and Henry is considered factually incorrect, methodologically unsound, and dangerous as a basis for social policy (174, 261). In a nationwide survey in the United States about people aged 65 years or older, 14% of all who had died within the past year were reported by survivors to have been *fully* functional in the last year of life; 10% were defined as severely restricted, related to health problems causing death, such as severe heart disease, stroke, cancer, or several diseases. It is possible that the last year of severe restriction follows a long period of being fully functional. As men generally live shorter lives, they are less likely to be impaired than women. It is possible that lifestyle changes will improve not only the life span but also the probability of remaining healthy (171). Sill's research (261) reveals that awareness of **finitude,** *estimate of time remaining before death,* and physical incapacity were more important than age in predicting level of activity. The person who perceives self as near death

begins to constrict life space; psychological preparation for death may lead to disengagement. The person may consciously or unconsciously be aware of **terminal drop,** *the period preceding the person's death from a few weeks up to 2 years,* which may account for some intellectual decline, changed verbal abilities, withdrawal from the world, and mood changes, as well as onset of physical illness (296).

Activity Theory, formulated by Havighurst, Maddox, and Palmore to refute Disengagement Theory, is the more popular of the two theories. *Basic concepts of the theory are that most elderly people maintain a level of activity and engagement commensurate with their earlier patterns of activity and past lifestyles and that the maintenance of physical, mental, and social activity is usually necessary for successful aging* (46, 183, 224).

Activity Theory implies that the older adult has essentially the same psychological and social needs as do middle-aged people. According to this theory, the older adult must compensate for the loss of roles experienced in later maturity. The older adult does not disengage but needs to maintain a moderately active lifestyle. In reality, the response to aging by most older adults is a combination of the two theories (174).

Sheehy found, in her study of women in their seventies, eighties, and nineties, that many are, indeed, very actively pursing a second adulthood. They have remained active, creative, involved in various organizations; they may be returning to college or acting as consultants. They are full of zest and have a passion and purpose in life. They may concentrate on a few priorities intensely or volunteer in a number of projects. They demonstrate wisdom, discussed by Erikson, and ego and spiritual transcendence rather than self-preoccupation, as discussed by Peck (259).

Mead first articulated the **Symbolic Interaction Theory** in 1934, from which many of our present theories have grown. This theory holds that *the person develops socially according to the continuous bombardment of self-reflections perceived from others.* The aged in our culture are generally seen as having little social validity, and if this attitude is perceived consistently, it can become a self-fulfilling prophecy. People may expect to become inept and forgetful. Social and cultural expectations may strongly color self-view and consequent behavior. Symbolic Interaction Theory attempts to consider the interrelationships of several dimensions of the aging process, including (201):

- Sociocultural dimensions that set the limits on available alternatives for the person.
- Contextual dimensions within which the individual's life course develops (e.g., includes biological change, past experiences).

- Personal evaluation of life experience, health status, and the future foci of energy and roles.

Biological changes, psychological changes, societal circumstances, and past and present experiences all are considered as relevant for explaining the aging process (201).

Brown developed the **Urban Ecologic Model of Aging,** which is based on *person–environment interaction and the fact that human behavior and subjective well-being are reflected in the social interaction that occurs between the individual and the environment* (41). Lawton and Nahemon first proposed the Ecologic Model of Aging. Their original model characterized the person as possessing various degrees of competence in four dimensions: (1) biological health, including chronic medical diseases; (2) sensorimotor function and ability to perform activities of daily living; (3) cognitive ability; and (4) ego strength or emotional function. Individual adaptive behavior and subjective well-being are balanced when demands of the environment do not exceed level of ability to manage the demands. The older person is more vulnerable than the younger counterpart, especially if the person is impoverished, experiences environmental stress or social problems, or has multiple problems or needs. The greater the individual vulnerability, the greater the environmental impact on the person (41).

Brown expanded the model to include (1) consideration of the suprapersonal environment and characteristics of the neighborhood, (2) personal characteristics of residents in the locale, (3) perceptions of the surrounding environment, (4) effects of media reports on the person's perception, (5) factual data about the surrounding environment, and (6) residential satisfaction and subjective well-being. The elder's personal experience or perception may differ from the factual reports of the neighborhood or environment, especially in urban, inner-city, or poverty-stricken areas (41).

FAMILY DEVELOPMENT AND RELATIONSHIPS

The changing demographic profile of developed countries has been associated with an increased number of four- and five-generation families. In such families it is common to have two generations at or near old age, with the oldest person frequently over 75 years. The "generation in the middle" may extend into retirement years in many families. Thus the "young-old," facing the potential of diminished personal resources, may be the group increasingly called on to give additional support to aged kin—the old-old and very or frail-old.

Several authors have written about aging in different cultures, family relationships between generations in different cultures and countries, and how worldwide social changes are affecting the elderly as family members (21, 46, 58, 68, 71, 85, 138, 189, 200, 237, 248, 268, 306).

Relationship With Spouse

In later life, responsibilities of parenthood and employment diminish with few formal responsibilities to take their place. There is usually a corresponding decline in social contacts and activities. The factors that affect the social life of the elderly are found in personal social skills and in resources available in the private life. Marital status remains a major organizing force for personal life. With children gone and without daily contact with co-workers provided by employment, the elderly lose the basis for social integration. Declining health, limited income, and fewer daily responsibilities may create greater needs for social support. Thus, having a spouse provides the possibility for increased companionship. Having a spouse also increases longevity, especially for older males, unless the male never married.

Interestingly, spouses may not increase in their support of each other into late life, perhaps because of increased **interiority** (introspection) with aging. Time may erode bases of respect, affection, and compatibility. Sometimes marriages have not been filled with mutual emotional or social support in earlier years, so there is no foundation for increasing mutual emotional support. Women are often the sole support for men. Older women tend to feel the husband is not supportive emotionally or in health care; however, women tend to rely on a more extensive network of family and friends for support (218).

The greater the number of adult children living nearby, the more likely the elderly mother is to have a weekly conversation or visit with at least one child. Women with two or more children are more likely than women with only one child to see the children as a source of potential help. Interestingly, adult children with siblings are more likely to report a higher-quality relationship with the mother than are adults who are only children (14, 280).

For the woman continually to have a spouse in the house or with her, wanting to share in her activities, can be distressing, even though it has been anticipated. The loss of privacy and solitude, doing tasks her own way and at her own pace, loss of independence, and loss of contact with friends may all be issues. The increased accommodation to meeting husband's needs, however, is offset by increased opportunities for nurturing and being nurtured and for sharing mutual interests (233).

Your listening and teaching may assist the elderly person in making the necessary adjustments to the spouse.

Relationships With Offspring and Other Family Members

Historical trends toward smaller families, longer life spans, increasing employment of women, and increasingly high mobility of both young and old have important implications for children being a primary resource in old age.

The number of children is related to the recency with which older parents have seen their child, the amount of assistance older parents receive, and factors influencing older parents' interaction with children. Parents with one child report fewer visits and less help received, especially if the only child is an employed daughter. Older parents expect children, especially the daughter(s), to assume an appreciable level of responsibility in meeting important health, economic, and emotional needs, regardless of how many offspring there are to share in the assistance. Assistance from children-in-law, grandchildren, siblings and siblings-in-law, and nieces and nephews increases as the number of offspring decreases. Geographic proximity is a stable predictor of older parent–child interaction, more than offspring gender or health status of the parent. Daughters who are primarily blue-collar workers provide more assistance to older parents and have more association with parents than corresponding sons. Parents receive more help from offspring as income for the offspring increases (46, 85).

Older parents receive and perceive their children's help in several ways. Younger parents receive more help with automobile maintenance and help in the form of gifts. Older parents receive help with shopping and transportation. Parents who most strongly valued family are most desirous of and satisfied with family support. Parents may tend to expect less help from children when they live at a distance or when they work outside the home. Further, they appreciate most the help that keeps them self-reliant or autonomous, maintains social integration, maximizes choice and expressive interactions, and forestalls reliance on more extensive services. Parents with a greater degree of ill health express less satisfaction with children's help, possibly because it symbolizes dependency and loss of social integration (140, 279).

Some elderly people have a limited number of family members; some couples have no children. The childless couple will probably have adapted to childlessness psychologically; however, they are especially vulnerable at crisis points such as episodes of poor health and death of spouse or housing companion. If those persons or couples cannot drive or have no transportation, they will have a greater need for help, although they may hesitate to ask for help.

Your teaching and referrals may enable the elderly person with few relatives or resources to manage more effectively.

Grandparenthood

Grandparenthood has multiple meanings for the person, depending in part on age at the initial time of grandparenthood, and the number and accomplishments of the grandchildren are probably a source of status (98, 140, 204, 243, 279). The stage of grandparenthood may come to middle-aged persons, depending on age of their own childbearing and age of their childrens' childbearing. The relatively young grandparent may either like and accept or resist the role and may not like the connection of age and being a grandparent. Relative youth of grandparents contributes to the complex patterns of help and relationships between the generations. Older African-American and Latino females are distinctive for extending their own households to children and grandchildren, bearing child-care and housekeeping responsibilities into old age. Traditionally, the central figure, especially in the poor African-American family, has been the mother or grandmother, who has been responsible for maintenance of family stability and a source of socialization (58). The increasing divorce rate also adds to the complexity of grandparent relationships. The child may have eight sets of grandparents. The grandparents may be the main caretakers for the child(ren), or there may be a part-time commitment, sharing child care with their adult children. Likewise, grandchildren have a special tie to grandparents (243, 263). Research indicates that even when there was divorce in the family, adult children from divorced families continued their relationships with grandparents (63).

Grandparents increasingly are the main caretaker of the child, often in the custodial role, although legal custody is unlikely even if the child has a permanent home. Sometimes the grandparents serve as babysitter or a day-care service. When mothers also live in the home, the grandmother's being the main caregiver may have a negative impact on both the mother's and grandmother's parenting (98, 137, 150, 157, 158, 263, 293).

Grandparents are often happy with their role in that they can enjoy the young person and enter into a playful, informal, companion, and confidant relationship (Fig. 14–2). The grandchild is seen as a source of leisure activity, someone for whom to purchase items that are also enjoyable to the grandparent. The grandparent typically does not want to take on an authoritarian or disciplinarian role but will, and has the experience to do so, if necessary. The number of **great-grandparents** and **great-great-grandparents** is increasing as more people live longer. The roles are emotionally fulfilling; these young family members provide a sense of personal and family renewal and transcendence; add diversion to conversations if not activities; and mark longevity. Great-grandparents may be as active in the grandparenting role as they were as grandparents, but advanced age, geographic distance, and cohabitation, divorce, and remarriage of family members tend to limit their participation. Also, this generation feels removed from the very young, whereas the grandparent generation feels a special tie with the very young (56, 75).

Social Relationships

Social networks of family, friends, and neighbors provide instrumental and expressive support. They contribute to well-being of the senior by promoting socialization and companionship, elevating morale and life satisfaction, buffering the effects of stressful events, providing a confidant, and facilitating coping skills and mastery. For example, social supports buffer the effects of stressful life events and represent more than the

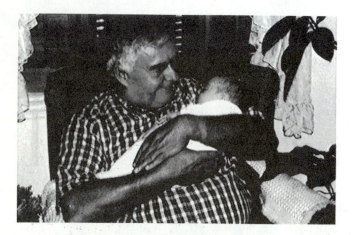

Figure 14–2. Grandparents often look forward to their role. *(From Sherwen, L.N., M.A. Scoloveno, and C.T. Weingarten,* Nursing Care of the Childbearing Family. *Stamford, CT: Appleton & Lange, 1991, p. 764.)*

quantity or proximity of social ties but also the extent to which social ties fulfill needs of the senior. Also, the components of informal support networks—spouses, children, close relatives, distant kin (cousins, aunts, uncles, nieces, nephews), co-workers, close friends, neighbors, and acquaintances—have a variety of functions and vary in importance to the senior. Instrumental help is given in the form of advice, information, financial aid, and assistance with tasks. Socioemotional aid is given in the form of affection, sympathy, understanding, acceptance, esteem, and referral to services (61, 272, 273). Planning for contact between the generations (e.g., with preschoolers or adolescents) also contributes to meaningful social interactions for both generations (56, 153, 166).

Frequency of use of social networks is not related to physical health. As income decreases, visiting with neighbors declines, but visits to close friends or relatives increase, as does the tendency to talk to family members about feelings and to talk to friends about events. The elderly rate helpfulness of children and other family members as important. Lower income increases the senior's reliance on friends and relatives and the value placed on their help. Higher income may provide resources that facilitate social visiting and a broader network of relationships. A higher frequency of social contacts and greater intensity of kin and friend relationships have been found for women in comparison to men. Apparently intimacy or close friendship ties and having a confidant are less important to the male (61).

Supportive ties become smaller and more unstable in old age, and social support may provide burdens for those who provide it to the senior. The closer the bond, the greater are the physical, emotional, and financial strains. Burdens and costs may result in being less willing or able to help, physical or psychological distancing, increasing the social isolation of the dependent senior, or becoming enmeshed in the caregiver role to the exclusion of other relationships or roles. Informal networks ideally are integrated with formal support services (140, 271).

An unregulated or informal social welfare system naturally exists in the average community or senior residence, which provides more services, security, and hope for the future than is provided by formal agencies. This system of informal assistance through family, friends, and neighbors is the major source of help for the elderly. Among and for seniors, there are three types of neighborhood exchange types: (1) high helpers, who exhibit a more formal quasi-professional style of helping without reciprocation; (2) mutual helpers, who show an interdependent style of give and take; and (3) neighborhood isolates, whose social ties and help sources are primarily outside the neighborhood. High helpers with neighbors are those who also do volunteer work or are active in self-help groups. Often these people have been in the helping professions in their work years; they also had a spiritual or religious orientation with serving others. Mutual helpers have more neighborhood contact and are generally quite outgoing. Isolates have little contact with others and view themselves as quiet people. They may be in poor health and in need of help themselves (140, 279).

Many of the events of later life are exit events, involving continuous threat, stress, and loss such as widow(er)hood, chronic or poor health, retirement, change in residence, and lower income. Thus, coping often becomes problem specific and also involves socialization, leaning how to perform new roles, adjusting to changing roles, and relinquishing old roles. Socialization contributes to well-being by lending continuity and structure to the transitions encountered by people.

Often you will be able to assist the elderly in asking for and accepting help from others, or in becoming familiar with community resources.

Caregiver Role

The role of the middle-aged offspring in caring for the elderly parent has been described in Chapter 13. Refer to Chapter 13 and references at the end of that chapter and at the end of this chapter for more information on the caregiver role (34, 108, 175, 272, 273). Even as elders are being cared for, they are also a source of support—emotionally, socially, and financially (by providing living arrangement)—for the adult child.

The caregiver in an elderly couple is most frequently the wife, as women live longer than men and are usually younger than spouses. If the woman is impaired, the husband is often the caregiver. The spouse is the primary source of help for married elderly with impaired capacity, and adult daughters are the major helpers when a spouse is not present or not able to sufficiently help. The probability of relying on friends is highest among impaired elderly who are unmarried and have few family members within an hour's travel. The more frail the person, the more likely a family member will be the primary caregiver rather than formal systems or nonrelated people (34, 39, 108, 175, 177, 271, 272, 273). The majority of noninstitutionalized elderly are self-sufficient.

When the spouse cannot manage care for the elderly parent, children try to assist. Sons tend to become caregivers only in the absence of an available female sibling and are more likely to rely on their own spouses for support and help. Sons tend to provide less direct care assistance and to be less involved; hence, they do not feel as stressed by the caregiving experience.

The elderly person who cares for a disabled spouse is a hidden victim, at risk for physical and emotional stresses of caregiving superimposed on stresses of the aging process. He or she is likely to experience a barrage of feelings and role overload, including being head of the household. The woman, as the spouse who is the caregiver, may also be chronically ill or disabled. Thus, the family caregiver of the noninstitutionalized elderly is in need of help from supportive services. These services for the spouse could include a wives' support group sponsored by a senior center; home health care; adult day-care; foster home placement; extended respite care; homemaker, transporter, and repairman services; and visitor or "relief" services. Sometimes the elder is caregiver for an adult child with developmental disability, mental retardation, or mental illness. The gratification, frustration, and stress are related to the adult child's diagnosis, size of the women's support system, the family's social climate, and adult child's participation in out-of-home programs (109).

Be aware of feelings of the middle-aged or elderly caregiver and the family; needs and feelings of the elderly person; issues and conflicts for the family; and ways to help families manage the caregiving experience. Education and support group programs appear to hold great promise as a means for assisting family caregivers of older relatives. You will have an important role in implementing both of those interventions. A number of strategies can be helpful to the caregiver both in preventing decline in the caregiver and in administering care to the elder (46, 85). Various programs can be effective for reducing stress for caregivers of elderly family members who are emotionally or physically disabled (70):

- Support groups, especially for caregivers of patients with Alzheimer's or other dementias, which offer practical solutions to problems as well as emotional support
- Respite care programs based at the person's home or in agencies, to care for the ill person when the caregiver needs time off (a day, weekend, or week)
- Education about stress management techniques that enhance abilities to care for the self as well as the family member

Widow(er)hood

Because widow(er)hood may occur before late life, the feelings, problems, and issues pertinent to the widow(er) have been discussed in Chapter 13. Refer to

Chapter 13 and the references at the end of this chapter for additional insights. Bereavement does not permanently affect health status for most seniors, although the grief reaction may induce physiologic symptoms initially. Stress appears to increase as the death approaches, and then health status may deteriorate. Regardless of the predeath mourning done by the survivor, the elderly widow(er) has great increase in psychological distress (22, 34, 81, 165, 175, 210).

Widow(er)hood disrupts couple-based relationships and obligations to a spouse and introduces emotional and material burdens on those relationships that outlive the marriage. Widow(er)hood, especially after a period of caregiving, may also introduce both a measure of freedom to make new contacts and a stimulus to do so. If the person moves to a smaller dwelling, increased housing density produces a greater increase in social contacts among the widowed than is seen in the married. Without the support that the spouse usually provides, the widowed may turn to friends and relatives as a source of replacement. The widowed may have greater intimacy with their friends than the married, for married people interact more with their spouses (213).

The elderly widowed are not more isolated than elderly married, and elderly women have some advantage over elderly men in their ability to develop or maintain social relationships. Patterns of social relationships established among the married apparently provide the parameters within which social relationships continue among the widowed. Both married and widowed women are more likely to talk to close friends and relatives and to talk to family about worries and to children about crises than are married or widowed men. Loss of spouse allows for expansion or addition of new roles; frequency of contact increases with widow(er)hood. Widow(er)hood results in greater involvement with informal social relationships than marriage.

The widow who lives alone in her own home may be in need of a great deal of help. Neighbors often provide this help, especially if children reside out of town. The childless widow, however, may not receive any more help from neighbors than widows with children despite greater needs. Perhaps adult children are able to elicit neighbor assistance; such requests for extra help are not forthcoming if there are no children.

Your teaching, emotional support, referral to services, and encouragement to continue as active a life as possible are important to the widow(er) as she or he adjusts to losses and new roles. A helpful book for the widow is *Suddenly Alone: A Woman's Guide to Widowhood,* by P. Gates, Harper Perennial Publishers, 1991.

Divorce and the Elderly

Those who are separated from their spouses and those who are legally divorced total slightly more than 5% of the population. The numbers of people who were ever divorced, who were divorced before age 65, and who are over age 65 when divorce occurs are increasing. Also, the proportion of older persons who have ever experienced a divorce is considerably larger than the proportion who are currently divorced, as many divorced people remarry. In the future fewer marriages will be terminated by death before old age. Also, an increased number of seniors will fall in the ever-divorced and currently divorced categories because those entering old age in the future will be more accepting of divorce as a solution to an unpleasant marriage. Further, in the future more elderly women will have economic independence because of their years in the work force, and this may encourage higher divorce rates (57, 281).

Being divorced in old age, or in any age, may negatively affect a person's economic position and may increase demands for social welfare support. Typically divorce is associated with a deterioration in the standard of living for women, although it has little effect for men. Further, family and kinship relationships are affected by divorce. The children or other relatives who would provide physical help and psychosocial support may not be available to one of the parents in his or her old age. Remarriage also establishes a new set of nuclear family relationships. The experience of being divorced can help the senior cope with bereavement. The person knows survival is possible after a marital relationship ends (57, 281).

Be prepared to give emotional support or crisis intervention to the older person who is encountering divorce or who is reworking the conflicts, dilemmas, and losses of having experienced divorce.

Singlehood

A small percentage (approximately 5%) of elderly people remain single and never marry. They have no spouse or children. They may or may not have living family members. They may or may not live alone. The never-married elderly do not constitute a single "social type"; their situations are more complex. Like other elderly, they are affected by social opportunities and restraints and the cultural values and changes that impinge on their life situations. Some older people are homosexual. Some live in locations in which women outnumber men, causing an imbalance in mate selection. Others may have chosen the single lifestyle as a means to some end such as a career. Some have had family responsibilities that precluded marriage or were otherwise unable to break out of their families of orientation. Others have been lifelong isolates and have had poor health or a stigmatized social identity. Possibly the factors for singlehood have been multiple.

In an interview study of 90 older women, the women discussed the meaning of childlessness over the life course. They realized the social system perceives the childless woman as marginal and incomplete. The women discussed that they missed having children but also believed the idealization of motherhood does not necessarily reflect reality, as children do not always take care of elderly parents and having children can be difficult and painful. Further, they felt satisfied with their lives; being childless did not negate their whole life because they had made other contributions (8).

Well-being in old age can be at least partly explained by a supportive relationship with the parent in early life. Elders who had a supportive relationship are more likely to be adaptive and cope with adversity effectively in old age (14, 26). As practitioners, we should be sensitive to these differences and to their effects on the lives and identities of never-married elderly (251).

There are five types of key personal relationships for never-married older women that help reduce social isolation and loneliness and increase life satisfaction and social support (see Chapter 13, p. 696).

Issues of attachment may be different for the widowed and the never married, but this does not mean that there are no loss issues, although it is clear that there are some never-married elderly who do not develop such attachments. There are a range of attachments and bereavement experiences for the never married in late life, not just an absence of personal loss issues (251). Having lived independently all during adult life, the person may have developed effective adaptive mechanisms and a supportive social network. The assumption is that being married provides social, emotional, and sustenance needs. In fact, the single person who has planned carefully for retirement may be as satisfied with self and life and as secure in all aspects as the married person. The single person may be no more lonely than the married person. He or she does not experience the desolation of widow(er)hood or divorce (250, 251).

Few studies have been done on health status of the single senior. They generally conclude that the well-being of single people is equivalent to that of married persons, whereas widowed, divorced, and separated persons have lower well-being. A decline in functional capacity greatly increases the likelihood that the unmar-

ried older person will move in with others or become institutionalized (250, 307).

Single women tend to have greater education, occupational status, and intellectual ability than married women, suggesting that career orientation makes marriage less attractive for women. Single women are likely to be first-born, which leads to a less romantic view of marriage because of early roles as surrogate parents. Single men do not display the higher educational and occupational attainment found with single women, but they are more likely to be only children, suggesting socialization for greater achievement. Psychological integrity and social independence are features of the single personality (251).

The single person views fluidity and variety in social relationships, rather than the exclusivity of marriage, as an advantage in promoting opportunities for personal growth while still protecting autonomy. Lifestyle is geared to preserving personal independence and the development of self, with privacy, self-expression through work, freedom of movement, and preoccupation with expanding experiences, philosophic insights, and imaginative conceptions of life as goals for the person. Single women are happier and better adjusted than single men; marital roles may be less beneficial and more stressful for women than for men. Although single women are happier than single men, they are nevertheless less happy than married women. The characteristic that best explains their relative unhappiness is greater dissatisfaction with family life. The lower well-being of the never married is attributable either to changes accompanying aging, which lessen the viability of single lifestyles, or to less support of single living among other older people (250, 251).

Be alert to special emotional and social needs of the single elderly, to their reticence at times to ask for help, and to the need for information about community resources. You may become a significant confidant.

Elderly and Pets

Pets are great companions for older people. In 1983, President Ronald Reagan signed a law guaranteeing the right to keep pets in government-assisted rental housing for the elderly and handicapped. A number of states have adopted laws to allow animals as permanent residents of hospitals and nursing homes. Pets are therapeutic in the home and in the center or institution for the elderly. They offer companionship and unconditional love, they soothe and lift the spirits, and a specially trained dog can offer assistance and security (e.g., as a brace for the neurologically impaired). Dogs can pull wheelchairs and even help load them into cars. Pets have a beneficial effect on physical health: they lower stress response and lower blood pressure. The touch from the pet and stroking the pet offer physiologic release and lower anxiety. Pets can promote verbal communication skills; birds can even talk back. Although animals and birds do carry disease, healthy pets can be obtained from well-run shelters and shops or the Humane Society. Canine Companions for Independence is a national organization that supplies highly trained service dogs for helping people who use wheelchairs or are hearing impaired/deaf, and social companions for people with disabilities. Pets are chosen for temperament, not breed. There is no charge for the dog. Contact the agency at PO Box 446, Santa Rosa, CA 95402–0446 (707–528–0830) (24, 302). The person or family may need help in keeping the pet immunized, cleaned, and given the care that prevents unnecessary decline in the pet's health. Care of pets, especially dogs, in the home can take lots of energy but is essential. A 1-in.-wide, soft leather leash is easier to grasp than a nylon leash. Leashes and collars should have a swivel-bolt clasp or a large buckle for ease of use. A brush with a leather strap that fits over the back of the hand or a grooming glove (Lawrence glove) that fits like a mitten can be attached to the correct kind of brushing materials (soft for cats, stiff for a long-haired dog). An automatic watering spa or pet feeder that holds supplies for several days can be used to eliminate need for daily attention. Mount the water and food container at a height and at a place that is good for the pet and the owner. A pet door can be installed to allow the pet to get in and out to save the owner movements if the person has great restrictions. Explore accessible pet services. Mobile veterinarians, grooming vans, and other services are available in some areas (24). You can be instrumental in promoting pet therapy (24, 160, 302).

The death of a pet can precipitate a deep grief, and mourning will result because of the loss. Crisis counseling, giving the person a helping hand and a shoulder to cry on, may help the person work through the pet's death or work through feelings related to having to put the pet to sleep. Be aware that the senior who is wanting euthanasia for an apparently healthy pet may be contemplating suicide or suicide may follow the death of a pet. Death of a pet can be the last straw in a series of stresses and losses.

Elder Abuse and Neglect

The Older Americans Act (Public Law 89–73), passed by Congress in 1965, was amended in 1987 (Public Law 100–175) to add services for prevention of elder abuse as a priority for government funding. In addition, state offices of aging were to identify nonprofit entities that were involved in prevention, identification, and treatment of abuse, neglect, and exploitation of older persons.

It is estimated that 2 million older Americans are abused annually; it is a problem that still remains hid-

---

► TYPES AND MANIFESTATIONS OF ELDER ABUSE

Physical Abuse

- Neglect of physical care (food, eyeglasses, hearing aid, or information withheld)
- Slap, bruise, push
- Beating
- Burns, broken bones
- Brandishing a knife, cutting, stabbing
- Restraint (chain to toilet or tie to bed), resulting in skin breakdown or decubitus ulcers, as well as fractures
- Sexual molestation, rape

Psychological Abuse

- Verbal abuse (curse, scream, insult, demean, treat like a child)
- Verbal threats, name calling
- Decision making, voting denied
- Exclusion from family activities, isolation
- Placement in nursing home without consent or knowledge

Financial Abuse

- Confiscation of Social Security or other income checks
- Person forced to sign over property or assets
- Other financial exploitation
- Theft of property and personal items for sale
- Takeover of trust, guardianship
- Exploitation of resources for profit

Social Abuse

- Forced isolation from family, friends
- Constant switching of doctors
- Refusal of home health care or other community resources (day-care, home health aide, Meals-on-Wheels
- Inability to accept help or acknowledge difficulty with care
- Geographic isolation, e.g., rural, inner city ghetto

▶ **CAUSES OF ELDER MALTREATMENT, ABUSE, OR NEGLECT**

- Elder becomes more dependent or disabled.
- Elder is cognitively impaired or has Alzheimer's disease.
- Family is under economic stress.
- Caregiver is exhausted or loses control.
- Adult offspring is unemployed, lives in parent's home, and expects to be cared for.
- Adult offspring is mentally ill or alcohol or drug addicted.
- Family interaction pattern of screaming, hitting, and violence has existed through lifetime of marriage or childrearing.
- Retirement and lack of role clarity for both spouses result in much frustration in retired man.
- Man who was abusive to co-workers now abuses most available person, the wife.
- Woman is financially dependent on spouse.
- Elder is abandoned or seldom visited by children.
- Victim is unwilling or unable to report the problem.

den from the public and even professionals. Any elder can be a victim, but the victim usually is a Caucasian female over 70 with moderate to severe physical or mental impairments. Usually the abuser is a relative (spouse moreso than offspring) residing with her. Refer to Types and Manifestations of Elder Abuse for further description (46, 86, 126, 206, 260).

Hypotheses about the causes of elder abuse are listed in Causes of Elder Maltreatment, Abuse, or Neglect (46, 86, 126, 206, 260, 300).

Ways to prevent or reduce abuse are listed in Tips for the Older Person for Preventing or Reducing Abuse.

Signs and symptoms of the abused or neglected elder include the following:

- Bruises, fractures, malnourished status
- Undue confusion not attributable to physiologic consequences of aging
- Conflicting explanation about the senior's condition
- Unusual fear exhibited by the senior in a presumed safe environment, in the home, or in the presence of the caregiver
- A report of the daily routine that has considerable gaps in the sequence
- Apparent impaired functioning or abnormal behavior in the caregiver
- Indifference or hostility displayed by caregiver in response to questions

During assessment of potential abuse or neglect, do not let stereotypes about the elder or caregiver(s), an emphasis on family privacy, or denial prevent you from identifying the problem. Avoid a censuring tone of voice or judgmental expression or stance. Show a willingness to listen to the caregiver's perspective. Solicit the caregiver's early memories of relationships with the senior to learn of long-term conflicts. Most abused seniors are reluctant and ashamed to report abuse or neglect because of (1) fear of retaliation, (2) exposure of offspring to community censure or legal punishment, and (3) fear of potential removal from their home.

In planning care and during intervention, be familiar with the reporting laws of your state and whether the law covers only known abuse or suspected abuse. In most states professionals who fail to report abuse may be fined, and they are accorded protection from civil and criminal liability if they report abuse.

Because the abused or neglected senior is an adult with full legal rights, intervention is not possible without the consent of the senior if the person is legally competent. If the client is in a life-threatening situation, is competent, and chooses to remain at home, the nurse must honor that decision after counseling the elder of the danger. If the person is legally incompetent and ap-

▶ **TIPS FOR THE OLDER PERSON FOR PREVENTING OR REDUCING ABUSE**

- Remain sociable and stay active in the community; enlarge your circle of friends; join local chapters of American Association of Retired Persons or Older Women's League.
- Plan for possible disability by completing an advance medical directive and arranging for power-of-attorney.
- Familiarize yourself with community resources that help older people remain as independent as possible.
- Do not share a household with anyone who has a history of violent behavior or substance abuse.
- Do not move in with a child or relative if your relationship is troubled.
- Avoid taking into your home new or unknown people in a live-in arrangement.
- Ask for help when you need it from a lawyer, physician, or trusted family member.
- Call Adult Protective Services or Elder Protective Services (found in State Government section of white pages) if you or someone you know suffers abuse.
- Call the ombudsman in State Office of Aging (or 1–800–677–1116) to investigate complaints against long-term care facilities in which you reside.

pears in immediate danger, the nurse should begin appropriate guardianship procedures.

Be aware that advocacy for the abused elder may be difficult; you may receive threats of harm from caregivers who resent the disruption of a previously convenient financial exploitation of an elderly relative. A common situation is when the elder refuses help and desires to remain in an environment that, by your standard, is unacceptable or unsafe. This can be very frustrating. Testifying in court to the nature of specific abusive situations can be anxiety provoking.

PHYSIOLOGIC CONCEPTS

Physical Characteristics

When we are born, regardless of our genetic background or external influences, we all have one thing in common—the element of aging. From the day of birth, we begin the aging process.

The rapidity and manifestations of aging in each individual depend on heredity, past illnesses, lifestyle, patterns of eating and exercise, presence of chronic illnesses, and level of lifetime stress. Some generalized physiologic changes do occur, however; they include a decrease in rate of cell mitosis, a deterioration of specialized nondividing cells, an increased rigidity and loss of elasticity in connective tissue, and a loss of reserve functional capacity (73, 85, 115, 279).

Certain other characteristics have been observed about aging (46, 73, 85, 219, 279):

- Time of onset, type, and degree of aging differ between men and women and are more distinctive between the sexes in middle life than in the later years.
- Senescent alterations in one organ or in the whole organism can be either premature or delayed in relation to the body's total chronology.
- The progression of aging in cellular tissues is asymmetric: the characteristics of old age may be displayed prominently in one system (brain, bone, cardiovascular apparatus, lungs) and be less obvious elsewhere (liver, pancreas, gastrointestinal tract, muscles).
- Certain pathology is a manifestation of aging.
- **Organ reserve,** *the extra capacity of the organs that is drawn on in times of stress or illness,* lessens with age. (In young adulthood, the body can put forth 4 to 10 times its usual effort when stressed.)
- A direct relationship exists between the sum of common aging traits and the length of survival.

General Appearance

The general appearance of the older adult is determined in part by the changes that occur in the skin, face, hair, and posture. Old women have significantly more body fat, greater truncal skinfolds, and greater circumferences than old men and young adult women (192, 279) and less fat-free body mass than young adult women (192).

Skin. The overall appearance of the skin changes dramatically (Table 14–2). Berliner's two articles (29, 30) are excellent references and also contain pictures of various conditions seen in the older adult.

Head. Even the appearance of the *face* changes as the nose and ears tend to become longer and broader and the chin line alters. Wrinkles on the face are pronounced because of the repeated stress produced by the activity of facial muscles. The predominant mood expressed by the facial muscles of the individual becomes permanently etched on the face in the form of wrinkles (smile or frown lines) above the eyebrows, around lips, over cheeks, and around the outer edges of the eye orbit. Shortening of the platysma muscle produces *neck* wrinkles (85, 115, 279).

Gray hair is the universal phenomenon associated with aging, but it is not a reliable indicator of age, as some individuals begin graying as early as their teen years. The hair gradually grays; the exact shade of gray depends on the original hair color. Eventually all the pigmented hair is replaced by nonpigmented hair; gradually the overall hair color turns pure white. Both males and females are affected. The loss of hair occurs on the scalp, in the pubic and axillary areas, and on the extremities. In most older adults there is also increased growth of facial hair due to the change in the androgen–estrogen ratio (73, 85, 115, 279).

Posture. The posture of the older adult is one of general flexion. The head is tilted forward; hips and knees are slightly flexed. Muscles in the torso are held rigidly. The older adult stands with the feet apart to provide a wide base of support. He or she takes shorter steps, which may produce a shuffling gait. A shift in the center of gravity occurs as well, which affects movement and balance (73, 85, 115, 122, 140, 279).

Neurologic System

Nervous System Changes. With aging there are major changes in the nervous system that occur normally and alter the individual's sensory response (38, 45, 69, 73, 83, 85, 86, 115, 140, 279):

TABLE 14–2. ALTERATIONS IN INTEGUMENTARY SYSTEM RELATED TO AGING

Tissue/Organ	Alteration and Rationale	Implications for Health Promotion
Epidermis	Skin manufactures less collagen, elastin, and other proteins. Cellular division decreases; thus, skin cells are replaced more slowly. (Skin cells live an average of 46 days in 70-year-old, compared with 100 days in 30-year-old.)	Wounds heal more slowly. Maintain nutrition and hygiene.
	Elastin fibers are more brittle. Loss of collagen fibers rearranged into thicker bundles causes decreased turgor and loss of elasticity, wrinkles, and creases. Permeability increases and cells are thinner. Ability to retain fluids decreases, causes skin to become drier, less flexible.	Use emollients/lotion to maintain moisture on skin. Avoid hot water baths, excessive soap. Rinse skin well; pat dry. Some medications make skin more fragile and susceptible to bruising: aspirin, prednisone, steroid topical cremes
	Fair-skinned persons lose pink tones, become more pale. **Lentigo senilis,** *irregular areas of dark pigmentation on dorsum of hands, arms, face,* and uneven pigmentation occur. Capillaries and small arteries on exposed skin surface become dilated.	Cosmetics may be used. Protect from direct sun; use sunscreen. Assist person in accepting appearance changes.
	Decreased response to pain sensation and temperature changes may cause accidents or burns.	Teach safety factors. Care with heating pads or hot water bottles and ice packs.
Subcutaneous tissue (hypodermic)	Loss of fat cells, especially in face and limbs, causes sagging and wrinkles. Lack of tissue over bony prominences contributes to decubitus ulcers.	Assist adjustment to appearance and changes. Protect bony prominences from pressure, abrasions, injury, and decubitus ulcers.
	Lower cutaneous blood flow and loss of fat contribute to decreased insulation and susceptibility to chilling.	Provide adequate clothing and heat control for comfort.
Dermis	Decreased fat, water, and matrix content causes translucent appearance of skin. Larger and coarser collagen fibers decrease flexibility of collagen, reduce elasticity, and cause sags and wrinkles.	Emollients/lotions and cosmetics may be used. Assist person in accepting appearance changes.
	Decreased number of fibroblasts and fibers cause thinning tissue.	Avoid bumps, scrapes, and lacerations of skin. Wear protective clothing.
Hair	Reduced melanin production causes graying. Thinning, stiffness, and loss of luster are due to change in germ center that produces hair follicles. Baldness is related to genetics.	Use hair coloring or cosmetic techniques if desired.
Women	Increased facial hair on upper lip and chin are related to diminished estrogen.	Assist person in integrating appearance changes into body image.
Sebaceous oil glands	Decreased lubrication with oil causes skin to be drier, rougher, scaly.	Use emollients/lotions. Avoid hot water, use minimal soap, rinse well. Pat dry. Use room humidifiers.
Sweat glands	Reduced number interferes with ability to sweat freely and regulate body temperature.	Prevent heat stroke. Drink adequate water. Dress in garments that allow heat transmission from body. Use fan or air conditioner as needed in hot weather.
Nails	Growth is slower. Increased calcium deposition causes ridges and thickening.	Encourage visit to podiatrist for care of toenails and cosmetologist for care of fingernails.

- Loss of nerve cells
- Decrease in neurotransmitters
- Slower nerve impulse transmission
- Decrease in nerve conduction velocity
- Decline in electric activity
- Increase in sensory threshold
- Decline in integration of sensory and motor function

All of these neurologic changes create problems for the older adult. For example, by age 70, upper body stiffness, slower voluntary movement, slower decision making, visual changes, and slowed startle response are seen. Because of these particular neurologic changes, older adults do not respond as quickly to changes in their external environment. This slower response affects many facets of their life (e.g., there is greater risk to overall safety, and drivers over 65 years of age are involved in a higher percentage of automobile accidents per mile driven than are drivers aged 25 to 54 years). The older adult's increase in sensory threshold affects pain and tactile perception and response to stimuli, resulting in increased susceptibility to burns or other injuries (85, 86, 115).

Brain. By age 90 the brain's weight has decreased 10% from its maximum and reduction in size is not uniform throughout the brain. This weight loss is accompanied by a reduction of cells in the cerebral cortex and a decrease in the number of functioning neurons in the gray matter, rather than in the brain stem. The white matter is not significantly different than in young people. The void left by these anatomic changes is filled by expanding ventricular volumes in the form of cerebrospinal fluid.

The amount of space between the skull and brain tissue doubles from ages 20 to 70. Reduced cerebral blood flow and oxygenation of the brain and reduced glucose metabolism may alter thought processes and perceptual function. Altered brain waves and sleep patterns, including reduced REM (dream) sleep, contribute to nighttime wakefulness. (Measures to reduce insomnia are discussed in Chapter 12.) Increased activity of monoamine oxidase enzymes may contribute to depression (cognitive therapy discussed in Chapter 5, medication, and measures discussed later in this chapter prevent or reduce depression (69, 83, 86, 140, 279). The anatomic and physiologic changes in the brain of the older adult are not always directly related to performance abilities. Declining human performance in advanced age may be due to deficits in systems peripheral to the central nervous system and/or to other behavioral factors (73, 85, 115, 279).

Vestibular and Kinesthetic Response. The response to vestibular and kinesthetic stimuli decreases with age. The vestibular division of the vestibulocochlear nerve is associated with balance and equilibrium. With aging there is a decrease in the number of nerve fibers, thus affecting balance and equilibrium. Reduction in the number of sensory cells in the utricle, saccule, and semicircular ducts further affects balance. These reductions may begin as early as 50 years of age but are especially noticeable after 70. Vestibular sense receptors are located in muscles and tendons; these receptors relay information about joint motion and body position in space to the

central nervous system. Loss of neurons in the cerebellum that receive the sensory information also contributes to diminished balance (73, 115, 279).

Vision. Visual changes occur. Loss of vision is gradual; fewer than 1% have extremely severe visual impairment. The number of fibers composing the optic fiber decreases over time. Lacrimal glands produce fewer tears, causing the cornea to become dry and irritated. The lens thickens and yellows; objects take on a yellowish hue; and the cells within the lens lose water and shrink. The diameter of the pupil decreases and the pupil is less able to accommodate to light changes. The lack of pupillary response, increased lens opacity, and irregular corneal surface, which causes light to scatter, together result in intolerance to glare and difficulty in adjusting from brightly to dimly light areas, or vice versa. Visual contrast sensitivity for size and light decreases. These changes interfere with the ability to transmit and refract light. Because of loss of elasticity in the lens and slower response in accommodation, **presbyopia,** *inability to change lens shape for near vision,* is present in most adults after age 45 or 50. Even with corrective lenses the individual may need longer to focus on near objects (38, 73, 83, 85).

Color vision is also altered after age 60, because of retinal changes (rods and cones), loss of sensitivity of photoreceptors, and slower transmission of visual impulses to the nervous system. The reception of short wavelengths (blue) is affected first, followed by middle-wavelength hues (green, greenish yellow), and, last, by the longwavelengths (red). Thus, for the older adult, colors such as green, blue, and violet are more difficult to see than are red, orange, and yellow. Pastels fade so that they are indistinguishable from each other; monotones, whites, and dark colors are also difficult to see. Brighter colors compensate for decline in color discrimination and yellowing and opacity of the lens (83, 85, 115)

Cataract development and glaucoma frequently occur in this age group. With **cataracts** the *lens becomes opaque,* accompanied by diminished vision and increased sensitivity to glare. **Glaucoma** is caused by damage to the optic nerve from increased intraocular pressure. These conditions and the other visual changes such as **arcus senilis,** the *accumulation of lipids on the cornea,* can be assessed during periodic eye examinations. The elderly with lens-opacifying disease have increased risk for macular degeneration, regardless of age, sex, or systolic blood pressure (38, 115, 151, 279).

See Table 14–3 for health promotion implications related to visual changes, as well as Guidelines for Helping the Blind Person (46, 69, 73, 83, 136, 140, 220).

TABLE 14–3. NEUROLOGIC CHANGES IN THE EYE: IMPLICATIONS FOR HEALTH PROMOTION

Change	Health Promotion Measure
Dry cornea	Use artificial tears if needed. Wear glasses to protect eyes from dust, flying debris.
Lens changes Presbyopia Spatial–depth vision changes	Wear corrective glasses or contact lens. Use hard lens to magnify print for reading. Obtain books and periodicals in large print or tape-recorded materials. Teach safety considerations; take time to focus for vision. Adapt to yellow vision; teach implications for selecting clothing, cosmetics, or interior decor. Teach safety factors related to doorways, space and objects. It is important for institutions to place color guards on stair steps, to clearly mark doorways; to avoid having carpet, furniture, walls, and drapes all of same or similar color; walls, floor, doors, door frames, and furniture should be clearly delineated.
Pupillary and lens changes: Decreased tolerance to glare or light changes	Wear tinted glass or brimmed hat to reduce glare or bright light. Turn on light in dark room before entering. Stand in doorway or at stairwell briefly to adjust to light changes from either bright light or dark. Teach need for more *indirect* but adequate illumination to perceive stimuli, do visual work. Avoid white or glossy surfaces. It is important for institutions to cover windows and avoid shiny wax on floor. Avoid glare on floor in bedroom, dining areas, lounges, or hallways. Teach safety considerations, especially with driving in bright sunlight or at night. Use night light to allow low-lighted visibility.
Retinal changes: Color vision altered	Teach implications for personal grooming and dress, enjoyment of colors in nature, interior decoration, and design of living environment. Brighter colors are enjoyed. Teach family implications for selecting greeting cards and gifts. It is important for institutions to use colors in interior decor that can readily be seen and enjoyed and not misinterpreted by elderly. Use sharp contrasting colors on doors, strips of contrasting color on bottom of wall, and colored or white strip at edge of each step to assist in distinguishing colors, space, and specific areas. Teach safety considerations to avoid misinterpretation of color or not seeing objects that are pale or light colors.

Hearing. With age, the pinna (external ear) becomes longer, wider, and less flexible; this change does not appear to affect hearing. As cerumen production diminishes and the wax becomes drier, however, blockage of the ear canal can occur. The presence of dried, packed wax can interfere with sound transmission. Any auditory changes that occurred in middle age continue through later life. Men are twice as likely as women to have hearing loss. The tympanic membrane becomes thinner and less resilient and may show some sclerotic changes. In some older adults calcification of the ossicles occurs. There are also changes in the organ of Corti, loss of nerve cells in the eighth cranial nerve, and an increased rate of time for passage of impulses in the auditory nerve. Because of the changes to the inner ear and cochlea, a hearing aid (many are small) or corrective surgery may partially improve hearing; however, a hearing aid magnifies all sounds. If there is **sensorineural deafness,** *damage to the auditory nerve, or the hearing center of the brain* from bacterial or viral infections, head injuries, or prolonged exposure to loud

► GUIDELINES FOR HELPING THE BLIND PERSON

- Talk to the blind person in a normal tone of voice. The fact that he or she cannot see is no indication that hearing is impaired.

- Be natural when talking with a blind person.

- Accept the normal things that a blind person might do such as consulting the watch for the correct time, dialing a telephone, or writing his or her name in longhand without calling attention to them.

- When you offer assistance to a blind person, do so directly. Ask, "May I be of help?" Speak in a normal, friendly tone.

- In guiding a blind person, permit him or her to take your arm. Never grab the blind person's arm, for he or she cannot anticipate your movements.

- In walking with a blind person, proceed at a normal pace. You may hesitate slightly before stepping up or down.

- Be explicit in giving verbal directions to a blind person.

- There is no need to avoid the use of the word *see* when talking with a blind person.

- When assisting a blind person to a chair, simply place his or her hand on the back or arm of the chair. This is enough to give location.

- When leaving the blind person abruptly after conversing with him or her in a crowd or where there is a noise that may obstruct hearing, quietly advise that you are leaving so that he or she will not be embarrassed by talking when no one is listening.

- Never leave a blind person in an open area. Instead, lead him or her to the side of a room, to a chair, or some landmark from which he or she can obtain direction.

- A half-open door is one of the most dangerous obstacles that blind people encounter.

- When serving food to a blind person who is eating without a sighted companion, offer to read the menu, including the price of each item. As you place each item on the table, call attention to food placement by using the numbers of an imaginary clock. ("The green beans are at 2 o'clock.") If he or she wants to cut up the food, he or she will tell you.

- Be sure to tell a blind person who the other guests are so that he or she may know of their presence.

noise, a hearing aid will not improve hearing (73, 83, 86, 140, 279).

About 75% of people in the United States 75 to 79 years of age have hearing loss. Of all individuals over 65, 13% suffer severe **presbycusis,** *progressive loss of hearing and sound discrimination.* The consonants, especially *s, sh, ch, th, dg, z* and *f,* and high-frequency sounds produce problems for the individual with presbycusis. The ability to locate the direction from which sound is coming diminishes, and older people have difficulty hearing individuals who speak rapidly or in high tones (38, 85, 86, 115, 140). For some helpful suggestions, see Guidelines for Communicating With the Hearing-impaired Person (46, 143, 215).

Tactile Acuity. There is a decreased number of nerve cells innervating the skin and thus a decreased response or sensitivity to touch. Even the soles of the feet have fewer sensory receptors and less responsivity. Two-point threshold is one of the oldest measures of spatial acuity of the skin. Age-related deterioration of tactile acuity, like visual and hearing changes, begins in late middle age. Acuity of touch, however, varies with different body regions; the fingertip has more acuity than the forearm for texture and temperature in old age. Acuity is also related to space between stimuli; for example, the fingertip may be sensitive to a single nodule but not as sensitive to the dots of Braille, to the glucose testing monitor used by the diabetic, or to other tactile aids

---

► GUIDELINES FOR COMMUNICATING WITH THE HEARING-IMPAIRED PERSON

- When you meet a person who seems inattentive or slow to understand you, consider the possibility that hearing, rather than manners or intellect, may be at fault. Some hard-of-hearing persons refuse to wear a hearing aid. Others wear aids so inconspicuous or clearly camouflaged that you may not spot them at first glance. Others cannot be helped by a hearing aid.

- Remember the hard-of-hearing may depend to a considerable extent on reading your lips. They do this even though they may be wearing a hearing aid, for no hearing aid can completely restore hearing. You can help by trying *always to speak in a good light* and by facing the person and the light as you speak.

- When in a group that includes a hard-of-hearing person, try to carry on your conversation with others in such a way that he or she can watch your lips. Never take advantage of the disability by carrying on a private conversation in his or her presence in low tones that cannot be heard.

- Speak distinctly but naturally. Shouting does not clarify speech sounds, and mouthing or exaggerating your words or speaking at a snail's pace makes you harder to understand. On the other hand, try not to speak too rapidly.

- Do not start to speak to a hard-of-hearing person abruptly. Attract his or her attention first by facing the person and looking straight into the eyes. If necessary, touch the hand or shoulder lightly. Help him or her grasp what you are talking about right away by starting with a key word or phrase, for example, "Let's plan our weekend now," "Speaking of teenagers. . . ." *If he or she does not understand you, do not repeat the same words.* Substitute synonyms: "It's time to make plans for Saturday," and so on.

- If the person to whom you are speaking has one "good" ear, always stand or sit on that side when you address him or her. Do not be afraid to ask a person with an obvious hearing loss whether he or she has a good ear and, if so, which one it is. The person will be grateful that you care enough to find out.

- Facial expressions are important clues to meaning. Remember that an affectionate or amused tone of voice may be lost on a hard-of-hearing person.

- In conversation with a person who is especially hard-of-hearing, do not be afraid occasionally to jot down key words on paper. If he or she is really having difficulty in understanding you, the person will be grateful for the courtesy.

- Many hard-of-hearing persons, especially teenagers, who hate to be different are unduly sensitive about their disability and will pretend to understand you even when they do not. When you detect this situation, tactfully repeat your meaning in different words until it gets across.

- Teach the family to avoid use of candles. Electric light will give the person a better chance to join the conversation because he or she can see the lips during conversation. Similarly, in choosing a restaurant or night club, remember that *dim lighting may make lipreading difficult.*

- Teach family members that they do not have to exclude the hard-of-hearing person from all forms of entertainment involving speech or music. Concerts and operas may present problems, but movies, plays, ballets, and dances are often just as enjoyable to people with a hearing loss as to those with normal hearing. (Even profoundly deaf persons can usually feel rhythm, and many are good and eager dancers.) For children, magic shows, pantomimes, and the circus are good choices.

- When sending a telegram to someone who does not hear well, instruct the telegraph company to deliver your message, not telephone it.

- The speech of a person who has been hard-of-hearing for years may be difficult to understand since natural pitch and inflection are the result of imitating the speech of others. To catch such a person's meaning more easily, watch the face while he or she talks.

- Do not say such things as "Why don't you get a hearing aid?" or "Why don't you see a specialist?" to a person who is hard-of-hearing. Chances are he or she has already explored these possibilities, and there is no need to emphasize the disability.

- *Use common sense* and tact in determining which of these suggestions apply to the particular hard-of-hearing person you meet. Some persons with only a slight loss might feel embarrassed by any special attention you pay them. Others whose loss is greater will be profoundly grateful for it.

used by the sensory handicapped (73). See Table 14–4 for health promotion implications related to tactile changes.

Taste and Smell. With aging, there is a general decrease in taste perception because of a decline in the actual number of taste buds (about half as many as in young adulthood, but women have more than men.) Diminished taste perception is linked to the changes in the processing of taste sensations in the central nervous system. Taste perception may also be affected by the diminished salivation that occurs in older persons. Usually older adults experience an increased preference for more sugar, salt, spices, and highly seasoned foods.

The sense of smell begins to decline in most people by middle age and continues a gradual decline into old age because the number and sensitivity of receptors decrease, especially after age 80. It is believed that the sense of smell decreases because the olfactory nerves have fewer cells. This diminished sense of smell combined with the decline in taste sensation may account for the loss of appetite experienced by many older adults. The inability to smell also presents hazards for the individual, as he or she cannot quickly detect leaking gas, spoiled food, smoke, or burning food (73, 85, 115, 186, 279).

See Table 14–4 for health promotion implications related to changes in taste and smell.

Cardiovascular System

Although the cardiovascular system undergoes considerable changes with aging (Table 14–5), in the absence of heart disease it is usually able to maintain the daily cardiac and circulatory functions of the older adult. However, the cardiovascular system may not be able to meet the needs of the body when a disease process is present or when there are excess demands caused by stress or excessive exercise. Obesity, physical inactivity, and abdominal fat distribution also reduce physiologic function. See Table 14–5 for cardiovascular changes and implications for health promotion (69, 73, 83, 86, 115, 279).

Respiratory System

Changes produced by aging affect both internal and external respiration; the older adult has difficulty taking oxygen from the atmosphere and delivering it to internal organs and tissues. See Table 14–6 for physiological changes and implications for health promotion (69, 73, 83, 86, 115, 140, 279). Be prepared to do the Heimlich maneuver if the person chokes because of a weaker gag reflex or musculature (see Fig. 14–3).

Musculoskeletal System

The major age-related change in the skeletal system is the loss of calcium from bone. Bone loss is accelerated with the loss of gonadal function at menopause. Therefore, bone loss is greater in females than in males and in older than younger females. Some studies have shown that by age 70 a woman's skeletal frame may have lost 30% or more of its calcium. With this change in bone composition comes a gradual decrease in height, on the average of 1.2 cm for each 20 years of life in both men and women and all races. Decreased synthesis of bone and increased decalcification, or osteoporosis in vertebrae, cause collapse, and loss of collagen and atrophy in intervertebral disks cause the spinal column to compress and posture to become curved or stooped and shorter. In addition to the decrease in height, bone strength is progressively lost because of loss of bone mineral content. Osteoporosis (which is discussed later) is seen as the extreme version of the universal process of adult bone loss (69, 73, 83, 115, 140, 192, 279).

TABLE 14–4. HEALTH PROMOTION IMPLICATIONS FOR OTHER NEUROLOGIC CHANGES

Change	Health Promotion Implication
Vestibular and kinesthetic	Teach safety factors, such as ways to maintain balance and safe walking. Canes, walking sticks, or walkers can be helpful.
Tactile	Use firm but gentle pressure on hand, arm, or shoulder to indicate your presence or soothe with touch. Teach safety factors: 1. Walk more slowly to allow feet to fully touch surface and to be cognizant of foot placement, e.g., on stairs, uneven surfaces, or outdoors. 2. Monitor use of hot water bottles, heating pads, or ice bags to avoid burns or frostbite. 3. Teach ways to avoid bumps or abrasions. Bed-ridden or chair-bound person *must* have position changed frequently to prevent decubitus ulcer.
Taste and smell	Teach need for more seasoning, preferably spices and herbs rather than sugar or salt, to better enjoy food and discriminate tastes. Encourage adequate nutrition. Teach safety factors related to reduced smell, e.g., how to monitor for burning food or gas leaks.

TABLE 14–5. CARDIOVASCULAR CHANGES WITH AGING AND HEALTH PROMOTION IMPLICATIONS

Organ/Tissue	Change and Rationale	Implication for Health Promotion
Heart Internal	At age 70, cardiac output at rest is 70% of that at age 30.	Medication may be needed to maintain adequate function. Exercise routine should be maintained.
	Number and size of cardiac muscle cells decrease, causing loss of cardiac muscle strength, reduction in stroke volume, and less efficient pumping and cardiac output.	Assess for myocardial damage, muscle damage, and congestive heart failure.
	Thickening of collagen in heart valves reduces efficiency of closure because of rigidity. Calcification of valves increases.	Assess for aortic and mitral murmurs, valve stenosis or insufficiency, and endocarditis.
	Thickness of left ventricle wall increases; left ventricle is unable to pump volume of blood in cardiac cycle. Blood flow is maintained to brain and coronary arteries to greater extent than other body parts.	Cognitive, visceral, and muscular functions may not be adequately maintained with less cardiac output and inadequate blood supply.
	Pacemaker cells in sinuatrial node and atrioventricular node are replaced by fibrous and connective tissue, causing delay in nerve transmission and more time to complete the cardiac cycle.	Assess for ectopic activity, arrhythmias, and conduction defects.
External	Increased amount and stiffening of collagen surrounding heart, causing inelasticity. Increased fat deposits on surface of heart, reducing oxygen supply to body.	Maintain fluid balance and adequate aeration; avoid standing too long or constipation to reduce strain on heart. Straining to defecate strains right side of heart as blood suddenly pours through vena cava after pressure is decreased.
Blood vessels	Reduced elastin content and increased collagenous connective tissue in arterial walls reduce elasticity of walls of peripheral vessels as well as aorta and other arteries.	Assess for increased systolic and diastolic blood pressure, abdominal pulsation, bruits, and aneurysms. Orthostatic hypotension may occur; blood pressure falls sharply upon standing. Instruct person to arise to sitting position from lying position; stand slowly to allow for adjustment.
	Atherosclerosis, *increased accumulation and calcification in arterial walls,* makes smaller lumen diameter; vessel walls harder, thicker, and resistant to blood flow; and less rebound to vessel after being stretched. Blood flow is reduced to vital organs; cerebrovascular accidents (strokes) and multifarct dementia may occur.	Low-cholesterol diet should begin in early life, as these changes may occur in early life. Moderately elevated blood pressure may have protective effect on brain. Assess for hypertension, and other circulatory problems.
	Walls of veins are thicker due to increased connective tissue and calcium deposits, decreasing elasticity.	Wear support hose to reduce varicose veins, beginning in early life. Sit with feet and lower legs elevated to enhance return blood flow to heart.
	Valves in large veins may become incompetent; varicose veins are common.	Avoid prolonged standing.

Decreased sensorimotor functions affect postural stability. Increased body sway is associated with reduced visual acuity, tactile sensitivity, vibration sense, joint position sense, ankle dorsiflexion strength, quadriceps muscle strength, and increased reaction time. Peripheral sensation ability is also a factor in sway and maintenance of postural stability (73).

Maintaining upright posture and balance is a complex task. As postural control mechanisms deteriorate with disease and age, the person is more susceptible to falls. Standing on one leg and tandem walking become more difficult. The center of pressure tends not to approach the edges of the base of support as closely as in younger years. One way to determine stability is to measure **functional reach,** *the maximum distance one can reach beyond arm's length while maintaining a fixed base of support in standing position.* Height and age affect reach, but the general ability to reach and the length of reach are related to ability to maintain stability when walking (80).

The older adult experiences a gradual loss of muscular strength and endurance. Muscle cells atrophy, and lean muscle mass is lost. Studies have shown a 30% loss in muscle fiber between ages 30 and 80. In addition, as the elastic fibers in the muscle tissues decrease, the muscles become less flexible, and stiffness is noted more frequently (73, 115, 279).

Changes in body weight also occur in the older adult. These changes follow definite patterns. Men usually exhibit an increase in weight until their middle

TABLE 14–6. RESPIRATORY SYSTEM CHANGES AND HEALTH PROMOTION IMPLICATIONS

Organ	Change and Rationale	Implication for Health Promotion
Nose	Reduced number and activity of cilia cause reduced bronchoelimination.	Less effective clearing of respiratory tract predisposes to infections. Avoid smoke-filled environment. Wear mask if air pollution exists. Avoid allergens. Maintain health status and avoid crowds in winter to prevent respiratory infections and pneumonia.
Throat	Cough reflex decreased. Sensitivity to stimuli decreased.	Teach safety factors, especially when eating (cut food into small portions, chew well, eat slowly).
Trachea	Flexibility is decreased; size of structure is increased.	
Rib cage and Respiratory Muscles	Calcification of chest wall causes rib cage to be less mobile. Decreased strength of intercostal and other respiratory muscles and diaphragm impairs breathing. Osteoporosis of ribs and vertebrae weakens chest wall and respiratory function. Calcification of vertebral cartilage and kyphosis stiffen chest wall and impair respiratory movements.	Maintain exercise, deep breathing, and erect posture to enhance respiratory muscle function. Avoid pressure to ribs to prevent rib fracture (e.g., leaning chest on edge of bath tub).
Lungs	Capacity to inhale, hold, and exhale breath decreases with age. Vital capacity at 85 is 50–65% of capacity at 30. Elastin and collagen changes cause loss of elasticity of lung tissue; lungs remain hyperinflated even on exhalation, and proportion of dead space increases. Decreased elasticity and increased size of alveoli. Increased diffusion and surface area across alveolar–capillary membrane.	Encourage deep breathing, full exhalation, and erect posture throughout life. Maintain exercise to enhance lung function. Activity should be adjusted to respiratory efficiency and ventilation–perfusion ratio.

fifties and then gradually lose weight. Women continue to gain weight until their sixties before beginning a gradual reduction in weight. The most significant weight loss occurs near 70 years of age and is probably due to decreased number of body cells, changes in cell composition, and decreased amounts of body tissue. See Table 14–7 for health promotion implications related to aging changes in the musculoskeletal system (69, 73, 83, 86, 115, 140, 279).

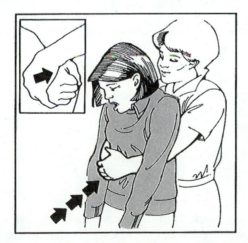

Figure 14–3. Heimlich maneuver. *(From Berger, K.J., and M.B. Williams. Fundamentals of Nursing: Collaborating for Optimal Health. Norwalk, CT: Appleton & Lange, 1992, p. 317.)*

Urinary System

As with the other body systems, major changes in structure and function of the urinary system are associated with aging. The kidneys, bladder, and ureters are all affected by the aging process.

Kidney. The aging kidney suffers a decrease in renal function as one ages. There is a loss of nephrons, the size of the kidney diminishes, and there is a loss of glomeruli—as much as 30 to 40% by age 70. Vascular changes affect the blood flow. Narrowing of blood vessels and vasoconstriction often due to arteriosclerosis and hypertension produce a decreased total renal blood flow. This is more significant than renal tissue loss (73, 129) and causes reduced glomerular filtration rate and tubular function. See Table 14–7 for health promotion implications.

TABLE 14–7. AGING CHANGES AND HEALTH PROMOTION IMPLICATIONS

System/Organ	Implication for Health Promotion
Musculoskeletal	Maintain calcium intake, normal nutrition, and exercise to slow degradation of bone or osteoporosis, to overcome stiffness, and to maintain strength, endurance, and joint mobility.
	Teach safety measures related to less coordination and strength, postural and structural changes, and slower reaction time to avoid falls and fractures.
	Teach ways to arrange the home environment and needed supplies to avoid excessive reach or climbing.
	Use devices to extend arm reach to obtain objects/supplies.
Renal	
Kidney	Avoid **polypharmacy** or *excess medication intake.*
	Assess for drug side effects and toxicity as kidneys are major route of excretion.
	Assess for renal insufficiency if person is dehydrated, hypotensive, feverish, or using diuretics.
Bladder	Maintain adequate fluid intake and frequent toileting.
	Avoid diuretic use afternoon or before long travel.
	Pads may be worn in underpants or lined pants can be worn as precaution.
	Assess for urinary tract infections.
	Explore self-esteem issues related to incontinence.
	Engage in bladder retraining.
Gastrointestinal	
Mouth	Encourage drinking 8 glasses of water daily to avoid dry mouth and dehydration.
	Maintain dental hygiene and care to prevent periodontal disease and loss of teeth.
	Teach new brushing techniques, daily flossing and use of tooth paste with fluoride additive.
	Teach safety factors related to prevention of choking and use of Heimlich maneuver if needed.
Stomach	Encourage adequate nutritional intake, adjusting food texture and taste, as necessary, and with vitamin–mineral supplements if necessary.
	Promote nutrition through programs like senior nutrition sites or Meals-on-Wheels, as needed.
Liver/gallbladder	Encourage adequate protein intake to overcome hepatic synthesis.
	Avoid excessive-fat foods.
	Avoid polypharmacy because of reduced metabolism and excretion.
Bowel	Encourage bulk, vegetables, fruits, and cereals; especially water; exercise; and regular toileting patterns to prevent constipation.
	Avoid daily laxatives if at all possible, but if self-administered for years, it will need to be continued. Mild stool softener is preferred.
Immune	Maintain nutrition, hygiene, and health status to overcome delayed immune response and trend to infections.
	Observe for masked signs of inflammation or infection; e.g., temperature or white blood count may not be as elevated as in middle age.
	Teach safety measures and stress management strategies to overcome delayed or inadequate body response to stress.
	Treat symptomatically for comfort if autoimmune processes occur.

Bladder. The bladder of an elderly person has a diminished capacity—less than 50% that of the young adult—because of atrophy, decreased size and elasticity, and reduced tone (73). Coupled with a delayed desire to void, the elderly often have problems with frequent urination and a severe urgency to void. Aged women are especially prone to incontinence as the pelvic muscles become more flaccid. It is estimated that the United States spends approximately $10 billion a year on this problem. The pelvic diaphragm is the muscle mass that helps maintain bladder tone and proper closure of the bladder outlet. Weakening of the pelvic diaphragm leads to stress incontinence. More that 20% of admissions to geriatric facilities are due to the inability to deal with incontinence (85).

The same factors involved in the problem, reduced urinary capacity resulting in frequency and retention of residual urine, often lead to chronic cystitis, skin irritation, frequent need for antibiotics, and withdrawal from society (149). Urinary tract infections (UTIs) are three times more prevalent in patients who are bowel incontinent. In a study done in a Veteran Affairs Medical Center, *Escherichia coli* was the main organism found in the urine cultures of patients with bowel incontinence. Nurses need to be aware of this when assisting the patient who may suffer from repeated UTIs (168). It may not stem from frank bowel incontinence but there may be sufficient staining to provide contamination, and therefore more frequent hygiene may be advisable. Measures to combat urinary incontinence include regulation of fluid intake, pelvic muscle exercises designed by the physiotherapist, a regular pattern of voiding, and the use of drugs that block the hyperactivity of voiding. Nurses can help immeasurably by establishing routines for toileting and reinforcing the patient with a positive attitude, helping to foster self-esteem and independence.

Hypertrophy of the prostate in the older male is very common and can begin as early as age 40. Irregular changes in the smooth muscle fibers and the prostate tissue occur with age. The problem consists of frequency, especially at night, difficulty starting the stream, dribbling, and retention with overflow. Cancer of the prostrate is the most prevalent malignancy in the male. Therefore, regular physical examinations should be encouraged to screen out the possibility of a malignancy. Some men are concerned about their sexual potency if surgery is to be performed (149). Care should be taken to explain that though external ejaculation will be absent, erection and orgasm will be unaffected.

See Table 14–7 for health promotion implications.

Gastrointestinal System

Changes occur throughout the gastrointestinal system.

Mouth. The oral mucosa atrophies; the connective tissue becomes less elastic; vascular tissue becomes calcified and fibrotic; and nerve cells diminish in number. Tooth decay, loss of teeth, degeneration of the jaw bone, progressive gum recession, and increased resorption of the dental arch interfere with the older adult's ability to chew food. Saliva flow decreases and becomes more alkaline as the salivary glands secrete less ptyalin and amylase. Thirst sensation decreases. All of these changes alter the digestive process at the onset (73, 115). See Table 14–7 for health promotion implications.

Gastrointestinal Tract. Because of decreased stimuli from the autonomic nervous system, peristalsis is slowed the entire length of the gastrointestinal tract. Emptying of the esophagus and stomach is delayed. The gastric mucosa shrinks, causing decreased secretion of pepsinogen and hydrochloric acid, which delays digestion. Digestion is decreased further by the reduction in secretion of hydrochloric acid and pancreatic enzymes. Bile tends to be thicker, and the gallbladder empties more slowly. Hepatic synthesis is reduced. These changes result in a decreased absorption of nutrients and drugs by the gastrointestinal tract. In addition, some older adults do not have enough intrinsic factor and develop pernicious anemia (73, 115).

Elimination of waste products is of equal importance to gastrointestinal function in the aged. The changes in the cell, and therefore in tissue structure, and the loss of muscle tone may decrease intestinal mobility. Elimination depends on fluid intake, muscle tone, regularity of habits, culture, state of health, and adequate nutrition—all of which interrelate. Alterations in many of these areas occur with aging. Poor nutrition and lack of exercise add to the problem.

In the majority of persons over age 65 there is some degree of immobility, either physical, social, or environmental. Physical changes in the tissues combine with this immobility to produce constipation or fecal impaction in circumstances that might not so affect a younger person.

See Table 14–7 for health promotion implications.

Endocrine System

During aging, the ability of endocrine glands to synthesize hormones appears to remain within normal limits, although one study revealed significantly lower total body potassium and total body water levels in older than younger females (192). The number or sensitivity of hormonal receptors, however, may decrease. This means that, even though blood levels remain adequate, there is a lack of response to some hormones; this is especially true of the hormones produced by the adrenal and thyroid glands. Failure to respond to these hormones decreases the individual's ability to respond to stress (73, 112).

Beta cell activity of the pancreas appears altered with age, although the extent varies among people. Decreased insulin response causes hyperglycemia. Aging is associated with elevated glucose levels after ingestion of glucose under the standard conditions of oral glucose tolerance testing. After ingestion of more physiologically mixed meals, a mild degree of postprandial hyperglycemia and hyperinsulinemia can still be demonstrated in the elderly compared with young adults. Postprandial elevations in glucose and insulin levels, however, are much lower after mixed meals compared with that observed during the standard glucose tolerance test. Increased circulating glucose and insulin levels are accompanied by a detectable elevation in hemoglobin A_I concentration. These modest abnormalities, sustained over many years, may contribute to the development of atherosclerosis or other manifestions of aging (73, 115).

The chemical composition of fluids surrounding body cells must be closely regulated, and when analysis of blood shows alterations in blood volume, acidity, osmotic pressure, or protein and sugar content, older adults require a longer time to recover internal chemical equilibrium. Insulin, secreted by cells in the pancreas, normally accelerates the removal of sugar from the blood. In older adults given intravenous insulin with extra glucose, the glucose is removed from the bloodstream at a slower rate than in younger people because of poorer hormone production. Stress intensifies glucose intolerance. Elderly persons undergoing the stress of surgery, illness, injury, or emotional stress may manifest diabetic symptoms; the elevated blood and urinary glucose levels usually return to normal when the stressor subsides (46, 73, 85, 131).

There is decreased metabolic clearance rate and plasma concentration of aldosterone. An increased response by antidiuretic hormone to hyperosomolarity contributes to hyponatremia (73, 112).

Growth hormone, estrogen, and testosterone blood levels do decrease in later maturity. Because of the decrease in estrogen levels after menopause, the breasts of the female have more connective tissue and fat and less glandular tissue. The breast tissues lose elasticity and begin to sag. The lack of estrogen causes the uterus and fallopian tubes to decrease in size. The fallopian tubes also become less motile. The decline of testosterone secretion is not abrupt like that of estrogen. Therefore the changes are less obvious; however, the gradual decline of hormone does increase the incidence of benign prostatic hypertrophy in the older adult male and affects physical reserves, as testosterone has a nitrogen-conserving effect (73, 115).

Immune System

During the aging process, the thymus gland starts to involute and degenerate; the total number of circulating lymphocytes decreases by approximately 15%, and anti-body–antigen reactions decline. In addition, lymphoid tissue decreases, and a general decline occurs in immune responses, including both cell-mediated and humoral immunity (115). The immune system becomes less efficient with aging because of reduced production and function of T and B cells. The reduced T cells may be a factor in increased malignancy rates. Autoimmune responses may increase, causing diseases such as rheumatoid arthritis and other collagen diseases (112). See Table 14–7 for health promotion implications.

Hematopoietic System

There are minor changes in the blood components of the older adult; hemoglobin level, red blood cell count, and circulatory blood volume are not significantly changed. Most of the changes that occur are related to specific pathologic conditions instead of normal aging (73, 115).

Reproductive System and Changes That Influence Sexual Function

Although the male and female experience some common changes as a result of aging, it is well to consider them separately because of certain particular physiologic changes relating to sexual response and vigor.

Male Changes. The production of testosterone continues throughout the man's lifetime, and this hormone is available longer and at a higher level than its counterpart, estrogen, in the woman. As the concentration of the male hormone diminishes, the testes become smaller and softer; the testicular tubes thicken and begin to degenerate; and sperm production decreases or is inhibited. In addition, the prostate gland enlarges, contractions weaken, force of ejaculation decreases, and volume and viscosity of seminal fluid are reduced (112, 115).

In 1970, Masters and Johnson found that as a sexual partner, the older male experiences reduction in the frequency of intercourse, the intensity of sensation, the speed of attaining erection, and the force of ejaculation. *Excitement phase* builds more slowly, and erection takes longer to attain; with diminished vasoconstriction of the scrotum, there is less elevation of the testes. The *plateau phase* preceding orgasm lasts longer, with less muscle tension. There is a reduced or absent secretory activity by Cowper's gland before ejaculation. The *orgasmic phase* is of shorter duration, and the expulsion of the seminal fluid is usually completed with one or two contractions as compared with four or more in the young male. In the *resolution stage,* loss of erection may take seconds as compared with the young man's minutes or hours (191). **Refractory time,** *time needed for another erection,* is extended from several to 24 hours.

Female Changes. In the older adult woman there is a decline in the blood level of estrogen because of reduced ovarian function after menopause. This reduction in hormone causes the vaginal wall to shrink and thin and the vaginal and cervical secretions to diminish and become more acid. These changes may produce pruritis as well as **dyspareunia** (*pain on intercourse*), which can restrict sexual activity. In addition, the size of the clitoris is slightly smaller, and lubrication from the Bartholin glands decreases. With the loss of subcutaneous body fat, the vulva and external genitalia shrink (73, 112, 115).

Female sexual performance in later maturity reveals no reduction in sexual desire or excitability with advancing age. Regular sexual stimulation and activity seem to overcome the effects of estrogen starvation. Studies reveal an increase in masturbation for relief of sexual tension in postmenopausal women into their sixth and seventh decades and for men over age 65. There may be an increased level of sexual desire among women after hysterectomies, indicating that there is no connection between fertility and libido. Studies have indicated that women who have been exclusively homemakers and mothers have greater difficulty in meeting the advancing physiologic changes than women who have combined the role of homemaker with a career (73, 85).

Yet neural and hormonal changes can combine to affect her sexual activity. In the *excitement phase* of coitus, vaginal lubrication is reduced and takes longer to appear. There are less flattening and separation of the labia major and decreased vasocongestion of the labia minora. Atrophy or thinning of vaginal walls causes the vagina to be less elastic (less depth and breadth). Muscle tension is reduced. During the *plateau phase,* there is less vasocongestion and less secretion from the Bartholin glands. All of these changes make penetration more difficult and less comfortable. During the *orgasmic phase,* there are fewer contractions of the uterus and vagina. During the *resolution phase,* the vasocongestion of the clitoris and orgasmic platform quickly subsides. Burning and frequency of urination may follow intercourse as the atrophic bladder and urethra are not adequately protected. Thus, the sex act may become less satisfying and even painful. A number of diseases and some medications can cause impotence. See References 144 and 191.

Sexuality. It is well known that stress, hormonal activity, general health, and aging can each be assessed according to measurable standards. The data are sufficient to infer that psychological influences can be exerted to produce physiologic change in young and old alike. Because of the relationships between the mind and body and the interdependence of all body systems, societal attitudes regarding the characteristics and needs of older citizens are crucial to their quality of life.

There is no doubt that normal aging of the reproductive system decreases efficiency and lengthens time for response for both men and women, but unlike other organ systems that perform more specific functions, the reproductive system extends far beyond procreation. It is deeply tied to the need for interpersonal communication, and it involves that warmth and comfort found only in body contact. When one is old, the yearning for intimacy, security, and belonging becomes intensified as other privations are felt keenly: loss of friends, job status, active participation in parenting or career, and decision making.

The older person is not a nonperson sexually. Research about sexuality in people between the ages of 60 and 91 years indicates the following:

- Ninety-seven percent like sexual activity.
- Seventy-five percent think intercourse feels as good now, or better, than it did when they were young.
- Seventy-two percent are satisfied by their sexual experiences.
- Ninety percent think sexual activity is good for their health.
- Women are more satisfied with activities such as sitting close to someone and talking and saying and hearing endearments if sexual intercourse is not a choice.
- Men are more satisfied with reading or watching erotic materials and caressing another person's body if sexual intercourse is not a choice.

The person's sense of self-worth and the partner's physical health status are positively related to the continuance of sexual intercourse (46, 85, 86).

Nutritional Needs

Special problems exist in the nutrition of older people. Factors that affect nutrition and their clinical manifestations are described in Tables 14–7 and 14–8. Although caloric requirements are lower than in earlier life, the elderly require somewhat greater amounts of some of the vitamins and trace elements. Ensuring enough protein in the diet each day is probably the greatest dietary problem in meal planning for the elderly person who lives alone, for he or she often wants foods that can be

TABLE 14–8. FACTORS THAT MAY AFFECT NUTRITION IN LATER MATURITY

Factor and Process	Effect	Clinical Manifestation
Ingestion		
Loss of teeth; poor dentures; atrophy of jaws	Improper mastication; deletion of important foods from diet	Irritable bowel syndrome; constipation; malnutrition
Dietary habits	Overeating; eccentric diets	Obesity; malnutrition
Psychological losses and changes; changes in social environment; lack of socialization	Poor appetite	Anorexia; weight loss
Reduced income; difficulty with food preparation and ingestion	Excessive ingestion of carbohydrates	Obesity; malnutrition
Decreased fluid intake	Dry feces	Impacted stools
Digestion and Absorption		
Decreased secretion of hydrochloric acid and digestive enzymes	Interference with digestion	Dietary deficiencies
Hepatic and biliary insufficiency	Poor absorption of fats	Fat-soluble vitamin deficiency; flatulence
Atrophy of intestinal mucosa and musculature	Poor absorption; slower movement of food through intestine	Vitamin and mineral deficiencies; constipation
Decreased secretion of intestinal mucus	Decreased lubrication of intestine	Constipation
Metabolism		
Impaired glucose metabolism and use	Diabetic-like response to glucose excesses	Hyperglycemia; hypoglycemia
Decrease in renal function	Inability to excrete excess alkali	Alkalosis
Impaired response to salt restriction	Salt depletion	Low-salt syndrome
Decline in basal metabolic rate	Lower caloric requirements but same amount of food eaten	Obesity
Changes in iron and calcium (phosphorus, magnesium) metabolism	Iron deficiency; increased requirements for calcium	Anemia; demineralization of bone; osteoporosis
Changes in vitamin metabolism	Deficiency in vitamins K and C especially	Peripheral neuropathy, sensorimotor changes; easy bruising and bleeding tendencies

prepared and chewed easily, and he or she may seldom eat meat. Milk products may be poorly tolerated, especially in dark-skinned people, because of decreased lactase, the enzyme for digesting lactose. Fermented products such as cheese, yogurt, and buttermilk may be tolerated well and supply needed calcium (299). There must be enough vitamin coenzymes to ensure metabolism of these three nutrients and absorption of enough bulk elements to maintain a balance of sodium, potassium, calcium, magnesium, and other trace element cofactors for metabolic needs. Because foods today are subjected to many refinement processes with the loss of some vitamins and essential elements, supplements are often recommended. The same food groups are the foundation of a balanced diet for the elderly as in any life stage. Plan a diet that is (65):

- Limited in total fat and cholesterol and that contains the recommended types of fat
- Relatively high in complex carbohydrates and fiber
- Moderately restricted in sodium, as appropriate
- Adequate in calcium (1000–1500 mg daily), other minerals, vitamins, and protein
- High in nutrient density, especially in the presence of anorexia or feeding difficulties

Sufficient water or other fluid intake is essential. Fluid intake is often reduced in seniors for several reasons:

- The aging process reduces the thirst sensation.
- The senior who has incontinence problems limits fluid intake to reduce output.
- Fewer meals are eaten; opportunity for fluid intake is less apparent.
- The senior who takes a diuretic wrongly assumes fluid intake should be reduced.

At least six or seven glasses (8 ounces) of water should be ingested daily to (1) soften stools; (2) maintain kidney function; (3) aid expectoration; (4) moisturize dry skin; and (5) aid absorption of medications, bulk laxatives, and high-fiber foods.

You can help *make mealtime pleasant* for the older person:

- Encourage the person to prepare menus that are economical and easy to shop for, prepare, and consume.
- Encourage the person to do meal preparation to the extent possible.
- The environment should be a comfortable temperature and well lighted so food can be seen.
- Place food where the person can smell, see, and reach it.
- If needed, open cartons and food packets of various sorts and help season the food.
- Keep the tray attractive, neat, and uncluttered to ensure an appetizing appearance.
- Use foods that can be easily chewed and digested.
- Ensure that dentures and eyeglasses are clean and in place on the person at mealtime, instead of in the drawer or on the bedside table.
- Oral hygiene is important and contributes to greater enjoyment of food. Mouth care also promotes healthy tissues in the mouth, thereby keeping the beginning of the alimentary canal intact and functional.
- Do not give medications with meals if avoidable, especially if the medication has an unpleasant taste.
- Offer foods when the person is hungry rather than only at set meal or snack times.
- If necessary, use adaptive feeding devices to help the person feed self.

The elderly are denied many pleasures, and food should not be one of them. Consult with other members of the health team, especially the dietitian and the physician, if there are problems. The family must be included, too, and can often be of great help when there are cultural, religious, or ethnic reasons for a poor appetite. Often the most important member of the team, the client, is not consulted enough; he or she should be the first one involved in planning nutritional needs if at all possible. These same principles can be used as a basis for helping the elderly maintain good nutrition in the home, where, as the community health nurse or primary care practitioner, you may need to make careful assessment of the home situation when problems of poor nutrition exist. Determine whether the problem stems from lack of funds, physical handicaps, family structure, cultural barriers, or any combination of similar unmet needs. Often you will be the one who helps the client contact community agencies, family, church, and whatever other means may be available.

Elderly persons living alone and unable to shop or to prepare food may need the assistance of a home health aide—available through some community agencies—to shop for them and assist with other routines of living. You might arrange to have meals sent in from agencies designed to give this type of service. These programs are discussed more fully later in this chapter under Community Planning.

The whole area of client teaching is affected by the changing needs of the older adult. Adapt your nutrition teaching to these changes and keep in mind the altered responses associated with the aging nervous system.

Rest and Sleep

Rest is of importance. Though older adults may not sleep as many hours as they once did, frequent rest periods and sensible pacing of activities provide the added energy for a full and active life. Rest may consist of listening to soft music, reading, thinking of happy experiences, napping, or merely lying with eyes closed. Some older adults have several 15- to 60-minute naps during the daylight hours.

With so much diversity among the individuals in this age group, it is difficult to state how many hours of *sleep* are recommended. Older adults in reasonably good health probably do not require any more sleep than was required during their middle adulthood.

Aging affects the process of sleep in three areas: length of sleep, distribution of sleep during the 24-hour day, and sleep stage patterns. The older adult requires a somewhat longer period to fall asleep, and sleep is lighter, with more frequent awakenings. The total amount of daily sleep declines as the spontaneous interruption of sleep increases. The older adult may actually spend more time in bed but sleep less, waking with the feeling of inadequate sleep. The time spent in stage IV, the deepest sleep period, and REM sleep decreases. This also contributes to feelings of fatigue (12, 73, 77, 294).

Sleep apnea, described in Chapter 12, occurs in many elderly adults. Persons with sleep apnea are more sleepy during the day than nonapneic individuals; apnea during sleep has a detrimental effect on the well-being of elderly adults, even if oxygen desaturation is mild or moderate. Greater levels of depression and cognitive impairment are seen in sleep apneic elders (12).

Insomnia is a common problem in the older adult. Many factors contribute to this. You can determine the person's usual sleeping patterns, the amount and type of daily activity, and the existence of disturbing environmental conditions. Assess the presence of pain, fear, anxiety, lack of exercise, or depression.

Exercise and Activity

Physical activity that is sensibly paced and gradually increased will promote and maintain health. In a longitudinal study of more than 1700 Caucasian adults over 80 years old, one-third had no difficulty walking $\frac{1}{4}$ mile; lifting 10 pounds; climbing 10 steps without resting; or stooping, crouching, or kneeling. Fifty percent of the women and 42% of the men remained healthy over a 5-year study period. Physical ability was associated with never having had cardiovascular disease or arthritic complaints, few fractures, a body mass less than 75th percentile, and 13 years or more of education. These results indicate that even the oldest old can participate in preventive exercise programs and postpone disability. See Table 14–9 for physical, psychological, and social benefits of exercise (33, 86, 91, 106, 298, 305).

One group of active people is farmers, and farmers age 65 or older generally enjoy better health then city or small-town dwellers of the same age. They have fewer medical conditions and excel at performing tasks. Farmers may be healthier because of their lifestyle, and 70% are married. If you are looking for a 75-year-old who still works, that person is more likely to farm than do anything else; 61% of farmers say they do not expect to stop working (140).

Even if the individual has a decreased exercise tolerance, with supervision a plan can be developed to help him or her achieve higher levels of physical fitness. It is, however, important that the older adult not start an exercise program without consulting the physician, who would be aware of any needed limitations. Table 14–10 lists consequences of not having sufficient exercise (279).

For the individual who is not especially interested in planned exercise programs, you can suggest walking, bowling, golf, swimming, dancing, games such as shuffleboard and horseshoes, and home and garden chores. All of these activities can improve the well-being of the older adult (Fig. 14–4).

An exercise program regularly followed may bring a dimension of dynamic fitness to life that helps him or her move vigorously and live energetically as long as possible. Histories of vigorous persons in their eighties and nineties and even over age 100 show that the majority have been physically and mentally active throughout their earlier lives (46). Movement therapy programs

TABLE 14–9. BENEFITS OF REGULAR EXERCISE

Physical
- Helps slow aging process, regardless of age
- Maintains good health and energy
- Improves general strength and body agility and balance
- Improves respiration and circulation
- Promotes muscle mass, strength, and endurance
- Protects against ligament injuries
- Promotes bone mass formation; slows loss of bone tissue
- Induces better sleep patterns
- Normalizes blood cholesterol levels
- Controls blood sugar
- Normalizes blood pressure
- Improves appetite and digestive processes
- Promotes weight control (moderate exercise burns 240–420 calories per hour)
- Reduces risk of heart disease

Psychological
- Reduces age-related decline in brain's oxidative capacity and improves memory and information processing
- Promotes faster reaction time
- Contributes to improved mood and morale
- Improves cognitive test scores
- Enhances self-confidence
- Maintains interest in life and alertness
- Contributes to sense of control

Social
- Promotes socialization when exercise is included in group activity
- Maintains independence

contribute to improved morale, self-esteem, and attitudes toward aging (106).

Health Promotion and Health Protection

Male and female differences in longevity result from hormones, genetic makeup, natural immunity, and lifestyle behavior. Because of the immunity effects of estrogen, women, statistically, develop heart disease 10 years later than men. In the past, life-style choices of women also gave them a biological advantage—less drinking of alcoholic beverages, less cigarette smoking, more attention to personal health care, and less exposure to risks at work and play. As women are changing their lifestyles, however, the gap between the sexes in health status and longevity is narrowing (86).

TABLE 14–10. CONSEQUENCES OF NOT EXERCISING/BEING SEDENTARY

- Decline in all body systems
- General weakness
- Lower energy level
- Stooped posture
- Muscle tissue replaced by fat tissue
- Atrophy of tissues and functions
- Lower self-concept, self-esteem
- Depressive mood

The focus of health care for individuals in this period of life should be on the prevention of disease and the promotion of health. Although numerous body changes occur with aging, many older adults live active, productive lives. Thorough assessment is essential. Several references are useful (44, 46, 85, 131, 144).

Immunizations

As older adults are more susceptible to acute illnesses, they should be encouraged to avail themselves of recommended immunizations against communicable dis-

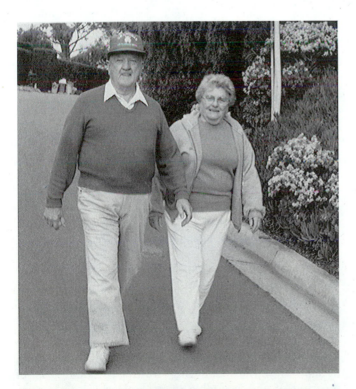

Figure 14–4. Older adults can maintain health and prevent illness by participating in regular exercise. *(From Berger, K.J., and M.B. Williams. Fundamentals of Nursing: Collaborating for Optimal Health. Stamford, CT: Appleton & Lange, 1992, p. 1317.)*

eases. Individuals who garden and participate in other outdoor activities should receive tetanus immunization as indicated. Immunization for influenza and pneumococcal pneumonia is recommended for older adults, especially those with chronic respiratory and cardiovascular diseases. Adults at risk for hepatitis should receive hepatitis B vaccination (see Chart 7 in Appendix IV) (53).

Safety Promotion and Accident Prevention

Older people have a disproportionate share of accidents that cause body injury or death. This is especially true for accidents that occur in the home. Many of these accidents are directly related to physiologic changes that result from normal aging.

Falls in the elderly may occur for a number of reasons:

- Improper use of or incorrectly fitted assistive devices
- Lower-extremity disability
- Decrease in functional base of support
- Vision and hearing impairment
- Arrhythmias, cardiovascular disease, strokes
- Kinesthetic changes, changes in postural reflexes, sway
- Vertigo and syncopal (fainting) episodes
- Peripheral neuropathy
- Inadequate swing foot clearance, tripping
- Depression, inattention
- Excess ingestion of alcohol
- Use of certain medications, e.g., diuretics, sedatives, antibiotics, antidepressants, antipsychotics
- Excess cigarette smoking or osteoporosis, which reduces bone mineral density and can cause fractures resulting in falls

Safety measures to be used by the elderly to avoid injury include the following (6, 7):

- Place padding on hard edges of wheelchairs and over rough or sharp corners or surfaces of furniture, tables, or countertops.
- Pad the wooden or metal arms of chairs used by the elderly.
- Wear gloves to wash dishes or work in the garden to protect hands.
- Wear long sleeves to protect arms.
- Wear long pants to protect the legs.
- Work and walk more slowly to avoid collisions with objects or falls.

Older adults are also particularly vulnerable to fraudulent sales pitches and seemingly honest requests

► SAFETY IN THE HOME: DO NOT BE A VICTIM OF THE CON GAME

- **Carpet cleaner:** Ad offers very low price to clean carpeting in one or more rooms of your house. Workers flood room, ruin carpet, and scheme to charge more than quoted to replace damaged material.

- **City inspector:** "Inspector" says he or she needs to check plumbing, furnace, heater, wiring, trees, or whatever. Once inside, he or she may rob you or insist something needs repair and charge excessively for the job.

- **Home repair or inspection:** "Contractor" offers, for example, to repair, inspect, or remodel your home, exterminate pests, or check for radon or offers work with leftover materials from another job in area. The person will find unnecessary work, resulting in unnecessary expense.

- **Product demonstration:** Agent offers to describe only (not sell) new product if you will sign paper "for my boss" proving he or she did it. Once inside the house, anything can happen.

- **Contest winner:** You are told you have won vacation, auto, or other prize but must send $5 for postage or registration or call 800 number for details.

- **Lottery:** Person offers to sell you winning lottery ticket he or she cannot cash because "I'm an illegal immigrant," or "I'm behind in my child-care payments." Or "law firm" says anonymous donor has bequeathed a winning lottery ticket to you, but first you must send $20 for a computer search to verify your identity.

- **Land sale:** You are promised cheap land or complete retirement and recreational facilities in sunny gorgeous site. The land may not exist, even if you paid for it.

- **Credit or phone card:** Person asks for your credit or phone card number to send you a product, check unauthorized charges, verify insurance, and so on. They can then use your number to charge items.

- **Government service.** Official-sounding firm (e.g., with "Social Security" in name) offers Social Security service that is "required" (e.g., plastic-coated identification cards), "critically needed" (e.g., to help keep agency solvent), or useful (e.g., earnings form). The money sent obtains no service.

- **Mail-order health care or laboratory tests:** You are promised medical care by mail or laboratory screening for AIDS, cholesterol, cancer, hair, and so on. The results are likely to be phony if received at all for the money you sent.

- **Medical products:** You buy health, beauty care, or "cure" product by mail, or you are sent newspaper clipping extolling magic diet with note scribbled across it, "It works—try it!" signed "J."

- **900 number:** Products are offered through special 900 number. (Such numbers are common and legitimate.)

- **Obituary:** You are recently widowed; COD box arrives for product "your husband (or wife) ordered."

- **Pigeon drop:** Person offers to share "found" money with you if you will put some of your own money "to show good faith."

- **Need help:** Man says his wife is sick, his car has been impounded, he has run out of gas, or some such tale; he needs just $10 or $20, promises to pay it back, and shows extensive identification.

- **Unknown callers:** Woman with child knocks on door and asks for some favor requiring entrance.

- **Travel club:** Firm offers bargain airfare or hotel package in glamorous foreign locale. You may never get where you are going or find the accommodations listed.

Modified from Marklein, M., Con Games Proliferate: New Threats Haunt City Folks, *AARP Bulletin*, 32, no. 2 (1991), 1, 16–17.

for help by strangers (see Safety in the Home: Do Not Be a Victim of the Con Game) (190).

Visual Changes. Changes in visual acuity produce numerous hazards for the older adult. The older adult's problems with color interpretation, light intensity, and depth perception should be considered in the home and institutional environment. See Table 14–3 for suggestions on how to assist the elder in maintaining vision comfort and safety. Other suggestions follow.

The environment should be kept free of hazards—no articles on the floor, no furniture with sharp edges, no scatter rugs. The baseboards should be painted a darker color than the walls. Signs should be prepared with dark backgrounds and light lettering. Blues and greens on signs should be avoided. Numbers on doors, elevators, and telephones should be large enough for the older adult to see (38, 120). Encourage use of a magnifying glass for close vision work, a small flashlight to illuminate dim areas, and having properly fitted and cared for eyeglasses. Teach proper care of contact lenses.

Television should be viewed with normal room illumination and at a distance at least 6 ft from the screen. Some persons with impaired vision may have to sit closer. Glasses correcting distance vision should be worn while watching television, and the set should be adjusted as clearly as possible.

Some signs and symptoms indicate the need for appropriate referral to an ophthalmologist:

- Pain in and around eyes
- Headaches, especially at night or early morning
- Mucous discharge from eyes
- Obvious inflammation or irritation of the eyes and surrounding tissue
- Avoidance of activities requiring sight
- Glasses not being worn, missing, or not fitting properly
- Change of previous visual habits (requiring different light or reading distance)

When you are caring for a blind person, follow the guidelines given on p. 713.

Hearing Impairment. Changes in hearing acuity may predispose the person to accident risks. Many elderly persons have been diagnosed as being mentally ill, whereas in reality they were suffering from a gradual loss of hearing. If one is unable to hear clearly, it is easy to imagine one is being talked about or ignored. This leads to depression, and then behavior often is categorized as irrational, suspicious, or hostile. This produces isolation and further frustrations, and the vicious cycle that ensues may in the end cause real paranoia to develop.

Refer to the suggestions on effective communication with the hearing impaired person given on p. 713. Encourage the hearing impaired person to consult with a physician about use of a hearing aid rather than going to a nonqualified practitioner.

Tactile Changes. Changes in *temperature regulation* and the inability to feel pain also produce safety problems. See Table 14–4 for health promotion implications. The elderly usually *feel cold* more easily and may require more covering when in bed; a room temperature somewhat higher than usual may be desirable. Most hospitals and nursing homes do not have thermometers that register body temperatures below 94°F (35°C). Therefore, statistics are not available on how many elderly persons suffer and die from hypothermia. Mildly cool temperatures of 60°F (15.5°C) to 65°F (18.3°C) can trigger hypothermia. A nighttime room temperature of 66°F (18.3°C) can be too low for an aged person. The victim may not be aware of the extreme loss of body heat, especially when supine and relatively inactive.

Clues to *hypothermia* risk or presence follow:

• Medications to treat anxiety or depression, hypothyroidism, vascular disease, alcoholism, and immobility reduce the body's response to cold.
• Living alone or anything that increases nighttime accidents can increase risk, as do poverty and poor housing.
• The elder may insist he or she is comfortable in a cool environment; the person is unaware of the temperature of surroundings.
• The person is not thinking clearly or acting as usual.
• Low body temperature, irregular or slow pulse, slurred speech, shallow respirations, hypotension, drowsiness, lack of coordination, and sluggishness may be present, singly or in combination.
• Coma may occur and is probable when the body temperature is 90°F (32.2°C) or less.

Severe hypothermia can cause complications of kidney, liver, or pancreatic disorders, ventricular fibrillation, and death. Recovery depends on severity and length of exposure, previous health, and the rewarming treatment (46, 85).

Teach the elderly person the following measures to *prevent hypothermia* in cold weather (46, 85):

1. Stay indoors as much as possible, especially on windy, wet, and cold days.

2. Wear layered clothing, and cover the head when outdoors.
3. Eat high-energy foods such as some fats and easily digested carbohydrates and protein daily.
4. Keep at least one room warm at 70°F (20°C) or above.
5. Use extra blankets, caps, socks, and layered clothing in bed.
6. Have contact with someone daily.
7. Avoid drinking alcoholic beverages.

Perception of and reaction to *painful stimuli* may be decreased with age. Because pain is an important warning device serving the safety of the organism, use caution when applying hot packs or other hot or cold applications. The elderly person may be burned or suffer frostbite before being aware of any discomfort. More accurate assessment of physical signs and symptoms may be necessary to alleviate conditions underlying complaints of pain such as abdominal discomfort and chest pain, which may be more serious than the older person's perception indicates.

Dulling of *tactile sensation* occurs because of a decrease in the number of areas of the body responding to all stimuli and in the number and sensitivity of sensory receptors (115). There may be clumsiness or difficulty in identifying objects by touch. The person may not respond to light touch but needs to be touched. Because fewer tactile cues are received from the bottom of the feet, the person may get confused about position and location. These factors, combined with sensitivity to glare, poorer peripheral vision, and a constricted visual field, may result in disorientation, especially at night when there is little or no light in the room (46). Because the aged person takes longer to recover visual sensitivity when moving from a light to a dark area, night lights and a safe and familiar arrangement of furniture are essential. Sensory alterations may require modification of the home environment and extra orientation to new surroundings. Simple explanations of routines, location of the bathroom, and the way the signal cord works in the hospital are just a few examples of information the older client needs. Objects in a familiar environment should not be moved. Use touch, if acceptable to the person. Increased hairbrushing or combing, back rubs, hugs, and touch of shoulders, arms, or hands increase tactile sensation.

Understand that some of the changed behavior, discussed later under Psychological Concepts, is directly related to physical changes in nerve and sensory tissue and influences nursing practice, whether you are giving physical care, establishing a relationship, providing a safe environment, or planning recreational needs. Research indicates that hand, foot, and eye preference becomes more right-sided and ear preference becomes more left-sided with advancing age. Adapt nursing care measures to accommodate these changes. The whole area of client teaching is also affected, because you must understand the altered responses and the changing needs of the elderly before beginning their health education.

Special Considerations in the Physical Examination of Older Patients

In carrying out any particular physical assessment in the older adult, the nurse may need to modify some procedures to glean the most information. Even helping the patient undress gives the nurse opportunity to observe the patient's ability to perform the task and to note anything unusual, for example, condition of clothing, personal hygiene, or clothing that may be inappropriate for the season or temperature (thermal underwear in August).

Orthostatic vital signs are valuable in the elderly, as heart rate response to postural change may alter decisions regarding hyper- or hypotension.

Attention needs to be given to avoid discomfort, maintain the patient's dignity, and distinguish signs of disease from changes typical of normal aging.

Another important observation is the palpation of temporal arteries. Checking for tenderness or thickening may raise the possibility of temporal arteritis, especially in a patient with jaw pain, temporal headaches, earache, or unexplained fever.

The following are specific ways to increase patient comfort:

- Warm the examining room sufficiently (75°F).
- Use chairs that are high enough to make rising easy.
- Provide a footstool for getting on and off the table.
- Place a pillow under the head and perhaps under the knees, as many elders feel a strain on the back when lying supine.
- Place grab bars near the scale.
- Minimize positional changes during the examination.

Other important areas of exploration in the elderly are hearing acuity; condition of dentures; suspicious lesions under the tongue; jugular venous pulse; carotid arteries for bruits; and breast examination, including the skin under pendulous breasts.

Suspected urinary incontinence can be tested by having the patient hold a small pad over the urethral area and coughing three times in a standing position. Cystocele, rectocele or uterine prolapse should be ruled out, and in the male a digital rectal examination should be done to check the prostate.

Examination of the elder patient's feet is most important; also, have the patient sit up and hang the feet down to check the venous flow. Are the patient's shoes appropriate for good balance and prevention of falls? The patient's gait can offer significant clues, for example, the Parkinsonian gait shown by short, shuffling steps, short or absent arm swing, and a stooped trunk (92).

Common Health Problems: Prevention and Treatment

The health problems of the older adult may be associated with the aging process, a disease state, or both. Yet more than 90% of the elderly need no help with activities of daily living (298). You should consider all of the aspects of aging before deciding on a course of action. Refer to a medical–surgical nursing text for in-depth information on health problems. Other references will also be useful (38, 46, 73, 85, 103, 131).

Table 14–11 summarizes common neurologic and respiratory diseases; blood dyscrasias; genitourinary, skeletal, and cardiovascular diseases; and tuberculosis. Sexual function diseases and substance abuse are also presented in overview (46, 73, 85).

Heart disease is the number one killer for men and women; however, men and women differ in the classic warning symptoms. Men are likely to experience **angina,** *a severe squeezing pain that radiates to the neck, upper abdomen, or left arm and occurs during stress or exertion.* Women are more likely to experience shortness of breath or profound fatigue that occurs in activities they previously found easy to do. Or they may have nausea, heartburn, or indigestion unrelated to anything recently eaten (95, 123).

Stroke (cardiovascular accident) is the third most common cause of death. Excessive adiposity in adults aged 65 to 74 seems to influence risk of stroke in conjunction with hypertension, diabetes, and other cardiovascular disease risk factors; therefore, control of weight and fat remains an important concern as people age (74).

Cancer is the second leading cause of death; pneumonia/influenza and chronic obstructive lung disease rank fourth and fifth as causes of death (123). Other prevalent disorders are arthritis, diabetes, hypertension, and osteoporosis (279). Elderly men are more likely to commit suicide than any other age group in the United States, and Caucasians, in contrast to other

TABLE 14–11 COMMON HEALTH PROBLEMS IN LATER MATURITY

Problem	Definition	Symptoms/Signs	Prevention/Treatment
Neurologic Diseases			
Herpes zoster (shingles)	Caused by same virus that causes chicken-pox Involves dorsal root ganglia	Unilateral vesicular eruption that follows dermatomes of affected nerve root Severe pain; rash that progresses from macules to crusting pustules	Analgesics; cool soaks; acyclovir (Zovirax) Investigation of underlying immunologic problems
Parkinson's disease	Slowly progressive degenerative disorder of nervous system	Resting tremor; masklike face; shuffling gait; forward flexion; muscle weakness; rigidity	Symptomatic; medicine to correct depleted dopamine and rid excessive acetylcholine
Alzheimer's disease	Presenile dementia or neural atrophy	Cognitive, physical, and emotional deterioration	Treatment extremely varied, depending on areas affected Much support and understanding needed from families and caretakers; in turn, families and caretakers need support
Respiratory Diseases			
Chronic obstructive pulmonary disease	Consists of three components: bronchitis, bronchoconstriction, and emphysema	Three components: (1) bronchitis—excessive mucous and sputum production with inflammation of the bronchi; (2) bronchoconstriction—narrowing airways; (3) emphysema—irreversible destruction of distal air space Shortness of breath, sputum production, wheezing, tachypnea, hyperinflation	Smoking cessation; increased fluids; yearly influenza vaccine; one-time pneumonia vaccine; bronchodilator; expectorants as necessary; avoidance of sedatives and cold, wet weather; postural drainage; antibiotics if infection General attention to proper nutrition, rest, and hygiene
Blood Dyscrasias			
Pernicious anemia	Progressive megaloblastic microcytic anemia that results from lack of intrinsic factor essential for absorption or vitamin B_{12}	Weakness, numbness, tingling of extremities; fever, pallor; anorexia, weight loss	Vitamin B_{12} injections; folic acid and iron medications
Secondary anemia	Reduced hemoglobin, hematocrit, and red blood cell counts, resulting from nutritional deficiency, blood loss, and primary problem	Fatigue, shortness of breath, lightheadedness, skin pallor; sometimes arrhythmia	Iron preparation or perhaps blood transfusion; maintenance or stable activities of daily living; attention to primary issue
Chronic lymphocytic leukemia	Neoplasm of blood-forming tissue	Characterized by small, long-lived lymphocytes, chiefly B cells in bone marrow, blood, liver, and lymphoid tissue	Complexity of disease dictates seeking medical–surgical text
Hodgkin's disease	Malignant disorder	Characterized by painless progressive enlargement of lymphoid tissue	Complexity of disease necessitates seeking medical–surgical text
Genitourinary Diseases			
Benign prostatic hypertrophy **(BPH)**	Overall enlargement of prostate gland via enlargement of fibrous and muscular tissue	Difficulty in stopping and starting urinary flow; voiding frequent small amounts Diffuse enlargement of prostate; landmarks preserved	No medical treatment; possible surgical intervention; rule out cancer
Skeletal Diseases			
Osteoporosis	Absence of normal quantity of bone Predisposes to fracture	Loss of normal cortisol thickness; increased porosity in cortical bone; thinning, fragmentation and loss of trabeculae in cancellous bone	Prevention: diet in earlier years containing adequate calcium, vitamin D, phosphorus, protein, and fluoride

(*continued*)

TABLE 14–11 COMMON HEALTH PROBLEMS IN LATER MATURITY (continued)

Problem	Definition	Symptoms/Signs	Prevention/Treatment
Osteoarthritis	Degeneration of articular cartilage and hypertrophy of bone	Pain and stiffness, mainly in weight-bearing joints and dorsal interphalangeal joints of fingers	Exercise to improve stiffness; rest to help pain; heat, antipyretic, adequate nutrition, physical therapy
Cardiovascular Diseases (Congestive) heart failure	Cardiac function altered so that there is not enough cardiac output to meet demands of tissue metabolism; consequently sodium and body water are retained	Arteriosclerotic heart disease and hypertension precursors; depressed breathing (unless sitting or standing); ankle swelling; frequent nighttime voiding; weight gain; distended neck veins; rales in lungs; heart with "gallop rhythm"	Low-sodium diet; correct high blood pressure with angiotensin-converting enzyme (ACE) inhibitors, nitrates, and other vasodilators; chemical trials being done with calcium channel blockers, prostacycline analogs, and oral inotropes; rate and rhythm regulated with digitalis preparation; urinary output increased with diuretics
Chronic occlusive arterial disease of the extremities	Because of partial or complete occlusion of one or more peripheral blood vessels, decreased blood flow to one or more extremities	Diabetes often a precursor; cramping pain in the muscles during exercise that is relieved by rest; sometimes nighttime cramping; extremity may feel cool; pulses may be decreased; skin may lose hair and appear shiny	Evaluate for revascularization; practice good skin care; avoid excess heat or cold; avoid tobacco and caffeine; drugs not effective
Stasis ulcer of the lower extremity	Chronic ulcerative skin lesion caused by venous stasis and consequent poor circulation	Peripheral pulses intact, **pitting edema** (*induration remains after pushing in skin and tissue with a finger*) or **brawny edema** (*thickened and hardened skin*) around ulcer site	Rest and elevation of involved leg; once or twice daily cleaning with povidone–iodine (Betadine) or hydrogen peroxide solution; occasionally application of moist heat or Unna boot; watch for widening of lesion and cellulitis
Infectious Diseases Tuberculosis (not yet common, but reemerging)	Infectious disease transmitted by airborne route and caused by *Mycobacterium tuberculosis;* infection refers to successful colonization in a host; active disease indicates pathogenic process	Chronic flulike cough, decreased appetite, weakness, weight loss, continued slightly elevated temperature, night sweats, dyspnea on exertion, pain with respiratory movements if pleura involved, rales over apex of lung, hoarseness if larynx involved, dysphagia if pharynx involved	TB skin testing, x-ray if indicated, sputum testing, multiple-drug therapies (isoniazid, rifampin, pyrazinamide, and ethambutol or streptomycin); appropriate infection control techniques for both patient and those in contact with patient

racial groups, are the most likely to use firearms for suicide (147).

Diseases That Affect Sexual Function

Health problems associated with the *sexual changes* of aging are of concern to the older adult. Certain diseases in the elderly female have been linked to estrogen deficiency. There is a statistical rise in atherosclerosis attacking the coronary arteries in aged females (and in younger women who have had ovaries removed); women treated with estrogen therapy have had fewer myocardial infarctions. Although there is no clear-cut case for a cause-and-effect relationship, the female hormones apparently are crucial to the enzymatic system in the metabolism of fats and proteins.

Factors that contribute to *sexual dysfunction* are essentially the same as those that affect performance at any age: disease or mutilating surgery of the genitourinary tract, diverse systemic diseases, and emotional disturbance coupled with societal attitudes. Treatment of

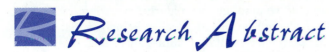

Research Abstract

Finfgeld, D., Becoming and Being Courageous in the Chronically Ill Elderly, Issues in Mental Health Nursing, *16, no. 1 (1995), 1–11.*

A sample of 21 persons, aged 67 to 94, were interviewed to learn about the courage that is developed in chronically ill elders as they deal with declining physical and mental ability and severe health care problems. The sample was composed of 10 men and 11 women, all Caucasian, Christian persons living in the community, who had varying educational and socioeconomic backgrounds. Cardiovascular problems were the most common. Grounded theory methodology and qualitative data analysis were used. Results indicated that becoming and being courageous involved a number of components, including learning as a result of a threatening experience, transforming a struggle into a challenge by problem solving, and courageous actions. Courageous behaviors involved a sense of acceptance, equanimity, and personal integrity that evolved as the person struggled with the stressors of chronic illness. The elders were determined to get on with their lives regardless of the hardships. Assuming responsibility for self-care was one of the struggles and necessitated problem solving. Over time, courageous behavior became part of the lifestyle. Courageous behavior was maintained through encouragment from significant others, role models who were struggling with similar issues, health care providers, and a personal value system and sense of hope.

You can promote becoming and being courageous through several interventions:

1. Assist clients to recognize that developing courage is lifelong.
2. Assist clients to maintain ties with friends and family members.
3. Foster a support group that will act as a role model for learning attributes of courage.
4. Provide clients with accurate information.
5. Sustain courage and enhance problem solving through realistic optimism.
6. Discuss the process of becoming and being courageous to help individuals identify their courageous behavior.
7. Be patient and nonjudgmental as elders use trial-and-error methods to develop courage.

the aged for a physical complaint often contributes to widespread use of drugs. Tranquilizers can give way to excessive use of alcohol or marijuana. They weaken erection, reduce desire, and delay ejaculation. Many of the metabolic disorders are overlooked and go untreated; anemia, diabetes, malnutrition, and fatigue may negatively affect the quality of life and cause impotence. Obesity may impose a hazard for cardiac and vascular integrity and at best is damaging to a healthy self-image.

Many older persons are under the false impression that any sexual activity will increase the danger of illness or even death because of stress on heart or blood pressure. In truth, oxygen consumption, heart rate, and blood pressure increase only moderately during intercourse and may actually afford a distinct therapeutic and preventive measure. In persons with arthritis, for example, the increase in adrenal corticosteroids during sexual activity relieves some of the symptoms. The present-day practice of prescribing exercise for cardiac patients attests that sexual intercourse need not be considered dangerous for anyone able to walk around a room.

Radical surgery or dysfunction of the genitourinary tract produces the most devastating effects on sexual capacity and libido. Extensive resectioning due to malignancy may make intercourse difficult if not impossible. Although a decline in desire and capacity for climax may follow hysterectomies, they are by no means inevitable. The loss of childbearing ability and the lack of an ejaculation are for some women and men psychologically traumatic, and these clients may need some support and guidance in adjusting to change.

Nursing care involves first a reexamination of one's own bias about sex and sexuality in the aged. Human sexuality covers a wide spectrum, and the pattern for each individual is a product of prenatal development and postnatal learning experiences coupled with one's inherent sense of personal identity within a sex classification. This basic pattern is not altered simply by age. It continues to mediate one's capacity for involvement in all life activities.

With this in mind, nursing care planning for the elderly can be made most effective. Realizing the need for sexual expression in some form or other, nurses can be open and nonjudgmental when clients display a desire for warmth, close contact, and companionship. Touch is particularly important to the older person who has been bereft of family ties, perhaps for many years. Some people require more relief from sexual tension than others. If incidents arise that seem unduly unorthodox, such as open masturbation or unusual behavior with the opposite sex, the nurse can be a support person if there is a sincere desire to be available for counseling. An atmosphere of trust must prevail in which the nurse focuses on the person and not on any specific act.

Exploring alternate lifestyles with persons who are single, alone, and old may be a way for the nurse to assist. Teaching that includes information about therapy available, such as estrogen replacement, when there are emotional or physiologic problems associated with the climacteric can help the elderly woman to choose treatment. A thorough knowledge of anatomy and physiology of normal aging is essential for the nurse who cares for the elderly. Only then can information be accurate and teaching effective. The nurse also has a responsibility to communicate to the families and friends of the older client and to colleagues the information that will help in dealing with their inability to understand the sexual needs of the aged.

Intervention can include the following:

- Becoming better educated about sexuality
- Increasing self-awareness
- Discussing openly sexuality with peers, staff, and students
- Attempting to manipulate the environment of the aged client to provide a healthier milieu in which relationships can be a source of comfort
- Evaluating own behavior in terms of intimacy, touch, friendships, and interest in the aged
- Above all, accepting the challenge ourselves to live fully and to assist the aged in our care to do the same

Pharmacokinetics and Aging Changes

Changes in brain structure and function in the aging process may potentiate the effects of alcohol and other psychoactive drugs. Total body water content decreases by 10 to 20% from ages 20 to 80, and extracellular fluid volume decreases by 35 to 40%. An increase of 18 to 36% in total body fat occurs in men and an increase of 33 to 45% occurs in women from 20 to 80 years. Alcohol, which distributes in body water, has a smaller water distribution volume in the elderly, resulting in higher blood alcohol levels. Medications that are fat soluble have a large distribution volume, lower serum levels for a single dose, longer elimination times, and, thereby, greater cumulative and toxic effects. Serum albumin decreases from a mean of 4.7 mg/dL in the young adult to 3.8 mg/dL in the elderly. Albumin is the major drug-binding protein; a decrease in albumin level may result in higher levels of free medication, less therapeutic effect, and increased drug–drug interactions. Aging affects both the liver and kidneys, reducing the rate of medication elimination and increasing the side effects or toxicity. Blood flow and oxidative enzyme levels decrease with age, which affects disposition of medications and contributes to less therapeutic effects (73).

Magnesium toxicity may occur in older people who regularly ingest large doses of magnesium-containing antacids for indigestion and constipation. Symptoms include muscle weakness and incoordination, drowsiness, and confusion; coma occurs in severe cases (18).

Table 14–12 lists magnesium-containing drugs that are often used by the elderly (18). This is just one example of how you need to be observant about medications ingested by the elderly and to educate about adverse effects.

Substance Abuse

Approximately 10 to 15% (more than 2 million) of elderly Americans suffer from alcoholism, and an increasing number are abusing not only prescription drugs, but also heroin, LSD, marijuana, and cocaine. Contrary to popular opinion, they can be successfully treated.

TABLE 14–12. MAGNESIUM-CONTAINING MEDICATIONS

Antacids	Laxatives
Gaviscon	Citrate of magnesia
Maalox Heartburn Relief	Epsom salts
Mylanta	Milk of Magnesia
Di-Gel	
Mylagen II	**Analgesics**
Milk of Magnesia	Backache Caplets
Simaal Gel	Doan's Arthritis Pain Formula
Mag-Ox-400	Bufferin
Uro-Mag	Bayer Select Backache Pain Formula
Riopan	

There are two types of elderly alcoholics: those who began alcohol abuse in their youth (approximately two-thirds of the elderly) and those whose minimum drinking habits increased in old age as a reaction to and way to cope with various problems and losses. Widowers constitute the largest proportion of late-onset elderly alcoholics (85).

Because alcohol is a central nervous system depressant, there are some adverse effects of alcohol abuse. With low blood levels, the person may feel relaxed and comfortable. With increased blood levels, the person may feel a sense of stimulation, but in reality the brain centers lose ability to check belligerent or antisocial behavior. Alcohol also interacts with various drugs, through either potentiation of or interference with medication action, as shown in Table 14–13. Other effects such as loss of coordination, slower reflex reaction time, and slower mental response cause the person to be accident prone, which may in turn cause injury, fractures, or death. Excess alcohol intake and, as a result, poor dietary intake, malabsorption, and progressive liver damage cause hypomagnesemia and hypocalcemia, resulting in osteoporosis and avitaminosis, causing various deficiency states. Esophagitis, erosive gastritis and ulcer formation, pancreatitis, and liver cirrhosis are serious diseases that may hasten death. Cancer of the mouth, pharynx, and esophagus is more common in the alcoholic. Finally, excessive alcohol intake may cause pneumonia, respiratory failure, or cardiac failure and death.

As a nurse, your acceptance of, listening to, and assessment of the elderly person in various health care sites can be critical for diagnosis and treatment. You are a liaison between the client and other professionals and can facilitate treatment of the alcoholism and prevention or treatment of various complications. Further, your education and support of the family and client can foster their acceptance of the diagnosis and pursuit of treatment. See Reference 215 for additional information on alcohol and drug abuse (signs and symptoms, treatment, and nursing care).

Failure-to-Thrive

Annually a small percentage of frail old elders are admitted to hospitals with the diagnosis, **failure-to-thrive,** *a complex presentation of symptoms causing gradual decline in physical and/or cognitive function that occurs without immediate explanation.* The weight loss, disability, and social withdrawal may be caused by hidden organic illness, polypharmacy, malnutrition, depression, age-related changes, an inadequate support system, accompanied by denial of symptoms, feelings of great loss and grief, helplessness, loneliness, and giving up. Without adequate care, the person is likely to die prematurely (28, 154).

A holistic focus, involving a multidisciplinary team, is needed in care and treatment. Besides the necessary physical measures, reminiscence and life review therapy, remotivation therapy, and promotion of a relationship and social support system will be necessary to help the person gain physical and emotional energy to survive (28, 154).

PSCYHOLOGICAL CONCEPTS

The psychological and socioeconomic concepts of aging are significant for all who work with the aged, and you will find older people concerned and needing to talk about the many changes to which they must adjust. Knowledge of the crises in this life stage is necessary if you are to aid clients and families in the attainment of

TABLE 14–13. ALCOHOL INTERACTIONS WITH MEDICATIONS

Alcohol Taken With Medication	Effect on Person
Antidiabetic agents	Increased hypoglycemia; increased effects of alcohol
Anticoagulants	Increased effect; possible hemorrhage
Barbiturates	
Tranquilizers	
Narcotics	Increased central nervous system depression, oversedation
Antidepressants	
Antihistamines	
Anesthetics	
Antibiotics	Inhibition of antimicrobial action

developmental tasks, in meeting the crises, and in the early or appropriate treatment of these crises.

Cognitive Development

One universal truth that concerns the process of aging is that its onset, rate, and pattern are singularly unique for each person. Within the individual, the cognitive functions do not change or decline at the same pace. Some will not decrease at all; for example, memorization of facts may be difficult but wisdom will be evident. This is especially true of psychological and mental changes, which generally have a later and more gradual onset than physical aging. Many factors must be considered when assessing the intellectual functioning of older people:

- Overall health status, as physical health can affect the level of psychological distress, life satisfaction, and cognitive ability (that is, anemia, lung disease, poor circulation, blood pressure or blood sugar changes, hypothyroidism, and fluid or nutritional imbalance can profoundly affect mental status).
- Medications (prescribed and over-the-counter) that are being taken (Some drugs slow or interfere with cognitive processes because of toxicity related to slower elimination from the body. Drug overdose or **polypharmacy,** taking *excess and unneeded combinations of drugs, may cause drug interactions, toxicity, confusion, or depression,* and must be avoided with careful monitoring and adjustments.
- Sensory impairments (vision, hearing) that interfere with integration of sensory input into proper perception, consequent learning, and appropriate behaviors
- Sociocultural influences
- Motivation
- Interest
- Educational level
- Time since school learning
- Isolation from others
- Deliberate caution
- Using more time to do something, which others may interpret as not knowing
- Adaptive mechanism of conserving time and emotional energy rather than showing assertion

The initial level of ability is important: a bright, 20-year-old will be a bright 70-year-old. Overall, mental ability is incremental (76, 176, 229, 254, 279).

The elder demonstrates **crystallized intelligence,** *knowledge and cognitive ability maintained over the lifetime, dependent on sociocultural influences, life experiences, and broad education, which involve the ability to perceive relationships, engage in formal operations, and understand the intellectual and cultural heritage.* Crystallized intelligence is measured by facility with numbers, verbal comprehension, general information, and integrative and interpretive ability. It is influenced by the amount the person has learned, the diversity and complexity of the environment, the person's openness to new information, and the extent of formal learning opportunities. Self-directed learning opportunities and educational opportunities to gain additional information increase crystallized intelligence after 60 years of age (254).

A decline occurs in many people after the late seventies. The loss of biological potential is offset by acquired wisdom, experience, and knowledge. In contrast, **fluid intelligence,** *independent of instruction, social or environmental influences, or acculturation and dependent on genetic endowment, is less apparent. It consists of ability to perceive complex relationships, use of short-term or rote memory, creation of concepts, and abstract reasoning.* Fluid intelligence is measured by ability to do tasks of memory span, inductive reasoning, and figural relations. (The fluid intelligence actually begins to decrease in middle age.) There is, however, no uniform pattern of age-related changes for all intellectual abilities, nor is there a consistent decline in all elders (254).

Intellectual plasticity refers to the fact that the *person's performance or ability can vary a great deal, depending on social, environmental, and physical conditions,* for example, time to do a task, anxiety about evaluation, attention to or motivation for task, amount of environmental stimulation, or cognitive training or education (279).

The senior performs certain cognitive tasks more slowly for several reasons:

- Decreased visual and auditory acuity.
- Slower motor response to sensory stimulation.
- Loss of recent memory.
- Divided attention.
- Greater amount of prior accumulated knowledge and learning that must be scanned and appropriately placed mentally.
- Perceived meaninglessness of task.
- Changed motivation.

He or she may be less interested in competing in timed intellectual tests. Reaction time is also slower when the person suffers significant environmental or social losses, is unable to engage in social contact, and is unable to plan daily routines. The person who is ill often endures environmental and social losses by virtue of being in the client role. Thus, he or she may respond more slowly to your questions or requests (46, 229, 254, 279).

Range of intellectual functioning is quite wide; although there is an average of decline in IQ test scores for people over 60, some people over 60 score higher than some of their younger counterparts. When retested in later life, there is typically little decline in test scores. Further, IQ test results are based on speed; they are timed tests. All research findings show that there is an age-related decrease in the speed of almost all behavioral processes. Thus, older people carry out the same processes as do younger adults, but at a slower rate. (Results of intelligence quotient tests may reflect the stress of having to cope with the test more than actual intelligence.) Overall, general and verbal intelligence, problem solving, coordination of ideas and facts, judgment, creativity, and other well-practiced cognitive skills and wisdom are maintained even into old age if there is no deterioration caused by extensive physical or neurologic changes. Further, *memory can be improved* with skills training and motivational incentives (140, 279).

Studies indicate that elderly adults are equivalent to young adults in cue use, encoding, specificity, decision-making speed, design recognition, and spatial memory or awareness of location, especially when distinctive cues are available. Other studies indicate that cognitive performances of young and old adults are comparable when the task is divided or attention has not been interrupted, on assessing contents and products of memory and on recall and recognition of factual information (69, 73, 83, 86, 140, 279).

Older women excel over men in verbal ability and speed of reaction. Older people are able to tolerate very extensive degenerative changes in the central nervous system without serious alteration of behavior if their social environments are sufficiently supportive. If their environment was restricted in early life, however, learning is inhibited in later life. Mental functions, especially vocabulary and other verbal abilities, do not deteriorate appreciably until 6 to 12 months before death (174).

Table 14–14 summarizes types of cognitive functions, characteristics of the elderly, and health promotion implications (69, 83, 86, 140, 279).

Cognition and intellectual development are part of maturity. It is in the last half of life that the person best draws on cumulative experiences to establish social, moral, and ethical standards; render decisions; assist in planning; erect social guideposts; and establish pacific relationships between oncoming generations. The judgmental functions of the mind are most highly developed after midlife (88, 174).

Creativity is evident in the later years. The following are important to remember as you teach, assist, and advocate for the elderly (279):

- People are not identical to others in creative output at any age. Expected age decrement in creativity varies across disciplines; in some there is scarcely a decline at all.
- Creative output of the person in her or his sixties or seventies will most often exceed that produced in the twenties as long as the person is healthy
- Creative output changes in relation to role changes in career or profession rather than in relation to age.
- The person with a late start in career or profession usually reaches a later peak and higher output in the last years.
- Reduced creative output does not mean corresponding loss of intellectual or motivational capabilities.
- Factors such as health and reduced vigor may interfere with creative output but can be overcome with individual motivation and assistance to the person.
- Creativity can resurge in life's last years.

In your care of the older person and in teaching about cognitive characteristics of later maturity, recognize that the normal aging brain, free of disease, may function as effectively and efficiently as the normal young adult brain except for speed and recent memory. Significant cognitive impairment is related to disease, not normal aging.

The elder can be taught to remember essential information (see Effective Memory Strategies) (140).

Use the following *suggestions when you teach:*

- Always approach the teaching situation in a way that enhances the person's self-concept and self-confidence.
- Keep in mind and assess the elder's experiences, current knowledge, needs, interests, questions, health status, and developmental level as you plan and implement teaching.
- Minimize distracting noise; select a comfortable setting.
- Tell the person that you are planning a teaching session, state the general topic, and emphasize importance. Get the person's attention and increase anticipation.
- Arrange for the person to be near the teacher, teaching aids, or demonstration.

TABLE 14–14. COGNITIVE DEVELOPMENT IN THE OLDER YEARS

Characteristic	Change During Aging	Implication for Health Care
Sensory memory	Large amount of information enters nervous system through the senses; selective attention occurs. Some information is sent to short-term memory for further processing; some is lost because nervous system cannot process.	Avoid sensory overload. Assist hearing, visual, and tactile functions. Recognize that person may be inattentive to your teaching or to their symptoms or situation. Use variety of teaching methods, include visual aids. Teach importance of health maintenance, as healthy elders maintain general intellectual function.
	First step of memory process involves recall that lasts a few minutes.	
Short-term memory	Brain holds information for immediate use: conceptualization, rehearsal, memorization, association with long-term memory. Deals with current activities or recent past of minutes to hours. Remains consistent with earlier abilities. Older person can repeat string of digits as well as younger person unless asked to repeat them backward; information about digits fades in about a minute unless person rehearses it. Overall mental status is poorly correlated with short-term memory. Recall is better for logically grouped, chunked, or sequenced information.	Give attention for memory abilities. Teach importance of continuing to use memory, memory retrieval tricks, or cues. Teach person to use variety of associational and memory strategies to enhance recall. Teach relaxation methods to reduce anxiety about memory and enhance attention, rehearsal, motivation, and general function. Teach cognitive tricks or use of lists or ways to organize information to improve memory or remember essential information. Teach person to overcome interferences. Let person set own pace to enhance learning and memory.
Long-term memory	Use of information acquired, transferred for storage, and stored over years. Unlimited, permanent storehouse of memories which may not have to pass through short-term memory. Involves images (mental pictures) and verbalization. Three encoding systems are used: visual–spatial, verbal sequential, and abstraction.	Give attention for memory abilities. Recognize that dysfunctions in short- and long-term memories occur independently. Encourage person to use memories and associations in tasks.
Declarative (episodic)	Conscious memory of specific persons, places, events, or facts that is acquired quickly, but may not be accurately or easily recalled. Requires intact hippocampus. Older person stores long-term memories, but does not retrieve as quickly as younger person unless he or she uses memory tricks.	Give person adequate time for recall. Encourage use of memory tricks and associations.
Recognition	Involves selecting correct response from incoming information rather than recall or retrieval. Ability is retained with age for words, background, familiar objects.	Give support and recognition for ability to recognize and use information.
Implicit (reflexive)	Unconscious learning of information or skill through experience or practice (e.g., playing piano, riding bicycle). Requires intact cerebellum. Ideas, concepts, or ability to perform readily remembered. Does not weaken with age in absence of pathology, as person can demonstrate if not discuss.	Use practice in learning new skills for self-care. Reinforce use of habits. Encourage reminiscence or life review. Use habits and well-practiced skills when possible in teaching or assisting them. Encourage continued practice of implicitly learned tasks or information.
Reaction time (RT)	Speed of response slows during life, and is more obvious after age 60 because of central nervous system changes; shorter duration of alpha rhythm in brain wave (RT fastest between ages 20 and 30). RT remains faster in males than females. RT remains accurate even if slower in both sexes in older adult.	If the person is hurried, response quality and quantity will be reduced. Allow person to proceed at own pace in learning, making decisions, or doing tasks. Do not consider slower response the same as confusion or dementia.
Attentional selectivity	Gradual reduced ability in focusing on a specific idea or event, especially as the information processing demands of the task increase. As capable as younger people in correcting unanticipated errors.	Call attention to specific tasks or ideas that the person must focus on when teaching or counseling. Recognize and reinforce capabilities.
Problem solving	Skills increase steadily into old age; performance unrelated to IQ test scores or formal education. Person adopts simpler judgmental strategies and relies on preexisting knowledge moreso than young adult. In low-memory-demand tasks, elder is more efficient than young adult. Is better at complex judgmental strategies than young adult.	Teach importance of continuing cognitive function. Engage person in goal setting and problem solving.

(continued)

TABLE 14–14. COGNITIVE DEVELOPMENT IN THE OLDER YEARS (continued)

Characteristic	Change During Aging	Implication for Health Care
Dialectical thinking	Older people better able to see all sides of a situation and come to conclusion that integrates different viewpoints and contradictory ideas when given time and when experience rather than memory is required. Is better at solving conditional-probability problems than young adult. Is better at telling integrated story than young adult.	Listen to what may appear to be rambling or loose associations as ideas are likely to be related and pertinent.
Social awareness	Increased knowledge and empathy related to culture, living, value systems, or application of ethical and moral principles. Social responsibility traits remain stable or increase in older adult.	Recognize and reinforce capabilities. Use older people as consultants and teachers of the culture.
Higher mental functions: Calculations, abstract reasoning	Involves integrity of several cognitive functions and exercising values and judgment in decision making and problem solving, logical thinking, future planning, comparison and evaluation of alternatives in context of reality and social responsibility, considering consequences of action. These functions are vulnerable to neurologic pathology; loss of abstraction ability may be first sign of disease or dementia.	Encourage person to remain active in situations or roles that require use of cognitive abilities, e.g., volunteer, mentor, teaching aide, organizational committees, political activities.
Creativity	Productivity continues into old age. Aesthetic sense and appreciation of beauty continue to develop.	Provide pleasing environment and opportunities for creativity. Teach family and elder that intellectual and creative mastery of the world exists in many forms and manifests itself daily.
General knowledge	Maintains or improves into old age, especially in vocabulary, verbal abilities, and verbal comprehension. General task-specific skills remain equal to those of young adult.	Encourage person to remain active in family and community; participation is a predictor of ability. Reinforce knowledge and wisdom and combat ageism. Teach health promotion as physical health can affect mental function.
Academic performance	Elderly students in college perform as well as younger students, tend to have fewer problems, and are able to use new technology and equipment.	Encourage elder to participate in classes, continue learning in credit or noncredit courses or in elder hostel.
Spatial discrimination	High-level cortical function related to (1) visual and kinesthetic senses; (2) frontal lobe (motor skill) and parietal lobe (association) functions; (3) ability to produce accurate representations of the way in which objects or parts of objects relate to each other in space; (4) interpretation of directions and top/bottom and visual and spatial cues. Loss of impairment occurs independent of altered sensory function, language dysfunction, or position sense. Older adult tends to need more time and be less accurate in case of maps or finding directions.	Teach spatial cues. Recognize impact on rehabilitation. Test for constructional ability (copy geometric figure or draw face of clock) and general orientation to determine early brain dysfunction. Observe for unilateral neglect of body, inattention to objects or people in left half of sensory field. Assist with and teach family about self-care and safety implications.
Wisdom	Superior knowledge and judgment with extraordinary scope, depth, and balance applicable to specific situations and the general life condition. Increases because of empathy and understanding developed over the years. Depends on cognitive and personality factors as well as virtue (character).	Acknowledge the elder's wisdom, creative ability, and productivity. Encourage family to use elder as confidante and consultant.

- Consider the aged person's difficulty with fine movement and failing vision when you are using visual aids.
- Provide adequate lighting without glare; do not have the person face outdoor or indirect light.
- Use sharp colors with a natural background and large print to offset visual difficulties.

- Explain procedures and directions with the person's possible hearing loss and slowed responses in mind.
- Use a low-pitched, clear speaking voice; face the person so he or she can lip read if necessary.
- Teach slowly and patiently, with sessions not too long or widely spaced and with repetition and reinforcement.

► **EFFECTIVE MEMORY STRATEGIES**

Selective Encoding (getting information into memory)

- Actively and creatively try to find meaning in facts
- Underline selectively; outline
- Distinguish between important and nonimportant points/facts
- Summarize main points
- Reconstruct facts; test self

Elaboration

- Use imagery, visualization of content
- Use metaphor
- Use analogy
- Paraphrase in own words
- Encode more than one strategy

Organization

- Understand how information is organized
- Choose appropriate and effective retrieval cues
- Be aware that related items may cue memory
- Reorganize information so new material better relates to prior knowledge

External Representation

- Take notes; outline
- Make charts, diagrams, tables, or graphs
- Make conceptual map

Monitoring

- Test self
- Check where errors are made; correct errors

- Give the aged person time to perceive and respond to stimuli, to learn, to move, to act.
- Help the person make associations between prior and new information and emphasize abilities that remain constant to enhance recall and application.
- Have the person actively use several sensory modalities to make motions and repeat the content aloud verbally while seeing or hearing it.
- Plan extra sessions for feedback and return demonstrations and extra time for these sessions.
- Whenever possible, include a significant other in the teaching session to ensure further interpretation and support in using the information.

Two forms of recall serve as therapeutic interventions: reminiscence and life review. Reminiscence and life review differ but share some characteristics: (1) both use memory and recall; (2) both can be structured or free-flowing; (3) both can involve happy or sad feelings; (4) both serve a therapeutic function; and (5) both are implemented primarily with elderly but can be used with middle-agers or young adults, especially in terminal illness. **Reminiscence** involves *informal sharing of bits and pieces of the past that surface to the consciousness and involves the feeling related to the memories. Thus, this memory process includes affective and cognitive functions*. It is an oral history.

Goals for *use of reminiscence* include the following:

- Provide pleasure and comfort (but sad memories also come forth)
- Improve self-confidence
- Improve communication skills
- Increase socialization, decrease isolation
- Improve alertness, connectedness with others
- Increase deeper friendships
- Promote role of confidante
- Promote ego integrity
- Obtain data

During *reminiscence therapy*, your role is to:

- Encourage informal, spontaneous discussion
- Be supportive, provide positive atmosphere
- Avoid probing or pushing for insight
- Allow repetition in the person's discussion
- Encourage the person to integrate the happy and sad memories
- Allow the person to evaluate implications or prior outcomes as memories are recalled, if desired
- Validate and support the meaningful contributions and activities of past life

- Mentally "walk through" or imagine a task through verbal explanation before it is to be done to enhance recall.
- Material should be short, concise, and concrete; present material in a logical sequence; summarize often.
- Break complex tasks or content into smaller and simpler units; focus on a single topic to promote concentration.
- Match your vocabulary to the learner's ability and define terms clearly and as frequently as needed.

- Use themes or props, if desired, to stimulate discussion, especially in a group
- Avoid focusing on issues or judgment of memories

Life review involves *deliberately recalling memories about life events; it is the life history or story in a structured autobiographical way. It is a guided or directed cognitive process, used with a goal in mind.* It may include reminiscence and affective functions.

Goals for use of life review include the following:

- Increase self-esteem
- Increase life satisfaction, or well-being
- Increase sense of wisdom, validate wisdom
- Increase sense of peace about life
- Decrease depression
- Integrate painful memories, crises, unmet needs, unfulfilled aspirations
- Promote ego integrity, resolve self-despair
- Work through prior crises, events, traumas, relationships

During *life review therapy,* your role is to:

- Accept the story but encourage a life span approach
- Convey empathy for experiences and feelings (happy and sad)
- Validate and support values being expressed
- Allow repetition to promote necessary catharsis
- Discuss issues that arise so they can be resolved
- Reframe events if the person cannot do so
- Encourage the person to evaluate prior responses, achievements, or ways of handling a situation
- Allow the focus to remain on the person's own self.
- Validate that which has been meaningful in life to the person
- Recognize that the person may not ever really resolve or accept the multiple losses that have occurred (Sadness may remain.)

These measures, combined as necessary, allow for comprehension and appropriate response and compensate for decline in perception, memory, and slower formation of associations and concepts.

Emotional Development

The older person experiences emotions at least as intensely as young adults (259). The physiologic response to emotional stress, for example, increased blood pressure, takes longer to return to baseline in older than younger adults. There is less variability in emotional responses within a day, probably an adaptive response. Further, because the older person's expectations about the ability to control events changes with age, the person is less likely to evidence negative affect than would be expected. Emotional responses become less unidimensional with age; for example, love may be less euphoric and become more bittersweet the second or third time around. Positive emotions acquire negative loading over time, and vice versa. Identical events may elicit different emotions over time, and events that elicited emotional response earlier may no longer do so. Multiple roles in old age are linked to greater psychological well-being and flexibility in emotional responses overall (69, 83, 140, 279).

Erikson (89), describing the eight stages of man, states the developmental or psychosexual task of the mature years is ego integrity versus despair. A complex set of factors combines to make the attainment of this task difficult for the elderly person.

Ego integrity is the *coming together of all previous phases of the life cycle* (89). Having accomplished the earlier tasks, the person accepts life as his or her own and as the only life for the self. He or she would wish for none other and would defend the meaning and the dignity of the lifestyle. The person has further refined the characteristics of maturity described for the middle-aged adult, achieving both wisdom and an enriched perspective about life and people. Even if earlier development tasks have not been completed, the aged person may overcome these handicaps by associating with younger persons and helping others resolve their own conflicts. Historical situation, family environment, marital status, and individual development all influence the integrity achievement (88, 174).

Use the consultative role to enhance ego integrity. Ask the person's counsel about various situations that relate to him or her personally or to ideas about politics, religion, or activities current in the residence or institution. Although you will not burden the person with your personal problems, the senior will be happy to be consulted about various affairs, even if his or her advice is not always taken. Acting as a consultant enhances ego integrity. Having the person reminisce also promotes ego integrity, and reintegration and recasting of life events put traumatic events into perspective.

The person who has achieved ego integrity remains creative. Decrement in achievement is rarely so substantial that the person becomes devoid of creativity at life's end. Even an octogenarian can expect to produce many notable contributions to any creative activity, as has been witnessed with artists, composers, and statesmen. Creativity in the late years depends on initial creative potential, but creativity may lie dormant during the demanding young adult years. The older adult has many of the necessary qualities for creativity: time, accumulated experience, knowledge, skills, and wisdom. Often the changes mandated by retirement and late life trigger new creative levels, including those in ordinary people (279).

Without a sense of ego integrity, the person feels a sense of **despair** and **self-disgust**. *Life has been too short and futile. The person wants another chance to redo life.* Refer to Consequences of Self-despair or Self-disgust for a list of feelings and behaviors that are part of self-despair (88, 89). Feelings of despair and disgust about self are compounded by the relationship losses suffered and the consequent loneliness and hopelessness that may occur. Having no confidant or companion and physical health status are both related to the emotional status (37, 86, 88, 276, 291). Suicidal thoughts or attempts may result; this is a growing problem (202). Jung (142) believed the old person could not face death in a healthy manner without some image of the hereafter. He believed the unconscious has an archetype of eternity that wells up from within the person as death nears.

Nursing care for the person in despair involves use of therapeutic communication and counseling principles, use of touch, and being a confidant so that the person can work through feelings from the past and present ones of sadness and loneliness. The maintenance phase of the nurse–client relationship is important, as the person needs time to resolve old conflicts and learn new patterns of thinking and relating. The person can move to a sense of ego integrity with the ongoing relating of at least one caring person—a person who listens; meets physical needs when the person cannot; nurtures and encourages emotionally; brings in spiritual insights; validates the senior's realistic concerns, fears, or points of anguish; and listens to the review of life, patching together life's experiences. Another reference furnishes more detail (215).

Personality Development and Characteristics

No specific personality changes occur as a result of aging: values, life orientation, and personality traits remain consistent from at least middle age onward. *The older person becomes more of what he or she was.* The older person continues to develop emotionally and in personality but adds on characteristics instead of making drastic changes (142, 182, 216, 254). If he or she were physically active and flexible in personality and participated in social activities in the young years, these characteristics will continue appropriate to physical status and life situation. If the person was hard to live with when younger, he or she will be harder to live with in old age. The garrulous, taciturn person becomes moreso, and problems of control and dominance are common. Stereotypes describe the older person as rigid, conservative, opinionated, self-centered, and disagreeable to be with. Such characteristics are not likely to be new; rather they are an exaggeration of lifelong traits that cannot be expressed or sublimated in another way.

Personality Types

Studies of large samples of seniors reaffirm their uniqueness, but researchers have categorized the variety of their behaviors.

Four personality types were described by Neugarten (216, 217): integrated, defended, passive dependent, and disintegrated.

The **integrated personality** type is characteristic of most elderly. These people function well and have a complex inner life, intact cognitive abilities, and competent ego. They are flexible, open to new stimuli, and mellow. They adjust to losses and are realistic about the past and present. They have a high sense of life satisfaction. The integrated group is made up of three sub-

► ## CONSEQUENCES OF SELF-DESPAIR OR SELF-DISGUST

- Discusses unresolved conflicts related to people or life situations
- Wishes to relive life, redo life course; fears death
- Suspicious or hypercritical of others; angry toward others, especially significant others
- Has a sense of overwhelming guilt, shame, self-doubt, self-disgust, inadequacy
- Disengages from others; withdraws from people or life's interests
- Feels worthless, a burden
- Demonstrates decreasing cognitive competence
- Discusses lack of accomplishments in life or unfinished endeavors
- Is lonely, has had few relationships
- Describes desire for relationships, a confidant, companion
- Feels hopeless, helpless, sad, depressed
- Has suicidal thoughts or behavior

types: reorganizers, focused, and disengaged. The *reorganizers* engage in a wide variety of activities; when they lose old roles and related activities, they substitute new ones. They are as active after retirement as before. The *focused* are selective in their activities; they devote energy to a few roles that are important to them rather than being involved in many organizations. The *disengaged* are well-integrated persons who have voluntarily moved away from role commitments. Activity level is low but not because of external losses or physical deficits. They are self-directed and interested in the world but have chosen the rocking-chair approach to life without guilt. They are calm, aloof, but contented. Thus, Neugarten defines the disengaged person differently from Cumming and Henry (216, 217).

The **defended personality** is seen in ambitious, achievement-oriented persons who have always driven themselves hard and who continue to do so. They have a number of defenses against anxiety and a tight control over impulses. This "armored" group has medium to high life satisfaction. The defended group is made up of two subtypes: those who hold on and the constricted. The *holding on* persons have a philosophy of, "I'll work until I drop." So long as they can keep busy, they can control their anxieties and feel worthwhile. The *constricted* are preoccupied with their losses and deficits. They have always shut out new experiences and have had minimum social interactions. Their caution continues as they try to defend themselves against aging. Nevertheless, they are satisfied with life, possibly because they know nothing different (216, 217). Most seniors are resourceful and psychologically healthy.

The **passive-dependent personality** type is divided into two patterns: succorance-seeking and apathetic. The *succorance-seeking* have strong dependency needs and seek help and support from others. They manage fairly well as long as they have one or two people on which to lean. They have medium levels of activity and medium life satisfaction. The *apathetic* have an extremely passive personality. They engage in few activities and little social interaction. They have little interest in the world around them. They believe that life has been and continues to be hard and that little can be done about it. They have low satisfaction with life (216, 217).

The **disintegrated** or **disorganized personality** type describes a small percentage of elderly who show gross defects in psychological functions and deterioration in thought processes. They may be severely neurotic or psychotic. Yet these elderly are not necessarily institutionalized. They may manage to live in the community because of the forbearance or protection of others around them.

Personality and Lifestyle Types

These types were categorized extensively for women and men in one longitudinal study. Results of the study showed a diversity of behavior in seniors. No correlations existed between personality and lifestyle, and spouses did not show similar personality types. Health status strongly influenced lifestyle and personality characteristics; healthy people were more active and involved in life roles. Evidence supports the general hypothesis that personality characteristics in old age are highly correlated with early life characteristics. Although early adult lifestyles are more likely to continue into old age for men than for women, the early life personality of women is more likely to continue into old age than the early personality type of men (182).

Although the popular stereotype is that women cannot cope effectively, this study revealed that *all* women, even those who were more rigid in ego defenses, were higher in ability to cope than in ego disorganization and women were more adaptable than men. Whenever defensiveness or ego disorganization does occur, it is related to general personality predisposition throughout life, outlook on life, and physical health (182).

Personality problems in old age are related to problems in early life. Even when the younger years are too narrowly lived or painfully overburdened, the later years may offer new opportunities. Different ways of living can be developed as the social environment changes and as the person also changes. Later maturity can provide a second and better chance at life (88, 182).

Authors cited personality trends that are commonly found in the elderly. Some difference is noted between the earlier and later decades of later maturity.

Young-Old Personality

In the *young-old* person (65 to 75 or 80 and sometimes beyond) (174), the personality is frequently flexible, shows characteristics commonly defined as mature, and is less vulnerable to the harsh reality of aging. The person manifests self-respect without conceit; tolerates personal weakness while using strengths to the fullest; and regulates, diverts, or sublimates basic drives and impulses instead of trying to suppress them. He or she is guided by principles but is not a slave to dogma; maintains a steady purpose without pursuing the impossible goal; respects others, even when not agreeing with their behavior; and directs energies and creativity to master the environment and overcome the vicissitudes of life (40, 43).

Motivations change; the senior wants different things from life than he or she did earlier. Concerns about appearance, standards of living, and family change. Stronger incentives, support, and encouragement are needed to do what used to be eagerly anticipated. He or she avoids risks or new challenges and is increasingly introspective and introverted.

The elderly are tough; they often endure against great physical and social odds. Experience has taught the senior to be somewhat suspicious as he or she is likely to be a victim of "borrowings," a fast-sell job for something he or she does not need, thievery, or physical attacks.

Yet generosity is a common trait of the elderly; the person gives of self fully and shares willingly with people who are loved and who seem genuinely interested in him or her.

The elderly person hopes to remain independent and useful as long as possible, to find contentment, and to die without being a burden to others. Increasingly, dependency may undermine self-esteem, especially if the person values independence.

Personality characteristics differ for men and women, especially in relation to assertiveness. The man becomes more dependent, passive, and submissive and more tolerant of his emerging nurturant and affiliative impulses. The woman becomes more dominant and assertive and less guilty about aggressive and egocentric impulses. Perhaps the reversal in overt behavior is caused by hormonal changes. Perhaps the man can be more open to his long-unfulfilled emotional needs when he is no longer in the role of chief provider and no longer has to compete in the work world. Perhaps the woman reciprocates in an effort to gratify needs for achievement and worth; she expresses more completely the previously hidden conflicts, abilities, or characteristics (217).

Old-Old Personality

Old-old age (80 or 85 years and beyond) (174) is a time for meditation and contemplation, not camaraderie. Camaraderie is for young people who have energy and similarities in background, development, and interest. Old-old people may be friendly and pleasant, but they are also egocentric. Egocentricity is a physiologic necessity, a protective mechanism for survival, not selfishness. Life space shrinks. When old-old people get together, certain factors block camaraderie, even if they want to be sociable: varying stages of deafness and blindness, other faulty sense perceptions, and the fact that they may have little in common other than age and past historical era. Old-old people are even more unique in the life pattern than young-old people because they have lived longer. Further, they have less energy to

deal with challenging situations, and relating to a group of oldsters can be challenging (40, 43). There is increased interiority in the personality (218).

The person in later maturity, especially in old-old age, may be called childish. Rather, the person is child-like; he or she pays attention to quality in others. He or she senses when another is not genuine or honest—as a person or in activities. The old-old person reacts with sometimes exasperating conduct because he or she sees clearly through the facade and lacks the emotional energy to be as polite as earlier. Self-control, willpower, and intellectual response are less effective in advanced age. Many of the negative emotional characteristics ascribed to the elderly may be based on this phenomenon. Only the very simple, those who have not grappled with the complexities of life, or the very ill and regressed will be infantile.

The old old have greater need than ever to hold onto others. They are often perceived as clingy, sticky, demanding, loquacioius, and repetitious. This often causes the younger person to want to be rid of the senior, which causes a vicious circle of increased demand and increased rejection.

Preoccupation with the body is a frequent topic of conversation, and other elderly people respond in kind. The behavior is analogous to the collective monologue and parallel play of young children. The talk about the body satisfies narcissistic needs, and it is an attempt magically to relieve anxiety about what is happening. This pattern alienates the young and the young old, and they tend to avoid or stop conversing with the aged.

Old-old persons intensely appreciate the richness of the moment, the joys or the sorrows. They realize the transience of life, and they are more likely to start each day with a feeling of expectancy, not neutrality or boredom. Their future is today. As a result, they become more tolerant of others' foibles, more thrilled over minor events, and more aware of their own needs, even if they cannot meet them.

Irritating behavior of the old-old person is frequently related to the frustration of being dependent on others or helpless and the fear that accompanies dependency and helplessness. The tangible issue at hand—coffee too hot or too cold, visitors too early, too late or not at all, or the fast pace of others—is often not really what is irritating, although the person attaches complaints to something that others can identify. The irritability is with the self, loss of control, lost powers, and present state of being.

Perhaps the *most frequent error in assessing* the elderly is the diagnosis of senility. Conditions labeled as such may actually be the result of physiologic imbalances, depression, inadequacy feelings, or unmet affectional and dependency needs. Psychological problems in the elderly are often manifested in disorientation, poor judgment, perceptual motor inaccuracy, intellectual dysfunction, and incontinence. These problems are frequently not chronic and may respond well to supportive therapy. Just as few young adults reach complete maturity, few older persons attain an ideal state of personality integration in keeping with their developmental stage.

Nursing needs a strong commitment to assist the elderly in maintaining adaptive mechanisms appropriate to this period of life, although each person will accomplish them in his or her unique way, pertinent to life experiences and cultural background. Cooper's study (64) of concentration camp survivors illustrates the impact of the experience on the person's adaptation. Carry out principles of care previously described to meet emotional and personality needs of the elderly.

Adaptive Mechanisms

Persons in their older years are capable of changes in behavior but find changing difficult. As new crises develop from social, economic, or family restructuring, new types of ego defenses may be needed. At the same time, the need to change may interfere with developing a sense of ego integrity.

Changing adaptive mechanisms must be developed for successful emotional transition in these later years. They help the person maintain a sense of self-worth and control over external forces, which in turn promotes a higher level of function (119, 174). Peck (228) lists three developmental tasks related to adaptation, and they serve to show not only the tasks involved but also the mechanisms undergoing change as the older personality strives to become integrated.

Ego differentiation *versus work-role preoccupation is involved in the adaptation to retirement, and its success depends on the ability to see self as worthwhile not just because of a job but because of the basic person he or she is.* **Body transcendence** *versus body preoccupation requires that happiness and comfort as concepts be redefined to overcome the changes in body structure and function* and, consequently, in body image and the decline of physical strength. The third task is **ego transcendence** *versus ego preoccupation, the task of accepting inevitable death.* Mechanisms for adapting to the task of facing death are those that protect against loss of inner contentment and help to develop a constructive impact on surrounding persons (228).

Certain adaptive or defensive mechanisms are used frequently by the aged. **Regression,** *returning to earlier behavior patterns,* should not be considered negative unless it is massive and the person is incapable of

self-care. A certain amount of regression is mandatory to survival as the person adapts to decreasing strength, changing body functions and roles, and often increasing frustration. Regression is an adaptive mechanism used by the older adult who is dying, and it is manifested differently than in younger years. The regression is a complex of behaviors not associated solely with a return to former levels of adaptation.

To integrate into self-concept and handle the anxiety created by a complex of losses, changes, and adaptation related to aging and dying, the older person behaves in a way that may be confused with dementia or drug reactions. Careful assessment is needed, using history of the person's normal patterns and history of illness (174, 244).

The dying elderly person may express regression in any or all of the following behaviors (46, 85, 174):

- Massive denial and projection
- Misuse of words, confusion about familiar concepts, fragmentation of speech, misinterpretation
- Preoccupation with minutiae, impaired ability to deal with simple abstractions
- Awkward childlike thinking

The dying elderly person will invest little emotionally into goal setting and care planning. Any goal must be short-term. Caregivers, including family, must provide physical and emotional support, recognizing the dying person's need to disengage from self-care and significant others. During the care process you must support the family caregivers and encourage them to talk about perceptions and feelings and to explain behavioral changes and needs of the dying person.

Other commonly used adaptive mechanisms are described in Table 14–15 (174, 215). McCrae (197) found in a study that controlled for types of stress that older persons did not consistently differ from younger ones in using 26 of 28 coping mechanisms, including rational action, expression of feelings, and seeking help. Middle-aged and older persons were less likely than younger ones to use immature and ineffective mechanisms of hostile responses and escapist fantasy. Health threats in all ages elicit wishful thinking, faith, and fatalism. Using **insight** (*intellectual understanding*) and reminiscence is also adaptive (174). Resilience is also a part of adaptation. *Characteristics of the successfully adjusted older woman* include the following (288):

- **Equanimity:** *balanced perspective of one's life and experiences*
- **Perseverance:** *persistence despite adversity or discouragement*
- **Self-reliance:** *belief in oneself and one's abilities*

TABLE 14–15. ADAPTIVE MECHANISMS USED BY THE OLDER ADULT

Mechanism	Description
Emotional Isolation	*By repressing the emotion associated with a situation or idea while intellectually describing it,* the person can cope with very threatening situations and ideas such as personal and another's disease, aging, and death and can begin to resolve the associated fears. Thus, the aged can appear relatively calm in the face of crisis.
Compartmentalization	*Narrowing of awareness and focusing on one thing at a time* so that the aged seem rigid, repetitive, and resistive.
Denial	*Blocking a thought or the inability to accept the situation* is used selectively when the person is under great stress and aids in maintaining a higher level of personality integration.
Rationalization	*Giving a logical sounding excuse for a situation* is often used to minimize weakness, symptoms, and various difficulties or to build self-esteem.
Somatization	*Complaints about physical symptoms and preoccupation with the body* may become an outlet for free-floating anxiety. The person can cope with vague insecurities and rapid life changes by having a tangible physical problem to deal with, especially because others seem more interested and concerned about disease symptoms than feelings about self.
Counterphobia	*Excessive behavior in an area of life to counter or negate fears about that area of life* is observed in the person who persists at activities such as calisthenics or youthful grooming or fashion to retain a youthful appearance.
Rigidity	*Resisting change or not being involved in decision making* is a common defense to help the person feel in control of self and life. A stubborn self-assertiveness is compensatory behavior for the person who has been insecure, rigid, and irritable.
Sublimation	*Channeling aggressive impulses into sociably acceptable activity* can be an effective defense to meet old age as a challenge and maintain vigor and creativity. Often the elderly desire to live vicariously through the younger generation, and they become involved with the young through mutual activities and listening or observing their activities.
Displacement	*Expressing frustration or anger onto another person or object that is not the source of the feelings* provides a safe release and disguises the real source of anxiety. The elder may blame another for his or her deficiencies, bang furniture, throw objects, or unjustly criticize family or health care workers.
Projection	*Attributing personal feelings or characteristics, usually negative, to another* allays anxiety, releases unpleasant feelings, or elevates self-esteem and self-concept. Projection is done unconsciously, usually to those closest to the person; a milieu free of counteraggression helps the person feel secure.

- **Meaningfulness:** *realization that life has purpose and the value of one's contribution*
- **Existential aloneness:** *realization that each person's path is unique and some experiences must be faced alone*

Hoarding may be an adaptive behavior, although it is usually regarded as a disagreeable, messy, and unsafe characteristic of the elderly or a sign of illness or dementia (it may be maladaptive behavior signaling illness at any age). The elderly may hoard and collect various or specific items for various *reasons:*

- It may be a lifelong habit; in the younger years the person was considered a "pack rat," or someone who always had what was needed in an emergency, or "someone who had everything handy." The behavior, if part of the person's self-concept and previously rewarded, is likely to continue to be valued and practiced.
- It may be the mark of a creative, intelligent person, an artist, or former teacher who keeps supplies that can be used in the vocation or hobby.

- The articles that are saved, potentially useful or likely to be used, represent security, especially if the person (a) lived through the Great Depression and World War II and remembers severe scarcity or poverty, and will not waste; (b) was an immigrant or displaced person from another country; or (c) buys food or supplies in large quantities to save money, even if not used.
- The articles may be symbolic of a happier past or represent a future.
- The gathered objects may represent a sense of control.
- The articles may compensate for loneliness and recent losses or be a way to keep in touch with family or friends now dead or relocated.
- Collecting, observing, handling, and sorting objects may be a pleasant diversion, especially for the old who are less socially active.
- Articles may be kept close at hand rather than stored in cabinets or closets to save energy in retrieving them when needed.
- When cognitive impairment occurs, the person may be unable to discriminate between needed

and unneeded objects and thereby keep everything.

Table 14–16 lists *interventions* that can be used by you, family, or friends, if the hoarding poses a problem. The following are *components of an adaptive old age* (85, 88):

- High mental status
- Absence of organic brain damage or disease
- High morale
- Counterphobic rather than passive-dependent behavior
- Denial of aging
- Vitality, interest, and enjoyment
- Adequate income
- Relatively good health
- Personal adaptability
- Available family
- Psychosocial stimulation
- Maintenance of meaningful goals
- Acceptance of death
- Sense of legacy

Characteristics of Successful Aging summarizes a holistic perspective about successful aging (246, 279).

TABLE 14–16. INTERVENTIONS FOR HOARDING BEHAVIOR

1. Discuss the situation with the person. Let the person show you collections and tell the stories; learn the meaning of behavior.
2. Offer to assist with cleanup, filing, or discarding if the person wishes and lacks energy or motivation. Never throw away objects without consent of the person unless dementia is present.
3. Set limits firmly if the hoarding is hazardous; e.g., help the person clean out the refrigerator with spoiled or unedible food, straighten up a room, and make a clear walkway to avoid falls.
4. Do not argue or nag about insignificant articles or out-of-the-way collections.
5. Discuss the need to discard some of the accumulation but tell the person he or she can decide what to discard, store, give to family or friends, and keep.
6. Reward behaviors that reduce hoarding.
7. Arrange for the person to engage in outside activities, groups, and relationships. Keep the person busy with interesting activities.
8. Evaluate the person's need for possible relocation to the home of a family member or to an assisted living retirement center for close supervision and assistance.
9. Refer the person, after consultation with family, guardian, or health care team, to a treatment facility if the behavior is indicative of depression, obsession–compulsion, paranoia, or dementia.
10. Assist family and friends, if necessary, in determining whether a legal guardian should be appointed.

► CHARACTERISTICS OF SUCCESSFUL AGING

High Degree of Life Satisfaction

- Feels life has been rewarding; has met goals
- Has few regrets
- Has positive attitude about past and future
- Feels life is stimulating, interesting; sets new goals
- Is able to relax; has good health habits

Harmonious Integration of Personality

- Has developed ego strength, unity, and maturity over the years
- Demonstrates self-actualization, satisfaction, individuation, authenticity
- Makes use of potentials and capabilities throughout life
- Has an accurate self-concept and body image
- Has meaningful value system

Maintenance of Meaningful Social System

- Keeps involved with caring network of family and friends
- Maintains interest in life through social attachments
- Feels affection for and from others and sense of belonging

Personal Control Over Life

- Feels independent and autonomous
- Makes own decisions, in charge of self to extent possible
- Maintains sense of dignity, self-worth, positive self-concept

Establishment of Financial Security

- Has made careful and effective financial plans
- Uses community resources to extent necessary

Acute illness at any age influences behavior, affective responses, and cognitive function. These aspects of the person are also affected by chronic illness, but their effects and adaptive mechanisms used are less well known.

Your approach during care can either increase or decrease *motivation to participate in treatment or rehabilitation*, even when the person already feels self-motivated. *Helpful approaches* include the following:

- Set a definite goal with the client.
- Reinforce and support the basic drives or character/personality structure of the client. Do not

label the preoccupation with achieving or the persistence in practice as obsession or compulsion. Realize that the former "toughness" or "survival traits" of the person are now an asset, not to be diminished by your traditional approach.

- Convey caring, be kind, share "power" or control with the client rather than trying to be the boss. In turn, the client will feel, and be, more "cooperative."
- Encourage or reinforce with attention to the attempts as well as achievements.
- Use humor gently and appropriately to release tension or encourage. Do not use sarcastic humor.
- Convey a positive attitude that the person can achieve the goal, at least to the extent possible. Avoid negative comments, an attitude that "puts down" the client, or nonverbal behavior that conveys you do not perceive capability.
- Avoid a power struggle, insistence on the client doing an activity your way, or domination of the client. Let the person go at his or her own pace and in a way that is safe but will still achieve results.

Body Image Development

Physical changes discussed earlier have both private and public components and combine to change the appearance and function of the older individual and thereby influence the self-image. In one study healthy elderly, when compared with healthy young adults, were more conscious of external physical appearance, possibly because of societal attitudes about youth and beauty. They also self-evaluated higher body competence; perhaps this was a result of their health status or a denial of aging. Both young and older adults revealed no differences in private body consciousness (246); however, as the person ages, loss of muscle strength and tone is reflected in a decline in the ability to perform tasks requiring strength. The old-old or frail person sees self as weakened and less worthwhile as a producer of work either in actual tasks for survival or in the use of energy for recreational activities.

The loss of skin tone, although not serious in itself, causes the aged in a society devoted to youth and beauty to feel stigmatized. Changing body contours accentuate sagging breasts, bulging abdomen, and the dowager's hump caused by osteoporosis. These changes all produce a marked negative effect. This stigma can also affect the sexual response of the older person because of perceived rejection by a partner.

Loss of sensory acuity causes alienation from the environment. Full sensory status cannot be regained once it is lost through aging. Although eyeglasses and better illumination are of great help in fading vision, the elderly recognize their inability to read fine print and to do handwork requiring good vision for small objects. The danger of injury caused by failure to see obstacles in their paths because of cataracts, glaucoma, or senile macular degeneration makes the elderly even more insecure about the relationship of their body to their environment. They often seek medical help too late because they do not understand the implications of the diagnosis or the chances for successful correction.

Hearing loss, the result of degeneration of the central and peripheral auditory mechanism and increased rigidity of the basilar membrane, is likely to cause even more negative personality changes in the older person than loss of sight. Behavior such as suspiciousness, irritability, and impatience, and paranoid tendencies may develop simply because hearing is impaired. Again the person may fear to admit the problem or to seek treatment, especially if he or she is unaware of the possibilities of help, through either hearing aids or corrective surgery.

Often the elderly view the hearing aid as another threat to body image. Eyeglasses are worn by all age groups and hence are more socially acceptable, but a hearing aid is conceived as overt evidence of advanced age. Adjustment to the hearing aid may be difficult for many people, and if motivation is also low, the idea may be rejected.

Be especially alert as you assess visual and auditory needs of the elderly. One of the modern medical miracles is lens implant surgery for those with cataracts. Seeing the senior before and after surgery allows you to share the joy of blindness-to-sight and to do necessary teaching. Surgery and discharge are usually the same day.

Hearing needs may not be met as easily, but astute observation can change the situation quickly. Consider the elderly woman who returned to her home after colostomy surgery. Although she had been pleasant and cooperative in the hospital, always nodding "Yes," she had failed to learn her colostomy irrigation routine. The visiting nurse learned, through being in the home and getting information from the family, that the client was nearly deaf. The client covered her loss by nodding pleasantly. Slow, distinct instructions allowed her to grasp the irrigation techniques, and within several days she was managing well. The nurse also had an opportunity to refer the woman for auditory assessment. There are a number of specific ways to modify the environment for persons with sensory impairments.

Jourard (141) speaks of *spirit-titre*. He thinks the way we perceive our body determines the degree to which our self-structure can be organized for optimum body defense against loss of energy. Jourard suggests that the term *spirit* be used to express the *titre,* or concentration of purpose, which may be encouraged in the aged to produce a well-integrated "personality-health."

Helping the senior keep an intact, positive body image will raise his or her *spirit-titre.* Encourage the senior to talk about feelings related to the changing body appearance, structure, and function. Provide a mirror so that he or she can look at self to integrate the overt changes into his or her mental image. Photographs can also be useful in reintegrating a changing appearance. Help the senior to stay well groomed and attractively dressed, and compliment efforts in that direction. Touch and tactile sensations are important measures to help the person continue to define body boundaries and integrate structural changes.

Moral–Spiritual Development

The elderly person with a mature religious outlook and philosophy still strives to incorporate broadened views of theology and religious action into the thinking. Self-transcendence is related to lower loneliness scores and to mental and spiritual health (236). Because the elderly person is a good listener, he or she is usually liked and respected by all ages. Although not adopting inappropriate aspects of a younger lifestyle, he or she can contemplate the fresh religious and philosophic views of adolescent thinking, thus trying to understand ideas previously missed or interpreted differently. Similarly, others listen to him or her. The elderly person feels a sense of worth while giving experienced views. He or she is concerned about moral dilemma and conflict and offers suggestions on ways to handle them. Basically he or she is satisfied with living personal beliefs, which can serve as a great comfort when he or she becomes temporarily despondent over life changes or changes in the family's life, or when confronting the idea of personal death.

A study of life satisfaction in 166 African-Americans ranging in age from 65 to 88 years (87 males and 79 females) revealed that men and women differed. High life satisfaction in women and men was related to church participation, religious faith, and family role involvements (often associated with the religious roles). High life satisfaction in men was also related to income and education levels (60).

Life experience that is meaningful has a spiritual quality. Four themes give life meaning and promote spiritual well-being (174):

1. Concern for the welfare of others
2. Opportunity to be helpful or useful as needed
3. Becoming involved in activity that is useful to someone else
4. Maintaining positive feelings about self and others

Religious belief and participation are important for most elders, regardless of ethnicity; however, different ethnic groups vary in how they participate, and they differ in the role religion plays in providing a resource for coping with adversities of aging. Nonorganizational religious participation includes reading religious materials, watching or listening to religious programs, prayer, and requests for prayer. Demographics, religious denomination, and health disability factors influence participation in these and organizational activities.

Elderly persons who have not matured religiously or philosophically may sense a spiritual impoverishment and despair as the drive for professional and economic success wanes. An immature outlook provides no solace, and, if church members, they may become bitter. They may believe that the church organization to which they gave long and dedicated service has forgotten them as they have less stamina for organizational work. They may feel cast aside in favor of the young who have so many activities planned for them. These persons need help to arrive at an adequate spiritual philosophy and to find some appropriate religious or altruistic activities that will help them gain feelings of acceptance, self-esteem, and worth.

Nursing Care to Meet Spiritual Needs

Care of clients' spiritual needs is an essential part of holistic care. This includes talking with the elderly, listening to statements that indicate religious beliefs or spiritual needs, and reading scriptures or praying with the person when indicated or requested. Giving spiritual care to the elderly person may involve providing prompt physical care to prevent angry outbursts and accepting apologies as the person seeks forgiveness for a fiery temper or sharp tongue. Quoting or reading favorite scripture verses, saying a prayer, providing religious music, or joining with the person in a religious song may calm inner storms. Acknowledging realistic losses and feeling with those who weep can provide a positive focus and hope. Helping the aged person remain an active participant in church, religious programs, or Bible study in the nursing home can maintain his or her self-esteem and sense of usefulness. Finally, in dying and near death, the religious person may want to practice beloved rituals and say, or have quoted, familiar religious or scriptural verses.

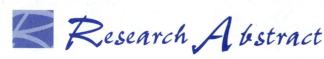

Research Abstract

Kay, J., and K. Robinson, Spirituality Among Caregivers, Image, *26 (1994), 218–221.*

A pilot study compared a convenience sample of 17 caregiver wives of men with dementia and 23 noncaregiver wives of healthy men for spiritual perspectives. In all areas tested, the caregiver wives, in contrast to the noncaregiver wives, used as coping strategies more spiritual symbols and behaviors, such as prayer, forgiveness, sharing of spiritual beliefs, and seeking spiritual guidance. Caregiver wives related to their concept of God and tended to share problems and joys of living according to their spiritual beliefs more often than did noncaregiver wives. Caregiver wives also used private prayer and spiritual guidance in making decisions in their everyday life more often than did noncaregiver wives. Findings suggest that nurses network with and intervene in churches to provide a natural network for caregivers. By using the spiritual interventions of prayer, sharing spiritual reading material, and encouraging experiences of faith and forgiveness, nurses can be helpful to caregivers.

Developmental Tasks

The following developmental tasks are to be achieved by the aging couple as a family and by the aging person living alone. You can assist the elderly person to meet these tasks (82, 88, 117):

- Recognize the aging process, define instrumental limitations, and adjust to societal views of aging.
- Adjust to decreasing physical strength and health changes.
- Decide where and how to live out the remaining years; redefine physical and social life space.
- Continue a supportive, close, warm relationship with the spouse or significant other, including a satisfying sexual relationship.
- Find a satisfactory home or living arrangement and establish a safe, comfortable household routine to fit health and economic status.
- Adjust living standards to retirement income and reduced purchasing power; supplement retirement income if possible with remunerative activity.
- Maintain culturally assigned functions and tasks.
- Maintain maximum level of health; care for self physically and emotionally by getting regular health examinations and needed medical or dental care, eating an adequate diet, and maintaining personal hygiene.
- Maintain contact with children, grandchildren, and other living relatives, finding emotional satisfaction with them.
- Establish explicit affiliation with members of own age group.
- Maintain interest in people outside the family and in social, civic, and political responsibility.
- Pursue alternate sources of need satisfaction and new interests and maintain former activities to gain status, recognition, and a feeling of being needed.
- Find meaning in life after retirement and in facing inevitable illness and death of oneself, spouse, and other loved ones.
- Work out values, life goals, and a significant philosophy of life, finding a comfort in a philosophy or religion.
- Reassess criteria for self-evaluation.
- Adjust to the death of spouse and other loved ones.

McCoy (195) describes similar developmental tasks for this era:

- Disengage from paid work.
- Reassess finances.
- Be concerned with personal health care.
- Search for new achievement outlets.
- Manage leisure time.
- Adjust to more constant marriage companion.
- Search for meaning of life.
- Adjust to single state.
- Problem solve.
- Manage stress accompanying change.
- Be reconciled to death.

Case Situation: Later Maturity

Mrs. Bertini, 78 years old, has been a widow for 20 years. She and her husband had no children, but two nieces and a nephew who live in another state visit occasionally. Mrs. Bertini has coped with arthritis for many years and, with the help of a home health agency and friends, has been able to remain in her home after suffering a broken hip. She has taken medication for cardiac disease and hypertension since experiencing a mild heart attack 10 years ago.

Despite increasing physical disability, Mrs. Bertini has maintained close ties with three female friends, two of whom had worked with her in a hat factory when they were young. These friends and their husbands were also friends of her husband. The four couples often played cards and attended social functions together.

Mrs. Bertini has begun to find it increasingly difficult to do her housework and shopping. Although the neighborhood pharmacy still delivers medication, the family-owned grocery on the block where she has lived for 20 years recently closed, and she cannot manage the four-block walk to the bus stop. She has admitted to her friends that she needs assistance, but on her limited income of a small pension from her husband and the minimum amount from Social Security, she cannot afford to hire help.

Although Mrs. Bertini has occasionally considered entering a nursing home, the decision is forced when her landlord announces a rent increase of $90 monthly. With great reluctance, she asks her closest friends to take her to several nursing homes in her area of the city. As a devout Catholic, her decision is immediate; she feels most comfortable with the home operated by The Sisters of the Poor. It is accredited, looks homey, and is clean. The sisters and other workers are friendly and kind. Her friends help her sell her furniture and move to the nursing home. She takes her television and stand, her favorite chair and footstool, and her most treasured mementos and clothes with her.

The first few days in the nursing home are eventful as Mrs. Bertini meets new people and attends the planned activities. Then she begins to feel confined by having only a small room. She misses her independence and occasionally feels lonely. In her own home she used to sleep until 9 AM, but now if she wants breakfast, she must be in the dining room no later than 8 AM. Although mobility is painful, slow, and possible only with aid of a walker, Mrs. Bertini makes a point to attend the activities given in the home and accepts invitations from her friends to go out to eat at favorite restaurants. She looks forward to the letters, gifts, and holiday visits from her nieces and nephews and writes short notes to keep in touch with them. She also attends chapel services weekly. She tells her visitors that she is not afraid of death; her only wish is that she does not suffer long.

Brown (40) refers to different developmental tasks for young-old and old-old persons because the changing life situations necessitate different attitudes, efforts, and behaviors. The tasks are listed as follows for each age group.

Young-Old

- Prepare for and adjust to retirement from active involvement in the work arena with its subsequent role change (especially for men).
- Anticipate and adjust to lower and fixed income after retirement.
- Establish satisfactory physical living arrangements as a result of role changes.
- Adjust to new relationships with one's adult children and their offspring.
- Learn or continue to develop leisure time activities to help in realignment of role losses.
- Anticipate and adjust to slower physical and intellectual responses in the activities of daily living.
- Deal with the death of parents, spouses, and friends.

Frail-Old or Old-Old

- Learn to combine new dependency needs with the continuing need for independence.
- Adapt to living alone in continued independence.
- Learn to accept and adjust to possible institutional living (nursing and/or proprietary homes).
- Establish an affiliation with one's age group.
- Learn to adjust to heightened vulnerability to physical and emotional stress.

- Adjust to loss of physical strength, illness, and approach of one's death.
- Adjust to losses of spouse, home, and friends.

SOCIOECONOMIC CONCEPTS

Retirement

Age, sex, health status, family background, ethnicity, type of job or profession, lifetime work experience, and economic incentives all influence when the person voluntarily or involuntarily ceases the career or job. As corporations reduce their work force numbers, the older worker is most likely to be released because of salary and pension costs, despite job discrimination legislation. Yet keeping the older worker may be less costly because of retraining costs and lower turnover and absenteeism. He or she is loyal and committed to the company, is flexible about accepting new assignments, and often is a better salesperson. Many people are living longer but are working shorter careers; yet the proportion of young to old people is diminishing. After the turn of the century, it is likely that more older people will be needed in the workplace to relieve the labor shortage (74).

Retirement affects all the other positions the person has held and the relationships with others. Retirement is a demotion in the work system. It will, for many people, mean a reduction in income, or the person may seek a new job, either part or full-time, for financial reasons but also for emotional and socialization reasons. Inability to keep up with the former activities of an organization or group may result, and a change in status may require a changing social life (36, 240, 309).

In a study of retirees in Israel, four developmental tasks were found to relate specifically to retirement (15):

- Remaining actively involved and having a sense of belonging unrelated to work
- Reevaluating life satisfaction related to family and social relations and spiritual life rather than to work
- Reevaluating the world's outlook, keeping a view of the world that is coherent and meaningful and a view that one's own world is meaningful
- Maintaining a sense of health, integrating mind and body to avoid complaints or illness when work is no longer the focus

Retirement Planning

Prior planning will help in the transition from worker to retiree. Nurses are often with persons nearing retirement and may be asked directly or through nonverbal cues and disguised statements to help them sort out their feelings as they face this adjustment. Although some persons who disliked their jobs, have an adequate income, and participate in a variety of activities eagerly look forward to a pleasurable retirement, many seniors would prefer and are able to work past 65 years.

Despite much work in recent years at both the national and local levels to develop comprehensive programs for the aged, few business organizations have recognized the many ways in which they might assist the potential retiree. Private organizations with large numbers of employees are, for the most part, the only ones having effective retirement preplanning programs. The federal government offers little in retirement planning for its employees, and this is true for almost all state and local governments as well. Those programs offered usually include lectures and discussions on financial security, health insurance, legal matters, Social Security benefits, company pension and retirement policies, and health maintenance information.

The retiree may be faced with these questions: Can I face loss of job satisfaction? Will I feel the separation from people close to me at work? If I need continued employment on a part-time basis to supplement Social Security payments, will the old organization provide it, or must I adjust to a new job? Shall I remain in my present home or seek a different one because of easier maintenance or reduced cost of upkeep? Might a different climate be better and, if so, will I miss my relatives and neighbors?

Whatever the elderly person's need, your role will be supportive. Advocate retirement planning. Recommend agencies that may be useful in making plans, and provide current information on Social Security benefits and Medicare coverage. Unless you are able to discuss these areas of concern and to answer questions, the needs of the person approaching retirement cannot be met. One of the most helpful resources is the large supply of government publications available at little or no cost from the Superintendent of Documents of the Government Printing Office in Washington, DC. Current lists of material pertinent to health and social programs may be obtained directly from the National Clearing House on Aging, U.S. Department of Health and Human Services, 330 Independence Avenue, SW, Washington, DC 20201.

Use of Leisure

The constructive use of free time is often a problem of aging. What a person does when he or she no longer works is related to past lifestyle, continuous core activities, accumulated experiences, and the way in which he or she perceives and reacts to the environment.

Leisure time, *having opportunity to pursue activities of interest without a sense of obligation, demand, or urgency,* is an important aspect of life satisfaction, expression of self, and emotional and social development. Leisure activity is chosen for its own sake and for the meaning it gives to life, but it involves both physical or mental activity and participation. It is a way to cope with change. Adults value most of the leisure activity that involves interaction with others and/or a pet, promotes development, or is expressive and maintains contact with the broader community. Most people have a core of activity that they enjoy. Reading and viewing television are popular pastimes; interestingly, television preferences are similar for older and younger adults, but reading preferences vary strongly with age and sex.

Use of leisure time by volunteering is rewarding but constrained by household income, education, and age. In a study of elders in Minnesota, 52% did volunteer work that could be classified as formal or informal, regular or occasional, and with either people, objects, or community system (93). Older Americans participate in many unpaid productive activities at levels commensurate to those reached by young and middle-aged adults. Elders who have been self-reliant and have always worked hard are more likely to incorporate service to others into their leisure and volunteer time (9, 140, 279).

The *elder can contribute in many ways to the community and society after his or her retirement:*

- Through volunteer or part-time work with hospital, community agency, or social, welfare, or conservation organization of choice
- Through a friendly visitor program to other old or homebound people
- Through a telephone reassurance program (calling the same person at the same time each day to determine the status)
- Through foster grandparent programs in nurseries, with failure-to-thrive children, and in preschool or day-care settings, homes for abused or orphaned children, or juvenile detention centers
- To homes for battered women or children, providing mothering or fathering skills
- To shelters for the homeless, providing counseling, teaching for General Education Development (GED) certification, or socializing
- To churches and church-related organizations in many capacities
- To Habitat for Humanity, an organization that builds or remodels homes for poor people in various rural and urban areas of the United States and in other underdeveloped nations
- As a volunteer for a crisis hot line (suicide, drug use, child care, prayer line)
- Through collaboration with police, clergy, or community leaders, working to create drug-free and gun-free neighborhoods and schools

Questions to Consider Before Volunteering lists questions to consider before assuming the volunteer role or questions the senior should ask key people in an agency that is being considered for a volunteer role. Explore these questions with the person.

Because Americans live in a society that has a high work priority, more training for leisure in middle age and earlier or more opportunity for continued employment in old age must be provided through public policy.

The American Association of Retired Persons (AARP) is studying the potential impact on people as

---

▶ **QUESTIONS TO CONSIDER BEFORE VOLUNTEERING**

- Do you have the time to give?
- Do you make punctuality a habit?
- Do you take responsibility seriously?
- Can you give reasonable advance notice if you must cancel plans or appointments?
- Do you consistently follow through on projects?
- Do you work well with others?
- Do you adhere to an organization's policies and procedures?
- Do you accomplish tasks that have been assigned?
- Would you receive orientation or training you want or need?
- Do you understand and agree with the details of the position and the demands it will place on you?
- Would you have enough responsibility or authority to challenge you if you desired the challenge?
- Is the organization respected in your community?
- Does the organization respect its volunteers' time?
- Are the current volunteers dedicated to the organization or cause?
- Would you be able to use your experience or educational background?

the United States moves from an industrialized mass society into a more technologically complex but fragmented society. Older people will be retained as consultants in the workplace. All people will need an education for a life of ceaseless change, for new activities, and for new roles with passing years. Older people can lead in creating a better society for all generations.

Materialism and productivity have been key American values. As population shifts occur and society becomes more technologically complex, causing earlier retirement for some workers, the definition of productivity must be changed from that which involves exchange of money. Toffler has coined the word **prosumers,** *people who produce goods and services for their families and friends but not for monetary gain.* Family roles are also likely to change, with an older family adopting or nurturing a younger family, giving assistance with child care or other tasks. The elderly will be needed as caregivers across family lines as home care becomes an important aspect of the health care system, and the caregiving role can give added meaning to life.

Federal Planning for the Aged in America

The United States is not alone in having to consider ways to provide care for the dependent elderly. Many countries throughout the world are experiencing a growing aging population. Some of the issues and approaches are similar across nations; some differences reflect basic national ethics and beliefs about how human services should be rendered. Kane and Kane (145) examine themes that transcend boundaries. We present issues related only to the United States.

Administration on Aging

In 1958 government interest in the older citizen inspired the formation of the President's Council on Aging, which later expanded and became the Administration on Aging (AOA). The AOA was established by the Older Americans Act of 1965 and operated as the central agency for assistance to the aged under the Department of Health and Human Services (DHHS).

The focus of AOA has been to identify the needs, concerns, and interests of older persons and to carry out the programs of the Older Americans Act. It was the principal agency for promoting coordination of the federal resources available to meet the needs of the elderly. Federal grants to state agencies on aging have been administered by AOA. The state agencies then acted as advocates and assisted in the establishment of comprehensive, coordinated service systems for older

Americans at the community level. State agencies, in turn, designated and funded area agencies, county or municipal, which then served the aged within their own communities. The various social and nutritional services were planned and managed by these local area agencies. Direct grants to Indian tribal organizations have been made by AOA for social and nutritional services to older American Indians. AOA has awarded grants for research, educational demonstrations, and manpower development projects. It has operated the National Information and Resource Clearinghouse for the Aged.

The Older Americans Act has promoted research to improve or expand social or nutritional services. It has also supported education of individuals working with aging. Multidisciplinary centers of gerontology established under AOA developed, employed, and disseminated models for teaching and training, conducted research, and operated experimental model service community laboratories in the areas of policy and program significance.

Under the amended Domestic Volunteer Service Act of 1973, special programs more geared to the development of a greater, more significant role in the society for older Americans were begun so that they could participate more fully in the life of their communities and the nation. One of them, the Foster Grandparents Program, had a dual purpose: (1) to provide part-time volunteer service opportunities for low-income persons age 60 and over, and (2) to give supportive, person-to-person assistance in health, human services, and educational and related agencies to help alleviate the physical, mental, and emotional problems of children having exceptional needs. Through grants, AOA provided the recruitment and training of the volunteers. The participants worked 4 hours a day, 5 days a week, and received a stipend equal to the federal minimum hourly wage. Everyone gained in this program: the elderly earned much-needed income along with a sense of dignity and achievement and the children blossomed in the warmth of personal attention (46).

The following are examples of projects developed under this program: work in a juvenile prison helping youth gain education, guidance, and companionship; work with severely burned children in whom the warmth and personal attention seemed to promote healing; assisting autistic children with basic tasks and encouraging performance through praise; providing care to infants while unwed mothers attend basic education classes; and helping teenagers prepare to move out of a mental health institution into a community setting such as a group home or foster home. In Babylon, New York, 10 mildly to moderately mentally retarded persons who were formerly institutionalized later served as foster grandparents themselves. Not only did they gain a feeling of self-worth, but the institutional cost to the public was eliminated.

Another program sponsored by AOA, the Retired Senior Volunteer Program (RSPV), afforded out-of-pocket expenses to persons over 60 who wished to participate in locally organized volunteer projects. The local service organization, the RSVP sponsor, developed a wide variety of service opportunities in the community in hospitals, courts, schools, day-care centers, libraries, and other volunteer settings. Grants were used primarily for travel expenses of the volunteers. The advantage in this program was that many older persons whose income might otherwise have limited their eligibility could participate as volunteers (52).

Knowing about the programs available to the elderly is helpful to professionals in several ways. In counseling, health teaching, and giving support, you will find this knowledge useful as older clients demonstrate a need for guidance in seeking help. Often the answer to loneliness is participation in a program to help others. In addition, you may have occasion through an employing health agency to apply for federal grant money either for supportive services or for research relevant to aging.

For more information about functions of state and local Area Agencies on Aging, see local AOA representatives.

Social Security

Under the Social Security Act were grouped Old Age Survivors Insurance, Medicare, and Supplemental Security Income for the Elderly.

Old Age Survivors Insurance provides a consistent monthly income to men 65 and older and to women 62 and older. Family payments are made to various dependents: wives 62 and older; dependent children; wives younger than 62 caring for dependent children; dependent husbands or widowers 62 or older; and dependent parents 62 or older after the death of the insured worker. Payments are made also to persons certified to be disabled (85).

The *Supplemental Security Income* program was begun as part of the Social Security Amendments of 1972. It guarantees that the annual income of an older or a disabled person will not fall below a minimum level. This redirected the responsibility for the aged, blind, and disabled poor from the states to the federal government. The program is administered by the Social Security Administration and had one standard for eligibility: low assets and specified low income.

Of public concern in our age is the ultimate viability of the Social Security system. Originally it was assumed that our expanding population and labor force would provide adequately for continued growth as an increasing wage base would provide greater taxes. On the contrary, zero population growth, decline of productivity, and inflation threaten the system. The problem is whether or not a diminishing work force of young and middle-aged persons will be willing to support the steadily growing numbers of retired persons. Population aging has created a concern that the projected number of elderly persons in the future will represent a crushing burden on the working population.

The general mandatory retirement age will continue to be raised in the future. Federal and some other sectors have already increased mandatory retirement age to 70. According to the Social Security Amendments of 1983, the general retirement age will be gradually raised to 67 from 65 in two stages. A major argument for raising the retirement age is that life expectancy at age 65 has been increasing over the years and is expected to continue to rise in the future. It will be difficult to determine how much to raise the retirement age. Many would consider it unfair to expect that all the years of life expectancy gained should be spent working. At the same time, it is probably unreasonable to expect that all the additional years of life expectancy should be spent in leisure (46). Even if retirement ages are postponed, the number of dependent elderly will continue to increase, and it will do so quite substantially around the end of the first quarter of the 21st century.

Although increasing longevity is also a factor, population aging during the first quarter of the next century will result primarily from (1) high birth rates from mid-1940s to mid-1960s and (2) subsequent declining birth rates in the 1970s and beyond. As fewer children are born, the age structure of the population changes: the young segment becomes smaller and the old larger. Decreased morbidity accompanies increased longevity; the elderly of the future could remain in or reenter the work force to compensate for the relatively smaller labor force in the traditional age groups. Then paying Social Security benefits could be postponed. Changes in the work environment, however, are the prerequisites for keeping older persons in the work force.

Understanding the problems that are developing in the Social Security system is important for all who care for the elderly. The elderly will need support when their fears arise, and they will benefit from the help of an informed professional, one who has taken the time, through the use of the media and numerous government publications, to keep abreast of the changing scene regarding Social Security.

Medicare

The federally financed health insurance program in the United States is called Medicare. It provides benefits to persons over age 65 who paid into Social Security, and since 1972 it has extended care to the disabled and some chronically ill persons. There are two parts to Medicare: Part A, hospital insurance, and for those who choose to have a nominal monthly fee deducted from their Social Security checks, Part B, medical insurance.

Under Part A, most hospital costs and costs for a specified period in a skilled nursing facility or home are covered after an annual deductible is met by the insured. Part B of Medicare covers 80% of allowable costs for physicians' services and outpatient care. If the charges for services rendered exceed that which Medicare Part A or B deems reasonable and proper for the particular service, the enrollee must pay the difference, although prospective payment regulations are changing this. Insurance programs specific for supplement to Medicare payments are available.

January 1992 marked the start of a new nationwide fee schedule for physicians who see Medicare clients. They cannot charge more than 20% of what Medicare allowed to charge clients.

As with Social Security, the nurse must be conversant with current public announcements and other information to help and assure the elderly who may have great concern when they are ill about their security and care under this program. The Social Security representative available in all cities and most hospitals can help the individual in planning for any problems arising in the areas of either Social Security or Medicare. Inform elders, if necessary, of the Medicare Catastrophic Insurance Act, which provides extra coverage.

Federal Role in Health Promotion

The major federal role in the area of health has been that of the Public Health Service, under the DHHS. All planning for health care has been filtered through the state, county, and city health departments. Under the U.S. Public Health Service are countless agencies with programs that include health services to veterans, control of food and drugs, construction of health facilities, medical services for retired civil service employees, rent supplements, and provision of public housing.

As part of the ongoing federal concern for the aged, the third decennial White House Conference on Aging was held in Washington, DC, in November–December 1981. Whereas the first conference in 1961 produced the concept of Medicare and the second in 1971 helped yield the Older Americans Act, this next conference was more general in its recommendations. The

conference empowered older persons to speak their minds. There was a positive stand taken on residents' rights in nursing homes, the need for staff training, and the upgrading of nursing assistants. Although no definitive policy was forthcoming, the conference of 1981 reflected a concern by the elderly for continued improvement and expansion of services, both in long-term care facilities and in the community.

As a nurse, your influence can be felt in these areas through your work and community activities and in civic affairs by participation in your professional organization.

Community Planning

As people become older, infirm, and less mobile, a battery of community services is needed, not only to provide social activities and a reason to remain interested in life, but also to enable them to live independently. Most of the federal programs operate at the local level in actual practice, but, in addition, there is much that each community can do to provide needed services, which are available through the local Council on Aging. In small communities these services may be limited, but further information is available through any county public health agency.

Community Services

Supportive services may include the following:

- Referral services
- Visiting and telephone-reassurance programs, sometimes offered through churches or private organizations
- Services that provide shopping aides
- Portable meals, sometimes known as Meals on Wheels, for those who cannot shop for or prepare their own food
- Transportation and handy-person services, including home upkeep
- Day-care or foster home placement for the elderly (patterned after services for young children but modified for older adults)
- Recreation facilities geared to the older person
- Senior citizen centers that provide recreation and a place for the lonely to belong
- Respite services so that the family can get relief from caregiving while the elderly person receives needed care (The AARP offers numerous benefits socially and financially through insurance and other programs.)

All of these services can be used to promote health, prevent dysfunction, enhance a sense of independence, and aid family caregivers. Adult day-care services allow the person to remain at home and avoid institutionalization; the elder has daytime supervision and care, and the family member can continue employment (Fig. 14–5). Home health care prevents lengthy hospitalization, assists families and the elder with the tasks of care, and permits respite for the family.

Another helpful community service for elders is the senior center. Senior centers are found in almost all communities and are based in a variety of settings. Some are operating in buildings built for this purpose, but most are housed in facilities originally planned for other purposes: church halls, community buildings, old schools, mobile home park clubhouses, and the like. Their programs are federally funded to some extent but rely heavily on community support. A small staff is maintained, and most of the help with programs, maintenance, and materials comes from volunteers among the older persons who attend the center. Programs include activities such as crafts, social events from cards to dancing, exercise classes, and a full meal served at noon most weekdays. Other services may be daily telephone calls to homebound elderly, information and referral services, home-delivered meals, minor profit-making endeavors, and discount programs in cooperation with local merchants.

Several approaches are being tried in various communities based on the principle that before helping maintain health in the aged or contributing toward restoration of health, those working with community health must understand this age group. Toward this end, many persons enrolled in educational programs for the health professions are carrying out visiting programs with the elderly. Most nursing students are ex-

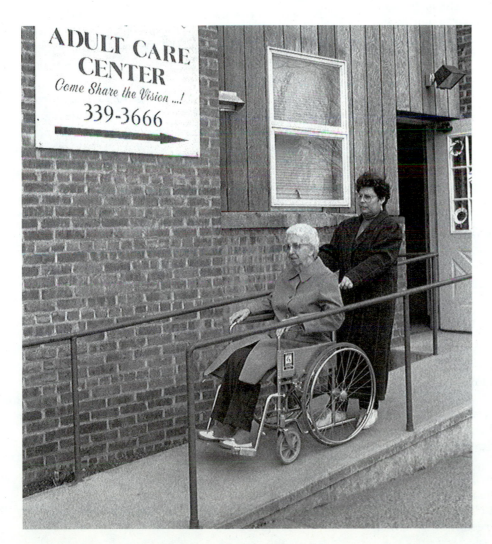

Figure 14–5. Adult day-care centers offer meals, nutritional counseling, mental health services, exercise classes, physical therapy, and social activities to elders. *(From Berger, K.J., and M.B. Williams,* Fundamentals of Nursing: Collaborating for Optimal Health. *Stamford, Conn: Appleton and Lange, 1992, p. 1717.)*

posed to elderly persons through visits to geriatric centers or by interviewing experinces designed to sharpen communication skills and afford opportunities to gain insight into the needs of older persons.

Group work among the aged has been done with much success in a number of communities and in a variety of settings. Some of this work has been initiated in centers operated for the elderly and has been used not only to encourage the individual to participate in a group activity, but also to carry out health teaching. Many types of groups can be developed for the elderly; some are described in Reference 215.

As a citizen of the community, you can be active in inititing and supporting local programs such as those described above and in Table 14–17.

Extended-Care Facility or Campus

The concept of long-term care for the elderly has broadened to be less custodial, more homelike, more holistic, and community focused. The names for the institutions vary: extended-care facility or campus or senior health care center. The term *nursing home* is used less frequently. The facility must be approved for skilled nursing, although it may have both skilled and intermediate care levels for residents. Criteria are set by Medicare as to what constitutes a person who needs skilled versus intermediate care. Medicare pays for 100 days of care when a client has been discharged directly from the hospital; Medicare does not pay for intermediate care. The person who needs intermediate care either will pay individually or, if he or she has a minimum amount of financial income or savings, Medicaid will pay for these services (310).

Certification of a nursing care facility is by a representative from the State Department of Aging who also represents standards set by the federal government. The main concern is the quality of care given. [The federal government may send out inspectors to check not only the nursing care facilities but also the state inspectors (310.)]

Licensing of a care facility is done by each state. For example, in South Carolina the organization is the Health and Education Council. The main concern is adequacy of the building and equipment (310).

The extended-care facility may serve as a transitional stop between hospital and home (generally for those over 65); in some cases, however, the stay is permanent.

The goals of the modern-day facility are to provide continuous supervision by a physician, 24-hour nursing services, hospital affiliation, written client care policies, and specialized services in dietary, restorative, pharma-ceutical, diagnostic, and social services. Unfortunately, these are sometimes hollow goals, even though the physical plant is new, licensing is current, and government funds are being used. Often the homes are operated for profit by those outside the nursing or medical profession. The residents are not always physically or mentally able to protest if care is poor, and often families of the residents do not monitor the care. National exposure of blatant neglect in some of the facilities has awakened public and government consciousness; perhaps this exposure will correct the most glaring problems and alert other facilities to their obligation to follow prescribed goals. If standards are met, the nursing home provides an excellent and needed service to society because the elderly must be discharged from expensive acute care hospital beds as soon as possible. Prolonged hospitalization can foster confusion, helplessness, and the hazards of immobility. Further, some elderly cannot care for self. There are ways to individualize care, give holistic care, and prevent neglect or abuse of residents in long-term care settings (46, 86).

Some even go beyond these concepts and provide independent living options. For example, the Methodist Retirement Community in Durham, North Carolina, starts with offering people meals and clinic access in a congregate (hotel type) setting. All services and living space are available in one facility. Or the residents may live in a free-standing house or apartment on campus. These independent residents come and go as they please. They choose this living option for the security of the campus and for the assurance that they will get whatever living facility and care that they will need for the rest of their lives.

Adult care, commonly known as assisted living or domiciliary care, is for residents who need help in taking medicines and in some activities of daily living. This care is managed by a registered nurse.

Skilled nursing care offers 24-hour nursing care. This particular retirement community also includes a dementia unit, which is licensed in the same way as adult care and is managed by a registered nurse. Unfortunately some facilities do not meet such a broad range of needs.

Selecting a Care Facility. When you help the family or senior select a nursing home, the following questions should be asked:

- What type of home is it, and what is its licensure status?
- What are the total costs, and what is included for the money?

TABLE 14–17 COMMUNITY RESOURCES FOR OLDER PEOPLE

Resource	Service
Adult congregate living facilities (ACLF)	Room, board, and personal services for elderly who would benefit from living in a group setting but do not require medical services; no nursing or medical services available
Adult day-care	Provision of comfortable, safe environment for functionally impaired adults, especially frail elderly, moderately handicapped, or slightly confused, who need care during the day, either because they live alone and cannot manage, or because family needs relief from the care to keep the elderly in the home
Adult foster care	Provision for continuous care to a functionally impaired older person in a private home with people who provide all services needed by the elderly individual
Aftercare	Posthospitalization rehabilitation such as cardiac or respiratory rehabilitation or occupational or physical therapy
American Association of Retired Persons (AARP)	Nationwide organization for people over 50 that offers discount drug purchases, health and auto insurance, publications, and other activities
Area Agency on Aging	Federal agency that provides information, referral services, planning, and coordination, but not direct or health care services, on a regional or countrywide basis
Congregate nutrition sites	Free or low-cost meals, social activities, and nutrition or health education provided in local churches or senior centers
Congregate living facility	Apartment complex that provides meals and social programs for older people
Elderhostel	An on-campus educational experience, living on campus for duration of the course that includes opportunity for new knowledge, travel to various campuses and national and international geographic areas, new experiences, meeting new people
Foster care	Placement of nonrelated elderly person in private residence for care
Foster Grandparents	Federal program paying people with low income who are over 60 a modest amount for working more than 20 hours a week with mentally or physically handicapped children
Friendly Visiting	Organized visiting services staffed by volunteers who visit homebound elderly once or twice weekly for companionship purposes if no relatives or friends are available
Gray Panthers	Nationwide politically oriented organization that works to raise awareness about issues affecting older people and to advocate and lobby on these issues in local, state, and national government
Home health services	Agency providing intermittent nursing, social work, physical, occupational, and speech-therapies, and other related services in the home via qualified health care professional or paraprofessionals to home-bound person
Homemaker/chore services	Agency providing help with light housekeeping, laundry, home chores, meal preparation, shopping for older people meeting income and other eligibility requirements
Hospice	Continuum of care systems for persons suffering from terminal disease and for their family, including home care, pain management, respite care, counseling, family support delivered in the home through outpatient and inpatient care—all within the same licensed program (It is medically directed, nurse coordinated, autonomously administered, and provides care for the physical, emotional, spiritual and social needs of client and family, using an interdisciplinary team approach.)
Long-term care ombudsman committees	Citizen committees appointed by the governor who volunteer their time to investigate and resolve grievances or problems of people in nursing homes and ACLFs
Meals on Wheels	Provision of hot or cold nutritious meals to a homebound elderly person, brought by another person or agency
Medicaid	Governmental coverage of health care and nursing home costs for older people with limited incomes who are eligible (People who receive Supplemental Security Income or Aid to Families with Dependent Children are automatically eligible.)
Medicare	National health insurance program for people age 65 and older or disabled, or in some special cases under 65, that is administered by the Social Security Administration (Part A is hospital insurance; Part B covers diagnostic tests, physician fees, outpatient and ambulance costs. Dental, vision, hearing, and preventive services are excluded.)
Protective services	Constellation of social services that assist older, noninstitutionalized people who manifest at least some incapacity to manage their money or their daily living or assist those who need protection of life or property
Respite care	Agency providing relief for specified hours, a weekend, or a week, for family caregivers, allowing time for the caregiver to shop, have the time for other reasons, or vacation while care is given to functionally impaired person residing in the home setting
Senior center	Program providing a combination of services; designed to be open 3 or more days a week, with meal, recreational, educational, and counseling services available (Sometimes medical services are provided.)
Senior Corp of Retired Executives	Agency of retired executives who volunteer their counseling services to small businesses and companies on request
Supplemental Security Income (SSI)	Minimum monthly to blind, disabled, and aged persons whose income falls below a specified level (Personal effects, household goods, and home ownership are not counted as assets, although savings, stocks, jewelry, or car would be.)
Telephone reassurance	Daily telephone calls to people who live alone, including the aged and disabled, or telephone crisis and information services provided by an agency

- Is the physical plant adequate, clean, and pleasant? How much space and furniture are allowed for each person?
- What safety features are evident? Are fire drills held?
- What types of care are offered (both acute and chronic)?
- What is the staff:resident ratio? What are the qualifications of the staff? What are staff attitudes toward the elderly?
- What are the physician services? Is a complete physical examination given periodically?
- What therapies are available?
- Are pharmacy services available?
- Are meals nutritionally sound and the food tasty? Is food refrigerated, prepared, distributed, and served under sanitary conditions? Is eating supervised or assisted?
- Are visitors welcomed warmly?
- Are residents aware of their Bill of Rights (see Bill of Rights for Residents of Extended Care Facilities)?
- Do residents appear content and appropriately occupied? (Observe on successive days and at different hours.) Are they treated with dignity and warmth by staff? Is privacy afforded during personal care?

► BILL OF RIGHTS FOR RESIDENTS OF EXTENDED CARE FACILITIES

- To choose your own doctor and help plan your course of treatment
- To be free of physical or mental abuse and from any restraints not medically required
- To use pharmacologic drugs by prescription and only for the symptoms for which they are prescribed
- To have privacy
- To be assured of confidentiality of records
- To have services tailored to individual needs and to be given notice before room or roommate is changed
- To voice grievances
- To organize and participate in resident groups
- To participate in social, religious, and community activities
- To examine the most recent survey of the facility and plans to correct deficiencies
- To obtain any other rights established by the Secretary of the Department of Health and Human Services

---

- Has the local Better Business Bureau received any complaints about this facility?
- Does the administrator have a current state license?
- Is the home certified to participate in government or other programs that provide financial assistance when needed?
- Is an ombudsman available to investigate complaints of residents or family?

Translocation. The elderly person who is moved to a nursing home or long-term care facility (often rest-of-the-lifetime care facility) or who is moved from one room to another within the same facility undergoes a crisis called **translocation syndrome,** *physical and emotional deterioration as a result of changes or movement.* A move may be made because of changes in health, in staffing, or in the residents or because families desire it. Such a move may be life threatening, however.

People at greater risk are those who are depressed, highly anxious, severely ill, intermittently confused, or over 85 years of age. People who need structure, who cannot stand changes, or who deny problems or feelings are also more likely to experience difficulty.

Reducing relocation's impact begins with enlisting the resident's understanding of the need for the move and participation. The person should be prepared for the move. When he or she can make decisions about the move and predict what will happen, the person maintains a sense of control, which diminishes the move's impact. Moving to a similar environment also reduces the problems. The ability to express fears, concerns, and anger helps. If the person to be moved to an institution is relatively young, has good morale, and has an opportunity to select and then feel satisfied with the new surroundings, the translocation syndrome may be minimum (208).

One way to reduce the crisis of admission to a nursing home or long-term care center or to reduce translocation shock is to have preschool or school children visit in the home. Both generations benefit from the exchange of affection. The youngsters bring stimulation to the elderly generation; the older generation can demonstrate stability, wisdom, and coping with adversities, and the qualities of ego integrity.

Elderly persons living alone or only with a spouse were, in one study, more likely than those who lived with a child, relative, or friend to prefer moving to an alternate setting such as a nursing home or senior housing when they were unable to care for self.

Taking one's frail loved one to a nursing home is not easy at that point in life when he or she can no longer care for self and home, at that point when the person has lost about everything that was precious and gave life meaning. Many family members have given poignant accounts of the pain for the elder and for the family and how the elder works to retain personal integrity and dignity despite the emotional assault.

Other Living Arrangements

For those elderly who want to live at home but need some degree of care, there are alternatives. A Florida agency is helping more than 10,000 persons stay out of institutions by delivering meals to them at home or shuttling them to community dining centers. Through the program, the elderly can hire helpers to wash windows or rake lawns and homemakers to shop or do light housekeeping. Transportation is provided to doctors' offices. Fees are based on ability to pay. The state of Florida estimates it saved $9.5 million in the past year by assisting these persons to live at home.

Senior day-care centers provide another alternative. The charges are reasonable per day, and they cater to persons not as able as those who may avail themselves of the usual senior center (see Criteria for Selecting Elder Day-care).

Some communities have set up centers to match roommates. Two persons may function better than alone, and the costs are shared. A Boston group has sponsored a project that arranges intergenerational living: 14 people ages 30 to 80 share a 19th-century townhouse. Everyone takes part in the chores and pays a nominal rent for their own room. Extended families have been created in some cities. A retired hospital administrator with arthritis now shares her four-bedroom home with a young couple and their newborn daughter, and each generation learns from the other.

Remotivation

Remotivation is one form of group therapy that can be conducted in a hospital, nursing home, or senior center for disengaged or regressed elderly. The training materials for instructing employees in the techniques are available from the American Psychiatric Association's central office in Washington, DC.

The goal of this therapy is to remotivate the unwounded areas in the personality of the older adult. It can be used by the average employee—nurse or ancillary—who is closest to the client or resident. It is designed to stimulate self-respect, self-reliance, and self-esteem in the older person who has become disengaged (102, 215, 235, 275). It encourages the person to focus attention on the simple, objective aspects of everyday life.

The method consists of a series of meetings, usually of about 12 clients, led by a person who has been trained in the technique. The sessions last about an hour. The leader guides the group through five steps (102, 215, 275):

1. Creating a climate of acceptance by greeting each person by name, making them welcome, and making remarks that encourage replies such as comments on the weather or a familiar incident
2. Creating a bridge to the world by relating a current event or referring to a topic of general interest (Each client is encouraged to comment.)
3. Sharing the world we live in, expanding step 2 through the use of appropriate visual aids
4. Appreciating the work of the world through discussion of jobs, how goods are produced, how jobs are done, or the type of work the clients have done in the past

---

► ## CRITERIA FOR SELECTING ELDER DAY-CARE

- Is agency certified or licensed? (Forty-two states now regulate elder day-care). Who sponsors the agency?

- Is the agency designed in space, furniture, decor and color, equipment, and safety features for the elderly, including frail but ambulatory elderly and the cognitively impaired?

- What meals are served? Are special diets served? Ask the attendees about food.

- Are nurses and social workers employed? Physical therapists? Occupational therapists? Are attendants certified? Professionals should be available to the extent that the agency enrolls elders with physical or cognitive problems. The staff:client ratio should be no more than 1:8, with fewer clients if they are impaired.

- Is transportation provided? Some agencies have van service to pick up and deliver the senior home—within a certain mile radius and at certain hours—for a nominal fee.

- How do staff members handle medical or psychiatric emergencies? What is the policy if the elder becomes ill during the day?

- What is the schedule for the day? Are a variety of activities available? Are trips taken to the community? Are there activities of interest to and for participation by individuals and groups?

- What is the cost per day? Is financial aid available? Are there extra fees for activities? For clients with special physical or cognitive problems?

- How do staff members interact with clients and families?

- What are the appearance and interaction of the clients? Talk with them. Are they satisfied?

5. Creating a climate of acceptance by showing pleasure in their attendance and speaking of plans for the next meeting

Remotivation increases communication and strengthens contact with everyday features of the world for the person who may still have areas of intact personality. You may use this as an adjunct to other interventions.

Reminiscence

This strategy can be a means of helping the older client to reaffirm and discover life through the act or process of recalling the past. It may be used with an individual client or in group therapy.

In individual reminiscence, benefits include improved mood, increased self-esteem, satisfaction with life, and maintenance of cognitive skills. As the older client faces major life crises, it can be helpful to review life achievements and recall old family relationships and friends. Putting relationships in order can be most satisfying. The recall of successes in the past can provide strength to face new life changes. An oral format can provide a release of anger against perceived injustices and allow for expressing memories to share.

Group reminiscence may help the individual to place events in their correct context and to attain a broader perspective. The group provides support as the client reflects on life and is able to resolve and reintegrate feelings. Sometimes groups of individuals of different ages in a family can be helpful in exploring family history and strengthening family ties. A formal group is not always necessary; the technique could be used within a family visit, for example.

The SolCos Reminiscence Model is one example of this technique. It includes processes, items, and outcomes. Processes include talking, listening, and touching to explore the client's historical perspective, education, ethnicity, and the like. The focus is on family, home, community, and life role. Items can be crafts, pictures, music, hobbies, and so on. Audio, video, or written records the client may have can be useful. Outcomes are benefits to the client such as a sense of identity, self-esteem, and communication skills, to name a few (264).

Group Action Among Older Citizens

Interest in civic, social, political, and economic issues is shown in various action groups that have been organized among older citizens through community projects. The Gray Panthers is a well-known organization, as is AARP, but there are other groups as well.

Older persons can help isolated elderly persons in their community. A survey of community services can determine which services are most and least used, which are inadequate, what changes are needed, and what sort of problems the elderly in the area have to face. In one community a one-to-one visiting service was needed; it brought joy and met needs of the isolated elderly. It also provided the elderly visitors with a sense of independence, social acceptability, recognition, status, and a sense of meaning in their lives at a time when losses of one sort or another had left them vulnerable.

Action groups have been formed in many of our major cities in recent years. Their members are elderly persons who are concerned about the needs of their peers and who believe that group action is effective in bringing about legislative change, especially in the area of financial assistance to meet rising costs. Many of these groups have sent representatives to the White House Conference on Aging and have exerted a considerable influence on federal and local planning. Such issues as tax relief, transportation, health care, and nutrition are of vital interest to many concerned elderly citizens who still feel responsible for themselves and their community.

You may have the opportunity to work with action groups in either an advisory, consultative, or direct participation role.

Retirement Communities

Retirement brings many changes, which are discussed by several authors (19, 46, 48, 121, 231, 268). Along with our increased life span and the development of social planning for retirement has come the emergence of a distinct social phenomenon: the retirement apartment complex community.

Apartment complexes are financed privately, by religious organizations, or by the government. The senior must be able to maintain self, although visiting nurse services are acceptable. These complexes may include a central dining room, a nurse and doctor on call, planned social events, transportation services, and religious services. Essentially all living needs are within easy access. Additionally, the seniors have the company of each other if they so desire.

In many cities, hotels have been converted to residence facilities for the elderly. Reminiscent of old-style rooming houses, they provide more supervision and services such as meals, laundry facilities, and shopping. In most of these residences each person is responsible for his or her own room, laundry, and breakfast.

Many couples opt for continuous care facilities. An example of this style of living is the type of community that has been built by the Life Care Services Corporation. Since 1961 this nonprofit organization has built 30 retirement communities in 17 states. One- or two-bedroom apartments or cottages are available for a one-time endowment and a monthly fee for two persons. Services include one meal a day, maid service, all utilities including local telephone bill, full maintenance, a full recreational and social program, and many extras. The residents have at their disposal a fully equipped health center with 24-hour nursing care service as long as needed in the intermediate or long-term care sections of the nursing home facility.

In many regions of the United States, especially in Florida, the desert Southwest, and California, planned communities have been built that are specifically designed for and restricted to those persons over 55. Some are carefully planned miniature cities of low cost with simply designed homes built around clubhouse activities, golf courses, and swimming and therapy pools. Activities such as bingo games, dance instruction, foreign-language study, crafts, and bridge lessons are offered. Other communities are mobile home parks in which often elaborate coaches cost as much as and are set up as permanent homes.

One sociologic aspect of these communities bearing such names as Sun City, Leisure World, and Carefree Village is the lifestyle adopted by the residents as they try to establish a secure base in a new life that is often far removed from family, former friends, and familiar patterns of living. They show concern for the safety, health, and well-being of each other by watching to see that lights are on at accustomed hours in each other's homes, signifying all is well. Celebration of birthdays with special parties and remembrances, entertaining for visiting friends and relatives of one's neighbors, visiting the sick members, and providing food and transportation to the hospital for the spouse of a sick resident all become part of the new life. The residents participate in activities that either are completely new or have not been indulged in for many years such as golf, bicycle riding, hiking, and dancing. Even clothes become gayer for both sexes, and the popularity of casual dress provides for the members of the snowbird set—those who have moved to a warm climate—a new freedom and a chance to try bright colors and styles they may not have worn in a former setting.

This phenomenon gives you insight into the needs for security, a sense of maximum personal effectiveness and belonging, and a feeling of self-actualization felt by older persons, especially when old patterns are put aside either by choice or because of circumstances mediated by health or socioeconomic conditions. Further, the older adult needs a suitable place to live, supportive relationships, a sense of community, financial security, and a sense of setting and achieving goals.

See Guidelines for Selecting a Retirement Community.

Impact of the Able Elderly

The emergence of a population group identified as the well elderly is the result of social and demographic progress in the industrial world. More people are living longer, and poverty, frailty, and dependence are not the common characteristics of most of these older people. In the future there will be more healthy elderly who are better educated and physically and emotionally capable. Our society can already use the elderly population's capabilities; in the future we shall have a rich human resource in larger numbers.

The elderly often give financial support and other kinds of assistance to their younger family members; most old people are not a drain on the family. An aging society offers expanding opportunities for family life. Four types of new potentials are present because of re-

---

▶ **GUIDELINES FOR SELECTING A RETIREMENT COMMUNITY**

- Check climate and cultural and recreational facilities in relation to your preferences and lifestyle.
- Visit the facility; talk with residents; eat a meal. Is it an active, lively community?
- Call state regulators, Chamber of Commerce, and Better Business Bureau to check track record of the developer or owner(s).
- Ask what insurance or bonding instruments will protect you in case the facility experiences financial difficulty. Get copies.
- Review all documents you are asked to sign and seek competent legal advice before signing.
- Ask about lease termination policies. How much notice must the owner give? What are the refund policies?
- Get terms of the deposit in writing. If it is refundable, how and at what percentage? Will interest be applied; if so, at what rate?
- Determine if monthly fees are tied to an index. If so, which one? Ask for a history of increases to date, and check the index at a library.
- If it is a lifetime or continuing care community, are nursing home costs prepaid? If not, what are the additional costs?
- Ask about restrictions and policies about visitors (overnight, for how long), parking a recreational vehicle, parking more than one car in the driveway, and use of facilities by visitors.
- Take your time to decide. Visit different facilities.

cent demographic change: (1) increased complexity of social networks, (2) increased duration of relationships, (3) prolonged opportunities to accumulate experience, and (4) new chances to complete or change role assignments.

The elder's accumulated shared experience builds family bonds but also helps others deal with a changing historical context. As the elder leaves certain roles behind, he or she can pick up new ones—whether as a grandparent; in a second career; as an activist in the political, social, or community arena; as a decision maker; as an advocate for ethical and moral actions; or as a participant in policy making or creative pursuits in the arts. Well elderly are and will be making contributions to society; it is important to perceive the well older person as a contributing resource.

Outlook for the Future

The current generation of older persons is where we shall all be one day; therefore planning for them is planning for all of us. Areas such as health care delivery, distribution of income over a long life span, sustaining adequate social involvement, coping with organizational systems, and use of leisure are all problems of now and the future. Intervention that seems costly now may be, in the long run, the most economical in terms of tax dollars.

In the face of increasing shortages that raise the cost of living and the change in age and sex distribution by that time, future planning for the elderly will include employment and the attendant problems usually associated with younger persons. Our society will need the experience and wisdom of the senior generation. If persons are employed as late as age 75, health maintenance programs, industrial planning, and awareness of safety needs are just a few of the necessary considerations.

For the older less active persons of the future, Burnside (46) suggests intervening in loneliness through listening, exploring what may be significant to the seniors, and helping them to compensate in some way for personal losses. In addition, she suggests that nurses record the experiences of the elderly for posterity. Day schools for the elderly might encourage research projects, family therapy, and the study of successful aging.

Thus you, the professional of the future, will be challenged to be the innovator. You will be called on to devise and use new treatment methods so that the elderly will function more effectively in society. It is your goal to help them (1) use the potential they have developed throughout life, (2) pass through the years of late

maturity with ego intact and satisfying memories, and (3) leave something of their philosophy for posterity.

▶ HEALTH CARE AND NURSING APPLICATIONS

Assessment and Nursing Diagnoses

Your role in caring for the elderly person or couple has been described throughout the chapter. Assessment, using knowledge presented about normal aging changes versus pathology in the elderly, provides the basis for *nursing diagnoses*. See Selected Nursing Diagnoses Related to Persons in Later Maturity.

Interventions

Interventions may involve direct care, use of verbal and nonverbal skills, availability of self and therapeutic relationship, support, counseling, education, spiritual care, use of remotivation techniques, or referral as you assist the person in later maturity to meet physical, emotional, cognitive, spiritual, or social needs.

You represent a whole cluster of psychological potentials for the elderly person; you become the supportive figure, interpreter of the unknown, symbol of the people close to him or her, and possessor of important secrets or privileged information. You become guide and companion. All this occurs if an empathic regard for the elderly person is reflected in your attitude and actions, even though your initial image of him or her may have been that of punitive parent. Of prime importance is your willingness to listen, explain, orient, reassure, and comfort the elderly person. Your role is crucial, for you are the one who is most likely to maintain personal contact with the client either in an institutional setting or in a community agency.

Involve the person's family if possible. The interest of a family member does much to increase motivation on the part of the elderly. Determine family attitudes and evaluate relationships during teaching–learning or visiting sessions at which the family is present. This procedure helps the family members alter their attitudes to a more realistic acceptance of their relative's health needs. Social support of family and friends is critical for maintaining lifestyle behaviors, emotional and physical health, and coping skills, including for the frail elderly (46, 85, 86, 97, 255).

The cognitive and emotional needs of the elderly person can be met in many ways. Adequate environmental conditions to overcome sensory impairment and

SELECTED NURSING DIAGNOSES RELATED TO PERSONS IN LATER MATURITY*

Pattern 1: Exchanging
Altered Nutrition: More than Body Requirements
Altered Nutrition: Less than Body Requirements
Hypothermia
Hyperthermia
Stress Incontinence
Risk for Injury
Risk for Trauma
Risk for Disuse Syndrome
Impaired Skin Integrity
Pattern 2: Communicating
Impaired Verbal Communication
Pattern 3: Relating
Impaired Social Interaction
Social Isolation
Altered Role Performance
Sexual Dysfunction
Altered Family Processes
Altered Sexuality Patterns
Pattern 4: Valuing
Spiritual Distress
Pattern 5: Choosing
Ineffective Individual Coping
Impaired Adjustment
Defensive Coping
Ineffective Denial
Ineffective Family Coping: Disabling
Ineffective Family Coping: Compromised
Family Coping: Potential for Growth
Decisional Conflict
Health-Seeking Behaviors

Pattern 6: Moving
Impaired Physical Mobility
Fatigue
Risk for Activity Intolerance
Sleep Pattern Disturbance
Diversional Activity Deficit
Impaired Home Maintenance Management
Altered Health Maintenance
Bathing/Hygiene Self-Care Deficit
Dressing/Grooming Self-Care Deficit
Pattern 7: Perceiving
Body Image Disturbance
Self-Esteem Disturbance
Chronic Low Self-Esteem
Situational Low Self-Esteem
Sensory/Perceptual Alterations
Unilateral Neglect
Hopelessness
Powerlessness
Pattern 8: Knowing
Knowledge Deficit
Altered Thought Processes
Pattern 9: Feeling
Pain
Chronic Pain
Dysfunctional Grieving
Anticipatory Grieving
Post-Trauma Response
Anxiety
Fear

*Other of the NANDA diagnoses related to physiologic phenomena are applicable to the ill individual in this group.
From *North American Nursing Diagnosis Association*, NANDA Nursing Diagnoses: Definitions & Classification 1995–1996. Philadelphia: *North American Nursing Diagnosis Association, 1994.*

clearly defined communication, including explanations of procedures and the necessity for them, are vital. Demonstration and written instructions along with the verbal message, divided into small units, are very effective for teaching skills related to self-care and should be combined with practice sessions. The older person seems to learn more easily when stimuli are logically grouped and sequential, when a larger amount of data is given rather than isolated bits, and when the essential information is relevant to needs, interests, and life experience. He or she is likely to recall this information when necessary. When planning for a new task is overlapped with the execution of a previous one, the older person works slowly and with care. The real situation should be simulated as much as possible so that essential steps of the task can be clearly perceived and the teaching can be adapted to the individual's pattern and ability. Allow the person ample time to respond to a task. Your understanding attitude is important if you are to prevent discouragement and depression.

As in all communication, false assurance can only inhibit the person's ability to develop a trusting attitude and suggest paternalism. The display of genuine interest and a receptive attitude will show the older person that he or she is not alone and will help immeasurably in allaying fear. Candor helps decrease anxiety, and the person's fear of death, the dark, or the unknown may be overcome to a great degree through your presence.

Encourage the senior to reminisce; it is an effective intervention for many reasons. Reminiscence helps the older person, through discussion or use of photographs, music, or literature, to do the following (46, 85, 160, 252, 289):

- Maintain a sense of identity and self-worth
- Stay oriented
- Remain aware of his or her environment
- Relive memorable times
- Acknowledge and explore changes in life
- Find meaning in relationships and life cycle events
- Facilitate grieving for losses
- Think in a logical fashion
- Socialize with others
- Work through previously unresolved conflicts
- Manage current stresses with validation of the past
- Reaffirm the worth of life
- Gain a new perspective on life and personal accomplishments
- Refine a sense of ego integrity

Ask questions about his or her early years, work experience, family, special events, travel, and hobbies. Listen as the person shares life philosophy and gives counsel. Look at family photographs and treasured objects with him or her. You may wish to establish a group of seniors whose main goal is to reminisce.

Loneliness is an outgrowth of age-related losses and psychological changes in the elderly (291). It implies a need to assess carefully situations to determine the signs as described in the following case study:

An elderly man living alone made no complaint of loneliness, but the astute community health nurse found his home in deplorable untidiness and unsafe clutter, his diet extremely limited, and his personal hygiene poor. After a homemaker was sent in to help him clean the house, sit with him during meals, and provide a chance for a trusting relationship with another person, he became receptive to suggestions for modifying his living habits and eventually began to visit a senior-citizen group regularly and to make new friends. He came to realize that adaptation to isolation had been unsafe. Interest and patience showed by others restored the feeling of being a valued and accepted human being again.

The authors know of other individuals who would not modify living habits but chose to remain (from a health care viewpoint) in unsafe and unsanitary conditions. Yet instead of giving the person up as a "hopeless case," the nurses continued to foster a relationship of trust, listened to reasons for remaining in the present situation, and helped the person live out the remaining life on his or her own terms.

Helping the elderly person to remain in contact with the environment may be as simple as providing devices such as clocks, watches, and calendars and letting him or her be the one who winds the clock and turns the calendar page each day. If a hearing aid is worn, check its effectiveness. Sudden moves, even within the same institution, increase mortality rates and psychological and physical deterioration. The person should be permitted to remain in familiar territory and with the desired clutter. If a move is essential, he or she should have some choice in the decision, an opportunity to keep valued possessions, and time to adjust to the idea. The person needs to have a personal lounging chair or specific place in the dining room. Room furniture should be arranged for physical safety and emotional security. Privacy must be respected.

Darkness is a cause of confusion. Night lights should be left on and call bell, tissues, and water placed within easy reach. In the hospital room contact should be available to the client through frequent, quietly made rounds at night. Sometimes a client remains oriented more easily if the room door is open so that he or she can see the nurses' station and be reassured of not being alone.

The use of touch is very beneficial, for the older person has little physical contact with others. The need for contact comfort is great in the human organism, and you can satisfy this need to a degree, provided you remember that touch is a language and has a special power. In giving medications, physical care, and treatments, touching is a crucial encounter. Often the person will pay close attention to instructions and cooperate more in his or her care when you use touch on the hand or shoulder while speaking. The success of this aid depends on what your hands are saying.

To the elderly, all things connected with food service have psychological implications. Food represents life; it nurtures. Mealtime is thought of as a time of fellowship with others and a sharing of pleasure, and this attitude should be retained as much as possible for older people. Making the food more attractive, talking with the person, comforting and touching, cajoling if need be, may help, especially if food is being refused. Appetizers and special drinks have been successfully used as an aid to therapy.

The overall loss of physical capacity, decreased resilience, and lowered capacity to resist stress cause most elderly people to view any illness as a potential major crisis in life. Although it may not be obvious, fear is ever present, and death seems to wait in the wings. Unfamiliar surroundings cause apprehension, and either temporary or permanent loss of contact with those who could give support—spouse, friends, relatives—may cause anxiety. Such anxiety can reduce recuperative powers and is sometimes more distressing than the illness itself.

During any crisis in which the organism is under stress, there are several alternatives: exhaustion, recuperation through the help of others, or despondency and dependency. Through the second alternative you may work toward resolution of the crisis. Share the following suggestions with the person:

- Acknowledge the sadness, anger, guilt, and other feelings that are a part of the loss. It is not a sign of weakness to have those feelings.
- Allow self to express the feelings; cry alone or talk and cry with someone who is understanding. If you have always been stoic, it is all right to show feelings. Others may feel more comfortable with you.
- Indulge self constructively. Feelings of fatigue, confusion, and even depression occur with grief. Pay attention to basic needs of nutrition, sleep, and exercise. Do something pleasurable for yourself. Resist artificial consolers such as alcohol, sleeping pills, other drugs, and cigarettes.
- Ask for support and accept it. Determine wishes, needs, and wants. It is all right to ask for help. You have done your share of nurturing; now is your time to allow others to help you.
- Say "No" to major stressors. Take your time in making major decisions. Do not undertake too many life-changing events at once.
- Move beyond regret—the "if only" or "I should have." Do what is needed in the situation. Learn from mistakes. Forgive self and others.
- Affirm your power to heal the wounds. Life will not be the same after a loss; however, life can go on. Talk to others. Call forth inner reserves and spiritual strength. Imagine the person is present.

- State aloud or in a letter or tape to the person that which was left unsaid.
- Focus memory on the valued or favorite times, the happy scenes, and the pleasant instead of the disease, death, or the traumatic.

The fine line between independence and dependence is difficult to maintain with clients of any age, but especially in the elderly because of society's view of them. Expectations of those around us generally foster behavior to match. Conflict between independent and dependent feelings can be avoided, usually first by assuming a firm control based on professional competence and then later by relaxing and allowing the client to emancipate self.

Working with the elderly person may be very rewarding if you are able to suspend youth-directed attitudes and not measure the person against standards that are inappropriate and perhaps too demanding. As with other age groups and in all our relationships, acceptance of the other person as he or she is, not as you wish him or her to be, is extremely important.

> ▶ **CONSIDERATIONS FOR THE EDLERLY CLIENT IN HEALTH CARE**

- Personal history
- Family ties; family history; widow(er)
- Cultural history
- Current responsibilities with a spouse or other family members
- Impact of physiologic changes on functional status and activities of daily living
- Behaviors or appearance that indicate person is being abused or neglected
- Implementation of safety measures, immunizations, and health practices
- Preexisting illness
- Risk factors, past or current measures used to reduce or prevent them
- Current illness
- Bahaviors that indicate age-appropriate cognitive status; ability to manage own affairs
- Behaviors that indicate age-appropriate emotional status, including ego integrity instead of self-despair, and moral–spiritual development
- Behaviors that indicate that retirement and losses that occur in late life have been grieved and integrated into the self-concept and life patterns
- Satisfactory living arrangements
- Involvement in the community to the extent possible
- Behavioral patterns that indicate adult has achieved development tasks

SUMMARY

Later maturity spans many years; thus, the era is divided into young- old, mid-old, and old- old, and frail-old. Certainly the person at 90 or 100 is different from the 70-year-old. Numerous changes occur over the life span; yet, the person maintains many characteristics and abilities typical of the younger years. Generally, the older person is more adaptive and able than is expressed in attitudes of ageism and stereotypes. Some changes may be the result of disease, rather than the aging process, and should be treated.

Considerations for the Elderly Client in Health Care and Chart 7 in Appendix IV summarize what you should consider in assessment and health promotion of the elderly. Chart 7 presents the American Academy of Family Physicians Periodic Health Examination Ages 65 and Over. It includes guidelines for screening, health counseling, immunization schedules, and high-risk categories (10).

► REFERENCES

1. Abraham, I., J. Fox, D. Harrington, D. Smystad, et al., A Psychogeriatric Nursing Assessment Protocol for Use in Multidisciplinary Practice, *Archives of Psychiatric Nursing,* 4 (1990), 242–259.
2. Achenbaum, W., and V. Bengston, Re-engaging the Disengagement Theory on Aging: On the History and Assessment of Theory Development in Gerontology, *The Gerontologist,* 34, no. 6 (1994), 756–763.
3. Adamchak, D., et al., Elderly Support and Intergenerational Transfer in Zimbabwe: An Analysis by Gender, Marital Status, and Place of Residence, *The Gerontologist,* 31, no. 4 (1991), 505–513.
4. Adelmann, P., Multiple Role and Psychological Well-being in a National Sample of Older Adults, *Journal of Gerontology: Social Sciences,* 49 (1994), S277–S285.
5. Aging Brain's Staying Power, *AARP Bulletin,* 37, no. 4 (1996), 1, 15.
6. Aging Skin: Handle With Care, *Harvard Health Letter,* 20, no. 10 (1995), 6–7.
7. Aging Skin, *Harvard Women's Health Watch,* 11, no. 10 (1995), 4–5.
8. Alexander, B., R. Rubinstein, M. Goodman, and M. Luborsky, A Path Not Taken: A Cultural Analysis of Regrets and Childlessness in the Lives of Older Women, *The Gerontologist,* 32 (1992), 618–626.
9. Allen, K., and V. Chin-Sang, A Lifetime of Work: The Context and Meanings of Leisure for Aging Black Women. *The Gerontologist,* 30, no. 6 (1990), 734–740.
10. American Academy of Family Physicians, *Age Charts for Periodic Health Examination.* Washington, DC: Author, 1995.
11. American Association of Retired Persons, *A Portrait of Older Minorities.* Long Beach, CA: Author, 1995.
12. American Nurses Association, *Integrating an Understanding of Sleep Knowledge Into Your Practice.* Washington, DC: Author, 1995.
13. American Psychiatric Association, *Diagnostic and Statistical Manual of Mental Disorders* (4th ed.). Washington, DC: American Psychiatric Association, 1994.
14. Anderson, L., and N. Stevens, Associations with Parents and Well-being in Old Age, *Journal of Gerontology: Psychological Sciences,* 48 (1993), P109–P118.
15. Antonovsky, A., and S. Sagy, Confronting Developmental Tasks in Retirement Transition, *The Gerontologist,* 30, no. 3 (1990), 362–368.
16. Assessing the Elderly System by System, Part I, *American Journal of Nursing,* 85, no. 9 (1985), 974–984.
17. Atchley, R., A Continuity Theory of Normal Aging, *The Gerontologist,* 29 (1989), 183–190.
18. Avoiding Magnesium Overdose, *Tufts University Diet and Nutrition Letter,* 13, no. 9 (1995), 7.
19. Bailey, L., and R. Hanssen, Psychological Obstacles to Job or Career Change in Late Life, *Journal of Gerontology: Psychological Sciences,* 50B (1995), P280–P288.
20. Balin, A., and A. Kligman, eds. *Aging and the Skin.* New York: Raven Press, 1988.
21. Baltes, M., H. Wahl, and U. Furstoss, The Daily Life of Elderly Germans: Activity Patterns. Personal Control, and Functional Health, *Journal of Gerontology: Psychological Sciences,* 45, no. 4 (1990), P173–P179.
22. Barusch, A., and W. Spaid, Gender Differences in Caregiving: Why Do Wives Report Greater Burden? *The Gerontologist,* 29, no. 5 (1989), 667–676.
23. Bass, D., and K. Bowman, The Transition From Caregiving to Bereavement: The Relationship of Care-related Strain and Adjustment to Death, *The Gerontologist,* 3, no. 1 (1990), 35–42.
24. Bassett, B., All Creatures Great and Small, *Arthritis Today,* March–April (1995), 28–34.
25. Beck, C., P. Heacock, S. Mercer, C. Walton, and J. Shook, Dressing for Success: Promoting Independence Among Cognitively Impaired Elderly, *Journal of Psychosocial Nursing,* 29 (1991), 30–38.
26. Bedford, V., Memories of Parental Favoritism and the Quality of Parent–Child Ties in Adulthood, *Journal of Gerontology: Social Sciences,* 47 (1992), S149–S155.
27. Bell, J., In Search of a Discourse on Aging: The Elderly on Television, *The Gerontologist,* 32 (1992), 305–311.
28. Berkman, B., L. Foster and E. Campion, Failure to Thrive: Paradigm for the Frail Elder, *The Gerontologist,* 29, no. 5 (1989), 654–659.
29. Berliner, H., Aging Skin, *American Journal of Nursing,* 86, no. 10 (1986), 1138–1141.
30. ———, Aging Skin: Part Two, *American Journal of Nursing,* 86, no. 11 (1986), 1259–1262.
31. Birren, J., *The Psychology of Aging.* Englewood Cliffs, NJ: Prentice-Hall, 1964.
32. Blackman, L., and M. Larsson, Recall of Organizable Words and Objects in Adulthood: Influences of Instructions, Retention Interval, and Retrieval Cues, *Journal of Gerontology: Psychological Sciences,* 47 (1992), P273–P278.
33. Blumenthal, J., et al., Long-term Effects of Exercise on Psychological Functioning in Older Men and Women, *Journal of Gerontology: Psychological Sciences,* 46, no. 6 (1991), P352–P361.
34. Boland, D., and S. Sims, Family Care Giving: Care at Home as a Solitary Journey, *IMAGE: Journal of Nursing Scholarship,* 28 (1996), 55–58.

35. Borysenko, J., *Minding the Body, Mending the Minds.* New York: Bantam New Age Books, 1988.

36. Bosse, R., et al., How Stressful is Retirement? Findings From the Normative Aging Study, *Journal of Gerontology: Psychological Sciences,* 46, no. 1 (1991), P9–P14.

37. Bowling, A., and P. Browne, Social Networks, Health and Emotional Well-being Among the Oldest-Old in London, *Journal of Gerontology: Social Sciences,* 46, no. 1 (1991), S20–S32.

38. Bozian, M., and H. Clark, Counteracting Sensory Changes in the Aging, *American Journal of Nursing,* 80, no. 3 (1980), 473–476.

39. Brody, E., et al., Caregiving Daughters and Their Local Siblings: Perceptions, Strains, and Interactions, *The Gerontologist,* 29, no. 4 (1989), 529–538.

40. Brown, M., *Readings in Gerontology.* St. Louis: C. V. Mosby, 1978.

41. Brown, V., The Effects of Poverty Environments on Elders' Subjective Well-being: A Conceptual Model, *The Gerontologist,* 35 (1995), 541–548.

42. Browne, C., and A. Broderick, Asian and Pacific Island Elders: Issues for Social Work Practice and Education, *Social Work,* 39 (1994), 252–259.

43. Buhler, C., The Developmental Structure of Goal Setting in Group and Individual Studies, in Buhler, C., and F. Massarik, eds., *The Course of Human Life.* New York: Spring, 1968.

44. Burggraf, V., and B. Donlon, Assessing the Elderly, *American Journal of Nursing,* 85, no. 9 (1985), 974–984.

45. Burke, J., and G. Kamen, Changes in Spinal Reflexes Preceding a Voluntary Movement in Young and Old Adults, *Journal of Gerontology: Medical Sciences,* 51A, no. 1 (1996), M17–M22.

46. Burnside, I., ed., *Nursing and the Aged* (3rd ed.). New York: McGraw-Hill, 1988.

47. Calasanti, T., Theorizing About Gender and Aging: Beginning with the Voices of Women, *The Gerontologist,* 32 (1992), 280–281.

48. ———, Gender and Life Satisfaction in Retirement: An Assessment of the Male Model, *Journal of Gerontology: Social Sciences,* 51B, no. 1 (1996), S18–S29.

49. Caplan, L., and P. Lipman, Age and Gender Differences in the Effectiveness of Map-like Learning Aids in Memory for Routes, *Journal of Gerontology: Psychological Sciences,* 50B (1995), P126–P133.

50. Carlson, S., When Grandmothers Take Care of Grandchildren, *American Journal of Maternal Child Nursing,* 18 (1993), 206–207.

51. Carmichael, C., and M. McGue, A Cross Sectional Examination of Height, Weight, and Body Mass Index in Adult Twins, *Journal of Gerontology: Biological Sciences,* 50A, M-4 (1995), B237–B244.

52. *Catalog of Federal Domestic Assistance.* Washington, DC: U.S. General Services Administration, January 1995.

53. Centers for Disease Control and Prevention General Recommendations on Immunization: Recommendations of the Advisory Committee on Immunization Practices (ACIP), *Morbidity and Mortality Weekly Report,* 43 (January 28, 1994), 23.

54. Chambre, S., Volunteerism by Elders: Past Trends and Future Prospects, *The Gerontologist,* 33 (1993), 221–228.

55. Changes in the Aging Heart, *American Journal of Nursing,* 91, no. 11 (1991), 27–30.

56. Chapman, N., and M. Neal, The Effects of Intergenerational Experiences on Adolescents and Older Adults, *The Gerontologist,* 30, no. 6 (1990), 825–832.

57. Chiriboga, D., Adaptation of Marital Separation in Later and Earlier Life, *Journal of Gerontology,* 37, no. 1 (1982), 109–114.

58. Choi, N., Racial Differences in the Determinants of Living Arrangements of Widowed and Divorced Elderly Women, *The Gerontologist,* 31, no. 4 (1991), 496–504.

59. Cockburn, J., and P. Smith, The Relative Influence of Intelligence and Age on Everyday Memory, *Journal of Gerontology: Psychological Sciences,* 46, (1991), P31–P36.

60. Coke, M., Correlates of Life Satisfaction Among Elderly African Americans, *Journal of Gerontology: Psychological Sciences,* 47, no. 5 (1992), P316–P320.

61. Connidis, I., and L. Davies, Confidants and Companions in Later Life: The Place of Family and Friends, *Journal of Gerontology: Social Sciences,* 45, no. 4 (1990), S141–S149.

62. ———, and J. McMullin, To Have or Have Not: Parent Status and the Subjective Well-being of Older Men and Women, *The Gerontologist,* 33 (1993), 630–636.

63. Cooney, T., and L. Smith, Young Adults' Relations with Grandparents Following Recent Parental Divorce, *Journal of Gerontology: Social Sciences,* 51B, no. 2 (1996), S91–S95.

64. Cooper, R., Concentration Camp Survivors: A Challenge for Geriatric Nursing, *Nursing Clinics of North America,* 14, no. 4 (1979), 621–627.

65. Craig, L., *Nutrition and Aging,* Columbus, OH: Ross Laboratories, 1991.

66. Crystal, S., and P. Beck, A Room of One's Own: The SRO and the Single Elderly, *The Gerontologist,* 32, (1992), 684–692.

67. Cumming, E., and W.E. Henry, *Growing Old: The Process of Disengagement.* New York: Basic Books, 1961.

68. Curb, J., et al., Health Status and Life Style in Elderly Japanese Men With a Long Life Expectancy, *Journal of Gerontology: Social Sciences,* 45, no. 5 (1990), S206–S211.

69. Dacey, J., and J. Travers, *Human Development Across the Lifespan* (3rd ed.). Madison, WI: Brown & Benchmark, 1996.

70. Dellasega, C., Coping with Caregiving: Stress Management for Caregivers of the Elderly, *Journal of Psychosocial Nursing,* 28, no. 1 (1990), 15–22.

71. DeVos, S., Extended Family Living Among Older People in Six Latin American Countries, *Journal of Gerontology: Social Sciences,* 45, no. 3 (1990), S87–S94.

72. Dickerson, A., and A. Fisher, Culture Relevant Functional Performance Assessment of the Hispanic Elderly, *Occupational Therapy Journal of Research,* 15, no. 1 (1995), 50–68.

73. Digiovanna, A. G., *Human Aging.* New York: McGraw-Hill, 1994.

74. DiPietro, L., A. Ostfeld, and G. Rosner, Adiposity and Stroke Among Older Adults of Low Socioeconomic Status: The Chicago Stroke Study, *American Journal of Public Health,* 84, no. 1 (1944), 14–18.

75. Doka, K., and M. Mertz, The Meaning and Significance of Great-grandparenthood, *The Gerontologist,* 28, no. 2 (1988), 192–197.

76. Doress, P., and D. Siegel, *Ourselves, Growing Older.* Boston: Simon & Schuster, 1987.

77. Dowling, G., Sleep Problems in Older Adults, *The American Nurse,* April-May (1995), 24–25.

78. Dracup, K., S. Dunbar, and D. Baker, Rethinking Heart Failure, *American Journal of Nursing,* 95, no. 7 (1995), 23–27.

79. Drug Metabolism: When Does Gender Matter? *Women's Health Advocate,* 2, no. 7 (1995), 4–5, 8.

80. Duncan, P., et al., Functional Reach: A New Clinical Measure of Balance, *Journal of Gerontology: Medical Sciences,* 45, no. 6 (1990), M192–M197.

81. Dura, J., E. Haywood-Niler, and J. Kiecolt-Glaser, Spousal Caregivers of Persons With Alzheimer's and Parkinson's Disease

Dementia: A Preliminary Comparison, *The Gerontologist,* 30, no. 3 (1990), 332–336.

82. Duvall, E., and B. Miller, *Marriage and Family Development* (6th ed.). Philadelphia: J.B. Lippincott, 1984.

83. Dworetzky, J., *Human Development: A Life Span Approach* (2nd ed.). St. Paul/Minneapolis: West, 1995.

84. Eaglstein, W., M. Mckay, and D. Pariser, The Problems That Plague Aging Skin, *Patient Care,* 28, no. 7 (1994), 89–92, 95–96, 101–107.

85. Ebersole, P., and P. Hess, *Toward Health Aging: Human Needs and Nursing Response* (3rd ed.). St. Louis: C. V. Mosby, 1990.

86. Edelman, C., and C. Mandle, *Health Promotion Throughout the Lifespan* (3rd ed.). St. Louis: C. V. Mosby, 1994.

87. Emerg, C., F. Huppert, and R. Schein, Relationships Among Age, Exercise, Health, and Cognitive Function in a British Sample, *The Gerontologist,* 35 (1995), 378–384.

88. Erikson, E. *Adulthood.* New York: W. W. Norton, 1978.

89. ———, *Childhood and Society* (2nd ed.). New York: W. W. Norton, 1963.

90. Estrogen and Bone Loss: A Matter of Timing, *American Journal of Nursing,* 94, no. 2 (1994), 9.

91. Exercise and Aging, *Women's Health Advocate Newsletter,* 2, no. 8 (1985), 1–3.

92. Fields, S. D. Special Considerations in the Physical Exam of Older Patients, *Geriatrics,* 46, no. 8 (August, 1991), P39–P44.

93. Fischer, L., D. Mueller, and P. Cooper, Older Volunteers: A Discussion of the Minnesota Senior Study, *The Gerontologist,* 31, no. 2 (1991), 183–194.

94. For Avoiding Broken Bones, More Vitamin D, *Tuft's University Diet and Nutrition Letter,* 13, no. 5 (1995), 1–2.

95. For Women Sick at Heart, *Tufts University Diet and Nutrition Letter,* 13, no. 9 (1995), 2.

96. Fozard, J., M. Vercrucyssen, S. Reynolds, P. Hancock, and R. Quilter, Age Differences and Changes in Reaction Time: The Baltimore Longitudinal Study of Aging, *Journal of Gerontology: Psychological Sciences,* 49, no. 4 (1994), P179–P189.

97. Fried, H., and H. Waxman, Stockholm's Cafe 84: A Unique Day Program for Jewish Survivors of Concentration Camps, *The Gerontologist,* 28, no. 2 (1988), 253–255.

98. Gardner, J., et al, Grandparents' Beliefs Regarding Their Role and Relationship With Special Needs Grandchildren, *Education and Treatment of Children,* 17, no. 2 (1994), 185–196.

99. Garfein, A., and R. Herzog, Robust Aging Among the Young-Old, Old-Old, and Oldest-Old, *Journal of Gerontology: Social Sciences,* 50B, S77–S87.

100. Gerace, L., Using Family Photographs to Explore Life Cycle Changes, *Nursing and Health Care,* 10, no. 5 (1989), 245–249.

101. Gerber, J., et al., *Lifetrends: The Future of Baby Boomers and Other Aging Americans.* New York: Macmillan, 1989.

102. Gershowitz, S., Adding Life to Years: Remotivating Elderly People in Institutions, *Nursing and Health Care,* 3, no. 3 (1982), 141–145.

103. Gioiella, E., Give the Older Person Space, *American Journal of Nursing,* 80, no. 5 (1980), 898–899.

104. Gladstone, J., The Marital Perceptions of Elderly Persons Living in or Having a Spouse Living in a Long-term Care Institution in Canada, *The Gerontologist,* 35 (1995), 52–59.

105. Glick, O., Normal Thought Processes, *Nursing Clinics of North America,* 28, no. 4 (1993), 715–727.

106. Goldberg, W., and J. Fitzpatrick, Movement Therapy With the Aged, *Nursing Research,* 29 (1980), 339–348.

107. Graber, M., R. Allen, and B. Levy, *University of Iowa: The Family Practice Handbook* (2nd ed.), St. Louis: C. V. Mosby, 1994.

108. Greenberg, J., and M. Becker, Aging Parents as Family Resources, *The Gerontologist,* 28, no. 6 (1988), 786–791.

109. Greenberg, J., M. Seltzer, and J. Greenley, Aging Parents of Adults with Disabilities: The Gratifications and Frustrations of Later-life Caregiving, *The Gerontologist,* 33, no. 4 (1993), 542–550.

110. Grimes, D., and R. Grimes, Tuberculosis: What Nurses Need to Know to Help Control the Epidemic, *Nursing Outlook,* 43, no. 4 (1995), 164–173.

111. Gutheil, I., Introduction: The Many Faces of Aging: Challenges for the Future, *The Gerontologist,* 36, no. 1 (1996), 13–14.

112. Guyton, A., *Textbook of Medical Physiology* (9th ed.). Philadelphia: W. B. Saunders, 1995.

113. Haight, B., and I. Burnside, Reminiscence and Life Review: Explaining the Differences, *Archives of Psychiatric Nursing,* 6, no. 2 (1993), 91–98.

114. Haimov, I., M. Laudon, N. Zisapel, et al., Sleep Disorders and Melatonin Rhythms in Elderly People, *British Medical Journal,* 309, no. 6948 (1994), 167.

115. Hampton, J., *The Biology of Human Aging.* San Luis Obispo, CA: Wm. C. Brown, 1991.

116. Harris, M., Growing Old Gracefully: Age Concealment and Gender, *Journal of Gerontology: Psychological Sciences,* 49, no. 4 (1994), P149–P158.

117. Havighurst, R., *Developmental Tasks and Education* (3rd ed.). New York: David McKay, 1972.

118. ———, A Social–Psychological Perspective on Aging, in Sze, W., ed., *Human Life Cycle,* New York: Jason Aronson, 1975, pp. 627–635.

119. Hayslip, B., Personality–Ability Relationships in Aged Adults, *Journal of Gerontology: Psychological Sciences,* 43, no. 3 (1988), P79–P84.

120. Hayter, J., Modifying the Environment to Help Older Persons, *Nursing and Health Care,* 4, no. 5 (1983), 265–269.

121. Hayward, M., S. Friedman, and H. Chen, Race Inequities in Men's Retirement, *Journal of Gerontology: Social Sciences,* 51B, no. 1 (1996), S1–S10.

122. Hazzard, W., et al., *Principles of Geriatric Medicine and Gerontology* (2nd ed.). New York: McGraw-Hill, 1990.

123. Health Risks: Perception and Reality, *Harvard Women's Health Watch,* 1, no. 10 (1994), 1.

124. Hill D., M. Storandt, and M. Malley, The Impact of Long-Term Exercise Training on Psychological Function in Older Adults, *Journal of Gerontology: Psychological Sciences,* 48, no. 1 (1993), P12–P17.

125. Himes, C., D. Hoban, and D. Eggeben, Living Arrangements of Minority Elders, *Journal of Gerontology: Social Sciences,* 51B, no. 1 (1996), S42–S48.

126. Hirst, S., and J. Miller, The Abused Elderly, *Journal of Psychosocial Nursing,* 24, no. 10 (1988), 28–34.

127. Hogstel, M., Understanding Hoarding Behavior, *American Journal of Nursing,* 93, no. 7 (1993), 42–45.

128. Hollenbeck, K., E. Barrett-Connor, S. Edelstein, and T. Holbrook, Cigarette Smoking and Bone Density in Older Men and Women, *American Journal of Public Health,* 83 (1993), 1265–1270.

129. Hollenberg, N. K., and T. J. Moore, Age and the Renal Blood Supply: Renal Vascular Responses to Angiotensin Converting Enzyme Inhibition in Healthy Humans, *Journal of the American Geriatrics Society,* 42, no. 8 (August 1994), P805–P808.

130. Hong, S., and P. Keith, The Status of the Aged in Korea: Are the Modern More Advantaged? *The Gerontologist,* 32 (1992), 197–202.

131. Hoole, J., C. Pickard, R. Ouimette, J. Lohr, and R. Greenberg, *Patient Care Guidelines for Nurse Practitioners* (4th ed.). Philadelphia: J.B. Lippincott, 1995.

132. Howard, J., P. Rechnitzer, D. Cunningham, and A. Donner, Change in Type A Behavior a Year After Retirement, *The Gerontologist,* 26 (1986), 643–649.

133. Hultsch, D., M. Hammer, and B. Small, Age Differences in Cognitive Performance in Later Life: Relationships to Self-reported Health and Activity Life Style, *Journal of Gerontology: Psychological Sciences,* 48 (1992), P1–P11.

134. Hummert, M., T. Garstka, J. Shaner, and S. Strahm, Stereotypes of the Elderly Held by Young, Middle-aged, and Elderly Adults, *Journal of Gerontology: Psychological Sciences,* 49 (1994), P240–P249.

135. Hunter, S., Adult Day Care: Promoting Quality of Life for the Elderly, *Journal of Gerontological Nursing,* 18, no. 2 (1992), 17–20.

136. Jacobson, W. H., *The Art and Science of Teaching Orientation and Mobility to Persons With Visual Impairments.* New York: American Foundation for the Blind, 1993.

137. Jendrek, M., Grandparents Who Parent Their Grandchildren: Circumstances and Decisions, *The Gerontologist,* 34, no. 2 (1994), 206–216.

138. Johnson, C., and B. Baker, Families and Networks Among Older Inner-city Blacks, *The Gerontologist,* 30, no. 6 (1990), 726–733.

139. ——, and L. Troll, Constraints and Facilitators to Friendships in Late Late Life, *The Gerontologist,* 34, no. 1 (1994), 79–87.

140. Jolley, J., and M. Mitchell, *Lifespan Development: A Topical Approach.* Madison, WI: Brown & Benchmark, 1996.

141. Jourard, S. M., *The Transparent Self.* Princeton, NJ: D. Van Nostrand, 1964.

142. Jung C., Psychological Types, in Adler, G., et al., eds., *Collected Works of Carl G. Jung,* Vol. 6. Princeton, NJ: Princeton University Press, 1971.

143. Kaakinen, J., Living With Silence, *The Gerontologist,* 32 (1992), 258–264.

144. Kain, C., N. Reilly, and E. Schultz, The Older Adult: A Comparative Assessment, *Nursing Clinics of North America,* 25, no. 4 (1990), 833–848.

145. Kane, R., and R. Kane, Delivering Long-term Care; Lessons From the Developed World, *Aging,* 2, no. 4 (1990), 337–345.

146. ——, et al., Adult Foster Care for the Elderly in Oregon: A Mainstream Alternative to Nursing Homes? *American Journal of Public Health,* 81, no. 9 (1991), 1113–1120.

147. Kaplan, M., M. Adamek, and S. Johnson, Trends in Firearm Suicide Among Older American Males: 1979–1988, *The Gerontologist,* 34, no. 1 (1994), 59–65.

148. Kapp, M., Health Care Decision Making by the Elderly: I Get By With a Little Help From My Family, *The Gerontologist,* 31, no. 5 (1991), 619–623.

149. Kart, S., E. K. Metress, and S. Metress, *Human Aging and Chronic Disease.* Boston/London: Jones & Bartlett, 1992.

150. Kelley, S., Caregiver Stress in Grandparents Raising Their Grandchildren, *IMAGE: Journal of Nursing Scholarship,* 25 (1993), 331–338.

151. Kelly, J., Visual Impairment Among Older People, *British Journal of Nursing,* 2, no. 2 (1993), 110, 112–113, 115–116.

152. Kendrick, Z., S. Nelson-Steen, and K. Scafidi, Exercise, Aging, and Nutrition, *Southern Medical Journal,* 87, no. 5 (1994), 550–560.

153. Kennedy, G., College Students' Expectations of Grandparent and Grandchild Role Behaviors, *The Gerontologist,* 30, no. 1 (1990), 43–48.

154. Kimball, M., and C. Williams-Burgess, Failure to Thrive: The Silent Epidemic of the Elderly, *Archives of Psychiatric Nursing,* 9, no. 2 (1995), 99–105.

155. King, M., J. Judge, and L. Wolfson, Functional Base of Support Decreases With Age, *Journal of Gerontology: Medical Sciences,* 49 (1994), M258–M263.

156. Kitzman, D., and W. Edwards, Age-related Changes in the Anatomy of the Normal Human Heart, *Journal of Gerontology: Medical Sciences,* 45 (1990), M33–M39.

157. Kivett, V., Centrality of the Grandfather Role Among Older Rural Black and White Men, *Journal of Gerontology: Social Sciences,* 46, no. 5 (1991), S250–S258.

158. ——, Racial Comparisons of the Grandmother Role: Implications for Strengthening the Family Support System of Older Black Women, *Family Relations,* 42, no. 2 (1993), 165–172.

159. Knollmueller, R. ed., *Prevention Across the Life Span: Healthy People for the Twenty-first Century.* Washington, DC: American Nurses Association Council of Community Health Nursing, 1993.

160. Kongable, L., K. Buckwalter, and J. Stolley, The Effects of Pet Therapy on the Social Behavior of Institutionalized Alzheimer's Clients, *Archives of Psychiatric Nursing,* 3, no. 4 (1989), 191–198.

161. Kowald, A., and T. Kirkwood, Towards a Network Theory of Aging: A Model Combining the Free Radical Theory and the Protein Error Theory, *Journal of Theoretical Biology,* 169, no. 1 (1994), 75–94.

162. Krause, N., Stressful Events and Life Satisfaction Among Elderly Men and Women, *Journal of Gerontology: Social Sciences,* 46, no. 2 (1991), 584–592.

163. ——, and E. Borowski-Clark, Social Class Differences in Social Support Among Older Adults, *The Gerontologist,* 35 (1995), 498–508.

164. Krueger, J., and J. Heckhausen, Personality Development Across the Adult Life Span: Subjective Conceptions vs Cross-sectional Contrasts, *Journal of Gerontology: Psychological Sciences,* 48, no. 3 (1993), P100–P108.

165. Kohlman, G., et al., Alzheimer's Disease and Family Caregiving: Critical Synthesis of the Literature and Research Agenda, *Nursing Research,* 40, no. 6 (1991), 331–337.

166. Lambert, D., M. Dellmann-Jenkins, and D. Fruit, Planning for Contact Between the Generations: An Effective Approach. *The Gerontologist,* 30, no. 4 (1990), 553–556.

167. Lankford, S., Sleep Loss in the Elderly: Understanding the Reasons, *Journal of Gerontological Nursing,* 20, no. 8 (1994), 49–52.

168. Lara, L. L., P. R. Troop, and M. Beadleson-Baird, The Risk of Urinary Infection in Bowel Incontinent Men, *Journal of Gerontological Nursing,* 16, no. 5 (1990), P24–P26.

169. Lashley, M., Reminiscence: A Biblical Basis for Telling Our Stories, *Journal of Christian Nursing,* Summer (1995), 4–8.

170. Laws, G., Understanding Ageism: Lessons From Feminism and Postmodernism, *The Gerontologist,* 35 (1995), 112–118.

171. Lentzer, H., E. Pamuk, E. Rhodenhiser, R. Rothenberg, and E. Powell-Griner, The Quality of Life in the Year Before Death, *American Journal of Public Health,* 82, (1992), 1093–1098.

172. Levine, J., and R. Taylor, Gender and Age Differences in Religiosity Among Black Americans, *The Gerontologist,* 33 (1993), 16–23.

173. Levinson, D., A Conception of Adult Development. *American Psychologist,* 41 (1986), 3–13.

174. Lidz, T., *The Person: His and Her Development Throughout the Life Cycle* (2nd ed.). New York: Basic Books, 1983.

175. Lindgren, C., The Caregiver Career, *IMAGE: Journal of Nursing Scholarship,* 25 (1993), 214–219.

176. Litchenberg, P., T. Ross, S. Mullis, and C. Manning, The Relationship Between Depression and Cognition in Older Adults: A Cross-validation Study, *Journal of Gerontology: Psychological Sciences,* 50B (1995), P25–P32.

177. Litvin, S., Status Transitions and Future Outlook as Determinants of Conflict: The Caregiver's and Care Receiver's Perspective, *The Gerontologist,* 32, no. 1 (1992), 68–76.

178. Lookinland, S., and K. Anson, Perpetuation of Ageism Attitudes Among Present and Future Health Care Personnel: Implications for Elder Care, *Journal of Advanced Nursing,* 21, no. 1 (1995), 47–56.

179. Lord, S., R. Clark, and I. Webster, Postural Stability and Associated Physiological Factors in a Population of Aged Persons, *Journal of Gerontology: Medical Sciences,* 46, no. 3 (1991), M69–M76.

180. D. Lloyd, M. Nirui, J. Raymond, P. Williams, and R. Stewart, The Effect of Exercise on Gait Patterns in Older Women: A Randomized Controlled Trial, *Journal of Gerontology: Medical Sciences,* 51A, no. 2 (1996), M64–M70.

181. Lowenthal, M., M. Thurnher, and D. Chiriboga, *Four Stages of Life.* San Francisco: Jossey-Bass, 1976.

182. Maas, H., and J. Kuypers, *From Thirty to Seventy.* San Francisco: Jossey-Bass, 1974.

183. Maddox, G. L., Disengagement Theory: A Critical Evaluation, *The Gerontologist,* 4, (1974), 80–83.

184. ———, Lives Through the Years Revisited, *The Gerontologist,* 34, no. 6 (1994), 764–767.

185. Maki, B., P. Holliday, and A. Topper, A Prospective Study of Postural Balance and Risk of Falling in an Ambulatory and Independent Elderly Population, *Journal of Gerontology: Medical Sciences,* 49, no. 2 (1994), M72–M84.

186. Making Sense of Taste and Smell, *Tufts University Diet and Nutrition Letter,* 13, no. 9 (1995), 3–6.

187. Malcolm J., Creative Spiritual Care for the Elderly, *Journal of Christian Nursing,* 4, no. 1 (Winter 1987), 24–26.

188. Mantylo, T., Remembering to Remember: Adult Age Differences in Prospective Memory, *Journal of Gerontology: Psychological Sciences,* 49 (1994), P276–P282.

189. Markides, K., and D. Lee, Predictors of Health Status in Middle-aged and Older Mexican Americans, *Journal of Gerontology: Social Sciences,* 46, no. 5 (1991), S243–S249.

190. Marklein, M., Con Games Proliferate: New Threats Haunt City Folk, *AARP Bulletin,* 32, no. 2 (1991), 1, 16–17.

191. Masters, W., V. Johnson, and R. Kolodny, *Masters and Johnson on Sex and Human Loving.* Boston: Little, Brown, 1988.

192. Mazariegos, M., Z. Wang, D. Gallagher, R. Baumgartner, D. Allison, J. Wang, R. Pierson, and S. Heymsfield, Differences Between Young and Old Females in the Five Levels of Body Composition and Their Relevance to the Two-compartment Chemical Model, *Journal of Gerontology: Medical Sciences,* 49, (1994), M201–M208.

193. McCartney, N., A. Hicks, J. Martin, and C. Webber, *Journal of Gerontology: Biological Sciences,* 50A (1995), B97–B104.

194. McConatha, D., J. McConatha, and R. Dermigny, The Use of Interactive Computer Services to Enhance the Quality of Life for Long-term Care Residents, *The Gerontologist,* 34 (1994), 553–556.

195. McCoy, V., Adult Life Cycle Tasks/Adult Continuing Education Program Response, *Lifelong Learning in the Adult Years,* October (1977), 16.

196. McCrae, R., Age Differences in the Use of Coping Mechanisms, *Journal of Gerontology,* 37 (1982), 454–460.

197. ———, and P. Costa, Age, Personality, and Spontaneous Self-concept, *Journal of Gerontology: Social Sciences,* 43, no. 6 (1988), S177–S185.

198. McDonald-Miszczak, L., A. Hubley, and D. Hultsch, Age Differences in Recall and Predicting Recall of Action Events and Words, *Journal of Gerontology: Psychological Sciences,* 51B, no. 2 (1996), P81–P90.

199. McDougall, S., A Critical Review of Research on Cognitive Function/Impairment in Older Adults, *Archives of Psychiatric Nursing,* 9 (1995), 22–33.

200. Mckenna, M., Twice in Need of Care: A Transcultural Nursing Analysis of Elderly Mexican Americans, *Journal of Transcultural Nursing,* 1, no. 1 (1989), 46–52.

201. Mead, G., Mind, Self, and Society, in Strauss, A. ed., *George Herbert Mead: On Social Psychology.* Chicago: University of Chicago Press, 1964.

202. Meehan, P., L. Saltzman, and R. Sattin, Suicides Among Older United States Residents: Epidemiologic Characteristics and Trends. *American Journal of Public Health,* 81, no. 9 (1991), 1198–1200.

203. Mikhail, M., Psychological Responses to Relocation to a Nursing Home, *Journal of Gerontological Nursing,* 18, no. 3 (1993), 35–39.

204. Miller, S., and J. Cavanaugh, The Meaning of Grandparenthood and Its Relationship to Demographic, Relationship, and Social Participation Variables, *Journal of Gerontology: Psychological Sciences,* 45, no. 6 (1990), P244–P246.

205. Mills, E., The Effect of Low-intensity Aerobic Exercise on Muscle Strength, Flexibility, and Balance Among Sedentary Elderly Persons, *Nursing Research,* 43, (1994), 207–211.

206. Minaker, K., and R. Frishman, Love Gone Wrong, *Harvard Health Letter,* Special Supplement, October (1995), 9–12.

207. Mion, L., J. McDowell, and L. Heaney, Nutritional Assessment of the Elderly in the Ambulatory Care Setting, *Nurse Practitioner Forum,* 5, no. 1 (1994), 46–51.

208. Mirotznik, J., and A. Ruskin, Inter-institutional Relocation and Its Effects on Psychosocial Status, *The Gerontologist,* 25, no. 3 (1988), 263–270.

209. Moloney, M., A Heideggerian Hermeneutical Analysis of Older Women's Stories of Being Strong, *IMAGE: Journal of Nursing Scholarship,* 27 (1995), 104–109.

210. Moritz, D., S. Kasl, and L. Berkman, The Health Impact of Living With a Cognitively Impaired Elderly Spouse: Depressive Symptoms and Social Functioning, *Journal of Gerontology: Social Sciences,* 44, no. 1 (1989), S17–S27.

211. Moon, A., and O. Williams, Perceptions of Elder Abuse and Help-seeking Patterns Among African-American, Caucasian American, and Korean-American Elderly Women, *The Gerontologist,* 33 (1993), 386–395.

212. Mor, V., K. Branco, J. Fleishman, C. Hawes, et al., The Structure of Social Engagement Among Nursing Home Residents, *Journal of Gerontology: Psychosocial Sciences,* 50B (1995), P1–P8.

213. Morgan, D., Adjusting to Widowhood: Do Social Networks Really Make it Easier? *The Gerontologist,* 29, no. 1 (1989), 101–107.

214. Mui, A. and D. Burnette, Long-term Care Service Use by Frail Elders: Is Ethnicity a Factor? *The Gerontologist,* 34 (1994), 190–198.

215. Murray, R., and M. Huelskoetter, *Psychiatric/Mental Health Nursing: Giving Emotional Care* (3rd ed.). Norwalk, CT: Appleton & Lange, 1991.

216. Neugarten, B., Grow Old Along With Me! The Best is Yet to Be, *Psychology Today,* 5, no. 7 (1971), 45ff.

217. ———, Adult Personality: A Developmental View, in Charles, D., and W. Looft, eds., *Readings in Psychological Development Through Life.* New York: Holt, Rinehart & Winston, 1973, pp. 356–366.

218. ———, Adaptation and the Life Cycle, *Counseling Psychologist,* 6, no. 1 (1976), 16–20.

219. ———, Development Perspective of Aging, in Karl, E., and B. Manard, eds., *Aging in America.* Sherman Oaks, CA: Alfred Publishers, 1981.

220. Norris, R., Commonsense Tips for Working With Blind Patients, *American Journal of Nursing,* 89, no. 3 (1989), 360–361.

221. O'Connor, P., Salient Themes in the Life Review of a Sample of Frail Elderly Respondents in London, *The Gerontologist,* 34, no. 2 (1994), 224–230.

222. O'Donnell, M., Assessing Fluid and Electrolyte Balance in Elders, *American Journal of Nursing,* 95, no. 11 (1995), 41–45.

223. Osguthorpe, N., and E. Morgan, An Immunization Update for Primary Health Care Providers, *Nurse Practitioner: American Journal of Primary Health Care,* 20, no. 6 (1995), 52, 54, 60–65.

224. Palmore, E., The Effects of Aging on Activities and Attitudes, *The Gerontologist,* 8 (1968), 259–263.

225. Parker, M., M. Thorslund, and O. Lundberg, Physical Function and Social Class Among Swedish Oldest-Old, *Journal of Gerontology: Social Sciences,* 48 (1994), S196–S201.

226. Parker, R., Reminiscence: A Continuity Theory Framework, *The Gerontologist,* 35, (1995), 515–520.

227. Peachey, N., Helping the Elderly Person Resolve Integrity Versus Despair, *Perspectives in Psychiatric Nursing,* 28, no. 2 (1992), 29–31.

228. Peck, R. C., Psychological Development in the Second Half of Life, in Neugarten, B., ed., *Middle Age and Aging.* Chicago: University of Chicago Press, 1968.

229. Perlmutter, M., and L. Nyquist, Relationships Between Self-reported Physical and Mental Health and Intelligence Performance Across Adulthood, *Journal of Gerontology: Psychological Sciences,* 45, no. 4 (1990), P145–P155.

230. Phillips, S., S. Bruce, D. Newton, and R. Woledge, The Weakness of Old Age Is Not Due to Failure of Muscle Activation, *Journal of Gerontology: Medical Sciences,* 47 (1992), M45–M49.

231. Pienta, A., J. Burr, and J. Mutchler, Women's Labor Force Participation in Later Life: The Effects of Early Work and Family Experiences, *The Journal of Gerontology,* 49 (1994), S231–S238.

232. Pietrukowicz, M., and M. Johnson, Using Life Histories to Individualize Nursing Home Staff Attitudes Toward Residents, *The Gerontologist,* 31, no. 1 (1991), 102–106.

233. Pina, D., and Bengston, V., Division of Household Labor and the Well-being of Retirement-aged Wives, *The Gerontologist,* 35 (1995), 308–317.

234. Porter, E., Older Widows' Experience Living Alone at Home, *IMAGE: Journal of Nursing Scholarship,* 26 (1994), 19–24.

235. Pullinger, W.F., Jr., A History of Remotivation, *Hospital and Community Psychiatry,* 18, no. 1 (1967), 35–39.

236. Reed, P., Self-transcendence and Mental Health in Oldest-old Adults, *Nursing Research,* 40, no. 1 (1991), 5–11.

237. Revicki, D., and J. Mitchell, Strain, Social Support, and Mental Health in Rural Elderly Individuals, *Journal of Gerontology: Social Sciences,* 45, no. 6 (1990), S267–S274.

238. Richard, H., F. Scogin, and S. Keith, A One-year Follow-up of Relaxation Training for Elders With Subjective Anxiety, *The Gerontologist,* 34 (1994), 121–122.

239. Richardson, J., and E. Hurvitz, Peripheral Neuropathy: A True Risk Factor for Falls, *Journal of Gerontology: Medical Sciences,* 50A, no. 4 (1995), M211–M215.

240. Richardson, V., and K. Kilty, Retirement Intentions Among Black Professionals: Implications for Practice With Older Black Adults, *The Gerontologist,* 32, no. 1 (1992), 7–16.

241. Richelman, B., L. Gallman, and H. Parra, Attachment and Quality of Life in Older, Community-residing Men, *Nursing Research,* 43 (1994), 68–72.

242. Richard, H., F. Scogin, and S. Keith, A One-year Follow-up of Relaxation Training for Elders With Subjective Anxiety, *The Gerontologist,* 34 (1994), 121–122.

243. Roberto, K., Grandchildren and Grandparents: Roles, Influences, and Relationships, *International Journal of Aging and Human Development,* 34 (1992), 227–239.

244. Roberts, B., R. Dunkle, and M. Haug, Physical, Psychological, and Social Resources as Moderators of the Relationship of Stress to Mental Health of the Very Old, *Journal of Gerontology: Social Sciences,* 49 (1994), S35–S43.

245. Rohan, E., B. Berkman, S. Walker, and W. Holmes, The Geriatric Oncology Patient: Ageism in Social Work Practice, *Journal of Gerontology: Social Work,* 23, no.1/2 (1994), 201–221.

246. Roos, N., and B. Havens, Predictors of Successful Aging: A 12 Year Study of Manitoba Elderly, *American Journal of Public Health,* 81, no. 1 (1991), 63–68.

247. Rose, M., Evolutionary Biology of Aging, *Human Biology,* 65, (1993), 844–847.

248. Rosenbaum, J., Cultural Care of Older Greek Canadian Widows Within Leininger's Theory of Culture Care, *Journal of Transcultural Nursing,* 2, no. 1 (1990), 37–47.

249. Ross, M., et al., Age Differences in Body Consciousness, *Journal of Gerontology: Psychological Sciences,* 44, no. 1 (1989), P23–P24.

250. Rubenstin, R., Never Married Elderly as a Social Type: Re-evaluating Some Images, *The Gerontologist,* 27, no. 1 (1987), 108–112.

251. ———, et al., Key Relationships of Never Married, Childless Older Women: A Cultural Analysis, *Journal of Gerontology: Social Sciences,* 46, no. 5 (1991), S270–S277.

252. Rybarczyk, B., and S. Auerbach, Reminiscence Interviews as Stress Management Interventions for Older Patients Undergoing Surgery, *The Gerontologist,* 30, no. 4 (1990), 522–528.

253. Salthouse, T., General and Specific Speed Mediation of Adult Age Differences in Memory, *Journal of Gerontology: Psychological Sciences,* 51B, no. 1 (1996), P30–P42.

254. Schaie, K., and S. Willis, Adult Personality and Psychomotor Performance: Cross-sectional and Longitudinal Analysis, *Journal of Gerontology: Psychological Sciences,* 46, no. 6 (1991), P275–P284.

255. Schank, M., and M. Lough, Profiles of Frail Elderly Women, Maintaining Independence, *Journal of Advanced Nursing,* 15, no. 6 (1990), 674–682.

256. Schneewind, E., Of Ageism, Suicide, and Limiting Life, *Journal of Gerontological Social Work,* 23, no.½ (1994), 135–150.

257. Schulz, R., Emotionality and Aging: A Theoretical and Empirical Analysis, *Journal of Gerontology,* 37, no. 1 (1982), 412–451.

258. Seeman, T., L. Berkman, P. Charpentier, D. Bluzer, M. Albert, and M. Tinetti, Behavioral and Psychosocial Predictors of Physical Performance: MacArthur Studies of Successful Aging, *Journal of Gerontology: Medical Sciences,* 50A, no. 4 (1995), M177–M183.

259. Sheehy, G., *New Passages.* New York: Random House, 1995.

260. Shiferaw, B., M. Mittelmark, J. Wofford, R. Anderson, P. Walls, and B. Rohrer, The Investigation and Outcome of Reported Cases of Elder Abuse: The Forsyth County Aging Study, *The Gerontologist,* 34 (1994), 123–125.

261. Sill, J., Disengagement Reconsidered: Awareness of Finitude, *The Gerontologist,* 20, no. 4 (1980), 457–462.

262. Small, B., D. Hulstch, and M. Masson, Adult Age Differences in Perceptually Based, But Not Conceptually Based Implicit Tests of Memory, *Journal of Gerontology: Psychology Sciences,* 50B, no. 3 (1995), P162–P170.

263. Solomon, J. and J. Marx, "To Grandmother's House We Go": Health and School Adjustment of Children Raised Solely by Grandparents, *The Gerontologist,* 35, no. 3 (1995), 386–394.

264. Soltys, F. G., and L. Coats, The SolCos Model: Facilitating Reminiscence Therapy, *Journal of Gerontological Nursing,* 20, no. 11 (1994), P11–16.

265. Steinmetz, H., and S. Hobson, Prevention of Falls Among the Community-dwelling Elderly: An Overview, *Physical and Occupational Therapy in Geriatrics,* 12, no. 4 (1994), 13–29.

266. Stelmack, G., J. Phillips, R. Fabio, and N. Teasdale, Age, Functional Postural Reflexes, and Voluntary Sway, *Journal of Gerontology: Biological Sciences,* 44 (1989), B100–B106.

267. Sung, K., Measures and Dimensions of Filial Deity in Korea, *The Gerontologist,* 35 (1995), 240–246.

268. Szinovacz, M., and C. Washo, Gender Differences in Exposure to Life Events and Adaptation to Retirement, *Journal of Gerontology: Social Sciences,* 47 (1992), S191–S196.

269. Tanjasiri, S., S. Wallace, and K. Shibata, Picture Imperfect: Hidden Problems Among Asian Pacific Islander Elderly, *The Gerontologist,* 35 (1995), 753–760.

270. Taylor, R., and L. Chatters, Extended Family Network of Older Black Adults, *Journal of Gerontology: Social Sciences,* 46 (1991), S210–S217.

271. Tennstedt, S., J. McKinlay, and L. Sullivan, Informal Care for Frail Elders: The Role of Secondary Caregivers, *The Gerontologist,* 29, no. 5 (1989), 677–683.

272. Thomas, J., Concerns Regarding Adult Children's Assistance: A Comparison of Young-old, and Old-old Parents, *Journal of Gerontology: Social Sciences,* 48 (1993), S315–S322.

273. Thompson, E., A. Futterman, D. Gallagher-Thompson, J. Rose, and S. Lovett, Social Support and Caregiving Burden in Family Caregivers of Frail Elders, *Journal of Gerontology: Social Sciences,* 48, no. 5 (1993), S245–S254.

274. Timiras, P., ed. *Physiological Basis of Geriatrics.* New York: Churchill Livingstone, 1990.

275. Tolbert, B. M., Reality Orientation and Remotivation in a Long-term Care Facility, *Nursing and Health Care,* 5, no. 1 (1984), 40–44.

276. Tran, T., Language Acculturation Among Older Vietnamese Refuge Adults, *The Gerontologist,* 30 (1990), 94–99.

277. Trentini, G., C. DeGaetami, and M. Criscuolo, Pineal Gland and Aging, *Aging,* 3 (1991), 103–116.

278. Tsuji, I., Y. Minami, A. Fukao, S. Hisamichi, H. Asano, and M. Sato, Active Life Expectancy Among Elderly Japanese, *Journal of Gerontology: Medical Sciences,* 50A, no. 3 (1995), M173–M176.

279. Turner, J., and D. Helms, *Lifespan Development* (5th ed.). Ft. Worth: Harcourt Brace College, 1995.

280. Uhlenberg, P., and T. Cooney, Family Size and Mother–Child Relations in Later Life, *The Gerontologist,* 30 (1990), 618–625.

281. Uhlenberg, P., and M. A. Myers. Divorce and the Elderly, *The Gerontologist,* 21, no. 3 (1981), 276–282.

282. Uphold, C., and M. Graham, *Clinical Guidelines in Family Practice* (2nd ed.). Gainesville, FL: Barmarrae Books, 1994.

283. Uriri, J., and R. Thatcher-Winger, Health Risk Appraisal and the Older Adult, *Journal of Gerontological Nursing,* 21, no. 5 (1995), 25–31.

284. U.S. Census Bureau, *Current Population Reports.* Washington, DC: U.S. government Printing Office, 1990.

285. Vaillant, G., The Association of Ancestral Longevity With Successful Aging, *Journal of Gerontology: Psychological Sciences,* 46, no. 6 (1991), P292–P298.

286. Verbrugge, L., A. Gruber-Baldini, and J. Fozard, Age Differences and Age Changes in Activities: Baltimore Longitudinal Study of Aging, *Journal of Gerontology: Social Sciences,* 51B, no. 1 (1996), S30–S41.

287. Vos, S., Extended Family Living Among Older People in Six Latin American Countries, *Journal of Gerontology: Social Sciences,* 45 (1990), S87–S94.

288. Wagnild, G., and H. Young, Resilience Among Older Women, *IMAGE: Journal of Nursing Scholarship,* 22, (1990), 252–255.

289. Wallace, J., Reconsidering the Life Review: The Social Construction of Talk About the Past, *The Gerontologist,* 32, no. 1 (1992), 120–125.

290. Walsh, K., Guideline for the Prevention and Control of Tuberculosis in the Elderly, *Nurse Practitioner,* 19, no. 11 (1994), 79–84.

291. Walton, C., et al., Psychological Correlates of Loneliness in the Older Adult, *Archives of Psychiatric Nursing,* 5, no. 3 (1991), 165–170.

292. Ward, M., H. Hubert, H. Shi, and D. Bloch, Physical Disability in Older Runners: Prevalence, Risk Factors, and Progression with Age, *Journal of Gerontology: Medical Sciences,* 50A (1995), M70–M77.

293. Warshaw, R., Can Grandparent Caregivers Find Help? *Modern Maturity,* July–August (1995), 28.

294. Werner, K., D. Christoph, J. Born, and H. Fehm, Changes in Cortisol and Growth Hormone Secretion During Nocturnal Sleep in the Course of Aging, *Journal of Gerontology: Medical Sciences,* 51A, no. 1 (1996), M3–M9.

295. Weilitz, P., and A. Lueckenotte, Respiratory Assessment of Older Adults: Part I, *Perspectives in Respiratory Nursing,* 6, no. 1 (1995), 1, 3–4.

296. White, N., and W. Cunningham, Is Terminal Drop Pervasive or Specific? *Journal of Gerontology,* 43, no. 6 (1988), 141–144.

297. Why We Forget, *Harvard Women's Health Watch,* 3, no. 1 (1995), 1.

298. Wiener, J., et al., Measuring the Activities of Daily Living: Comparisons Across National Surveys, *Journal of Gerontology: Social Sciences,* 45, no. 6 (1990), 229–237.

299. Williams, S., *Nutrition and Diet Therapy* (10th ed.). St. Louis: C. V. Mosby, 1995.

300. Williams-Burgess, C., and M. Kimball, The Neglected Elder: A Family Systems Approach, *Journal of Psychosocial Nursing,* 30, no. 10 (1992), 21–25.

301. Wilson, P., K. Anderson, T. Harris, W. Kannel and W. Castelle, Determinants of Change in Total Cholesterol and HDL-C with Age: The Framingham Study, *Journal of Gerontology,* 49, no. 6 (1994), M252–M257.

302. Winkler, A., et al., The Impact of a Resident Dog on an Institution for the Elderly: Effects on Perceptions and Social Interactions, *The Gerontologist,* 29, no. 2 (1989), 216–223.

303. Wister, A., Environmental Adaptation by Persons in Their Later Life, *Research on Aging,* 11, (1989), 267–291.

304. Wolf, D., Changes in the Living Arrangements of Older Women: An International Study, *The Gerontologist,* 35 (1995), 724–731.

305. Wolinski, F., T. Stump, and D. Clark, Antecedents and Consequences of Physical Activity and Exercise Among Older Adults, *The Gerontologist,* 35, no. 4 (1995), 451–462.

306. Worach-Kardas, H., The Polish Family Tradition, *The Gerontologist,* 23, no. 6 (1983), 593–596.

307. Worobey, J., and R. Angel, Functional Capacity and Living Arrangements of Unmarried Elderly Persons, *Journal of Gerontology: Social Sciences,* 45, no. 3 (1990), S95–S101.

308. Wykle, M., E. Kahana, and J. Kowal, eds., *Stress & Health Among the Elderly.* New York: Springer, 1992.

309. Zsembik, B., and A. Singer, The Problem of Defining Retirement Among Minorities: The Mexican Americans, *The Gerontologist,* 30, no. 6 (1990), 749–757.

► INTERVIEW

310. Alverson, P., Jr., Nursing Home Administrator, Greenwood, SC, March 15, 1995.

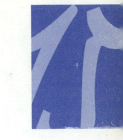

chapter fifteen

Death, the Last Developmental Stage

Death is universal, but there is no universal meaning to death. Meaning comes from a merging of philosophical, spiritual, emotional, sociocultural, historical and geographical factors.
—Ruth Beckmann Murray

 Key Terms

Death	Physician-assisted suicide	Psychological isolation	Psychic death
Coma	Near-death experience	Anger	Karoshi
Euthanasia	Out-of-body experience	Bargaining	Delayed grief response
Active	Nearing-death awareness	Depression	Complicated grief response
Passive	Closed awareness	Preparatory depression	Dysfunctional grief response
Living will	Suspicious awareness	Acceptance	Pathologic grief response
Durable power of attorney for	Mutual pretense	Anniversary reaction	
health care	Open awareness	Predilection to death	
Assisted suicide	Denial and isolation	Scared-to-death individual	

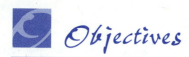 *Objectives*

1. Explore personal reactions to active and passive euthanasia and the right-to-die movement versus extraordinary measures to prolong life. Contrast home or hospice care with hospital or nursing home care.

2. Contrast the child's, adolescent's, and adult's concept of death.

3. Discuss personal feelings about death and the dying person.

4. Discuss the stages of awareness and related behavior as the person adapts to the crisis of approaching death.

5. Discuss the sequence of reactions when the person and family are aware of terminal illness.

6. Talk with another about how to plan for eventual death.

7. Assess reactions and needs of a dying client and family members with supervision.

8. Plan and give care, with supervision, to a client based on understanding of his or her awareness of eventual death, behavioral and emotional reactions, and physical needs.

9. Intervene appropriately to meet needs of family members of a dying person.

10. Evaluate the effectiveness of care given.

Death has been avoided in name and understanding. There may be no harm in saying "he passed" instead of "he died." There is harm in suddenly facing a client's death without sufficient emotional preparation.

ISSUES RELATED TO DYING AND DEATH

Definitions of Death

The aged differ from persons in other life areas in that their concept of future is realistically limited. The younger person may not live many years into the future but generally thinks of many years of life ahead. The older person knows that, despite medical and technical advances, life is limited.

Death is the last developmental stage. It is more than simply an end process; it can be viewed as a goal and as fulfillment. If the person has spent his or her years unfettered by fear, if he or she has lived richly and productively, and if he or she has achieved the developmental task of ego integrity, he or she can accept the realization that the self will cease to be and that dying has an onset long before the actual death. Research on near-death experiences also conveys that death is another stage (15, 26, 28, 59, 83, 91, 95).

If death is considered the last developmental phase, it is worth the kind of preparation that goes into any developmental phase, perhaps physically, certainly emotionally, socially, philosophically, or spiritually.

Until this century death usually occurred in the home, but at present more than 70% of deaths in American cities occur in institutions so that death has become remote and impersonal.

Because of technologic advances, the determination of **death** is *changing from the traditional concept that death occurs when the heart stops beating*. The neurologic criteria for death are as valid as the cardiopulmonary criteria. The Uniform Determination of Death Act (UDDA), or similar legislation, is recognized in all 50 states. The Act defines death as *irreversible cessation of circulatory and respiratory functions, or irreversible cessation of all functions of the brain, including the brain stem*. Death based on neurologic criteria is true death (21).

Medically accepted standards for *brain death* include the following neurologic criteria (21, 94):

- Underlying cause of condition or brain injury must be known and diagnosed as irreversible.
- Declaration of death can be made only if patient is not suffering from hypothermia (32.2°C) or receiving central nervous system depressants, either of which present appearance of brain death.
- Person must manifest cerebral unresponsiveness and no reflexes.
- Apnea testing must not produce spontaneous respiration.

Institutions may also have other criteria for their policies and procedures for pronouncing brain death. Most institutions require an electroencephalogram (EEG) to confirm absence of brain activity. Some require a cerebral radionuclide scan or four-vessel arteriogram to verify absence of blood flow (21).

Thus, brain death is differentiated from **coma,** a *persistent vegetative state* in which the person, not assistive devices, maintains basic vital homeostatic functions and therefore is not dead, even though he or she is not responding verbally or nonverbally. In brain death, the appearance of life continues when the ventilator is used to deliver enough oxygen to keep the heart beating and skin warm. The ventilation is maintained until there is a decision about tissue or organ donation. If there is no organ procurement, the ventilator is discontinued (21).

The sophisticated machinery has caused some to ask questions such as, "If we declare someone entirely dead when the brain is 'dead,' even though some of the body continues to function with the help of life supports, then doesn't that body lose its sanctity and become the object of transplant organ harvesting?" The opposition might answer. "Without the present life-support systems, this person would certainly have been dead. Why not take the opportunity to save another person's life with the needed organ(s)?" Some people believe organ donation gives meaning to their own life and death (or that of the family member). Depending on the belief system, the organ donation that allows another to live a long, productive life may be viewed as a kind of immortality.

The current issue is not only "When is someone dead?" but "Who decides when to turn off the machines?" Is it the client, medical personnel, a lawyer, the clergy, or the courts?

The family, more than anyone else, must live with the memories of their loved ones and the events surrounding death. It is a violation of the family's dignity to rush death. Even though a lesser involved person might say, "Why don't they turn the machines off!" this person should be ignored until all those closely involved with the client can say with acceptance and assurance, "Now is the time." Increasingly, the *person* is saying that he or she has a right to decide how long machines should maintain personal life or that of a loved one.

The moral, ethical, and legal dilemmas of maintaining or withdrawing life support (ventilator, fluids, antibiotics) are debated, especially when the patient can respond verbally or nonverbally, knows his or her name, and says she or he either does or does not want to die. Family, health care providers, ethical committee, and hospital legal counsel may all be involved in conversations about when to end life. The nurse may advocate for the patient when he or she cannot speak for self (82, 96).

Organ and Tissue Donation

As a nurse, you have significant responsibilities regarding declaration of brain death. You help collect, review, and evaluate data that are essential to declaration of death or maintenance on the ventilator. Comfort and support the family as they anticipate death of the loved one. You continue to observe and give thorough care to the person who is being evaluated as if the person was indeed going to live. Identifying a potential donor and referring to an appropriate procurement agency are crucial steps. Until the donor status is confirmed, you continue to administer care and assist in comfort measures and fluid and ventilatory management (21).

The family must clearly understand the person is dead before they are informed of their legal right to the option of donating, or not donating, tissues or organs. Local organ procurement organizations and tissue and eye banks can supply information and have trained personnel available 24 hours a day to assist families in counseling related to the options. The family needs sensitive communication and a thorough knowledge of the step-by-step process (24).

The procurement coordinator will be the best person to talk with the family about donation because he or she is specially trained. A caring, gentle expression of sorrow for the family is necessary. After they have had time to grieve and realize death has occurred, information and support can be given and questions answered. The coordinator can handle cultural or religious considerations. No major religious denomination opposes organ donation; some ethnic or cultural groups may. The family should not be coerced but should be given an opportunity to make an informed decision that is best for them. The family are to be told about the need for organ and tissue donation and how people are helped and that the donation will not disfigure the person, will cost them nothing, and will not delay the funeral (21).

Words are chosen carefully. For example, the coordinator describes the procurement process as receiving, removing, or retrieving organs or tissues, not with the unacceptable term *harvesting*. The ventilator is not a life support machine to "keep the patient alive." The patient is referred to as "dead," not as "nearly dead." The patient is referred to by name, not as donor. If family members disagree, they need time to resolve the conflict (21).

When the family agree to donation, you will focus on physical care for the donor, especially eye and skin care, and emotional support for the family. For a grief-stricken family, participating in donation can be a comfort. They will remember your kind and considerate care and be grateful for the opportunity to contribute life to another, or several persons (21).

The National Organ Procurement and Transplantation Network, established in 1986, is administered by the United Network for Organ Sharing and, in turn, works with staff from local organ procurement organizations who work with local health care providers. A national waiting list is maintained of people in need of transplantation; the Network oversees equitable allocation of organs. About 35,000 people are on the waiting list, an increase in the past few years. Age is no longer a factor for the donor, but donor tissues or organs must be healthy. Thus, patients with extracerebral malignancies or unresolved transmittable infections, such as AIDS and hepatitis B, cannot be donors (21).

The following organs can be transplanted: heart, kidney (can be donated by living donor); liver, lung and pancreas (segments can be donated by living donor); small bowel; and stomach. A number of tissues can be donated, including cornea, skin, dura, fascia, cartilage, tendons, saphenous veins, heart valves, bone marrow, and bones (ribs, femurs, tibias, fibulas, ilium) (21).

Euthanasia

Euthansia is legally defined as the *act or practice of painlessly putting to death persons suffering from incurable or distressing diseases.*

Although maintaining life beyond all reason is an ethical dilemma for the nurse, an equally taxing ethical dilemma occurs when the doctor deliberately hastens the client's death by increasing the dose of a narcotic analgesic such as morphine to the point of lethality. Responsible, moral caregivers promote quality of life and right to die with dignity. If each human life is seen as of infinite value, it will be worth the efforts to ease pain and help the person find meaning in the current situation.

Euthanasia is not new. It was practiced in Greece. African bushmen and North American primitive tribes abandoned their infirm elderly to die; there was insufficient food for anyone who could not produce his or her own food. Eskimo tribal elders cut a hole in the ice and disappeared when they became burdensome.

Euthanasia is illegal throughout the world; in The Netherlands, immunity is granted to the physician who follows specific guidelines. Most nurses do not support active euthanasia; support for it is based on patient autonomy, informed consent, and suffering. Religious beliefs may be the most accurate predictor of the person's stance on euthanasia. Nurses who are opposed to active euthanasia do so on the basis of sanctity of life and limits to autonomy and are worried about the double effect of giving medication for pain that may also shorten life and their own professional integrity and responsibility. Nurses who support active euthanasia define professional integrity and responsibility as being an advocate for patients who make a decision to end their life (26).

To withdraw a patient from life support may allow the patient to die; however, the patient may not die (26).

Most Western countries consider **active euthanasia,** *deliberately hastening death,* as first-degree murder. On the other hand, court decisions have been inconsistent about **passive euthanasia,** *omission of care or inaction to prolong life.*

The development of Judeo-Christian law from the beliefs of St. Augustine and St. Thomas Aquinas held that suicide was a sin and against natural law. In the past in American institutions, physiologic aspects only were considered in prolonging life. Today sociologic and economic aspects are also being considered. The value or quality of life when the person is kept alive by artificial support systems is considered. Costs to client, family, and society are being considered. Ordinary care is the prevailing standard, not extraordinary means, although what constitutes ordinary care is debated.

Euthanasia is based on two fundamental legal premises: the right to privacy and the right to refuse treatment when informed. The competent client may decline treatment for religious reasons, fear of pain or suffering, exhaustion of finances, and unlikelihood of recovery. The incompetent client is not allowed the right to refuse in similar situations for fear of an irrational choice. Medical practice defers to wishes of the family. Those who are disabled, elderly, retarded, or insane may not receive the treatment ordinarily given to others.

Nurses and other health care workers must explore their personal beliefs and stance in active euthanasia, passive euthanasia, and physician-assisted death; their professional obligations to patients who request these; and ethical principles that balance the conflicting moral claims (3, 25, 40, 44, 55, 63, 73, 74, 82, 85, 96, 98).

Leininger (68) believes quality of life is culturally defined and patterned, and issues related to life, death, health, and well-being must be studied from a transcultural rather than individual perspective.

Right-to-Die Movement and the Patient Self-determination Act

Another increasingly publicized facet with moral and ethical aspects is the right-to-die movement, which was first begun in England, Holland, and the Scandanavian countries and which has gained momentum in the United States. Originally the Right-to-Die Society and the movement insisted that people should have the last word about their own lives, either to maintain or to discontinue treatment when ill or dying. The District of Columbia and many states have adopted Living Will laws (right-to-die or natural death laws) that permit mentally competent adults to declare, before they are ill, that they do not want life prolonged artificially or by heroic measures (see Fig. 15–1 pp. 805–806). In states with no formal legislation, living wills have been upheld in courts. Many states have brain death laws that allow withdrawal of respirators when a client no longer shows signs of brain activity. In the case of a lingering, comatose, incompetent person, the relatives, hospital ethics committee, or courts must make decisions about not instituting or withdrawing life-prolonging measures; or the person may have designated someone to have durable power of attorney, available in all states, who can make decisions about health care, finances, and property in the event of incapacity. Please note that Figures 15–1 through 15–6 cited in the following section may be found at the end of this chapter on the indicated pages.

The Patient Self-determination Act became effective in December 1991. All health care institutions or agencies receiving Medicare or Medicaid funds are required to give clients written information about these rights to allow them to make decisions about medical care, to formulate advanced directives, and to refuse treatment (see Figures 15–2, 15–3, pp. 807–810) These agencies must (1) educate staff about how to talk with patients/clients or families about these issues, (2) maintain written policies and procedures for adhering to these requirements, (3) document the person's status on the medical record, and (4) not neglect or withhold treatment from the person based on the decision. This legislation has forced states to develop mechanisms for Durable Power of Attorney for Health Care (Fig. 15–4, pp. 811–813).It has created dilemmas when caring for people who are mentally incompetent (another person then makes the decision as surrogate); in cases of minors needing treatment; when the outcome of an illness is unlikely to be death or in need of heroic measures; or when the person is extremely anxious of facing unexpected death. Will the decision be too hasty? Is sufficient support given to the patient/client, surrogate, and family members? Are qualified witnesses available? Staff also need support as they implement the requirements in unusual or difficult situations (98).

Weber (98) discusses tips on implementing the Patient Self-determination Act, including the nurse's role in formulating directives and how to be effective in talking with the patient/client and family. The roles of advocate and educator are crucial (see Fig. 15–5, p. 814, sample of a Medical Directive, and Fig. 15–6, p. 815, Declaration of Desire for a Natural Death).

Various types of treatment directives that a person must consider are (1) the **Living Will** (Figs. 15–1, 15–3), which *states what medical treatment a person chooses to omit or refuse in case he or she cannot make a decision at the time of the illness* and which indicates that the person would rather die than be kept alive by artificial or heroic measures if there is no reasonable expectation of recovery; (2) a **Surrogate** or **Durable Power of Attorney for Health Care** (Figs. 15–2, 15–4); (3) a **Medical Directive** (Fig. 15–5); or (4) a **Declaration of Desire for a Natural Death** (Fig. 15–6).

Anyone interested in having a Living Will drawn up can request the free forms appropriate to his or her state from Choice in Dying—The National Council for the Right to Die, 200 Varick St., New York, NY 10014 (1–800–989–WILL).

Additionally, an Electronic Living Will Registry is now available. Choice in Dying and the National Electronic Archives of Advance Directives (NEAAD) have collaborated to offer the storage of exact images of patients' advance directives in computer files. The staff will ensure that the directives meet legal requirements of state law. The forms are accessible 24 hours a day, 7 days a week. The forms can be faxed to the individual's family, health care provider, or hospital within 15 minutes of request. For further information call NEAAD at 800–397–6866 (5).

The consequences of ignoring the Living Will and the inconsistency that can arise are explained by Edwards (35). Henderson's study showed that having instructions about and planning for the Living Will can decrease death anxiety (55).

Physicians fear indictment for homicide or aiding suicide even when following the living will, although these laws in all states grant immunity to health care professionals who comply with the declaration. Further, in some states there is a penalty if the physician does not comply. Relatives may sue the physician and/or hospital that refuses to follow the client's wishes reflected in the living will. (Legally, the physician may be charged with battery.)

Nurses are increasingly having to face questions of conscience, ethics, morals, and legalities in relation to what to say to the client and relatives and whether to assist with initiating heroic measures when it is known that the client does not want them or whether to disconnect life-support machines.

Assisted Suicide

The patient may ask you to assist in the committing of suicide. **Assisted suicide** is defined by the American Nurses Association (ANA) *as making a means of suicide* *available to the patient with the knowledge of the person's intended use of the equipment, medication, object, or weapon.* It differs from euthanasia, where the professional directly ends the patient's life. The ANA has issued a statement against assisted suicide or acting deliberately to terminate a patient's life. And in most states such action is illegal. The nurse's role is to assist the person, to comfort, and to be present and available as a support (40, 64).

Certain measures are not considered assisted suicide or euthanasia (40):

- Giving a patient who is hypotensive enough morphine to control his or her pain (Here the principle of double effect applies, in which an action intended to reduce pain and suffering is permissible even if it may have the unintended effect of death.)
- Giving a dyspneic patient enough morphine to control her or his pain symptoms (Again, double effect applies.)
- Sedating a symptomatic or distressed patient at his or her request (The principle of autonomy applies.)
- Withholding or withdrawing nutrition or hydration at the request of a patient (Autonomy applies.)

It is possible to buy manuals on how to commit suicide. The demand for these books is increasing as the public realizes it is illegal for doctors to practice euthanasia and that often doctors feel forced to prolong life, in whatever condition. The manuals argue against suicide when the problem is a distortion of judgment or a psychiatric disorder but give a factual guide about the least painful and most effective measures. Violent methods such as shooting, jumping, and hanging are counseled against because they are too traumatic for the survivors.

In contrast, the Samaritans, an international suicide prevention group, and professionals who work in hospice care and the Medical Association of each country have been sharply critical of such manuals, believing that they may pressure terminally ill, depressed, or elderly people to exit early because they believe they are a burden and unwanted. It is as if society fosters rejection instead of seeking solutions to the problem.

Withholding food and water or discontinuing a feeding tube and intravenous fluids to the chronically or terminally ill or those in a persistent vegetative state is a form of passive euthanasia or assisted suicide and is of growing ethical concern for nurses. The nurse is taught to be an advocate for the client—a very special charge and a difficult but committed kind of caring related to client's needs and rights (103).

Benner describes the conflict between heart and conscience when her father, terminally ill with chronic obstructive pulmonary disease and unable to live without a ventilator, made it known he did not want to live that way and wanted the ventilator removed. The family respected his wishes and remained with him. Versed and morphine were given to ease anxiety and pain and to enable him to rest until he died. Death did not come quickly. A new lung infection was not treated. Other medications (heparin, digoxin, and theophylline) were discontinued. A compassionate and competent staff were valued by the family. Both the staff and family continued to talk with the father, although he was in deep sleep, to treat him as a person with dignity and worth. The final pain, twinges of guilt, and self-doubt are poignantly described even though the family had followed the father's wishes. It took him 10 days to die of respiratory failure. Respect for the father as an intelligent man, capable of deciding the difference between living and lingering, respect for his sense of pride and dignity, and respect for him as a person helped to ease the pain for the family (9).

Several legal cases concerning clients in a persistent vegetative state surviving solely because of the use of respirators and tube feeding have come before the courts, beginning with the Karen Quinlan case in 1977. At least two-thirds of the court rulings in these cases have allowed the removal of the life-support equipment. Many of these people were chronically ill. The cases of Nancy Cruzan and Christine Busalacchi in Missouri are two cases involving discontinuance of feeding and hydration. Nancy Cruzan died in 1990, 12 days after a Missouri judge ruled that her feeding tube be discontinued; three previous co-workers had testified that she had said she "never wanted to live life as a vegetable." In 1991 the Missouri legislature began to study bills that would legalize euthanasia for an expanded group of physically and chronically ill clients. These bills include the Durable Power of Attorney, Health Care Surrogate, and Health Care Consent bills.

The Hemlock Society believes people should be allowed to die. In fact, the society advocates lethal injection as more humane with less suffering. The international Anti-Euthanasia Task Force believes such action is the forerunner of outright killing of sick, disabled, and vulnerable people, rather than having a society and professionals committed to caring for these people. The questions to decide concern who will die when and who will decide (3, 4).

Ferdinand discusses *guidelines to help you determine reasons for a patient's desire to die and how to respond without compromising professional principles* (40):

- Talk with the patient about suicidal statements.
- Assess emotional as well as physical pain and work to reduce both through a variety of pain management methods.
- Allow the patient to express fears about "losing his (or her) mind" as a result of the disease or aging process and how this can be prevented, prepared for, or coped with in late stages of AIDS, brain cancer, or liver or kidney disease.
- Assess and treat underlying depression, which is likely to remove the desire to die.
- Explore losses with the patient and how to cope with or overcome these, and enhance the person's autonomy and control to the extent possible.
- Discuss the patient's idea of death with her or him. Encourage the person to make plans via advance directives or options of hospice care.
- Encourage the patient to discuss faith, hope, and meaning of life. Refer to pastoral care.
- Listen nonjudgmentally, with compassion and concern.
- Encourage the person to do what he or she can for self and to ask others for help when necessary.
- When thoughts of suicide persist, the principle of confidentiality does not prevent you from sharing the patient's disclosure with the physician and health care team, or from facilitating discussion between the patient and family.

As people live longer, they fear there may be a longer period of frailty, disability, depression, and social disconnectedness. Some will choose death rather than survive with pain, isolation, tubes, and machines. There is an increasing movement for the person who is mentally alert but in great pain or disability to make a life termination decision (20, 40, 71, 106). When caring for such ill clients, the clients and the nurses often see meaning in the person's life; to terminate that life would be against what nursing represents. What will be the effects on the nurse of carrying out euthanasia orders? What if the nurse refuses? Nursing is a caring profession. Can caring nurses be educated to participate in planned killing?

The nursing profession and all health care providers have a great deal at stake. Members of the American Nurses Association (and the nurses who are not members) need to speak out. Nurses must decide the meaning of being a nurse and how that meaning applies to caring for the seriously, chronically, terminally, or vegetatively ill. Further, nurses must:

- Listen carefully to clients and families about their concerns.
- Educate society to think and act rationally.
- Act on spiritual convictions about the sanctity of life and health.
- Engage in research about the life promotion effects of imagery, faith, prayer, anointing with oil, and other spiritual or emotional methods of healing.
- Publicize healing events, including the "miracles" so that clients and families can be encouraged and believe in remission and recovery.
- Let live and let die, discerning when the fight must be for life and when death is inevitable, acceptable and natural, discerning when to engage in life extension and when to continue life support.

Recently **physician-assisted suicide,** *prescription of medication or counseling of an ill patient so that he or she may use a drug overdose to end his or her own life,* has been in the news. Dr. Jack Kevorkian had attended at least 25 deaths by suicide by August 1995. He is responsible for developing the "suicide machine" to inject lethal drugs into those seeking his help in dying (62).

This issue encompasses the autonomy/individual rights of the patient, the nurse's or physician's role, and society's stake. Each perspective is a complicated issue. We need to establish safeguards so that the true wishes of the patient can be expressed and legally accounted for. Many people know they can write living will directives but do not do so.

The health care professional role has seen so much technology for life support that much of the human perspective on dying can be lost. So much emphasis has been placed on scarce resources (e.g., organs), being a gatekeeper, and being an entrepreneur that the concept of aggressive, compassionate, palliative care has been lost, except in Hospice. Terminal illness and suffering must be seen as a challenge and a responsibility no matter how the health care professional interprets the euthanasia issue.

Our society in the mid-1990s shows that we still hope for the quick fix with technology, but the aging population reminds us otherwise. We are faced with Oregon Ballot Measure 16 (Oregon Death with Dignity Act of 1994). We are looking at The Netherlands' experience, referred to as the "slippery slope" where, in 1990, there were 8100 intentional opiate overdoses, 1000 lethal injections *without request*, and physician-assisted suicides of which only 41% met regulatory requirements (76). We must remember that a society is defined by how it meets the needs of its least fortunate (62).

Case Situation: Issues in Death and Dying

Mrs. Morton is a 94-year-old widow who has resided in the same farmhouse since her marriage in the early 1920s. She has a history of cardiac disease for approximately 45 years. She now has a pacemaker and daily takes medication for her heart. She has had a bilateral modified mastectomy but has had no further recurrence of cancer. Several times she has been hospitalized, and during the last two hospitalizations she required resuscitation after suffering cardiac arrest.

Mrs. Morton is a very determined, devout, Christian woman, and each time she has been gravely ill, she has proclaimed her faith and has been discharged to her home. She firmly refused admittance to a senior residence center after the last hospitalization, insisting that if she had a visiting nurse and continued help from her grandson, she could live alone in her farm home. Her grandson, who has shopped for her for the last 10 years agreed to do more tasks as necessary. Reluctantly, her physician agreed and ordered home health aide and nurse services. Because of her grave condition and inability to walk except for a few steps, the physician also made occasional home visits.

Mrs. Morton is chronically ill. In fact, her cardiovascular condition is so grave that she is considered terminally ill. According to the euthanasia movement, she should have been allowed to die the last time she required resuscitation. *How wrong that perspective would have been.*

In the 9 months since her discharge, Mrs. Morton has regained her strength, and her circulation has improved. She now walks in her home with a walker and cooks meals for herself and her grandson. She does receive help with bathing and vacuuming. Thus she contributes to the employment of several people. Recently her divorced granddaughter, Jean, and two great-grandchildren have come to live with her because Jean is on welfare and cannot pay the rent and other expenses.

Mrs. Morton acknowledges that having three more people in her home is stressful but says she believes she must help them. She has loaned, or given, considerable money from her farm income and Social Security check to all three of her grandchildren and several of her great-grandchildren. Thus she contributes to the economic support of three, and sometimes more, people. She doubts that anyone will ever repay her.

Because Mrs. Morton is very alert, friendly, indeed very wise, she is a joy to visit. When her many friends come to visit, she shares a piece of cake she has baked and chats about local news. She reminisces some, but not excessively. She seldom complains, even briefly. Although her physical condition is marginal, her mental health is excellent. Possibly because of those healthy components, her physical condition has improved. Mrs. Morton is very much alive and looking forward to her 95th birthday. It is fortunate the emergency team responded by resuscitating Mrs. Morton during her last hospitalization. Indeed, many people would have felt the loss.

It is important for you to struggle with the values and issues of death—accidental death, long-term dying, active or passive euthanasia, and right-to-die choices—and consequently the issues and values of life. You will often be asked about your thoughts and beliefs; it is impossible to be value-free, but you can be nonjudgmental and accepting of another's values. How you proceed with nursing care of the chronically ill or dying person will be influenced by your beliefs. Do not force your beliefs and values on another, but often the client will appreciate your open sharing of values and beliefs. Such sharing may even give him or her energy to continue to live, with quality of life, against overwhelming odds (28, 83, 95, 106). *Certainly do all possible so that the person does not face dying and death alone.*

For more information on the types of euthanasia and the moral–ethical issues, see the references at the end of this chapter (3, 4, 9, 20, 24, 26, 29, 44, 47, 55, 56, 63, 71, 74, 76, 83, 95, 96, 100, 103, 106). Many other references are available for much has been written about dying and death; this chapter provides only an overview of the subject.

DEVELOPMENTAL CONCEPTS OF DEATH

To understand how adults and aged persons perceive death, a review is given here of how the child, adolescent, and adult perceive death. The concept of death is understood differently by persons in the different life eras because of general maturity, experience, ability to form ideas, and understanding of cause and effect.

Children's Concepts of Death

Nagy (79) found three stages in the child's concept of death: (1) death is reversible, until age 5 years; (2) death is personified, ages 5 to 9; and (3) death is final and inevitable, after age 9 or 10.

The *child less than 5* sees death as reversible, a temporary departure like sleep, being less alive, very still, or unable to move. There is much curiosity about what happens to the person after death. The child connects death with funerals, cemeteries, and absence. He or she thinks dead persons are still capable of growth, that they can breathe and eat and feel, and that they know what is happening on earth. Death is disturbing because it separates people from each other and because life in the grave seems dull and unpleasant. Fear of death in the child of this age may be related to parental expression of anger; presence of intrafamily stress such as arguing and fighting; physical restraints, especially during illness; or punishment for misdeeds. At times the child feels anger toward the parents because of their restrictions and wishes they would go away or be dead. Guilt feelings arising from these thoughts may add to the fear of death (72, 79). De Arteaga (27) discusses how to help a young child deal with death, answer questions, and grieve.

The *child from ages 5 to 9* accepts the existence of death as final and not likelife. He or she thinks of death as a person such as an angel, a frightening clown, or monster who carries off people, usually bad people, in the night. Personal death can be avoided; he or she will not die if he or she runs faster than Death, locks the door, or tricks Death unless there is bad luck. Parental disciplining techniques inadvertently add to this belief if they threaten that bad things will happen to the child. Traumatic situations also can arouse fear of death (79).

The *child after age 9 or 10* realizes that death is inevitable, final, happens according to certain laws, and will one day happen to him or her. If he or she is terminally ill, the child may acknowledge approaching death before the parents do (73). Death is the end of life, like the withering of flowers or falling of leaves, and results from internal processes. Death is associated with being enclosed in a coffin without air, being slowly eaten by bugs, and slow rotting unless cremation is taught. The child may express thoughts about an afterlife, depending on ideas expressed by parents and other adults and their religious philosophy (72, 79, 80, 102).

Death is an abstract concept, and Nagy's stages offer a guide; however, not all children's thinking about death fits into those stages. Children (and adults) may have a concept of death that contains ideas from all three stages. The ability to think abstractly is acquired slowly and to varying degrees by different people. Usually the child is unable to understand death until he or she is preadolescent or in the chum stage, for until then he or she has not learned to care for someone else as much as for self.

The child's ideas and anxiety about separation and death and the ability to handle loss are influenced by many factors: experiences with rejecting or punitive parents; strong sibling rivalry; violence; loss, illness, or death in the family; the reaction and teaching of adults to separation or death; and ability to conceptualize and assimilate the experience (31).

The child may think of the parent's death as deliberate abandonment for which he or she is responsible and expect death to get him or her next. The child may fear death is catching and for that reason avoid a friend whose parent has just died. If the child perceives death as sleep, he or she may fear sleep to the point of being unable to go to bed at night or even to nap. He or she may blame the surviving parent for the other parent's death, a feeling that is compounded when the surviving parent is so absorbed in personal grief that little attention is given to the child. The child may use magical thinking, believing that wishing to have the parent return will bring the parent back (31).

The child's fascination with and fear of death may be expressed through the games he or she plays or concern about sick pets or a dead person. Short-lived pets such as fish or gerbils help the child deal with death. Parents should handle these concerns and the related questions in a relaxed, loving manner (31, 73, 80).

Self-Knowledge of Death

Can the sick child realize personal approaching death? Waechter's study (97) showed that despite widespread efforts by adults to shield sick children from awareness of their diagnosis of cancer and the inevitability of death, the school-aged children in her study knew of their impending death, although they might not say so directly to their parents. The evasiveness and false cheerfulness of the adults, either parents or staff, did not hide their real feelings from the child.

Often children know more about death than adults may realize. Children are harmed by what they do not know, by what they are not told, and by their misconceptions. Parents should monitor the child's television viewing carefully, for programs often give an unrealistic impression of death, for example, cartoons and movies that show that death is reversible (or that there is survival or no harmful effects after obviously lethal injuries) (97).

Children's Attendance at Funerals

There are age-based guidelines for a child's involvement in a funeral. Children from 2 to 3 can view the body or be given a brief explanation, depending on their level of understanding and relationship to the deceased. But 3- to 6-year-olds benefit from a short private funeral home visit or the service itself. Seven- to 9-year-old children should attend the funeral unless they resist. Eleven- and 12-year-olds should be included in making the arrangements and the funeral service itself. In the teen years friends of the adolescent should be encouraged to share the grief, and all should be treated as adults (see Dos and Don'ts for Discussing Death with Children).

Other research is finding similar results about children and the subject of death (27, 30, 31, 39, 56, 72, 73, 77, 80, 102). Although it s not easy for adults to talk with children about death, the book, *Talking About Death: A Dialogue Between Parent and Child,* by Grollman (53), is a helpful reference.

Adolescents' Concept of Death

The adolescent is concerned about a personal future and is relatively realistic in thinking, but because of dependency–independency conflicts with parents and efforts to establish individuality, he or she has a low tolerance for accepting death. The healthy young person seldom thinks about death, particularly as something that will happen to the self. He or she fears a lingering death and usually views death in religious or philosophic terms. He or she believes death means lack of fulfillment; there is too much to lose with death (39, 56, 72).

Because of inexperience in coping with crisis and the viewpoints of death, the adolescent may not cry at the death of a loved one or parent. Instead he or she may continue to play games, listen to records, withdraw into seclusion or vigorous study, or go about usual activities. If the young person cannot talk, such activities provide a catharsis. Mastery of feelings sometimes comes through a detailed account of the parent's death to a peer or by displacing grief feelings onto a pet. Also, the adolescent may fantasize the dead parent as perfect or feel much the way a child would about loss of a parent. Often the adolescent's behavior hides the fact that he or she is in mourning. Be attuned to the thoughts and feelings of the adolescent who has faced death of a loved one so that you can be approachable and helpful. One study found that the father had a more accurate view of the adolescent child's grief than did the mother (56).

Adult Concepts of Death

The adult's attitudes toward and concept about dying and death are influenced by cultural and religious backgrounds. A number of references provide information (2, 13, 19, 25, 39, 54, 60, 65). The adult's reactions to death are also influenced by whether the death event is sudden or has been anticipated. Fear of death is often more related to the process of dying than to the fact of death—to mutilation, deformity, isolation, pain, loss of control over body functions and one's life, fear of the unknown, and permanent collapse and disintegration. Premonitions about coming death, sometimes correct, may occur.

▶ DOS AND DON'TS FOR DISCUSSING DEATH WITH CHILDREN

Do

- Ask the child what he or she is feeling: Bring up the subject of death naturally in the context of a dead pet, a book character, television show, movie, or news item.
- Help the child have a funeral for a dead pet.
- Help the child realize he or she is not responsible for the death.
- Tell the child what has happened on his or her level (but not in morbid detail).
- Explain the funeral service briefly beforehand; attendance depends on the child's age and wishes.
- Answer questions honestly, with responses geared to the child's age.
- Remember that expressions of pain, anger, loneliness or aloneness do not constitute symptoms of an illness but are part of a natural process of grieving.
- Help the child realize that the adults are also grieving and feel upset, anger, despair, and guilt.

Do not

- Admonish the child not to cry; it is a universal way to show grief and anxiety.
- Tell a mystical story about the loss of the person; it could cause confusion and anxiety.
- Give long, exclusively detailed explanations beyond the level of understanding.
- Associate death with sleep, which could result in chronic sleep disturbances.
- Force the child to attend funerals or ignore signs of grieving in the child.

Anticipation of Death

There are four responses to viewing death: positivist, negativist, activist, and passivist. Fear of death is less in the person who believes that most of the valued goals have been attained. This person is likely to reflect positively on present activities and death as an aspect of the future and is referred to as a *positivist*. If the person believes that the time left is short, fears loss of ego integration, wishes that he or she could relive part of life, and fears death, the person is referred to as a *negativist*. A person may perceive death as diminishing the opportunity for continued fulfillment of goals. The achieved goals do not offset the fear of death. Death as a foreclosing of ambition is more distasteful than the prospect of loss of life. A person with such an attitude is referred to as an *activist*. Finally, the person may not view death with concern or fear but as a respite from disappointments of life because attempts to attain life goals may have been so overshadowed by failure. Death may be accepted as a positive adjustment to life. Such a person is referred to as a *passivist* (94).

Women are more likely to integrate widowhood than are men, and greater stability of friendships through the life cycle eases adaptation to loss of spouse. The widow is likely to seek intimacy with same-sex friends, who replace family ties in late life.

The importance of will to live, or lack of it, has been recognized by nurses and others for many years. The person may not be terminally ill yet, but because of loss of a loved one, loss of feelings of self-worth and usefulness, boredom, or disillusionment with life, may lose the will to live and rapidly decline and die. Often there are few or no causes for death apparent on autopsy. Some individuals, despite impending death, maintain hope and endurance and apparently refuse to die and live beyond the time of expected death. A person can program, through unconscious or conscious will, onset of illness, recovery from severe illness, or time of death. A strong will to live is often associated with the person's being interested, involved, or active in life or having a loved one, spouse, or dependent whom he or she desires to be with or for whom he or she feels responsible. For some the death month is related to the birth month in that some people postpone death to witness their birthdays or another important holiday. The person with excessive fear of death may be unable to die until able to express and work through conscious fears or phobias (32, 94).

Meaning of Death

To the adult facing death because of illness, particularly the elderly, death may have many meanings. Death may convey some positive meanings: a teacher of transcendental truths uncomprehended during life; an adventure; a friend who brings an end to pain and suffering; or an escape from an unbearable situation into a new life without the present difficulties. The great destroyer who is to be fought, punishment and separation, and a means of vengeance to force others to give more affection than they were willing to give in the past are examples of negative meanings (39).

The person who is dying may have suicidal thoughts or attempt suicide. Suicide is a rebellion against death, a way to cheat death's control over him or her.

One woman who had breast cancer spent 15 months planning her suicide. She wrote a book on her right to die when and as she wished, made a videotape, collected her mementos for preservation after her death. He last meal before she took a lethal dose of medicine included champagne and special sharing with her husband and son. This approach is repulsive and anti-Christian to some; see *The Illusion of Rational Suicide* published by the Hastings Center Report, December 1982, for a counterattack.

Cox (23) writes a poignant account of how one person made a choice about where and how he would die—making his death and the events leading to it a triumph—in a society in which society and health care professionals believe that the system is more important than the individual. She writes also of her feelings and beliefs and the ethical decision-making process involved in ensuring that his choice was carried out.

The time comes in an illness or in later life when both the person and the survivors-to-be believe death would be better than continuing to suffer. The client has the conviction that death is inevitable and desirable and works through feelings until finally he or she has little or no anxiety, depression, or conflicts about dying. The body becomes a burden, and death holds a promise. There is little incentive to live.

Recently in the United States the concept of death has been investigated by adults who are not necessarily facing immediate death of themselves or their loved ones. The stigma that formerly caused people to use euphemisms has been replaced with research involving attitudes toward death and classes on dying and death. For example, one study concluded that highly creative artists and scientists who believe they have successfully contributed their talents to society have little fear of death. Another example involves a religion professor who for several years has taught courses on death at two universities and has had to limit class size because of the subject's popularity. The students face their own concepts and fears about death, study various religious views and myths surrounding death, examine the possible stages of dying, and interview a dying person.

A phenomenon that has gained public interest through Moody's publication *Life After Life* (75) is the **near-death experience (NDE)** of *"coming back to life" after just being declared clinically dead or near dead.* The stories (those told to Moody and those heard before and since) have a sameness, although details and interpretation depend on the personality and beliefs of the person (15, 75, 84, 87, 91, 95, 104). *Embraced by the Light* by Betty J. Eadie wih Curtis Taylor had been on the *New York Times* best seller list for nearly a year in August 1995 (33).

There is additional publicity about men and women of a wide range of age, education, background, religious and nonreligious belief, and temperament who came close to death or had a near-death experience or who had an **out-of-body experience (OBE),** *a feeling that one's consciousness or center of awareness is at a different location than one's body,* often reported in relation to being resuscitated. Olson (84) compares these experiences with other normal states of consciousness, such as dreams, reverie, hypnotic states or hallucinations on falling asleep or awakening, and pathologic states such as hallucinations and depersonalization. When they recall what happened to them after they returned to consciousness, the people describe a sense of comfort, beauty, peace, and bliss. For example, Groff writes of his experience of falling into a mountain crevasse, buried by snow and ice, and the rush of feelings experienced in the few minutes before loss of consciousness when he thought he was dying. He then describes the behavior and feelings on being unearthed from the crevasse 25 minutes later by frantically digging friends. As a result of this experience he finds compelling meaning and reason in innumerable small experiences of life. There is a new and deeper spiritual dimension. Nothing is taken for granted. The routine or trivial aspects of life are seen and heard more clearly; and dying and death are viewed from a different perspective than before (52).

Research with people who have been successfully resuscitated or who have been nearly dead and then lived shows that *features of the near-death experience* include the following (14, 15, 91, 94):

- Feeling of being drawn through a long, dark tunnel or passage at the end of which is a bright light
- Looking down from a spiritual body on the resuscitation efforts of the health care team on one's own physical body
- Awareness of loud noises or vibrations
- Recognizing the presence of and communicating with dead relatives or other deceased loved ones who were there to help make the transition from life to death
- Seeing one's own life in review; watching one's own life pass before him or her in color, three dimensions, and third person
- Being met or confronted by a brilliant light or many intense colors and the Creator, God, Jesus, a light or Being of Love who asks the person to provide a review of his or her life.
- Being given acceptance in the presence of the brilliant light, being in the presence of great love, even though the person may feel embarrassment or rejection about the past life
- Reaching a threshold but drawing back because of a sense of responsibility for others on earth

The person may have difficulty describing the feelings; as there has been more researched and written, individuals are more willing to share what several decades ago was not talked about readily. People who have experienced a positive near-death experience speak of a spiritual encounter that parallels the writings in the Bible in relation to the afterlife, a paradise, heaven, and express a stronger spiritual faith and no fear of death. They report a feeling of bliss about a life to come and new meaning in this life. Some people have had a negative, unpleasant or fear-producing near-death experience; they remain afraid to die unless they turn their life around spiritually (94).

Researchers Michael Sabon, a cardiologist at Emory University in Atlanta, Kenneth Ring, Bruce Greyson, and Ian Stevenson, all psychiatrists, Fred Shoenmaker, physician in charge of Cardiovascular Services at St. Luke's Hospital in Denver, and Dr. Raymond Moody, Jr., have accumulated several thousand case studies to verify near-death experiences. Anesthesia, drugs, hallucinations, or wishful fantasies do not account for these experiences. Clinical death has been recorded by absence of electric activity in the brain for 3 to 30 minutes in hundreds of subjects, although at times adequate brain function continued when heart function stopped. Often the person describes exactly what happened when the medical team was working to revive him or her as if the person were looking on from above.

Papowitz (87) describes near-death experiences that have been recounted by various people. She describes guidelines for caring for the person who is being resuscitated in light of the fact that the person may be able to hear and see what is happening. She describes ways to help the person talk about the near-death experience if it is recalled and the importance of listening and taking the necessary time to allow the person to express emotions. Respect that some people view this as a religious experience; some do not. Ask for permission to share the account with family members as a way to enrich their understanding.

This trend toward talking about, investigating, and studying death points to a willingness to confront finally an absolute fact: Each of us will die.

There is evidence of life after death. Each person must integrate this information and come to terms with it in his or her own life.

Nearing-Death Awareness

Nearing-death awareness (NDA) differs from near-death experiences. It is an *extraordinary awareness of how death will unfold and what the person will need to die well*. This awareness is often communicated symbolically or in obscure messages by people who are dying slowly. Typically the person describes seeing or being visited by a dead loved one(s) or a spiritual figure, and may be heard talking with this visitor. (These are not pathologic hallucinations.) The person may talk of getting in line for a journey (departure from this life) while lying in the hospital bed. (The person is not confused.) Family may think the person is losing his or her mind; reassure them by explaining the nearing-death awareness phenomenon and the need to stay with and talk to the person, and listen and learn. The person may speak of a reunion or a wonderful place, describe heaven or Jesus, talk about having a dream, or talk about a certain day being sad (and die on that day). The person may call to someone, seeking reconciliation and forgiveness. A spiritual care provider should be called (16).

If the patient dies alone, family and staff often express guilt. The patient may have chosen to die alone to spare his or her loved ones. Let the family know this was the dying person's gift to them (16).

The patient may need the family to acknowledge what's happening and give permission to die. If the patient is restless, picking at self or clothing, or struggling, it is often helpful to tell her or him "it's OK to let go," to convey the person will be missed but the family will be allright (16).

Use the following *principles when caring for the patient who is manifesting a nearing-death awareness* and teach these to the family and friends as well (16):

- Pay attention to everything the dying person says. All communication has meaning. Keep a pen and pad at the bedside so notes can be jotted down on any unusual comments or gestures made by the patient.

- Watch for signs in the patient's behavior that may indicate nearing-death awareness: glassy-eyed look, distractedness, strange gestures (pointing at or waving to someone you cannot see), efforts to get out of bed for no apparent reason.

- Respond to the patient's statements with gentle, open-ended questions that encourage her or him to explain. When a patient whose mother died long ago says, "My mother's waiting for me," say, "I'm so glad she's close to you. Tell me about it."

- Accept what the patient says; do not argue. Do not insist on reality, for example, "Your mother died 10 years ago." When a patient speaks in metaphors, respond in kind. If the patient says, "I've got to catch a train," you might say, "Do you want to get on?" "Do you know anyone on the train?" "Where are you going?"

- If you do not understand what the patient is saying, admit it. You might say, "I think you're telling me something important, but I'm not getting it. Don't give up trying—I want to know."

Keep in mind that dying patients in any setting—intensive care unit, emergency department, home, or hospice—may express nearing-death awareness. Talk to co-workers about this phenomenon, and make sure to chart patients' comments and behavior suggesting it. If we listen with care to our dying patients, we may be able to comprehend their special awareness and help loved ones to share in it—to receive the parting gifts the dying want to give. We, too, may benefit. We have much to learn about dying. Our patients are the best possible teachers.

BEHAVIOR AND FEELINGS OF THE PERSON FACING DEATH

When death comes accidentally and swiftly, there is no time to prepare for death. However, death is a normal, expected event to the old, and studies show that most old people anticipate death with equanimity and without fear. The crisis is not death but where and how the person will die. Studies show that old persons living in their own homes or having adjusted to living in an institution do not fear death. Those who are close to death and are on a waiting list for admission to an institution score the highest for fear of death. The prospect of dying in nonnormal, unexpected circumstances creates the crisis (86, 103, 105).

Widowhood is more expected after age 65; thus women who are over 65 show less mental or physical illness or immediate mortality than widows who are under 65. Mental illness in the widow is associated with self-blame, with reports of having missed opportunities and having failed to live up to potentials, and with unexpected death of spouse (94). When the person approaches death gradually by virtue of many years lived or from a terminal illness, he or she will go through a predictable sequence of feelings and behavior.

Awareness of Dying

Glaser and Strauss (49) describe the stages of awareness that the terminally ill or dying person may experience depending on the behavior of the health team and family, which, in turn, influences interaction with others. He or she may not be aware of the prognosis, may suspect approaching death, or may be totally aware of diagnosis and prognosis.

Closed Awareness

Closed awareness *occurs when the person is dying but has neither been informed nor made the discovery.* He or she may not be knowledgeable about the signs of terminal illness, and the health team and family may not want the person to know for fear that "he will go to pieces."

Hospitals are designed to keep information from the client. Even other clients who know are likely to keep the information from him or her. The doctor and nursing staff spend less time with this client than other clients; topics of conversation are brief, direct, superficial, and about the present.

Maintaining closed awareness is less likely to occur if the dying person is at home. In the hospital it is maintained primarily to protect the health team and the family; yet the burden of keeping the prognosis a secret from the client becomes an ever-increasing strain. The only person who really is protected is the doctor, for the nurses who are with this client throughout the day find being deceitful increasingly difficult. The family may continue to pretend, but they are robbed of the opportunity to express openly and share the burden of grief with their loved one and helpful others. The client and family cannot support each other, nor can the staff fully support the client. The client and family have no opportunity to review their lives, plan realistically for the family's future, and close life with the proper rituals. Even legal and business transactions of the client may suffer as he or she tries to carry on life as usual, starts unrealistic plans, and works less feverishly on unfinished business than he or she would if the prognosis were known.

Despite the intentions and efforts of the health team and family, however, the client may become increasingly aware. He or she has a lot of time to observe the surroundings, even when very ill. Clients no doubt spend more time assessing the personnel and environment than the staff spends assessing them. He or she has time to think about the nonverbal cues and indirect comments from the staff, the inconsistent answers, the new and perplexing symptoms that do not get better despite reassurance that they will improve. Privileges that were previously denied are granted, and the client is subjected to a barrage of diagnostic and treatment procedures. At times the staff may relax their guard when they think he or she does not understand and say something about the prognosis that is understood. All these things help the person formulate the conclusion that he or she is very sick and perhaps even dying. Of course, if the person is kept sedated, as much to relieve the staff from having to face the client as to relieve the client's suffering, he or she may be less aware of the external cues.

Suspicious Awareness

Suspicious awareness *develops for the reasons previously described. The person may or may not voice suspicions to others, and they are likely to deny his or her verbal suspicions.* A contest for control develops, with the client on the offensive and the staff on the defensive.

The client watches more closely for signs to confirm suspicions. The changing physical status; the nonverbal and verbal communications of others, with their hidden meanings; the silence; the intensity of or challenges in care; and the briskness of conversation usually will inadvertently tell or imply what he or she suspects.

Now deceitfulness has fully developed. The client knows that he or she is dying but realizes that others do not know he or she knows.

Mutual Pretense

Mutual pretense *occurs when staff and family become aware that the client knows he or she is dying, but all continue to pretend otherwise.* There is no conversation about impending death unless the client initiates it, although on occasion staff members may purposely drop cues because they believe the client has a right to know.

Although the client now knows and can plan for the remaining life, this measure of dignity is offset because intimate relationships are denied. There is no one to talk with honestly, although all persons involved could benefit. Neither anticipatory grieving nor other preparation for death can be accomplished very well.

There has been a movement toward no pretense, where there is frank discussion between patient and health care providers. The talks may indicate the family are reluctant to let go or are letting go prematurely. The patient and family are helped to resolve the mutual pretense (14, 16).

Open Awareness

Open awareness *exists when the person and family are fully aware of the terminal condition, although neither may realize the nearness nor all the complications of the condition and the mode of death.*

With the certainty of death established, the person may plan to end life in accord with personal ideas about proper dying, finish important work, and make appropriate plans for and farewells with the family. He or she and the family can talk frankly, make plans, share grief, and support each other. The anguish is not reduced but can be faced together.

The health team in the hospital has ideas, although not always verbalized, about how the person ought to die morally and stylistically. These ideas may conflict with or differ from the ideas of the client and family. The wishes of the client and the family should always have priority, particularly when they ask that no heroic measures be taken to prolong life. Extra privileges, special requests, or the client's discharge to the family can be granted. Most people wish to die without pain, with dignity, in privacy, and with loved ones nearby. Often dying in the hospital precludes both privacy and dignity, and the health team should continuously work to provide these rights.

But how? Research physicians, students, and other team members hover over the client as they attempt to learn more and to develop future treatments. Clients sometimes feel more like experimental animals than dignified human beings. Do you follow orders to prolong life with gadgetry or to hasten death with a lethal dose of medication? How do you decide what the client's rights are? What if they conflict with the doctor's orders? Does the health team work together on these matters?

One way to work through feelings, clarify ideas, and collaborate with other health team members would be to suggest a seminar, or series of them, on the topic of death, to be attended by the team. Certain general guidelines could be set, based on the premise that the client should be granted the right to die as he or she wishes.

Sequence of Reactions to Approaching Death

When the person becomes aware of the diagnosis and prognosis, whether he or she is told directly or learns by advancing through the stages of awareness discussed previously, he or she and the family usually go through a predictable sequence of reactions described by Kübler-Ross (65, 66).

Denial and Isolation

Denial and **isolation** are the *initial and natural reactions when the person learns of terminal illness:* "It can't be true. I don't believe it's me." The person may go through a number of rituals to support this denial, even to the point of finding another doctor. He or she needs time to mobilize resources. Denial serves as a necessary buffer against overwhelming anxiety.

The person is denying when he or she talks about the future; avoids talking about the illness or the death of self or others; or persistently pursues cheery topics. Recognize the client's need; respond to this behavior, and let him or her set the pace in conversation. Later the person will gradually consider the possibility of the prognosis; anxiety will lessen; and the need to deny will diminish.

Psychological isolation occurs when the *client talks about the illness, death, or mortality intellectually but without emotion as if these topics were not relevant.* Initially the idea of death is recognized, although the feeling is repressed. Gradually feelings about death will be less isolated, and the client will begin to face death but still maintain hope.

If the client continues to deny for a prolonged time despite advancing symptoms, he or she will need much warmth, compassion, and support as death comes closer. Your contacts with the client may consist of sitting in silence, using touch communication, giving meticulous physical care, conveying acceptance and security, and looking in on him or her frequently. If denial is extensive, he or she cannot grieve or face the inevitable separation. Yet Kübler-Ross (66) found that few persons maintain denial to the end of life.

Anger

The second reaction, **anger,** *occurs with acknowledgment of the reality of the prognosis.* It is necessary for an eventual acceptance of approaching death. As denial and isolation decrease, anger, envy, and resentment of the living are felt. In the United States, direct expression of anger is unacceptable, so this stage is difficult for the client and others. Anger is displaced onto things or people: "The doctor is no good," "the food is no good," "the hospital is no good," "the nurses are neglectful," and "people don't care." The family also bears the brunt of the anger.

Anger results when the person realizes life will be interrupted before he or she finishes everything planned. Everything reminds the person of life while he or she is dying, and he or she feels soon-to-be-forgotten. He or she may make angry demands, frequently ring the bell, manipulate and control others, and generally make the self heard. He or she is convincing self and others that he or she is not yet dead and forgotten.

Do not take the anger personally. The dying person whose life will soon end needs empathy. The person who is respected, understood, and given time and attention will soon lower the angry voice and decrease demands. The person will realize he or she is considered a valuable person who will be cared for and yet allowed to function at maximum potential as long as possible. Your calm approach will lower anxiety and defensive anger.

Bargaining

The third reaction, **bargaining,** occurs when *the person tries to enter into some kind of agreement that may postpone death.* He or she may try to be on the best behavior. He or she knows the bargaining procedure and hopes to be granted the special wish—an extension of life, preferably without pain. Although the person will initially ask for no more than one deadline or postponement of death, he or she will continue the good behavior and will promise to devote life to some special cause if he or she lives.

Bargaining may be life promoting. As the person continues to hope for life, to express faith in God's willingness to let him or her live, and to engage actively in positive, health-promoting practices, the body's physical defenses may be enhanced by mental or emotional processes yet unknown. This process may account for those not-so-uncommon cases in which the person has a prolonged, unexpected remission during a malignant disease process. Hope, which is involved in bargaining and which you can support, gives each person a chance for more effective treatment and care as new discoveries are made.

Depression

Depression is the fourth reaction and occurs when *the person gets weaker, needs increasing treatment, and worries about mounting medical costs and even necessities.* Role reversal and related problems add to the strain.

Depression about past losses and the present condition; feelings of shame about the illness, sometimes interpreted as punishment for past deeds; and hopelessness enshroud the person and extend to the loved ones.

Depression is normal. The family and staff need to encourage the person by giving realistic praise and recognition, letting him or her express feelings of guilt, work through earlier losses, finish mourning, and build self-esteem. You will need to give more physical and emotional help as the person grows weaker. He or she should stay involved with the family as long as possible.

Preparatory Depression

Preparatory depression is the next stage and differs from the previous depression. Now *the person realizes the inevitability of death and comes to desire the release from suffering that death can bring.* He or she wishes to be a burden no more and recognizes that there is no hope of getting well. The person needs a time of preparatory grief to get ready for the final separation of impending loss: not only are loved ones going to lose him or her, but the person is losing all significant objects and relationships. The person reviews the meaning of life and searches for ways to share insights with the people most significant to him or her, sometimes including the staff. Often the fear that he or she cannot share aspects of life or valued material objects with people of his or her own choosing will cause greater concern than the diagnosis of a terminal illness or the knowledge of certain death. As the person thinks of what life has meant, he or she begins to get ready to release life, but not without feelings of grief. Often he or she will talk repetitiously to find a meaning in life.

The family and health team can either inhibit the person during this stage or promote emotional comfort and serene acceptance of death. The first reaction to depressed, grieving behavior and life review is to cheer him or her. This meets your needs but not those of the client. When the person is preparing for the impending loss of all love objects and relationships, behavior should be accepted and not changed. Acceptance of the final separation in life will not be reached unless he or she is allowed to express a life review and sorrow. There may be no need for words if rapport, trust, and a working nurse–client relationship have been previously established. A touch of the hand and a warm accepting silence are therapeutic. Too much interference with words, sensory stimuli, or burdensome visitors hinders rather than helps emotional preparation for death. If the person is ready to release life and die and others expect him or her to want to continue to live and be concerned about things, the person's own depression, grief, and turmoil are increased. He or she wishes quietly and gradually to disengage self from life and all that represents life. He or she may request few or no visitors and modifications in the routines of care and repeatedly request no heroic measures to prolong life.

Honor the client's requests but at the same time promote optimum physical and emotional comfort and well-being. Explain the feelings and needs of the client to the family and other members of the health team so that they can better understand his or her behavior. The family should know that this depression is beneficial if the client is to die peacefully and that it is unrelated to their past or present behavior.

Acceptance

The final reaction, **acceptance** or a *kind of resolution,* comes if the person is given enough time, does not have a sudden, unexpected death, and is given some help in working through the previous reactions. He or she will no longer be angry or depressed about the fate and will no longer be envious or resentful of the living. He or

she will have mourned the loss of many people and things and will contemplate the end with a certain degree of quiet expectation. Now the ultimate of ego integrity, described by Erikson (38) becomes evident. Acceptance is difficult and takes time. It depends in part on the client's awareness of the prognosis of illness so that he or she can plan ahead—religiously, philosophically, financially, socially, and emotionally. This last stage is almost devoid of feeling.

The healthy aged person will also go through some aspects of the reactions discussed previously, for as the person grows old, he or she contemplates more frequently personal mortality and begins to work through feelings about it.

Whereas Kübler-Ross looks at the dying *person* with the family implied, Giacquinta (46) looks at the *family* with the dying person implied. Table 15–1 outlines the four main stages and the 10 phases the family will experience from the time of diagnosis through the postdeath period.

Both the Kübler-Ross (65, 66) and the Giacquinta (46) models are helpful. They are built on observations of hundreds of dying persons and families, but you

TABLE 15–1. FAMILY'S RESPONSE TO DYING AND DEATH

Four Main Stages	Family Experiences:	Nurse Can Foster:
Living With Terminal Illness Person learns diagnosis, tries to carry on as usual, undergoes treatment	*Impact:* emotional shock, despair, disorganized behavior	
	Functional disruption: much time spent at hospital (if traditional surgery or treatment chosen), ignoring of home tasks and emotional needs, weakening of family structure, emotional isolation	Hope as different treatment methods are used, communication, seeking helpful resources, family cohesiveness
	Search for meaning: questioning why this happened; casting blame on various persons, deity, institutions, habits; realization that "Someday I will die too"	Security
	Informing others (family and friends): ascent from isolation, with moral and practical support—or feeling of rejection: others do not understand, do not care, or are afraid; possible need to retreat again into emotional isolation	Courage, reliable help, understanding of why some people cannot help
	Engaging emotions: beginning grieving, fearing loss of emotional control, assumption of roles once carried by dying person	Problem solving; idea that life will change but will be ongoing
Living–Dying Interval Person ceases to perform family roles, is cared for either at home or in hospital; person needs to come to terms with accomplishments and failures and to find renewed meaning in life	*Reorganization:* firmer division of family tasks	Cooperation instead of competition; analysis to see if new role distribution is workable
	Framing memories: reviewing life of dying person—what he or she has meant and accomplished, new sense of family history, relinquishment of dependency on dying member	Focus on life review rather than only on what person is now
Bereavement Death occurs	*Separation:* absorption in loneliness of separation as person becomes unconscious	Intimacy among family members; release of grief as normal
	Mourning: guilt, "Could I have done more?"	
Reestablishment	*Expansion of the social network:* overcoming feelings of alienation and guilt	Looking back with acceptance and forward to new growth and socialization with a reunited, normally functioning family

must not stereotype responses into these stages. Do not assume that everyone is experiencing each stage as the research results describe. Sometimes the person or family will not go through every one of these stages, and the stages will not always follow in this sequence. The person or family may remain in a certain stage or revert to earlier stages. Feelings related to several of the researched stages may exist; the person who has been told he or she has cancer and a limited time to live feels fear, loss of control over destiny, a discontinuity in life goals, a sense of future time being meaningless, and a sense of isolation. A magazine subscription is chosen 1 year at a time; the 20,000-mile guarantee on tires seems more appropriate than the 40,000-mile guarantee. Friends may react out of fear of disease contagion. Professional colleagues, relatives, and friends avoid talking about the condition, and the person does not bring up the subject out of deference not to burden them, or that may be all friends or relatives seem to want to discuss. Priorities change; family and close friends become more important. Gradually the person is able to plan for the not-too-far future. Money is less important. Negative friends are avoided. The person must adjust to fatigue, changes in body function or structure, effects of chemotherapy or radiation, the continuing treatment appointments, and loss of control. Do not convey that the client or family should be in a certain stage or reacting a certain way. Avoid social and religious clichés. Rather, be a caring, concerned, available person, willing to do nondramatic, simple, but helpful tasks such as bringing the family member something to drink, watering the flowers sent by a friend, and offering to call a significant person. Equally important will be doing physical care procedures in a thorough but efficient manner so that visiting family members can spend as much time with their dying loved one as possible. Listen to feelings when the person wants to talk but do not probe. Benner (9) writes a personal account of the difficulties of terminal illness and death for the surviving family members and suggests how health care professionals can help.

Anniversary Reaction and Emotionally Invested Deadlines

The classic **anniversary reaction** or **emotionally invested date or event** is a psychodynamic pattern in a child who is sensitized by some emotional event, most severely by the death of the parent of the same sex when the child is between the ages of 2 and 16. The specific age of this child at the time of the trauma is the key time marker. When the traumatized child grows into adulthood and has a child the same age as he or she was when originally traumatized, the stressful reaction occurs. This reaction also typically involves the age of the parent at the time the event occurred and the exact date (day, month, year) of the event; these factors function as related emotionally invested markers. For example, a 54-year-old man who suffered a coronary occlusion after apparent good health revealed that when he was 18 his 54-year-old father had died of a heart attack. He had experienced hostilities toward his father, describing him as having a vicious temper and being responsible for the family's poverty. Now he was 54 and had an 18-year-old son. He blamed his heart attack on the hatred and tension between himself and his relatives. In short, this man had repeated the experience of his father and perhaps subconsciously brought it on himself through his unresolved feelings toward his father (41).

Emotionally invested deadlines are the result of the emotional investment of the individual into specific dates, events, and anniversaries. When such an emotionally invested date is reached, the person may react with varying degrees of psychological stress, ranging from illness to death. Emotionally invested occasions are unique for each person, yet a characteristic in common is that all these dates and events have long-standing emotional meaning for these individuals. The choice of the date or event for the time of death seems fitting to the uniqueness of the person (41). For example, two of the first four presidents died on July 4, undoubtedly an emotionally invested event for them. The person appears to have psychological vulnerability on an emotionally charged occasion; it is well known and accepted that an emotionally depressed or brooding client is a poor surgical risk.

Although anniversary reaction is classically seen in the middle-aged or aging person, emotionally invested deadlines may be seen at any age. Both phenomena, however, tend to increase with age as one accumulates more and more emotionally charged experiences.

Predilection to Death

The phenomenon of **predilection to death** is seen in *people who, although lacking any signs of emotional conflict, suicidal tendencies, severe depression, or panic, correctly anticipate their own deaths* (23). These persons are firmly convinced of their impending death yet feel no depression or anxiety toward it, regarding it as completely appropriate. Such clients are resigned to death; to fight against it is unthinkable, for death is a release from the burden of their life or body. It is significant that predilection clients experience a lack of close human relationships and emotional isolation from significant others during their terminal period. Death holds more appeal than life because it promises either a reunion with lost love, resolution of long conflict, or respite from anguish. Death is perceived as a release from continuing in a world in which there are no longer any emotional bonds; thus there is no fear, anxiety, or depression regarding its approach, but rather a distinctly eager and expectant attitude toward its swift occurrence. Research shows that death comes to the predilection clients just as they have anticipated it would, although medically their condition does not warrant such a quick demise or, in some cases, any death at all (12, 20, 31, 41, 74, 99).

Another form is the person who holds onto life until a specific event has passed, or certain persons have arrived, or who dies just before entry into a nursing home from his or her own residence or the hospital. The person has chosen to die, or has timed his or her death (74).

"Scared to Death" (Death by Autosuggestion)

Unlike the predilection client, who, convinced of impending death, anticipates it, the **scared-to-death individual** does not see death as appropriate (6, 17, 36, 51, 89, 90). He or she *believes self the victim of a curse, hex, or prediction and therefore cannot be saved by anyone or by any means.* **Psychic death** is said to occur when *a person is convinced of and accurately predicts his or her own death when no medical cause for death exists.* Autosuggestion is the most accurate description for the cause of psychic death; it implies that the person responded in such a way as to convince self of imminent death. A synonym for autosuggestion might be "self-hypnosis." Death without any apparent organic cause has been documented to have occurred as a result of belief in hexing, voodoo, curses, predictions (fortune tellers, psychics, clairvoyants), premonitions, and dreams predicting death. Two types of behavior are exhibited by persons who are scared to death: (1) some individuals, after a suggestion of impending death, experience a panic reaction and literally die of fright; or (2) they may take the suggestion calmly, believe it to be useless to resist, give up, and simply die. Death by fright or autosuggestion can occur at any age; Baker (6) cites the case of a 3-year-old boy who died of fright after being caught in a rainstorm.

Fear is one of the strongest of emotions and has very definite and demonstrable effects on body homeostasis, particularly the cardiovascular and endocrine systems, which prepare the body to defend itself physically or to escape. Several physiologic causes have been suggested for voodoo and other deaths resulting solely from the conviction of death. Cannon (17), one of the first researchers of voodoo death, proposed that death was the result of a state of shock due to persistent overactivity of the sympathicoadrenal system, with continuous outpouring of adrenaline and rapid depletion of the adrenal corticosteroid hormones. Cannon reviewed voodoo deaths in primitive cultures in South America, Africa, Australia, New Zealand, Haiti, and some Pacific Islands. Richter (90) and Engel (36, 37) assumed such deaths were the result of complete surrender and loss of hope, the expectation of death, the giving up–given up phenomenon with parasympathetic system failure. Rahe and Romo (89) have correlated illness and death with overwhelming life events. Sudden deaths do not occur only in primitive societies. They occur in more developed societies as the result of acute or accumulating stress after rejection, separation, or loss and the consequent feelings of hopelessness and helplessness. Beliefs may be planted by the family or culture during the formative years and later in life as posthypnotic suggestions that are acted out. Removal of support systems and the violation of shared belief systems may cause a sense of rejection, abandonment, and hopelessness, with death as the consequence. Immaturity, suggestibility, infantile dependency, external locus of control, and fatalistic orientation are individual variables observed in relation to sudden death. Sudden death may be the result of a complex of psychological, social, and biological factors (36, 37, 51, 90). Richter (90) proposed that death from autosuggestion resulted from overstimulation of the parasympathetic, rather than the sympathetic, autonomic nervous system and that cardiac arrest resulted from excessive stimulation of the vagus nerves. Rigidity is one of the first human responses to fear; hence intense panic could lead to a state of body rigidity, with cessation of respiration leading to cerebral anoxia, cardiac arrest, and death (6).

Be aware that voodoo, hexes, premonitions, dreams, and predictions are taken seriously by some people and are practiced as a part of health care in some cultures. Do not discount the impact of such phenomena. Listen carefully to what the client and family say and do.

Being Worked to Death

Although we may frequently say, "This job is killing me," or "I'm being worked to death," such statements are said in jest or as a metaphor for feelings of being too busy, stressed, or overwhelmed. Yet, one can be worked to death. In Japan, **Karoshi** *the phenomenon of death from overwork,* occurs among nurses and other employees working many days without a day off along with irregular and long shifts, contributing to severe health problems and death at an early age. The woman who does all the homemaking tasks as well as remains employed, again at irregular shifts for many days in sequence (11 days straight in a 2-week period), may also die early (1). Anders and Kanai-Pak (1) describe influences of Japanese culture on the professional role of the nurse, such as man–woman or doctor–nurse relationships, the stereotyped sex-defined roles, the strong work ethic, and the lack of opportunity to talk about feelings or conflicts, as factors that contribute to having ill effects from the workplace. They describe the first acknowledged fatality of a nurse attributed to Karoshi.

People in the United States also suffer health effects or die before the expected age because of occupational or environmental hazards (see Chapter 2).

Legal Planning for Death

While the person is still healthy and capable of making the many decisions in relation to death, he or she can do much to relieve worries and take the burden of those decisions off others. You are in a position to give the following information to others as indicated.

Although not legally binding, the Living Will (see Fig. 15–1) is being used by increasing numbers of people (see Right-to-Die Movement section in this chapter).

Representatives from some nursing and funeral homes and cemeteries are educating people to keep a folder, revised periodically, of all information that will be used by those making arrangements at the time of death. Such a folder might include names of advisors such as attorney, banker, life insurance broker, and accountant. Personal and vital information should be included such as birth certificate, marriage license, military discharge papers, and copies of wills, including willing of body parts to various organizations. Financial records (or a copy of those held in a safety deposit box), estimated assets and liabilities, and insurance and social security information should be there. Personal requests and wishes, listing who gets what, should be written along with funeral arrangements and cemetery deeds.

Having this information written assumes that the person has made a legal will, has some knowledge of the purposes and functions of probate court, has access to Social Security information, and has decided on a funeral home and burial plot.

Knowledge of matters such as how to claim survivor's benefits from Social Security and how to claim the government burial allowance for honorably discharged veterans can ease the loved one's confusion at time of death.

These are intellectual preparations. They cannot ease the sense of loss in the living, but they can foster peace of mind, realizing that the deceased's wishes were carried out.

► HEALTH CARE AND NURSING APPLICATIONS

Death is an intensely poignant event, one that causes deep anguish, but one you may frequently encounter in client care.

Self-Assessment

Personal assessment, being aware of and coping with your personal feelings about death, is essential to assess accurately or intervene helpfully with the client, family, or other health care providers. How do you protect yourself from anxiety and despair resulting from repeated exposure to personal sufferings? The defenses of isolation, denial, and "professional" behavior are common in an attempt to cope with feelings of helplessness, guilt, frustration, and ambivalence about the client's not getting well or the secret wish for the client to die. It takes courage and maturity to undergo the experience of death with clients and families and yet remain an open, compassionate human being. You are a product of the culture as much as is the client and the family and hence will experience many of the same kinds of reactions. Religious, philosophic, educational, and family experiences and general maturity also affect your ability to cope with feelings related to death.

You may see, consciously or unconsciously, yourself in the dying person. The more believable the identification with the person or family, the more devastating the experience will be as you are forced to recognize personal vulnerability to death. The client may remind you of your grandfather, aunt, or friend, and you may react to the dying client as though he or she were that person.

The dying client may seek an identification and partnership with someone, and often this person is the nurse. You may be unwilling to share the relationship or respond to the dying client. The sense of guilt that results may be as burdensome as the actual involvement.

Dying in the hospital has become so organized and care so fragmented that you are not necessarily vulnerable to personal involvement in the client's death. However, you are more likely to be personally affected by and feel a sense of loss from the client's death if an attachment has been formed to the client and family because of prolonged hospitalization and if the death is unexpected. Also, if you perform nursing measures you believe might have contributed to the client's death, if you have worked hard to save a life, or if the client's social or personal characteristics are similar to your own, you will feel the loss (2, 26, 34, 45, 49, 54, 92).

Glaser and Strauss (49) describe how the nurse judges a client's value according to social status and responds accordingly. The client's death is considered less a social loss and is therefore less mourned by the nursing staff if he or she is elderly, comatose, or confused, of a lower socioeconomic class or a minority group, poorly educated, not famous, or unattractive. The dying client in these categories is likely to receive less care or only routine care. The client with high social value, whose death is mourned and who receives optimum care by the nursing staff is the person who is young, alert, or likable, has prominent family status, has a high-status occupation or profession, is from the middle or upper socioeconomic class, or is considered talented or pretty.

If the client's death is very painful or disfiguring, you may avoid the client because of feelings of guilt or helplessness. In addition, you may be aware of the callous attitudes of health team members or of the decision of the family and doctor about prolonging life with heroic measures or not prolonging life. These situations can provoke intense negative reactions if you disapprove of the approaches of other members of the health team.

You must attempt to deal with the various pitfalls of working with the dying: withdrawal from the client, isolation of emotions, failure to perceive own feelings or feelings of client and family, displacing own feelings onto other team members, "burning out" from intense emotional involvement, and fearing illness and death.

Support for Nurses

The nurse should be able to say, "I need help in dealing with my feelings about this dying client" just as easily as she or he would say, "I need help in starting this respirator."

A support system should be available. Specific times should be set aside for staff members to share emotional needs related to a specific dying client or to learn specifics of the dying process. Often nurses can help each other, but there should also be a specialist with whom to confer: a nurse with additional training, a religious leader, a nun, a psychologist, or a psychiatrist. The specialist should also be available for spontaneous sessions.

The administration may also encourage and sponsor the nurses in taking courses other than in nursing (sociology, philosophy, religion) to gain different perspectives, joining professional organizations in which they can share problems or solutions and gain support, changing departments either temporarily or permanently to feel the accomplishment of working with those who recover, and arranging for two primary care nurses (if that is the system) to work together so that they can share emotions and support each other.

If you work with cancer clients exclusively, you may also need special assistance. Although cancer does not always cause death, many people still equate cancer with death. Optimism and logical thinking must be encouraged in the client and maintained in yourself. The cause(s) of cancer is(are) not definitely known, and some people still worry about "catching cancer." You may hear many opinions about helpful treatment, both inside and outside the medical establishment; and you may see that some of the established treatments have unpleasant side effects. The question arises: Why must the client endure so much?

If you can think of death as the last stage of life and as fulfillment, you can mature and learn from the client as he or she comes to terms with personal illness. The meaning of death can serve as an important organizing principle in determining how the person conducts his or her life, and it is as significant for you as for the client. With time and experience, you will view the role of comforter as being as important as that of promoting care. Then the client who is dying will be less of a personal threat.

Some *guidelines for the nurse working with dying clients* are presented:

- Individual staff members should be encouraged to gain personal insight and acknowledge their own limits. One's limits vary over time, and extra support or time off may be necessary when staff members are under a high degree of stress. The needs of clients deserve priority, however; if certain staff members constantly require considerable support, they may be encouraged to seek employment elsewhere.
- A healthy balance must be maintained between work and an outside life. Although this type of work demands considerable personal involvement, there must be times when staff is totally off call and left to pursue own life-affirming activities.
- The individual must be careful when the "need to be needed" becomes too great and he or she attempts to be everything to everyone. This work is probably best accomplished by a team.

- The individual must maintain a support system at work and outside the work setting. Hospice units must make provision for ongoing staff support through the use of visitation, psychiatric consultants for the staff, weekly staff support meetings, or other models that seem appropriate to a given unit. In addition, individuals should be encouraged to seek relationships outside the work setting for additional support.
- For those working in isolation, it may be wise to consider seriously ongoing contact with an outside consultant and therapist who can offer guidance as needed and provide support as well.

Assessment of Client and Family

Assessment of the client and family is done according to the standard methods of assessment. The total person (physical, intellectual, emotional, social, and spiritual needs and status) must be assessed to plan effective care. Learn what the client and family know about the client's condition and what the doctor has told them, to plan for a consistent approach.

Recognize also that people differ in the way they express feelings about dying and death. Mourning may be private or public. Listen to the topics of conversation the person discusses, observe for rituals in behavior, and learn of typical behavior in health from him or her or the family to get clues to what is important. The routines that are important in life may become more important now, and they may assist in preparation for death. Observe family members for pathologic responses—physical or emotional—as grief after loss from death increases the risk of mortality for the survivor, especially for the male spouse or relative who is in late middle age or older.

Nursing Diagnoses

See Nursing Diagnoses Related to the Dying Person for a list of diagnoses that may be pertinent to the dying person and are related to assessment and need for holistic care. Stepnick and Perry (93) relate the phase of resolving death according to the Kübler-Ross format to what could be nursing diagnoses. They list four stages of spiritual development (chaotic, formal, skeptic, and mystic) and nursing strategies to assist the client at each stage of spiritual development as the client approaches death.

Intervention With the Family

The family will be comforted as they see *compassionate care being given to their loved one.* Your attitude is important, for both family members and clients are very perceptive about your real feelings, whether you are interested and available, giving false reassurance, or just going about a job. Family members often judge your personal relationship with the loved one as more important than your technical skill. Being interested and available takes emotional energy. Without this component in your personality, perhaps you should not be in the profession of nursing.

Try to *help the relatives compensate for their feelings of helplessness, frustration, or guilt.* Their assisting the client with feeding or grooming or other time-consuming but nontechnical aspects of care can be helpful to them, the client, and the nursing staff. The family may be acting toward or caring for the client in a way that seems strange or even nontherapeutic to the nursing staff. Yet these measures or the approach may seem fine to the client because of the family pattern or ritual. It is not for you to judge or interfere unless what the family is doing is unsafe for the client's welfare or is clearly annoying to the client. In turn, recognize when family members are fatigued or anxious and relieve them of responsibility at that point. Encourage the family to take time to rest and to meet needs adequately. A lounge or other place where the family can alternately rest and yet be near the client is helpful.

Show acceptance of grief. By helping the family members express their grief and by giving support to them, you are helping them, in turn, to support the client.

Prepare the family for sudden, worsening changes in the client's condition or appearance to avoid shock and feelings of being overwhelmed.

The crisis of death of the loved one may result in a life *crisis for the surviving family members.* The problems with changes in daily routines of living, living arrangements, leisure-time activities, role reversal and assuming additional responsibilities, communicating with other family members, or meeting financial obligations can seem overwhelming. The failure of relatives and friends to help or the insistence by relatives and friends on giving help that is not needed is equally problematic. Advice from others may add to rather than decrease the burdens. The fatigue that a long illness causes in a family member may remain for some time after the loved one's death and may interfere with adaptive capacities. You can help by being a listener, exploring with the family ways in which to cope with their problems, and making referrals or encouraging them to

► NURSING DIAGNOSES RELATED TO THE DYING PERSON*

Pattern 1: Exchanging
Altered Nutrition: Less than Body Requirements
Risk for Infection
Ineffective Thermoregulation
Constipation
Diarrhea
Bowel Incontinence
Altered Urinary Elimination
Altered (specify type) Tissue Perfusion
Risk for Injury
Impaired Tissue Integrity
Impaired Skin Integrity
Impaired Skin Integrity
Pattern 2: Communicating
Impaired Verbal Communication
Pattern 3: Relating
Impaired Social Interaction
Social Isolation
Altered Role Performance
Altered Family Processes
Altered Sexuality Patterns
Pattern 4: Valuing
Spiritual Distress
Pattern 5: Choosing
Ineffective Individual Coping
Impaired Adjustment
Defensive Coping
Ineffective Denial
Ineffective Family Coping: Disabling
Ineffective Family Coping: Compromised

Family Coping: Potential for Growth
Decisional Conflict
Health-Seeking Behaviors
Pattern 6: Moving
Impaired Physical Mobility
Activity Intolerance
Fatigue
Risk for Activity Intolerance
Sleep Pattern Disturbance
Diversional Activity Deficit
Impaired Home Maintenance Management
Altered Health Maintenance
Bathing/Hygiene Self-Care Deficit
Dressing/Grooming Self-Care Deficit
Toileting Self-Care Deficit
Pattern 7: Perceiving
Body Image Disturbance
Self-Esteem Disturbance
Sensory/Perceptual Alterations
Hopelessness
Powerlessness
Pattern 8: Knowing
Knowledge Deficit
Pattern 9: Feeling
Pain
Chronic Pain
Anticipatory Grieving
Anxiety
Fear

*Other NANDA diagnoses are applicable to the dying person.
From North American Nursing Diagnosis Association, NANDA Nursing Diagnoses: Definitions & Classification 1195–1996. Philadelphia: North American Nursing Diagnosis Association, 1994.

seek other persons or agencies for help. Often your willingness to accept and share their feelings of loss and other concerns can be enough to help the family mobilize their strengths and energies to cope with remaining problems.

The most heartbreaking time for the family may be the time *when the client is disengaging from life* and from them. The *family will need help to understand this process* and recognize it as normal behavior. The dying person has found peace. His or her circle of interests has narrowed, and he or she wishes to be left alone and not disturbed by any news of the outside world. Behavior with others may be so withdrawn that he or she seems unreachable and uncooperative. He or she prefers short visits and is not likely to be in a talkative mood. The television set remains off. Communication is primarily nonverbal. This behavior can cause the family to feel rejected, unloved, and guilty about not doing enough for the client. They should understand that the client can no longer hold onto former relationships as he or she accepts the inevitability of death. The family needs help in realizing that their silent presence can be

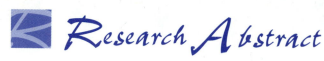

Research Abstract

Constantino, R., Comparison of Two Group Interventions for the Bereaved, IMAGE: Journal of Nursing Scholarship, *20, (1988), 83–87.*

Approximately 5% of the population in the United States is widowed. This group includes more women than men as women outlive men by 7 or 8 years and usually marry men older than themselves.

The experimental study sought to test the helpfulness of two types of group interventions, a bereavement crisis intervention and a social adjustment intervention, in reducing depression and increasing socialization among widows aged 50 to 79. The Beck Depression Inventory, the Depression Adjective Check Test, and the Revised Social Adjustment Scale were used to test two experimental groups and a control group. Participants were randomly assigned to each type of group. Levels of depression and socialization were tested initially and at 6 weeks, 5 months, 9 months, and 12 months after the group interventions.

In the bereavement crisis intervention group the leader was active in leading discussion, planned a theme for discussion, gave mental health education, and provided insight into each member's plight. The group lasted 6 weeks, with ½ hour sessions weekly. In the social adjustment group the leader was an inactive person, a timekeeper, gathering the group weekly for 6 weeks for a social activity. The group was task oriented, discussing current problems and planning an outing for each week. Each leader was a doctoral student and was prepared to do group leading.

The participants (44 in crisis group, 36 in social group, and 37 in control group) had been widowed from less than 1 year to 29 years. Causes of husband's deaths included accidents, acute and chronic illness, and suicide. A two-way repeated measures analysis of variance (ANOVA) test was used to analyze the changes in level of depression over time. The mean score for depression decreased over time in the crisis group and remained the same in the social and the control groups. The results in social adjustment were similar.

The implications are that 6 weeks of group bereavement crisis intervention are effective in lowering depression and increasing social adjustment; however, the results are greatest while the group is being conducted, according to test scores. Thus group intervention for widows should be longer and in two stages: (1) to deal with the crisis of loss and emerging physical, emotional, and social problems and reactions; and (2) to continue a support program focusing on education and reorientation to the internal and external resources.

a very real comfort and shows that he or she is loved and not forgotten. Concurrently, the family can learn that dying is not a horrible thing to be avoided.

This may be the time when family insist on additional life-sustaining or heroic measures, although they will only prolong suffering. The nurse can listen to their desire to prolong life, explain the needs and what is happening to the patient, act as a mediator when various family members make contradictory statements, calm angry tempers, and start a rational discussion about what's best for the patient. Having a meeting that includes family, nurse, pastoral care, the physician, members of an ethics committee, and other health care workers or significant others is useful. Keeping lines of communication open and maintaining a bond with the family, being nonjudgmental, and encouraging family contact with the patient are essential and challenging, even difficult at times (35, 78, 88, 95, 96, 103, 105, 106).

News of impending or actual death is best communicated to a family unit or group rather than to a lone individual to allow the people involved to give mutual support to each other. This should be done in privacy so they can express grief without the restraints imposed by public observation. Stay and comfort the person facing death, at least until a religious leader or other close friends can come.

Requests by an individual or family to see the dead person should *not* be denied on the grounds that it would be too upsetting. The person who needs a leave taking to realize the reality of the situation will ask for it; those for whom it would be overwhelming will not request it.

Sometimes the survivor of an accident may ask about people who were with him or her at the time of the accident. The health team should confer on when and how to answer these questions; *well-timed honesty is the healthiest approach;* otherwise the person cannot adapt to the reality of the accidental death. The person's initial response of shock, denial, and tears or later grief will neither surprise nor upset the medical team who understand the normal steps in resolving crisis and loss. Cutting off the person's questions or keeping him or her sedated may protect the staff, but it does not help the survivor.

The parents who grieve for their dying or fatally injured child must be respected, be given the opportunity to minister to the child when indicated, and be relieved of responsibilities at times (30). Encourage the parents to share feelings, and work to complement, not compete with, the parents in caring for the child. Also, remember that grandparents, siblings, peers, and sometimes the babysitter will need understanding in their grieving. The timing and type of support given after accidental death of a child are important (77). Nelson gives some practical suggestions for care of the parents (80).

Accident, suicide, and homicide are the leading causes of death before age 40. Thus, survivors often include children and adolescents. The grief and mourning that surrounds each of these death events differ from an anticipated death. The suddenness of each causes shock, confusion, helplessness, emptiness, and intense sadness. With suicide comes guilt and shame, a sense of being responsible, as well as anger at the person who committed suicide. With homicide comes the feelings of intense anger, rage, revenge, with the sadness intensified by the imagery related to brutality and what the person suffered in the last moments alive. With each of these types of death, the family longs to undo certain acts and to be able to say goodbye in a loving way. Long-term therapy is often needed.

Other Grief Responses

As you care for the family of the dying person, or interact with the family after death, you may perceive that they are not grieving in what you consider the usual or normal way. You may label their grief and mourning, both in anticipation of and at the time of death as absent or delayed, as complicated, pathologic, neurotic, and dysfunctional, or as a clinical depression (40).

Delayed grief response may be identified when *there is no anticipatory grieving or no expression of grief at death.* Later, there may be manifestations of not having grieved the loss (40):

- Continuing to act as if the person still lives, or looking for them

- Various physical symptoms, such as insomnia, loss of appetite and weight, pain, and actual malfunction of the body
- Expressions of frustration or anger that is out of context or excessive, or personality changes
- Complaints of excessive stress at work or home
- Increased smoking and use of alcohol or other drugs
- Difficulty in interpersonal and family relationships
- Nightmares, illusions of seeing the person and then realizing the person was someone else, or hallucinations of the person
- Statements about "shutting down at the time of death"

Complicated grief response may occur *when the person is experiencing unresolved grief associated with the past.* It is manifested in several ways (40, 67):

- Multiple physical complaints, often with no significant findings or physical examination (Often the symptoms mimic those of the deceased.)
- Suicidal ideas or attempts, wanting to join the dead person
- Intense grief when speaking of the deceased, or inappropriate, angry affect, or the mechanism of emotional isolation, e.g., smiling while talking about the dead person
- Withdrawal from others, failure to participate in the usual family or social activities, radical life changes
- Inability to talk about the deceased without intense grief expressions
- Intense grief reactions triggered by minor events
- Repeated verbalization of themes of loss
- Extreme sadness at certain times of the year, e.g., anniversary dates or special holidays

Through counseling, the person may remember past losses or rejections and grieve these as well as the current loss.

Dysfunctional grief response may occur when (1) *the person had a very dependent or ambivalent relationship with the deceased;* (2) *the circumstances surrounding death were uncertain, sudden, or overwhelming,* such as homicide, *or complicated with assault,* such as rape or violent attack; *or* (3) *a loss that is socially unspeakable or socially negated,* such as capital punishment or death or murder of someone who had been a gang member or molestor of children or had a criminal history. If there has been a history of mental illness or suicide, or if the person has minimal support systems, another loss will be more difficult to handle (8, 40, 58, 67).

Pathologic grief response is an *intensification of grief to the point that the person is overwhelmed, demonstrates prolonged maladaptive behavior, manifests excessive symptoms and extensive interruptions in healing,* and does not progress to integration of the loss, finding meaning in the loss, and resolution of the mourning process (40).

Intervention for the Dying Person

Care of the dying client falls primarily on the nurse. You have sustained contact with the client and understand dying and the many needs of the dying person. You know the value of compassionate service of mind and hands. You can protect the vulnerable person and understand some of the distress felt by client and family. You have an opportunity to help the client bring life to a satisfactory close, truly to live until he or she dies, and to promote comfort. The client needs your unqualified interest and response to help decrease loneliness and make the pain and physical care or treatment bearable.

You will encounter *frustrations during the care of the dying person* for many reasons. There is the challenge of talking with or listening to the client. Will he or she talk about death? Pain may be constant and difficult to relieve, causing you to feel incompetent. He or she may be demanding, nonconforming to the client role, or disfigured and offensive to touch or smell. The family may visit so often and long that they interfere with necessary care of the client. Accusations from the client or family about neglect may occur or be feared. It is no wonder that despite good intentions, religious convictions, and educational programs, you may avoid the dying client and family. They are left to face the crisis of death alone. As you rework personal feelings about crisis, dying, and death and become more comfortable with personal negative feelings and emotional upset, you will be able to serve more spontaneously and openly in situations previously avoided. You will be able to admit, without guilt feelings, personal limits in providing care, to use other helpers, and yet to do as much as possible for the client and family without showing shock or repugnance about the client's condition.

Physical care of the dying person includes providing for nutrition, hygiene, rest, elimination, relief of pain or other symptoms; care of the mouth, nose, eyes, skin, and peripheral circulation; positioning; and environmental considerations. Hospital personnel should not focus exclusively on the client's complaints of pain or other physical symptoms or need to avoid the subject of death. Complaints may be a camouflage for anxiety, depression, or other feelings and covertly indicate a desire to talk with someone about the feelings. Analgesics and comfort measures to promote rest can be used along with crisis therapy. Spend sufficient time with the client to establish a relationship that is supportive. Provide continuity of care. Try to exchange information realistically within the whole medical team, including client and family, to reduce uncertainty and feelings of neglect. Clients can withstand much pain and distress as long as they feel wanted or believe their life has meaning.

Thorough, meticulous physical care is essential to promote physical well-being but also to help prevent emotional distress. During the prolonged and close contact physical care provides, you can listen, counsel, and teach, using principles of effective communication. But let the client sleep often, without sedation if possible. The many physical measures to promote comfort and optimum well-being can be found in texts describing physical care skills. *Nursing care is not less important because the person is dying.*

Avoid too strict a routine in care. Let the client make some decisions about what he or she is going to do as long as safe limits are set. Modify care procedures as necessary for comfort. Through consistent, comprehensive care you tell the client you are available and will do everything possible for continued well-being.

During care, conversation should be directed to the client. Explain nursing procedures, even though the client is comatose, as hearing is the last sense lost. Response to questions should be simple, encouraging, but as honest as possible. Offer the person opportunities to talk about self and feelings through open-ended questions. When the client indicates a desire to talk about death, listen. There is no reason to expound your philosophy, beliefs, or opinions. Focus your conversation on the present and the client. Help the client maintain the role that is important to him or her. Convey that what he or she says has meaning for you. You can learn by listening to the wisdom shared by the client, and add to feelings of worth and generativity. Recognize when the client is unable to express feelings verbally, and help him or her reduce tension and depression through other means—physical activity, crying, or sublimative activities.

If the client has an intense desire to live and is denying or fearful of death, be accepting but help him or her maintain a sense of balance. Do not rob the person of hope or force him or her to talk about death. Follow the conversational lead; if the topics are concerned with life, respond accordingly.

Encourage communication among the doctor, client, and family. Encourage the client to ask questions and state needs and feelings instead of doing it for him or her, but be an advocate if the person cannot speak for self.

Explore with family members the ways they can communicate with and support the client. Explain to the family that because the comatose client can probably understand what is being said, they should talk in ways that promote security and should avoid whispering, which can increase the person's fears and suspicions.

Psychological care includes showing genuine concern, acceptance, understanding, and promoting a sense of trust, dignity, or realistic body image and self-concept. Being an attentive listener and providing for privacy, optimum sensory stimulation, independence, and participation in self-care and decision making are helpful. You will nonverbally provide a feeling of security and trust by looking in frequently on the client and using touch communication.

Spiritual needs of the dying person, regardless of the spiritual beliefs, can be categorized as follows (22):

- Search for meaning and purpose in life and in suffering, including to integrate dying with personal goals and values, to make dying and death less fearful, to affirm the value of life, and to cope with the frustration caused by anticipated death.
- Sense of forgiveness in the face of guilt about unfulfilled expectations for self, accepting non-fulfillment or incompleteness and making the most of remaining life, acts of omission or acts of commission toward others, resolving human differences.
- Need for love through others' words and acts of kindness and silent, compassionate presence. If family and friends are not present, the nurse may be the primary source of love.
- Need for hope, which connotes the possibility of future good. Concrete hope consists of objects of hope within the person's experience such as freedom from pain or other symptoms or ability to perform certain tasks or to travel. Abstract hope or transcendent hope is characterized by distant and abstract goals and incorporates philosophic or religious meanings. Hope may be expressed as belief about afterlife, reunion with deceased loved ones, and union with God, a superior alternative to present existence. If there is no belief in the afterlife, hope may be expressed as belief about transfer of physical energy from the deceased body, belief about contributing to another's life through an organ donation, or belief in leaving a legacy in his or her children or community or organizational contributions.

You may assist with meeting the person's spiritual needs if requested and if you feel comfortable in doing so. Certainly you should know whom to contact if you feel inadequate. The religious advisor is a member of the health team. If the client has no religious affiliation and indicates no desire for one, avoid proselytizing.

Consider the social needs of the client until he or she is comatose or wishes to be left alone. Visitors, family, or friends can contribute significantly to the client's welfare when visiting hours are flexible. If possible, help the client dress appropriately and groom to receive visitors, go out of the room to a lounge, meet and socialize with other clients, or eat in a client's dining room or the unit.

Community health nurses have found two distinct attitudes in families of dying clients. The first attitude is, "If he is going to die soon, let's get him to the hospital!" For these families the thought of watching the actual death is abhorrent. They feel personally unable to handle the situation and feel comforted by the thought of their loved one's dying in a place where qualified professionals can manage all the details. If possible, these families should have their wishes met.

The second attitude is, "I want her to die at home. This is the place she loved. I can do everything that the hospital personnel can do." This attitude can be supported by the visiting nurse. The visiting nurse can usually coordinate community resources so that a home health aide, homemaker services, proper drug and nutrition supplies, and necessary equipment can be available in the home. Even the comatose client who requires a hospital bed, tube feedings, catheter change and irrigation, daily bed bath, feces removal, and frequent turning can be cared for in the home if the health team, family, and friends will share efforts. The families who desire this approach and who are helped to carry out their wishes seem to derive great satisfaction from giving this care.

Clients and family members often select the *home as the place of care in the terminal stages of disease and as the place to die*. Being with family and friends and living in their own home are often high priorities for clients. Home represents their life's work and helps to maintain a sense of dignity, identity, and control over dying. They realize at home they would not have to battle extraordinary measures. The family wants the client at home because it is his or her wish and because they believe they would desire to be at home if they were dying. Clients and families who choose the hospital as the place of death believe clients would receive better care there. Clients do not want to burden families. Families are concerned about their loved one's comfort (24, 29, 45, 48, 71, 76, 82, 86, 105).

The *hospice* is an institution and a concept that gives the dying person homelike care either at home with the help of an interdisciplinary team or in an institution with a homelike atmosphere and special attention to the needs of the dying and their families. The hospice concept is indeed a "care system" that coexists with a "cure system." In the United States the definition of what constitutes hospice care varies from region to region; the goal, however, is essentially the same. The hospice concept originated in the Middle Ages; St. Christopher's Hospice in England has been the most famous to date. In some hospitals one unit is designated as the hospice area. A modern, freestanding hospice was opened in 1980 in Branford, Connecticut. Connecticut was the first state to regulate the licensing of hospices. In other states licensing depends on the types of facilities and services a hospice provides (105). More information about hospice care, especially ways that the nurse can help the client accept and cope with the dying process, foster communication between client and family, enhance the client's autonomy, relieve physical pain and other common symptoms, and work with the psychological aspects of late-stage cancer or other disease is found in several references (29, 45, 46, 86, 105).

Most hospice care programs enable the family to care for the dying person through a team approach: (1) a visiting nurse does multiple interventions, (2) home health aides do morning household chores, (3) a family physician enables pain control through effective use of medications, (4) a physical therapist helps the person maintain mobility and later teaches the family various transfer techniques, (5) a music therapist brings diversion and suggests exercise to music, and (6) the clergy and church choir visit the home.

At times the client needs to be alone, either at home or in the hospital, as he or she goes through the preparatory depression discussed by Kübler-Ross and is disengaging self from life, loved ones, and all that has been important to him or her. For you to impose yourself at these times might complicate the emotional tasks near the end of life You should not, however, abandon the client; give the necessary care but go at his or her pace in conversation and care.

Although most people who are about to die have made peace with themselves, some bargain or fight to the end. Accept this behavior, but do not encourage the client to fight for life when the last days are near with no chance for continuing life. *Instead, let him or her know that accepting the inevitable is not cowardly.* Remember that fear of death is often found more in the living than in the dying and that this fear is more for the impending separation of intimate relationships than of death itself.

After the death of the client, your relationship with the family need not end immediately. Explore with them how they will manage. Follow-up intervention in the form of a telephone call or home visit by a nurse, minister, social worker, or nursing care coordinator would be a way of more gradually terminating a close relationship and performing further crisis intervention as needed. Use this opportunity to evaluate the effectiveness of care given to the family throughout the client's terminal care period.

Evaluation

Throughout intervention with the dying client or his or her family you must continually consider whether your intervention is appropriate and effective, based on their needs rather than yours. Observation alone of their condition or behavior will not provide adequate evaluation. Ask yourself and others how you could be more effective, whether a certain measure was comforting and skillfully administered, and how the client and family perceived your approach and attitude. Assigning a person unknown to the client and family to ask these questions will help obtain an objective evaluation. Because of your involvement, you may be told only what people think you want to hear. If you and the client have established open, honest communication that encompasses various aspects of dying and if the client's condition warrants it, perhaps you will be able to interview the dying to get evaluation answers. You might ask if and how each member of the health team has added physically, intellectually, emotionally, practically, and spiritually to the person's care. You may also ask how each member of the health team has hindered in these areas.

Through careful and objective evaluation you can learn how to be more skillful at intervention in similar situations in the future.

SUMMARY

The concept of and reaction to dying and death depend on the person's cultural background and developmental level, the kind of death, the extent of support from significant others, and the quality of care given by nurses and other health care providers. Nurses and other health care workers must work through their own feelings as they face ethical and moral dilemmas related to use of technology and either prolonging or shortening life deliberately. There is much to learn from people who have nearing-death awareness, near-death experience, premonitions about death, or other kinds of dying experiences. The dying process and the afterlife are indeed the last stage of development.

REFERENCES

1. Anders, R. , and M. Kanai-Pak, Karoshi—Death From Overwork: A Nursing Problem in Japan? *Nursing and Health Care,*13, no. 4 (1992), 186–191.

2. Aries, P., *Western Attitudes Toward Death.* Baltimore: Johns Hopkins University Press, 1974.

3. Aroskar, M., Legal and Ethical Concerns: Nursing and the Euthanasia Debate, *Journal of Professional Nursing,* 10, no. 1 (1994), 5.

4. ———, The Aftermath of the Cruzan Decision: Dying in a Twilight Zone, *Nursing Outlook,* 38, no. 6 (1990), 256–261.

5. Association News, *N.P. News,* 3, no. 5 (1995), 100.

6. Baker, J.C., *Scared to Death, An Examination of Fear—Its Cause and Effects.* London: Frederic Muller, 1968.

7. Barbus, A.J., The Dying Person's Bill of Rights, *American Journal of Nursing,* 75 (1975), 99.

8. Bateman, A., D. Broderick, L. Gleason, R. Kardon, C. Flaherty, and S. Anderson, Dysfunctional Grieving, *Journal of Psychosocial Nursing,* 30, no. 12 (1992), 5–9.

9. Benner, K., Terminal Weaning: A Loved One's Vigil, *American Journal of Nursing,* 93, no. 5 (1993), 22–25.

10. Bereavement After Homicide for a Loved One, *The Menninger Letter,* 3, no. 6 (1995), 3.

11. Brown, M., Lifting the Burden of Silence, *American Journal of Nursing,* 94, no. 9 (1994), 62–63.

12. Burgess, K., The Influence of Will on Life and Death, *Nursing Forum,* 15, no. 3 (1976), 238–258.

13. Butler, R., The Roman Catholic Way in Death and Mourning, in Grollman, E., ed., *Concerning Death: A Practical Guide for the Living.* Boston: Beacon Press, 1974, pp. 101–118.

14. Callahan, M., Breaking the Silence, *American Journal of Nursing,* 94, no. 1 (1994), 22–23.

15. ———, Back from Beyond, *American Journal of Nursing,* 94, no. 3 (1994), 20–23.

16. ———, Farewell Messages, *American Journal of Nursing,* 94, no. 5 (1994), 18–19.

17. Cannon, W., Voodoo Death, *Psychosomatic Medicine,* 19 (1957), 182.

18. Carpenito, L., *Handbook of Nursing Diagnosis* (4th ed.). New York: J.B. Lippincott, 1991.

19. Cassini, N., Care of the Dying Person, in Grollman, E., ed., *Concerning Death: A Practical Guide for the Living.* Boston: Beacon Press, 1974, pp. 13–48.

20. Cate, S., Death by Choice, *American Journal of Nursing,* 91, no. 7 (1991), 33–34.

21. Chalalewski, F., and M. Norris, The Gift of Life: Talking to Families About Organ and Tissue Donation, *American Journal of Nursing,* 94, no. 6 (1994), 28–33.

22. Conrad, N., Spiritual Support for the Dying, *Nursing Clinics of North America,* 20, no. 2 (1985), 415–426.

23. Cox, C., The Choice, *American Journal of Nursing,* 81, no. 9 (1981), 1627–1628.

24. Coyle, N., The Last Four Weeks of Life, *American Journal of Nursing,* 90, no. 12 (1990).

25. Davis, A., L. Phillips, T. Drought, S. Sellin, K. Ronsman, and A. Hershberger, Nurses' Attitudes Toward Active Euthanasia, *Nursing Outlook,* 43, no. 4 (1995), 174–179.

26. ———, and P. Slater, U.S. and Australian Nurses' Attitudes and Beliefs About the Good Death, *IMAGE: Journal of Nursing Scholarship,* 21, no. 1 (1989), 34–39.

27. De Arteaga, C., Helping Children Deal With Death, *Journal of Christian Nursing,* 10, no. 1 (1993), 28–31.

28. De Vries, B., S. Bluck, and J. Birren, The Understanding of Death and Dying in a Life-span Perspective, *The Gerontologist,* 33, no. 3 (1993), 366–372.

29. Devich, L., B. Fields, and R. Carlson, Supportive Care for the Hopelessly Ill, *Nursing Outlook,* 36, no. 3 (1990), 140–142.

30. Diaz, M., When a Baby Dies, *American Journal of Nursing,* 95, no. 11 (1995), 54–56.

31. Dunton, H., The Child's Concept of Death, in Schoenberg, B., et al., eds., *Loss and Grief.* New York: Columbia University Press, 1970, pp. 355–361.

32. Dworetzky, J., *Human Development: A Life Span Approach* (2nd ed.). St. Paul/Minneapolis: West, 1995.

33. Eadie, B., and C. Taylor, *Embraced by the Light.* Riverside, NJ: McMillan, 1992.

34. Eakes, G., Grief Resolution in Hospice Nurses, *Nursing and Health Care,* 11, no. 5 (1990), 243–248.

35. Edwards, B., When the Family Won't Let Go, *American Journal of Nursing,* 94, no. 1 (1994), 52–56.

36. Engel, G., Sudden and Rapid Death During Psychological Stress: Folklore or Folk Wisdom? *Annals of Internal Medicine,* 74 (1971), 771–792.

37. ———, Psychological Stress, Vasodepressor (Vasovagal) Syncope, and Sudden Death, *Annals of Internal Medicine,* 89 (1978), 405–412.

38. Erikson, E.H., *Childhood and Society* (2nd ed.). New York: W.W. Norton, 1963.

39. Feifel, H., ed., *The Meaning of Death.* New York: McGraw-Hill, 1959.

40. Ferdinand, R., I'd Rather Die Than Live This Way, *American Journal of Nursing,* 95, no. 12 (1995), 42–47.

41. Fischer, H.K., and B.M. Dlin, Man's Determination of His Time of Illness or Death, *Geriatrics,* 26, no. 7 (1971).

42. *Florida Designation of Health Care Surrogate.* New York: Choice in Dying, 1995.

43. *Florida Living Will.* New York: Choice in Dying, 1995.

44. Fuller, J., Lethal Dose: Should a Nurse Resist Doctor's Orders, *Journal of Christian Nursing,* 3, no. 4 (Fall 1986), 4–8.

45. Gates, M.F., Transcultural Comparison of Hospital and Hospice as Caring Environments for Dying Patients, *Journal of Transcultural Nursing,* 2, no. 2 (1991), 3–15.

46. Giacquinta, B., Helping Families Face the Crises of Cancer, *American Journal of Nursing,* 77, no. 10 (October 1977), 1585–1588.

47. Gianelli, D., Would Aiding in Dying Make MDs Hired Killers? *American Medical News,* February 16 (1990), 1.

48. Gifford, B. and B. Cleary, Supporting the Bereaved, *American Journal of Nursing,* 90, no. 2 (1990), 49–53.

49. Glaser, B., and A. Strauss, The Social Loss of Dying Patients, *American Journal of Nursing,* 64, no. 6 (1964), 119ff.

50. ———, *Awareness of Dying.* Chicago: Aldine, 1965.

51. Gomez, E., and N. Carazos, Was Hexing the Cause of Death? *American Journal of Psychiatry,* 1, no. 1 (April 1981), 50–52.

52. Groff, B,. "Death and I," *American Journal of Nursing,* 82, no. 7 (1982), 1080–1083.

53. Grollman, E., *Talking About Death: A Dialogue Between Parent and Child* (3rd ed.). Boston: Beacon Press, 1990.

54. Gyulay, J., The Forgotten Grievers, *American Journal of Nursing,* 75, no. 9 (1975), 1476–1479.

55. Henderson, M., Beyond the Living Will, *Gerontologist,* 30. no. 4(1990), 480–485.

56. Hogan, N., and D. Balk, Adolescents' Reactions to Situational Death: Perceptions of Mothers, Fathers, and Teenagers, *Nursing Research,* 39, no. 2 (1990), 103–106.

57. Jecker, N., and L. Schneiderman, Is Dying Young Worse Than Dying Old? *The Gerontologist,* 34, no. 1 (1994), 66–71.

58. Joffrion, L., and T. Douglas, Grief Resolution: Facilitating Self-transcendence in the Bereaved, *Journal of Psychosocial Nursing,* 32, no. 3 (1994), 13–19.

59. Jolley, J., and M. Mitchell, *Lifespan Development: A Topical Approach.* Madison, WI: Brown & Benchmark, 1996.

60. Jordon, M., The Protestant Way in Death and Mourning, in Grollman E., ed., *Concerning Death: A Practical Guide for the Living.* Boston: Beacon Press, 1974, pp. 81–100.

61. Kaprio, J., M. Koskenvao, and H. Rita, Mortality After Bereavement: A Prospective Study of 95,647 Widowed Persons, *American Journal of Public Health,* 77, no. 3 (1987), 283–287.

62. Kevorkian Attends Suicide, *Hickory Daily Record,* August 21 (1995), 5–B.

63. Killian, W., Knowledge of Living Will Laws Essential, *American Nurse,* July–August (1990), 33.

64. Kowalski, S., Assisted Suicide: Where do Nurses Draw the Line? *Nursing and Health Care,* 14, no. 4 (1993), 70–76.

65. Kübler-Ross, E., ed., *On Death and Dying.* New York: Collier-Macmillan, 1969.

66. ———, *Death, the Final Stage of Growth.* Englewood Cliffs, NJ: Prentice-Hall, 1975.

67. Lazare, A., Breavement and Unresolved Grief, in Lazare, A., ed., *Outpatient Psychiatry: Diagnosis and Treatment* (2nd ed.). Baltimore: Williams & Wilkins, 1989.

68. Leininger, M., Quality of Life From a Transcultural Nursing Perspective, *Nursing Science Quarterly,* 7, no. 1 (1994), 22–28.

69. Libbus, M.K., and C. Russell, Congruence of Decisions Between Patients and Their Potential Surrogates About Life-sustaining Therapies, *IMAGE: Journal of Nursing Scholarship, Journal of Nursing Scholarship,* 27, no. 2 (1995), 135–140.

70. MacGregor, P., Grief: The Unrecognized Parental Response to Mental Illness in a Child, *Social Work,* 39, no. 2 (1994), 160–166.

71. Malcolm, A., The Right to Die, *New Choices,* July/August (1991), 68–70.

72. McIntire, M., C. Angle, and L. Struempler, The Concept of Death in Midwestern Children and Youth. *American Journal of Diseases of Children,* 123 (June 1972), 527–532.

73. Miles, A., Am I Going to Die? *American Journal of Nursing,* 94, no. 7 (1994), 20.

74. Montalvo, B., The Patient Chose to Die: Why? *The Gerontologist,* 31, no. 5 (1991), 700–703.

75. Moody, R.A., *Life After Life.* New York: Bantam Books, 1975.

76. Moore, M., Ethical Dilemmas in Managing Terminally Ill Patients, NCAPA Conference, Myrtle Beach, SC, August 16, 1995.

77. Murphy, S., Preventive Intervention Following Accidental Death of a Child, *IMAGE: Journal of Nursing Scholarship,* 22, (1990), 174–179.

78. Murray, R., and M. Huelskoetter, *Psychiatric Mental Health Nursing: Giving Emotional Care* (3d ed.). Norwalk, CT: Appleton & Lange, 1991.

79. Nagy, M., The Child's View of Death. In Fiefel, H., ed., *The Meaning of Death.* New York: McGraw-Hill, 1959.

80. Nelson, L., When a Child Dies, *American Journal of Nursing,* 95, no. 3 (1995), 61–64.

81. Norris, P., Organ Donations: Precious Gift or Market Commodity? *Ethical Issues in Health Care,* 14 (no. 3), 1992, 1–2.

82. ———, Disregarding Patients' Wishes: A Closer Look, *Ethical Issues in Health Care,* 14, no. 6 (1993), 1–2.

83. Oleson, M., Subjectively Perceived Quality of Life, *IMAGE: Journal of Nursing Scholarship,* 22, no. 3 (1990), 187–190.

84. Olson, M., The Out-of-Body Experiences and Other States of Conscious, *Archives of Psychiatric Nursing,* 1, no. 3 (1987), 201–207.

85. O'Rourke, K., Baby K: Is It Time to Take a Stand? *Ethical Issues in Health Care,* 15, no. 7 (March 1994), 1–2.

86. Palker, N., and B. Nettles-Carlson, The Prevalence of Advance Directives: Lessons from a Nursing Home, *Nurse Practitioner,* 20, no. 2 (1995), 7–21.

87. Papowitz, L., Life/Death/Life, *American Journal of Nursing,* 86, no. 4 (1986), 416–418.

88. Potter, P., and A. Perry, *Fundamentals of Nursing: Concepts, Process, and Practice* (2nd ed.), St. Louis: C.V. Mosby, 1989.

89. Rahe, R., and M. Romo, Recent Life Changes and the Onset of Myocardial Infarction and Sudden Death in Helsinki, in Gunderson, E., and R. Rahe, eds., *Life, Stress, and Illness.* Springfield, IL: Charles C Thomas, 1974, pp. 105–120.

90. Richter, G., On the Phenomenon of Sudden Death in Animals and Man, *Psychosomatic Medicine,* 19 (1959), 191.

91. Schoenbeck, S., Exploring the Mystery of Near-death Experiences, *American Journal of Nursing,* 93, no. 5 (1993), 43–46.

92. Stephany, T., A Death in the Family, *American Journal of Nursing,* 90, no. 4 (1990), 54–56.

93. Stepnick, A., and T. Perry, Preventing Spiritual Distress in the Dying Client, *Journal of Psychosocial Nursing,* 30, no. 1 (1992), 17–24.

94. Turner, J., and D. Helms, *Lifespan Development* (5th ed.). Ft. Worth: Harcourt Brace College, 1995.

95. Van Ora, L., Terminal Is a Relative Term, *Nursing and Health Care,* 10, no. 2 (1989), 97–100.

96. Vergara, M., and D. Lynn-McHale, Withdrawing Life Support: Who Decides? *American Journal of Nursing,* 95, no. 11 (1995), 47–52.

97. Waechter, E., Children's Awareness of Fatal Illness, *American Journal of Nursing,* 71, no. 6 (1971), 1168–1172.

98. Weber, G., Tips in Implementing the Patient Self-determination Act, *Nursing and Health Care,* 14, no. 2 (1993), 86–90.

99. Weisman, A., and T. Hackett, Predilection to Death, *Psychosomatic Medicine,* 23, no. 3 (1961).

100. West, J., Civilized Societies Don't Kill Coma Victims, *San Francisco Chronicle,* January 9, 1989.

101. When a Living Will Is Ignored, *American Journal of Nursing,* 94, no. 7 (1994), 62, 64.

102. White, A., The Needs of Dying Children and Their Families, *Health Visitor,* 62, no. 6 (1989), 176–178.

103. Wilson, D., Ethical Concerns in a Long-term Tube Feeding Study, *IMAGE: Journal of Nursing Scholarship,* 24 (1992), 195–199.

104. Zentner, R., Personal Story of Life After Life, March 1971.

105. Zerwekh, J., The Truth-tellers: How Hospice Nurses Help Patients Confront Death, *American Journal of Nursing,* 94, no. 2 (1994), 31–34.

106. Zimbelman, J., Good Life, Good Death, and the Right to Die: Ethical Considerations for Decisions at the End of Life, *Journal of Professional Nursing,* 10, no. 1 (1994), 22–37.

THE FOLLOWING IS AN EXAMPLE OF A LIVING WILL FOR THE STATE OF FLORIDA. PLEASE CONTACT CHOICE IN DYING AT (800) 989-WILL TO RECEIVE A FREE COPY OF APPROPRIATE ADVANCE DIRECTIVES FOR YOUR STATE.

FLORIDA LIVING WILL

INSTRUCTIONS

PRINT THE DATE

PRINT YOUR NAME

Declaration made this _____ day of _____, 19 ____ .

I, _____ , willfully and voluntarily make known my desire that my dying not be artifically prolonged under the circumstances set forth below, and I do hereby declare:

If at any time I have a terminal condition and if my attending or treating physician and another consulting physician have determined that there is no medical probability of my recovery from such condition, I direct that life-prolonging procedures be withheld or withdrawn when the application of such procedures would serve only to prolong artificially the process of dying, and that I be permitted to die naturally with only the administration of medication or the performance of any medical procedure deemed necessary to provide me with comfort care or to alleviate pain.

It is my intention that this declaration be honored by my family and physician as the final expression of my legal right to refuse medical or surgical treatment and to accept the consequences for such refusal.

In the event that I have been determined to be unable to provide express and informed consent regarding the withholding, withdrawal, or continuation of life-prolonging procedures, I wish to designate, as my surrogate to carry out the provisions of this declaration:

PRINT THE NAME, HOME ADDRESS, AND TELEPHONE NUMBER OF YOUR SURROGATE

© 1995 CHOICE IN DYING, INC.

Name: _____

Address _____

_____ Zip Code: _____

Phone _____

Figure 15–1. Sample living will. (*Reprinted by permission of Choice in Dying, 200 Varick Street, 10014, New York, NY, 212-336-5540*)

FLORIDA LIVING WILL — PAGE 2 OF 2

I wish to designate the following person as my alternate surrogate, to carry out the provisions of this declaration should my surrogate be unwilling or unable to act on my behalf:

PRINT NAME, HOME ADDRESS, AND TELEPHONE NUMBER OF YOUR ALTERNATE SURROGATE

Name: _____

Address: _____

_____ Zip Code: _____

Phone: _____

ADD PERSONAL INSTRUCTIONS (IF ANY)

Additional instructions (optional):

I understand the full importance of this declaration, and I am emotionally and mentally competent to make this declaration.

SIGN THE DOCUMENT

Signed: _____

WITNESSING PROCEDURE

Witness 1:

Signed: _____

TWO WITNESSES MUST SIGN AND PRINT THEIR ADDRESSES

Address: _____

Witness 2:

Signed: _____

Address: _____

© 1995
CHOICE IN DYING, INC.

*Courtesy of **Choice In Dying***
200 Varick Street, New York, NY 10014 1-800-989-WILL

9/95

Figure 15–1. Sample living will. (continued)

FLORIDA DESIGNATION OF HEALTH CARE SURROGATE

INSTRUCTIONS

PRINT YOUR NAME

Name: _____
       (Last)   *(First)*   *(Middle Initial)*

In the event that I have been determined to be incapacitated to provide informed consent for medical treatment and surgical and diagnostic procedures, I wish to designate as my surrogate for health care decisions:

PRINT THE NAME, HOME ADDRESS, AND TELEPHONE NUMBER OF YOUR SURROGATE

Name: _____

Address: _____

_____ Zip Code: _____

Phone: _____

If my surrogate is unwilling or unable to perform his duties, I wish to designate as my alternate surrogate:

PRINT THE NAME, HOME ADDRESS, AND TELEPHONE NUMBER OF YOUR ALTERNATE SURROGATE

Name: _____

Address: _____

_____ Zip Code: _____

Phone: _____

I fully understand that this designation will permit my designee to make health care decisions and to provide, withhold, or withdraw consent on my behalf; to apply for public benefits to defray the cost of health care; and to authorize my admission to or transfer from a health care facility.

© 1995 CHOICE IN DYING, INC.

Figure 15–2. Florida designation of a health care surrogate. (*Reprinted by permission of Choice in Dying, 200 Varick Street, 10014, New York, NY, 212-336-5540*)

FLORIDA DESIGNATION OF HEALTH CARE SURROGATE — PAGE 2 OF 2

ADD PERSONAL INSTRUCTIONS (IF ANY)

Additional instructions (optional):

I further affirm that this designation is not being made as a condition of treatment or admission to a health care facility. I will notify and send a copy of this document to the following persons other than my surrogate, so they may know who my surrogate is:

PRINT THE NAMES AND ADDRESSES OF THOSE WHO YOU WANT TO KEEP COPIES OF THIS DOCUMENT

Name: _____

Address: _____

Name: _____

Address: _____

SIGN AND DATE THE DOCUMENT

Signed: _____

Date: _____

WITNESSING PROCEDURE

TWO WITNESSES MUST SIGN AND PRINT THEIR ADDRESSES

Witness 1:

   Signed: _____

   Address: _____

Witness 2:

   Signed: _____

   Address: _____

© 1995
CHOICE IN DYING, INC.

*Courtesy of **Choice In Dying***
200 Varick Street, New York, NY 10014 1-800-989-WILL

9/95

Figure 15–2. Florida designation of a health care surrogate. (continued)

ADVANCE DIRECTIVE
Living Will and Health Care Proxy

Death is a part of life. It is a reality like birth, growth and aging. I am using this advance directive to convey my wishes about medical care to my doctors and other people looking after me at the end of my life. It is called an advance directive because it gives instructions in advance about what I want to happen to me in the future. It expresses my wishes about medical treatment that might keep me alive. I want this to be legally binding.

If I cannot make or communicate decisions about my medical care, those around me should rely on this document for instruction about measures that could keep me alive.

I do not want medical treatment (including feeding and water by tube) that will keep me alive if:
- I am unconscious and there is no reasonable prospect that I will ever be conscious again (even if I am not going to die soon in my medical condition), *or*
- I am near death from an illness or injury with no reasonable prospect of recovery.

I do want medical and other care to make me more comfortable and to take care of pain and suffering. I want this even if the pain medicine makes me die sooner.

I want to give some extra instructions: [*Here list any special instructions, e.g., some people fear being kept alive after a debilitating stroke. If you have wishes about this, or any other conditions, please write them here.*]

The legal language in the box that follows is a health care proxy.
It gives another person the power to make medical decisions for me.

I name _____ , who lives at_____
_____ , phone number _____ ,
to make medical decisions for me if I cannot make them myself. This person is called a health care "surrogate," "agent," "proxy," or "attorney in fact." This power or attorney shall become effective when I become incapable of making or communicating decisions about my medical care. This means that this document stays legal when and if I lose the power to speak for myself, for instance, if I am in a coma or have Alzheimer's disease.

My health care proxy has power to tell others what my advance directives means. This person also has power to make decisions for me, based either on what I would have wanted, or, if this is not known, on what he or she thinks is best for me.

If my first choice health care proxy cannot or decides not to act for me, I name _____
_____ , address _____ ,
phone number_____ , as my second choice.

(continued on other side)

Figure 15–3. Advance directive, living will, and health care proxy. (*Courtesy of Dr. Reid and Mrs. Judith Zentner.*)

I have discussed my wishes with my health care proxy, and with my second choice if I have chosen to appoint a second person. My proxy(ies) has(have) agreed to act for me.

I have thought about this advance directive carefully. I know what it means and want to sign it. I have chosen two witnesses, neither of whom is a member of my family, nor will inherit from me when I die. My witnesses are not the same people as those I named as my health care proxies. I understand that this form should be notarized if I use the box to name (a) health care proxy(ies).

Signature _____

Date _____

Address _____

Witness' signature _____

Witness' printed name _____

Address _____

Witness' signature _____

Witness' printed name _____

Address _____

Notary [to be used if proxy is appointed] _____

Drafted and distributed by Choice In Dying, Inc. — the national council for the right to die. Choice In Dying is a national not-for-profit organization which works for the rights of patients at the end of life. In addition to this generic advance directive, Choice In Dying distributes advance directives that conform to each state's specific legal requirements and maintains a national Living Will Registry for completed documents.

CHOICE IN DYING, INC. —
the national council for the right to die
(formerly Concern for Dying/Society for the Right to Die)
200 Varick Street, New York, NY 10014 (212) 366-5540

Figure 15–3. Advance directive, living will, and health care proxy. (continued)

STATE OF NORTH CAROLINA
COUNTY OF CATAWBA

HEALTH CARE POWER OF ATTORNEY

NOTICE: This document gives the person you designate your health care agent broad powers to make health care decisions for you, including the power to consent to your doctor not giving treatment or stopping treatment necessary to keep you alive. This power exists only as to those health care decisions for which you are unable to give informed consent.

This form does not impose a duty on your health care agent to exercise granted powers, but when a power is exercised, your health care agent will have to use due care to act in your best interests and in accordance with this document. Because the powers granted by this document are broad and sweeping, you should discuss your wishes concerning life-sustaining procedures with your health care agent.

I, _____
being of sound mind, hereby execute this Health Care Power of Attorney as follows:

1. Designation of Health Care Agent. I hereby appoint:
   Name: _____
   Home Address: _____
   Home Telephone No.: _____
   Work Telephone No.: _____

as my health care attorney-in-fact (herein referred to as my "Health Care Agent") to act for me and in my name (in any way I could act in person) to make health care decisions for me as authorized in this document.

If the person named as my Health Care Agent is not reasonably available or is unable or unwilling to act as my Agent, then I appoint the following persons (each to act alone and successively, in the order named), to serve in that capacity:

   A. Name: _____
      Home Address: _____
      Home Telephone No.: _____
      Work Telephone No.: _____
   B. Name: _____
      Home Address: _____
      Home Telephone No.: _____
      Work Telephone No.: _____

Each successor Health Care Agent designated shall be vested with the same power and duties as if originally named as my Health Care Agent.

2. Effectiveness of Appointment. ***Notice: This Health Care Power of Attorney may be revoked by you at any time in any manner by which you are able to communicate your intent to revoke to your Health Care Agent and your attending physician.***

Absent revocation, the authority granted in this document shall become effective when and if the physician (or Physicians) designated below determine that I lack sufficient understanding or capacity to make or communicate decisions relating to my health care and will continue in effect during my incapacity, until my death. This determination shall be made by the following physician (or physicians). (You may include here a designation of your choice, including your attending physician, or any other physician. You may also name two or more physicians, if desired, both of whom must make this determination before the authority granted to the Health Care Agent becomes effective.)

   A. First Physician's Name: _____
      Address: _____
      Work Telephone No.: _____
      Home Telephone No.: _____
   B. Second Physician's Name: _____
      Address: _____
      Work Telephone No.: _____
      Home Telephone No.: _____

3. General Statement of Authority Granted. I hereby grant to my Health Care Agent named above full power and authority to make health care decisions on my behalf.

My Health Care Agent is authorized in my Health Care Agent's sole and absolute discretion to exercise the powers granted herein relating to matters involving health and medical care. In exercising such powers, my Health Care Agent should first try to discuss with me the specifics of any proposed decision regarding my medical care and treatment if I am able to communicate in any manner, however rudimentary. My Health Care Agent is further instructed to give, withhold or withdraw consent to any medical treatment for me based upon any treatment choices that I have expressed while competent, whether under this document or otherwise. If my Health Care Agent cannot determine the treatment choice I would want made under the circumstances, then my Health Care Agent should make such choice for me based upon what my Health Care Agent believes to be in my best interests.

My Health Care Agent shall have the following powers and authority:

   A. To request, review, and receive any information, verbal or written, regarding my physical or mental health, including, but not limited to, medical and hospital records, and to consent to the disclosure of this information.

   B. To employ and discharge medical personnel including physicians, psychiatrists, dentists, nurses, and therapists as my Health Care Agent shall deem necessary for my physical, mental and emotional well-being, and to pay them (or cause to be paid to them) reasonable compensation.

   C. To consent to and authorize my admission to and discharge from a hospital, nursing or convalescent home, or other institution.

   D. To give consent for, to withdraw consent for, or to withhold consent for x-ray, anesthesia, medication, surgery, and all other diagnostic and treatment procedures ordered by or under the authorization of a licensed physician, dentist or podiatrist. This authorization specifically includes the power to consent to measures for relief of pain.

Figure 15–4. Sample health care power of attorney, state of North Carolina. (*Courtesy of Dr. Reid and Mrs. Judith Zentner.*)

E. To authorize the withholding or withdrawal of life-sustaining procedures when and if my physician determines that I am terminally ill, permanently in a coma, suffer severe dementia, or am in a persistent vegetative state. Life-sustaining procedures are those forms of medical care that only serve to artifically prolong the dying process and may include mechanical ventilation, dialysis, antibiotics, artifical nutrition and hydration, and other forms of medical treatment which sustain, restore or supplant vital bodily functions. Life-sustaining procedures do not include care necessary to provide comfort or alleviate pain.

I DESIRE THAT MY LIFE NOT BE PROLONGED BY LIFE-SUSTAINING PROCEDURES IF I AM TERMINALLY ILL, PERMANENTLY IN A COMA, SUFFER SEVERE DEMENTIA OR AM IN A PERSISTENT VEGETATIVE STATE.

F. To exercise my right of privacy and my right to make decisions regarding my medical treatment even though the exercise of my rights might hasten my death or be against conventional medical advice.

G. To consent to and arrange for the administration of pain-relieving drugs of any kind or other surgical or medical procedures calculated to relieve my pain, including unconventional pain-relief therapies which my Health Care Agent believes may be helpful, even though such drugs or procedures may lead to permanent physical damage, addiction or hasten the moment of (but not intentionally cause) my death.

H. To exercise any right I may have to make a disposition of any part or all of my body for medical purposes, to donate my organs, to authorize an autopsy, and to direct the disposition of my remains.

I. To take any lawful actions that may be necessary to carry out these decisions, including the granting of releases of liability to medical providers.

4. Special Provisions and Limitations. *Notice:* **The above grant of power is intended to be as broad as possible so that your Health Care Agent will have authority to make any decisions you could make to obtain or terminate any type of health care. If you wish to limit the scope of your Health Care Agent's powers, you may do so in this section.**

In exercising the authority to make health care decisions on my behalf, the authority of my Health Care Agent is subject to the following special provisions and limitations: (Here you may include any specific limitations you deem appropriate such as your own definition of when life-sustaining teratment should be withheld or discontinued, or instructions to refuse any specific types of treatment that are inconsistent with your religious beliefs, or unacceptable to you for any other reason)

_____

_____

_____

_____

5. Guardianship Provision. If it becomes necessary for a court to appoint a guardian of my person, I nominate my Health Care Agent acting under this document to be the guardian of my person, to serve without bond or security.

6. Reliance of Third Parties on Health Care Agent.

A. No person who relies in good faith upon the authority of or any representations by my Health Care Agent shall be liable to me, my estate, my heirs, successors, assigns, or personal representatives, for actions or omissions by my Health Care Agent.

B. The powers conferred on my Health Care Agent by this document may be exercised by my Health Care Agent alone, and my Health Care Agent's signature or act under the authority granted in this document may be accepted by persons as fully authorized by me and with the same force and effect as if I were personally present, competent, and acting on my own behalf. All acts performed in good faith by my Health Care Agent pursuant to this Power of Attorney are done with my consent and shall have the same validity and effect as if I were present and exercised the powers myself and shall inure to the benefit of and bind me, my estate, my heirs, successors, assigns, and personal representatives. The authority of my Health Care Agent pursuant to this Power of Attorney shall be superior to and bind upon my family, relatives, friends and others.

7. Miscellaneous Provisions.

A. I revoke any prior health care Power of Attorney.

B. My Health Care Agent shall be entitled to sign, execute, deliver, and acknowledge any contract or other document that may be necessary, desirable, convenient, or proper in order to exercise and carry out any of the powers described in this document and to incur reasonable costs on my behalf incident to the exercise of these powers; provided, however, that except as shall be necessary in order to exercise the powers described in this document relating to my health care, my Health Care Agent shall not have any authority over my property or financial affairs.

C. My Health Care Agent and my Health Care Agent's estate, heirs, successors and assigns are hereby released and forever discharged by me, my estate, my heirs, successors, and assigns and personal representatives from all liability from and all claims or demands of all kinds arising out of the acts or omissions of my Health Care Agent pursuant to this document, except for the willful misconduct or gross negligence.

D. No act or omission of my Health Care Agent, or of any other person, institutions, or facility acting in good faith in reliance on the authority of my Health Care Agent pursuant to this Health Care Power of Attorney shall be considered suicide, nor the cause of my death for any civil or criminal purposes, nor shall it be considered unprofessional conduct or as lack of professional competence. Any person, institution, or facility against whom criminal or civil liability is asserted because of conduct authorized by this Health Care Power of Attorney may interpose this document as a defense.

8. Signature of Principal. By signing here, I indicate that I am mentally alert and competent, fully informed as to the contents of this document, and understand the full import of this grant of powers to my Health Care Agent.

_____   _____
Date   (SEAL)

Figure 15–4. Sample health care power of attorney, state of North Carolina. (continued)

9. Signature of Witnesses. I hereby state that the Principal, _____ being of sound mind, signed the foregoing Health Care Power of Attorney in my presence, and that I am not related to the principal by blood or marriage, and I would not be entitled to any portion of the state of the principal under any existing will or codicil of the principal or as an heir under the Interstate Succession Act, if the principal died on this date without a will. I also state that I am not the principal's attending physician, nor an employee of the principal's attending physician, nor an employee of the health facility in which the principal is a patient, nor an employee of a nursing home or any group care home where the principal resides. I further state that I do not have any claim against the principal.

_____   _____ (SEAL)
Date   Witness

_____   _____ (SEAL)
Date   Witness

STATE OF NORTH CAROLINA

COUNTY OF MECKLENBURG   CERTIFICATE

I, _____ , a Notary Public for Mecklenburg County, North Carolina, hereby certify that
_____ appeared before me and swore to me and to the witnesses in my presence that this instrument is a Health Care Power of Attorney, and that she willingly and voluntarily made and executed it as her free act and deed for the purposes expressed in it.
    I further certify that _____ and _____ , witnesses, appeared before me and swore that they witnessed _____ sign the attached Health Care Power of Attorney, believing her to be of sound mind; and also swore that at the time they witnessed the signing (i) they were not related within the third degree to her or her spouse, and (ii) they did not know nor have a reasonable expectation that they would be entitled to any portion of her estate upon her death under any will or codicil thereto then existing or under the Interstate Succession Act as it provided at that time, and (iii) they were not a physician attending her, nor an employee of an attending physician, nor an employee of a health facility in which she was a patient, nor an employee of a nursing home or any group-care home in which she resided, and (iv) they did not have a claim against her. I further certify that I am satisfied as to the genuineness and due execution of the instrument.
    This the _____ day of _____ , 1991.

(NOTARY SEAL)   Notary Public _____
                                       My Commission expires: _____

NOTICE: A copy of this form should be given to your Health Care Agent and any alternate named in this Power of Attorney and to your physician and family members.

I, _____ agree to act as Health Care Agent for _____ pursuant to this Health Care Power of Attorney.
This the _____ day of _____ , 1991.

                                       _____ (SEAL)
                                       Health Care Agent

I, _____ agree to act as Health Care Agent for _____ pursuant to this Health Care Power of Attorney.
This the _____ day of _____ , 1991.

                                       _____ (SEAL)
                                       Health Care Agent

I, _____ agree to act as Health Care Agent for _____ pursuant to this Health Care Power of Attorney.
This the _____ day of _____ , 1991.

                                       _____ (SEAL)
                                       Health Care Agent

Figure 15–4. Sample health care power of attorney, state of North Carolina. (continued)

MEDICAL DIRECTIVE

I, _____ being of sound mind, make this statement as a directive to be followed if I am ever unable to participate in decisions regarding my medical care. Should I become mentally incompetent because of a medical condition like a coma or persistent vegetative state or severe dementia and my doctors do not expect me to recover, I direct the following treatment decisions be made in my behalf. These directions express my legal right to refuse treatment.

	YES	NO	UNSURE
1. **CPR:** Use drugs, electric shock and artificial breathing to bring me back to life when my heart stops.	___	___	___
2. **Mechanical breathing:** Use a machine to do my breathing for me when I cannot breathe unaided.	___	___	___
3. **Artificial nutrition:** Give me food through a tube in my vein or my stomach.	___	___	___
4. **Artificial hydration:** Give me liquid through a tube in my vein.	___	___	___
5. **Hospitalization:** Move me from home or hospice or nursing home to a hospital.	___	___	___
6. **Major surgery:** Operate on something like a blockage in my stomach or remove my gall baldder.	___	___	___
7. **Kidney dialysis:** Have a machine do the work of my kidneys - cleansing my blood - when they stop working on their own.	___	___	___
8. **Chemotherapy:** Give me drugs to fight cancer.	___	___	___
9. **Minor Surgery:** Operate on something minor like an infected toe.	___	___	___
10. **Major tests:** Do tests like heart catheterization or colonoscopy to see what's wrong inside me.	___	___	___
11. **Blood:** Transfuse blood or blood products into me if I am in need of them.	___	___	___
12. **Antibiotics:** Give me drugs to fight diseases like pneumonia or a kidney infection.	___	___	___
13. **Minor tests:** Do an x-ray or a blood test to see what's wrong with me.	___	___	___
14. **Pain medication:** Give me enough medication so that I am not in pain.	___	___	___
15. **Home:** Move me from the hospital so that I can die at home	___	___	___

16. **Other:** _____
_____
_____
_____
_____   ___ ___ ___

I provide this directive in addition to my living will.

Signed _____ Date _____

Witness _____

Witness _____

Figure 15–5. Sample medical directive. (*Courtesy of Dr. Reid and Mrs. Judith Zentner*)

DECLARATION OF A DESIRE FOR A NATURAL DEATH

I, _____ being of sound mind, desire that, as specified below, my life not be prolonged by extraordinary means or by artificial nutrition or hydration if my condition is determined to be terminal and incurable or if I am diagnosed as being in a persistent vegetative state. I am aware and understand that this writing authorizes a physician to withhold or discontinue extraordinary means or artificial nutrition or hydration, in accordance with my specifications set forth below:

(Initial any of the following as desired):

If my condition is determined to be terminal and incurable, I authorize the following:

_____   My physician may withhold or discontinue extraordinary means only.

In addition to withholding or discontinuing extraordinary means if such means are necessary, my physician may withhold or discontinue either artificial nutrition or hydration, or both.

If my physician determines that I am in a persistent vegetative state, I authorize the following:

_____   My physician may withhold or discontinue extraordinary means only.

In addition to withholding or discontinuing extraordinary means if such means are necessary, my physician may withhold or discontinue either artificial nutrition or hydration, or both.

This the _____ day of _____ , 1991.

I hereby state that the Declarant, _____ being of sound mind, signed the above Declaration in my presence and that I am not related to the Declarant by blood or marriage and that I do not know or have a reasonable expectation that I would be entitled to any portion of the estate of the Declarant under any existing Will or Codicil of the Declarant or as an heir under the Interstate Succession Act if the Declarant died on this date without a Will. I also state that I am not the Declarant's physician, or an employee of any health facility in which the Declarant is a patient or an employee of a nursing home or any group-care home where the Declarant resides. I further state that I do not now have any claim against the Declarant.

WITNESS our hands and seals this the _____ day of _____ , 1991.

_____ (SEAL)
Witness

_____ (SEAL)
Witness

CERTIFICATE

I, _____ , Notary Public for Mecklenburg County, North Carolina, hereby certify that _____ the Declarant, appeared before me and swore to me and to the witnesses in my presence that this instrument is her Declaration of a Desire For a Natural Death, and that she had willingly and voluntarily made and executed it as her free act and deed for the purposes therein expressed.

I further certify that _____ and _____ , witnesses, appeared before me and swore that they witnessed _____ the Declarant, sign the attached Declaration, believing her to be of sound mind; and also swore that at the time they witnessed the Declaration (i) they were not related within the third degree to the declarant or to the Declarant's spouse, and (ii) they did not know or have a reasonable expectation that they would be entitled to any portion of the estate of the Declarant upon the Declarant's death under any Will of the Declarant or Codicil thereto then existing or under the Intestate Succession Act as it provides at that time, and (iii) they were not a physician attending the Declarant or an employee of an attending physician or an employee of a nursing home or any group-care home in which the Declarant resided, and (iv) they did not have a claim against the Declarant. I further certify that I am satisfied as to the genuineness and due execution of the Declaration.

This the _____ day of _____ ,

_____
Notary Public for Mecklenburg
County, North Carolina

(Notary Seal)

My Commission expires: _____

Figure 15–6. Declaration of a desire for a natural death. (*Courtesy of Dr. Reid and Mrs. Judith Zentner.*)

Appendices

Appendix I

A. Recommended U.S. Dietary Allowances, Revised 1989

B. Recommended Nutrient Intakes for Canadians

A. RECOMMENDED U.S. DIETARY ALLOWANCES,[a] REVISED 1989

Category	Age (years) or Condition	Weight[b] kg	Weight[b] lb	Height[b] cm	Height[b] in.	Protein (g)	Fat-soluble Vitamins Vitamin A (μg RE)[c]	Vitamin D (μg)[d]	Vitamin E (mg α-TE)[e]	Vitamin K (μg)
Infants	0.0–0.5	6	13	60	24	13	375	7.5	3	5
	0.5–1.0	9	20	71	28	14	375	10	4	10
Children	1–3	13	29	90	35	16	400	10	6	15
	4–6	20	44	112	44	24	500	10	7	20
	7–10	28	62	132	52	28	700	10	7	30
Males	11–14	45	99	157	62	45	1000	10	10	45
	15–18	66	145	176	69	59	1000	10	10	65
	19–24	72	160	177	70	58	1000	10	10	70
	25–50	79	174	176	70	63	1000	5	10	80
	51+	77	170	173	68	63	1000	5	10	80
Females	11–14	46	101	157	62	46	800	10	8	45
	15–18	55	120	163	64	44	800	10	8	55
	19–24	58	128	164	65	46	800	10	8	60
	25–50	63	138	163	64	50	800	5	8	65
	51+	65	143	160	63	50	800	5	8	65
Pregnant						60	800	10	10	65
Lactating	First 6 months					65	1300	10	12	65
	Second 6 months					62	1200	10	11	65

[a]The allowances, expressed as average daily intakes over time, are intended to provide for individual variations among most normal persons as they live in the United States under usual environmental stresses. Diets should be based on a variety of common foods to provide other nutrients for which human requirements have been less well defined. See text for detailed discussion of allowances and of nutrients not tabulated.

[b]Weights and heights of reference adults are actual medians for the U.S. population of the designated age as reported by NHANES II. The use of these figures does not imply that the height-to-weight ratios are ideal.

[c]Retinol equivalents. 1 retinol equivalent = 1 μg retinol or 6 μg β-carotene.

[d]As cholecalciferol, 10 μg cholecalciferol = 400 IU of vitamin D.

[e]Tocopherol equivalents. 1 mg d-α tocopherol = 1 α-TE.

[f]1 NE (niacin equivalent) is equal to 1 mg of niacin or 60-mg of dietary tryptophan.

Reprinted with permission from Recommended Dietary Allowances, *10th Edition, © 1989 by the National Academy of Sciences. Courtesy of National Academy Press, Washington, DC.*

A.   RECOMMENDED U.S. DIETARY ALLOWANCES[a], REVISED 1989 (continued)

Water-soluble Vitamins							Minerals						
Vita- min C (mg)	Thia- min (mg)	Ribo- flavin (mg)	Niacin (mg NE>[f]	Vita- min B_6 (mg)	Fo- late (µg)	Vita- min B_{12} (µg)	Cal- cium (mg)	Phos- phorus (mg)	Mag- nesium (mg)	Iron (mg)	Zinc (mg)	Iodine (µg)	Sele- nium (µg)
30	0.3	0.4	5	0.3	25	0.3	400	300	40	6	5	40	10
35	0.4	0.5	6	0.6	35	0.5	600	500	60	10	5	50	15
40	0.7	0.8	9	1.0	50	0.7	800	800	80	10	10	70	20
45	0.9	1.1	12	1.1	75	1.0	800	800	120	10	10	90	20
45	1.0	1.2	13	1.4	100	1.4	800	800	170	10	10	120	30
50	1.3	1.5	17	1.7	150	2.0	1200	1200	270	12	15	150	40
60	1.5	1.8	20	2.0	200	2.0	1200	1200	400	12	15	150	50
60	1.5	1.7	19	2.0	200	2.0	1200	1200	350	10	15	150	70
60	1.5	1.7	19	2.0	200	2.0	800	800	350	10	15	150	70
60	1.2	1.4	15	2.0	200	2.0	800	800	350	10	15	150	70
50	1.1	1.3	15	1.4	150	2.0	1200	1200	280	15	12	150	45
60	1.1	1.3	15	1.5	180	2.0	1200	1200	300	15	12	150	50
60	1.1	1.3	15	1.6	180	2.0	1200	1200	280	15	12	150	55
60	1.1	1.3	15	1.6	180	2.0	800	800	280	15	12	150	55
60	1.0	1.2	13	1.6	180	2.0	800	800	280	10	12	150	55
70	1.5	1.6	17	2.2	400	2.2	1200	1200	300	30	15	175	65
95	1.6	1.8	20	2.1	280	2.6	1200	1200	355	15	19	200	75
90	1.6	1.7	20	2.1	260	2.6	1200	1200	340	15	16	200	75

B. RECOMMENDED NUTRIENT INTAKES FOR CANADIANS: AVERAGE ENERGY REQUIREMENTS AND SUMMARY EXAMPLES OF RECOMMENDED NUTRIENT INTAKES

Age	Sex	Average Height (cm)[c]	Average Weight (kg)[c]	Requirements[a,b]					
				kcal/kg[c,d]	MJ/kg[d]	kcal/day[e]	MJ/d[f]	kcal/cm[g]	MJ/cm[f]
Months									
0–2	Both	55	4.5	120–100	0.50–0.42	500	3.0	9	0.04
3–5	Both	63	7.0	100–95	0.42–0.40	700	2.8	11	0.05
6–8	Both	69	8.5	95–97	0.40–0.41	800	3.4	11.5	0.05
9–11	Both	73	9.5	97–99	0.41	950	3.8	12.5	0.05
Years									
1	Both	82	11	101	0.42	1100	4.8	13.5	0.06
2–3	Both	95	14	94	0.39	1300	5.6	13.5	0.06
4–6	Both	107	18	100	0.42	1800	7.6	17	0.07
7–9	M	126	25	88	0.37	2200	9.2	17.5	0.07
	F	125	25	76	0.32	1900	8.0	15	0.06
10–12	M	141	34	73	0.30	2500	10.4	17.5	0.07
	F	143	36	61	0.25	2200	9.2	15.5	0.06
13–15	M	159	50	57	0.24	2800	12.0	17.5	0.07
	F	157	48	46	0.19	2200	9.2	14	0.06
16–18	M	172	62	51	0.21	3200	13.2	18.5	0.08
	F	160	53	40	0.17	2100	8.8	13	0.05
19–24	M	175	71	42	0.18	3000	12.4		
	F	160	58	36	0.15	2100	8.8		
25–49	M	172	74	36	0.15	2700	11.2		
	F	160	59	32	0.13	1900	8.0		
50–74	M	170	73	31	0.13	2300	9.6		
	F	158	63	29	0.12	1800	7.6		
75+	M	168	69	29	0.12	2000	8.4		
	F	155	64	23	0.10	1500	6.0		

Pregnancy (additional)[h]

Lactation (additional)[h]

[a]Recommened nutrient intakes for Canadians, 1982—Committee for the Revision of the Dietary Standard for Canada, Bureau of Nutritional Sciences, Department of National Health and Welfare. Recommended intakes of energy and of certain nutrients are not listed in this table because of the nature of the variables on which they are based. The figures for energy are estimates of average requirements for expected patterns of activity. For nutrients not shown the following amounts are recommended: thiamine, 0.4 mg/100 kcal (0.48 mg/5000 kJ); riboflavin, 0.5 mg/1000 kcal (0.6 mg/5000 kJ); niacin, 6.6 NE/1000 kcal (7.9 NE/5000 kJ); vitamin B_6, 15 μg, as pyridoxine, per gram of protein intake; phosphorus, same as calcium. Recommended intakes during periods of growth are taken as appropriate for individual representative of the midpoint in each age group. All recommended intakes are designed to cover individual variations in essentially all of a healthy population subsisting on a variety of common foods available in Canada. It is emphasized that these are examples of the application of the RNI to particular classes of individuals and/or particular situations.

[b]Requirements can be expected to vary within a range of ±30%.

[c]Figures rounded to the closest whole number when ≥10 and to the closest 0.5 when <10.

[d]First and last figures are averages of those at the beginning and the end of the 3-month period.

[e]Figures rounded to the nearest 50 when <1000 and to the nearest 100 when ≥1000.

[f]Figures include two decimals if value is <1 and one decimal if ≥1.

[g]Figures rounded to the nearest 0.5.

[h]Pregnancy: add 100 kcal during the first trimester and 300 for the second and third trimesters; lactation: add 450 kcal/day.

[i]The primary units are grams per kilogram of body weight. The figures shown here are only examples.

[j]One retinol equivalent (RE) corresponds to the biological activity of 1 μg of retinol, 6 μg of β-carotene, or 12 μg of other carotenes.

[k]Expressed as cholecalciferol or ergocalciferol.

[l]Expressed as d-α-tocopherol equivalents, relative to which β- and γ-tocopherol and α-tocotrienol have activities of 0.5, 0.1, and 0.3 respectively.

[m]Expressed as total folate.

[n]Assumption that the protein is from breast milk or is of the same biologic value as that of breast milk and that between 3 and 9 months adjustment for the quality of the protein is made.

[o]For the infant it is assumed that breast milk is the source of iron up to 2 months of age.

[p]Based on the assumption that breast milk is the source of iron up to 2 months of age.

[q]After menopause the recommended intake is 7 mg/day.

From Bureau of Nutritional Sciences, Department of National Health and Welfare, Ottawa, Canada, 1982. Reproduced with permission of the Minister of Supply and Services, Canada, 1996.

B. RECOMMENDED NUTRIENT INTAKES FOR CANADIANS: AVERAGE ENERGY REQUIREMENTS AND SUMMARY EXAMPLES OF RECOMMENDED NUTRIENT INTAKES (continued)

Protein (g/day)[i]	Fat-soluble Vitamins			Water-soluble Vitamins			Minerals				
	Vit A (RE/day)[i]	Vit D (μg/day)[k]	Vit E (mg/day)[l]	Vit C (mg/day)	Folacin (μg/day)[m]	Vit B_{12} (μg/day)	CA (mg/day)	MG (mg/day)	FE (mg/day)	I (μg/day)	Z in (mg/day)
11[n]	400	10	3	20	50	0.3	350	30	0.4[o]	25	2[p]
14[n]	400	10	3	20	50	0.3	350	40	5	35	3
16[n]	400	10	3	20	50	0.3	400	45	7	40	3
18	400	10	3	20	55	0.3	400	50	7	45	3
18	400	10	3	20	65	0.3	500	55	6	55	4
20	400	5	4	20	80	0.4	500	65	6	65	4
25	500	5	5	25	90	0.5	600	90	6	85	5
31	700	2.5	7	35	125	0.8	700	110	7	110	6
29	700	2.5	6	30	125	0.8	700	110	7	95	7
38	800	2.5	8	40	170	1.0	900	150	10	125	6
39	800	2.5	7	40	170	1.0	1000	160	10	110	7
49	900	2.5	9	50	160	1.5	1100	220	12	160	9
43	800	2.5	7	45	160	1.5	800	190	13	160	8
54	1000	2.5	10	55	190	1.9	900	240	10	160	9
47	800	2.5	7	45	160	1.9	700	220	14	160	8
57	1000	2.5	10	60	210	2.0	800	240	8	160	9
41	800	2.5	7	45	165	2.0	700	190	14	160	8
57	1000	2.5	9	60	210	2.0	800	240	8	160	9
41[n]	800	2.5	6	45	165	2.0	700	190	14[q]	160	8
57	1000	2.5	7	60	210	2.0	800	240	8	160	9
41	800	2.5	6	45	165	2.0	800	190	7	160	8
57	1000	2.5	6	60	210	2.0	800	240	8	160	9
41	800	2.5	5	45	165	2.0	800	190	7	160	8
15	100	2.5	2	0	305	1.0	500	15	6	25	0
20	100	2.5	2	20	305	1.0	500	20	6	25	1
25	100	2.5	2	20	305	1.0	500	25	6	25	2
20	400	2.5	3	30	120	0.5	500	80	0	50	6

Appendix II

Major Sources and Functions of Primary Nutrients

Nutrient	Major Sources	Major Functions
Protein	Meat; poultry, fish; dried beans and peas; eggs; nuts; cheese; milk. Whole grain cereals are incomplete and must be combined with animal protein. Animal and vegetable protein combined increase use by body of all amino acids.	Builds, maintains, and repairs body cells; is required for amino acids (eight are essential). Constitutes part of the structure of every cell such as muscle, blood, bones, and ligaments. Supports growth and maintains healthy body cells. Maintains pH balance of blood; acts as buffer system. Regulates osmotic pressure. Constitutes part of enzymes, some hormones, body fluids, antibodies that increase resistance to infection, hemoglobin, plasma proteins. Is source of energy and fuel when inadequate carbohydrate and fat unavailable. Because protein and other nitrogenous compounds are degraded and resynthesized continually, daily intake is needed. Essential for nitrogen balance; excess excreted in urea and urine.
Carbohydrate	Bread, potatoes, pasta, dried beans, corn, rice, fruit, vegetables, sugar, desserts, candy, jam, syrup, honey.	Supplies energy and forms ATP so protein can be used for growth; maintenance of body cells and metabolic processes. Maintains body temperature. Supplies fiber in unrefined products—complex carbohydrates in fruits, vegetables, and whole grains—for regular elimination. Assists in fat utilization.
Fat	Animal fat, shortening, vegetable oil, butter, margarine, salad dressing, mayonnaise, sausages, lunch meats, whole milk and milk products, nuts. No more than 30% of total calories should be from fat. No more than 10% of fat intake should be saturated fat.	Provides concentrated source of energy. Constitutes part of the structure of every cell. Helps control cell permeability. Supplies essential fatty acids. Necessary for absorption of (carrier for) fat-soluble vitamins (A, D, E, and K). Maintains adipose tissue, which insulates and protects inner organs from trauma. Is component of thromboplastin, used in blood clotting. Adds to food taste, texture, and appearance. Provides reserve supply of phosphate ions. Excess animal fat is linked to cancer of gastrointestinal tract and possibly cancer of breast and prostate.

Major Sources and Functions of Primary Nutrients (continued)

Nutrient	Major Sources	Major Functions
Vitamins		
Vitamin C (ascorbic acid) (water soluble)	Citrus fruits such as orange, grapefruit, lime, lemon, papaya; mango, kiwi, cantaloupe, pineapple, rose hips, strawberries, raspberries, blackberries, black currants, melons, cherries, alfalfa sprouts, watercress, parsley, tomatoes, broccoli, sweet peppers, raw potatoes, raw leafy vegetables, kale, brussel sprouts, cabbage, cauliflower, asparagus, bok choy, thyme, horehound root, celery seed, sarsaparillo root, dandelion root.	Forms cementing substances such as collagen that hold body cells together, thus strengthening blood vessels, hastening healing of wounds and bone fractures, and increasing resistance to infection. Helps develop and maintain healthy bones, teeth, gums, skin, muscles, and blood vessels. Prevents scurvy. Regulates mitochondria and microsomal respiratory cycle. Aids use of iron and folic acid metabolism. Normalizes body cholesterol. Decreases risk of cancer of esophagus and stomach; aspirin prevents absorption.
Thiamine (B_1) (water soluble)	Pork, lean meat, nuts, liver, fish, oysters, crabmeat, dried yeast, milk, whole grains, enriched bread and cereals, pasta, dry beans, peas, lima beans, soybeans, sunflower seeds, brown rice, asparagus, raisins, alfalfa.	Functions as part of coenzyme to promote use of carbohydrate and protein and release of energy. Reduces fatigue and weakness. Promotes normal appetite. Contributes to normal functioning of nervous, muscle, and digestive systems. Prevents beriberi.
Riboflavin (B_2) (water soluble)	Liver and other organ meats, ham, poultry, milk and milk products, yogurt, cottage cheese, egg yolk, green leafy vegetables, lean meat, whole grains, soybeans, peas, beans, nuts, enriched bread and cereal, brewer's yeast, blackstrap molasses, sunflower seeds, wheat germ, alfalfa.	Is component of flavoprotein involved in biological oxidation. Is essential for building and maintaining body tissues, antibodies, and red blood cells. Functions as part of a coenzyme in the production of energy within body cells. Promotes carbohydrate, fat, and protein metabolism. Maintains nitrogen balance. Is essential for use of oxygen in cells. Promotes healthy skin, eyes, tongue, lips, mucous membranes. Prevents sensitivity of eyes to light.
Niacin (water soluble)	Liver, meat, rabbit, poultry, fish, peanuts, whole grains, brewer's yeast, fortified cereal and bread products, wheat germ, gentian root, licorice root, alfalfa.	Aids use of vitamins B_1 and B_2. Is essential for tissue respiration. Functions as part of a coenzyme in fat synthesis, protein use, glycolysis and use of carbohydrate, and release of energy. Promotes healthy skin, nerves, digestive tract, blood vessels. Aids digestion and fosters normal appetite. Is required for formation of certain hormones and nerve-regulating substances. Prevents pellagra.
Pyridoxine (B_6) (water soluble)	Liver, meat, fish, poultry, whole-grain bread and cereals, wheat germ, brewer's yeast, sunflower seeds, soybeans, nuts, brown rice, bananas, avocado, sweet potato, white potato, corn, white beans, green leafy vegetables, alfalfa.	Is coenzyme in basic reactions of amino acid, fat metabolism, protein metabolism. Assists antibody, hormone, and red blood cell formation. Is involved with function of neurotransmitters. Helps maintain balance of sodium and phosphorus and metabolism of iron and potassium.
Cyanocolabalamin (B_{12}) (water soluble)	Organ meats such as liver, kidney, and heart; lean meat; poultry; fish; oysters; clams; sea vegetables (kelp, dulse, komba); eggs; milk; cheese; brewer's yeast; angelica root; alfalfa.	Is essential for all blood cell formation. Is coenzyme for synthesis of materials for nucleus of all cells. Is essential for synthesis of nucleic acids; metabolism of certain amino acids, protein, carbohydrate, fat; and generally normal cell function. Converts folic acid to folinic acid. Is especially important for cells of bone marrow, intestinal tract, central nervous system. Strict vegetarian at risk for deficiency, pernicious anemia.

Major Sources and Functions of Primary Nutrients (continued)

Nutrient	Major Sources	Major Functions
Folacin (folic acid) (water soluble)	Dark green, leafy vegetables such as collards, mustard greens, turnip greens, kale; organ meats, dried beans, root vegetables, whole grains, brewer's yeast, oysters, salmon, milk, black-eyed peas, lima beans, watermelon, cantaloupe.	Synthesizes nucleic acid and proteins. Acts with B_{12} in making genetic material. Assists metabolism of certain amino acids. Assists in hemoglobin, red blood cell, protein formation. Is necessary for normal cell division. Prevents anemia.
Vitamin A (retinol) (fat soluble)	Liver; orange-colored fruits; orange, yellow, and dark green vegetables such as carrots, winter squash, sweet potatoes, broccoli, and greens; eggs; fortified milk, butter, margarine, cheese; horehound root; celery seed; dandelion root; red peppers.	Assists formation, maintenance, and repair of normal skin, hair, mucous membranes that line body cavities and tracts such as nasal passages and intestinal tract, thus increasing resistance to infection. Maintains mitochondrial and liposomal membranes. Functions in visual processes, forms visual purple, thus promoting healthy eye tissue and eye adaptation in dim light or at night. Increases resistance to infection. Decreases risk of cancer of lung, thyroid, esophagus, bladder because it aids in controlling cell differentiation.
Vitamin D (fat soluble)	Fortified milk, butter, margarine, fish liver oil, salmon, tuna, egg yolk, liver, bone meal, sunshine, thyme.	Regulates calcium and phosphorus metabolism; promotes intestinal absorption of calcium and phosphorus. Promotes bone mineralization (prevents rickets) and tooth formation.
Vitamin E (fat soluble)	Vegetable oils, liver, wheat germ, whole-grain cereals, rice, oats, brewer's yeast, peanuts, foods high in poly-unsaturated fatty acids, eggs, molasses, sweet potatoes, leafy vegetables, lettuce, spinach, asparagus, cauliflower, broccoli, angelica root, horehound root.	Is essential in cellular respiration. Is antioxidant at tissue level; maintains tissue. Prevents abnormal fat breakdown in tissues. Assists in formation of normal red blood cells and muscle. Functions in reproductive system. Prevents buildup of cholesterol plaque and blood clot formation in blood vessels, thus preventing coronary disease. Protects against exposure to radiation.
Vitamin K (fat soluble)	K_1 is found in lean meat, liver, green plants, green leafy vegetables, tomatoes, cauliflower, peas, carrots, potato, cabbage, soybean and safflower oil, egg yolk, blackstrap molasses, wheat germ. K_3 is synthetic therapeutic form. Half of vitamin K in body synthesized by intestinal bacteria as K_2.	Is essential for synthesis of blood-clotting factors: prothrombin (factor I), factors VII, IX, X. Stimulates coagulation proenzymes II, VII, IX, X.
Biotin	Egg yolk, organ meats, fish, brewer's yeast, whole grains, legumes, sardines, most fresh vegetables, lima beans, mushrooms, peanuts, bananas, yogurt.	Is necessary for formation of folic acid. Is necessary for carbohydrate, protein, fat metabolism. Aids in use of other B vitamins.
Pantothenic acid	Organ meats, lobster, oyster, salmon, brewer's yeast, egg yolk, legumes, whole grains, wheat germ, nuts, soy flour, sunflower and sesame seeds, green leafy vegetables, broccoli, cauliflower, potato, licorice root.	Aids in formation of some fats, hormones. Aids in metabolism and release of energy from carbohydrates, fats, proteins. Aids in use of some vitamins. Improves resistance to stress and infection.
Choline	Egg yolk, organ meat, fish, salmon, brewer's yeast, wheat germ, soybeans, legumes.	Aids normal nerve transmission. Aids metabolism and transport of fats.
Inositol	Citrus fruits, whole grains, brewer's yeast, molasses, meat, milk, nuts, vegetables, gentian root.	Is necessary for formation of lecithin. Aids hair growth.
para-Aminobenzoic acid (PABA)	Organ meats, wheat germ, yogurt, molasses, green leafy vegetables.	Aids bacteria producing folic acid. Acts as a coenzyme in use of proteins. Aids in formation of red blood cells. Acts as sunscreen.
Pangamic acid	Brewer's yeast, brown rice, sunflower, pumpkin, and sesame seeds.	Helps eliminate hypoxia. Promotes protein metabolism. Stimulates nervous and glandular systems.

Major Sources and Functions of Primary Nutrients (continued)

Nutrient	Major Sources	Major Functions
Minerals		
Calcium	Milk and milk products, chowder, cream soups, puddings made with milk, custards, yogurt, shellfish, salmon, sardines, bone meal, dark green leafy vegetables, kale, egg yolk, whole grains, legumes, nuts, tofu, molasses, broccoli, tomatoes, chamomille flower, cascara sagrada, angelica root, passion flower.	Works with phosphorus, magnesium, vitamin D, other minerals, protein to build bones and teeth. Assists blood clotting. Is necessary for nerve transmission, heart function, muscle contraction and relaxation, cell wall permeability. Activates enzyme ATPase. Intestinal absorption of vitamin D, which decreases with age, necessary for calcium metabolism. Oxylates and phytates in green leafy vegetables, and grains interfere with calcium absorption by combining with calcium and creating insoluble compound. Fiber may combine with calcium and limit absorption. Alcohol intake interferes with metabolism. Caffeine and excess salt intake cause calcium excretion.
Phosphorus	Milk and milk products, meat, liver, seafood, whole grains, wheat germ, nuts, egg yolk, legumes, peas, beans, lentils, brown rice, sunflower seeds, brewer's yeast.	Helps formation of nucleic acids. Works with calcium and vitamin D to build and maintain healthy bones, teeth, cell membranes. Aids absorption of glucose and glycerol. Transports fatty acids. Acts as buffer system. Aids energy metabolism.
Potassium	Lean meat, chicken, whole grains, bananas, oranges, apricots, dried fruits, potato, vegetables, broccoli, spinach, raw cabbage, swiss chard, okra, legumes, lima beans, sunflower seeds, molasses, wheat germ, skim milk, roasted chestnuts, cascara sagrada, horehound root.	Controls activity of heart, muscles, nervous system, kidneys. Regulates neuromuscular excitability and muscle contraction. Is major intracellular fluid cation. Promotes acid–base balance. Is necessary for glycogen formation and protein synthesis.
Magnesium	Whole grains, cereals, nuts, citrus fruits, figs, green leafy vegetables, swiss chard, dried beans and peas, soybeans, meat, milk, brown rice, wheat germ, chamomile flower, passion flower, sevega root.	Promotes healthy nerve and muscle tissue and function. Is component of bones and teeth. Is activator and coenzyme in carbohydrate, fat, protein metabolism. Acts as catalyst in use of calcium and phosphorus. Is essential intracellular fluid cation.
Iodine	Iodized salt, seafood, kelp, green leafy vegetables.	Is necessary for thyroid gland to control cell activities and metabolism. Synthesizes thyroxine, the thyroid hormones, which regulates cell oxidation. Promotes growth. Prevents goiter.
Sodium	Table salt, fish, seafood, kelp, baking powder and baking soda, milk, cheese, meat, eggs, celery, carrots, beets, spinach, cucumber, asparagus, turnips, stringbeans, coconut, processed foods and cereals, snack foods such as potato chips, pretzels, salted nuts.	Maintains normal fluid level and osmotic pressure in cells. Is major extracellular fluid cation. Maintains health of nervous, muscular, blood, lymph systems. Promotes cell permeability and absorption of glucose. Transmits electrochemical impulse in muscle, resulting in contraction. Promtoes acid–base balance; acts with potassium, magnesium, chlorine; buffers carbon dioxide and ketones.
Cobalt	Organ meats, oysters, clams, poultry, milk, green leafy vegetables, fruits, supplied by preformed vitamin B_{12}.	Is component of vitamin B_{12}. Is essential for red blood cell formation. Activates a number of body enzymes.

Major Sources and Functions of Primary Nutrients (continued)

Nutrient	Major Sources	Major Functions
Chlorine	Table salt, seafood, meats, liver, fish, ripe olives, rye flour, soybeans, egg yolks, peanuts, wheat germ.	Regulates acid–base balance and chlorine–bicarbonate shift. Is major extracellular fluid anion. Maintains osmotic pressure. Stimulates production of hydrochloric acid. Helps maintain joints and tendons.
Sulfur	Fish, shrimp, eggs, meat, cabbage, brussels sprouts, asparagus, milk, cheese, nuts, legumes, peas, beans, mustard greens, cauliflower, mashed potatoes.	Is component of amino acids and B vitamins. Is essential for formation of body tissues, collagen, skin, bones, tendons, cartilage. Assists in tissue respiration. Required for oxidation–reduction reactions. Activates enzymes. Aids in detoxification reactions.
Fluorine	Natural supply in water in some areas of United States; fluoridated water, seafood, bone meal, tea.	Is deposited in teeth and bones. May reduce tooth decay by discouraging growth of acid-forming bacteria.
Molybdenum	Legumes, whole-grain cereals, milk, liver, dark green vegetables.	Acts in oxidation of fat and aldehydes. Aids in mobilization of iron from liver reserves. Assists in conversion of purine to uric acid.
Vanadium	Fish, whole grains, root vegetables, nuts, vegetable oils.	Inhibits cholesterol formation. May assist in tooth and bone formation.

Trace Minerals

Nutrient	Major Sources	Major Functions
Iron	Organ and red meats, fish, poultry, beef, pork, lamb, dried and canned beans and peas, enriched whole-grain breads and cereals, dark green leafy vegetables, mustard and dandelion greens, egg yolk, blackstrap molasses, cherry and prune juice, legumes, nuts, dried fruits (raisins, apricots), chamomile flower, horehound root, sevega root, celery seed.	Is essential for hemoglobin and myoglobin formation. Helps protein metabolism. Is used by cells as component for oxidation of glucose in production of energy. Aids tissue respiration. Promotes growth. Increases resistance to infection. Is more readily used by body when ascorbic acid, copper, folic acid, vitamin B_{12} available. Excess calcium intake interferes with iron absorption.
Zinc	Organ and red meats, sunflower seeds, oysters, herring, seafood, eggs, mushrooms, brewer's yeast, soybeans, wheat germ.	Is component of insulin, serum proteins, reproductive fluid, bone, muscle, eyes, hair, teeth, liver. Aids digestion and metabolism of phosphorus. Necessary for adequate respiration and digestion. Important for sensory functioning, normal growth, hair, complexion, sexual function, wound healing. Aids healing and resistance to infection; excess or deficiency interferes with immune function.
Copper	Organ and lean meats, seafood, nuts, legumes, molasses, raisins, bone meal, cocoa, food cooked in copperware.	Absorbs and transports iron and aids in formation of red blood cells. Is component of many enzymes, which, in turn, are necessary for development and maintenance of skeletal, cardiovascular, and central nervous systems. Works with vitamin C to form elastin.
Manganese	Whole grains, green leafy vegetables, legumes, nuts, pineapple, grapefruit, egg yolk, tea, coffee, cascara sagrada, licorice root.	Is enzyme activator for urea formation, protein and fat metabolism, glucose oxidation, synthesis of fatty acids. Is necessary for normal skeletal formation, brain function. Maintains sex hormone production. May protect against pancreatic cancer.

Major Sources and Functions of Primary Nutrients (continued)

Nutrient	Major Sources	Major Functions
Chromium	Corn oil, clams, whole-grain cereals, meat, liver, wheat germ, brewer's yeast, drinking water in some areas of United States.	Stimulates enzymes in metabolism of energy and synthesis of fatty acids, cholesterol, protein. Increases effectiveness of action of insulin in cell, which improves glucose uptake by body tissues.
Selenium	Seafood; tuna; herring; organ and red meat; brewer's yeast; wheat germ; bran; asparagus; mushrooms; broccoli; whole grains; bread; cereals; garlic.	Acts as cofactor in cell oxidation enzyme systems. Is constituent of factor III, which acts with vitamin E to prevent fatty liver. Preserves tissue elasticity. Protects against heart disease. May prevent liver, colon, breast cancer.
Water	Water, coffee, tea, milk, soup, fruit juices, flavored gelatin, fruits, vegetables.	Is part of blood, lymph, body secretions. Aids digestion. Dissolves nutrients and enables them to pass through intestinal wall. Regulates body temperature. Transports body wastes for elimination.

Appendix III

Stress Management Strategies

STRESS MANAGEMENT

Stress management involves not only a variety of techniques, but also knowledge of the stress level at which response is harmful, avoidance of excess stress, and involvement with other people and groups. (See Chapter 5)

Assessment

Stressful life events interfere with health promotion and precede many health problems. Stress encounters in life and their potential impact on health can be assessed by using the *Social Readjustment Rating Scale* (see Table 5–16) developed by Holmes and Rahe (22).

You may have the person do a stress charting exercise, listing all current stressors and the areas of life impacted by these stressors (e.g., spouse, children, relatives, friends, work or profession, personal health effects, finances, social concerns, recreation or leisure, church, other organizational activity, other areas). Then each stressor should be rated as to the impact it is having, using a scale of 1 to 5, with the number 5 indicating severe impact. Awareness gained from this exercise may motivate the person to use stress management and relaxation techniques.

Intervention

Strategies for adaptation to stressors include biological mechanisms, psychological adaptive mechanisms, and coping behaviors. There are intrapsychic, interpersonal, and system or institutionalized ways of coping with stressors. You will assist clients to develop and use these strategies through (1) direct care, (2) exploration with the person, (3) teaching or counseling of the person, or (4) creating changes in the person, family, group, health care agency, or client's environment. Approach intervention from a *holistic* philosophy; mind, body, spirit, and culture are a fully unified system. A variety of approaches can be used to prevent or treat illness.

Physical Methods of Relaxation/Stress Management

Relaxation and stress management techniques can be used with people of any age, including school-age children (6, 29).

Progressive Relaxation. **Progressive relaxation** was developed by Jacobson in 1938 and *involves tightening and relaxing muscle groups* of the body for 5 to 7 seconds each, beginning with the hand and moving to the upper and lower arm, forehead and face, neck, upper back, abdomen, buttocks, thigh, calf, and foot. Or relaxation may progress from the feet, legs, buttocks, torso, shoulders, and neck, arms and hands, to face. The person is encouraged to check for relaxation before moving to the next major muscle group. In a relaxation session you and the individual can agree that if he or she is tense, the index finger of the right or left hand will be raised when relaxation is felt (2, 10, 13, 16, 38).

The person may be able to relax through breathing techniques that use deep, slow inhalation and full exhalation, with the person focusing mentally on the body part to which the inhalation is directed. Rapid, shallow breathing is often induced by stress. Thus concentration on proper breathing, especially abdominal breathing can help relieve stress. Music can be used with the breathing exercises (3).

A careful assessment of the person is essential before using relaxation techniques. Baseline and post-treatment vital sign measures will validate physiologic changes associated with relaxation. *Essential components of the pretreatment interview include assessing (2, 10, 13, 16, 38):*

- Client's identification of the most bothersome symptom(s), including onset, duration, and full description
- Family history of similar complaints
- Client interventions and description of the results, including use of current and recent medications, including over-the-counter drugs
- Physical limitations or illnesses
- Previous experience with relaxation training
- Use of alcohol or mind-altering drugs to relax
- Dietary patterns, especially use of caffeine, sugar, and foods that connote relaxation and are eaten at stressful times
- Sleep and exercise patterns
- Overview of daily routine, including stressors
- Psychiatric history, including screening for major depressive or psychotic disorders
- Willingness to learn techniques and to practice at home

Although progressive relaxation has proved effective in most studies, *precautions* should be taken for persons in the following categories:

- Depressed or withdrawn persons: Relaxation may cause further withdrawal.
- Persons who are experiencing hallucinations and delusions: They may lose contact with reality.
- Persons with cardiac conditions: They should use nontensing relaxation exercises as tightly tensing muscles can increase blood pressure.
- Persons on medications: The toxic effects of some medications can be increased by the relaxation state.

A number of *techniques,* as described below, can be used to foster the relaxation response.

A change of pace or scenery can bring about immediate stress relief. Take a brief walk outside; look at the sky, flowers, or birds; carefully wash hands and face; massage the face and forearms briefly; listen to music for a few minutes; and look out a window at a tree or clouds in the sky. Eliminate activities that are unnecessary, excessive, or generally insignificant. Make no attempt to "finish everything" by a set time. Do only one activity at a time (33).

Postural release of tension is the most basic movement of the body and helps the body to regain natural movement patterns and balance and to integrate all body parts. At the beginning of any movement or act, pull the head upward and away from the body and let the whole body lengthen by following that upward direction (33).

Deep abdominal breathing is done by standing in a comfortable position, head up and level, neck relaxed, arms and shoulders relaxed, knee joints straight but not locked, and feet a little more than shoulder width apart. Close the eyes and practice slow, deep, abdominal breathing for ten cycles. The chest should be relaxed and ribs allowed to move naturally. As the diaphragm moves downward on inhalation, the abdomen will move outward. Conscious control of breathing patterns helps to maintain a calm but alert mental state and control over body movement (33).

Tense and relax muscles systematically while sitting in a comfortable position. Contrast the sensation of tension with that of letting go. Eventually learn to tense and release body muscles from head to toe. Practice this technique to feel the rippling effect (33).

Exercise can be used to relax the neck and back muscles and the lumbar spine (Table A–1). The exercise is done in three parts (33).

Exercise or massage of a specific body area can also promote relaxation. **Rotation of the head in a circular motion** while maintaining relaxed shoulders with arms hanging at the side may allow relaxation of the neck muscles and can relieve a headache. You can also rotate the shoulders backward in a circular, shrugging motion. This will stretch the muscles of the chest that tend to shorten and cause round shoulders. Back, shoulder, neck, and foot massage promotes relaxed muscles and a calm mind (33).

Additionally, the use of **touch** can be perceived as supportive, calming, and strengthening. Holistic health workers emphasize the importance of touch, massage, and anywhere from 4 to 20 hugs daily for mental and physical health (33).

Some relaxation methods can be done simultaneously with other tasks or while at work. For example, while sitting, raise your legs until they are parallel with the floor. Then alternate bringing your feet back toward the upper torso and pointing them straight out while curling your toes. When talking on the telephone or reading, elevate your feet. This will aid circulation by redistributing the blood that tends to pool in the legs and feet after prolonged sitting. Stand up and stretch two or three times each day, perhaps when breaking for coffee and lunch (33).

TABLE A–1. EXERCISE ROUTINE FOR RELAXATION OF NECK AND BACK MUSCLES

Part 1

First, lie on your back on the floor. Lift your knees so your feet are flat on the floor. Arms lie comfortably a little less than 90° from the sides of your body. Cross your right leg over your left leg at the knee. Take in a deep abdominal breath; on exhalation, allow your legs to drop by gravity to the right. Relax for a moment. With the next inhalation, bring your legs up to a crossed knee position. Repeat five or ten times. Switch leg positions and repeat to the other side. Slowly extend your legs to lie flat on the floor. Notice that the lumbar region of your back is now touching the floor, or is not as arched as before the exercise.

Part 2

Next, lie flat and lift both arms above your chest and clasp your fingers together. A triangle is formed by your arms at each side with your shoulders and chest as the base. Maintain this triangle as you repeat the exercise in part 1. Your shoulders will be gently pulled off the floor during the exercise. Notice more of a stretch from shoulder to hip this time. Repeat 5 to 10 times with crossed knees and legs falling first to the right, then to the left.

Part 3

Finally, bring your arms back to a central position above your body, unfold your hands, and allow your elbows and forearms to slowly touch the floor. Allow both knees to fall to the side and extend legs slowly to the floor. Move to a side-lying position and then push to a sitting position. (Do not sit erect by pulling the torso vertically after this or any exercise that is done while lying on the floor.)

TABLE A–2. CLIENT INSTRUCTIONS FOR RELAXATION

1. This relaxation session will last from 20 to 40 minutes depending on your comfort level. You may want to go to the bathroom or get a drink of water before beginning.
2. The setting should be as quiet and distraction free as possible. The lights will be dimmed.
3. Loosen any clothing that is tight or uncomfortable. You will probably want to remove your shoes.
4. You will want to get as fully comfortable as possible, preferably on a bed, a mat, or in a reclining chair.
5. The best position is lying on your back with your legs extended. Do not cross your knees or ankles as this restricts your blood circulation. Let your arms rest loosely at your sides with your fingers gently extended.
6. If you feel cool ask the therapist to tuck a light blanket around you.
7. As you relax, you may notice brief tingling sensations and warmth in your arms and legs.
8. You will find this experience more helpful if you close your eyes but you may open them if you feel a need.
9. During the session feel free to get more comfortable, to scratch or swallow if you need to, and then resume following the therapist's instructions.
10. If any of the therapist's instructions feel uncomfortable to you, then you may want to ignore them. You will only be able to relax with directions in which you feel trust and confidence.
11. You may want the therapist to tape record this session so that you can use it when the therapist is not present.

Instructions for progressive relaxation are given in Tables A–2 and A–3.

Acupuncture. **Acupuncture** is a *treatment method based on the Chinese philosophy that all life is a microcosm of a vast, constantly changing flowing circle of energy,* without beginning or end, that flows through the karma (fate) of our lives. This circle is divided into a rising energy, *yang,* seen as positive and male, and a descending energy, *yin,* seen as negative and female. Yet yang and yin are symbolic rather than superior or inferior to each other. The body can reach a balanced state only if both forces are flowing smoothly. The energy of yin and yang together is called *qi* (chee), and in the body it is called *true qi.* Illness occurs when the flow of true qi around the 12 main channels or meridians of the body is impeded or blocked and the energy balance becomes disturbed. The 12 meridians are named after 12 organs as defined by Chinese acupuncturists: lung, large intestine, pericardium, bladder, small intestine, triple warmer, stomach, heart, gallbladder, spleen, kidney, and liver (1, 5).

Acupressure. **Acupressure** is the *predecessor of acupuncture.* The term is applied to a *number of techniques of applying pressure to stimulate acupuncture points on the body.* Acupressure releases tension and relieves pain. It is a preventive treatment used to balance energy by applying pressures to specific points (1, 5, 10).

Shiatsu. **Shiatsu** is an *ancient, simple treatment method whereby a form of manipulation is administered by the thumbs, fingers, and palms, without any use of instruments,* mechanical or otherwise, to apply pressure to the human skin, correct internal malfunctioning, promote and maintain health, and treat specific disease. Shiatsu is a fusion of the ancient Japanese manipulation therapy, *anma,* and the Chinese concept of acupuncture; however, no needles are used, only pressure. The philosophy is similar to that of Chinese acupuncture. Illness occurs as a result of excess or deficiency of yin and yang energy or a block of true qi. Gentle pressure along the meridian lines restores the balance (1).

Tai Chi. **Tai Chi Chuan** is a *routine of synchronized, yoga-like, nonstrenuous movements and postures that are slowly done, involving the whole body.* Concepts of yin

TABLE A–3. PROGRESSIVE RELAXATION

Give the instructions in a calm, slow, even voice. Pause for 5 to 20 seconds wherever you see the pause dots (. . .) to allow the client to follow directions and experience the sensations. Inhalation should occur with tensing and exhalation should occur with relaxing of muscles.

1. Close your eyes. Take a moment to examine any sensations you are experiencing. (. . .) Let your thoughts and body movements follow my suggestions so that you can fully experience the contrast between tense and relaxed muscles.

2. Tense the muscles in your feet and legs by pulling your toes back toward your head. Hold. (. . .) Feel the spots where tension is present. Notice where any uncomfortable tenseness is present. (. . .) Now, relax. (. . .) Let your feet relax completely. Do you experience any unusual sensations in the muscles that you just tensed? Do they feel warm or tingly? Do you find that you do not want to move your toes from this relaxed position? These are signs of relaxation. They are pleasant feelings that will increase as your muscles become more and more relaxed.

3. Tense the thigh muscles as tightly together as you can. Hold. (. . .) Notice the rigidity and hardness of tight muscles. (. . .) Relax. Let the tension of your thighs drain away down into the chair or bed. (. . .) Let looseness replace tightness. Notice the comfort of relaxed muscles. Check if your lower legs and feet are still relaxed.

4. Keep your legs and feet totally relaxed. Tense your abdomen and stomach. Pull the muscles in your abdomen taut. As you do this you will feel yourself pushing down into the bed or chair. Push hard and hold this pressure. (. . .) Notice the difference between the tightness of your abdomen and the relaxation of your legs and feet. Now relax. Let wave after wave of gentle relaxation sweep over your abdomen. Let your abdomen become relaxed and soft.

5. Straighten your back. Pull yourself up tightly. Feel the tightness in your back. Hold that tense, uncomfortable position while remembering to keep your legs and feet relaxed. (. . .) Then let your back collapse comfortably while all of the tension flows away. Let the bed or chair support you totally.

6. Keep your legs, feet, abdomen, and back relaxed. Squeeze your hands into tight, tight fists. Tense your forearms and upper arms as well. (. . .) Now let go. Open your hands and let your fingers dangle. Let all of the stress pour out of your fingertips and allow a warm, gentle, massaging relaxation to sweep over your arms and hands. Allow tension everywhere to simply disappear.

7. Lift your shoulders, as if you are trying to touch your ears with your shoulders. Pull tight. Notice the tension across your shoulder blades. Feel the tightness of the muscles on top of your shoulders and in your neck. (. . .) Drop your shoulders and let them relax. Let them slide back down, relieving all the stress in the neck and shoulders. Let your shoulder blades snuggle back into the bed or chair comfortably.

8. Keep relaxing your arms, your body, and your legs. Let everything become loose and limp. While you are relaxing, tense up your facial muscles. Scrunch up your face. Wrinkle and tighten your forehead. Wrinkle your eyes and nose. Clamp your jaw shut. Notice the tension beside your ears from clenching your jaws. Hold all this tension. (. . .) Now let go. Let your jaw drop slack. Let your forehead slide into comfort. Let your eyelids gently smooth out. Concentrate on whether your whole face is smooth and wrinkle free. Move your jaw slightly from side to side to clear any residual tension and then let it hang loosely. Let your tongue lie passively in your mouth. It feels so good to relax the entire body.

9. You have experienced tension and relaxation in the major muscles of your body. Now while you are very relaxed, check your body to see if any tension or stress remains. Wriggle your toes gently, then let them relax. Take a deep breath. As I name each body area check for any residual tension or discomfort. Allow for total relaxation. You might imagine someone gently massaging every inch of your body. (. . .) Become aware of the relaxed sensations in your legs. (. . .) your abdomen. (. . .) your back. (. . .) your arms. (. . .) your hands and fingers. (. . .) your neck. (. . .) shoulders. (. . .) jaw. (. . .) eyes. (. . .) forehead. (. . .) If you find some tension in any area, gently tighten that area and then let it relax completely. Continue to monitor your body for any place where tension is trying to remain. (Pause for 30 seconds.)

10. By repeating this exercise each day, or on any occasion when you are very tense, you will improve your health for both your mind and your body. Just now you may feel a bit tired from all the tensing. For the next few minutes just remain quiet, savoring the relaxed sensations. (Pause for 2 to 4 minutes.) Now gently open your eyes and softly stretch as you would when awakening. Be slow in coming to a full sitting position. Maintain your relaxed state as you return to regular awareness of today and any events yet to come. Whenever you become aware of tension, consciously tighten those muscles for a few seconds and then allow total relaxation.

---

and yang are incorporated. **Chi** (*energy*) is to flow unchecked. Movements and postures are performed in a sequence without stopping so that each melts smoothly into the next. The body receives a sensation like pushing the hand against onrushing air outside a moving car window or swimming on dry land. A Tai Chi workout leads to relaxed muscles, improved balance and coordination, lower blood pressure, and fewer aches or less intense pain (1).

Biofeedback. **Biofeedback** is a *means of receiving feedback or a message from the body about internal physio-* *logic processes, using specific techniques or equipment.* It involves use of instruments to develop the ability to read tension in various body systems and to learn ways of releasing the tension when cues of stress response are identified.

Biofeedback permits a person to become familiar with internal functions such as moving index of body temperature or a reading of brain waves. As with externally directed behavior, the person is able with practice to learn how to control internal behavior (10). Most people have experienced the physician's interpreting for them, in an illness–wellness context, the results of physiologic tests. If the person is able to read the same information as it is occurring within him or her, he or she is using biofeedback.

Biofeedback has two aspects: (1) the actual use of biomedical devices capable of taking a reading of one's physiologic activity such as temperature or heart rate, and (2) the training in which one learns what to do with the devices. The client is linked to the instruments, which are modified to display the body information as visual or auditory signals, by delicate wires or tubes connected to special sensing materials taped to the skin. The body information is carried back to the devices, which continually read the signals, reflecting the constantly changing activity within. As the person continues to work with biofeedback instrumentation, an association develops between changes in body signals and various subjective feelings that are either consciously or subconsciously recognized. The monitor gives information about the degree of success. Dependence on the instrumentation is temporary. Eventually the person should be able to monitor the fluctuations and thereby exercise some conscious control over physiologic adaptation. Once learned, control over a physiologic function is retained in the person's memory for a long time (1, 10). Biofeedback has been used successfully to treat tension headaches, migraine headaches, hypertension, insomnia, peptic ulcers, colitis, muscle spasms or pain, epilepsy, asthma, anxiety states, panic disorders, phobic reactions, stuttering, and teeth grinding.

A directory of certified feedback practitioners is available from the Association for Applied Psychophysiology and Biofeedback, 10200 44th Ave, Suite 304, Wheat Ridge, CO 80033.

Massage. The effects of massage are psychological, mechanical, physiologic, and reflexive. **Massage** is an art (a unique way of communicating without words and showing caring) and a science; a *systematic manipulation of the body tissue* produces beneficial effects on the nervous and muscular systems, local and general circulation, skin, viscera, and metabolism (1, 10).

During massage the hands stimulate the sensory receptors of the skin and subcutaneous tissues, causing a series of reflex effects, including capillary vasodilation or constriction, relaxation or stimulation of voluntary muscle contraction, and possible sedation or stimulation of pain in an area remote from the area being touched, depending on the type of massage or stroking movements (1, 10).

Yoga. The word **yoga** means *to unite, implying the balance or harmony that can exist within the individual.*

Yoga is an Indian philosophic system that emphasizes the practice of special techniques to attain the highest degree of physical, emotional, and spiritual integration. *Hatha-yoga* is the branch that emphasizes physical postures and breathing practices to attain body–mind balance.

Studies of the effects of hatha-yoga have shown it especially beneficial to optimum functioning of the endocrine, circulatory, musculoskeletal, respiratory, and nervous systems. Yoga reduces blood pressure, lowers pulse rate, reduces serum cholesterol, regulates menstrual flow and thyroid function, increases range of motion in joints, reduces join pain, and increases feeling of well-being (1, 10).

Autogenics. **Autogenics** is a *form of self-hypnosis that allows the person to induce the feeling of warmth and heaviness associated with a trance state.* The method was developed by Johannes H. Schultz, a Berlin psychiatrist. Autosuggestion with some yoga techniques was developed into a system of autogenic training. The system is effective in treatment of disorders of the respiratory and gastrointestinal tracts and of the circulatory and endocrine systems and for anxiety and fatigue. The exercises can be used to increase resistance to stressors, reduce or eliminate sleep disorders, and modify pain reactions. Autogenic therapy is not recommended for children less than 5 years old or for adults who lack motivation or have severe emotional disorders. Those with diabetes, hypoglycemic conditions, or heart conditions should discuss the use of the method with their physicians. Occasionally, a client experiences a sharp rise or drop in blood pressure when doing the exercises; blood pressure should be taken to ensure the exercises are useful. The exercise can be completed in a comfortable sitting or lying position in which the person assumes an attitude of passive concentration. It may take up to 10 months to master the six exercises. Ninety-second sessions five to eight times a day are recommended for mastery. Clark (10) describes in detail the technique to follow. See also Table A–4 (33).

Krieger's Theory of Therapeutic Touch

Dolores Krieger (27) draws on Eastern beliefs and literature in her theory of therapeutic touch. She theorizes that *prana* (Sanskrit term for energy) is transferred in the healing act; the source of prana in Eastern thinking is the sun. Eastern thinking contends that well people have an excess of prana; Western physiology texts state there is a great deal of energy in the human body. Krieger pictures the healer as a person with excess

TABLE A–4. AUTOGENIC THERAPY

Guidelines

1. Sit or lie in a relaxed state with eyes closed.
2. Have an attitude of passive concentration.
3. Imagine mental contact with the part of the body on which you are concentrating.
4. Keep repeating the instructions to yourself, either in words or in mental pictures.
5. Have a casual attitude toward achieving results.

Exercises

There are six standard, 60-second autogenic exercises.

1. Concentrate on a feeling of heaviness in your arms and legs. Start with the dominant hand. Simultaneously imagine a peaceful scene or verbally repeat to yourself, "I am at peace." *Produces relaxation.*
2. Concentrate on feelings of warmth in feet, legs, arms, and hands. *Relaxes blood vessels and increases peripheral blood flow.*
3. Become aware of your heartbeat. Repeat, "Heartbeat calm and regular." *Strengthens self-regulation of heart.*
4. Focus on calm and regular breathing.
5. Focus on warming your solar plexus. (The solar plexus is deep in your abdomen, below your waist and above the navel.) You should not do this activity if you are having any kind of problem that would be affected by increased abdominal blood flow. *Calms the nervous system, improves muscle relaxation, and improves sleep.*
6. Focus on cooling your forehead.

These exercises can be used as introductions to other meditations or visualizations.

---

prana or energy who has a strong sense of commitment and intention to help people. Healing entails channeling of this energy flow by the healer for the well-being of the sick individual. Healers do not become depleted of energy, however, because they are in a constant state of energy input. Healers become depleted of energy only if they draw on their own energy rather than being a channel of energy. Healers are thought to accelerate the healing process by giving the client an extra boost to his or her recuperative system.

Krieger presents physiologic data to support her theory. There is evidence that therapeutic touch raises hemoglobin levels and influences electroencephalogram (EEG) patterns. The healer's EEG changes to a high-amplitude beta state, indicative of deep concentration similar to meditation, and the person's brain waves are typically low-amplitude alpha waves, correlated with a state of calmness and well-being. The person experiences slower, deeper respirations and a sense of warmth and relaxation (27).

According to Krieger (27), therapeutic touch works well with all stress-related diseases, having a sig-

nificant effect on the autonomic nervous system and reducing nausea, dyspnea, tachycardia, pallor, and peristalsis. Use of therapeutic touch has also been successful with children and with the terminally ill.

The healer centers and uses the hands (placed 2 to 3 in. from the person's skin) to move quickly over the body, reading signals of illness or blockage of energy flow. The feeling of pressure sensed in the hands when congestion or blockage is present is explained biophysically; as the healer moves the hands over the body, positive ions are sensed. Positive ions are associated with feelings of lethargy, headache, irritability, and inflammation of the mucosal tissues. Negative ions are noted when the person has a feeling of well-being (27, 40).

Krieger (27) refers to the pressure as a "ruffling in the field"; the healer can move the positive ions by shaking or wiping the hands. When the healer's hands are placed in the area of a "ruffle" and the hands are moved away from the body in a sweeping gesture, the pressure is reduced, and the feeling of energy flow is sensed; this is called "unruffling the field." The unruffling motion can be used to soothe babies or reduce pain and tension. A 2- to 3-minute treatment is sufficient for children or the debilitated. With others the healer stops when the body feels balanced (21, 27, 40).

The object of therapeutic touch is to balance the healer's "field" so that symmetry of energy flow is restored. With practice the hands begin to move toward areas of unbalanced energy flow as they become more sensitive to changes in the field of another person's body. Therapeutic touch can raise hemoglobin levels, reduce anxiety, relieve headache, and promote other physical well-being and healing by redirecting energy fields and enabling the sick person to mobilize personal healing powers (21, 27, 40).

The spiritual implications of therapeutic touch are discussed by two nurses, Wuthnow (47) and Miller (32). Wuthnow believes that the technique can be used by nurses of all faiths who are trained in the technique and that it can be used with or without Christian beliefs. Miller believes that Christian nurses cannot use the technique because it represents a wrong relationship with the Holy Spirit and assumes a manipulating role of God. (This same argument is used by some Christian nurses against use of guided imagery, visualization, and other cognitive techniques for healing.) Some nurses combine emotional and Christian spiritual components when using touch to heal.

Clark (10) describes in detail various touch and healing interventions that can be used by the nurse, including (1) behavioral kinesiology interventions, (2) therapeutic touch interventions, (3) yoga interventions, (4) massage interventions, (5) acupressure interventions, and (6) reflexology interventions.

COGNITIVE METHODS OF COPING, RELAXATION, AND STRESS MANAGEMENT

Both you and your clients need to take time for play, leisure, or diversional activities and spiritual pursuits that (1) are rewarding emotionally, (2) are done voluntarily rather than out of obligation, (3) are outside of ordinary life routines, (4) absorb attention, (5) are not necessarily productive in earnings, and (6) have definite time and space boundaries. Laughter, pleasant thoughts, and relaxing activities stimulate production of endorphins and enkephalins, chemical pain relievers. Adrenaline and other hormones are also produced, stimulating body function. The body's production of immune cells increases. Arteries and muscles relax, reducing blood pressure.

Transcendental meditation, from which other meditation methods derive, *combines physical and cognitive methods and involves self-mastery of mental functioning.* Meditation is practiced for 15 to 20 minutes twice daily, preferably in the early morning and in the evening before meals. The technique can be practiced by anyone from any culture, religion, or belief. Meditation causes decreased oxygen consumption and increased skin resistance and alpha brain waves, indicating a state of deep relaxation and rest, different from sleep in that the person remains aware of surroundings. When the body is at optimum rest, the muscles are relaxed and the mind becomes more clear, alert, creative, stable, and less tense and depressed. Decreased anxiety, greater resistance to stress and pain, increased inner control, better job performance and interpersonal relationships, and a sense of joy about life can result. Physical health improves. Psychophysiologic illnesses, such as peptic ulcer and hypertension, are reduced. The resulting relaxation may help the person to reduce gradually his or her need for alcohol, drugs, and cigarettes. Research studies indicate a faster reaction time, more energy, and higher scores on self-actualization in persons who meditate (20). The method described in Table A–5 is only one of several effective techniques on meditation (33).

Thought Stopping

Thought stopping is a *behavioral modification technique useful when nagging, repetitive thoughts interfere with behavior and wellness. Unwanted thoughts are interrupted with the command "stop."* An image of the letters of the word *stop,* a loud noise (e.g., a buzzer or bell), or a negative stimulus such as wearing a rubber band around the wrist and snapping it when the unwanted

TABLE A–5. A MEDITATION TECHNIQUE

1. Find a quiet place. Avoid interruptions.
2. Sit in a comfortable position in a chair or on the floor. Maintain good posture with your back straight.
3. Select a sound or word to use as a mental device (*mantra*) (God, One, Allah, Buddha).
4. Gently close your eyes and notice how extraneous thoughts leave the mind. Passively disregard distracting thoughts in favor of the mantra. Continue to disregard any distracting thoughts; now is not the time to deal with them.
5. After about 15 or 20 minutes have passed, allow the mantra to fade away. As the mind increases its activity and thoughts come freely, sit quietly for a few minutes before slowly opening your eyes.
6. Remain seated and observe the changes that have taken place, including the following:
   a. Changes in breath rate or heart rate
   b. Shift in the quality of mental functioning, perhaps more perceptive and relaxed
   c. Loss of sense of time
   d. Release of physical tensions
   e. Shift in sense of body boundaries

thought occurs is used with the command. Then a thought that is positive, healthful, or desirable is substituted. Thought stopping may work because (1) distraction occurs, (2) the interruption behaviors serve as a punishment, (3) an assertive response can be followed by reassuring of self-accepting comments, and (4) a chain of negative and frightening thoughts leading to negative and frightening feelings is interrupted, thus reducing the stress level. Regular practice for 3 to 7 days is necessary for the person to learn to interrupt quickly a negative thought with a positive, constructive alternative thought (7, 10).

Refuting Irrational Ideas

People engage in almost continuous self-talk during waking hours. **Self-talk** is the *internal language used to describe and interpret the world.* When self-talk is accurate and realistic, wellness is enhanced; when it is irrational and untrue, stress and emotional disturbance occur.

Centering

Centering refers to *separating or differentiating from others so that there is an inner reference or thought of stability, calm, and self-awareness; a place of quietude* *within self where one can feel integrated, focused, and emotionally and spiritually calm.* As a result, you can communicate more openly and listen to self and others more effectively (27).

Centering reduces fatigue, stress, depression, or anger when working with a client. Centering takes little time once the idea is mastered and can be helpful to use before any anxiety-provoking situation in the hospital, at home, in social situations, or at work. Centering can also be taught to people to help them gain self-control. Centering can be achieved while standing or sitting, but beginning efforts produce the best results in a sitting position. The method is as follows (10):

1. Sit in a comfortable chair with feet flat on the floor and hands resting quietly in your lap; close your eyes.
2. Check out your body for tension spots and relax these areas as you exhale.
3. Inhale easily, filling your body with relaxation.
4. Exhale deeply.
5. Continue breathing in this matter until you feel calm, integrated, and focused.
6. (Optional) Picture the body surrounded by a protective shield that allows positive energy in but keeps negative energy out. The shield may be conceived as a color, light source, or spiritual sense.

Assertive Communication or Behavior

Assertiveness is the *ability to express personal thoughts, feelings, and desires, defining and making known personal rights that are reasonable, while being respectful to the other person and of his or her rights.* Expressing honest feelings, being willing to act on rational thoughts and controlled feelings to achieve a goal, and taking responsibility for consequences are part of assertive communication and behavior. Using "I . . . " statements to express feelings and ideas rather than "You make me feel . . . " or "You should . . . " statements will increase self-confidence, enhance relationships with others, reduce anxiety and stress, and control fear and anger (7, 10).

Assertive communication comes with practice with another, in a group, in front of a mirror, and/or using a tape recorder. Assertiveness includes paying attention to facial expression, voice tone, posture, use of gestures, congruity between words and appearance, and the way statements are phrased.

Various techniques are useful in assertive communication and behavior. You can use them in your personal and professional life and can teach them to clients. A summary of several techniques follows:

1. *Acknowledgment:* When you are criticized, you acknowledge the comment of the other, the feeling implied, and whatever part of the criticism is applicable to you. Avoid giving excuses or apologies.

   "Yes, I was late to work this morning. I punched in the time clock 10 minutes after 7:00, so I was 10 minutes late."

   "Yes, I overlooked carrying out the garbage last night, and I can appreciate your sense of frustration."

2. *Clouding:* When you are given a nonconstructive, manipulative criticism with which you disagree, you can stand your ground, implying that there could be other reasons for your action, while continuing to listen and communicate. You agree to the part of the criticism that is true without agreeing to any specific action plan.

   a. *Agreeing in part:*
Parent:	"You always have an excuse to get out of work around home."
Teen:	"I do have a lot of school and church group responsibilities."
Parent:	"You don't seem to care anything about your family."
Teen:	"You're right. I guess it does seem that way."

   b. *Agreeing in probability:*
Parent:	"You're putting on a lot of weight."
Teen:	"I may have gained a few extra pounds."
Parent:	"You'd better go on a diet."
Teen:	"Perhaps it is time for starting a diet."

   c. *Agreeing in principle:*
Parent:	"If you don't study more, you're not going to pass this semester."
Teen:	"You're right. If I don't study, I will fail."

3. *Probing:* This response can determine whether criticism is constructive or manipulative and clarifies unclear comments. First you isolate the part of the criticism that is most bothersome to the other and then ask what specifically is bothersome about the behavior.
   Assertive Probing:

Supervisor:	"Your work is not satisfactory."

Nurse:	"What about my work bothers you?"
Supervisor:	"Everyone else works overtime when necessary; you always leave on time."
Nurse:	"What is it about my leaving on time that bothers you?"
Supervisor:	"It's not right that you work only by the clock when the rest of us work overtime. None of us likes to work overtime, but the work has to be done."
Nurse:	"What bothers you about me working by the clock?"
Supervisor:	"When you leave, someone else has to finish your work. The rule here is that no one leaves until the shift's work is done.

4. *Broken record:* This technique can be used when another is not listening to you, when it is necessary to clarify limits about what should be done, or when explanation would provide the other with an opportunity to continue a pointless discussion.
   a. Give a short, specific statement about what is desired, without giving excuses.
   b. Use body language that shows you are calm and in control of your feelings: stand or sit erect, maintain eye contact, keep hands and arms quiet at the side.
   c. Calmly and firmly repeat the chosen statements as many times as necessary until the other person realizes negotiation is not possible. Ignore the other's excuses, ramblings, curses, or false accusations.

Situation: Driver A pulls out of a parking place, very fast, with a too sharp turn, managing to pull loose the back bumper of the car in the next parking place (Driver B), which is parked right on the line. Driver A pulls forward into the parking place, gets out of the car, and proceeds toward Driver B. Driver B stays in the car. Driver A stands by the car door, yelling how stupid Driver B is to park on the line.

| Driver B: | Rolling down the window slightly, "Yes, you are right; I am parked on the line." |
| Driver A: | Continues to accuse Driver B, yelling invectives. |

Driver B:	Maintains eye contact, every 1 minute rolls down the window slightly and says, "When you are ready, I'll talk about what can be done about the bumper." This is repeated for approximately 10 minutes.
Driver A:	Begins to calm down, finally smiles, and says, "OK, what do you want?".
Driver B:	"I want you to pay for repair of my ripped bumper."
Driver A:	"OK." Proceeds to give telephone number, with an adequate down payment (in cash) toward bumper repair, and promises to pay more if cost is greater. "I just don't want my insurance company to get hold of this. Call if it costs more."

5. *Content to process shift:* When focus of conversation drifts from the original topic, conversation can be purposefully shifted from the subject (content) being discussed to the feelings between the two speakers (process). The statement should be made with a calm voice and demeanor, defusing anger that has arisen. Attack is avoided.

   "We're off the subject; let's get back to what we agreed to discuss."
   "I'm feeling uncomfortable about the drift of our conversation, and I notice we both appear tense."
   "We seem to be getting into a battle. I sense we are both talking about the same thing but are coming from a different perspective."

6. *Momentary delay:* When a situation is compelling or another gives a command or implies an answer right away, it is important not to be swayed by the emotion of the moment. After a deep breath and a moment of delay, the comment could be:

   "I'll need more information before I can act."
   "There may be something to what you say, I need a few minutes to think about this."
   "I can understand your feeling. I need a minute to sort out what you are saying."

7. *Time-out:* If the conversation is important but has reached an impasse because of angry feelings or bias, conversation can be delayed and

continued later by setting a near-future time to continue talking when both parties are more calm.

"We've been talking about this for quite a while, and I don't think we're getting anywhere. I'd like to sleep on it and talk more with you about it tomorrow morning. Let's meet to talk at 8:30 AM.

(Designate a mutually neutral place if possible.)

8. *Joining and circling the attacker:* This technique is derived from the martial art of akido, in which the attacked person accepts and turns with the attack, then lets the attacker pass on. The focus of the intervention is to resolve conflict, restore harmony, and problem solve. There are four alternative responses:

   a. *Do nothing.* This is a conscious choice, not a response of fear, when (I) the attack makes no sense, (II) the attacked does not want to dignify the attack by reacting, and (III) more information is needed to determine the reason for the attack

   b. *Use humor or deflection.* Give an absurd reason or a surprise line as a reason for not accomplishing something that should have been done.

   c. *Joining the attacker.* The attack is not taken personally and the attacker agrees, then moves to resolve the problem.

   "I don't blame you for feeling the way you do."
   "My job is to work with you. If you think we can work together, I want to hear your complaints."

   d. *Parley.* This technique is useful if you have been engaged in a no-win situation; the other person has defined the encounter as a competition or contest.

Various mental strategies to handle stress are listed and described in Table A–6 (33).

Laughter, Humor, Play, Tears

Laughter, humor, play, and tears are natural ways of handling stress and releasing tension. The psychological effects of a deep laugh or of a playful attitude work against the stress response: muscles in the face, diaphragm, abdomen, and blood vessels relax; blood pressure decreases; respirations normalize; the brain releases endorphins; and the immune system is strengthened. Tears and nasal secretions, excreted during both laughing and crying, contain hormones, steroids, and toxins that accumulate in the body during stress when there are feelings of anger, fear, frustration, sadness, and tedium. When these substances are secreted, the negative effects of the General Adaptation Syndrome are counteracted.

Emotionally and cognitively, humor, comedy, cartoons, and playing games help us to develop another perspective, to see the absurdity of a situation, to clarify the situation and be better able to think clearly, to problem-solve, and to cope. Laughing at personal foibles and mistakes enables others to laugh with us, not at us. Inanimate objects such as computers can be safe targets for humor about peoples' behavior and life's ironies. The catharsis that comes with both laughter and tears brings not only emotional release, but a sharing of feelings and consequent support from others. Without crying, healing cannot occur. Without laughter, forgiveness, and thereby healing, is impossible (8, 9, 11, 12, 15, 28, 31, 34, 35, 39, 41, 44, 45).

Norman Cousins (11) conquered his own illness and pain through comedy, humor, and laughter. Sometimes people have to cry before they can laugh. There is no way to force either. In some cultures the value is to be stoic; the person may not cry in front of others, and a cheerful countenance is practiced. In other cultures if you do not cry with the person during troubled times, you are considered unfeeling, uncaring—not a friend.

Nurses can integrate laughter and tears appropriately into nursing care. To do so means that the nurse must integrate them into self. Hutchinson (24) found that humor was a self-care strategy that facilitated other strategies of assertion, catharsis, cultivating relationships by offering help to others, and withdrawal—becoming aloof and rising above the situation or resigning self to it. These are strategies nurses use to handle job stress; these strategies can also be taught to clients to handle their stress. Buxman (8, 9) presents details about how to use humor and laughter for client recovery, staff morale, and hospital regulation. She lists specific resources for a "humor room," including books, magazines, newsletters, audiocassettes, movies, and videocassettes. Further, she describes how to establish a humor room administratively so that clients, families, and staff can use the resources.

Clients, especially those suffering the greatest pain or fear, often express a joke, a sarcastic remark, a flippant line, a pun, cynicism, or dry humor. Acknowledge these statements. Be prepared both to laugh and to cry with the person as the need for both may be implied.

Guided Imagery

Guided imagery can be defined as *focused attention on an inner, mental picture or a statement of belief of what the individual wants to accomplish by being open to and*

TABLE A–6   VARIOUS THOUGHT STRATEGIES TO HANDLE STRESS AND THEIR RATIONALE

Mental Response	Definition and Rationale
Use of knowledge	Learn causes of stress and ways to prevent/manage situation. Know personal limits. If problem is beyond your control and cannot be changed now, accept the situation until it can be changed.
Objectivity (reality orientation)	Sort out, compare, and validate events, ideas, and emotions to gain a total perspective and better understanding on basis of facts, not just feelings; maintain realistic perception.
Analysis	Study logically and systematically the component parts of a situation to arrive at realistic explanations and answers; manage part if not all of situation.
Concentration (mental self-control)	Set aside deliberately thoughts and feelings unrelated to the situation to master tension, save energy, find answers, and make necessary decisions for the task at hand.
Planning	Think through situation before acting to release tension, promote problem solving, and avoid unnecessary use of energy, error, and consequent frustration. Avoid too many deadlines. Decide on what drudgery chore you want to complete and do it as quickly as possible so it does not become a focus. Make a list of tasks and check off as they are accomplished.
Reconstruction	Review recent stressful event, writing ways it could have been better and ways it could have been worse. Write what could have been done to make it better, thus improving sense of challenge and control.
Fantasize (daydream)	Visualize release of tension and successful achievement rather than dwelling on fear of failure to plan strategy, ensure goal-directed action, cope with stressors, and relieve tension.
Rehearsal	Fantasize or anticipate event or another's response before stressful event to practice coping mentally or behaviorally and to gain confidence in ability to manage.
Substitution of thoughts and emotions	State ideas and feelings that are different than real ones to avoid adding to stressful situation or to meet demands of the situation. Focus on one good thing that happened during the day.
Suppression	Hold thoughts and emotions in abeyance or momentarily forget to wait until it is more timely to change behavior, attack a problem, or implement a solution. Deliberately push all stress-producing thoughts aside for 60 seconds.
Valuing	Establish or reaffirm religious or sociocultural values to foster sense of balance and relaxation in face of stressors. Value and believe in yourself. Take an hour each day for yourself.
Empathy	Imagine how others in the situation are feeling so that behavior can take these feelings into account.
Humor	Point out inconsistencies in situation, laugh at self, and use past feelings, ideas, and behavior to be playful, keep objective distance from a problem, reduce anxiety, maintain self-identity, enrich solution, and add enjoyment to life.
Tolerance of ambiguity	Function in a way that lays the basis for eventual effective solutions when the situation is so complex that it cannot be fully understood or clear choices cannot be made now.

responding to the language of the unconscious or the deeper body levels. Other terms are used for imagery: imagination, visualization, autosuggestion, mental programming, and self-hypnosis. The term *imagination* or *visualization* is not totally descriptive of guided imagery. The term *self-hypnosis* is frightening to some. Thus the term that is used in the literature and is effective with clients is *guided imagery, imagery,* or *use of imaging.*

Imagery is not new. Some people say, without diminishing God the creator, that the first record of what could be considered a mental image producing results is written in Genesis with the creation. God said, "Light, be," and there was light. There are a number of accounts in the Old and New Testaments of the *Bible* of how people accomplished what was mentally visualized. For example, records of the fall of the walls of Jericho and the miracles of Jesus convey the power of the mental image. Whenever faith is involved, for example, in the healings of today, the person visualizes what is to be before it comes.

Guided imagery is not the same as a trance, play acting, use of fantasy or denial, raising of false hope, or claiming to work miracles. Rather, it is the purposeful use of a technique that requires time and effort to accomplish a purpose.

Physiologic Mechanisms Involved in Imagery

Much is still unknown about the private physiologic mechanisms that occur during private processes that allow for the manifestation of various results.

Imagery is a covert process whose characteristics, while observed, must be inferred. Imaging activity apparently is a complex blend of receptive-perceptual processes and efferent activity. Imagery can be conditioned in certain circumstances; it can show properties of skill learning; it is responsive to motivation; and it has properties of passive receptivity similar to those of reverie, dreams, and hypnosis (17, 42, 43, 46).

Muscle activity changes occur in response to the content of the image. For example, images of lifting an object were associated with increased activity in the arm muscles that would be involved in the actual movement, although the magnitude of the muscular changes is less during imagery than it would be during the overt movement (42, 43, 46). Imagery can reduce muscular tension as measured by electromyographic recording from the frontalis muscles on the forehead.

Images of moving objects are associated with greater oculomotor activity than images of stationary objects. Skin conduction responses during vividly imagined stressful scenes are more frequent, of greater magnitude, and slower to habituate than are skin conduction responses of nonvivid imagers. Different levels of activity of facial muscles have been measured during imagery of different emotional states, representational of changes that actually occur with different emotional states in real life (17, 42, 43, 46).

Studies using physiologic measures of imagery have employed a wide range of measures. They are heart rate, respiration, EEG, alpha activity, skin temperature, electromyographic activity in a number of different muscle groups, diastolic and systolic blood pressure, salivation, eye movements and pupillary responses, vasomotor responses, and measure of electrodermal activity such as the galvanic skin response, skin conductance, and skin resistance. Furthermore, significant effects have been reported, at least sometimes, for each measure that has been used. In general, it appears that heart rate is the most sensitive measure in that changes in heart rate associated with imagery have been the most consistently reported. Studies also show an increase in thymosin and white blood count with imagery (17, 43, 46).

Images, especially those without external representation, are apparently processed by the right hemisphere, which has a passive-receptive quality to the type of function it sustains. Right brain hemisphere function is concerned with intuition, visual and spatial events, imagination, and emotion. Receptive, representational, and spatial imagery is linked to right hemisphere functioning. The right hemisphere mediates analogic thinking and perceives the whole experience or "gestalt." In contrast, the left brain is logical and reasoning; it breaks down experience into sequential units, compartmentalizes and interprets information, and deals with verbal images. The right brain is stimulated by and receptive to imagery and, in turn, promotes release of chemicals and enzymes in the body that result in relaxation, healing, and well-being. Positive feelings release endorphins, which promote well-being and healing. Brain wave changes occur when the person is in a relaxed state (14, 17, 42, 43, 46). When these physiologic changes are facilitated regularly and over time, changes occur in body tissues, individual feelings and reactions, cognition, and life patterns.

Symbols useful in guiding imagery experiences are listed in Table A–7.

Technique of Guided Imagery

First, a rapport and a climate of trust must be established between the client and you, the nurse or therapist. After initial assessment and exploration of the problem and often after trying other techniques, guided imagery is proposed to the client as another way to promote healing or change. An explanation is given of what is involved: (1) sitting in a quiet, comfortable environment without distractions; (2) beginning with a technique to obtain total body relaxation; (3) envisioning a peaceful, soothing scene that can maintain relaxation and a positive attitude; (4) focusing attention on what is desired or to be accomplished; (5) telling the therapist what thoughts or feelings come to mind, answering questions, describing the healing; and (6) repeating the process regularly three or four times a day for 15 to 20 minutes. In that way the body learns to respond to the mind.

The nature of the instructions presented to the client appears to have an important impact on the response. Instructions must be clear, suggestive, and encouraging. Instructions that emphasize involvement of the person in the experience and the goals to be attained facilitate the process. Imagery works best when the person is motivated to try the technique, when there is confidence in the nurse or therapist, and when there is expectation of success. Some people need more time to relax and engage in the imagery process. The person should feel it is acceptable if he or she is unable initially to use imagery; however, if you suggest success, the person likely will be able to image. Use fun imagery exercises initially to help the person realize that he or she can engage in imagery. Then if the person believes that he or she wants to try imagery further as a method, continue with more introduction to and use of the technique.

As the person purposefully sets aside negative or sick images and images the positive, healthy, desired results while in a relaxed state, he or she is told that changes within the body and mind have been activated, which will be seen externally. The immune system, as

TABLE A–7 SYMBOLS USEFUL IN GUIDING IMAGERY EXPERIENCES

Ascending	Overcoming or transcending, climbing. Can use symbols such as a ladder, staircase, and mountain in which you have the client note any obstacles that appear. (Be sensitive to phobias of the person.)
Air	Creativity, breath, freedom, movement, freshness.
Birds	Freedom from the earthbound. Transcendence. Many birds will have specific symbolic associations such as the eagle, hawk, raven, vulture, dove, owl, and goose.
Cave	Hidden. A creature or figure that emerges from a cave can represent undeveloped qualities in the personality. If the emergent creature is frightening support the client in confronting, changing, or banishing the creature.
Chapel/Church	Place for facing basic questions of existence. Use any spiritual structure appropriate for the client.
Circle	Unity, eternity, oneness, completeness.
Cross	Tree of life, struggle, martyrdom, spiritual growth, salvation.
Dark	Undeveloped or uncreated, chaos, not visible, past wrongs, sin.
Descending	Moving toward the unconscious or potentialities of being, animal nature, instincts. Can have client descend in an elevator, down a deep well. (Be sensitive to phobias of the person.)
Egg	Self-contained completeness. Origin of life.
Eye	Understanding, intelligence, the inner self, soul.
House	Self, personality.
Lake	Mystery, depth, unconscious.
Light	Spirit, clarification, illumination, healing.
Magic potions	Use to relieve pain or reveal hidden answers.
Meadow	Serenity, space, freshness, childhood, happiness.
Moon	Femininity, influencer of vegetation and fruitfulness.
Monsters	Fears, power, death. Many creatures, such as the serpent, can have either positive or negative meanings, depending on cultural associations and the context in which the image occurs. Others, such as the lamb, are almost universally archetypal and will represent such qualities as gentleness, trust, purity, humility, simplicity, sacrifice, and atonement or forgiveness.
Rectangle	Rationality, security.
Space	Nothingness, void, empty, or heaven, spiritual force, hereafter.
Spiral	Evolution, growth, emotional development.
Square	Firmness, stability, solidity, earth.
Sun	Masculinity, life force, knowledge, fire, warmth, happiness.
Swamp	Repressed area, fears, chaos, prior harm done to person, sin.
Tree	Rooted in earth but reaching into heaven, tree of life or cosmic tree. A forest can represent ignorance, the dark side of nature, feeling lost.
Triangle	Communication, fire, trinity, movement upward.
Volcano	An erupting volcano can represent inner tension, panic, severe physical symptoms.
Water	The intuitive feminine aspect of the creative unconscious. A stream can represent psychic energy. A bubbling fountain is symbolic of the energy source of life (the soul).

A number of symbolic figures can be used as a way to see our own reflections. These include wise man, savior, angelic or guardian beings, image from a recent dream, an inner guide, a specific mythical god or goddess, a legendary hero or heroine, and a wise old woman. You can use child images in search of the inner child. You can have the client "hear" the name of a person, visualize that person, and describe that person as an Ideal personality. You can guide the client on a vision quest in which he or she leaves the world he or she is in; goes to a depth, a distance, or a height; and discovers what was missing in his or her consciousness.

well as other body systems, responds to mental visualizations.

It may take one time or many times for the person to gain an image of the desired goal. Have the person talk about the problem as imaged (e.g., physical, emotional, interpersonal, job) and the feelings and thoughts that come spontaneously and then allow the mind (the deep unconscious) to tell him or her what it would take to correct, heal, or overcome the problem and, thus, to reach the goal. It may take a number of sessions to get to this point. You may suggest a way for the person to image relief from a symptom or situation.

Before the initial session is ended, emphasize that this technique is totally under the control of the person and therefore can be used in the home or office at will. *Encourage regular daily use of imaging, following the same routine each time for the most effective outcome. The imaging can be combined with prayer, devotional reading, or meditation.* This method frees the person to make choices, to accomplish goals, to have a sense of mastery. The person is not under the control of the therapist. One full explanation and run-through of the method with the client may be enough to have the person successfully continue on his or her own, or it may take several times. Thus the method may be useful if you have only one contact with the person; or this method may be repeated in following sessions with the person, especially if there is a deep-seated or long-term problem.

In guided imagery use of the *inner advisor* after relaxation and a comfortable mental peace have been achieved can be helpful. It is a way of gaining access to the feelings, anxiety, guilt, and intuitions in the right hemisphere of the brain or the unconscious. The inner advisor is an imaginary creature drawn from the person's subconscious mind that can be questioned about physical and emotional feelings and through which dialogue can be continued that can resolve conflicts and aid decision making. The inner advisor may be expressed as the Holy Spirit or a religious figure; it may be a parent or spouse (living or dead); or it may be a friend, relative, or work colleague. Some people have a pet or favorite animal such as a squirrel, dog, cat, or pony (21).

Guided imagery can be used alone or with other therapies, whether these therapies involve use of medication, surgery, biofeedback, or individual counseling. Tapes, records, cassettes, disks, posters, and board games that can be used to create a background or an environment for relaxation, meditation, imagery, or just a peaceful mood can be obtained from Music Design, 207 E. Buffalo Street, Milwaukee, WI 53202. The catalog is available on request and features many artists and a variety of selections in type of music and instrumentation. Other such catalogs are also available.

Clinical Application of Imagery

If the person believes and participates regularly in the process of guided imagery, there would be a point at which there may be no need for other relaxation therapies.

Guided imagery can be used to promote emotional health by (1) building self-awareness; (2) helping the person to face issues and facilitating mood change; (3) clarifying the meaning of the situation; (4) assisting in dyadic communications and expression of feelings; (5) promoting a sense of strength and self-control, including overcoming phobias; (6) overcoming negative attitudes about self; and (7) increasing coping resources by releasing unconscious energies (30, 36).

TABLE A–8. MUSIC SELECTION FOR RELAXATION AND OTHER IMAGERY

Relaxation Imagery

1. Choose music with steady slow rhythm.
2. Choose a melody that is long, flowing, comforting, serene and without an easily identifiable tune or strong musical accents.
3. Match your imagery suggestions to variations in the music composition. You may want to match your opening music with the presenting mood or feeling of the client and then, during the imagery session, change the music to assist the client in changing mood. (The client should be informed about this before beginning. Do not use music unethically to manipulate client emotions.)
4. Music of the baroque, classic, romantic, impressionistic, or modern composers may be indicated because of its dynamic and mood qualities.
5. Avoid music with words or instrumental versions of songs with known lyrics as these may overengage the left brain.
6. The human voice doing chants or vocalizing in chorales or lullaby style may work best for some clients as it may encourage feelings of closeness and humanness.
7. Rising or descending melodic lines may suggest comparable imagery.
8. Some music therapists suggest using primarily stringed instruments such as harp, piano, guitar, cello, and violin.

Research increasingly shows that the body responds to our mental picture of it. The body may develop a full-blown infection, remain ill or less functional, or return to a healthy or normally functioning state, depending on the mental image we hold and what we continue to say about the body to self or others. Imagery can be used to enhance healing either by using a general image or by picturing what the impaired or diseased area would look like if it were normal. Table A–7 describes universal and specific images that can be used for various conditions after the person becomes relaxed. Table A–8 describes how music can be used with imagery (33). These are only suggestions. Each person can produce the image that is uniquely applicable and possible to achieve. Both universal and specific images can be held by the person in relation to a body part. And music must be carefully selected; the person may wish to choose the music to accompany the imagery session or may choose not to use music. Guided imagery can be used to *promote physical health* by (30, 36, 42, 43, 45, 46):

- Reducing the intensity of the stress response
- Assisting in control of various body symptoms
- Reducing and controlling pain symptoms
- Promoting weight loss in the obese person
- Helping the person to control or stop habits of smoking, alcohol or drug abuse

- Promoting healing after surgery or from cancer or various chronic conditions
- Increasing mobility and reducing tension, such as in arthritic conditions.

Guided imagery can be used to help the person overcome illness, achieve healing, and gain cognitive control—to make choices, to make decisions, to change life pattern and behavior, to respond to a situation by imaging and portraying a role, to reduce anxiety and fear, and to reduce depression. Tables A–9 and A–10 summarize use of imagery for these purposes. Allow sufficient time, free of distractions, to carry out the process (30, 36, 43, 45, 46).

When you have experienced guided imagery and used it with yourself and others under the supervision

TABLE A–9. USE OF IMAGERY TO PROMOTE HEATH AND HEALING

Symptom/Disorder	Universal Image	Specific Image
Sore throat	Image of cool air or moisture flowing over throat	Image of normally pink throat color; that normal color overtaking red, inflamed area
Fever	Image of coolness	Image of cool breeze, waterfall, fountain around self, with overall environment a comfortable temperature; image of self standing erect and feeling strong, invigorated, comfortable
Upper chest congestion, asthmatic attack	Image of cool throat and warm chest	Image of cool; normally pink throat and respiratory tree; lung sacs and bronchi expanding; airflow (seen as arrows, bubbles, streams of clouds) moving in and out (Hold image while breathing in relaxed manner.)
Chronic sinus problem	Image of tubes opening and draining	Image of sinus compartment as a sink, that you pulled the plug, and that draining is occurring: if persistent congestion, picture of self like a plunger at top of sinus compartment, pushing down the drainage through open drain pipe
Headache	Image of hole in head in area of headache; on exhalation, pain goes through hole as a color	Image of pain shooting out of head like a volcano with each exhalation and of a color that denotes calmness setting in and taking over the brain and head area
Itch or pain	Image of coolness to area	Image of ice cube on the area; as ice melts, itch or pain melts away; depending on location, may picture pain or itch as sliding off the body area
Low back pain	Image of heavy spine	Image of pain dropping down to the floor and walking away from it; image of self as erect, strong, active as pain is dropping away
Tight, tense muscle area	Image of muscles in area getting wider and longer, unknotting	Image that with deep, slow inhalation, breath is directed to the muscle area, breath soaks up the tension, and tension is removed with exhalation; picture of muscle stretching and smoothing out; picture of self in a calm, relaxing environment such as being surrounded by flower beds, the ocean, a lake, and meadow and that the body is stretched out; a relaxed, happy mood
Fatigue	Image of energy flow entering the body area	Image of self as light in weight; image of self surrounded by warmth, color, and music that represents happiness, energy, joy; picture of self as full of joy and dancing or skipping lightly in a meadow, lane, by the seashore
Stiff, painful joint; arthritis	Image of warmth	Image of self in warm sunlight at a relaxing place (seashore, field of grass or flowers) and moving freely; image of rising sun with warm rays aimed at joint or total body; picture of joint as normal in size; picture of self as light, moving at desired pace
Diarrhea, colitis	Image of coolness, control	Image of intestine as a tube that is set, firm, not moving and smooth, without bumps, rough areas, irritation; picture of self at activities and being in control; image of intestine as a pipe with plug firmly in place at lower end
Infection, cancer	Image of white cells carrying off abnormal cells	Image of white cells surrounding infectious area of cancer growth, eating up the abdominal area; image of area of infection or growth becoming smaller and smaller; image of antibiotic, chemotherapy, or radiation as an arrow piercing infectious or cancer area and causing abnormal cells to fall apart and be excreted by body; image of medication like Pacman, gobbling up the abnormal cells
Anger, resentment	Image of peace or harmony	Image of feeling as a ball of color; place it in front of you, kick it away; picture of self in control and solving the problem that is creating anger; picture of self in an area that was the happiest or most pleasant or most relaxing place you were ever in (vacation area, favorite childhood spot, most comfortable chair in your home, lovely garden area); soak up the calm and beauty and feel anger drain away; image of calming music—see yourself relaxed, light, dancing

TABLE A–10. USING IMAGERY TO SOLVE PROBLEMS

1. Find a quiet place and sit in a relaxed position; close the eyes.

2. Clearly and succinctly define the problem; picture telling the problem to a friend.

3. Mentally ask, "Am I ready to solve this problem?" If yes is the inner answer, proceed.

4. Place the clearly defined problem in a frame or a box.

5. Visualize the situation you desire and place it in a frame or box.

6. Visualize the steps that will be necessary to achieve the solution. Differentiate each step; continue to think until each step is clearly pictured.

7. Any barriers that come to mind in relation to any step of the solution can be looked at and then moved from the pathway to be cast off into space or to be placed in a locked box. Do this for each barrier that presents itself. Take a deep breath to relax as you do this so that you feel fully in control of handling barriers.

8. Mentally review each step that moves to a solution and picture yourself with the final desired solution. Hold the image.

9. Slowly open the eyes.

10. In the days or weeks that follow, repeat this process as necessary with your moving toward the goal or solution. See yourself with the solution or goal at hand in the frame or box. If certain intermediary steps have already been finished, omit them from the mental picture.

Note: Imagery can also be used quickly for an immediate situation with which you must cope or which must be mastered. The above method would be done in one sitting.

of someone who knows how to use the technique and when you believe in the results, you will see results.

You may wish to ask the client to verbalize the process by which healing was enhanced or may allow the person to complete the process without verbalizing unless he or she wishes to do so. The verbalization does not aid in the process for the client but can give clues about his or her ability to visualize and further issues with which you can be of assistance.

Plus Factor

Norman Vincent Peale (37) the first person to advocate the concept of positive thinking (which became the basis for the concept and practice of imagery), has formulated the concept of the "plus factor." According to Peale, the **plus factor** is a *power within the person that can transform and create a stronger, more confident, better balanced, more energetic and resilient, and more capable individual.* It is a special manifestation of the life force that animates everything in the universe. Attitudes and actions that are important to activate the plus factor and develop its power are faith, positive thinking, persistence, confidence, positive imaging, prayer, affirmation, belief, love, and work. Table A–11 lists several principles of the plus factor (37, 44).

TABLE A–11. POSITIVE THINKING/PLUS FACTOR PRINCIPLES TO TURN SETBACKS INTO COMEBACKS

- Expect and image good health. See yourself as vigorous and energetic.
- Develop spirit and soul health.
- Do not let a sense of guilt or anger fester in you.
- Stand up to your fear. Faith is bigger and stronger than fear.
- Think positively, especially when you feel the lowest. In the setback may be the answer to your comeback.
- Remind yourself that you are bigger than anything that can happen to you.
- Keep elasticity in your attitude. Change occurs, and you need to change also. Do not abandon basic principles, but listen to different points of view.
- Live one day at a time. See each day as precious. See opportunity.

Time Management

Symptoms of inappropriate time management include chronic rushing, fatigue, listlessness with many slack hours of nonproductive activity, vacillation between unpleasant alternatives, missing of deadlines, insufficient time for rest or personal relationships, and the sense of being overwhelmed by demands and details (13).

Most *methods of time management* include these steps:

- Keep a detailed log of each activity and time spent on each for 5 days.
- Establish priorities about what to accomplish.
- Eliminate low-priority tasks.
- Write specific goals for 1 month and 1 year.
- Learn to make and follow through with decisions.

Effective time management is useful in minimizing anxiety and job fatigue. To avoid being overwhelmed by goals, priorities, and decisions, work on one at a time (10, 13).

Other rules also help for making time (10, 13):

- Learn to say "no"; remind yourself that this is your life and your time to spend as best befits you. Only when your boss asks should you spend time on bottom-priority items.
- Build time into your schedule for unscheduled events, interruptions, and unforeseen occurrences.
- Set aside several periods during the day for structured relaxation; being relaxed allows you to use the time you have more efficiently.
- Keep a list of tasks that can be done in a few minutes any time you are waiting or are between other tasks.

- Learn to do two things at once; plan dinner while driving home or organize an important letter or list while waiting in line at the bank.
- Delegate low-priority tasks to others, if possible.
- Get up 15 to 30 minutes earlier every day than in the past to have a time for meditation or a hobby.
- Allow no more than 1 hour of television watching for yourself daily. Use it as a reward for your accomplishing high-priority items.

Part of time management is the ability to make decisions. Procrastination is the great time robber. Procrastination can often be overcome by (10, 13):

- Recognizing the unpleasantness of doing a task versus the unpleasantness of putting it off; analyzing the cost and risks of delay
- Examining the payoffs you receive by procrastinating (e.g., you will not have to do the task; you will not have to face the possibility of failure; you can be taken care of by others; you can gain attention); examining payoffs for finishing the task; building a special reward for completing an unpleasant task
- Exaggerating whatever you are doing to put off the decision; keeping it up until you are bored and making the decision seems more attractive than procrastination
- Taking responsibility for your delaying tactics by writing down how long each delay took; writing down how long it took to actually complete the task; comparing
- When making unimportant decisions, using a formula to choose—south or east over north or west, left over right or smooth over rough, easiest, shortest, or closest, the one that comes first alphabetically; then deciding a formula for making major decisions
- Taking small steps toward a major decision; listing each step; crossing it off the list as it is accomplished
- Avoiding beginning a new task until you have completed a predecided segment of the current one; allowing yourself to experience fully the reward of finishing something

You can practice some of the following *ways to adapt to stress* and teach these methods to others:

- Identify stressful aspects of your lifestyle to reduce frequency of the stress response or to avoid stressors when possible.
- Analyze what is making you tense or anxious and try to lessen the stressfulness of the situation.

- Develop spiritual and philosophic resources by talking to others who are wiser than you and by using literature and prayer.
- Keep something as the central core of your life and being, as your shelter or haven (e.g., a religious, philosophic, moral, or ethical belief; a special place in your home to relax; a specific time for doing certain pleasurable activities; or a person who is a confidant and friend).
- Try to slow your hectic pace. Do one thing at a time.
- Use temporary avoidance of identified stressors at times for regaining strength, energy, and ideas about fun in order to cope.
- Assume a more passive attitude toward irritating or frustrating events. Consciously work to remain calm or avoid the problem until you are in a better emotional condition to cope with it.
- Determine ways to enjoy selected stressors as a challenge by adjusting personal philosophy or behavior patterns.
- Accept love and support and encouragement and suggestions from others; be willing to receive help.
- Set aside time for relaxation each day. You may want to try relaxation techniques such as transcendental meditation, yoga, biofeedback, and the relaxation response or seek sources of joy and humor.
- Talk about your feelings with friends, family, or a counselor to gain objectivity about the problem, validate ideas and possible solutions, and affirm what you need and want to do.
- Accept things you cannot change. Do not expect too much from others. Accept your own normal irritation, anger, or crying.
- Try to correct aspects of your life that cause stress or worry or change a role that does not suit you.
- Do not push yourself beyond your limits of achievement or expect too much of yourself. Be satisfied with less while you do your best.
- Use physical exercise and recreation to work off the energy of anxiety and to relieve tension. Find a fulfilling hobby or try doing something helpful for someone. Books and audiotapes are available describing relaxation techniques and recreational activities or hobbies.
- Use visualization, imagery, or faith to affirm the answer to the problem until the solution is reached.
- Use conscious cognitive coping responses such as those described in this chapter.

- Seek psychotherapy if stress keeps you from functioning at your full capacity.
- Carry out health promotion measures described in each chapter.
- Realize that stressors are inevitable and can be handled and that some are necessary for survival, learning, development, and self-actualization.

EVALUATION

To determine your effectiveness in promoting stress reduction, see the criteria in Table A–12. Evaluate where the client is on the health–illness continuum, but realize that factors within the client or his or her situation may prevent restoration to or maintenance of an improved health status. Any of the criteria given in Table A–12 could assist with evaluation of the effectiveness of your assessment, teaching, counseling, goal setting, and other nursing interventions. You may think of other criteria (33).

TABLE A–12. CRITERIA FOR EVALUATION OF INTERVENTION RELATED TO STRESS MANAGEMENT

1. Client can identify stressors, stressful relationships, and lifestyle that interfered with personal functioning and interpersonal relationships.
2. Client can identify physical (psychosomatic) manifestations of stress that warrant self or other intervention.
3. Client can describe feelings related to anxiety state and can accept assistance in coping with anxiety as necessary.
4. Client can describe and use at least one strategy to reduce frequency of stress response.
5. Client can describe and demonstrate at least one strategy to avoid a stressor.
6. Client can describe at least one situation whereby he or she has changed perspective about life and stressful situations, so that a situation is perceived as challenging or positive rather than distressful.
7. Client practices at least one of each of the following: (a) conscious mental coping mechanism, (b) verbal response to release tension, (c) physical relaxation method, (d) emotional method of relaxation.
8. Client describes and practices one positive health habit and one other method to prevent disease and promote health.
9. Client demonstrates behaviors that reflect tasks of convalescence: (a) reassessment of life's meaning, (b) reintegration of body image, (c) role resolution.
10. Client demonstrates _____ taught in preparation for discharge.
    (SPECIFIC TASKS)
11. Client functions in impaired role, using maximum potential as indicated by demonstration of strategies to cope with disability/chronic disease.
12. Client's behavior changes from panic or severe anxiety to behavior typical of moderate or mild anxiety.
13. Client describes positive characteristics about self and lifestyle.
14. Client demonstrates improved interpersonal relationships; changed behavior is validated by significant others.
15. Client sets priorities and goals appropriate to developmental stage and life situation and that do not predispose to excessive stress.

REFERENCES

1. Alster, K., *The Holistic Health Movement.* Tuscaloosa, AL: University of Alabama Press, 1989.
2. Benson, H., *Beyond the Relaxation Response.* New York: Times Books, 1988.
3. ———, and W. Proctor, Your Maximum Mind. New York: Avon, 1989.
4. Bigbee, J., and N. Jansa, Strategies for Promoting Health Protection, *Nursing Clinics of North America,* 26, no. 4 (1991), 895–913.
5. Box, D., Putting on the Pressure, *Nursing Mirror,* 60, no. 21 (May 22, 1985), 28–29.
6. Brenner, A., *Helping Children Cope With Stress.* Lexington, MA: D.C. Heath, 1985.
7. Burns, D., *The Feeling Good Handbook: Using the New Mood Therapy in Everyday Life.* New York: William Morrow, 1989.
8. Buxman, K., Make Way for Laughter, *American Journal of Nursing,* 91, no. 12 (1991), 46–51.
9. ———, and A. LeMoine, *Nursing Perspectives in Humor.* Staten Island, NY: Power, 1995.
10. Clark, C., *Wellness Nursing: Concepts, Theory, Research, and Practice.* New York: Springer, 1986.
11. Cousins, N., *The Anatomy of an Illness as Perceived by the Patient's Reflections on Healing and Regeneration.* New York: Bantam, 1983.
12. Davidhizar, R., and M. Bowen, The Dynamics of Laughter, *Archives of Psychiatric Nursing,* 6 (1992), 132–137.
13. Davis, M., M. McKay, and E. Eshelman, *The Relaxation and Stress Reduction Workbook* (2nd ed.). Oakland, CA: New Harbinger, 1982.
14. Dossey, B., Awakening the Inner Healer, *American Journal of Nursing,* 91, no. 8 (1991), 31–32, 34.
15. Dugan, D., Laughter and Tears: Best Medicine for Stress, *Nursing Forum,* 24, no. 1 (1989), 18–26.
16. Edelman, C., and C. Mandle, *Health Promotion Throughout the Lifespan* (2nd ed.). St. Louis: C.V. Mosby, 1990.
17. Epstein, G., *Healing Visualization.* New York: Bantam, 1989.
18. Griffin, M., In the Mind's Eye, *American Journal of Nursing,* 86, no. 7 (1986), 804–806.
19. Grossman, J., The Quest for Quiet, *Health* (February 1990), 57–61, 84.
20. Guyton, A., *Textbook of Medical Physiology* (8th ed.). Philadelphia: W.B. Saunders, 1991.
21. Heidt, P., Openness: A Qualitative Analysis of Nurses' and Patients' Experiences of Therapeutic Touch, *Image,* 22, no. 3 (1990), 190–196.
22. Holmes, J., and R. Rahe, The Social Readjustment Rating Scale, *Journal of Psychosomatic Research,* 11 (1967), 213.
23. Hutchins, D., and C. Cole, *Helping Relationships and Strategies* (2nd ed.). Belmont, CA: Brooks/Cole, 1992.

24. Hutchinson, S., Self-care and Job Stress, *IMAGE: Journal Nursing Scholarship,* 19, no. 4 (1987), 192–196.

25. Kabut-Zinn, J., *Full Catastrophe Living: Using the Wisdom of Your Body and Mind to Face Stress, Pain, and Illness.* New York: Delacorte Press, 1990.

26. Keller, E., and V. Bzdek, Effects of Therapeutic Touch on Tension Headache Pain, *Nursing Research,* 35, no. 2 (1986), 101–105.

27. Krieger, D., *The Therapeutic Touch.* Englewood Cliffs, NJ: Prentice-Hall, 1979.

28. Lally, S., Laugh Your Stress Away, *Prevention,* June (1991), 50–55.

29. Lamontagne, L., K. Mason, and J. Hepworth, Effects of Relaxation on Anxiety in Children: Implications for Coping With Stress, *Nursing Research,* 34, no. 5 (1986), 289–292.

30. Mast, D., Effects of Imagery, *Image,* 8, no. 3 (1986), 118–120.

31. McHale, M., Getting the Joke: Interpreting Humor in Group Therapy, *Journal of Psychosocial Nursing,* 27, no. 9 (1989), 24–28.

32. Miller, A., Should Christian Nurses Practice Therapeutic Touching? No, *Journal of Christian Nursing,* 4, no. 4 (1987), 15ff.

33. Murray, R., and M. Huelskoetter, *Psychiatric/Mental Health Nursing: Giving Emotional Care* (3rd ed.). Norwalk, CT: Appleton-Lange, 1991.

34. Parish, A., It Only Hurts When I Don't Laugh, *American Journal of Nursing,* 94, no. 8 (1994), 46–47.

35. Pasquali, E., Learning to Laugh: Humor as Therapy, *Journal of Psychosocial Nursing,* 28, no. 3 (1990), 31–35.

36. Peale, N.V., *Imaging: The Powerful Way to Change Your Life.* Carmel, NY: Guideposts, 1982.

37. ———, *Power of the Plus Factor.* Old Tappan, NJ: Fleming H. Revell, 1987.

38. Pender, N., *Health Promotion in Nursing Practice* (2nd ed.). Norwalk, CT: Appleton & Lange, 1987.

39. Prerost, F., Use of Humor and Guided Imagery in Therapy to Alleviate Stress, *Journal of Mental Health Counseling,* 10, no. 1 (1988), 16–22.

40. Quinn, J., Therapeutic Touch as Energy Exchange: Testing the Theory, *Advance in Nursing Science,* 42 (1984), 49.

41. Raber, W., The Caring Role of the Nurse in the Application of Humor Therapy to the Patient Experiencing Helplessness, *Clinical Gerontologist,* 7, no. 1 (1987), 3–11.

42. Sheikh, A.A., ed., *Imagination and Healing.* New York: Baywood Press, 1984.

43. Shorr, G., et al., eds., *Imagery.* New York: Plenum Press, 1980.

44. Siegel, B., *Love, Medicine, and Miracles.* New York: Harper & Row, 1986.

45. Simonton, O.C., S. Matthews-Simonton, and J. Creighton, *Getting Well Again.* Los Angeles: J.P. Tarcher, 1978.

46. Singer, J., Towards the Scientific Study of Imagination, in Shorr, J., et al., eds., *Imagery: Theoretical and Clinical Applications,* Vol. 3. New York: Plenum Press, 1983.

47. Wuthnow, S., Should Christian Nurses Practice Therapeutic Touch? Yes, *Journal of Christian Nursing,* 4, no. 4 (1987), 15ff.

▶ SELECTED REFERENCES ON STRESS MANAGEMENT

Alderman, L., How to Tell the Boss You're Getting Worked to Death Without Killing Your Career, *Money,* May (1995), 41, 44.

Badger. K., Tips for Managing Stress on the Job, *American Journal of Nursing,* 95, no. 9 (1995), 31–34.

Bennett, C., Expanding the Mind–Body Connection: Working Women and Stress, *Capsules and Comments in Psychiatric Nursing,* 2, no. 4 (1996), 249–254.

Clark, S., D. Fontaine, and T.T. Simpson, Recognition, Assessment, and Treatment of Anxiety in the Critical Care Setting, *Critical Care Nurse,* August (1994, suppl.), 2–14.

Duffy, M., Determinants of Health-Promoting Lifestyles in Older Persons, *IMAGE: Journal of Nursing Scholarship,* 25 (1993), 23–28.

Field, T.C. Morrow, C. Valdeon, et al., Massage Reduces Anxiety in Child and Adolescent Psychiatric Patients, *Journal of American Academy of Child and Adolescent Psychiatry,* 31 (1992), 125–131.

Gift, A., T. Moore, and K. Soeken, Relaxation to Reduce Dyspnea and Anxiety in COPD Patients, *Nursing Research,* 41 (1992), 242–248.

Gillespie, B., and R. Eisler, Development of the Feminine Role Stress Scale, *Behavior Modification,* 16 (1992), 426–438.

Goleman, D., and J. Gurin, *Mind–Body Medicine.* Yonkers, NY: Consumer Report Books, 1993.

Healthier, Trimmer, Younger—in Just 90 Minutes a Week, *Tufts' University Diet and Nutrition Letter,* 13, no. 1 (1995), 3–5.

Jacobson, G., The Meaning of Stressful Life Experiences in Nine to Eleven-year-old Children: A Phenomenological Study. *Nursing Research,* 43 (1994), 95–99.

Knoop, R., Relieving Work Through Value-rich Work, *Journal of Social Psychology,* 134 (1994), 829–836.

Kulbok, P.A., and J.H., Baldwin, From Preventive Health Behavior to Health Promotion: Advancing a Positive Construct of a Health, *Advances in Nursing Science,* 14, no. 4 (1992), 50–64.

Lee, K., M. Lentz, D. Taylor, E. Mitchell, and N. Woods, Fatigue as a Response to Environmental Demands in Women's Lives, *IMAGE: Journal of Nursing Scholarship,* 26 (1994), 149–154.

Lerner, D., S. Levine, S. Malspeis, and R. D'Agostino, Job Strain and Health-related Quality of Life in a National Sample, *American Journal of Public Health,* 84 (1994), 1580–1585.

Maton, K., The Stress Buffering Role of Spiritual Support: Cross-sectional and Prospective Investigations, *Journal for the Scientific Study of Religion,* 28 (1988), 310–323.

McCain, N., and J. Smith, Stress and Coping in the Context of Psychoneuroimmunology: A Holistic Framework for Nursing Practice and Research, *Archieves of Psychiatric Nursing,* 7 (1994), 221–227.

McGinnis, A., *The Power of Optimism.* New York: Harper & Row, 1990.

Meyer, I., Minority Stress and Mental Health in Gay Men, *Journal of Health and Social Behavior,* 36 (1995), 38–56.

O'Leary, A., Stress, Emotion, and Human Immune Function, *American Psychologist,* 108 (1990), 363–382.

Peale, V., Be a Believer, Be an Achiever, *Possibilities,* January–February (1991), 21–25.

Pelletier, K., and R. Lutz, Healthy People, Healthy Business, *American Journal of Health Promotion,* 2 (1988), 5–12.

Research Links Health, Religion, *St. Louis Post Dispatch,* February 12 (1996), Sect. A, p. 9.

Researchers Say Anger May Make Headaches Worse, *First Page,* March (1993), 2.

Seligman, M., *Learned Optimism.* New York: Knopf, 1991.

Stress and Work, *Harvard Women's Health Watch,* 2, no. 1 (1994), 1.

Thomas, S., and R. Williams, Perceived Stress, Trait, Anger, Modes of Anger Expression, and Health Status of College Men and Women, *Nursing Research,* 40 (1991), 303–307.

U.S. Department of Health, Education, & Welfare, Public Health Service, Healthy People: The Surgeon General's Report on Health Promotion and Disease Prevention. DHEW Publication No. (PHS) 79-55071. Washington, DC: Government Printing Office, 1979.

Vogt, T., C. Pope, J. Mullvoly, and J. Hollis, Mental Health Status as a Predictor of Morbidity and Mortality: A 15-Year Follow-up of Members of a Health Maintenance Organization, *American Journal of Public Health,* 84 (1994), 222–231.

Walker, S., K. Volkan, K. Sechrist, and N. Pender, Health-promoting Life Styles of Older Adults: Comparisons With Young and Middle-aged Adults, Correlates and Patterns, *Advances in Nursing Science,* 11, no. 1 (1988), 76–90.

Yeo, S., Exercise Guidelines for Pregnant Women, *IMAGE: Journal of Nursing Scholarship,* 26 (1994), 265–270.

American Academy of Family Physicians·Age Charts For Periodic Health Examination

These Age Charts contain recommendations based on the *First Edition of the Guide to Clinical Preventive Services* (1989) and other outcomes-based recommendations, as well as the CDC Advisory Committee on Immunization Practices and the AAFP Commission on Public Health and Scientific Affairs through September 1995. A second revision of these age charts is anticipated in 1996 because of publication of the *Second Edition of the Guide to Clinical Preventive Services,* December 1995.

Preamble
- Chart 1   Ages Birth–18 Months
- Chart 2   Ages 19 Months–6 Years
- Chart 3   Ages 7–12 Years
- Chart 4   Ages 13–18 Years
- Chart 5   Ages 19–39 Years
- Chart 6   Ages 40–64 Years
- Chart 7   65 Years and Older

These recommendations are provided only as an assistance for physicians making clinical decisions regarding the care of their patients. As such, they cannot substitute for the individual judgment brought to each clinical situation by the patient's family physician. As with all clinical reference resources, they reflect the best understanding of the science of medicine at the time of publication, but they should be used with the clear understanding that continued research may result in new knowledge and recommendations.

Preamble to Age Charts
for
Periodic Health Examination

Periodic health examination, including immunizations, counseling, and other preventive services, are a part of continuing, comprehensive care in family practice. The content and frequency of these health examinations should be tailored to the patient's age, sex, and risk factors. Delivery of clinical preventive services should not be limited only to visits for health maintenance but also should be provided as a part of visits for other reasons such as acute and chronic care. For many patients, these visits provide the only opportunity to receive preventive services.

The following age-specific charts for periodic health examination are recommended by the Subcommittee on Periodic Health Intervention of the Commission on Public Health and Scientific Affairs as the minimum clinical preventive services to be provided for asymptomatic patients. They are based on the *First Edition of the Guide to Clinical Preventive Services: Report of the U.S. Preventive Services Task Force,* the American College of Physicians outcomes-based recommendations on hormone replacement therapy and recommendations of the Commission on Public Health Scientific Affairs. In making these recommendations, the subcommittee notes:

A) That all patients new to a medical practice should be urged to receive a comprehensive history and physical as well as the screening, laboratory and diagnostic procedures, counseling, immunizations and chemoprophylaxis appropriate for the patient's age, sex, and risk. Subsequent visits may be used in completion of workup.

B) That former health records should be obtained for review and avoidance of duplications of laboratory testing.

C) That the charts are not exhaustive and the physicians may add other preventive services either routinely or for individual patients based on clinical judgement.

D) That as new scientific findings become available, the subcommittee anticipates changes in the recommendations.

E) That the subcommittee has added interventions beyond the recommendations of the U.S. Preventive Services Task Force and other explicitly developed guidelines that it feels are necessary. These are noted with footnotes on the charts and shown in italics.

F) The date in the lower left hand corner identifies the most recent update of these charts. The date in the lower right hand corner is the most recent printing. This document is updated annually.

Chart 1
Periodic Health Examination* Birth to 18 Months
Schedule: 2, 4, 6, (12), 15, 18 Months† (See Preamble)

Leading Causes of Death

- Conditions originating in perinatal period
- Congenital anomalies
- Heart disease
- Injuries (nonmotor vehicle)
- Pneumonia/influenza

Remain Alert for

- Ocular misalignment
- Tooth decay
- Signs of child abuse or neglect

FIRST WEEK

- Ophthalmic antibiotics[1]
- Hemoglobin electrophoresis (HR1)[1]
- T4/TSH[2]
- Phenylalanine[2]
- Hearing (HR2)

SCREENING

History

- Interval medical and family history[3]

Physical

- Height and weight

Laboratory/Diagnostic Procedures

- Hemoglobin and/*or* hematocrit[4]

High-Risk Groups

- Hearing[5] (HR2)
- *Whole blood lead* (HR3)

HIGH-RISK CATEGORIES

HR1 Newborns of Caribbean, Latin American, Asian, Mediterranean, or African descent.

HR2 Infants with a family history of childhood hearing impairment or a personal history of congenital perinatal infection with herpes, syphilis, rubella, cytomegalovirus, or toxoplasmosis; malformations involving the head or neck (e.g., dysmorphic and syndromal abnormalities, cleft palate, abnormal pinna); birthweight below 1500 g; bacterial meningitis, hyperbilirubinemia requiring exchange transfusion; or severe perinatal asphyxia (Apgar scores of 0–3, absence of spontaneous respirations for 10 minutes, or hypotonia at 2 hours of age).

HR3 Infants who live in or frequently visit housing built before 1950 that is dilapidated or undergoing renovation; who come in contact with other children with known lead toxicity; who live near lead processing plants or whose parents or household members work in a lead-related occupation; or who live near busy highways or hazardous waste sites. Does your child: a. Live in or regularly visit a house built before 1960? This could include a day-care center, preschool, the home of a baby—sitter or a relative, etc. b. Have a brother or sister, housemate, or playmate being followed or treated for lead poisoning (that is, blood lead ≥ 15 µg/dL)? c. Live with an adult whose job or hobby involves exposure to lead? d. Live near an active lead smelter, battery recycling plant, or other industry likely to release lead?

---

[1]At birth
[2]Days 3 to 6 preferred for testing
[3]*An updating of the previously obtained medical and family medical history is recommended by the subcommittee.*
[4]Once during infancy. *The subcommittee believes either test is acceptable.*
[5]*By age 18 months, if not tested earlier.*

(continued)

Chart 1 (continued)

PARENT COUNSELING

Diet and Exercise

- Breastfeeding
- Nutrient intake, especially iron-rich foods

Substance Use

Sexual

Injury Prevention

- Child safety seats
- Smoke detector
- Hot water heater temperature (≤120°F)
- Stairway gates, window guards, pool fence
- Storage of drugs and toxic chemicals
- Syrup of ipecac, poison control telephone number

Dental Health

- Baby bottle tooth decay

Other Primary Preventive Measures

- Effects of passive smoking
- *Assess risk of lead exposure* (HR4)

IMMUNIZATIONS AND CHEMOPROPHYLAXIS

- Diphtheria-tetanus-pertussis (DTP) vaccine[6]
- Oral poliovirus vaccine (OPV)[7]
- Measles-mumps-rubella (MMR) vaccine[8]
- *Haemophilus influenzae* type b (Hib) conjugate vaccine[9]
- *Hepatitis B vaccine* (HBv)[10]
- *Varicella* (*Var*)[11]

High-Risk Groups

- Fluoride supplements (HR5)
- *Influenza vaccine* (HR6)

HIGH-RISK CATEGORIES

HR4 Infants who live in or frequently visit housing built before 1950 that is dilapidated or undergoing renovation; who come in contact with other children who known lead toxicity; who live near lead processing plants or whose parents or household members work in a lead-related occupation; or who live near busy highways or hazardous waste sites. Does your child: a. Live in or regularly visit a house built before 1960? This could include a day-care center, preschool, the home of a babysitter or a relative, etc. b. Have a brother or sister, housemate, or playmate being followed or treated for lead poisoning (that is, blood lead ≥ 15 µg/dL)? c. Live with an adult whose job or hobby involves exposure to lead? d. Live near an active lead smelter, battery recycling plant, or other industry likely to release lead?

HR5 Infants living in areas with inadequate water fluoridation (less than 0.7 parts per million).

HR6 Children over 6 months of age with chronic pulmonary or cardiovascular problems including asthma; or who required medical followup or hospitalization during the past year for chronic metabolic disease (including diabetes mellitus), renal dysfunction, hemoglobinopathies, or immunosuppression (including immunosuppression caused by medications).

---

[6] At ages 2, 4, 6, and *12–18* months. *Acellular pertussis vaccine may be used for the fourth and fifth doses. (DTP-HbOC or DTP-PRP-T may be used instead of DTP alone.)*

[7] Ages 2, 4, and 6 *to 18 months*

[8] At age 12–15 months

[9] *If using HbOC, PRP-T or combined DTP-HbOC or DTP-PRP-T, at ages 2, 4, 6, and 12–15 months. If using PRP-OMP, then at ages 2, 4, and 12–15 months.*

[10] The recommended option for administration is birth (before discharge from hospital), 1–2 months, 6–8 months. A second option is 1–2 months, 4 months and 6–18 months.

[11] *Between ages 12–18 months preferably at same visit as MMR is administered*

---

*This list of preventive services is not exhaustive. It reflects only those topics reviewed by the U.S. Preventive Services Task Force *and the AAFP Commission on Public Health and Scientific Affairs.* Clinicians may wish to add other preventive services on a routine basis and after considering the patient's medical history and other individual circumstances. Examples of target conditions not specifically examined by the Task Force include:

- Developmental disorders
- Musculoskeletal malformations
- Cardiac anomalies
- Genitourinary disorders
- Metabolic disorders
- Speech problems
- Behavioral disorders
- Parent/family dysfunction

†Schedule: 2, 4, 6, (*12*), 15, 18 Months At least five visits are required for immunizations. Because of lack of data and differing patient risk profiles, the scheduling of additional visits and the frequency of the individual preventive services listed in this table are left to clinical discretion (except as indicated in other footnotes).

Chart 2
Periodic Health Examination* Ages: 19 Months–6 Years
Schedule: See Footnote† (See Preamble)

Leading Causes of Death

- Injuries (nonmotor vehicle)
- Motor vehicle crashes
- Congenital anomalies
- Homicide
- Heart disease

Remain Alert for

- Vision disorders
- Dental decay, malalignment, premature loss of teeth, mouth breathing
- Signs of child abuse or neglect
- Abnormal bereavement

SCREENING

History

- *Interval medical and family history*[1]
- *Developmental/behavioral assessment*

Physical Examination†

- Height and weight
- Blood pressure
- Eye exam for amblyopia and strabismus[2]

Laboratory/Diagnostic Procedures

- Urinalysis for bacteriuria[3]

High-Risk Groups

- *Whole blood lead* (HR1)
- Tuberculin skin test (PPD) (HR2)
- Hearing[4] (HR3)

HIGH-RISK CATEGORIES

HR1 Infants who live in or frequently visit housing built before 1950 that is dilapidated or undergoing renovation; who come in contact with other children with known lead toxicity; who live near lead processing plants or whose parents or household members work in a lead-related occupation; or who live near busy highways or hazardous waste sites. Does your child: a. Live in or regularly visit a house built before 1960? This could include a day-care center, preschool, the home of a babysitter or a relative, etc. b. Have a brother or sister, housemate, or playmate being followed or treated for lead poisoning (that is, blood lead ≥ 15 µg/dL)? c. Live with an adult whose job or hobby involves exposure to lead? d. Live near an active lead smelter, battery recycling plant, or other industry likely to release lead?

HR2 Household members of persons with tuberculosis or others at risk for close contact with the disease; recent immigrants or refugees from countries in which tuberculosis is common (e.g., Asia, Africa, Central and South America, Pacific Islands); family members of migrant workers; residents of homeless shelters; or persons with certain underlying medical disorders.

HR3 Children with a family history of childhood hearing impairment or a personal history of congenital perinatal infection with herpes, syphilis, rubella, cytomegalovirus, or toxoplasmosis; malformations involving the head or neck (e.g., dysmorphic and syndromal abnormalities, cleft palate, abnormal pinna); birthweight below 1500 g; bacterial meningitis; hyperbilirubinemia requiring exchange transfusion; or severe perinatal asphyxia (Apgar scores of 0–3, absence of spontaneous respirations for 10 minutes, or hypotonia at 2 hours of age).

[1] *An updating of the previously obtained medical and family medical history is recommended by the subcommittee.*
[2] Ages 3–4
[3] *The optimal frequency for urine testing has not been determined and is left to clinical discretion. In general, dipsticks combining the leukocyte esterase and nitrite tests should be used to detect asymptomatic bacteriuria.*
[4] Before age 3, if not tested earlier

American Academy of Family Physicians Policy Action June 1995

(*continued*)

Chart 2 (continued)

PATIENT & PARENT COUNSELING

Diet and Exercise

- Sweets and between-meal snacks, iron-enriched foods, sodium
- *Nutritional assessment*
- Selection of exercise program

Substance Use

Sexual

- *Initiate sex education*

Injury Prevention

- Safety belts
- Smoke detector
- Hot water heater temperature (≤120°F)
- *Burn protection*
- *Electrical cords and outlets*
- *Warning about strangers*
- Window guards and pool fence
- Bicycle safety helmets
- Storage of drugs, toxic chemicals, matches and firearms
- Syrup of ipecac, poison control telephone number

Dental Health

- Tooth brushing
- Dental visits *starting at age 3*

Other Primary Preventive Measures

- Effects of passive smoking
- *Assess risk of lead exposure* (HR4)

High-Risk Groups

- Skin protection from ultraviolet light (HR5)

IMMUNIZATIONS AND CHEMOPROPHYLAXIS

- Diphtheria-tetanus-pertussis (DTP) vaccine[5]
- Oral poliovirus vaccine (OPV)[5]
- *Measles-mumps-rubella (MMR) vaccine*[6]
- *Review Haemophilus influenzae type b (Hib) conjugate vaccine immunization status*
- *Review hepatitis B vaccine (HBv) status*
- *Review Varicella (Var)*[7] *status*

High-Risk Groups

- Fluoride supplements (HR6)
- *Influenza vaccine* (HR7)
- *Pneumococcal vaccine* (HR8)

HIGH-RISK CATEGORIES

HR4   Infants who live in or frequently visit housing built before 1950 that is dilapidated or undergoing renovation; who come in contact with other children with known lead toxicity; who live near lead processing plants or whose parents or household members work in a lead-related occupation; or who live near busy highways or hazardous waste sites. Does your child: a. Live in or regularly visit a house built before 1960? This could include a day-care center, preschool, the home of a babysitter or a relative, etc. b. Have a brother or sister, housemate, or playmate being followed or treated for lead poisoning (that is, blood lead ≥ 15 µg/dL)? c. Live with an adult whose job or hobby involves exposure to lead? d. Live near an active lead smelter, battery recycling plant, or other industry likely to release lead?

HR5   Children with increased exposure to sunlight.

HR6   Children living in areas with inadequate water fluoridation (less than 0.7 parts per million).

HR7   Children with chronic pulmonary or cardiovascular problems including asthma; or who required medical followup or hospitalization during the past year for chronic metabolic disease (including diabetes mellitus), renal dysfunction, hemoglobinopathies, or immunosuppression (including immunosuppression caused by medications).

HR8   Children aged two and over with chronic illnesses specifically associated with pneumococcal disease or its complications, anatomic or functional asplenia, sickle cell disease, nephrotic syndrome or chronic renal failure, cerebrospinal fluid leaks, or conditions associated with immunosuppression (including HIV).

---

[5]Once between ages 4 and 6
[6]*MMR can be given either at 4–6 or 11–12 years depending on school entry requirements.*
[7]*For children between 18 months and 12 years if not previously administered and child does not have history of chickenpox*

---

*This list of preventive services is not exhaustive. It reflects only those topics reviewed by the U.S. Preventive Services Task Force *and the AAFP Commission on Public Health and Scientific Affairs.* Clinicians may wish to add other preventive services on a routine basis, and after considering the patient's medical history and other individual circumstances. Examples of target conditions not specifically examined by the Task Force include:

- Developmental disorders
- Speech problems
- Behavioral and learning disorders
- Parent/family dysfunction

†One visit is required for immunizations. Because of lack of data and differing patient risk profiles, the scheduling of additional visits and the frequency of the individual preventive services listed in this table are left to clinical discretion (except as indicated in other footnotes).

Chart 3
Periodic Health Examination* Ages: 7–12 Years†
Schedule: See Footnote† (See Preamble)

Leading Causes of Death

- Motor vehicle crashes
- Injuries (nonmotor vehicle)
- Congenital anomalies
- Leukemia
- Homicide
- Heart disease

Remain Alert for

- Vision disorders
- Diminished hearing
- Dental decay, malalignment, mouth breathing
- Signs of child abuse or neglect
- Abnormal bereavement
- *Depressive symptoms*

SCREENING

History

- *Interval medical and family history*[1]

Physical

- Height and weight
- Blood pressure
- *Tanner staging*[2]

Laboratory/Diagnostic Procedures

High-Risk Groups

- *Total cholesterol*[3,5]
- *Lipoprotein analysis*[4,5]
- Tuberculin skin test (PPD) (HR1)

HIGH-RISK CATEGORIES

HR1 Household members of persons with tuberculosis or others at risk for close contact with the disease; recent immigrants or refugees from countries in which tuberculosis is common (e.g., Asia, Africa, Central and South America, Pacific Islands); family members of migrant workers; residents of homeless shelters; or persons with certain underlying medical disorders.

---

[1]*An updating of the previously obtained medical and family medical history is recommended by the subcommittee.*
[2]*A physical examination including Tanner stage is recommended at least once in this age group by the subcommittee.*
[3]*Child of a parent with a blood cholesterol of 240 mg/dL or higher*
[4]*Child of a parent or grandparent with a documented history of premature (age less than 55 years) cardiovascular disease*
[5]*The exact frequency is not determined. It should be performed at least once.*

American Academy of Family Physicians Policy Action June 1995

(*continued*)

Chart 3 (continued)

PATIENT & PARENT COUNSELING

Diet and Exercise

- Fat (especially saturated fat), cholersterol, sweets and between-meal snacks, sodium
- *Nutritional assessment*
- Selection of exercise program

Substance Use

- *Tobacco, alcohol, and other drugs: primary prevention*

Sexual Practices

- *Sex education*

Injury Prevention

- Safety belts
- Smoke detector
- Storage of firearms, drugs, toxic chemicals, matches
- Bicycle safety helmets

Dental Health

- Regular tooth brushing and dental visits

Other Primary Preventive Measures

High-Risk Groups

- Skin protection from ultraviolet light (HR2)

IMMUNIZATIONS AND CHEMOPROPHYLAXIS

- *At age 11–12, check immunization status for Varicella (Var)[1], Hepatitis B vaccine (HBv)[2], Tetanus and diphtheria toxoids, adsorbed (Td)[3], Oral poliovirus vaccine (OPV), Measles-mumps-rubella (MMR)*

High-Risk Groups

- Fluoride supplements (HR3)
- *Influenza vaccine (HR4)*
- *Pneumococcal vaccine (HR5)*

HIGH-RISK CATEGORIES

HR2   Children with increased exposure to sunlight.

HR3   Children living in areas with inadequate water fluoridation (less than 0.7 parts per million).

HR4   Children with chronic pulmonary or cardiovascular problems including asthma; or who required medical followup or hospitalization during the past year for chronic metabolic disease (including diabetes mellitus), renal dysfunction, hemoglobinopathies, or immunosuppression (including immunosuppression caused by medications).

HR5   Children aged two and over with chronic illnesses specifically associated with pneumococcal disease or its complications, anatomic or functional asplenia, sickle cell disease, nephrotic syndrome or chronic renal failure, cerebrospinal fluid leaks, or conditions associated with immunosuppression (including HIV).

---

[1]*For children between 18 months and 12 years, if not previously administered and child does not have history of chickenpox*

[2]*HBv should be administered as a 3 dose series to all 11–12 year olds who have not previously received it.*

[3]*After age 6 Td should be administered*

---

*This list of preventive services is not exhaustive. It reflects only those topics reviewed by the U.S. Preventive Services Task Force *and the AAFP Commission on Public Health and Scientific Affairs*. Clinicians may wish to add other preventive services on a routine basis, and after considering the patient's medical history and other individual circumstances. Examples of target conditions not specifically examined by the Task Force include:

- Developmental disorders
- Behavioral and learning disorders
- Parent/family dysfunction

†Because of lack of data and differing patient risk profiles, the scheduling of visits and the frequency of the individual preventive services listed in this table are left to clinical discretion *(except as indicated in other footnotes). Additional visits should occur as risk factors are determined. Achievement of developmental or social milestones, such as entry to junior high school, may also warrant a visit. Each visit by patients in this age group should be considered an opportunity to assess and address risks.*

Chart 4
Periodic Health Examination* Ages: 13–18 Years
Schedule: At least one visit for preventive services should occur† (See Preamble)

Leading Causes of Death

- Motor vehicle crashes
- Homicide
- Suicide
- Injuries (nonmotor vehicle)
- Heart disease

Remain Alert for

- Depressive symptoms
- Suicide risk factors (HR1)
- Abnormal bereavement
- Tooth decay, malalignment, gingivitis
- Signs of child abuse and neglect

SCREENING

History

- Interval medical and family history[1]
- Dietary intake
- Physical activity
- Tobacco/alcohol/drug use
- Sexual practices

Physical

- Height and weight
- Blood pressure
- Tanner staging[2]

High-Risk Groups

- Complete skin exam (HR2)
- Clinical testicular exam (HR3)

Laboratory/Diagnostic Procedures

High-Risk Groups

- Rubella antibodies (HR4)
- VDRL/RPR (HR5)
- Chlamydial testing (HR6)
- Gonorrhea culture (HR7)
- Counseling and testing for HIV (HR8)
- Tuberculin skin test (PPD) (HR9)
- Hearing (HR10)
- Papanicolaou smear[3]
- Total cholesterol[4,5]
- Lipoprotein analysis[5]

HIGH-RISK CATEGORIES

HR1 Recent divorce, separation, unemployment, depression, alcohol or other drug abuse, serious medical illnesses, living alone, or recent bereavement.

HR2 Persons with increased recreational or occupational exposure to sunlight, a family or personal history of skin cancer, or clinical evidence of precursor lesions (e.g., dysplastic nevi, certain congenial nevi).

HR3 Males with a history of cryptorchidism, orchiopexy, or testicular atrophy.

HR4 Females of childbearing age lacking evidence of immunity.

HR5 Persons who enage in sex with multiple partners in areas in which syphilis is prevalent, prostitutes, or contacts of person with active syphilis.

HR6 Persons who attend clinics for sexually transmitted diseases; attend other high-risk health care facilities (e.g., adolescent and family planning clinics); or have other risk factors for chlamydial infection (e.g., multiple sexual partners or a sexual partner with multiple sexual contacts).

HR7 Persons with multiple sexual partners or a sexual partner with multiple contacts, sexual contacts of persons with culture-proven gonorrhea or persons with a history of repeated episodes of gonorrhea.

HR8 Persons seeing treatment for sexually transmitted diseases; homosexual and bisexual men; past or present intravenous (IV) drug users; persons with a history of prostitution or multiple sexual partners; women whose past or present sexual partners were HIV-infected, bisexual or IV drug users; persons with long-term residence or birth in an area with high prevalence of HIV infection; or persons with a history of transfusion between 1978 and 1985.

HR9 Household members of persons with tuberculosis or others at risk for close contact with the disease; recent immigrants or refugees from countries in which tuberculosis is common (e.g., Asia, Africa, Central and South America, Pacific Islands); migrant workers; residents of correctional institutions or homeless shelters; or persons with certain underlying medical disorders.

HR10 Persons exposed regularly to excessive noise in recreational or other settings.

[1]An updating of the previously obtained medical and family medical history is recommended by the subcommittee.
[2]A physical examination including Tanner stage is recommended at least once in this age group by the subcommittee.
[3]All women 18 years of age should have an annual Pap test and pelvic examination. All women between 13 and 18 who are or who have been sexually active, should also have an annual pap test and pelvic examination. After a woman has had three or more consecutive satisfactory normal annual examinations, the Pap test may be performed at the discretion of the physician based on the assessment of patient risk but not less frequently than every three years.
[4]Child of a parent with a blood cholesterol of 240 mg/dL or higher.
[5]Child of a parent or grandparent with a documented history of premature (age less than 55 years) cardiovascular disease.

(continued)

Chart 4 (continued)

COUNSELING

Diet and Exercise

- Fat (especially saturated fat), cholersterol, sodium, iron[6], calcium[6]
- *Nutritional assessment*
- Selection of exercise program

Substance Use

- Tobacco: cessation/primary prevention
- Alcohol and other drugs: cessation/primary prevention
- Driving/other dangerous activities while under the influence
- Treatment for abuse

High-Risk Groups

- Sharing/using unsterilized needles and syringes (HR11)

Sexual Practices

- Sex development and behavior[7]
- Sexually transmitted diseases: partner selection, condoms
- Unintended pregnancy and contraceptive options

Injury Prevention

- Safety belts
- Safety helmets
- Violent behavior[8]
- Firearms[8]
- Smoke detector
- *Noise induced hearing loss*[9]

Dental Health

- Regular tooth brushing, flossing, and dental visits

Other Primary Preventive Measures

- *Breast self-examination*[10]
- *Testicular self-examination*[11]

High-Risk Groups

- Discussion of hemoglobin testing (HR12)
- Skin protection from ultraviolet light (HR13)

IMMUNIZATIONS AND CHEMOPROPHYLAXIS

- Tetanus-diphtheria (Td) booster[12]
- *Hepatitis B vaccine (HBv)*[13]

High-Risk Groups

- *Measles-mumps-rubella (MMR) vaccine*[14]
- Fluoride supplements (HR14)
- *Influenza vaccine* (HR15)
- *Pneumococcal vaccine* (HR16)
- *Hepatitis B vaccine (HBv)* (HR17)

HIGH-RISK CATEGORIES

HR11 Intravenous drug users.

HR12 Persons of Caribbean, Latin America, Asian, Mediterranean or African descent.

HR13 Persons with increased exposure to sunlight.

HR14 Persons living in areas with inadequate water fluoridation (less than 0.7 parts per million).

HR15 Children with chronic pulmonary or cardiovascular problems including asthma; or who required medical followup or hospitalization during the past year for chronic metabolic disease (including diabetes mellitus), renal dysfunction, hemoglobinopathies, or immunosuppression (including immunosuppression caused by medications).

HR16 Children aged two and over with chronic illnesses specifically associated with pneumococcal disease or its complications, anatomic or functional asplenia, sickle cell disease, nephrotic syndrome or chronic renal failure, cerebrospinal fluid leaks, or conditions associated with immunosuppression (including HIV).

HR17 Homosexually and bisexually active men, intravenous drug users, recipients of some blood products, persons in health-related jobs with frequent exposure to blood or blood products, household and sexual contacts of HBV carriers, sexually active heterosexual persons with multiple sexual partners diagnosed as having recently acquired sexually transmitted disease, prostitutes, and persons who have a history of sexual activity with multiple partners in the previous six months.

[6]For females

[7]Often best performed early in adolescence and with the involvement of parents

[8]Especially for males

[9]*Education regarding hearing loss from recreational and personal listening devices is recommended by the subcommittee.*

[10]*The teaching of self-breast examination is recommended by the subcommittee at the time of initiation of pelvic examinations.*

[11]*The teaching of self-testicular examination is recommended by the subcommittee for male patients.*

[12]*If not given at ages 11–12 and at least 5 years since last Td or DTP*

[13]*May opt to immunize all adolescents based on level of risk in community*

[14]*A second measles immunization, preferably as MMR (Measles, Mumps, and Rubella Vaccine, Live), is recommended by the subcommittee for all patients unable to show proof of immunity who are entering post secondary school education and for those becoming employed in medical occupations with direct patient care.*

*This list of preventive services is not exhaustive. It reflects only those topics reviewed by the U.S. Preventive Services Task Force *and the AAFP Commission on Public Health and Scientific Affairs.* Clinicians may wish to add other preventive services on a routine basis and after considering the patient's medical history and other individual circumstances. Examples of target conditions not specifically examined by the Task Force include:

- Developmental disorders
- Behavioral and learning disorders
- Parent/family dysfunction

†*Additional visits should occur as other risk factors are determined such as initiation of sexual activity, experimentation with alcohol or other drugs, or licensure for operating a motor vehicle. Achievement of developmental milestones such as entry to high school may also warrant a visit. Each visit by patients in this age group should be considered an opportunity to assess and address risks.*

Leading Causes of Death

- Motor vehicle crashes
- Homicide
- Suicide
- Injuries (nonmotor vehicle)
- Heart disease
- *HIV infection* (males)[1]

Remain Alert for

- Depressive symptoms
- Suicide risk factors (HR1)
- Abnormal bereavement
- Malignant skin lesions
- Tooth decay, gingivitis
- Signs of physical abuse

SCREENING

History

- *Interval medical and family history*[2]
- Dietary intake
- Physical activity
- Tobacco/alcohol/drug use
- Sexual practices

Physical

- Height and weight
- Blood pressure[3]
- *Pelvic examination (for women)*
- *Clinical breast exam (for women)*[4]
- *Clinical testicular exam (for men)* (HR2)

High-Risk Groups

- Complete oral cavity exam (HR3)
- Palpation for thyroid nodules (HR4)
- Complete skin exam (HR5)

Laboratory/Diagnostic Procedures

- Nonfasting *or fasting* total blood cholesterol[5]
- Papanicolaou smear[6]

High-Risk Groups

- Fasting plasma glucose (HR6)
- Rubella antibodies (HR7)
- VDRL/RPR (HR8)
- Urinalysis for bacteriuria[7] (HR9)
- Chlamydial testing (HR10)
- Gonorrhea culture (HR11)
- Counseling and testing for HIV (HR12)
- Hearing (HR13)
- Tuberculin skin test (HR14)
- Electrocardiogram (HR15)
- Mammogram (HR16)
- Colonoscopy (HR17)

HIGH-RISK CATEGORIES

HR1 Recent divorce, separation, unemployment, depression, alcohol or other drug abuse, serious medical illnesses, living alone, or recent bereavement.

HR2 Men with a history of cryptorchidism, orchiopexy, or testicular atrophy.

HR3 Persons with exposure to tobacco or excessive amounts of alcohol, or those with suspicious symptoms or lesions detected through self-examination.

HR4 Persons with a history of upper-body irradiation.

HR5 Persons with a family or personal history of skin cancer, increased occupational or recreational exposure to sunlight, or clinical evidence of precursor lesions (e.g., dysplastic nevi, certain congenital nevi).

HR6 The markedly obese, persons with a family history of diabetes, or women with a history of gestational diabetes.

HR7 Women lacking evidence of immunity.

HR8 Prostitutes, persons who engage in sex with multiple partners in areas in which syphilis is prevalent, or contacts of persons with active syphilis.

HR9 Persons with diabetes.

HR10 Persons who attend clinics for sexually transmitted diseases; attend other high-risk health care facilities (e.g., adolescent and family planning clinics); or have other risk factors for chlamydial infection (e.g., multiple sexual partners or a sexual partner with multiple sexual contacts, age less than 20).

HR11 Prostitutes, persons with multiple sexual partners or a sexual partner with multiple contacts, sexual contacts of persons with culture-proven gonorrhea, or persons with a history of repeated episodes of gonorrhea.

HR12 Persons seeking treatment for sexually transmitted diseases; homosexual and bisexual men; past or present intravenous (IV) drug users; persons with a history of prostitution or multiple sexual partners; women whose past or present sexual partners were HIV-infected, bisexual, or IV drug users; persons with long-term residence or birth in an area with high prevalence of HIV infection; or persons with a history of transfusion between 1978 and 1985.

HR13 Persons exposed regularly to excessive noise.

HR14 Household members of persons with tuberculosis or others at risk for close contact with the disease (e.g., staff or tuberculosis clinics, shelters for the homeless, nursing homes, substance abuse treatment facilities, dialysis units, correctional institutions); recent immigrants or refugees from countries in which tuberculosis is common; migrant workers; residents of nursing homes, correctional institutions, or homeless shelters; or persons with certain underlying medical disorders (e.g., HIV infection).

HR15 Men who would endanger public safety were they to experience sudden cardiac events (e.g., commercial airline pilots).

HR16 Women aged 35 and older with a family history of premenopausally diagnosed breast cancer in a first-degree relative.

HR17 Persons with a family history of familial polyposis coli or cancer family syndrome.

---

[1]*HIV infection as leading cause of death among young adults in U.S. cities and states. JAMA 1993;269:2991–2994.*

[2]*An updating of the previously obtained medical and family medical history is recommended by the subcommittee.*

[3]*At every physician visit, with a minimum of every two years*

[4]*Every 1–3 years, starting at age 30 until age 40*

[5]*At least every five years*

[6]*All women 18 years of age and over should have an annual Pap test and pelvic examination. After a woman has had three or more consecutive satisfactory normal annual examinations, the Pap test may be performed at the discretion of the physician based on the assessment of patient risk but not less frequently than every three years.*

[7]*The optimal frequency for urine testing has not been determined. In general, dipsticks combining the leukocyte esterase and nitrite tests should be used to detect asymptomatic bacteriuria.*

Chart 5 (continued)

COUNSELING

Diet and Exercise

- Fat (especially saturated fat), cholesterol, complex carbohydrates, fiber, sodium, iron[8], calcium[8]
- *Nutritional assessment*
- Selection of exercise program

Substance Use

- Tobacco: cessation/primary prevention
- Alcohol and other drugs: Limiting alcohol consumption
  Driving/other dangerous activities while under the influence
- Treatment for abuse

High-Risk Groups

- Sharing/using unsterilized needles and syringes (HR18)

Sexual Practices

- Sexually transmitted diseases: partner selection, condoms, anal intercourse
- Unintended pregnancy and contraceptive options *for men and women*

Injury Prevention

- Safety belts
- Safety helmets
- Violent behavior[9]
- Firearms[9]
- Smoke detector
- Smoking near bedding or upholstery

High-Risk Groups

- Back-conditioning exercises (HR19)
- Prevention of childhood injuries (HR20)
- Falls in the elderly (HR21)

Dental Health

- Regular tooth brushing and dental visits

Other Primary Preventive Measures

- *Breast self-examination*[10]
- *Testicular self-examination*[11]

High-Risk Groups

- Discussion of hemoglobin testing (HR22)
- Skin protection from ultraviolet light (HR23)

IMMUNIZATIONS AND CHEMOPROPHYLAXIS

- Tetanus-diphtheria (Td) booster[12]

High-Risk Groups

- Hepatitis B vaccine *(HBv)* (HR24)
- Pneumococcal vaccine (HR25)
- Influenza vaccine[13] (HR26)
- Measles-mumps-rubella vaccine (MMR) (HR27)

HIGH-RISK CATEGORIES

HR18   Intravenous drug users.

HR19   Persons at increased risk for low back injury because of past history, body configuration, or type of activities.

HR20   Persons with children in the home or automobile.

HR21   Persons with older adults in the home.

HR22   Young adults of Caribbean, Latin America, Asian, Mediterranean, or African descent.

HR23   Persons with increased exposure to sunlight.

HR24   Homosexually *and bisexually* active men, intravenous drug users, recipients of some blood products, persons in health-related jobs with frequent exposure to blood or blood products, *household and sexual contacts of HBV carriers, sexually active heterosexual persons with multiple sexual partners diagnosed as having recently acquired sexually transmitted disease, prostitutes, and persons who have a history of sexual activity with multiple partners in the previous six months.*

HR25   Persons with medical conditions that increase the risk of pneumococcal infection (e.g., chronic cardiac or pulmonary disease, sickle cell disease, nephrotic syndrome, Hodgkin's disease, asplenia, diabetes mellitus, alcoholism, cirrhosis, multiple myeloma, renal disease or conditions associated with immunosuppression).

HR26   Residents of chronic care facilities or persons suffering from chronic cardiopulmonary disorders, metabolic diseases (including diabetes mellitus), hemoglobinopathies, immunosuppression, or renal dysfunction.

HR27   Persons born after 1956 who lack evidence of immunity to measles (receipt of live vaccine on or after first birthday, laboratory evidence of immunity, or a history of physician-diagnosed measles).

[8]For women
[9]Especially for young males
[10]*The teaching of self-breast examination is recommended by the subcommittee at the time of initiation of pelvic examinations.*
[11]*The teaching of self-testicular examination is recommended by the subcommittee for male patients.*
[12]Every 10 years
[13]Annually

*This list of preventive services is not exhaustive. It reflects only those topics reviewed by the U.S. Preventive Services Task Force *and the AAFP Commission on Public Health and Scientific Affairs.* Clinicians may wish to add other preventive services on a routine basis and after considering the patient's medical history and other individual circumstances. Examples of target conditions not specifically examined by the Task Force include:

- Chronic obstructive pulmonary disease
- Hepatobiliary disease
- Bladder cancer
- Endometrial disease
- Travel-related illness
- Prescription drug abuse
- Occupational illness and injuries

†The recommended schedule applies only to the periodic visit itself. The frequency of the individual preventive services listed in this table is left to clinical discretion, except as indicated in other footnotes.

Chart 6
Periodic Health Examination* Ages: 40–64 Years
Schedule: Every 1–3 Years† (See Preamble)

Leading Causes of Death

- Heart disease
- Lung cancer
- Cerebrovascular disease
- Breast cancer
- Colorectal cancer
- Obstructive lung disease
- *HIV infection* (males)[1]

Remain Alert for

- Depressive symptoms
- Suicide risk factors (HR1)
- Abnormal bereavement
- Signs of physical abuse or neglect
- Malignant skin lesions
- Peripheral arterial disease (HR2)
- Tooth decay, gingivitis, loose teeth

SCREENING

History

- *Interval medical and family history*[2]
- Dietary intake
- Physical activity
- Tobacco/alcohol/drug use
- Sexual practices

Physical

- Height and weight
- Blood pressure[3]
- Clinical breast exam[4]
- *Pelvic exam*
- *Digital rectal exam*[5]

High-Risk Groups

- Complete skin exam (HR3)
- Complete oral cavity exam (HR4)
- Palpation for thyroid nodules (HR5)
- Auscultation for carotid bruits (HR6)

Laboratory/Diagnostic Procedures

- Nonfasting *or fasting* total blood cholesterol[5]
- Papanicolaou smear[6]
- Mammogram[7]

High-Risk Groups

- Fasting plasma glucose (HR7)
- VDRL/RPR (HR8)
- Urinalysis for bacteriuria (HR9)
- Chlamydial testing (HR10)
- Gonorrhea culture (HR11)
- Counseling and testing for HIV (HR12)
- Tuberculin skin test (HR13)
- Hearing (HR14)
- Electrocardiogram (HR15)
- Fecal occult blood/sigmoidoscopy (HR16)
- Fecal occult blood/colonscopy (HR17)
- Bone mineral content (HR18)

HIGH-RISK CATEGORIES

HR1 Recent divorce, separation, unemployment, depression, alcohol or other drug abuse, serious medical illnesses, living alone, or recent bereavement.

HR2 Persons over age 50, smokers, or persons with diabetes mellitus.

HR3 Persons with a family or personal history of skin cancer, increased occupational or recreational exposure to sunlight, or clinical evidence of precursor lesions (e.g., dysplastic nevi, certain congenital nevi).

HR4 Persons with exposure to tobacco or excessive amounts of alcohol, or those with suspicious symptoms or lesions detected through self-examination.

HR5 Persons with a history of upper-body irradiation.

HR6 Persons with risk factors for cerebrovascular or cardiovascular disease (e.g., hypertension, smoking, CAD, atrial fibrillation, diabetes) or those with neurologic symptoms (e.g., transient ischemic attacks) or a history of cerebrovascular disease.

HR7 The markedly obese, persons with a family history of diabetes, or women with a history of gestational diabetes.

HR8 Prostitutes, persons who engage in sex with multiple partners in areas in which syphilis is prevalent, or contacts of persons with active syphilis.

HR9 Persons with diabetes.

HR10 Persons who attend clinics for sexually transmitted diseases, attend other high-risk health care facilities (e.g., adolescent and family planning clinics), or have other risk factors for chlamydial infection (e.g., multiple sexual partners or a sexual partner with multiple sexual contacts).

HR11 Prostitutes, persons with multiple sexual partners or a sexual partner with multiple contacts, sexual contacts of persons with culture-proven gonorrhea, or persons with a history of repeated episodes of gonorrhea.

HR12 Persons seeking treatment for sexually transmitted diseases; homosexual and bisexual men; past or present intravenous (IV) drug users; persons with a history of prostitution or mutliple sexual partners; women whose past or present sexual partners were HIV-infected, bisexual, or IV drug users; persons with long-term residence or birth in an area with high prevalence of HIV infection; or persons with a history of transfusion between 1978 and 1985.

HR13 Household members of persons with tuberculosis or others at risk for close contact with the disease (e.g., staff of tuberculosis clinics, shelters for the homeless, nursing homes, substance abuse treatment facilities, dialysis units, correctional institutions); recent immigrants or refugees from countries in which tuberculosis is common (e.g., Asia, Africa, Central and South America, Pacific Islands); migrant workers; residents of nursing homes, correctional institutions, or homeless shelters; or persons with certain underlying medical disorders (e.g., HIV infection).

HR14 Persons exposed regularly to excessive noise.

HR15 Men with two or more cardiac risk factors (high blood cholesterol, hypertension, cigarette smoking, diabetes mellitus, family history of CAD); men who would endanger public safety were they to experience sudden cardiac events (e.g., commercial airline pilots); or sedentary or high-risk males planning to begin a vigorous exercise program.

HR16 Persons aged 50 and older who have first-degree relatives with colorectal cancer; a personal history of endometrial, ovarian, or breast cancer, or a previous diagnosis of inflammatory bowel disease, adenomatous polyps, or colorectal cancer.

HR17 Persons with a family history of familial polyposis coli or cancer family syndrome.

HR18 Perimenopausal women at increased risk for osteoporosis (e.g., Caucasian race, bilateral oophorectomy before menopause, slender build) and for whom estrogen replacement therapy would otherwise not be recommended.

---

[1]*HIV infection as leading cause of death among young adults in U.S. cities and states. JAMA 1993;269:2991–2994.*

[2]*An updating of the previously obtained medical and family medical history is recommended by the subcommittee.*

[3]*At every physician visit with a minimum of once every two years*

[4]Annually for women

[5]*The subcommittee recommends this procedure but recognizes that the scientific evidence may not be conclusive to support.*

[6]*At least every five years*

[7]*All women who are, or who have been sexually active, should have an annual Pap test and pelvic examination. After a woman has had three or more consecutive satisfactory normal annual examinations, the Pap test may be performed at the discretion of the physician and the patient, but not less frequently than every three years.*

[8]*It is recommended that mammography be performed annually for all women beginning at age 50.*

Chart 6 (continued)

COUNSELING

Diet and Exercise

- Fat (especially saturated fat), cholersterol, complex carbohydrates, fiber, sodium, calcium[9]
- *Nutritional assessment*
- Selection of exercise program

Substance Use

- Tobacco cessation
- Alcohol and other drugs: Limiting alcohol consumption Driving/other dangerous activities while under the influence
- Treatment for abuse

High-Risk Groups

- Sharing/using unsterilized needles & syringes (HR19)

Sexual Practices

- Sexually transmitted diseases: partner selection, condoms, anal intercourse
- Unintended pregnancy and contraceptive options

Injury Prevention

- Safety belts
- Safety helmets
- Smoke detector
- Smoking near bedding or upholstery

High-Risk Groups

- Back-conditioning exercises (HR20)
- Prevention of childhood injuries (HR21)
- Falls in the elderly (HR22)

Dental Health

- Regular tooth brushing and dental visits

Other Primary Preventive Measures

- Discussion of hormone repalcement therapy in women

High-Risk Groups

- Skin protection from ultraviolet light (HR23)
- Discussion of hemoglobin testing (HR24)

IMMUNIZATIONS AND CHEMOPROPHYLAXIS

- *Immunization status check at age 50*
- Tetanus-diphtheria (Td) booster[10]

High-Risk Groups

- Hepatitis B vaccine *(HBv)* (HR25)
- Pneumococcal vaccine (HR26)
- Influenza vaccine (HR27)[11]

HIGH-RISK CATEGORIES

HR19   Intravenous drug users.

HR20   Persons at increased risk for low back injury because of past history, body configuration, or type of activities.

HR21   Persons with children in the home or automobile.

HR22   Persons with older adults in the home.

HR23   Persons with increased exposure to sunlight.

HR24   Men who have risk factors for myocardial infarction (e.g., high blood cholesterol, smoking, diabetes mellitus, family history of early-onset CAD) and who lack a history of gastrointestinal or other bleeding problems, and other risk factors for bleeding or cerebral hemorrhage.

HR25   Homosexually *and bisexually* active men, intravenous drug users, recipients of some blood products, persons in health-related jobs with frequent exposure to blood or blood products, *household and sexual contacts of HBV carriers, sexually active heterosexual persons with multiple sexual partners diagnosed as having recently acquired sexually transmitted disease, prostitutes, and persons who have a history of sexual activity with multiple partners in the previous six months.*

HR26   Persons with medical conditions that increase the risk of pneumococcal infection (e.g., chronic cardiac or pulmonary disease, sickle cell disease, nephrotic syndrome, Hodgkin's disease, asplenia, diabetes mellitus, alcoholism, cirrhosis, multiple myeloma, renal disease, or conditions associated with immunosuppression).

HR27   Residents of chronic care facilities and persons suffering from chronic cardiopulmonary disorders, metabolic diseases (including diabetes mellitus), hemoglobinopathies, immunosuppression, or renal dysfunction.

---

[9]For women
[10]Every 10 years
[11]Annually

---

*This list of preventive Services is not exhaustive. It reflects only those topics reviewed by the U.S. Preventive Services Task Force *and the AAFP Commission on Public Health and Scientific Affairs.* Clinicians may wish to add other preventive services on a routine basis and after considering the patient's medical history and other individual circumstances. Examples of target conditions not specifically examined by the Task Force include:

- Chronic obstructive pulmonary disease
- Hepatobiliary disease
- Bladder cancer
- Endometrial disease
- Travel-related illness
- Prescription drug abuse
- Occupational illness and injuries

†The recommended schedule applies only to the periodic visit itself. The frequency of the individual preventive services listed in this table is left to clinical discretion, except as indicated in other footnotes.

Chart 7
Periodic Health Examination* Ages: 65 Years and Over
Schedule: Every Year[†] (See Preamble)

Leading Causes of Death

- Heart disease
- Cerebrovascular disease
- Obstructive lung disease
- Pneumonia/influenza
- Lung cancer
- Colorectal cancer

Remain Alert for

- Depression symptoms
- Suicide risk factors (HR1)
- Abnormal bereavement
- Changes in cognitive function
- Medications that increase risk of falls
- Signs of physical abuse or neglect
- Malignant skin lesions
- Peripheral skin lesions
- Tooth decay, gingivitis, loose teeth

SCREENING

History

- *Interval medical and family history[1]*
- *Medication use (prescription and non-prescription)*
- Prior symptoms of transient ischemic attack
- Dietary intake
- Physical activity
- Tobacco/alcohol/drug use
- Functional status at home

Physical

- Height and weight
- Blood pressure[2]
- Visual acuity
- Hearing and hearing aids
- Clinical breast exam[3]
- *Pelvic exam*
- *Cardiac auscultation*
- *Digital rectal exam[4]*

High-Risk Groups

- Auscultation for carotid bruits (HR2)
- Complete skin exam (HR3)
- Complete oral cavity exam (HR4)
- Palpation for thyroid nodules (HR5)

Laboratory/Diagnostic Procedures

- Nonfasting *or fasting[5]* total blood cholesterol
- Dipstick urinalysis
- Mammogram[6]
- Thyroid function tests[7]

High-Risk Groups

- Fasting plasma glucose (HR7)
- Tuberculin skin test (PPD) (HR7)
- Electrocardiogram (HR8)
- Papanicolaou smear[8] (HR9)
- Fecal occult blood/sigmoidoscopy (HR10)
- Fecal occult blood/colonoscopy (HR11)

HIGH-RISK CATEGORIES

HR1 Recent divorce, separation, unemployment, depression, alcohol or other drug abuse, serious medical illnesses, living alone, or recent bereavement.

HR2 Persons with risk factors for cerebrovascular or cardiovascular disease (e.g., hypertension, smoking, CAD, atrial fibrillation, diabetes) or those with neurologic symptoms (e.g., transient ischemic attacks) or a history of cerebrovascular disease.

HR3 Persons with a family or personal history of skin cancer, increased occupational or recreational exposure to sunlight, or clinical evidence of precursor lesions (e.g., dysplastic nevi, certain congenital nevi).

HR4 Persons with exposure to tobacco or excessive amounts of alcohol, or those with suspicious symptoms or lesions detected through self-examination.

HR5 Persons with a history of upper-body irradiation.

HR6 The markedly obese, persons with a family history of diabetes, or women with a history of gestational diabetes.

HR7 Household members of persons with tuberculosis or others at risk for close contact with the disease (e.g., staff of tuberculosis clinics, shelters for the homeless, nursing homes, substance abuse treatment facilities, dialysis units, correctional institutions); recent immigrants or refugees from countries in which tuberculosis is common (e.g., Asia, Africa, Central and South America, Pacific Islands); migrant workers; residents of nursing homes, correctional institutions, or homeless shelters; or persons with certain underlying medical disorders (e.g., HIV infection).

HR8 Men with two or more cardiac risk factors (high blood cholesterol, hypertension, cigarette smoking, diabetes mellitus, family history of CAD); men who would endanger public safety were they to experience sudden cardiac events (e.g., commercial airline pilots); or sedentary or high-risk males planning to begin a vigorous exercise program.

HR9 Women who have not had previous documented screening in which smears have been consistently negative.

HR10 Persons who have first-degree relatives with colorectal cancer; a personal history of endometrial, ovarian, or breast cancer; or a previous diagnosis of inflammatory bowel disease, adenomatous polyps, or colorectal cancer.

HR11 Persons with a family history of familial polyposis coli or cancer family syndrome.

---

[1]*An updating of the previously obtained medical and family medical history is recommended by the subcommittee.*
[2]*At every physician visit with a minimum of every two years*
[3]Annually
[4]*The subcommittee recommends this procedure but recognizes the scientific evidence supporting it may not be conclusive.*
[5]*At least every five years*
[6]*It is recommended that mammography be performed annually for all women beginning at age 50.*
[7]For women
[8]Every 1–3 years

(continued)

Chart 7 (continued)

COUNSELING

Diet and Exercise

- Fat (especially saturated fat), cholersterol, complex carbohydrates, fiber, sodium, calcium[9]
- *Nutritional assessment*
- Selection of exercise program

Substance Use

- Tobacco: cessation
- Alcohol and other drugs: Limiting alcohol consumption Driving/other dangerous activities while under the influence
- Treatment for abuse

Sexual Practices

- *Sexuality*

Injury Prevention

- Prevention of falls
- Safety belts
- Smoke detector
- Smoking near bedding or upholstery
- Hot water heater temperature ($\leq 120°F$)
- Safety helmets

High-Risk Groups

- Prevention of childhood injuries (HR12)

Dental Health

- Regular tooth brushing, flossing, and dental visits

Other Primary Preventive Measures

- Glaucoma testing
- *Advance directives/living will/durable power of attorney*
- Discussion of hormone repalcement therapy in women

High-Risk Groups

- Discussion of aspirin therapy (HR13)
- Skin protection from ultraviolet light (HR14)

IMMUNIZATIONS AND CHEMOPROPHYLAXIS

- Tetanus-diphtheria (Td) booster[10]
- Influenza vaccine[11]
- Pneumococcal vaccine

High-Risk Groups

- Hepatitis B vaccine *(HBv)* (HR15)

HIGH-RISK CATEGORIES

HR12 Persons with children in the home or automobile.

HR13 Men who have risk factors for myocardial infarction (e.g., high blood cholesterol, smoking, diabetes mellitus, family history of early-onset CAD) and who lack a history of gastrointestinal or other bleeding problems, and other risk factors for bleeding or cerebral hemorrhage.

HR14 Persons with increased exposure to sunlight.

HR15 Homosexually *and bisexually* active men, intravenous drug users, recipients of some blood products, persons in health-related jobs with frequent exposure to blood or blood products, *household and sexual contacts of HBV carriers, sexually active heterosexual persons with multiple sexual partners diagnosed as having recently acquired sexually transmitted disease, prostitutes, and persons who have a history of sexual activity with multiple partners in the previous six months.*

---

[9]For women
[10]Every 10 years
[11]Annually

---

*This list of preventive services is not exhaustive. It reflects only those topics reviewed by the U.S. Preventive Services Task Force *and the AAFP Commission on Public Health and Scientific Affairs.* Clinicians may wish to add other preventive services on a routine basis and after considering the patient's medical history and other individual circumstances. Examples of target conditions not specifically examined by the Task Force include:

- Chronic obstructive pulmonary disease
- Hepatobiliary disease
- Bladder cancer
- Endometrial disease
- Travel-related illness
- Prescription drug abuse
- Occupational illness and injuries

†The recommended schedule applies only to the periodic visit itself. The frequency of the individual preventive services listed in this table is left to clinical discretion, except as indicated in other footnotes.

Index